Handbook of Substance Misuse and Addictions

Vinood B. Patel • Victor R. Preedy
Editors

Handbook of Substance Misuse and Addictions

From Biology to Public Health

Volume 2

With 432 Figures and 210 Tables

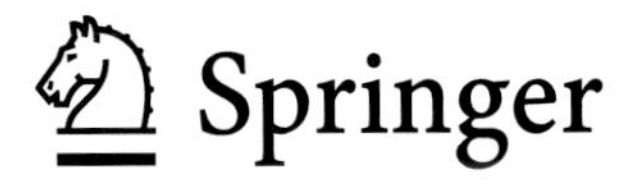

Editors
Vinood B. Patel
School of Life Sciences
University of Westminster
London, UK

Victor R. Preedy
School of Life Course and Population Sciences
Faculty of Life Sciences and Medicine
King's College London
London, UK

ISBN 978-3-030-92391-4 ISBN 978-3-030-92392-1 (eBook)
https://doi.org/10.1007/978-3-030-92392-1

This Springer imprint is published by the registered company Springer Nature Switzerland AG
The registered company address is: Gewerbestrasse 11, 6330 Cham, Switzerland

Preface

Worldwide there are several billion individuals who are either addicted to substances or misuse them. They can cause bodily or society-related harm. Globally, about 250 million people have an addiction to alcohol and more than 4 times that amount smoke tobacco-related products. In the USA, there are an estimated 25 million illegal drug users. In addition, there are millions who misuse prescription or over-the-counter medications. Addiction to khat and betel nut may also be considered problematic in some communities and countries.

Substance misuse and addictions have consequences not only for organs (e.g., the liver in alcohol misuse and the lungs in tobacco usage) but for the individual, community, and society at large. At the personal level, addictions may have long-term behavioral effects, and withdrawal symptoms may also cause a range of adverse physiological and psychological reactions. At the community and societal levels, there may be adverse effects, such as the impact on employment, accidents, divorce, crime, and breakup of family units. Crime itself is a societal event which will involve enforcement agencies, the judiciary, and councilors. The financial cost of addictions can also be considerable. For example, in the UK alone with a population of 65 million, the annual cost of alcohol misuse is reported to be the equivalent to 25 billion dollars.

Substance misuse and addictions are a public health issue. They affect the wellbeing of each community and nation as a whole. It is therefore necessary to identify, educate, and treat individuals who are addicted to such substances. Policies and procedures go hand in hand with public health education and safety. They encompass detection, prevention, treatment, assessment, as well as epidemiology and etiology. The science behind the public health issues of one drug may be applicable to other drugs as well. For example, the strategies to curb the usage of tobacco-related products have in some places been adopted to curb the excessive consumption of alcohol.

Apart from active agents which have a plant or chemical basis, there is a need to consider that there are other forms of addiction which may have common modes of causality or prevention. These include, for example, food addiction, gaming, Internet usage, and gambling.

Overall, a holistic understanding of the relationships between public health and substance misuse provides a common platform upon which other forms of addiction can be researched. This requires an understanding of the biological processes as well as the involvement of behavior, psychology, and sociology. All these processes are interlinked. However, marshalling all the aforementioned information into a single source is somewhat difficult due to the wide array of material. To address this, the Editors have compiled ***The Handbook of Substance Misuse and Addictions: From Biology to Public Health***.

There are 18 different sections as follows:

Foundations of Understanding and Setting the Scene
Brain, Neuroscience, and Neurobiology
Tobacco
Alcohol
Cannabinoids
Caffeine
Areca and Khat
Prescription Medications and Opioids
Stimulants
Club Drugs
Dissociative Drugs
Hallucinogens
Steroids and Inhalants
International Aspects
Dual and Polydrug Misuse and Addictions
Non-Drug Addictions
Emerging Addictions and Agents of Misuse
Screening Tools, Analytical Methods, and Resources

Each chapter has the following subsections:

Abstract (published on line)
Mini-Dictionary of Terms
Key Facts
Applications to Other Areas of Addiction
Applications to Other Areas of Public Health
Summary Points

These subsections are unique features of the book, which bridge the trans-intellectual and transdisciplinary divides. Thus, experts in one addiction area may become more knowledgeable in other areas. These features are also very useful for the non-expert such as students or newly qualified health-care professionals. The subheadings on ***Applications to Other Areas of Addiction or Other Areas of Public Health*** are intended to provide translational information of a practical or speculative nature. This is particularly useful when applied to those addictions where there is a paucity of scientific material.

Contributors are authors who are international and national experts, from respected institutions. Leaders in the field and trendsetters are also contributors. Emerging areas of addictions and substance misuse are also incorporated in ***The Handbook of Substance Misuse and Addictions: From Biology to Public Health***.

London, UK
October 2022

Dr. Vinood B. Patel
Prof Victor R. Preedy

Contents

Volume 1

Part I Introduction **1**

1 **Substance Misuse and Addictions in Context** 3
Rajkumar Rajendram, Vinood B. Patel, and Victor R. Preedy

Part II Foundations of Understanding and Setting the Scene **17**

2 **Linking Attitudes to Substance Misuse** 19
Nurcan Hamzaoglu and Sevcan Karatas

3 **The Gut-Brain Axis and Addictions** 35
Elisabet Jerlhag

4 **The Reward Deficiency Syndrome and Links with Addictive and Related Behaviors** 59
Eszter Kótyuk, Marc N. Potenza, Kenneth Blum, and Zsolt Demetrovics

5 **Linking Addictive and Obsessive-Compulsive Behaviors** 75
Lucy Albertella, Samuel R. Chamberlain, Leonardo F. Fontenelle, and R. Frederick Westbrook

6 **Cognitive Assessment, Management, and Training in Addiction Treatment** 93
Victoria Manning and Georgia Bolt

7 **Attachment and Behavioral Addictions** 123
Ana Estévez, Laura Macía, Janire Momeñe, and Nerea Etxaburu

8 **Disease and Addictions** 145
Diptadhi Mukherjee and Arun Kandasamy

9 **Facts Versus Fiction in Adolescent Substance Use: Implications for Public Health** 161
Melissa R. Schick, Tessa Nalven, Michael C. Crawford, Katelyn T. Kirk-Provencher, and Nichea S. Spillane

10 **Relapse Rates in Substance Misuse and the Role of Family** 187
Liang-Jen Wang and Sheng-Yu Lee

11 **People with Intellectual Disabilities, Drug Misuse, and Addiction** 209
Ram Lakhan and Manoj Sharma

12 **Long-Term Drug Use** 227
Ángel Romero-Martínez

13 **Public Health Impacts of Drug Overdose and Mental Health** 243
Satish Kedia, Patrick J. Dillon, Michael Schmidt, Coree Entwistle, and Hassan Arshad

14 **Linking Addictions and Health** 267
Ayşe Özdemir and Cenk Aypak

15 **Gender and Drug Policy** 289
Natalie Thomas and Jennifer Juckel

16 **Substance Use Disorder Treatment in the Age of COVID-19: Challenges, Responses, and Lessons for the Future** 305
Barak Shapira and Yehuda Neumark

17 **Socioeconomic Status and Drug Use Among Students** 327
Beata Gavurova, Boris Popesko, and Viera Ivankova

18 **Revolving Door** 353
Giuseppe Di Martino

19 **Substance Use in Older Adolescence: Overcoming the Prevention Paradox** 365
Jennifer Debenham, Nicola C. Newton, Katrina E. Champion, and Maree Teesson

20 **Medicinal Plants and Addiction Treatment** 389
Sahar Jaffal and Husam Abazid

Part III Brain, Neuroscience, and Neurobiology **415**

21 **Basic Structure of the Brain and Neurology** 417
R. A. Armstrong

22 **The Hippocampus and Addiction: Focus on Plasticity and Circuitry in the Hippocampus** 437
Chitra D. Mandyam

23 **The Medial Prefrontal Cortex (mPFC) and Addictions** 459
Marta Perez-Rando and Ramón Guirado

24 **Linking the Features of Food Addiction and Drug Addiction** 475
Poliana Guiomar Brasiel and Sheila Cristina Potente Dutra Luquetti

25 **The Left Frontoparietal Brain Network in Addictions** 489
Víctor Costumero and Alfonso Barrós-Loscertales

26 **Linking the Neural Correlates of Addiction and Negative Urgency** 513
Meredith Halcomb, Karmen Yoder, and Melissa Cyders

27 **Impulsivity, Decision-Making, and Reward System as Key Factors in Addiction** 537
Giacomo Grassi, Chiara Cecchelli, and Luisa Vignozzi

28 **Trace Amine-Associated Receptor 1 and Its Links to Addictions** 557
Jianfeng Liu

29 **Linking fMRI, Pain, and Addictions** 577
Semra A. Aytur, Grace Roy, Marcy Doyle, Kimberly L. Ray, Sarah K. Meier, and Donald A. Robin

30 **The Effects of Drugs of Abuse on ABC Transporters** 609
Noor A. Hussein, Dawn E. Muskiewicz, David Terrero, Saloni Malla, F. Scott Hall, and Amit K. Tiwari

31 **The Role of ABC Transporters in the Actions of Drugs of Abuse** 635
Saloni Malla, Dawn E. Muskiewicz, Noor A. Hussein, F. Scott Hall, and Amit K. Tiwari

Part IV Tobacco **653**

32 **Smoking and Genetics** 655
Shoaib Afzal

33 **Cigarette Smoke and the NLRP3 Inflammasome** 681
Sakshi Mehta and Veena Dhawan

34 **The Impact of Tobacco Smoke in the Home** 701
Siyu Dai and Kate C. Chan

35 **E-cigarette Polysubstance Vaping in Youth** 721
Lynnette Nathalie Lyzwinski and Mark J. Eisenberg

36 **Knowledge and Perceptions of Tobacco Harm Reduction: EU Aspects** 743
Josep M. Ramon-Torrell

37 **Smoking Cessation in Those with Mental Illness** 757
P. V. Asharani and Mythily Subramaniam

38 **Mental Illness and Tobacco Usage** 775
P. V. Asharani and Mythily Subramaniam

39 **Adolescents and Their Perception of Packaging on Tobacco Products** 801
Aaron Drovandi

40 **A Critical Analysis of the Prohibition of Electronic Nicotine Delivery Systems** 825
Kylie Morphett and Coral Gartner

41 **Features of Ex-Smokers** 851
Marta Manczuk and Magdalena Cedzynska

42 **Combustible and Electronic Cigarette Usage, Puff Protocols, and Topography Standards** 873
Risa Robinson and Edward Hensel

43 **Smoking and Lung Cancer: Public Health Perspectives** 899
Lynnette Nathalie Lyzwinski

Volume 2

Part V Alcohol **915**

44 **Fetal Alcohol Spectrum Disorder** 917
Jasmine M. Noble and Andrew J. Greenshaw

45 **Chronic Alcohol and Skeletal Muscle** 943
Brianna L. Bourgeois, Danielle E. Levitt, Patricia E. Molina, and Liz Simon

46 **Neuroimaging and Alcohol-Use Disorder (AUD)** 969
Andriana Kakanakova

47 **Alcohol as Prodrug of Salsolinol** 983
Valentina Bassareo, Riccardo Maccioni, Rossana Migheli, Alessandra T. Peana, Pierluigi Caboni, and Elio Acquas

48 **Linking Stress, Depression, and Alcohol Use** 1007
Beata Gavurova, Viera Ivankova, and Martin Rigelsky

49 **Alcohol and Disease** 1033
Mihir P. Rupani

50 **Using New Technology and Concepts on the Oldest Addiction on Earth, Alcoholism** 1059
Eric Merrell and Brian Johnson

51 **Google, Public Health, and Alcohol and Drug Policy** 1077
Abhishek Ghosh, Shinjini Choudhury, and Venkata Lakshmi Narasimha

52 **Alcohol Consumption in Low- and Middle-Income Settings** 1111
Jane Brandt Sørensen, Shali Tayebi, Amalie Brokhattingen, and Bishal Gyawali

53 **Metals in Alcoholic Beverages and Public Health Implications** 1131
Yasir A. Shah and Dirk W. Lachenmeier

54 **Alcohol Consumption and Suicidal Behavior: Current Research Evidence and Potential for Prevention** 1151
Kairi Kõlves, Rose Crossin, and Katrina Witt

55 **Interventions for Children and Adolescents with Fetal Alcohol Spectrum Disorders (FASD)** 1177
Gro Christine Christensen Løhaugen, Anne Cecilie Tveiten, and Jon Skranes

56 **Mothers of Children with Fetal Alcohol Spectrum Disorder** 1205
Larry Burd and Svetlana Popova

57 **Childhood Alcohol Use: Global Insights** 1223
Ingunn Marie Stadskleiv Engebretsen and Vilde Skylstad

58 **Alcohol Use Disorders and Neurological Illnesses** 1247
Lekhansh Shukla, Venkata Lakshmi Narasimha, and Arun Kandasamy

59 **Alcohol and Brain-Derived Neurotrophic Factor (BDNF)** 1273
Candelaria Martín-González, Emilio González-Arnay, Camino María Fernández-Rodríguez, Alen García-Rodríguez, and Emilio González-Reimers

60 **Alcohol and Cirrhosis** 1301
Beata Gavurova and Viera Ivankova

Part VI Cannabinoids **1319**

61 **Synthetic Cannabinoids and Neurodevelopment** 1321
João Pedro Silva, Helena Carmo, and Félix Carvalho

62 **Cannabis and Organ Damage: A Focus on Pancreatitis (to Include Different Scenarios)** 1343
Angela Saviano

63 **Cannabidiol (CBD) and Its Biological Toxicity** 1353
M. M. Dziwenka and R. W. Coppock

64 **Cannabis Use and Sleep** 1369
Renée Martin-Willett, Ashley Master, L. Cinnamon Bidwell, and Sharon R. Sznitman

65 **The Reward System: What It Is and How It Is Altered in Cannabis Users** 1399
Natasha L. Mason, Peter van Ruitenbeek, and Johannes G. Ramaekers

66 **Attitudes and Cannabis Legalization** 1441
Jennifer D. Ellis and Stella M. Resko

67 **Impact of Parental Cannabis** 1457
Nicolas Berthelot, Maude Morneau, and Carl Lacharité

68 **Public Health Issues of Legalizing Cannabis** 1471
Steven R. Boomhower

69 **Over-the-Counter Cannabidiol (CBD)** 1489
Leticia Shea

70 **Linking Cannabis and Homicide: Comparison with Alcohol** 1519
Oybek Nazarov and Guohua Li

Part VII Caffeine **1533**

71 **Caffeine Consumption over Time** 1535
Gabrielle Rabelo Quadra, Emília Marques Brovini, Joyce Andreia dos Santos, and José R. Paranaíba

72 **Caffeine and Alcohol** 1553
Laura Dazzi, Alessandra T. Peana, Rossana Migheli, Riccardo Maccioni, Romina Vargiu, Biancamaria Baroli, Elio Acquas, and Valentina Bassareo

73 **Caffeine and Anxiety-Like Behavior** 1573
Anderson Ribeiro-Carvalho, Ana C. Dutra-Tavares, Cláudio C. Filgueiras, Alex C. Manhães, and Yael Abreu-Villaça

74 **Caffeinated Beverages and Diabetes** 1591
Muneera Qassim Al-Mssallem and Salah M. Aleid

75 **Caffeine as an Active Adulterant: Implication for Drugs of Abuse Consumption** 1605
Cecilia Scorza, José Pedro Prieto, and Sara Fabius

Part VIII Areca and Khat **1617**

76 Areca Nut, Morbidity, and Cardiovascular Disease (Acute Coronary Syndrome): Implications for Policy and Prevention 1619
Kashif Shafique and Sumaira Nasim

77 Carcinogenic Alkaloids Present in Areca Nut 1637
Nisha Thakur and Ravi Mehrotra

78 Naturally Occurring Cathinone from Khat, Synthetic Cathinones, and Cytochrome P450 1659
Sharoen Yu Ming Lim, Mustafa Ahmed Alshagga, Chin Eng Ong, and Yan Pan

79 Cognitive Deficits and Synthetic Khat-Related Cathinones 1681
Vincent Carfagno, Jonna M. Leyrer-Jackson, and M. Foster Olive

80 Khat Use in Defined Population 1705
Yimenu Yitayih

81 Khat Consumption and Household Economies 1717
Zerihun Girma Gudata

82 Cytotoxicity and Genotoxicity of Khat (*Catha edulis* Forsk) 1739
Maged El-Setouhy and Ashraf A. Hassan

83 Khat (*Catha edulis*) and Oral Health 1751
Mir Faeq Ali Quadri and Syam Mohan

Volume 3

Part IX Prescriptions, Over-the-Counter Medications, and Opioids **1767**

84 The Orexin System, Prescription Opioid Use Disorder, and Orexin Receptors Blockade 1769
Alessandra Matzeu and Rémi Martin-Fardon

85 Prescription Stimulants: Use for Weight Control and Associations with Disordered Eating 1787
Sara Nutley

86 Heroin Use in China and the United States 1805
Elizabeth Monk-Turner, Hongyun Fu, and Xiushi Yang

87 Cognitive Enhancers: What They Are and How They Are Used in Heroin Addiction 1831
Wenwen Shen, Disen Mei, Yue Liu, and Wenhua Zhou

88 Fatalities in Patients with Opioid Use Disorders 1851
Erin Kelty, Agata Chrzanowska, and David B. Preen

89 Over-the-Counter Medications and Their Misuse 1869
Megan Weier, Naomi Weier, and Ben O'Mara

90 Opioid Reinforcement: What It Is and How It Can Be Modulated by Cannabinoids 1893
Cristina Cadoni

91 Drug Misuse as an Epidemic: A Focus on the Synthetic Opioid Fentanyl 1921
Anneli Uusküla, Jonathan Feelemyer, and Don C. Des Jarlais

92 Over-the-Counter Sinonasal Medicines and Potential for Misuse 1941
Thomas C. Flowers and Edward McCoul

93 The Biology of Morphine and Oxidative Stress 1955
Jinjing Jia, Guangtao Xu, and Xiansi Zeng

94 Prescription Drug Misuse and Women 1977
B. Peteet, V. Watts, E. Tucker, M. Hanna, A. Saddlemire, and P. Brown

Part X Stimulants **2001**

95 Amphetamine in Biological Specimens: Impact and Implications for Public Health 2003
Ana Y. Simão, Mónica Antunes, Hernâni Marques, Tiago Rosado, Sofia Soares, Joana Gonçalves, Mário Barroso, and Eugenia Gallardo

96 Transcriptomics and Cocaine Addiction 2029
Yorkiris Mármol Contreras and Thomas A. Green

97 Impact of Amphetamine Exposure During Adolescence on Neurobehavioral Endpoints 2053
Steven R. Boomhower

98 Sensitization to Amphetamine 2071
Jaanus Harro and Aet O'Leary

99 Methamphetamine Use Among Sexual Minority Men 2097
William Lodge II, Katie Biello, Pablo K. Valente, and Matthew J. Mimiaga

100 Chronic Methamphetamine and Psychosis Pathways 2121
Samuel Hogarth, Elizabeth Manning, and Maarten van den Buuse

101 Gene Variants and Cocaine Use Disorder 2147
Luis F. Alguacil

102 Amphetamine and the Biology of Neuronal Morphology 2169
Hiram Tendilla-Beltrán, Luis Enrique Arroyo-García, and Gonzalo Flores

Part XI Club Drugs **2193**

103 3,4-Methylenedioxymethamphetamine (MDMA) and Synaptic Dopamine 2195
Francesca Romana Rizzo, Antonio Bruno, Mauro Federici, and Nicola Biagio Mercuri

104 Life-Threatening 3,4-Methylenedioxyamphetamine (MDMA) Usage 2215
Francis Kin Chiu Chu

105 GHB and Driving Performance 2225
Arianna Giorgetti, Raffaele Giorgetti, and Giuseppe Basile

106 Drug and MDMA Interactions Implications for Public Health 2243
Esther Papaseit, Magí Farré, and Clara Pérez-Mañá

107 Effects of Amphetamine-Type Stimulants on the Metabolome 2269
Andrea E. Steuer

108 The Biology of Nitric Oxide Signaling and MDMA 2337
M. Pilar García-Pardo, Claudia Calpe-López, M. Ángeles Martínez-Caballero, and María A. Aguilar

109 Flunitrazepam as a Club Drug 2365
Mustafa Atilla Akgül and Cenk Aypak

Part XII Dissociative Drugs **2383**

110 Ketamine Misuse and Adverse Body Effects: A Focus on Uropathy 2385
Daniele Castellani

111 Addictions and Polymorphism 2409
Ying Yan, Minling Zhang, and Ni Fan

Part XIII Hallucinogens **2425**

112 **Psilocybin and Magic Mushrooms: Patterns of Abuse and Consequences of Recreational Misuse** 2427
Andreia Machado Brito-da-Costa, Diana Dias da Silva, Áurea Madureira-Carvalho, and Ricardo Jorge Dinis-Oliveira

113 **Pharmacological Action of LSD** 2457
Monika Herian

Part XIV Steroids and Inhalants **2477**

114 **Alkyl Nitrite Inhalants (Poppers)** 2479
Nicole Pepper

115 **Toluene Abuse** 2499
Beáta Hubková, Anna Birková, and Beáta Čižmárová

116 **Unsafe Behaviors and Anabolic Steroid Use** 2523
Eric J. Ip and Madeline D. Silva

117 **High Testosterone Levels: Impact on the Heart** 2543
Takayuki Matsumoto, Josiane F. Silva, and Rita C. Tostes

118 **Synaptic and Extrasynaptic Mitochondria** 2571
Vitória Girelli de Oliveira, Jijo Stebin Justus, Luis Valmor Cruz Portela, and Marcelo Salimen Rodolphi

119 **Toluene Abuse: A Medicolegal Perspective** 2591
Guido Pelletti

Volume 4

Part XV International Aspects **2611**

120 **Indian Aspects of Nondrug Addiction** 2613
Anuradha Dave and S. Dave

121 **Drug Abuse in the Middle East** 2629
Husam Abazid

122 **Co-occurrence of (Online) Gaming and Substance Use** 2649
Julian Strizek

123 **Drug Abuse in Pakistan** 2667
Shagufta Jabeen, Uzma Abdullah, Muhammad Sheeraz Ahmad, Muhammad Mobeen Zafar, Julia K. Pinsonneault, Wolfgang Sadee, and Ghazala Kaukab Raja

124 **Methamphetamine Use and Chemsex: An Emerging Threat for Gender and Sexually Diverse People** 2689
Sharful Islam Khan, Samira Dishti Irfan, and Mohammad Niaz Morshed Khan

125 **The Opioid Substitution Therapy (OST) Program for the People Who Inject Drugs (PWID) in Bangladesh: Lessons Learned and Way Forward** 2715
Sharful Islam Khan, Tanveer Khan Ibne Shafiq, Samira Dishti Irfan, and Mohammad Niaz Morshed Khan

Part XVI Dual and Polydrug Use and Addictions 2739

126 **Nandrolone Decanoate (Nan) Abusers and Concomitant Cannabis Use** 2741
Rabab H. Sayed and Mostafa A. Rabie

127 **Concomitant Δ-9-Tetrahydrocannabinol and Alcohol Use: Impact on Cognitive Function and Ingestive Behavior** 2755
Nu-Chu Liang

128 **Alcohol and Methamphetamine Interactions and Co-abuse** 2775
Amanda L. Sharpe, Marta Trzeciak, Kylie Handa, and Michael J. Beckstead

129 **Alcohol and Cocaine Co-usage** 2797
Alaa M. Hammad, Rinda D. Bachu, Dawn E. Muskiewicz, F. Scott Hall, and Amit K. Tiwari

130 **Linking Polysubstance Use, Glutamate, and the Nucleus Accumbens** 2817
Lori Knackstedt

131 **Prenatal Illicit Drug and Polysubstance Exposure and Impact on Developmental Outcome** 2833
Jon Skranes and Gro C. C. Løhaugen

132 **Buprenorphine, Polydrug Use, and Deaths** 2863
Ilkka Ojanperä, Claudia Mariottini, and Pirkko Kriikku

Part XVII Non-drug Addictions 2883

133 **Gambling Disorder as an Addiction** 2885
Grace Macdonald-Gagnon and Marc N. Potenza

134 **Food Addiction and Policy** 2903
Vincent A. Santiago, Stephanie E. Cassin, Sanjeev Sockalingam, and Adrian Carter

135 **Food Addiction** 2927
Julia Simkus, Mark S. Gold, Kenneth Blum, and Nicole M. Avena

136 **Behavioral Addictions in Children: A Focus on Gambling, Gaming, Internet Addiction, and Excessive Smartphone Use** 2941
Jeffrey Derevensky, Loredana Marchica, Lynette Gilbeau, and Jeremie Richard

137 **Nondrug Addictions** 2965
Javier Bueno-Antequera and Miguel Ángel Oviedo-Caro

138 **Non-drug Addiction: Addiction to Work** 2981
Paweł A. Atroszko

Part XVIII Emerging Addictions and Agents of Misuse **3013**

139 **Pathological Effects and Adverse Events Associated with the Phenylethylamine Derivative NBOMe** 3015
Patricia Pia Wadowski, Henriette Löffler-Stastka, and Renate Koppensteiner

140 **Piperazine Designer Drugs of Abuse** 3031
Sarah Eller and Marcelo Dutra Arbo

141 **The Use and Abuse of Synthetic Cathinones (aka "Bath Salts")** 3041
Hayley N. Manke, Katharine H. Nelson, and Anthony L. Riley

142 **The Toll of Benzofurans in the Context of Drug Abuse** 3065
Rita Roque Bravo, João Pedro Silva, Helena Carmo, Félix Carvalho, and Diana Dias da Silva

Part XIX Selective Screening Tools, Analytical Methods, and Resources **3089**

143 **The Indonesian Internet Addiction Questionnaires** 3091
Kristiana Siste, Enjeline Hanafi, Lee Thung Sen, Salma Kyana, and Peter Alison Lie

144 **The Addiction-Like Eating Behavior Scale: Features and Applications** 3115
Tiago Queiroz Cardoso and Lívia Shirahige

145 **The Karolinska Psychodynamic Profile** 3127
Elisabeth Punzi

146 Recommended Resources and Online Material for Investigating Substance Misuse and Addictions 3143
Rajkumar Rajendram, Vinood B. Patel, and Victor R. Preedy

147 Inventory for Early Screening of Work Addiction-Related Behaviors in High School and Undergraduate Students 3157
Paweł A. Atroszko

148 The Abbreviated Self Completion Teen-Addiction Severity Index (ASC T-ASI) 3199
Vivian Reckers-Droog, Leona Hakkaart-van Roijen, and Yifrah Kaminer

149 Stigma and Quality of Life in Substance Users: Methods and Applications 3217
Xavier C. C. Fung, Kun-Chia Chang, Chih-Cheng Chang, and Chung-Ying Lin

Index 3253

About the Editors

Vinood B. Patel, BSc, PhD, FRSC, is currently a Reader in Clinical Biochemistry at the University of Westminster. He presently directs studies on metabolic pathways involved in liver disease, particularly related to mitochondrial energy regulation and cell death. Research is being undertaken to study the role of nutrients, antioxidants, phytochemicals, iron, alcohol, and fatty acids in the pathophysiology of liver disease. Other areas of interest are identifying new biomarkers that can be used for the diagnosis and prognosis of liver disease and understanding mitochondrial oxidative stress in Alzheimer's disease and gastrointestinal dysfunction in autism. Dr. Patel graduated from the University of Portsmouth with a degree in Pharmacology and completed his PhD in protein metabolism from King's College London in 1997. His postdoctoral work was carried out at Wake Forest University Baptist Medical School studying structural-functional alterations to mitochondrial ribosomes. Dr. Patel is a nationally and internationally recognized researcher and was involved in several NIH-funded biomedical grants related to alcoholic liver disease. Dr. Patel has edited biomedical books in the area of toxic agents (alcohol), including *Biomarkers in Toxicology*, *Molecular Aspects of Alcohol and Nutrition*, and *Toxicology: Oxidative Stress and Dietary Antioxidants*, and health prevention, including the *Handbook of Nutrition, Diet, and Epigenetics* and *Diet Quality: An Evidence-Based Approach.* He has published over 150 articles. In 2014, he was elected as a Fellow to The Royal Society of Chemistry.

Victor R. Preedy, BSc, PhD, DSc, FRSB, FRSPH, FRCPath, FRSC, is Professor of Clinical Biochemistry (Hon) at King's College Hospital, London, and Emeritus Professor of Nutritional Biochemistry at King's College London. He has an Honorary Professorship at the University of Hull and was the long-term Director of the Genomics Centre at King's College London from 2006 to 2020. Professor Preedy graduated in 1974 with an Honours Degree in Biology and Physiology with Pharmacology. He gained his University of London PhD in 1981. In 1992, he received his Membership of the Royal College of Pathologists and in 1993 he gained his second doctorate (DSc), for his outstanding contribution to protein metabolism in health and disease. Professor Preedy was elected as a Fellow of the Institute of Biology in 1995 and the Royal College of Pathologists in 2000. He was elected as a

Fellow of the Royal Society for the Promotion of Health (2004) and The Royal Institute of Public Health (2004). In 2009, Professor Preedy became a Fellow of the Royal Society for Public Health and in 2012 a Fellow of the Royal Society of Chemistry. Professor Preedy has carried out research when attached to The National Heart Hospital (Imperial College London), The School of Pharmacy (now part of University College London), and the MRC Research Centre at Northwick Park Hospital. He has collaborated with research groups in Finland, Japan, Australia, USA, and Germany. Professor Preedy is a leading expert in the biomedical sciences and public health and has edited several books on addictions, including *The Neuroscience of Alcohol*, *The Neuroscience of Cocaine*, *The Handbook of Cannabis and Related Pathologies*, as well as the three-volume set *Neuropathology of Drug Addictions and Substance Misuse.* To his credit, Professor Preedy has published over 700 articles, which includes peer-reviewed manuscripts based on original research, abstracts and symposium presentations, reviews, and numerous books and volumes.

Contributors

Husam Abazid Department of Clinical Pharmacy and Therapeutics, Faculty of Pharmacy, Applied Science Private University, Amman, Jordan

Uzma Abdullah University Institute of Biochemistry and Biotechnology, Pir Mehr Ali Shah Arid Agriculture University Rawalpindi, Rawalpindi, Pakistan

Yael Abreu-Villaça Departamento de Ciências Fisiológicas, Instituto de Biologia Roberto Alcantara Gomes, Universidade do Estado do Rio de Janeiro, Rio de Janeiro, Brazil

Elio Acquas Department of Life and Environmental Sciences, Center of Excellence for the Study of Neurobiology of Addiction, University of Cagliari, Cagliari, Italy

Shoaib Afzal Department of Clinical Biochemistry, Copenhagen University Hospital – Herlev and Gentofte Hospital, Copenhagen, Denmark

Department of Clinical Medicine, University of Copenhagen, Copenhagen, Denmark

María A. Aguilar Unit of Research "Neurobehavioural Mechanisms and Endophenotypes of Addictive Behaviour", Department of Psychobiology, Faculty of Psychology, University of Valencia, Valencia, Spain

Muhammad Sheeraz Ahmad University Institute of Biochemistry and Biotechnology, Pir Mehr Ali Shah Arid Agriculture University Rawalpindi, Rawalpindi, Pakistan

Mustafa Atilla Akgül Department of Family Medicine, University of Health Sciences, Ankara Dışkapı Yıldırım Beyazıt Training and Research Hospital, Ankara, Turkey

Lucy Albertella BrainPark, Turner Institute for Brain and Mental Health, Monash University, Clayton, VIC, Australia

Salah M. Aleid Department of Food Sciences and Nutrition, College of Agriculture and Food Sciences, King Faisal University, Al-Ahsa, Saudi Arabia

Luis F. Alguacil Institute of Studies on Addictions IEA-CEU, San Pablo-CEU University, Alcorcón, Spain

Mir Faeq Ali Quadri Dental Public Health, Department of Preventive Dental Sciences, College of Dentistry, Jazan University, Jazan, Saudi Arabia

Muneera Qassim Al-Mssallem Department of Food Sciences and Nutrition, College of Agriculture and Food Sciences, King Faisal University, Al-Ahsa, Saudi Arabia

Mustafa Ahmed Alshagga Division of Biomedical Science, School of Pharmacy, University of Nottingham Malaysia, Semenyih, Malaysia

Mónica Antunes Centro de Investigação em Ciências da Saúde, Laboratório de Fármaco-Toxicologia, UBIMedical, Universidade da Beira Interior, Covilhã, Portugal

Marcelo Dutra Arbo Department of Analysis, Faculty of Pharmacy, Universidade Federal do Rio Grande do Sul, Porto Alegre, Brazil

R. A. Armstrong Vision Sciences, School of Life & Health Science, Aston University, Birmingham, UK

Luis Enrique Arroyo-García Division of Neurogeriatrics, Neuronal Oscillations Laboratory, Center for Alzheimer Research, NVS Karolinska Institutet, Solna, Sweden

Hassan Arshad Division of Social and Behavioral Sciences, School of Public Health, University of Memphis, Memphis, TN, USA

P. V. Asharani Research Division, Institute of Mental Health, Singapore, Singapore

Paweł A. Atroszko Department of Psychometrics and Statistics, Institute of Psychology, Faculty of Social Sciences, University of Gdańsk, Gdańsk, Poland

Nicole M. Avena Department of Psychology, Princeton University, Princeton, NJ, USA

Department of Neuroscience, Icahn School of Medicine at Mount Sinai, New York, NY, USA

Cenk Aypak Department of Family Medicine, University of Health Sciences, Ankara Dışkapı Yıldırım Beyazıt Training and Research Hospital, Ankara, Turkey

Semra A. Aytur Department of Health Management and Policy, University of New Hampshire, Durham, NH, USA

Rinda D. Bachu Department of Pharmacology and Experimental Therapeutics, College of Pharmacy and Pharmaceutical Sciences, University of Toledo College of Pharmacy, Toledo, OH, USA

Biancamaria Baroli Department of Life and Environmental Sciences, University of Cagliari, Cagliari, Italy

Alfonso Barrós-Loscertales Departamento de Psicología Básica, Clínica y Psicobiología, Universitat Jaume I, Castellón de la Plana, Spain

Mário Barroso Serviço de Química e Toxicologia Forenses, Instituto Nacional de Medicina Legal e Ciências Forenses, I.P., Delegação Sul, Lisbon, Portugal

Giuseppe Basile IRCCS Orthopedic Institute Galeazzi, Milan, Italy

Valentina Bassareo Department of Biomedical Sciences and Center of Excellence for the Study of Neurobiology of Addiction, University of Cagliari, Cagliari, Italy

Michael J. Beckstead Aging & Metabolism Research Program, Oklahoma Medical Research Foundation, Oklahoma City, OK, USA

Nicolas Berthelot Department of Nursing Sciences, Université du Québec à Trois-Rivières, Trois-Rivières, QC, Canada

L. Cinnamon Bidwell Department of Psychology and Neuroscience, University of Colorado Boulder, Boulder, CO, USA

Institute of Cognitive Science, University of Colorado Boulder, Boulder, CO, USA

Katie Biello Department of Behavioral & Social Sciences, School of Public Health, Brown University, Providence, RI, USA

Department of Epidemiology, School of Public Health, Brown University, Providence, RI, USA

The Fenway Institute, Fenway Health, Boston, MA, USA

Anna Birková Department of Medical and Clinical Biochemistry, Pavol Jozef Šafárik University in Košice, Faculty of Medicine, Košice, Slovakia

Kenneth Blum Division of Addiction Research and Education, Center for Psychiatry Medicine and Primary Care (Office of Provost), Western University Health Sciences, Pomona, CA, USA

Georgia Bolt Clinical Neuropsychologist, Turning Point, Eastern Health Clinical School, Richmond, VIC, Australia

Steven R. Boomhower Gradient, Boston, MA, USA

Harvard Division of Continuing Education, Harvard University, Cambridge, MA, USA

Brianna L. Bourgeois Department of Physiology, Comprehensive Alcohol HIV/AIDS Research Center, Louisiana State University Health Sciences Center, New Orleans, LA, USA

Poliana Guiomar Brasiel Department of Nutrition, Institute of Biological Sciences, Federal University of Juiz de Fora, Juiz de Fora, MG, Brazil

Andreia Machado Brito-da-Costa TOXRUN – Toxicology Research Unit, University Institute of Health Sciences, CESPU, CRL, Gandra, Portugal

UCIBIO-REQUIMTE, Laboratory of Toxicology, Department of Biological Sciences, Faculty of Pharmacy, University of Porto, Porto, Portugal

Associate Laboratory i4HB – Institute for Health and Bioeconomy, Faculty of Pharmacy, University of Porto, Porto, Portugal

Amalie Brokhattingen Global Health Section, Department of Public Health, University of Copenhagen, Copenhagen, Denmark

Emília Marques Brovini Laboratório de Química Tecnológica e Ambiental (LQTA), Programa de Pós-Graduação em Engenharia Ambiental, Universidade Federal de Ouro Preto, Ouro Preto, Brazil

P. Brown Department of Psychology, Loma Linda University, Loma Linda, CA, USA

Antonio Bruno IRCCS Neuromed, Pozzilli, Italy

Javier Bueno-Antequera Section of Physical Education and Sports, Department of Sports and Computer Science, Faculty of Sports Sciences, Physical Performance and Sports Research Center, Universidad Pablo de Olavide, Seville, Spain

Research Group in Development Movimiento Humano, Universidad de Zaragoza, Zaragoza, Spain

Larry Burd Department of Pediatrics, University of North Dakota School of Medicine and Health Sciences, Grand Forks, ND, USA

Pierluigi Caboni Department of Life and Environmental Sciences, University of Cagliari, Cagliari, Italy

Cristina Cadoni Department of Biomedical Sciences, Institute of Neuroscience, National Research Council of Italy, Cagliari, Italy

Claudia Calpe-López Unit of Research "Neurobehavioural Mechanisms and Endophenotypes of Addictive Behaviour", Department of Psychobiology, Faculty of Psychology, University of Valencia, Valencia, Spain

Tiago Queiroz Cardoso Instituto Dr. Tiago Queiroz, Recife, Brazil

Vincent Carfagno Midwestern University School of Medicine, Glendale, AZ, USA

Helena Carmo Associate Laboratory i4HB – Institute for Health and Bioeconomy, Faculty of Pharmacy, University of Porto, Porto, Portugal

UCIBIO, Laboratory of Toxicology, Department of Biological Sciences, Faculty of Pharmacy, University of Porto, Porto, Portugal

Adrian Carter School of Psychological Sciences, Monash University Clayton Campus, Clayton, VIC, Australia

Félix Carvalho Associate Laboratory i4HB – Institute for Health and Bioeconomy, Faculty of Pharmacy, University of Porto, Porto, Portugal

UCIBIO, Laboratory of Toxicology, Department of Biological Sciences, Faculty of Pharmacy, University of Porto, Porto, Portugal

Stephanie E. Cassin Department of Psychology, Ryerson University, Toronto, ON, Canada

Daniele Castellani Urology Unit, Azienda Ospedaliero-Universitaria Ospedali Riuniti di Ancona, Università Politecnica delle Marche, Ancona, Italy

Chiara Cecchelli Brain Center Firenze, Florence, Italy

Anne Cecilie Tveiten Department of Pediatrics, Sørlandet Hospital, Arendal, Norway

Magdalena Cedzynska Department of Cancer Epidemiology and Primary Prevention, Maria Sklodowska-Curie National Research Institute of Oncology, Warsaw, Poland

Samuel R. Chamberlain Department of Psychiatry, University of Southampton, Southampton, UK

Katrina E. Champion The Matilda Centre for Research in Mental Health & Substance Use, The University of Sydney, Camperdown, NSW, Australia

Kate C. Chan Department of Paediatrics, Faculty of Medicine, The Chinese University of Hong Kong, Hong Kong, China

Chih-Cheng Chang Division of Addiction Psychiatry, Department of Psychiatry, Chi Mei Medical Center, Tainan, Taiwan

Kun-Chia Chang Jianan Psychiatric Center, Ministry of Health and Welfare, Tainan, Taiwan

Department of Natural Biotechnology, Nan Hua University, Chiayi, Taiwan

Shinjini Choudhury Department of Psychiatry, All India Institute of Medical Sciences, Rishikesh, India

Gro Christine Christensen Løhaugen Department of Pediatrics, Sørlandet Hospital, Arendal, Norway

Agata Chrzanowska National Drug and Alcohol Research Centre, University of New South Wales, Randwick, NSW, Australia

Francis Kin Chiu Chu Accident and Emergency Department, Queen Elizabeth Hospital, Kowloon, Hong Kong, China

Beáta Čižmárová Department of Medical and Clinical Biochemistry, Pavol Jozef Šafárik University in Košice, Faculty of Medicine, Košice, Slovakia

Yorkiris Mármol Contreras Department of Pharmacology, University of Texas Medical Branch, Galveston, TX, USA

R. W. Coppock DVM, Toxicologist and Associates Ltd., Vegreville, AB, Canada

Víctor Costumero Departamento de Psicología Básica, Clínica y Psicobiología, Universitat Jaume I, Castellón de la Plana, Spain

Michael C. Crawford PATHS Lab, University of Rhode Island Department of Psychology, Kingston, RI, USA

Rose Crossin Department of Population Health, University of Otago, Christchurch, New Zealand

Melissa Cyders Department of Psychology, Indiana University – Purdue University Indianapolis, Indianapolis, IN, USA

Siyu Dai School of Clinical Medicine, Hangzhou Normal University, Hangzhou, China

Anuradha Dave Department of Community Medicine, Subharti Medical College, Swami Vivekanand Subharti University, Meerut, India

S. Dave Government Medical College, Saharanpur, India

Laura Dazzi Department of Life and Environmental Sciences, University of Cagliari, Cagliari, Italy

Vitória Girelli de Oliveira Laboratory of Neurotrauma and Biomarkers, Department of Biochemistry, ICBS, Universidade Federal do Rio Grande do Sul – UFRGS, Porto Alegre, Brazil

Jennifer Debenham The Matilda Centre for Research in Mental Health & Substance Use, The University of Sydney, Camperdown, NSW, Australia

Zsolt Demetrovics Institute of Psychology, ELTE Eötvös Loránd University, Budapest, Hungary

Centre of Excellence in Responsible Gaming, University of Gibraltar, Gibraltar, Spain

Jeffrey Derevensky International Centre for Youth Gambling Problems and High Risk Behaviors, McGill University, Montreal, QC, Canada

Don C. Des Jarlais Department of Epidemiology, New York University School of Global Public Health, New York, NY, USA

Veena Dhawan Department of Experimental Medicine and Biotechnology, Postgraduate Institute of Medical Education and Research, Chandigarh, India

Giuseppe Di Martino Unit of Hygiene, Epidemiology and Public Health, Local Health Autority of Pescara, Abruzzo, Italy

Department of Medicine and Ageing Sciences, "G. d'Annunzio" University of Chieti-Pescara, Abruzzo, Italy

Diana Dias da Silva UCIBIO/REQUIMTE, Laboratory of Toxicology, Faculty of Pharmacy, The University of Porto, Porto, Portugal

Associate Laboratory i4HB–Institute for Health and Bioeconomy, Faculty of Pharmacy, University of Porto, Porto, Portugal

TOXRUN – Toxicology Research Unit, University Institute of Health Sciences, IUCS-CESPU, Gandra PRD, Portugal

Patrick J. Dillon School of Communication Studies, Kent State University at Stark, North Canton, OH, USA

Ricardo Jorge Dinis-Oliveira TOXRUN – Toxicology Research Unit, University Institute of Health Sciences, CESPU, CRL, Gandra, Portugal

UCIBIO-REQUIMTE, Laboratory of Toxicology, Department of Biological Sciences, Faculty of Pharmacy, University of Porto, Porto, Portugal

Associate Laboratory i4HB – Institute for Health and Bioeconomy, Faculty of Pharmacy, University of Porto, Porto, Portugal

Department of Public Health and Forensic Sciences, and Medicinal Education, Faculty of Medicine, University of Porto, Porto, Portugal

Joyce Andreia dos Santos Departamento de Biologia, Laboratório de Ecologia Aquática, Programa de Pós-Graduação em Biodiversidade e Conservação da Natureza, Universidade Federal de Juiz de Fora, Juiz de Fora, Brazil

Marcy Doyle Institute for Health Policy and Practice, University of New Hampshire, Concord, NH, USA

Aaron Drovandi Queensland Research Centre for Peripheral Vascular Disease, College of Medicine and Dentistry, James Cook University, Townsville, QLD, Australia

Ana C. Dutra-Tavares Departamento de Ciências Fisiológicas, Instituto de Biologia Roberto Alcantara Gomes, Universidade do Estado do Rio de Janeiro, Rio de Janeiro, Brazil

M. M. Dziwenka Toxalta Consulting Ltd., Vegreville, AB, Canada

Mark J. Eisenberg Center for Clinical Epidemiology, Lady Davis Institute, Jewish General Hospital, Montreal, QC, Canada

McGill University, Medical School, Montreal, QC, Canada

Departments of Medicine and of Epidemiology, Biostatistics and Occupational Health, McGill University, Montreal, QC, Canada

Division of Cardiology and Clinical Epidemiology, Jewish General Hospital, McGill University, Montreal, QC, Canada

Sarah Eller Pharmacosciences Department, Federal University of Health Sciences of Porto Alegre, Porto Alegre, Brazil

Jennifer D. Ellis Department of Psychiatry, Johns Hopkins University, Baltimore, MD, USA

Maged El-Setouhy Department of Family and Community Medicine, Faculty of Medicine, Jazan University, Jazan, Saudi Arabia

Ingunn Marie Stadskleiv Engebretsen Centre for International Health, Department of Global Public Health and Primary Care, Medical Faculty, University of Bergen, Bergen, Norway

Coree Entwistle Division of Social and Behavioral Sciences, School of Public Health, University of Memphis, Memphis, TN, USA

Ana Estévez Psychology Department, University of Deusto, Bilbao, Spain

Nerea Etxaburu Psychology Department, University of Deusto, Bilbao, Spain

Sara Fabius Department of Experimental Neuropharmacology, Instituto de Investigaciones Biológicas Clemente Estable, Montevideo, Uruguay

Ni Fan The Affiliated Brain Hospital of Guangzhou Medical University, Guangzhou, China

Magí Farré Clinical Pharmacology Unit, Hospital Universitari Germans Trias i Pujol, Institut de Recerca Germans Trias i Pujol (HUGTiP-IGTP), Badalona, Spain

Department of Pharmacology, Therapeutics and Toxicology, Universitat Autònoma de Barcelona (UAB), Cerdanyola del Vallés, Spain

Mauro Federici IRCCS Fondazione Santa Lucia, Rome, Italy

Jonathan Feelemyer Department of Epidemiology, New York University School of Global Public Health, New York, NY, USA

Camino María Fernández-Rodríguez Servicio de Medicina Interna, Universidad de La Laguna. Hospital Universitario de Canarias, Canary Islands, Spain

Cláudio C. Filgueiras Departamento de Ciências Fisiológicas, Instituto de Biologia Roberto Alcantara Gomes, Universidade do Estado do Rio de Janeiro, Rio de Janeiro, Brazil

Gonzalo Flores Neuropsychiatry Laboratory, Instituto de Fisiología, Benemérita Universidad Autónoma de Puebla (BUAP), Puebla, Mexico

Thomas C. Flowers Department of Otolaryngology-Head and Neck Surgery, Tulane University, New Orleans, LA, USA

Leonardo F. Fontenelle Institute of Psychiatry, Federal University of Rio de Janeiro, Rio de Janeiro, Brazil

D'Or Institute for Research and Education, Rio de Janeiro, Brazil

Hongyun Fu Community Health and Research Division, Eastern Virginia Medical School, Norfolk, VA, USA

Xavier C. C. Fung Department of Rehabilitation Sciences, Faculty of Health and Social Sciences, The Hong Kong Polytechnic University, Hung Hom, Hong Kong

Eugenia Gallardo Centro de Investigação em Ciências da Saúde, Laboratório de Fármaco-Toxicologia, UBIMedical, Universidade da Beira Interior, Covilhã, Portugal

M. Pilar García-Pardo Department of Psychology and Sociology, Development Psychology Area, Faculty of Social and Human Sciences, University of Zaragoza, Campus Teruel, Teruel, Spain

Alen García-Rodríguez Servicio de Medicina Interna, Universidad de La Laguna. Hospital Universitario de Canarias, Canary Islands, Spain

Coral Gartner Faculty of Medicine, School of Public Health, The University of Queensland, Brisbane, QLD, Australia

Beata Gavurova Department of Addictology, First Faculty of Medicine, Charles University and General University Hospital in Prague, Prague, Czechia

Abhishek Ghosh Department of Psychiatry & Drug De-addiction and Treatment Centre, Postgraduate Institute of Medical Education and Research, Chandigarh, India

Lynette Gilbeau International Centre for Youth Gambling Problems and High Risk Behaviors, McGill University, Montreal, QC, Canada

Arianna Giorgetti Department of Medical and Surgical Sciences, Unit of Legal Medicine, University of Bologna, Bologna, Italy

Raffaele Giorgetti Department of Excellence of Biomedical Sciences and Public Health, Università Politecnica delle Marche, Ancona, Italy

Mark S. Gold Department of Psychiatry, School of Medicine, Washington University in St. Louis, St. Louis, MO, USA

Joana Gonçalves Centro de Investigação em Ciências da Saúde, Laboratório de Fármaco-Toxicologia, UBIMedical, Universidade da Beira Interior, Covilhã, Portugal

Emilio González-Arnay Departamento de Ciencias Básicas, Sección de Anatomía, Universidad de La Laguna, Hospital Universitario de Canarias, Canary Islands, Spain

Emilio González-Reimers Servicio de Medicina Interna, Universidad de La Laguna. Hospital Universitario de Canarias, Canary Islands, Spain

Giacomo Grassi Brain Center Firenze, Florence, Italy

Thomas A. Green Department of Pharmacology, University of Texas Medical Branch, Galveston, TX, USA

Andrew J. Greenshaw Department of Psychiatry, University of Alberta, Edmonton, Alberta, Canada

Zerihun Girma Gudata Haramaya University, Hararghe Health Research Project, CHAMPS Ethiopia, Harar, Ethiopia

Ramón Guirado Neurobiology Unit, Program in Neurosciences and University Institute of Biotechnology and Biomedicine (BIOTECMED), Universitat de València, Burjassot, Spain

Bishal Gyawali Global Health Section, Department of Public Health, University of Copenhagen, Copenhagen, Denmark

Leona Hakkaart-van Roijen Department of Health Technology Assessment, Erasmus School of Health Policy & Management, Erasmus University Rotterdam, Rotterdam, The Netherlands

Meredith Halcomb Department of Radiology and Imaging Sciences, Indiana University School of Medicine, Indianapolis, IN, USA

F. Scott Hall Department of Pharmacology and Experimental Therapeutics, College of Pharmacy & Pharmaceutical Sciences, University of Toledo, Toledo, OH, USA

Alaa M. Hammad Department of Pharmacy, Faculty of Pharmacy, Al-Zaytoonah University of Jordan, Amman, Jordan

Nurcan Hamzaoglu Institution of Medical Science, Istanbul Yeni Yuzyil University, Istanbul, Turkey

Enjeline Hanafi Department of Psychiatry, Faculty of Medicine, Universitas Indonesia – Dr. Cipto Mangunkusumo General Hospital, Jakarta, Indonesia

Kylie Handa Aging & Metabolism Research Program, Oklahoma Medical Research Foundation, Oklahoma City, OK, USA

M. Hanna Department of Psychology, Loma Linda University, Loma Linda, CA, USA

Jaanus Harro Institute of Chemistry, University of Tartu, Tartu, Estonia

Psychiatry Clinic, North Estonia Medical Centre, Tallinn, Estonia

Ashraf A. Hassan Department of Medical Laboratory Technology, Faculty of Applied Medical Sciences, Jazan University, Jazan, Saudi Arabia

Edward Hensel Department of Mechanical Engineering, Kate Gleason College of Engineering, Rochester Institute of Technology, Rochester, NY, USA

Monika Herian Department of Pharmacology, Maj Institute of Pharmacology, Polish Academy of Sciences, Cracow, Poland

Samuel Hogarth Department of Psychology and Counselling, School of Psychology and Public Health, La Trobe University, Melbourne, VIC, Australia

Beáta Hubková Department of Medical and Clinical Biochemistry, Pavol Jozef Šafárik University in Košice, Faculty of Medicine, Košice, Slovakia

Noor A. Hussein Department of Pharmacology and Experimental Therapeutics, College of Pharmacy & Pharmaceutical Sciences, University of Toledo, Toledo, OH, USA

Department of Pediatrics, Human Gene Therapy, Stanford University, School of Medicine, Stanford, CA, USA

Eric J. Ip Clinical Sciences Department, Touro University California College of Pharmacy, Vallejo, CA, USA

Department of Medicine, Stanford University School of Medicine, Stanford, CA, USA

Samira Dishti Irfan Program for HIV and AIDS, Infectious Diseases Division, International Centre for Diarrhoeal Diseases Research, Dhaka, Bangladesh

Viera Ivankova Institute of Earth Resources, Faculty of Mining, Ecology, Process Control and Geotechnologies, Technical University of Košice, Košice, Slovak Republic

Shagufta Jabeen Islamabad Model College for Boys, Islamabad, Pakistan

Sahar Jaffal Department of Biological Sciences, Faculty of Science, University of Jordan, Amman, Jordan

Elisabet Jerlhag Institute of Neuroscience and Physiology, Department of Pharmacology, The Sahlgrenska Academy at the University of Gothenburg, Gothenburg, Sweden

Jinjing Jia Department of Physiology, Jiaxing University Medical College, Jiaxing, China

Brian Johnson Department of Psychiatry, State University of New York (SUNY) Upstate Medical University, Syracuse, NY, USA

Jennifer Juckel Institute for Social Science Research, University of Queensland, Indooroopilly, Australia

Jijo Stebin Justus Laboratory of Neurotrauma and Biomarkers, Department of Biochemistry, ICBS, Universidade Federal do Rio Grande do Sul – UFRGS, Porto Alegre, Brazil

Andriana Kakanakova Department of Psychiatry and Medical Psychology, Medical University Plovdiv, Plovdiv, Bulgaria

Yifrah Kaminer Departments of Psychiatry and Pediatrics, Alcohol Research Center, University of Connecticut School of Medicine, Farmington, CT, USA

Arun Kandasamy Centre for Addiction Medicine, Department of Psychiatry, National Institute of Mental Health and Neurosciences, Bangalore, India

Sevcan Karatas First and Emergency Aid Program, Istanbul Yeni Yuzyil University, Istanbul, Turkey

Satish Kedia Division of Social and Behavioral Sciences, School of Public Health, University of Memphis, Memphis, TN, USA

Erin Kelty School of Population & Global Health, University of Western Australia, Crawley, WA, Australia

Mohammad Niaz Morshed Khan Program for HIV and AIDS, Infectious Diseases Division, International Centre for Diarrhoeal Disease Research, Dhaka, Bangladesh

Sharful Islam Khan Program for HIV and AIDS, Infectious Diseases Division, International Centre for Diarrhoeal Diseases Research, Dhaka, Bangladesh

Katelyn T. Kirk-Provencher PATHS Lab, University of Rhode Island Department of Psychology, Kingston, RI, USA

Lori Knackstedt Psychology Department, University of Florida, Gainesville, FL, USA

Kairi Kõlves Australian Institute for Suicide Research and Prevention, WHO Collaborating Centre for Research and Training in Suicide Prevention, School of Applied Psychology, Griffith University, Brisbane, QLD, Australia

Renate Koppensteiner Department of Internal Medicine II, Division of Angiology, Medical University of Vienna, Vienna, Austria

Eszter Kótyuk Institute of Psychology, ELTE Eötvös Loránd University, Budapest, Hungary

Pirkko Kriikku Department of Forensic Medicine, University of Helsinki, Helsinki, Finland

Forensic Toxicology Unit, Finnish Institute for Health and Welfare, Helsinki, Finland

Salma Kyana Department of Psychiatry, Faculty of Medicine, Universitas Indonesia – Dr. Cipto Mangunkusumo General Hospital, Jakarta, Indonesia

Carl Lacharité Department of Psychology, Université du Québec à Trois-Rivières, Trois-Rivières, QC, Canada

Dirk W. Lachenmeier Chemisches und Veterinäruntersuchungsamt Karlsruhe, Karlsruhe, Germany

Ram Lakhan Department of Health and Human Performance, Berea College, Berea, KY, USA

Sheng-Yu Lee Department of Psychiatry, Kaohsiung Veterans General Hospital, Kaohsiung, Taiwan

Danielle E. Levitt Department of Physiology, Comprehensive Alcohol HIV/AIDS Research Center, Louisiana State University Health Sciences Center, New Orleans, LA, USA

Jonna M. Leyrer-Jackson Department of Psychology, Arizona State University, Tempe, AZ, USA

Guohua Li Department of Anesthesiology, Vagelos College of Physicians and Surgeons, Columbia University, New York, NY, USA

Nu-Chu Liang Department of Psychology, University of Illinois at Urbana-Champaign, Champaign, IL, USA

Peter Alison Lie Department of Psychiatry, Faculty of Medicine, Universitas Indonesia – Dr. Cipto Mangunkusumo General Hospital, Jakarta, Indonesia

Sharoen Yu Ming Lim Division of Biomedical Science, School of Pharmacy, University of Nottingham Malaysia, Semenyih, Malaysia

Chung-Ying Lin Institute of Allied Health Sciences, College of Medicine, National Cheng Kung University, Tainan, Taiwan

Jianfeng Liu Brain Science and Advanced Technology Institute, Wuhan University of Science and Technology, Wuhan, People's Republic of China

Yue Liu Laboratory of Behavioral Neuroscience, Ningbo Kangning Hospital, School of Medicine, Ningbo University, Ningbo, People's Republic of China

Key Laboratory of Addiction Research of Zhejiang Province, Ningbo, People's Republic of China

William Lodge II Department of Behavioral & Social Sciences, School of Public Health, Brown University, Providence, RI, USA

Henriette Löffler-Stastka Department of Psychoanalysis and Psychotherapy, Medical University of Vienna, Vienna, Austria

Gro C. C. Løhaugen Department of Pediatrics, Sørlandet Hospital Arendal, Arendal, Norway

Sheila Cristina Potente Dutra Luquetti Department of Nutrition, Institute of Biological Sciences, Federal University of Juiz de Fora, Juiz de Fora, MG, Brazil

Lynnette Nathalie Lyzwinski Department of Medicine and of Epidemiology, Biostatistics and Occupational Health, McGill University, Montreal, QC, Canada

Centre for Clinical Epidemiology, McGill University, Montreal, QC, Canada

Center for Clinical Epidemiology, Lady Davis Institute, Jewish General Hospital, Montreal, QC, Canada

McGill University, Medical School, Montreal, QC, Canada

Laura Macía Psychology Department, University of Deusto, Bilbao, Spain

Riccardo Maccioni Department of Life and Environmental Sciences, University of Cagliari, Cagliari, Italy

Grace Macdonald-Gagnon Department of Psychiatry, Yale University School of Medicine, New Haven, CT, USA

Áurea Madureira-Carvalho TOXRUN – Toxicology Research Unit, University Institute of Health Sciences, CESPU, CRL, Gandra, Portugal

LAQV-REQUIMTE, Laboratory of Pharmacognosy, Department of Chemistry, Faculty of Pharmacy, University of Porto, Porto, Portugal

Saloni Malla Department of Pharmacology and Experimental Therapeutics, College of Pharmacy & Pharmaceutical Sciences, University of Toledo, Toledo, OH, USA

Marta Manczuk Department of Cancer Epidemiology and Primary Prevention, Maria Sklodowska-Curie National Research Institute of Oncology, Warsaw, Poland

Chitra D. Mandyam VA San Diego Healthcare System, San Diego, CA, USA

Department of Anesthesiology, University of California San Diego, San Diego, CA, USA

Alex C. Manhães Departamento de Ciências Fisiológicas, Instituto de Biologia Roberto Alcantara Gomes, Universidade do Estado do Rio de Janeiro, Rio de Janeiro, Brazil

Hayley N. Manke Psychopharmacology Laboratory, Department of Neuroscience, American University, Washington, DC, USA

Elizabeth Manning School of Biomedical Sciences and Pharmacy, University of Newcastle, Callaghan, NSW, Australia

Victoria Manning Research and Workforce Development, Turning Point, Eastern Health Clinical School, Monash University, Richmond, VIC, Australia

Loredana Marchica Department of Psychology, Montreal Children's Hospital, Montreal, QC, Canada

Claudia Mariottini Department of Forensic Medicine, University of Helsinki, Helsinki, Finland

Forensic Toxicology Unit, Finnish Institute for Health and Welfare, Helsinki, Finland

Hernâni Marques Centro de Investigação em Ciências da Saúde, Laboratório de Fármaco-Toxicologia, UBIMedical, Universidade da Beira Interior, Covilhã, Portugal

Candelaria Martín-González Servicio de Medicina Interna, Universidad de La Laguna. Hospital Universitario de Canarias, Canary Islands, Spain

Rémi Martin-Fardon Department of Molecular Medicine, The Scripps Research Institute, La Jolla, CA, USA

Renée Martin-Willett Department of Psychology and Neuroscience, University of Colorado Boulder, Boulder, CO, USA

M. Ángeles Martínez-Caballero Unit of Research "Neurobehavioural Mechanisms and Endophenotypes of Addictive Behaviour", Department of Psychobiology, Faculty of Psychology, University of Valencia, Valencia, Spain

Natasha L. Mason Department of Neuropsychology and Psychopharmacology, Faculty of Psychology and Neuroscience, Maastricht University, Maastricht, Netherlands

Ashley Master Department of Psychology and Neuroscience, University of Colorado Boulder, Boulder, CO, USA

Takayuki Matsumoto Department of Physiology and Morphology, Institute of Medicinal Chemistry, Hoshi University, Shinagawa-ku, Tokyo, Japan

Alessandra Matzeu Department of Molecular Medicine, The Scripps Research Institute, La Jolla, CA, USA

Edward McCoul Department of Otorhinolaryngology, Ochsner Clinic, New Orleans, LA, USA

Ravi Mehrotra Department of Epidemiology, Rollins School of Public Health, Emory University, Atlanta, GA, USA

School of Health Sciences, University of York, York, UK

Centre for Health Innovation and Policy (CHIP) Foundation, Noida, Uttar Pradesh, India

Sakshi Mehta Department of Experimental Medicine and Biotechnology, Postgraduate Institute of Medical Education and Research, Chandigarh, India

Adduct Healthcare Pvt. Ltd., Mohali, Punjab, India

Disen Mei School of Medicine, Ningbo University, Ningbo, People's Republic of China

Sarah K. Meier Department of Communication Sciences and Disorders, University of New Hampshire, Durham, NH, USA

Nicola Biagio Mercuri IRCCS Fondazione Santa Lucia, Rome, Italy

Department of System Medicine, University of Rome Tor Vergata, Rome, Italy

Eric Merrell Department of Medicine, SUNY Upstate Medical University, Syracuse, NY, USA

Rossana Migheli Department of Experimental Medical and Surgical Sciences, University of Sassari, Sassari, Italy

Matthew J. Mimiaga UCLA Center for LGBTQ+ Advocacy, Research & Health, Los Angeles, CA, USA

Department of Epidemiology, UCLA Fielding School of Public Health, Los Angeles, CA, USA

Department of Psychiatry & Biobehavioral Sciences, UCLA David Geffen School of Medicine, Los Angeles, CA, USA

Syam Mohan Substance Abuse and Toxicology Research Center, Jazan University, Jazan, Saudi Arabia

Patricia E. Molina Department of Physiology, Comprehensive Alcohol HIV/AIDS Research Center, Louisiana State University Health Sciences Center, New Orleans, LA, USA

Janire Momeñe Psychology Department, University of Deusto, Bilbao, Spain

Elizabeth Monk-Turner Department of Sociology and Criminal Justice, College of Arts and Letters, Old Dominion University, Norfolk, VA, USA

Maude Morneau Department of Psychology, Université du Québec à Trois-Rivières, Trois-Rivières, QC, Canada

Kylie Morphett Faculty of Medicine, School of Public Health, The University of Queensland, Brisbane, QLD, Australia

Diptadhi Mukherjee Department of Addiction Medicine, Department of Psychiatry, LGB Regional Institute of Mental Health, Tezpur, India

Dawn E. Muskiewicz Department of Pharmacology and Experimental Therapeutics, College of Pharmacy & Pharmaceutical Sciences, University of Toledo, Toledo, OH, USA

Tessa Nalven PATHS Lab, University of Rhode Island Department of Psychology, Kingston, RI, USA

Venkata Lakshmi Narasimha Department of Psychiatry, All India Institute of Medical Sciences (AIIMS), Panchayat Training Institute, Daburgram Jasidih, Deoghar, Jharkhand, India

Sumaira Nasim School of Public Health, Dow University of Health Sciences, Karachi, Pakistan

Oybek Nazarov The University of Queensland, School of Medicine, Mayne Medical Reception, Herston, QLD, Australia

Katharine H. Nelson Reichel Laboratory, Department of Neuroscience, The Medical University of South Carolina, Charleston, SC, USA

Yehuda Neumark Braun School of Public Health and Community Medicine, Faculty of Medicine, Hebrew University of Jerusalem, Jerusalem, Israel

Nicola C. Newton The Matilda Centre for Research in Mental Health & Substance Use, The University of Sydney, Camperdown, NSW, Australia

Jasmine M. Noble Department of Computing Science, University of Alberta, Edmonton, Alberta, Canada

Department of Psychiatry, University of Alberta, Edmonton, Alberta, Canada

Sara Nutley Department of Epidemiology, College of Public Health and Health Professions, College of Medicine, University of Florida, Gainesville, FL, USA

Ilkka Ojanperä Department of Forensic Medicine, University of Helsinki, Helsinki, Finland

Forensic Toxicology Unit, Finnish Institute for Health and Welfare, Helsinki, Finland

Aet O'Leary Neuropsychopharmacology, Institute of Chemistry, University of Tartu, Tartu, Estonia

Laboratory of Translational Psychiatry, Department of Psychiatry, Psychosomatics, and Psychotherapy, University Hospital Frankfurt, Frankfurt am Main, Germany

M. Foster Olive Department of Psychology, Arizona State University, Tempe, AZ, USA

Ben O'Mara Centre for Social Impact, University of New South Wales, Sydney, NSW, Australia

Chin Eng Ong School of Pharmacy, International Medical University, Kuala Lumpur, Malaysia

Miguel Ángel Oviedo-Caro Research Group in Development Movimiento Humano, Universidad de Zaragoza, Zaragoza, Spain

Department of Physical Education and Sport, University of Seville, Seville, Spain

Ayşe Özdemir Department of Family Medicine, University of Health Sciences, Ankara Dışkapı Yıldırım Beyazıt Training and Research Hospital, Ankara, Turkey

Yan Pan Division of Biomedical Science, School of Pharmacy, University of Nottingham Malaysia, Semenyih, Malaysia

Esther Papaseit Clinical Pharmacology Unit, Hospital Universitari Germans Trias i Pujol, Institut de Recerca Germans Trias i Pujol (HUGTiP-IGTP), Badalona, Spain

Department of Pharmacology, Therapeutics and Toxicology, Universitat Autònoma de Barcelona (UAB), Cerdanyola del Vallés, Spain

José R. Paranaíba Departamento de Biologia, Laboratório de Ecologia Aquática, Programa de Pós-Graduação em Biodiversidade e Conservação da Natureza, Universidade Federal de Juiz de Fora, Juiz de Fora, Brazil

Vinood B. Patel School of Life Sciences, University of Westminster, London, UK

Alessandra T. Peana Department of Chemistry and Pharmacy, University of Sassari, Sassari, Italy

Guido Pelletti Department of Medical and Surgical Sciences, Unit of Legal Medicine, University of Bologna, Bologna, Italy

Nicole Pepper University of California San Diego, San Diego, CA, USA

Clara Pérez-Mañá Clinical Pharmacology Unit, Hospital Universitari Germans Trias i Pujol, Institut de Recerca Germans Trias i Pujol (HUGTiP-IGTP), Badalona, Spain

Department of Pharmacology, Therapeutics and Toxicology, Universitat Autònoma de Barcelona (UAB), Cerdanyola del Vallés, Spain

Marta Perez-Rando Neurobiology Unit, Program in Neurosciences and University Institute of Biotechnology and Biomedicine (BIOTECMED), Universitat de València, Burjassot, Spain

B. Peteet Department of Psychology, Loma Linda University, Loma Linda, CA, USA

Julia K. Pinsonneault The Ohio State University Comprehensive Cancer Center, Columbus, OH, USA

Boris Popesko Faculty of Management and Economics, Tomas Bata University in Zlin, Zlin, Czech Republic

Svetlana Popova Centre for Addiction and Mental Health, Toronto, ON, Canada

Luis Valmor Cruz Portela Laboratory of Neurotrauma and Biomarkers, Department of Biochemistry, ICBS, Universidade Federal do Rio Grande do Sul – UFRGS, Porto Alegre, Brazil

Marc N. Potenza Departments of Psychiatry, Neuroscience and Child Study Center, Yale University School of Medicine, New Haven, CT, USA

Victor R. Preedy School of Life Course and Population Sciences, Faculty of Life Sciences and Medicine, King's College London, London, UK

David B. Preen School of Population & Global Health, University of Western Australia, Crawley, WA, Australia

José Pedro Prieto Department of Experimental Neuropharmacology, Instituto de Investigaciones Biológicas Clemente Estable, Montevideo, Uruguay

Elisabeth Punzi Department of Social Work, University of Gothenburg, Göteborg, Sweden

Gabrielle Rabelo Quadra Departamento de Biologia, Laboratório de Ecologia Aquática, Programa de Pós-Graduação em Biodiversidade e Conservação da Natureza, Universidade Federal de Juiz de Fora, Juiz de Fora, Brazil

Mostafa A. Rabie Department of Pharmacology and Toxicology, Faculty of Pharmacy, Cairo University, Cairo, Egypt

Ghazala Kaukab Raja University Institute of Biochemistry and Biotechnology, Pir Mehr Ali Shah Arid Agriculture University Rawalpindi, Rawalpindi, Pakistan

Rajkumar Rajendram College of Medicine, King Saud bin Abdulaziz University for Health Sciences, Riyadh, Saudi Arabia

Department of Medicine, King Abdulaziz Medical City, King Abdullah International Medical Research Center, Riyadh, Saudi Arabia

Johannes G. Ramaekers Department of Neuropsychology and Psychopharmacology, Faculty of Psychology and Neuroscience, Maastricht University, Maastricht, Netherlands

Josep M. Ramon-Torrell Bellvitge University Hospital, Barcelona, Spain

Kimberly L. Ray Department of Psychology, The University of Texas at Austin, Austin, TX, USA

Vivian Reckers-Droog Department of Health Economics, Erasmus School of Health Policy & Management, Erasmus University Rotterdam, Rotterdam, The Netherlands

Stella M. Resko School of Social Work, Wayne State University, Detroit, MI, USA

Anderson Ribeiro-Carvalho Departamento de Ciências, Faculdade de Formação de Professores, Universidade do Estado do Rio de Janeiro, São Gonçalo, Brazil

Jeremie Richard International Centre for Youth Gambling Problems and High Risk Behaviors, McGill University, Montreal, QC, Canada

Martin Rigelsky Faculty of Management and Business, University of Prešov, Prešov, Slovakia

Anthony L. Riley Psychopharmacology Laboratory, Department of Neuroscience, American University, Washington, DC, USA

Francesca Romana Rizzo IRCCS Neuromed, Pozzilli, Italy

Donald A. Robin Department of Communication Sciences and Disorders, University of New Hampshire, Durham, NH, USA

Risa Robinson Department of Mechanical Engineering, Kate Gleason College of Engineering, Rochester Institute of Technology, Rochester, NY, USA

Marcelo Salimen Rodolphi Laboratory of Neurotrauma and Biomarkers, Department of Biochemistry, ICBS, Universidade Federal do Rio Grande do Sul – UFRGS, Porto Alegre, Brazil

Ángel Romero-Martínez Department of Psychobiology, Faculty of Psychology, University of Valencia, Valencia, Spain

Rita Roque Bravo UCIBIO/REQUIMTE, Laboratory of Toxicology, Faculty of Pharmacy, The University of Porto, Porto, Portugal

Associate Laboratory i4HB–Institute for Health and Bioeconomy, Faculty of Pharmacy, University of Porto, Porto, Portugal

Tiago Rosado Centro de Investigação em Ciências da Saúde, Laboratório de Fármaco-Toxicologia, UBIMedical, Universidade da Beira Interior, Covilhã, Portugal

Grace Roy Department of Health Management and Policy, University of New Hampshire, Durham, NH, USA

Mihir P. Rupani Department of Clinical Epidemiology, Division of Health Sciences, ICMR – National Institute of Occupational Health (ICMR-NIOH), Ahmedabad, Gujarat, India

Department of Community Medicine, Government Medical College Bhavnagar (Maharaja Krishnakumarsinhji Bhavnagar University), Bhavnagar, Gujarat, India

A. Saddlemire Department of Psychology, Loma Linda University, Loma Linda, CA, USA

Wolfgang Sadee The Ohio State University, Columbus, OH, USA

Vincent A. Santiago Department of Psychology, Ryerson University, Toronto, ON, Canada

Angela Saviano Department of Emergency Medicine, Catholic University of the Sacred Heart, Rome, Italy

Rabab H. Sayed Department of Pharmacology and Toxicology, Faculty of Pharmacy, Cairo University, Cairo, Egypt

Melissa R. Schick PATHS Lab, University of Rhode Island Department of Psychology, Kingston, RI, USA

Michael Schmidt Graphic Design, Department of Art, Affiliate Faculty, Social and Behavioral Sciences, School of Public Health, University of Memphis, Memphis, TN, USA

Cecilia Scorza Department of Experimental Neuropharmacology, Instituto de Investigaciones Biológicas Clemente Estable, Montevideo, Uruguay

Lee Thung Sen Department of Psychiatry, Faculty of Medicine, Universitas Indonesia – Dr. Cipto Mangunkusumo General Hospital, Jakarta, Indonesia

Tanveer Khan Ibne Shafiq Program for HIV and AIDS, Infectious Diseases Division, International Centre for Diarrhoeal Disease Research, Dhaka, Bangladesh

Kashif Shafique School of Public Health, Dow University of Health Sciences, Karachi, Pakistan

Yasir A. Shah Department of Food Sciences, Government College University Faisalabad, Faisalabad, Pakistan

Barak Shapira Division of Enforcement and Inspection, Israel Ministry of Health, Jerusalem, Israel

Manoj Sharma Department of Social and Behavioral Health, School of Public Health, University of Nevada, Las Vegas, NV, USA

Amanda L. Sharpe Department of Pharmaceutical Sciences, University of Oklahoma College of Pharmacy, Oklahoma City, OK, USA

Leticia Shea Department of Pharmacy Practice, School of Pharmacy, Regis University, Denver, CO, USA

Wenwen Shen Laboratory of Behavioral Neuroscience, Ningbo Kangning Hospital, School of Medicine, Ningbo University, Ningbo, People's Republic of China

Key Laboratory of Addiction Research of Zhejiang Province, Ningbo, People's Republic of China

Lívia Shirahige Applied Neuroscience Laboratory, Universidade Federal de Pernambuco, Recife, Brazil

Lekhansh Shukla Centre for Addiction Medicine Office, Female Wing, NIMHANS Campus, Bangalore, India

João Pedro Silva Associate Laboratory i4HB – Institute for Health and Bioeconomy, Faculty of Pharmacy, University of Porto, Porto, Portugal

UCIBIO, Laboratory of Toxicology, Department of Biological Sciences, Faculty of Pharmacy, University of Porto, Porto, Portugal

Josiane F. Silva Department of Pharmacology, Ribeirao Preto Medical School University of Sao Paulo, Ribeirao Preto, Brazil

Madeline D. Silva Clinical Sciences Department, Touro University California College of Pharmacy, Vallejo, CA, USA

Ana Y. Simão Centro de Investigação em Ciências da Saúde, Laboratório de Fármaco-Toxicologia, UBIMedical, Universidade da Beira Interior, Covilhã, Portugal

Julia Simkus Department of Psychology, Princeton University, Princeton, NJ, USA

Liz Simon Department of Physiology, Comprehensive Alcohol HIV/AIDS Research Center, Louisiana State University Health Sciences Center, New Orleans, LA, USA

Kristiana Siste Department of Psychiatry, Faculty of Medicine, Universitas Indonesia – Dr. Cipto Mangunkusumo General Hospital, Jakarta, Indonesia

Jon Skranes Department of Pediatrics, Sørlandet Hospital Arendal, Arendal, Norway

Department of Clinical and Molecular Medicine, Faculty of Medicine and Health Sciences, Norwegian University of Science and Technology, Trondheim, Norway

Vilde Skylstad Centre for International Health, Department of Global Public Health and Primary Care, Medical Faculty, University of Bergen, Bergen, Norway

Sofia Soares Centro de Investigação em Ciências da Saúde, Laboratório de Fármaco-Toxicologia, UBIMedical, Universidade da Beira Interior, Covilhã, Portugal

Sanjeev Sockalingam Department of Psychiatry, University of Toronto, Centre for Addiction and Mental Health, Toronto, ON, Canada

Jane Brandt Sørensen Global Health Section, Department of Public Health, University of Copenhagen, Copenhagen, Denmark

Nichea S. Spillane PATHS Lab, University of Rhode Island Department of Psychology, Kingston, RI, USA

Andrea E. Steuer Department of Forensic Pharmacology and Toxicology, Zurich Institute of Forensic Medicine, University of Zurich, Zurich, Switzerland

Julian Strizek Kompetenzzentrum Sucht, Austrian Public Health Institute, Vienna, Austria

Mythily Subramaniam Research Division, Institute of Mental Health, Singapore, Singapore

Sharon R. Sznitman School of Public Health, University of Haifa, Faculty of Social Welfare and Health Sciences, Haifa, Israel

Shali Tayebi Global Health Section, Department of Public Health, University of Copenhagen, Copenhagen, Denmark

Maree Teesson The Matilda Centre for Research in Mental Health & Substance Use, The University of Sydney, Camperdown, NSW, Australia

Hiram Tendilla-Beltrán Neuropsychiatry Laboratory, Instituto de Fisiología, Benemérita Universidad Autónoma de Puebla (BUAP), Puebla, Mexico

David Terrero Department of Pharmacology and Experimental Therapeutics, College of Pharmacy & Pharmaceutical Sciences, University of Toledo, Toledo, OH, USA

Nisha Thakur Division of Non-communicable Diseases (NCD), ICMR-National Institute of Research in Tribal Health (NIRTH), Department of Health Research (DHR), Ministry of Health and Family Welfare (Govt. of India), Jabalpur, Madhya Pradesh, India

Natalie Thomas Institute for Social Science Research, University of Queensland, Indooroopilly, Australia

Amit K. Tiwari Department of Pharmacology and Experimental Therapeutics, College of Pharmacy and Pharmaceutical Sciences, University of Toledo College of Pharmacy, Toledo, OH, USA

Center of Medical and Bio-allied Health Sciences Research, Ajman University, Ajman, UAE

Department of Cell and Cancer Biology, College of Medicine and Life Sciences, University of Toledo, Toledo, OH, USA

Rita C. Tostes Department of Pharmacology, Ribeirao Preto Medical School University of Sao Paulo, Ribeirao Preto, Brazil

Marta Trzeciak Aging & Metabolism Research Program, Oklahoma Medical Research Foundation, Oklahoma City, OK, USA

E. Tucker Department of Psychology, Loma Linda University, Loma Linda, CA, USA

Anneli Uusküla Department of Family Medicine and Public Health, University of Tartu, Tartu, Estonia

Pablo K. Valente Department of Behavioral & Social Sciences, School of Public Health, Brown University, Providence, RI, USA

Maarten van den Buuse Department of Psychology and Counselling, School of Psychology and Public Health, La Trobe University, Melbourne, VIC, Australia

Peter van Ruitenbeek Department of Neuropsychology and Psychopharmacology, Faculty of Psychology and Neuroscience, Maastricht University, Maastricht, Netherlands

Romina Vargiu Department of Biomedical Sciences, University of Cagliari, Cagliari, Italy

Luisa Vignozzi Brain Center Firenze, Florence, Italy

Patricia Pia Wadowski Department of Internal Medicine II, Division of Angiology, Medical University of Vienna, Vienna, Austria

Liang-Jen Wang Department of Child and Adolescent Psychiatry, Kaohsiung Chang Gung Memorial Hospital, Kaohsiung City, Taiwan

V. Watts Department of Psychology, Loma Linda University, Loma Linda, CA, USA

Megan Weier Centre for Social Impact, University of New South Wales, Sydney, NSW, Australia

Naomi Weier School of Pharmacy and Pharmacology, University of Tasmania, Hobart, TAS, Australia

R. Frederick Westbrook School of Psychology, UNSW, Kensington, NSW, Australia

Katrina Witt Orygen, Melbourne, VIC, Australia

Centre for Youth Mental Health, The University of Melbourne, Parkville, VIC, Australia

Guangtao Xu Forensic and Pathology Laboratory, Jiaxing University Medical College, Jiaxing, China

Ying Yan The Affiliated Brain Hospital of Guangzhou Medical University, Guangzhou, China

Xiushi Yang Department of Sociology and Criminal Justice, College of Arts and Letters, Old Dominion University, Norfolk, VA, USA

Yimenu Yitayih Department of Psychiatry, Jimma University, Jimma, Ethiopia

Karmen Yoder Department of Radiology and Imaging Sciences, Indiana University School of Medicine, Indianapolis, IN, USA

Muhammad Mobeen Zafar University Institute of Biochemistry and Biotechnology, Pir Mehr Ali Shah Arid Agriculture University Rawalpindi, Rawalpindi, Pakistan

Xiansi Zeng Department of Biochemistry, Jiaxing University Medical College, Jiaxing, China

Minling Zhang The Affiliated Brain Hospital of Guangzhou Medical University, Guangzhou, China

Wenhua Zhou Laboratory of Behavioral Neuroscience, Ningbo Kangning Hospital, School of Medicine, Ningbo University, Ningbo, People's Republic of China

Key Laboratory of Addiction Research of Zhejiang Province, Ningbo, People's Republic of China

School of Medicine, Ningbo University, Ningbo, People's Republic of China

Part V

Alcohol

Fetal Alcohol Spectrum Disorder

44

A Focus on Biology

Jasmine M. Noble and Andrew J. Greenshaw

Contents

Introduction 919
The Epidemiology of FASD 919
Economic Implications of FASD 919
FASD Diagnostic Criteria 919
FASD Diagnostic Systems 920
The Biological Underpinnings of Fetal Alcohol Spectrum Disorder 921
General Neurological Differences Between Children with PAE and Healthy Control 927
Longitudinal and Cross-sectional Analyses of the Neurological Development of Children with PAE at Different Time/Age Intervals 928
The Teratogenic Vulnerability of a Fetus 929
Timing of Exposure 929
Social Determinants of Health and FASD 930
Genetic Predisposition 930
Treatments 931
Identifying and Measuring Prenatal Alcohol Exposure 931
Biomarkers 932
Surveys, Interviews, and Clinical Observations 932
Stigma 933
Applications to Other Areas of Addiction and Mental Health 933
Maternal Alcohol Consumption 933
Comorbidity Between FASD and Other Psychiatric Disorders 934

J. M. Noble (✉)
Department of Computing Science, University of Alberta, Edmonton, Alberta, Canada

Department of Psychiatry, University of Alberta, Edmonton, Alberta, Canada
e-mail: J.M.Noble@ualberta.ca; JMBrown1@ualberta.ca

V. B. Patel, V. R. Preedy (eds.), *Handbook of Substance Misuse and Addictions*,
https://doi.org/10.1007/978-3-030-92392-1_48

Application to Other Areas of Public Health ... 934
Mini-Dictionary of Terms ... 935
Key Facts of Fetal Alcohol Spectrum Disorder ... 936
Summary Points ... 936
Bibliography ... 937

Abstract

Maternal alcohol consumption can lead to a pattern of neurological, behavioral, and physical disabilities, termed fetal alcohol spectrum disorder (FASD). Fetal alcohol syndrome (FAS), the most severe form of FASD, is considered the leading preventable mental disability in Canada and the United States.

This chapter seeks to describe the biological underpinnings of FASD, as well as the predominant tools used to diagnose individuals suffering from the disorder. Following this, we will discuss the public health implications caused by the lack of the standardization of diagnostic tools and their implications on research, clinical practice, and public health.

Keywords

Fetal alcohol spectrum disorder · Fetal alcohol syndrome · Diagnostic guidelines · Diagnosis phenotypes · Biological · Genetic · Neuroimaging

Abbreviations

ADHD	Attention Deficit Hyperactivity Disorder
ARBD	Alcohol-Related Birth Defects
ARND	Alcohol-Related Neurodevelopmental Disorders
CDC	Centers for Disease Control
CNS	Central Nervous System
DSM	Diagnostic and Statistical Manual of Mental Disorders
FAS	Fetal Alcohol Syndrome
FASD	Fetal Alcohol Spectrum Disorder
FDA	US Food and Drug Administrator
ICD	International Classification of Diseases
IOM	Institute of Medicine
IQ	Intelligence Quotient
ND-PAE	Neurodevelopmental Disorder Associated with Prenatal Alcohol Exposure
pFAS	Partial FAS
T-ACE	"Tolerance, Annoyed, Cut down, Eye-opener" Screening Tool
TWEAK	"Tolerance, Worry, Eye-opener, Amnesia, Cut down" Screening Tool
CpGs	Cytosine-Phosphate-Guanines
PAE	Prenatal Alcohol Exposure

Introduction

The Epidemiology of FASD

It has been recognized for more than half a decade by health and public policy experts that prenatal alcohol, more specifically ethanol, exposure is teratogenic, with variable impacts on fetal development, and can lead to a constellation of neurological, behavioral, social, and physical disabilities (Ospina and Dennet 2013; Brown et al. 2019a; b; Jones et al. 1974; Lemoine et al. 1968). These constellations are termed "fetal alcohol spectrum disorder" (FASD). Globally, the prevalence of FASD among children and youth is estimated to be 7.7 per 1000 (Lange et al. 2017). In Canada and the United States, fetal alcohol syndrome (FAS), the most severe subtype of FASD, is considered the leading cause of preventable mental disability with a prevalence estimate of 1.46 per 1000 (Sebastiani et al. 2018; Popova et al. 2017).

Economic Implications of FASD

There is an incremental lifetime economic cost resulting from FASD. Additionally, individuals with FASD often face social issues due to neurobehavioral conditions such as withdrawal from school, family and care placement breakdown, homelessness, unemployment, alcohol and drug misuse, and involvement with the criminal justice system (Streissguth et al. 2004). Inclusive of the indirect (e.g., productivity losses) and direct costs (e.g., health, educational, social, correctional services) of FASD, the incremental fiscal cost per new case was estimated in excess of 800,000 CAD in 2011 (Thanh et al. 2011), now around 1.1M CAD in 2021, adjusting for cumulative price index changes. The total cost of FASD in Canada based on 2015 estimates will be in excess of 10 billion CAD per year in 2021 (Thanh and Jonsson n.d.). On a similar basis in the United States, for 2021, the estimated incremental cost will now be around 2.9 M USD for each individual with FAS (Lupton et al. 2004) (see Greenmyer et al. (2018), for a recent multi-country review (Greenmyer et al. 2018)).

FASD Diagnostic Criteria

The multiple subtypes of FASD can be described, in order of severity, as fetal alcohol syndrome (FAS), partial FAS (pFAS), alcohol-related neurodevelopmental disorder (ARND), and alcohol-related birth defect (ARBD). Another term used when seeking to emphasize only the psychometric measurements that are characteristic of FASD is "neurodevelopmental disorder associated with prenatal alcohol exposure" (ND-PAE). In relation to diagnostic tools, this term was introduced in the Diagnostic and Statistical Manual of Mental Disorders (5th edition). Although FASD is a recognized disorder, no standardized diagnostic tool yet exists for FASD. This is because the teratogenic impact of alcohol on fetal development, although clinical established, needs to be further elucidated from a dose-response perspective for low to moderate alcohol consumption. As such, diagnostic tools vary in terms of specificity for less severe forms of the disorder in terms of criteria, clinical cutoffs, and nomenclature (Campo and Jones 2017) (Stratton 1996) (Chudley et al. 2005) (Kable and Mukherjee 2017). Accepted diagnostic tools include the Institute of Medicine (IOM) criteria for FASD diagnosis; the Centers for Disease Control and Prevention (CDC) FAS: Guidelines for referral and diagnosis; the 4-Digit Diagnostic Code; the Canadian guidelines for diagnosis; the Diagnostic Statistical Manual for Psychiatric Disorders, 5th Edition (DSM-5) (code under "Other Specified Neurodevelopmental Disorder" and proposed criteria as a condition for further study); and ICD-9 and ICD-10 (Cook et al. 2015; Campo and Jones 2017; Stratton 1996; Hoyme et al. 2016; Astley and Clarren 2004; Chudley et al. 2005; Centers for Disease Control and Prevention 2004; World Health Organization 2016; American Psychiatric Association 2013).

Although nomenclature and clinical cutoffs differ between diagnostic tools for less severe forms of FASD, the core features of FAS are commonly described across tools as "...with growth deficiency, with height or weight below the 10th percentile, facial characteristics (e.g., small eyes, smooth philtrum, and thin upper lip), Central Nervous System (CNS) damage (structural, neurological, and/or functional impairment)" (Stratton K, 1996).

Less severe forms of FASD are pFAS, which may include some of the physiological symptoms of FAS, but not the full suite of criteria; ARND which includes symptoms of CNS damage associated with FAS but is absent of facial deformities; and ARBD which includes physical defects, such as malformations of the heart, bone, kidneys, eyes, or ears (Stratton K, 1996).

As noted above, the term neurodevelopmental disorder associated with prenatal alcohol exposure (ND-PAE) was introduced by DSM-5 and seeks to reflect only the psychometrically measured aspects of FASD.

FASD Diagnostic Systems

The recognition of a pattern of symptoms characteristic of FASD was first made by Lemoine (France) in 1964 and 1968, followed by Jones and Smith (United States) in 1973, who are attributed to having coined the term FAS. In light of contention that followed, extensive human and animal research were then conducted to verify the assertions around alcohol as a teratogen. The subsequent findings supported the conclusions identified by Lemoine, and Jones and Smith.

Since 1970, due to the lack of clarity around the detrimental effects of low levels of fetal alcohol exposure, and the lack of existing biomarker to definitively diagnose FASD, multiple diagnostic tools have been developed, and many are used actively to diagnose FASD. Frequently cited tools include the Institute of Medicine (IOM) Criteria for FASD Diagnosis; the CDC FAS: Guidelines for referral and diagnosis;

the 4-Digit Diagnostic Code; and the Canadian guidelines for diagnosis. Although mentioned under "conditions needing further study" in the DSM-5, the criteria noted are believed to be widely used, albeit not yet validated. The lack of a standardized diagnostic tool and discrepancies between existing tools complicate the comparability across research findings conducted within this field.

In the absence of a biomarker, the various diagnostic tools yield disagreement around which specific combination of criteria can most reliably be used to identify a child with FASD. This disagreement becomes more pronounced in consideration of less severe forms of the disorder. More specifically, there are significant differences in how neurobehavioral deficits and physical features of FASD are defined by each tool (Coles et al. 2016).

Additional areas of incongruity exist around the use of facial deformities characteristic of FASD in its diagnosis and confirmation of maternal alcohol consumption and/or estimated concentration of prenatal exposure to alcohol. Some diagnostic tools, like the DSM-5, emphasize the need to measure only neurocognitive impairments, while others like the IOM, 4-Digit Diagnostic Code, the Canadian guidelines, and the CDC guidelines consider physical features of FASD. The DSM-5 arguably chooses not to measure physical deformations in reflection of the complexities of defining what is "normal" in terms of physical measurement among diverse population groups (Coles et al. 2016). Of the tools that use physical features, some only require the identification of two, while others require three, facial features (Coles et al. 2016). The DSM-5 requires the need to document maternal alcohol consumption for diagnosis, while others like the IOM do not (Coles et al. 2016). For an overview of existing frequently cited diagnostic tools, as well as their differences, please see Table 1.

Regardless of which diagnostic tool is under consideration, FASD has been long accepted as a clinical disorder, and damage to the CNS is recognized across diagnostic platforms and linked to all subtypes (Campo and Jones 2017; Chudley et al. 2005). Nevertheless, the lack of standardization of diagnostic tools and terms used within the field of FASD has increased discordance and variability in research, clinical ambiguity in practice, and inconsistent government messaging in the public domain.

The Biological Underpinnings of Fetal Alcohol Spectrum Disorder

Although the recognition for FASD has had a contentious history prior to 1970, it has now been recognized medically as a clinical disorder for more than 50 years (Brown et al. 2019a,b; Lemoine et al. 1968; Jones and Smith 1973). As noted, damage to the CNS is characteristic of all subtypes of FASD and reflected in all diagnostic tools (Campo and Jones 2017; Chudley et al. 2005; Brown et al. 2019a,b). As children are exposed to alcohol during prenatal stage, this damage can manifest in a variety of ways, such as reduced IQ and executive functioning, difficulties maintaining attention, hyperactivity, impulsivity, emotional dysregulation, sleep problems, disruptive behavior, and mood problems that lead to difficulties with learning, memory, and social communication (O'Connor and Paley 2009; Mattson et al. 2019; Lees et al. 2020; Cook et al. 2015; Riley and McGee 2005; Glass et al. 2014). These deficits can also manifest

Table 1 Summary and comparison of the various diagnostic schemas for prenatal alcohol-related disorders

	4-Digit Code[5]	Revised IOM[6]	Canadian[7]	CDC Task Force on FAS/FAE[8]	DSM-5[9]
Fetal alcohol syndrome (FAS)					
Facial characteristics	Simultaneous presentation of short palpebral fissures (≤ 2 SDs), thin vermillion border, smooth philtrum	Two of the following: short palpebral fissures (≤10th percentile), thin vermillion border, smooth philtrum	Simultaneous presentation of short palpebral fissures (≤ 2 SDs), thin vermillion border, smooth philtrum	Simultaneous presentation of short palpebral fissures (≤10th percentile), thin vermillion border, smooth philtrum	
Growth retardation	Height or weight ≤10th percentile	Height or weight ≤10th percentile	Height or weight or disproportionately low weight-to-height ratio (≤10th percentile)	Height or weight ≤ 10th percentile	
Central nervous system (CNS) involvement	Head circumference (occipital-frontal circumference [OFC]) ≥ 2 SDs below norm or significant abnormalities in brain structure or evidence of hard neurological findings or significant impairment in three or more domains of brain function (≥2 SDs below the mean) as assessed by validated and standardized tools	Head circumference (OFC) ≤10th percentile or structural brain abnormality	Evidence of three or more impairments in the following CNS domains: hard and soft neurologic signs; brain structure; cognition; communication; academic achievement; memory; executive functioning and abstract reasoning; attention deficit/hyperactivity; adaptive behavior, social skills, social communication	Head circumference (OFC) ≤10th percentile or structural brain abnormality or neurological problems or other soft neurological signs outside normal limits or functional impairment as evidenced by global cognitive or intellectual deficits, below the 3rd percentile (2 SDs) below the mean or functional deficits below the 16th percentile (1 SD) below the mean in at least three domains: cognitive or	

				developmental markers, executive functioning, motor, social skills, attention/hyperactivity, and others (i.e., sensory, memory, language)	
Alcohol exposure	Confirmed or not confirmed	Confirmed or not confirmed	Confirmed or not confirmed	Confirmed or not confirmed	
Partial FAS					
Facial characteristics	Short palpebral fissures (≤2 SDs) and either a smooth philtrum or thin vermillion border, with the other being normal OR palpebral fissure (≤1 SD) and both a smooth philtrum and thin vermillion	Two or more of the following: short palpebral fissures (≤10th percentile), thin vermillion border, smooth philtrum	Two or more of the following: short palpebral fissures, thin vermillion border, smooth philtrum	Not applicable	
Growth retardation	Not required	Either height or weight ≤10th percentile OR (see CNS involvement)	Not required	Not applicable	
Central nervous system (CNS) involvement	Same as for FAS	Head circumference ≤10th percentile or structural brain abnormality or behavioral and cognitive abnormalities inconsistent with developmental level	Same as for FAS	Not applicable	

(continued)

Table 1 (continued)

	4-Digit Code[5]	Revised IOM[6]	Canadian[7]	CDC Task Force on FAS/FAE[8]	DSM-5[9]
Alcohol exposure	Confirmed	Confirmed or not confirmed	Confirmed	Felt that there was insufficient data to provide guidance for this diagnosis. Formed group to discuss	
Alcohol-related neurodevelopmental disorder (ARND)					
	Does not propose this diagnostic category but rather has several categories assessing functional deficits			Not applicable	
Central nervous system involvement	Same as for FAS	Either (1) structural brain anomaly or OFC ≤10th percentile or 2) evidence of a complex pattern of behavioral or cognitive abnormalities inconsistent with developmental level that cannot be explained by genetics, family background, or environment alone	Same as for FAS	Not applicable	

Alcohol exposure	Confirmed	Confirmed	Confirmed	Not applicable	
Neurodevelopmental disorder associated with prenatal alcohol exposure					
Central nervous system involvement	Only the DSM-5 uses the term "neurodevelopmental disorder associated with prenatal alcohol exposure"				Evidence of impaired neurocognitive functioning (≥ 1), self-regulation (≥ 1), adaptive functioning (≥ 2)
Alcohol exposure					Confirmed
Other					Onset in childhood; clinically significant distress or impairment
Notes	The 4-Digit Code provides an assessment of effects in four areas (growth, face, CNS, and alcohol exposure) that results in 256 different codes and 22 diagnostic categories. A specific pattern or level of alcohol exposure is not required, just that alcohol exposure is confirmed or not	Alcohol exposure is defined as a pattern of excessive intake or heavy episodic drinking Other behavioral characteristics are assessed, but it is unclear how they fit into the diagnosis for FAS	Alcohol exposure is defined as a pattern of excessive intake or heavy episodic drinkingA domain is considered "impaired" when on a standardized measure: scores are $\geq$ 2 SDs below the mean, or there is a discrepancy of at least 1 SD between subdomains or there is a discrepancy of at least 1.5–2 SD among subtests on a measure	Alcohol exposure levels are not defined, but the authors cite evidence of alcohol exposure based upon clinical observation; self-report; reports of heavy alcohol use during pregnancy by a reliable informant; medical records documenting positive blood alcohol levels or alcohol treatment; or other social, legal, or medical problems related to drinking during pregnancy	Although alcohol exposure levels are not defined, this tool notes confirmation of "more than minimal exposure" through self-report or medical or other records, or clinical observation are required for diagnosis. They define low levels of alcohol consumption to be "1–13 drinks per month during pregnancy with no more than 2 of these drinks consumed on any 1 drinking occasion"

(continued)

Table 1 (continued)

	4-Digit Code[5]	Revised IOM[6]	Canadian[7]	CDC Task Force on FAS/FAE[8]	DSM-5[9]

1. All of the diagnostic schemes assume that genetic or medical causes have been ruled out and that appropriate norms are used when available
2. All of the diagnostic schemes use the University of Washington Lip-Philtrum Guide (http://depts.washington.edu/fasdpn/htmls/lip-philtrum-guides.htm)
3. For palpebral fissure norms, the 4-Digit Code utilizes Hall et al.'s (1989) study, Hoyme utilizes Thomas et al.'s (1987) study, and Chudley provides both the Thomas and Hall charts; the National Task Force guidelines do not mention which chart to use. Hall recently wrote that her charts underrepresented normal palpebral fissure length (Hall 2010) and should be replaced by those from Clarren et al. (2010)
4. Note that < 2 SD $= 2.3$rd percentile in a normal distribution
5. Astley and Clarren 2000
6. Hoyme et al. 2005
7. Chudley et al. 2005
8. Bertrand et al. 2004
9. DSM-5

Adapted from Riley EP, Infante, MA, Warren, KR, Fetal Alcohol Spectrum Disorders: An Overview, Neuropsychol Rev, 2011, 21:73–80 (original), and Warren, KR, Hewitt, BG, Thomas, JD, Fetal Alcohol Spectrum Disorders: Research challenges and opportunities, Alcohol Res Health, 2011, 34(1): 4–14 (modified original)

physically, such as tremors, weak grasp, poor hand-eye coordination, and challenges with balance (Riley and McGee 2005). The prevalence of epilepsy is also higher for children with FASD (5.9%) than for the general population (1%) (Bell et al. 2010).

Both animal and human research can be used to describe the way in which alcohol works as a teratogen. We will begin with the exploration of these mechanisms at a cellular level via animal studies, following which we will review longitudinal, neuroimaging studies in order to describe the overall altered trajectory of brain development in children with FASD.

Laboratory animal studies have contributed greatly to our understanding of the biological, cellular underpinnings of prenatal exposure to alcohol (Goodlett et al. 2005; Driscoll et al. 1990; Patten and Fontaine 2003; Barron et al. 2016). This research reveals that alcohol may affect several neurological mechanisms and structures within the brain, including neuronal function and degradation, and genetic alteration, leading to structural and functional neural impairment. With regard to cellular function and neurodegenerative effects, alcohol may disrupt calcium signaling pathways and glutamate receptor function (Kumada et al. 2007; Hughes et al. 1998). The resulting increased oxidative stress leads to apoptotic neurodegeneration (Goodlett et al. 2005; Ikonomidou et al. 2001). Epigenetic alterations may also occur, including changes in DNA methylation patterns: these include "histone modifications, enrichment of histone acetylation and methylation, and increased expression of histone acetyltransferases and methyltransferases" (Coles et al. 2016; Laufer et al. 2016; Chater-Diehl et al. 2017; Jarmasz et al. 2019). These changes ultimately impact neuronal structure, impairing healthy neuronal proliferation and neuronal migration during brain development (Goodlett et al. 2005; Miller 1986) leading to widespread neuronal malformations and altered neurodevelopmental trajectories. In this context, changes in whole genome methylation and cytosine-phosphate-guanines (CpGs) have been found for numerous genes and buccal cells have exhibited differential methylation in babies with prenatal alcohol exposure (PAE) (Laufer et al. 2015; Portales-Casamar et al. 2016). One neurodevelopmental region that may be particularly vulnerable to insult is the midline tissues of the neural tube during prenatal development, which, if exposed to alcohol during the embryogenesis of early pregnancy, may underlie the cluster of abnormalities observed in the medial brain region of children with FASD (Beaulieu et al. 2014; Riley and McGee 2005; Beaulieu et al. 2013; Meintjes et al. 2014).

General Neurological Differences Between Children with PAE and Healthy Control

Children with FAS are at higher risk of microcephaly and structural anomalies in the cerebellum, brainstem, basal ganglia, and corpus callosum (Jones and Smith 1973; Clarren 1986; Mattson and Riley 1996). More specifically, children with FASD tend to have reductions in total gray matter volume globally, as well as in the hippocampus, thalamus, and globus pallidus (Sowell et al. 2001; Nardelli et al. 2011). Gray matter density however may be higher in areas such as the temporal and parietal cortices (Sowell et al. 2001; Sowell et al. 2002). Cortical thickness is higher in the frontal, parietal, and temporal lobes of children with FASD, and dysmorphic and cognitive features of FAS correlate with variances in the left inferior frontal and right superior and middle temporal cortices (Sowell et al. 2008; Fernandez-Jaen et al. 2011; Yang et al. 2012).

There is less white matter volume in frontal, parietal, and temporal lobes and less neuronal density in the posterior temporoparietal cortex for children with FASD (Bjorkquist et al. 2010; Fennema-Notestine et al. 2001; Sowell et al. 2002; Astley et al. 2009; Sowell et al. 2001; Riikonen et al. 1999). There may also be decreases in the occipital horns and parieto-occipital regions; however, further research is warranted (Riikonen et al. 1999).

Longitudinal and Cross-sectional Analyses of the Neurological Development of Children with PAE at Different Time/Age Intervals

Longitudinal studies of children with FASD in comparison with children who have not been exposed to alcohol during pregnancy suggest alterations in brain development revealed through neuroimaging studies in both gray and white matter structure. Additionally, there are brain activation differences, that is, in children with healthy development, we typically observe increases in functional MRI signal intensity over time. For children with FASD, the opposite pattern is observed, with decreases in functional MRI signal intensity. Neuronal recruitment patterns between groups are also different (Gautam et al. 2015).

Whereas gray matter development in healthy children follows an inverted “U” pattern, likely reflecting the proliferation of connective tissue, followed by synaptic pruning and refinement, brain development in children with FASD follows a linear and downward trajectory (Lenroot et al. 2007) (Giedd et al. 1999). Additionally, whereas the decrease in gray matter associated with these developmental changes in childhood in healthy brains often correlates with increased IQ, the opposite is true for children with FASD, where decreases in gray matter are associated with decreases in IQ (Shaw et al. 2006; Sowell et al. 2004; Beaulieu et al. 2014). In white matter, brain diffusivity, likely reflecting neural refinement and axonal myelination, is observed earlier in the developmental patterns of healthy children than for those with FASD, suggesting that these mechanisms are delayed (Beaulieu et al. 2013).

Although research is limited on the deviations from typical brain maturation following childhood and adolescence (i.e., from adolescence through to adulthood) in individuals with FASD, a recent cross-sectional study of 13–30-year-olds with FASD in comparison to healthy controls observed that various sub-regions of the brain (corpus callosum, caudate, and cerebellum) in adolescents with FASD, albeit delayed, increased in volume to match healthy controls, but followed with a premature decline in young adulthood. This premature decline in early adulthood is observed in other populations as well, such as those exposed to childhood maltreatment and children with Down’s syndrome (trisomy 21) (Inkelis et al. 2020). With FASD, the putamen and pallidum, although lower in volume compared to controls, followed a normal developmental trajectory in growth patterns (Inkelis et al. 2020). For that study, generally greater shape variability in the shape of sub-regions was also observed, which in theory could cause differences in neurobehavioral function. Important limitation to note is that the study was cross-sectional, which increases the possible influence of confounding variables such as environmental differences (e.g., maternal nutrition, childhood trauma, etc.) or changing public sentiment or awareness around the detrimental effects of drinking during pregnancy (Inkelis et al. 2020).

The Teratogenic Vulnerability of a Fetus

There are numerous factors which increase or reduce the level of fetal vulnerability to PAE including the amount, timing, type, and pattern of exposure in utero, social determinants of health, and genetic predisposition (Riley and McGee 2005).

Timing of Exposure

Using animal models, researchers have been able to explore what detrimental effects alcohol exposure has on a fetus at various points of prenatal development. Within the first trimester, damage may occur to neuronal migration, proliferation, and organization and can manifest as severe craniofacial malformations (e.g., cleft lip, smooth philtrum) as a result of midline tissue vulnerability (as described above) (Cook et al. 1990; Miller 1993; Miller 1996; Kotch and Sulik 1992). Additionally, exposure in the first and second trimesters may trigger alterations in neural tube midline tissue perforation, decreased neurogenesis, and delays in the differentiation in serotonergic neurons and closure of the ventral canal, which is associated with neurological abnormalities such as microencephaly, ventricular enlargement, and cortical thinning (Goodlett et al. 2005). In the third trimester, global brain structures are believed to be at risk for insult, including the hippocampus, cerebellum, and prefrontal cortex (Coles et al. 1991; Livy et al. 2003; Sutherland et al. 1997; West and Pierce 1986). Additionally, vulnerability may increase for specific structures temporarily based on gestational day. For example, in mouse studies, postnatal day 7 is associated with the activation of the "executioner" protease caspase-3 in cortical neurons, which is activated during neuronal cell death via apoptosis (Goodlett et al. 2005).

The lack of a dose-response relationship connecting maternal alcohol consumption to FASD or FAS is a major limitation in our understanding in this field. Although it is very clear that high levels of drinking, whether acute exposure or in the context of binge drinking, convey high risk, even low dose exposures may be sufficient to result in teratogenic consequences of drinking (Hamilton et al. 2014; Day et al. 2013).

Nevertheless, the status of the pregnant mother during alcohol consumption is a relevant determinant of risk, likely affecting the functional dose of alcohol consumed. These factors include poor maternal nutrition, multiparous pregnancy status, smaller physical stature and BMI, older age during pregnancy, and family history of heavy drinking/drinkers. From a simple perspective, these factors relate to risk of alcohol misuse, tolerance of the mother to alcohol (relating to pharmacodynamic profile in relation to alcohol dehydrogenase levels), and health in terms of availability of nutrients that may be somewhat protective for the fetal environment, with a focus on choline and multivitamin supplements (Erng et al. 2020).

Social Determinants of Health and FASD

The social determinant of the constellation of disorders resulting from prenatal exposure to alcohol, here we refer to FASD for a singular label, is one consequence of a general set of problems that connect biological and social determinants of health as a basis for responses to adversity (May 1995; May and Gossage 2011; Singal et al. 2017). A recent systematic review of factors related to alcohol use in pregnancy has provided a useful conceptual framework (Lyall et al. 2021).

Applying a qualitative lens, these authors identified five themes of particular interest.

These are (i) "social relationships and norms," (ii) "stigma," (iii) "trauma and other stressors," (iv) "alcohol information and messaging," and (v) "access to trusted equitable care and essential resources."

It is of interest that these themes overlap with factors that are not only relevant for substance misuse but various aspects of psychopathology. Since this chapter has a main focus on biological underpinnings in the context of FASD, we want to point out simply that there is an increasingly rich literature on trauma-informed care that includes a consideration of neurodevelopmental challenges due to adverse childhood experience as a key determinant of psychopathology, including substance misuse (Alvanzo et al. 2020). Alcohol misuse is a difficult to treat condition in many cases, and its consequences include disruption of social relationships, experience of stigma, and limitations in access to equitable care and essential resources. In the longer term or intense consumption cases, there are significant adverse effects on brain structure and function associated with limitations in cognitive decisions and emotional regulation (Carbia et al. 2021) (Carbia et al. 2021).

Genetic Predisposition

The genetic dysregulation that is consequent to prenatal exposure to alcohol includes epigenetic disruption. This combination of alteration of gene expression through modification of the structure of chromatin and metabolic disruption through cellular oxidative stress has major impacts on the developing fetus. There is also the development of key HPA axis changes that will alter normally adaptive responses to stress – a pattern that will extend to adulthood and parallels effects of other adverse experiences postnatally and is highly relevant to the psychiatric comorbidities seen in FASD patients (Ciafrè et al. 2020).

As we know, both genetic and environmental factors determine the outcome of the FASD developmental trajectory, and genetic and epigenetic cascades of interaction result in many different individual phenotypes within the FASD categories for individual patients. As with many other areas of medicine, greater knowledge of the underlying biological determinants of FASD may yield the promise of prevention strategies (other than abstinence – which although the simplest strategy is clearly not yet effective) (Kaminen-Ahola 2020). Some recent studies are pointing to potential genetic biomarkers that may signal specific FASD phenotypes, as in the case of genes involved in N-glycosylation (de la Morena-Barrio et al. 2018) (de la Morena-Barrio et al. 2018). Nevertheless, given the complexity of the scientific problem, a precise health approach is likely necessary – with implementation of large datasets and application of machine learning algorithms (Zhang et al. 2019; Lussier et al. 2018; Fang et al. 2008) (Zhang et al. 2019; Lussier et al. 2018; Fang et al. 2008).

Treatments

As a result of the complicated neurological developmental restructuring of circuitry and the complexity of presentation of this spectrum disorder (elaborated upon below), there are no standardized approaches to treatment. Personalized care programming is often warranted, where a suite of psychopharmacological treatments is considered alongside behavioral and educational interventions (Ritfeld et al. 2021).

Identifying and Measuring Prenatal Alcohol Exposure

Early identification and intervention have been found to improve health outcomes for individuals with FASD (Streissguth et al. 1997). A solution to resolve issues with diagnostic discrepancies lies in our ability to measure biomarkers, in order to definitively diagnose individuals with FASD and/or accurately measure the dose-response relationship between alcohol and CNS damage from mild to moderate alcohol consumption, which would allow for early identification and care of individuals with FASD, as well as for the standardization of a singular diagnostic tool for FASD for use by the medical and academic community for research and clinical practice.

Nevertheless, there are a variety of ways in which prenatal alcohol exposure is measured. One method of measurement is via biomarkers such as newborn blood, urine, hair, and meconium or through the mother's blood, sweat, saliva, hair, and placenta (Caprara et al. 2007; McQuire et al. 2016). A second approach is through maternal surveys and interviews, as well as clinical observations and medical records (Caprara et al. 2007; McQuire et al. 2016). Most, except for T-ACE and TWEAK questionnaires, are considered to lack sufficient evidence to support their use. As such, some researchers advocate for the use of a multimethod approach in measuring

PAE, including a combination of questionnaires and/or self-reporting and biomarker testing (Montag 2016) (Lange et al. 2014).

Biomarkers

Existing biomarkers currently have limited evidence to support their use in clinical and research settings (McQuire et al. 2016), as they are considered cumbersome, require repeated application, and to date have been found to provide limited information about alcohol consumption (Montag 2016; McQuire et al. 2016). In addition to the recent status of potential genetic and epigenetic biomarkers outlined earlier (Kaminen-Ahola 2020), recent systematic review in this area has indicated a significant body of data that may provide further insight from the metabolic biomarker perspective (Ehrhart et al. 2019). Taking the long view and considering advances that are now evident from a "big data" perspective, we agree with Erhart and colleagues that data-driven analysis, in our view likely applying machine learning techniques, has potential for identifying accessible cellular FASD biomarkers for early identification and assessment of projected severity, which may point to drug targets for intervention.

The pioneering work of Lebel and colleagues (Lebel et al. 2011) has been highly impactful in relation to our thinking about biomarkers – using the power of modern neuroimaging. This team provided an unprecedented window on how the teratogenic consequences of maternal ethanol exposure result in rewiring of neural pathways in developing brains using diffusion tensor imaging. Their recent work has described differences between prenatally alcohol exposed children and controls using functional MRI (Long et al. 2019). The value of this type of neuroimaging work overall is twofold. From a scientific perspective, this group and several others are demonstrating clear associations of observable brain circuit changes with neuropsychological deficits in children with prenatal alcohol exposure. Such studies are also exploiting machine learning techniques to use neuroimaging data toward clinical prognostic value (Rodriguez et al. 2021) (Rodriguez et al. 2021). From a knowledge dissemination point of view, neuroimaging results are a high impact stimulus for informing the public about the actual impact of alcohol on the brain in utero: given the persistence of drinking during pregnancy, this has potential for application in preventative public health communications.

Surveys, Interviews, and Clinical Observations

There is limited evidence to support the use of surveys, interviews, and clinical observations in attempting to measure PAE. First, existing survey tools are not able to capture all at-risk women, nor do they provide a descriptive account of maternal alcohol consumption and PAE (e.g., frequency, concentration, and/or developmental stage of exposure). This is believed to be due in part to underreporting and/or recall bias (Czeizel et al. 2004), as well as an apprehension by women to participate in surveys and/or interviews due to stigma (see below). Additionally, how questions are posed, the environment for which the interviews/surveys take place, and how questions are structured may influence the validity of responses (Midanik 1988). Of note, however, is that the T-ACE and TWEAK questionnaires, which have similar sensitivities and specificities, have been found to be efficient screening tools for maternal consumption of alcohol (Burns et al. 2010; British Medical Association Report 2007).

Stigma

Largely attributed to the significant stigma surrounding alcohol use during pregnancy, women may avoid disclosing accurate information about their drinking and/or avoid situations, such as participating in research, where their alcohol consumption is measured. Research examining this population group suggest that hesitancies may be due to fears of negative stereotyping, over-identification of marginalized populations, embarrassment, guilt, a perceived lack of benefit of FAS diagnosis and confirmation of PAE, and fear of reprisals such as child apprehension (Zadunayski et al. 2006; Zelner et al. 2012; Zelner et al. 2012; Zizzo et al. 2013). This is further elaborated upon in the below subsection.

Applications to Other Areas of Addiction and Mental Health

Maternal Alcohol Consumption

FASD is a completely preventable mental disorder. Nevertheless, alcohol use during pregnancy continues to occur. This may be attributed to several challenging considerations including negative maternal environmental factors leading mothers to problematic alcohol use (including experiencing trauma, violence, poverty, and stigma), general social acceptability of widespread alcohol consumption, and inconsistent public messaging around alcohol use during pregnancy since it was clinically recognized in the 1970s. The global prevalence of maternal alcohol use is believed to be approximately 9.8% among the general public (Popova et al. 2017). When biomarkers are used to assess maternal alcohol use (such as neonatal meconium or maternal hair), that estimate increases to 45% (Chiandetti et al. 2017; Lange et al. 2014). Women with higher rates of alcohol consumption, such as those suffering from alcohol use disorder (AUD) are at greater risk of having a baby with FASD. The prevalence of AUD among women who have given birth to a child with FASD is estimated to be as high as 771 per 1000 (Huebert and Raftis 1996). Therefore, pregnancy offers an opportunity for intervention and window for change and therefore is often targeted in prevention interventions for FASD.

There is, however, significant stigma around maternal alcoholism, and women often struggle to find support they need and/or face barriers to care. Women may lack support from partners and family members while juggling existing caregiving responsibilities (Poole and Isaac 2001). Fears around child apprehension, stereotyping, and shame may also reduce help-seeking (Montag 2016; Lange et al. 2014; Brown et al. 2019a,b; Midanik 1988). Additionally, the prevalence of individuals with problematic substance use who choose not to seek help generally (pregnant or not) is high (Room et al. 1989). Women are also believed to be underrepresented for prevalence of risky drinking as men are often flagged for engaging in problematic alcohol use more frequently than women (Dawson and Dadheich 1992). This topic will be further elaborated upon in Popova's chapter here.

Comorbidity Between FASD and Other Psychiatric Disorders

FASD often presents with other psychiatric disorders (Weyrauch et al. 2017; Lange et al. 2018). Evidence suggests that children with PAE are more likely to be diagnosed with higher rates of ADHD, oppositional defiant disorder, depressive disorder, and anxiety disorder (Glass et al. 2014; Ritfeld et al. 2021). One study examining the rate of attention deficit hyperactivity disorder (ADHD) reported a diagnosis rate of 95% among a PAE group, versus only 30% in a non-PAE group (Fryer et al. 2007), highlighting the weight of the prevalence of this comorbidity. Comorbidity can complicate treatment as pharmaceuticals interact differently with an individual with FASD than other disorders due to the tissue and functional neurological differences resulting from PAE. For example, although stimulant use, as well as selective norepinephrine reuptake inhibitors and alpha-2 agonists, used in the treatment of idiopathic ADHD are considered effective options, evidence to support their use for FASD is limited, mixed, or even controversial (Ritfeld et al. 2021). Equally, analysis on the effectiveness of selective serotonin reuptake inhibitors for use in FASD to treat depressive and anxiety related disorders, and antipsychotics such as risperidone for emotional outbursts, is limited (Schneider et al. 2005; Riikonen et al. 2005). Research in the determination of appropriate treatment is complicated as a result of difficulty of reproducing the neurobehavioral symptoms in mouse models that include some of the underpinnings of neurological circuitry to mimic executive functional differences associated with FASD (Ritfeld et al. 2021). Not surprising, and very much part of the negative cycle of causality in the FASD story, is the association of FAS and FASD with increased risk of substance misuse. Suffice it to say that there are genetic, epigenetic, and environmental components to this association, many aspects of which resonate with the constellation of features of FASD and what we understand about the antecedents of substance misuse (Popova et al. 2021).

Application to Other Areas of Public Health

Although FAS and FASD have been recognized by scientific and medical communities as clinical disorders since the 1970s, it was arguably socially documented or observed by various groups for hundreds of years. Regardless, incidence rates remain high. This is undoubtedly the result of general social acceptability and popularity of widespread alcohol consumption and inconsistent public messaging around alcohol use during pregnancy (Brown et al. 2019a,b), supported further by ambiguity regarding alcohol's dose-response relationship with fetal development. It is sobering that there was a UK governmental backlash when Professor David Nutt and colleagues in the UK published an, now highly publicized, article in *The Lancet* indicating that alcohol is the substance of abuse associated with the greatest harm in society at large (Nutt et al. 2010), a result echoed for Europe in 2015 (van Amsterdam et al. 2015) (van Amsterdam et al. 2015) and Australia in 2019 (Bonomo et al. 2019).

Government messaging in Canada and the United States currently recommend no alcohol consumption during pregnancy (Butt et al. 2011; Centers for Disease Control and Prevention 2021). However, it took 4 years following recognition for the American FDA to release their first public health warning on alcohol during pregnancy, recommending at the time that two to a maximum of six drinks a day was safe for pregnant women to consume (Warren 2015). This advisory at the time was endorsed by various professional bodies, including the American Academy of Pediatrics, the American Medical Association, and the American Congress of Obstetricians and Gynecologists (Warren 2015).

When consideration is given to the social acceptability and popularity of alcohol use among the general public, and in reflection that most pregnancies are unplanned (Finer and Zolna 2011) and women often do not know they are pregnant until 4–6 weeks after conception (Floyd et al. 1999), the true maternal alcohol consumption rate may be much higher than current estimates. For example, in a cross-sectional survey, almost half of women surveyed reported consuming alcohol in the 3 months before they discovered they were pregnant. The majority of these women surveyed (60%) did not discover they were pregnant until after the fourth week of gestation, suggesting that they may have consumed alcohol during those weeks prior (Floyd et al. 1999).

Mini-Dictionary of Terms

Fetal alcohol spectrum disorder (FASD): A term used to describe a constellation of physical, cognitive, and behavioral ailments associated with prenatal alcohol exposure.

Fetal alcohol syndrome: FAS is the most severe form of FASD. It is typically described as presenting with facial deformities, growth retardation, and central nervous system damage.

Neurodevelopmental disorder associated with prenatal alcohol exposure: A diagnostic term used in DSM-5, which includes only the psychometric measurements of FASD.

Partial FAS: How pFAS is defined differs between diagnostic tools, but generally it presents with most, but not all, of the diagnostic characteristics of FAS. Confirmation of maternal alcohol consumption is a required criterion by some tools.

Alcohol-related neurodevelopmental disorders: ARND presents with CNS-related symptoms but does not include facial deformities that are characteristic of more severe forms of FASD like FAS. Confirmation of material alcohol consumption is required.

Alcohol-related birth defects: ARBD includes physical defects, such as malformations of the heart, bone, kidney, eyes, or ears. Confirmation of material alcohol consumption is required.

Key Facts of Fetal Alcohol Spectrum Disorder

The prevalence rate for FASD among children and youth is estimated to be 7.7 per 1000.

The prevalence rate for FAS, the most severe subset of FASD, among the general public is estimated to be 1.46 per 1000.

The incremental cost per new case of FASD in Canada and the United States in 2021, inclusive of indirect and direct costs, is believed to be approximately $1.1M and $2.9M respectively.

Neurological damage may include volume and structural anomalies in both white and gray matter.

CNS damage can manifest through reduced IQ, executive functioning, difficulties maintaining attention, hyperactivity, impulsivity, emotional dysregulation, sleep problems, disruptive behavior, and mood problems that lead to difficulties with learning, memory, and social communication.

Physical manifestations include tremors, seizures, weak grasp, poor hand-eye coordination, and challenges with balance.

Fetal vulnerability to alcohol exposure may be influenced by factors such as the amount, timing, type, and pattern of exposure in utero, social determinants of health, and genetic predisposition.

Currently, researchers and clinicians use biomarkers such as newborn blood, urine, hair and meconium, maternal blood, sweat, saliva, hair, and placenta, and/or maternal surveys and interviews, as well as clinical observations and medical records, to assess timing and level of PAE. These tools, however, are largely considered unreliable as they require repeated application, may be cumbersome, and are subject to recall bias (in the case of interviews and questionnaires).

Summary Points

Fetal alcohol spectrum disorder (FASD) is a leading, preventable mental disorder, caused by maternal alcohol consumption.

Alcohol is teratogenic, and the consumption of alcohol during pregnancy can negatively impact fetal development, which presents as various neurological, behavioral, social, and physical disabilities.

There are a variety of subsets of FASD including fetal alcohol syndrome (FAS), partial FAS (pFAS), alcohol-related neurodevelopmental disorder (ARND), alcohol-related birth defect (ARBD). The term neurodevelopmental disorder associated with prenatal alcohol exposure (ND-PAE), emphasizing the psychometric measurements of FASD, may also be used.

Alterations in the trajectory of brain development, as well as structural anomalies in gray and white matter, have been observed in children with FASD.

There are multiple factors which may play a role in increasing or reducing the level of fetal vulnerability to prenatal alcohol exposure, including the amount, timing, type, and pattern of exposure in utero, social determinants of health, and genetic predisposition.

No standardized diagnostic tool exists for FASD.

Existing tools differ mostly in terms of less severe forms of FASD, which lead to negative implications on research, clinical practice, and public health.

Identifying a reliable biomarker may support early identification and intervention, which may help improve health outcomes for individuals with FASD.

Bibliography

Alvanzo A et al (2020) Adverse childhood experiences (ACEs) and transitions in stages of alcohol involvement among US adults: progression and regression. *Child Abuse Negl* 107:104624

American Psychiatric Association (2013) *Diagnostic and statistical manual of mental disorders*, 5th edn. APA, Arlington

Astley SJ, Clarren SK (2000) Diagnosing the full spectrum of fetal alcohol-exposed individuals: introducing the 4-digit diagnostic code. *Alcohol Alcohol* 35(4):400–410

Astley S, Aylward E, Carmichael Olson H et al (2009) Magnetic resonance imaging outcomes from a comprehensive magnetic resonance study of children with fetal alcohol spectrum disorders. Alcohol Clin Exp Res 33:1671–1689

Astley S, Clarren S (2004) *Diagnostic guide for fetal alcohol syndrome and related conditions: the 4-digit diagnostic code*, 3rd edn. University of Washington, Seattle

Barron S, Hawkey A, Fields L, Littleton JM (2016) Animal models for medication development and application to treat fetal alcohol effects. In: *International review of neurobiology: animal models for medications screening to treat addiction*. Academic Press, Cambridge, pp 423–440

Beaulieu C, Lebel C, Treit S et al (2013) Longitudinal MRI reveals altered trajectory of brain development during childhood and adolescence in fetal alcohol spectrum disorders. *J Neurosci* 33(24):10098–10109

Beaulieu C, Lebel C, Treit S et al (2014) Longitudinal MRI reveals impaired cortical thinning in children and adolescents prenatally exposed to alcohol. *Hum Brain Mapp* 35(9):4892–4903

Bell S, Stade B, Reynolds J et al (2010) The remarkably high prevalence of epilepsy and seizure history in fetal alcohol spectrum disorders. *Alcohol Clin Exp Res* 34:1084–1089

Bertrand J, Floyd RL, Weber MK et al (2004) *Fetal alcohol syndrome: guidelines for referral and diagnosis*. Centers for Disease Control and Prevention (CDC), Atlanta, GA. National Task Force on Fetal Alcohol Syndrome and Fetal Alcohol Effect

Bjorkquist O, Fryer S, Reiss A et al (2010) Cingulate gyrus morphology in children and adolescents with fetal alcohol spectrum disorders. *Psychiatry Res Neuroimaging* 181:101–107

Bonomo Y et al (2019) The Australian drug harms ranking study. *J Psychopharmacol* 33(7):759–768

British Medical Association Report (2007) *Alcohol and pregnancy: preventing and managing fetal alcohol spectrum disorders*. BMA, London

Brown J, Bland R, Jonsson E, Greenshaw A (2019a) A brief history of awareness of the link between alcohol and fetal alcohol spectrum disorder. *Can J Psychiatry* 64(3):164–168
Brown J, Bland R, Jonsson E, Greenshaw A (2019b) The standardization of diagnostic criteria for fetal alcohol spectrum disorder (FASD): implications for research, clinical practice and population health. *Can J Psychiatr* 64(3):169–176
Burns E, Gray R, Smith L (2010) Brief screening questionnaires to identify problem drinking during pregnancy: a systematic review. *Addiction* 105(4):601–614
Butt P, Beirness D, Stockwell T et al (2011) Alcohol and health in Canada: a summary of evidence and guidelines for low-risk drinking. *Can Centre on Subst Abus*
Campo MD, Jones KL (2017) A review of the physical features of the fetal alcohol spectrum disorders. *Eur J Med Genet* 60:55–64
Caprara DL, Nash K, Greenbaum R (2007) Novel approaches to the diagnosis of fetal alcohol spectrum disorder. *Neurosci Biobehav Rev* 254–260
Carbia C et al (2021) A biological framework for emotional dysregulation in alcohol misuse: from gut to brain. *Mol Psychiatry* 26(4):1098–1118
Centers for Disease Control and Prevention (2004) *Fetal alcohol syndrome: guidelines for referral and diagnosis*. U.S. Department of Health and Human Services, Atlanta
Centers for Disease Control and Prevention (2021) *Fetal alcohol spectrum disorders (FASDs)*. [Online] Available at: https://www.cdc.gov/ncbddd/fasd/alcohol-use.html Accessed 31 July 2021
Chater-Diehl EJ, Laufer BI, Singh SM (2017) Changes to histone modifications following prenatal alcohol exposure: an emerging picture. *Alcohol*
Chiandetti A et al (2017) Prevalence of prenatal exposure to substances of abuse: questionnaire versus biomarkers. *Reprod Health* 14:1–12
Chudley AE et al (2005) Fetal alcohol spectrum disorder: Canadian guidelines for diagnosis. *CMAJ* 172(5):S1–S21
Ciafrè S et al (2020) Alcohol as an early life stressor: epigenetics, metabolic, neuroendocrine and neurobehavioral implications. *Neurosci Biobehav Rev* 118:654–668
Clarren S (1986) Neuropathology in fetal alcohol syndrome. In: *Alcohol and brain development*. Oxford University Press, New York, pp 158–166
Clarren SK, Chudley AE, Wong L, Friesen J, Brant R (2010) Normal distribution of palpebral fissure lengths in Canadian school age children. *Can J Clin Pharmacol* 17:e67–e78
Coles CD, Gailey AR, Mulle JG et al (2016) A comparison among 5 methods for the clinical diagnosis of fetal alcohol spectrum disorders. *Alcohol Clin Exp Res* 40(5):1000–1009
Coles C et al (1991) Effects of prenatal alcohol exposure at school age, I: physical and cognitive development. *Neurotoxicol Teratol* 13:357–367
Cook R, Keiner J, Yen A (1990) Ethanol causes accelerated G1 arrest in differentiating HL-60 cells. Alcohol Clin Exp Res 14:695–703
Cook JL et al (2015) Fetal alcohol spectrum disorder: a guideline for diagnosis across the lifespan. *CMAJ* 1–7
Czeizel A, Petik D, Puhó E (2004) Smoking and alcohol drinking during pregnancy. The reliability of retrospective maternal self-reported information. *Cent Eur J Public Health* 12:179–183
Dawson N, Dadheich G (1992) The effect of gender on the prevalence and recognition of alcoholism on a general medicine inpatient service. J Gen Intern Med 7:38–45
Day N, Helsel A, Sonon K, Goldschmidt L (2013) The association between prenatal alcohol exposure and behavior at 22 years of age. *Alcohol Clin Exp Res* 37(7):1171–1178
de la Morena-Barrio M et al (2018) Genetic predisposition to fetal alcohol syndrome: association with congenital disorders of N-glycosylation. *Pediatr Res* 83(1-1):119–127
Driscoll CD, Streissguth AP, Riley EP (1990) Prenatal alcohol exposure: comparability of effects in humans and animal models. *Neurotoxicol Teratol* 12(3):231–237
Ehrhart F et al (2019) Review and gap analysis: molecular pathways leading to fetal alcohol spectrum disorders. *Mol Psychiatry* 24(1):10–17

Erng M, Smirnov A, Reid N (2020) Prevention of alcohol-exposed pregnancies and fetal alcohol spectrum disorder among pregnant and postpartum women: a systematic review. *Alcohol Clin Exp Res* 44(12):2431–2448

Fang S et al (2008) Collaborative initiative on fetal alcohol spectrum disorders. Automated diagnosis of fetal alcohol syndrome using 3D facial image analysis. *Orthod Craniofacial Res* 11(3):162–171

Fennema-Notestine C, Gamst A et al (2001) Brain dysmorphology in individuals with severe prenatal alcohol exposure. *Dev Med Child Neurol* 43:148–154

Fernandez-Jaen A, Fernandez-Mayoralas D, Quinones Tapia D et al (2011) Cortical thickness in fetal alcohol syndrome and attention deficit disorder. *Pediatr Neurol* 45:387–391

Finer LB, Zolna MR (2011) Unintended pregnancy in the United States: incidence and disparities 2006. *Contraception* 84(5):478–485

Floyd RL, Decoufle P, Hungerford DW (1999) Alcohol use prior to pregnancy recognition. *Am J Prev Med* 17(2):101–107

Fryer S et al (2007) Evaluation of psychopathological conditions in children with heavy prenatal alcohol exposure. *Pediatrics* 119:e733–e741

Gautam P et al (2015) Developmental trajectories for visuo-spatial attention are altered by prenatal alcohol exposure: a longitudinal FMRI study. *Cereb Cortex* 25:4761–4771

Giedd JN et al (1999) Brain development during childhood and adolescence: a longitudinal MRI study. *Nat Neurosci* 2:861–863

Glass L, Ware A, Mattson S (2014) Neurobehavioral, neurologic, and neuroimaging characteristics of fetal alcohol spectrum disorders. *Handb Clin Neurol* 125:435–462

Goodlett CR, Horn KH, Zhou FC (2005) Alcohol teratogenesis: mechanisms of damage and strategies for intervention. *Exp Biol Med* 230:394–406

Greenmyer J et al (2018) A multicountry updated assessment of the economic impact of fetal alcohol spectrum disorder: costs for children and adults. *J Addict Med* 12(6):466–473

Hall JG (2010) New palpebral fissure measurements. *Am J Med Genet Part A* 152A:1870.

Hamilton D et al (2014) Effects of moderate prenatal alcohol exposure and age on social behavior, spatial response perseveration errors and motor behavior. *Behav Brain Res* 269:44–54

Hoyme HE, May PA, Kalberg WO et al (2005) A practical clinical approach to diagnosis of fetal alcohol spectrum disorders: clarification of the 1996 Institute of Medicine criteria. Pediatrics 115 (1):39–47

Hoyme H, Kalberg WO, Elliott AJ et al (2016) Updated clinical guidelines for diagnosing fetal alcohol spectrum disorders. *Pediatrics* 138(2)

Huebert K, Raftis C (1996) *Fetal alcohol syndrome and other alcohol-related birth defects*, 2nd edn. Alcohol and Drug AbuseCommission, Edmonton: Alberta

Hughes PD, Kim YN, Randall PK, Leslie SW (1998) Effect of prenatal ethanol exposure on the development profile of the NMDA receptor subunits in rat forebrain and hippocampus. *Alcohol Clin Exp Res* 22:1255–1261

Ikonomidou C et al (2001) Neurotransmitters and apoptosis in the developing brain. *Biochem Pharmacol* 62:401–405

Inkelis S, Moore E, Bischoff-Grethe A, Riley E (2020) Neurodevelopment in adolescents and adults with Fetal Alcohol Spectrum Disorders (FASD): a magnetic resonance region of interest analysis. *Brain Res* 1732:146654

Jarmasz J et al (2019) Global DNA methylation and histone posttranslational modifications in human and nonhuman primate brain in association with prenatal alcohol exposure. *Alcohol Clin Exp Res* 43(6):1145–1162

Jones K, Smith D (1973) Recognition of the fetal alcohol syndrome in early infancy. *Lancet* 2: 999–1001

Jones KL, Smith DW, Streissguth AP, Myrianthopoulos NC (1974) Outcome in offspring of chronic alcoholic mothers. *Lancet* 1(866):1076–1271

Kable JA, Mukherjee RAS (2017) Neurodevelopmental disorder associated with prenatal exposure to alcohol (ND-PAE): A proposed diagnostic method of capturing the neurocognitive phenotype of FASD. *Eur J Med Genet* 60:49–54

Kaminen-Ahola N (2020) Fetal alcohol spectrum disorders: genetic and epigenetic mechanisms. *Prenat Diagn* 40(9):1185–1192

Kotch L, Sulik K (1992) Experimental fetal alcohol syndrome: proposed pathogenic basis for a variety of associated facial and brain anomalies. *Am J Med Genet* 44:168–176

Kumada T, Jiang Y, Cameron DB, Komuro H (2007) How does alcohol impair neuronal migration? *J Neurosci Res* 85:465–470

Lange S, Rehm J, Anagnostou E, Popova S (2018) Prevalence of externalizing disorders and autism spectrum disorders among children with fetal alcohol spectrum disorder: systematic review and meta-analysis. *Biochem Cell Biol* 96(2):241–251

Lange S et al (2014) A comparison of the prevalence of prenatal alcohol exposure obtained via maternal self-reports versus meconium testing: a systematic literature review and meta-analysis. *BMC Pregnancy Childbirth* 14:127

Lange S et al (2017) Global prevalence of fetal alcohol spectrum disorder among children and youth: a systematic review and meta-analysis. *JAMA Pediatr* 948–956

Laufer BI, Chater-Diehl EJ, Kapalanga J, Singh SM (2016) Long-term alterations to DNA methylation as a biomarker of prenatal alcohol exposure: from mouse models to human children with fetal alcohol spectrum disorders. *Alcohol* 1–9

Laufer B et al (2015) Associative DNA methylation changes in children with prenatal alcohol exposure. *Epigenomics* 7:1259–1274

Lebel C, Roussotte F, Sowell E (2011) Imaging the impact of prenatal alcohol exposure on the structure of the developing human brain. *Neuropsychol Rev* 21(2):102–118

Lees B et al (2020) Association of prenatal alcohol exposure with psychological, behavioral, and neurodevelopmental outcomes in children from the adolescent brain cognitive development study. *Am J Psychiatry* 177:1060–1072

Lemoine P, Haronsseau H, Borteyu J, Menuet JC (1968) Les enfants de parents alcooliques: anomalies observes a propos de 127 cas (children of alcoholic parents: abnormalities observed in 127 cases). *Ouest Med* 32:476–482

Lenroot RK et al (2007) Sexual dimorphism of brain developmental trajectories during childhood and adolescence. *NeuroImage* 36:1065–1073

Livy D, Miller E, Maier S, West J (2003) Fetal alcohol exposure and temporal vulnerability: effects of binge-like alcohol exposure on the developing rat hippocampus. *Neurotoxicol Teratol* 25: 447–458

Long X et al (2019) The brain's functional connectome in young children with prenatal alcohol exposure. *Neuroimage Clin* 24:102082

Lupton C, Burd L, Harwood R (2004) Cost of fetal alcohol spectrum disorders. *Am J Med Genet* 127C:42–50

Lussier A et al (2018) DNA methylation as a predictor of fetal alcohol spectrum disorder. *Clin Epigenetics* 10:5

Lyall V et al (2021) "The problem is that we hear a bit of everything. . .": A qualitative systematic review of factors associated with alcohol use, reduction, and abstinence in pregnancy. *Int J Environ Res Public Health* 18(7):3445

Mattson S, Bernes G, Doyle L (2019) Fetal alcohol spectrum disorders: a review of the neurobehavioral deficits associated with prenatal alcohol exposure. *Alcohol Clin Exp Res* 43: 1046–1062

Mattson S, Riley E (1996) Brain anomalies in fetal alcohol syndrome. In: *Fetal alcohol syndrome: from mechanism to prevention*. CRC Press, Boca Raton, pp 61–68

May P (1995) A multiple-level, comprehensive approach to the prevention of Fetal Alcohol Syndrome (FAS) and other Alcohol-Related Birth Defects (ARBD). *Int J Addict* 30:1549–1602

May P, Gossage J (2011) Maternal risk factors for fetal alcohol spectrum disorder: not as simple as it may seem. *Alcohol Res Health* 34(1):15–26

McQuire C et al (2016) Objective measures of prenatal alcohol exposure: a systematic review. *Pediatrics* 138(3):e20160517
Meintjes EM et al (2014) A tensor-based morphometry analysis of regional differences in brain volume in relation to prenatal alcohol exposure. *NeuroImage: Clinical* 5:152–160
Midanik L (1988) Validity of self-reported alcohol use: a literature review and assessment. *Br J Addict* 83(9):1019–1029
Miller MW (1986) Effects of alcohol on the generation and migration of cerebral cortical neurons. *Science* 233:1308–1311
Miller M (1993) Migration of cortical neurons is altered by gestational exposure to ethanol. *Alcohol Clin Exp Res* 17:304–314
Miller M (1996) Limited ethanol exposure selectively alters the proliferation of precursor cells in the cerebral cortex. *Alcohol Clin Exp Res* 20:139–143
Montag AC (2016) Fetal alcohol-spectrum disorders: identifying at-risk mothers. *Int J Women's Health* 8:311–323
Nardelli A, Lebel C, Rasmussen C et al (2011) Extensive deep gray matter volume reductions in children and adolescents with fetal alcohol spectrum disorders. *Alcohol Clin Exp Res* 35: 1404–1417
Nutt D, King L, Phillips L (2010) Independent scientific committee on drugs. Drug harms in the UK: a multicriteria decision analysis. *Lancet* 376(9752):1558–1565
O'Connor M, Paley B (2009) Psychiatric conditions associated with prenatal alcohol exposure. *Dev Disabil Res Rev* 15:225–234
Ospina M, Dennet L (2013) *Systematic review on the prevalence of fetal alcohol spectrum disorders*. Institute of Health Economics, Edmonton
Patten AR, Fontaine CJCBR (2003) A comparison of the different animal models of fetal alcohol spectrum disorders and their use in studying complex behaviors. *Front Pediatr* 2:1–19
Poole N, Isaac B (2001) *Apprehensions: barrier to treatment for substance-using mothers*. British Columbia Centre of Excellence for Women's Health, Vancouver
Popova S et al (2017) Estimation of national, regional, and global prevalence of alcohol use during pregnancy and fetal alcohol syndrome: a systematic review and meta-analysis. *Lancet* 5: e290–e299
Popova S et al (2021) Health, social and legal outcomes of individuals with diagnosed or at risk for fetal alcohol spectrum disorder: Canadian example. *Drug Alcohol Depend* 219:108487
Portales-Casamar E, Lussier AA, Jones MJ et al (2016) DNA methylation signature of human fetal alcohol spectrum disorder. *Epigenetics Chromatin* 9(25):25
Riikonen R, Salonen I, Partanen K et al (1999) Brain perfusion SPECT and MRI in foetal alcohol syndrome. *Dev Med Child Neurol* 41:652–659
Riikonen R et al (2005) Deep serotonergic and dopaminergic structures in fetal alcoholic syndrome: a study with nor-beta-CIT-single-photon emission computed tomography and magnetic resonance imaging volumetry. *Biol Psychiatry* 57:1565–1572
Riley EP, McGee CL (2005) Fetal alcohol spectrum disorders: an overview with emphasis on changes in brain and behavior'. *Exp Biol Med* 230(6):357–365
Ritfeld G, Kable J, Holton J, Coles C (2021) Psychopharmacological treatments in children with fetal alcohol spectrum disorders: a review. *Child Psychiatry Hum Dev.* p. Preprint
Rodriguez C et al (2021) Detection of prenatal alcohol exposure using machine learning classification of resting-state functional network connectivity data. *Alcohol* 93:25–34
Room R, Bondy S, Ferris J (1989) The risk of harm to one self from drinking, Canada. *Addiction* 90 (4):499–513
Schneider M et al (2005) Moderate-level prenatal alcohol exposure alters striatal dopamine system function in rhesus monkeys. *Alcohol Clin Exp Res* 29:1685–1697
Sebastiani G et al (2018) The effects of alcohol and drugs of abuse on maternal nutritional profile during pregnancy. *Nutrients* 10:1008
Shaw P et al (2006) Intellectual ability and cortical development in children and adolescents. *Nature* 440:676–679

Singal D, Brownell M, Chateau D et al (2017) The psychiatric morbidity of women who give birth to children with fetal alcohol spectrum disorder (FASD): results of the Manitoba mothers and FASD study. *Can J Psychiatr* 62(8):531–542

Sowell E, Mattson S, Kan E et al (2008) Abnormal cortical thickness and brain-behavior correlation patterns in individuals with heavy prenatal alcohol exposure. *Cereb Cortex* 18:136–144

Sowell E, Thompson P, Mattson S et al (2001) Voxel-based morphometric analyses of the brain in children and adolescents prenatally exposed to alcohol. *Neuroreport* 12:515–523

Sowell E, Thompson P, Mattson S et al (2002) Regional brain shape abnormalities persist into adolescence after heavy prenatal alcohol exposure. *Cereb Cortex* 12:856–865

Sowell ER et al (2004) Longitudinal mapping of cortical thickness and brain growth in normal children. *J Neurosci* 24:8223–8231

Stratton K et al (1996) *Fetal alcohol syndrome: diagnosis, epidemiology, prevention, and treatment.* National Academy Press, Washington

Streissguth A, Barr H, Kogan J, Bookstein F (1997) Primary and secondary disabilities. In: *Fetal alcohol syndrome in the challenge of fetal alcohol syndrome: overcoming secondary disabilities*. University of Washington, Seattle, pp 25–39

Streissguth AP et al (2004) Risk factors for adverse life outcomes in fetal alcohol syndrome and fetal alcohol effects. *J Dev Behav Pediatr* 25(4):228–238

Sutherland R, McDonald R, Savage D (1997) Prenatal exposure to moderate levels of ethanol can have long-lasting effects on hippo-campal synaptic plasticity in adult offspring. *Hippocampus* 7: 232–238

Thanh N, Jonsson E (n.d.) Chapter 4: Total cost of FASD including the economics of FASD associated with crimes. In: *Ethical and legal perspectives in fetal alcohol spectrum disorders (FASD)*. Springer, Berlin

Thanh NX, Jonsson E, Dennett L et al (2011) *Fetal alcohol spectrum disorder—management and policy perspectives of FASD*. Wiley-Blackwell, Edmonton

van Amsterdam J, Nutt D, Phillips L, van den Brink W (2015) European rating of drug harms. *J Psychopharmacol* 29(6):655–660

Warren KR (2015) A review of the history of attitudes toward drinking in pregnancy. *Alcohol Clin Exp Res* 39(7)

West J, Pierce D (1986) Perinatal alcohol exposure and neuronal damage. In: *Alcohol and brain development*. Oxford University Press, New York

Weyrauch D et al (2017) Comorbid mental disorders in fetal alcohol spectrum disorders: a systematic review. *J Dev Behav Pediatr* 38(4):283–291

World Health Organization (2016) *International classification of diseases and related health problems, 10th revision*. WHO, Geneva

Yang Y, Roussotte F, Kan E et al (2012) Abnormal cortical thickness alterations in fetal alcohol spectrum disorders and their relationships with facial dysmorphology. *Cereb Cortex* 22: 1170–1179

Zadunayski A, Hicks M, Gibbard B, Godlovitch G (2006) Behind the screen: legal and ethical considerations in neonatal screening for prenatal exposure to alcohol. *Health Law* 14:105–127

Zelner I et al (2012) Neonatal screening for prenatal alcohol exposure: assessment of voluntary maternal participation in an open meconium screening program. *Alcohol* 46:269–276

Zhang C et al (2019) Detection of children/youth with fetal alcohol spectrum disorder through eye movement, psychometric, and neuroimaging data. *Front Neuro* 10:80

Zizzo N et al (2013) Comments and reflections on ethics in screening for biomarkers of prenatal alcohol exposure. *Alcohol Clin Exp Res* 37(9):1451–1455

Chronic Alcohol and Skeletal Muscle

45

Brianna L. Bourgeois, Danielle E. Levitt, Patricia E. Molina, and Liz Simon

Contents

Introduction 944
Mechanisms of Alcohol-Mediated Skeletal Muscle Pathology 946
  Stem Cells and Regeneration 946
  Structure and Function 947
Protein Synthesis and Breakdown 948
Muscle Processes Affected by Alcohol 951
  Mitochondria: Bioenergetics, Dynamics, and Oxidative Stress 951
  Epigenetics 953
Alcohol-Mediated Muscle Changes in Exercise and Interorgan Communication 954
  Exercise 954
Interorgan Cross Talk 957
Applications to Public Health: The Aging Population 958
Key Facts 960
Mini-dictionary 960
Summary Points 961
Future Issues 961
References 962

Abstract

At-risk alcohol use is associated with tissue pathophysiology with significant adverse effects on multiple organ systems. Chronic alcoholic myopathy affects 40–60%, while alcohol-related liver injury affects only about 10–15% of people with at-risk alcohol use. Alcohol-induced mechanisms of dysfunctional muscle mass are multifactorial, complex, and interrelated. Alcohol decreases differentiation potential of muscle stem cells and dysregulates extracellular matrix remodeling decreasing muscle regenerative capacity in response to injury and atrophy. Alcohol-induced muscle loss is mediated by altering the balance of

B. L. Bourgeois · D. E. Levitt · P. E. Molina · L. Simon (✉)
Department of Physiology, Comprehensive Alcohol HIV/AIDS Research Center, Louisiana State University Health Sciences Center, New Orleans, LA, USA
e-mail: bboul1@lsuhsc.edu; dlevit@lsuhsc.edu; pmolin@lsuhsc.edu; lsimo2@lsuhsc.edu

V. B. Patel, V. R. Preedy (eds.), *Handbook of Substance Misuse and Addictions*,
https://doi.org/10.1007/978-3-030-92392-1_49

anabolic and catabolic pathways of muscle mass maintenance and mitochondrial dysfunction. Adaptations to exercise could directly reduce alcohol-associated myopathy; however, peri-exercise alcohol consumption may interfere with exercise performance and adaptive physiological processes. Emerging evidence indicates that epigenomic adaptations mediate this alcohol-induced myopathy. Muscle cross talk with multiple organs via myokines and extracellular vesicles is emerging as novel endocrine and paracrine mechanisms. How alcohol modulates this interorgan communication is under active investigation. In this chapter, we review the current understanding of pathophysiological mechanisms involved in alcohol-mediated myopathy together with emerging areas of research focus.

Keywords

Skeletal muscle · Regenerative capacity · Muscle stem cells · Muscle protein synthesis · Muscle protein breakdown · Mitochondrial function · Epigenetics · Exercise · Interorgan communication

Introduction

Alcohol use disorder (AUD) is the most prevalent mental disorder characterized by the inability to control alcohol consumption leading to physical and emotional dependence (Carvalho et al. 2019). AUD is defined by having two or more symptoms as outlined in the fifth edition of the *Diagnostic and Statistical Manual of Mental Disorders* (Association 2013). The National Epidemiologic Survey on Alcohol and Related Conditions reported a 49% increase in the 12-month prevalence of AUD between 2002 and 2013 (Hasin and Grant 2015). While men previously had a higher incidence of AUD, the gender gap is rapidly narrowing with more women exhibiting at-risk alcohol use (Grant et al. 2017). The 18–29 age-group continues to have the highest prevalence of alcohol use; however, binge drinking is increasing in the 50–74 age-group (Hasin and Grant 2015). This increase in middle-aged and older-adult binge drinking leads to an increase in alcohol-related morbidity and mortality (Grucza et al. 2018). AUD leads to or exacerbates liver disease, cardiovascular and digestive diseases, neuropsychiatric disorders, infections, and cancers (Simon et al. 2017a). While alcohol-related liver disease affects 10–15% of individuals with AUD, alcoholic myopathy affects 40–60% of people with AUD (Simon et al. 2017a).

One of the major detrimental effects of alcohol results from its metabolic breakdown primarily in the liver. The first step in alcohol metabolism is the conversion of ethanol to acetaldehyde, a short-lived but highly toxic metabolite, by the enzyme alcohol dehydrogenase (ADH). Aldehyde dehydrogenase (ALDH) converts acetaldehyde to acetate, which can be broken down further to carbon dioxide and water. Acetaldehyde is responsible for many of the damaging effects of alcohol. ADH is the predominant enzyme responsible for the conversion of ethanol to acetaldehyde; however, catalase and cytochrome P450 2E1 (CYP2E1) can also catalyze this reaction. CYP2E1 is activated with heavy alcohol consumption and produces reactive oxygen species (ROS). ROS and acetaldehyde are byproducts of alcohol metabolism that cause damage to DNA and proteins and contribute to overall toxic effects of alcohol (Cederbaum 2012).

One tissue affected by alcohol's toxic metabolites is the skeletal muscle (SKM), which plays a significant role in multiple body functions. SKM converts chemical energy to mechanical energy generating the force necessary for daily life activities, postural maintenance, and overall functional independence. From a metabolic perspective, SKM contributes to glucose homeostasis, stores amino acids, and maintains core body temperature. SKM is the predominant site for insulin-dependent glucose uptake, and skeletal muscle insulin resistance occurs decades before pancreatic beta cell failure during the development of type 2 diabetes (DeFronzo and Tripathy 2009). Thus, dysfunctional SKM contributes to the burden of chronic disease morbidity, frailty syndrome, and mortality.

Alcoholic myopathy can be classified as acute or chronic. Acute alcohol-related myopathy occurs in less than 5% of at-risk alcohol users and is characterized by abrupt rhabdomyolysis, or skeletal muscle destruction, that can lead to severe kidney injury. Acute alcohol-related myopathy presents with painful swollen skeletal muscle at the affected site, increased serum creatine kinase, and myoglobinuria (Preedy et al. 2001a). Increased deposition of myoglobin in the kidneys can lead to necrosis and kidney failure. Acute alcohol-related myopathy can occur with a single binge alcohol session (i.e., blood alcohol reaching 0.08 g/dl), and muscle-related symptoms will generally subside in 1–2 weeks of abstinence (Preedy et al. 2001a).

Chronic alcohol-related myopathy is characterized by muscle weakness beginning in the proximal muscles including quadriceps and deltoids and generally is not accompanied with pain. It results from selective atrophy of type 2 muscle fibers, although all fibers can be affected, leading up to a 20% reduction in muscle mass. Clinically this presents as a reduction in urine creatinine and body mass index (Preedy et al. 2001a) and decreased handgrip strength (González-Reimers et al. 2019). Chronic alcohol-related myopathy is largely underdiagnosed even though it is the most prevalent of alcohol-related diseases and is seen in up to 60% of muscle biopsies from people with at-risk alcohol use (González-Reimers et al. 2019). Its severity is associated with cumulative lifetime alcohol consumption and is most prevalent in people between 40 and 60 years of age (Simon et al. 2017a). While malnutrition seen with at-risk alcohol use may contribute to muscle pathology, chronic alcohol-related myopathy occurs independent of folate, protein, pyridoxine, riboflavin, thiamine, and vitamin B12 nutritional status (Nicolas et al. 2003; Preedy et al. 2001b).

Chronic alcohol-related myopathy can exacerbate other alcohol-associated comorbidities and worsen quality of life. Alcohol-related liver disease prognosis (i.e., survival, quality of life, and posttransplant outcomes) is worsened by alcohol-induced myopathy (Dasarathy et al. 2017). Binge alcohol consumption increases the prevalence of sarcopenia among women (Yoo et al. 2017), and sarcopenia is a predictor of chronic disease progression and poor patient outcomes in clinical and surgical settings. With the high prevalence of alcohol-related myopathy in people with AUD and the potential implications of this disease, the chapter outlines pathophysiologic factors associated with alcohol-induced SKM dysfunction.

Mechanisms of Alcohol-Mediated Skeletal Muscle Pathology

Stem Cells and Regeneration

The contractile functional units of SKM are myofibers. These myofibers are surrounded by connective tissue, the extracellular matrix (ECM) or matrisome, that house capillaries and nerves that supply the muscle. SKM atrophy or injuries, whether from routine wear and tear or trauma, result in regeneration in a healthy individual through a process including inflammation, regeneration, and remodeling (Yin et al. 2013). Muscle stem cells, satellite cells (SCs), and the ECM play principal roles in SKM maintenance and repair.

Satellite cells are located under the basal lamina of SKM, are typically quiescent, and account for 2–5% of nuclei of adult SKM (Dumont et al. 2015). Following SKM injury, tissue necrosis initiates an acute inflammatory response during initial hours, characterized by early infiltration of neutrophils followed by monocytes that transform into macrophages as they enter damaged tissue and clear tissue debris. These macrophages undergo a gradual shift from an early pro-inflammatory (M1)-dominant to an anti-inflammatory (M2)-dominant phenotype (Arnold et al. 2007; Tidball 2017). Subsequently, inflammation subsides, and the secretion of growth factors and cytokines triggers regeneration and repair by activating SCs. Acute alcohol is largely anti-inflammatory (Afshar et al. 2015; Mandrekar et al. 2007), while chronic alcohol promotes a systemic pro-inflammatory state (Mandrekar et al. 2009; Szabo et al. 2007). The pro-inflammatory milieu in chronic at-risk alcohol use impairs regenerative and repair processes (Dekeyser et al. 2013). Activated SCs proliferate and commit to form myogenic progenitor cells, myoblasts, that in turn proliferate and differentiate to fuse with each other or damaged fibers (Dumont et al. 2015). Myoblasts develop from mesodermal stem cells and express the paired box 7 gene (*Pax7*). When it is activated, SC *Pax7* expression decreases with a concomitant increase in myoblast determination protein (*MyoD*) and myogenic factor 5 gene expression, which is the hallmark for the cell's commitment to become a myogenic progenitor.

The fate of SCs is highly dependent on the environment (Yin et al. 2013), and alcohol impairs the regenerative capacity of SCs. In a preclinical model of hind-limb immobilization and recovery, skeletal muscle *MyoD* gene expression was significantly lower 3 days following hind-limb immobilization in alcohol-fed rats (Levitt et al. 2020a). Myoblasts from chronic binge alcohol-administered macaques had decreased expression of myogenic transcription factor genes and decreased myoblast fusion and myotube formation (Simon et al. 2014). In a mouse model of chronic alcohol use, delays in regeneration after barium chloride-induced injury were associated with increased inflammatory gene expression (e.g., tumor necrosis factor-α [*Tnfa*], interleukin [Il]-1β, and *Il6*), increased ECM accumulation, altered timing of transforming growth factor-β (*Tgfb*) gene expression, and increased tissue fibrosis during recovery (7 and 14 days post-injury) (Dekeyser et al. 2013). Together, these preclinical studies establish that alcohol has adverse effects on SKM regenerative capacity.

While the activation, proliferation, and differentiation of SCs are necessary for proper SKM regeneration, the ECM plays an important role in maintaining the SKM structure that is vital for regeneration and function. Several secreted factors and cytokines play a role in enhancing muscle fibrosis including myostatin and *Tgfb1*, which lead to fibroblast proliferation and activation, respectively (Mahdy 2019). Fibroblasts are profibrotic cells responsible for the production of collagen proteins that are important for the structural function of the ECM (Mahdy 2019). While the maintenance of ECM is necessary, at-risk alcohol use can lead to a state of tissue inflammation that results in an abnormal increase in profibrotic genes and collagen deposition. In an end-stage rhesus macaque model of simian immunodeficiency virus (SIV) infection, chronic binge alcohol administration increased hydroxyproline content and picrosirius red staining indicating increased collagen deposition in SKM (Dodd et al. 2014). This may partially underlie the chronic alcohol-mediated accentuated muscle wasting (Molina et al. 2008). Chronic alcohol also increased *Tgfb* and myostatin gene expression in an HIV-1 transgenic rat model (Clary et al. 2011). Similar chronic alcohol-mediated inductions in *Tnfa* and *Tgfb* gene expression have also been observed in SKM 14 days into recovery from hind-limb immobilization (Levitt et al. 2020a). The dysregulation of these secreted factors and cytokines may explain why alcohol feeding increases the expression of collagen and hydroxyproline in SKM (Steiner et al. 2015a). Excess collagen deposition with at-risk alcohol use can reduce the ability for the skeletal muscle to regenerate by limiting the available area for muscle growth. Thus, a reduction in SC differentiation potential and/or an increase in ECM fibrosis contributes to alcohol-induced impaired skeletal muscle regeneration (Fig. 1).

Structure and Function

The SKM maintains posture and performs movements through its ability to contract when stimulated by the somatic nervous system. The ability for the SKM to contract results from its striated structure of repeating sarcomere units composed of thick and thin filaments. Thick and thin filaments form cross-links through the binding of actin and myosin. Chronic alcohol consumption results in reduced expression of myosin heavy chain (MHC), a major motor protein in the thick filament, and troponin T, necessary for myosin and actin positioning (Crowell et al. 2019). Alcohol administration reduces titin and nebulin, proteins that contribute to sarcomere structure, proportional to MHC in rats (Hunter et al. 2003). Additionally, chronic alcohol consumption, but not acute binge alcohol, reduces post-fatigue contractile function. This occurs independent of loss in muscle mass indicating that chronic alcohol directly affects the intrinsic contractile function of SKM (Crowell et al. 2019).

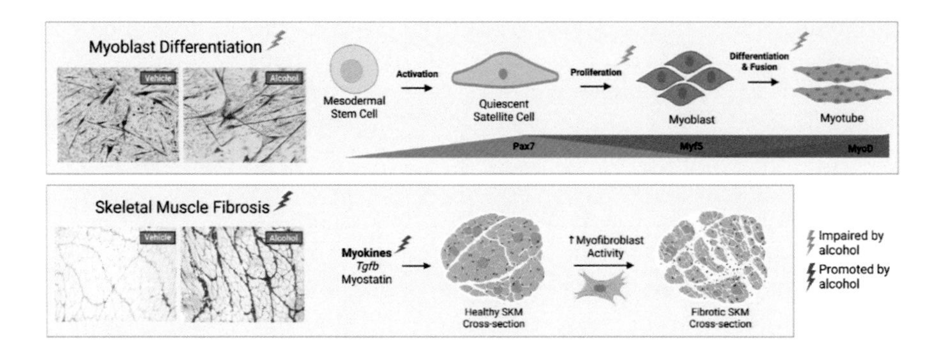

Fig. 1 Alcohol decreases skeletal muscle regenerative capacity. Alcohol decreases proliferation and differentiation of muscle stem cells and decreases myotube formation. Alcohol increases collagen deposition in the extracellular matrix by increasing the release of myostatin and transforming growth factor B, thus increasing fibrosis. A decrease in stem cell differentiation together with dysregulated extracellular matrix remodeling decreases regenerative capacity of the muscle after injury and atrophy. Created with BioRender.com

In addition to serving as contractile units, SKM serves a vital role in glucose homeostasis. Making up about 40% of body mass, SKM reduces circulating glucose levels through insulin-dependent mechanisms. While alcohol's effect on glucose disposal under basal conditions reveals inconsistent results, convincing clinical and preclinical evidence suggests that alcohol induces a decrease in insulin-dependent SKM glucose uptake (Steiner et al. 2015b). The exact mechanism by which alcohol decreases insulin-dependent glucose uptake is unknown, though a decrease in glucose transporter 4 translocation to the muscle cell membrane is one of the accepted downstream effects of alcohol (Steiner et al. 2015b) (Fig. 2). In a preclinical rat model of alcohol-related myopathy, chronic ethanol feeding reduced gastrocnemius expression of proteins in the insulin signaling pathway including IRS-1, Akt, and p70S6K (Nguyen et al. 2012). Additionally, chronic alcohol increases triglyceride deposition in SKM (Koh et al. 2020), which can further lead to metabolic dysregulation.

These intrinsic alcohol-mediated effects on SKM structure, contractility, and metabolic function can be exacerbated by an overall reduction in SKM mass that is common in at-risk alcohol users. Thus, people with at-risk alcohol use should be monitored for signs of SKM dysfunction, including insulin resistance.

Protein Synthesis and Breakdown

Changes in SKM mass are determined by the balance of muscle protein synthesis and protein breakdown. Anabolic stimuli (e.g., amino acids, hormones such as insulin and insulin-like growth factor [IGF] 1, and mechanical loading) shift the overall balance toward protein synthesis (Hodson et al. 2019), whereas catabolic stimuli (e.g., insufficient nutrition, cortisol, and mechanical unloading) shift the

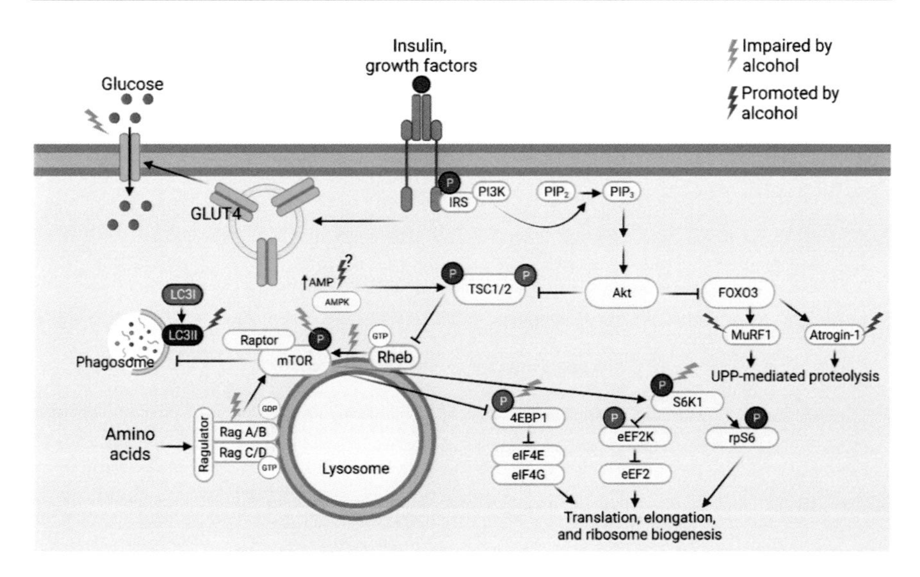

Fig. 2 Alcohol alters the balance of muscle protein synthesis and breakdown. Alcohol decreases expression and activity of proteins involved in the insulin and mammalian target of rapamycin (mTOR) signaling pathways, thus decreasing muscle protein synthesis. Alcohol may increase expression of proteins involved in the ubiquitin proteasome pathway (UPP) and increases autophagy, promoting protein breakdown. Created with BioRender.com

balance toward muscle protein breakdown (Bodine 2013). Evidence suggests that anti-anabolic and catabolic processes promoted by high-dose and/or chronic at-risk alcohol are major contributors to alcohol-related myopathy (Simon et al. 2017a).

Anabolic stimuli converge on the mammalian target of rapamycin (mTOR) signaling pathway, critical to protein synthesis (Bodine et al. 2001). mTOR is a protein kinase within two complexes, 1 and 2, and activation of mTOR within complex 1 is central to protein synthesis. Upstream regulation of mTOR is mediated by growth factors via phosphoinositide 3-kinase (PI3K)/protein kinase B (Akt) and by cellular metabolic state via AMP-activated protein kinase (AMPK). Akt inhibits, whereas AMPK activates, tuberous sclerosis complex (TSC)1/tuberous sclerosis complex 2 by either removing or promoting its inhibition of Ras homolog enriched in brain (Rheb) GTPase, respectively. When it is active, Rheb binds and activates mTOR (Jewell et al. 2013). The Ragulator-Rag complex is an alternative means of mTOR activation that is independent of TSC1/TSC2 and Rheb and is required for amino acid-mediated mTOR activation. Downstream of mTOR (Jewell et al. 2013), phosphorylation of eukaryotic initiation factor 4E (eIF4E)-binding protein (4EBP1) releases its inhibition of translation initiation factor eIF4E, allowing eIF4E to form an active complex with eIF4G and initiate 5' terminal oligopyrimidine tract (TOP)-dependent translation. Activation of S6 kinase 1 (S6K1) by mTOR initiates phosphorylation and suppression of eukaryotic elongation factor 2 kinase (eEF2k), disinhibiting its target eEF2 which has a critical role in peptide chain elongation. S6K1 also activates ribosomal protein S6 (rpS6), a component of the 40S subunit of the ribosome that is required for ribosomal RNA biogenesis (Jewell et al. 2013), contributing to translational machinery.

Acute and chronic alcohol reduce muscle protein synthesis, and although the understanding of underlying mechanisms is incomplete, alterations in mTOR pathway signaling are key contributors (Steiner and Lang 2015; Steiner and Lang 2019). Alcohol decreases phosphorylation of mTOR, S6K1, and 4EBP1, and the decreased association of Rheb with mTOR may partially underlie these signaling changes (Hong-Brown et al. 2012). Although results from in vitro work indicate that ethanol may activate AMPK leading to TSC1-/TSC2-mediated suppression of mTOR (Hong-Brown et al. 2012), this finding has not been replicated in vivo (Korzick et al. 2013) and thus is an unlikely contributor to alcohol-mediated decreased mTOR pathway signaling. Regardless, acute and chronic alcohol not only decrease muscle protein synthesis in the basal state but also prevent the increase in protein synthesis in response to anabolic stimuli including leucine (Hong-Brown et al. 2012; Lang 2018). Inhibition of Rag signaling is implicated as a mechanism by which alcohol blunts anabolic effects of leucine, and the constitutive activation of RagA and RagC rescues this effect (Hong-Brown et al. 2012). Overall, alcohol inhibits mTOR pathway signaling at several points both upstream and downstream of mTOR resulting in decreased muscle protein synthesis (Fig. 2).

Mechanisms of muscle protein breakdown include ubiquitin proteasome pathway (UPP) system activation and autophagy. Atrogin-1 and muscle ring finger (MuRF1), known collectively as atrogenes, are often used as markers of UPP system activation. Though the mRNA expression of atrogenes is increased in acute alcohol-administered adult rodents (Korzick et al. 2013; Vary et al. 2008), this does not necessarily result in increased protein breakdwon (Vary et al. 2008). Furthermore, atrogene expression was not increased by alcohol in older rats (Dekeyser et al. 2013). However, with another catabolic stimulus, SIV infection, chronic alcohol increased UPP activation and produced marked dysregulation of multiple components of the UPP system (LeCapitaine et al. 2011). In contrast to UPP signaling, a growing body of evidence supports a role for autophagy in alcohol-mediated SKM proteolysis. When C2C12 myotubes were cultured with 100-mM ethanol, proteolysis increased, and this was unchanged by MG132, a proteasome inhibitor (Thapaliya et al. 2014). However, 3-methyladenine, an inhibitor of autophagy, prevented the ethanol-mediated increase in proteolysis (Korzick et al. 2013), strongly suggesting a role for autophagy in alcohol-mediated muscle protein breakdown. This ethanol concentration increased autophagy markers (LC3II/LC3I and beclin1) in myotubes, and the increase in beclin1 was prevented by mitochondrial-targeted antioxidant MitoTEMPO (Kumar et al. 2019), suggesting that oxidative stress may be at least partially responsible for alcohol-mediated increases in autophagy. Complementing results from in vitro work, increased autophagy markers in SKM were observed in alcohol-fed mice and individuals with alcohol-related cirrhosis (Thapaliya et al. 2014). The dose and duration of alcohol consumption required to observe increased autophagy in humans in the absence of cirrhosis are unclear. Finally, increased SKM expression of inflammatory and fibrotic genes is observed with chronic alcohol consumption in the absence of underlying disease or injury (Clary et al. 2011) and can contribute to changes in muscle protein balance. *Tnfa* is of particular interest as it is consistently increased in SKM with chronic alcohol and knocking out *Tnfa* prevented the alcohol-mediated decrease in muscle protein synthesis and increases in myostatin and muscle protein breakdown markers (Li et al. 2020) (Fig. 2).

Muscle Processes Affected by Alcohol

Mitochondria: Bioenergetics, Dynamics, and Oxidative Stress

SKM is highly energetic and relies heavily on mitochondria to meet ATP demands, and mitochondria are critical in the maintenance of functional SKM mass. Thus, adverse effects of alcohol on SKM mitochondria could contribute to myopathy observed in individuals with chronic at-risk alcohol use. A key early study histologically examining SKM in volunteers fed a 42% alcohol diet for 28 days reported significantly enlarged mitochondria together with elevated serum creatine kinase, indicating alcohol-mediated mitochondrial dysregulation and SKM damage (Song and Rubin 1972). Despite this finding, early studies of the impact of alcohol on isolated mitochondria remained equivocal, with some reporting no effects (Cardellach et al. 1992) and others reporting decreased mitochondrial respiration and cytochrome content after chronic alcohol (Farrar et al. 1982).

More recently, alcohol was reported to interfere with several mitochondrial parameters including bioenergetics, dynamics, and redox state. Whereas treatment of C2C12 myoblasts with 100-mM ethanol for 6 h decreased basal, ATP-linked, maximal respiration and spare respiratory capacity (Kumar et al. 2019; Singh et al. 2021), treatment of primary myoblasts with 50-mM ethanol for 3 days increased maximal respiration and spare respiratory capacity with a concomitant decrease in glycolytic function (Levitt et al. 2020b). These results suggest dose- and time-dependent effects of ethanol on myoblast mitochondrial function, where a physiologically relevant ethanol concentration applied for a longer time may induce a mitohormetic response that is not seen with higher-concentration, shorter-duration exposure. However, chronic binge alcohol (50–60-mM peak BAC) in SIV-infected antiretroviral-treated male macaques decreased maximal myoblast respiration during asymptomatic infection (Duplanty et al. 2018) and dysregulated SKM mitochondrial gene expression at end-stage simian acquired immunodeficiency syndrome (Duplanty et al. 2017a). In the context of an additional mitochondrial stressor, chronic binge alcohol may be sufficient to impair SKM mitochondrial function (Fig. 3).

Together with bioenergetic function, mitochondrial quality control mechanisms are affected by alcohol. Chronic (6–11 months) consumption of a 36% alcohol diet decreased SKM mitochondrial fusion activity and decreased mitofusin (Mfn)1, but not Mfn2 or optic atrophy (Opa)1 in rodents (Eisner et al. 2014). This decreased fusion was associated with rapid decreases in calcium transients indicating enhanced SKM fatigability. However, Mfn1 overexpression did not rescue this response, demonstrating that aberrant mitochondrial fusion and calcium signaling are distinct but concurrent alcohol-mediated phenomena (Eisner et al. 2014). In addition to

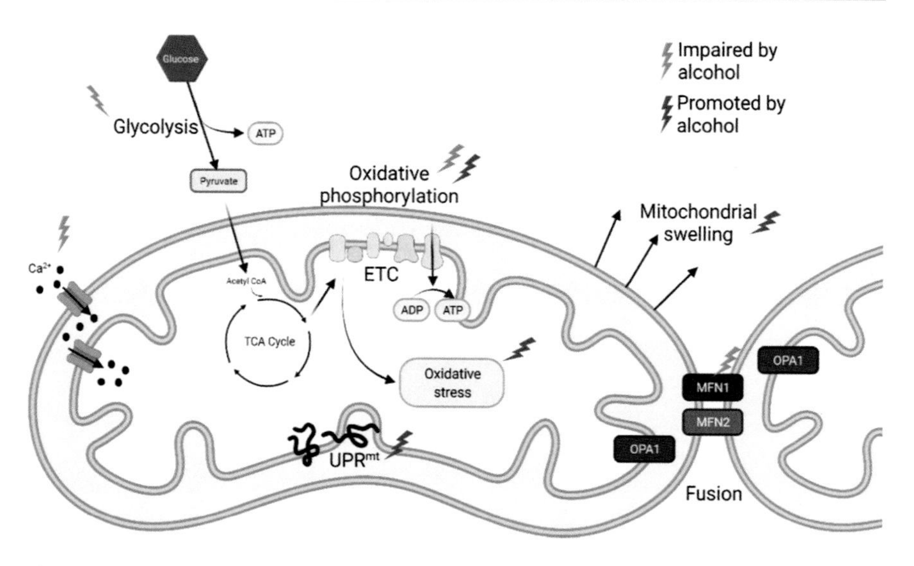

Fig. 3 Alcohol dysregulates mitochondrial function. Alcohol impairs mitochondrial bioenergetics by dysregulating oxidative phosphorylation, likely in a dose- and time-dependent manner, and decreasing glycolytic function during myoblast differentiation. Alcohol dysregulates mitochondrial dynamics by decreasing proteins implicated in mitochondrial fusion. The mitochondrial unfolded protein response (UPR^{mt}) appears to increase in response to alcohol and may partially protect against alcohol-mediated pathology. Alcohol induces oxidative stress in the skeletal muscle. Created with BioRender.com

decreased fusion, increased mitochondrial fragmentation is observed in alcohol-fed *C. elegans* (Oh et al. 2020). This fragmentation was coupled to the activation of the mitochondrial unfolded protein response (UPR^{mt}). A gain-of-function mutant for a master UPR^{mt} regulator, atfs-1, protected against alcohol-mediated muscle dysfunction (Oh et al. 2020), demonstrating the importance of the UPR^{mt} in mitochondrial and SKM homeostasis (Fig. 3).

Alcohol metabolism reduces nicotinamide adenine dinucleotide (NAD) to NADH and thus shifts the cellular redox state in many cell types. Although incubation of myocytes with 4-methylpyrazole, an ADH antagonist, demonstrated that adverse effects of alcohol on protein synthesis are independent of alcohol metabolism (Lang et al. 2004), other works demonstrate that SKM expresses ADH (Davuluri et al. 2021) and thus the shift in redox state may contribute to adverse effects of alcohol on SKM, particularly SKM mitochondria. Mechanisms underlying mitochondrial dysfunction with high-concentration (100 mM) ethanol treatment appear to include oxidative stress since antioxidants at least partially restore aberrant function (Kumar et al. 2019; Singh et al. 2021). Increased mitochondrial H_2O_2 emission has been observed in ethanol-treated C2C12 myotubes, and this increased emission was prevented by peroxisome proliferator-activated receptor (PPAR)δ activation (Koh et al. 2020). This increased PPARδ activation increased catalase in SKM of alcohol-fed rodents providing a mechanism by which PPARδ may protect against alcohol-induced oxidative stress. Overall, recent work has demonstrated multiple adverse effects of alcohol on SKM mitochondria although mechanisms remain to be elucidated. Oxidative stress appears to be a promising therapeutic target (Fig. 3).

Epigenetics

Epigenetics is the study of alterations in gene expression that occur independently of alterations in the genome. Epigenetic modifications include DNA methylation, histone modifications, and noncoding RNAs that can alter the transcription or translation of genes and lead to altered gene expression. Drugs, toxins, and environmental factors can influence the epigenome. Alcohol is a major contributor for epigenomic modifications affecting cells and tissues (Shukla and Zakhari 2013).

The most studied epigenetic modification is DNA methylation. DNA methylation involves the conversion of cytosine to 5-methylcytosine by DNA methyltransferase typically at a cytosine-phosphate-guanine (CpG) site. Methylated DNA is less likely to be transcribed into mRNA. S-adenosylmethionine (SAM) donates the methyl group for this reaction, and folate is essential for SAM synthesis. Chronic heavy drinking decreases folate levels through decreased folate consumption, intestinal malabsorption, or reduced liver uptake (Preedy et al. 2001a). This decrease in SAM can lead to DNA hypomethylation and overexpression of multiple genes. In an end-stage macaque model of SIV infection, chronic binge alcohol exacerbated muscle wasting, and this was associated with changes in promoter methylation of genes involved in SKM function (Simon et al. 2015). Dysregulated methylation seen with SKM wasting suggests a potential role of DNA methylation in alcohol-related myopathy.

An additional epigenetic modification is histone acetylation and deacetylation. Histone acetyltransferase (HAT) adds an acetyl group to lysine on histones, while histone deacetylase (HDAC) removes the acetyl group. An acetyl group on the lysine of histone causes chromatin to be more "open," and acetylation leads to an increase in gene transcription. The alcohol metabolite acetate can be converted to acetyl-CoA which is used by histone acetyltransferase to acetylate lysine residues on histones (Bodine 2013). Acetylation of histone H3 is affected by alcohol metabolites in the liver, lung, and spleen (Bodine et al. 2001), but the effect in the skeletal muscle is unknown. Nevertheless, ethanol-treated myoblasts have increased HDAC4 expression and decreased differentiation potential, and an HDAC4 inhibitor can restore differentiation in ethanol-treated myoblasts (Adler et al. 2019; Simon et al. 2017b; Steiner and Lang 2019).

microRNAs (miRNAs) and other noncoding RNAs can also interfere with gene transcription and translation. miRNAs are typically 21–23 nucleotides long and bind to mRNA leading to repressed translation of mRNA or mRNA degradation. miRNAs can be measured in serum or tissues, and alcohol dysregulates miRNA expression in SKM. Alcohol-treated zebra fish have reduced muscle fiber cross-sectional area and dysregulated expression of miRNAs associated with the *Notch* pathway that suppresses myogenesis (Khayrullin et al. 2016). In a rhesus macaque model of SIV infection, chronic binge alcohol decreases expression of miR-206, a muscle-specific miRNA, and inhibition of miR-206 leads to decreased myoblast differentiation (Simon et al. 2017b). Additionally, a clinical study of people living with HIV reveals differentially expressed circulating miRNAs in people with AUD compared to controls (Wyczechowska et al. 2017). Numerous other studies demonstrate the role of miRNAs in SKM insulin resistance (Chen et al. 2012; Esteves et al. 2017; Lee et al. 2016). While miRNAs evidently contribute to alcohol-mediated suppression of myogenesis, more studies are needed to elucidate how miRNAs mechanistically contribute to alcohol-mediated SKM pathologies.

DNA methylation, histone acetylation, and noncoding RNAs are implicated in multiple disease states including those linked to muscle pathology such as insulin resistance and sarcopenia. However, most of the studies regarding epigenetic mechanisms on alcohol-related pathologies are in the liver and neuronal systems (Lang 2018), and research on the role of epigenetic alterations on alcohol-induced skeletal muscle dysfunction is warranted.

Alcohol-Mediated Muscle Changes in Exercise and Interorgan Communication

Exercise

Regular exercise training confers wide-ranging, whole-body health benefits and is a powerful tool to decrease risk of many chronic conditions through adaptations such as improved SKM mass and function, SKM insulin sensitivity, and secretion of muscle-derived factors (Physical Activity Guidelines for Americans 2018; Severinsen and Pedersen 2020); **these adaptations make exercise an attractive lifestyle intervention to combat alcohol-associated myopathy**. However, findings from epidemiological studies demonstrate that individuals who participate in regular physical activity, especially vigorous intensity or strength exercise, consume alcohol more frequently and binge drink more often than sedentary individuals (Barry and Piazza-Gardner 2012; Dodge et al. 2017; French et al. 2009). Depending on exercise modality and acute programming variables (e.g., intensity, duration, rest periods, etc.), SKM adaptations to exercise training include increased muscular endurance, hypertrophy, strength, and power. In endurance-type exercise, exercise can be low, moderate, or high intensity. High-intensity exercise is further divided into heavy, severe, or exhaustive. SKM energy substrates and mechanisms of fatigue differ between these intensity domains. Skeletal muscle recovery from adaptation to exercise involves many of the processes discussed previously in this chapter and, as such, can be adversely affected by alcohol. Alcohol consumed prior to exercise may alter SKM metabolism and exercise capacity (Karvinen et al. 1962; Shaw et al. 2021) and, when it is consumed regularly throughout a training period, may adversely affect training adaptations such as muscle regeneration, hypertrophy, and function by mechanisms described above. Several variables including but not limited to alcohol timing, dose, nutritional status, sex, and exercise stimulus may influence effects of alcohol on exercise and recovery measures. Elucidation of such factors is essential to inform exercise prescription for individuals who consume alcohol or are recovering from AUD.

Much of the current body of literature regarding exercise and alcohol utilizes acute alcohol administration the day prior to or immediately following exercise sessions to examine influences on physiological responses and physical performance. Beer or Ethanol Effects on the Response to High Intensity Interval Training: A Controlled Study in Healthy Individuals (BEER-HIIT) study, examined muscle mass and performance parameters in humans when a moderate amount of alcohol was consumed regularly throughout training (~1 standard drink per day for women, 2 for men), and regular moderate alcohol intake did not affect lean mass accretion (Molina-Hidalgo et al. 2019) or increases in aerobic fitness, grip strength, or muscular power after 10 weeks of high-intensity interval training (Molina-Hidalgo et al. 2020).

Alcohol consumed the day prior to exercise may affect next-day exercise performance. An examination of heavy episodic drinking on next-day athletic performance in male rugby players revealed that the combination of self-selected alcohol intake (range of 6–20+ standard drinks) and sleep loss (~3 h) decreased lower body power performance but not isometric strength or sprint performance (Prentice et al. 2015). In the morning after a standardized dose of alcohol in active men and women (1.09 g ethanol/kg fat-free mass), muscle power, static and dynamic strength, and muscle fatigability were unaffected by alcohol; however, time to exhaustion in a severe-intensity cycling trial was decreased, with a combination of anaerobic and aerobic factors likely contributing to the observed decrease (Shaw et al. 2021). Decreased time to exhaustion in severe-intensity cycling has previously been observed after alcohol intake ranging from 1.0 to 2.4 g ethanol/kg body mass (Karvinen et al. 1962). A similar decrease in running performance was not observed the morning after women consumed two, four, or six bottles of beer (Kruisselbrink et al. 2006); differences in results may be explained by differences in exercise intensity. Combined, these studies demonstrate that binge drinking appears to negatively affect next-day severe-intensity exercise performance, but not muscular strength or power. Severe-intensity exercise is above maximal lactate steady state and relies heavily on anaerobic ATP production; therefore, decreased glycolytic function observed in vitro in alcohol-treated myoblasts (Levitt et al. 2020b) may be a potential mechanism of decreased severe-intensity exercise performance. Importantly, the role of hangover, or negative physical and mental symptoms following a single drinking episode that is often experienced the day after alcohol consumption (Verster et al. 2020), on exercise performance is unknown. More studies will aid in elucidating effects of alcohol consumption on next-day performance, relationship with hangover severity, and possible sex differences.

Alcohol is also often consumed following exercise or athletic performance. When men consume alcohol after resistance exercise, muscular strength and power recovery appears unaffected at doses ranging from 0.7 to 1.4 g ethanol/kg body mass (Levitt et al. 2020c). However, alcohol consumed after muscle-damaging exercise delays strength recovery in men at a higher (1.0 g ethanol/kg body mass) (Barnes et al. 2010) but not a lower (0.5 g ethanol/kg body mass) (Barnes et al. 2011) dose. In contrast, even at higher doses, delayed strength recovery was not observed among women (Levitt et al. 2017; McLeay et al. 2017). Exact mechanisms underlying these apparent sex differences in performance recovery when alcohol is consumed after muscle-damaging exercise are unknown but may involve potential protective effects of estrogens on muscle injury (Minahan et al. 2015; Williams et al. 2015).

As discussed, muscle damage, including exercise-induced muscle damage, requires an inflammatory response for repair. Acute binge alcohol consumption after resistance exercise decreased the early (3–5 h) inflammatory response during the postexercise period in a cohort of trained men and women (Levitt et al. 2016). When women consumed the same dose of alcohol after muscle-damaging resistance exercise involving a smaller amount of activated muscle, no significant decreases in inflammatory capacity were observed 5–48 h postexercise although moderate effect sizes for alcohol to prevent the increase in IL-1β and IL-6 suggest attenuation of inflammation in the postexercise period (Levitt et al. 2017). Whether alcohol modulates inflammatory capacity during the later (5–48 h) postexercise period in men remains to be observed; such sex differences are likely since alcohol delays strength recovery in men but not women as discussed previously. Although these changes in inflammatory capacity may impact the early muscle repair process, alcohol-mediated changes in intramuscular inflammation following exercise and impacts on tissue repair remain to be studied.

It is well known that an acute increase in hormones (e.g., testosterone, growth hormone, and cortisol) exists after moderately heavy, higher-volume resistance exercise (Kraemer and Ratamess 2005), but evidence regarding the importance of this acute hormonal response to resistance exercise adaptations is conflicting (Ronnestad et al. 2011; West and Phillips 2012; West et al. 2010). A systematic review found that alcohol consumed during exercise recovery augments postexercise cortisol and decreases testosterone (Lakicevic 2019), although results in the literature are incongruent. Most studies investigating the effect of alcohol on exercise-mediated hormonal responses are performed in young men. Binge alcohol consumed after resistance exercise consistently prolongs or augments the exercise-induced increase in cortisol (Haugvad et al. 2014; Koziris et al. 2000), indicating a potentially extended catabolic state. However, acute binge alcohol decreases the postexercise testosterone to cortisol ratio (Haugvad et al. 2014), does not affect circulating testosterone levels (Koziris et al. 2000), or prolongs the resistance exercise-induced elevation in free and total testosterone (Vingren et al. 2013). Mechanisms underlying the latter result are unknown, and whether alcohol simultaneously decreased intramuscular androgen receptor expression or nuclear translocation of activated androgen receptor, preventing the increased testosterone from exerting effects on gene expression, is unknown. Disparate findings between studies are likely due to differences in alcohol dosage, acute programming variables, and timing of measurement. Because testosterone and growth hormone can stimulate muscle protein synthesis and cortisol can stimulate muscle protein breakdown, it is thought that their elevation may contribute to increased protein turnover after resistance exercise, so alcohol-mediated changes in postexercise hormone levels could alter protein balance.

Furthermore, expression of *MyoD* in SKM at 12-h postexercise was increased in response to an exercise-induced acute hormonal response after muscle damage in men but not women (Luk et al. 2019). Therefore, antagonism of the anabolic hormonal milieu by postexercise alcohol may negatively affect not only muscle protein balance but also muscle regeneration after exercise-induced muscle damage, particularly in men. Effects of postexercise alcohol on the resistance exercise-induced hormonal response in women and long-term physiological consequences of observed changes remain unexplored.

SKM protein turnover increases after exercise, and with proper postexercise nutrition, muscle protein synthesis exceeds breakdown contributing to muscle protein accretion. As discussed, the mTOR signaling pathway is central to protein synthesis. mTOR signaling is activated after exercise, particularly resistance exercise that requires SKM to generate high force. When it is consumed postexercise, alcohol attenuated mTOR signaling (Duplanty et al. 2017b; Parr et al. 2014) and increased protein synthesis (Parr et al. 2014). Importantly, the alcohol-mediated attenuation in mTOR and S6K1 phosphorylation was observed in men but not in women (Duplanty et al. 2017b). Whether more severe impacts on postexercise mTOR pathway signaling would be observed with higher doses of alcohol remains to be determined.

Interorgan Cross Talk

Alcohol-induced SKM pathology extends well beyond the SKM. For instance, effects of alcohol on SKM wasting significantly contribute to alcohol-related liver disease mortality (Vary et al. 2008). SKM is heavily involved in whole-body metabolism and secretes bioactive material allowing for communication with itself or other tissues in an autocrine, paracrine, or endocrine manner.

Cytokines and growth factors are released from SKM according to muscle status (e.g., exercise, trauma, or disuse). These cytokines and growth factors are referred to as myokines but are not necessarily muscle specific. Myokines facilitate communication between skeletal muscle and multiple tissues including the adipose tissue, bone, liver, pancreas, intestine, vasculature, skin, and brain (Severinsen and Pedersen 2020) and can affect lipid and glucose metabolism, bone formation, and cognition. IL-6 and IL-15 are myokines expressed in SKM and are dysregulated in people with AUD (Gonzalez-Reimers et al. 2011). IL-15 is implicated in both bone and fat metabolism (Kaji 2016), while IL-6 has a number of effects on multiple tissues such as browning of white adipose tissue, increasing insulin-dependent glucose uptake, anti-inflammatory effects, regulation of bone formation, and appetite suppression (Severinsen and Pedersen 2020).

In addition to myokines, extracellular vesicles (EVs) can mediate interorgan communication. EVs are nanometer-sized particles with a lipid bilayer that prevents nucleases and proteases from degrading their cargo in circulation. EVs are divided into three main categories based on size and mechanism of biogenesis including exosomes (50–150 nm), microvesicles (100–1000 nm), and apoptotic bodies (50–5000 nm). It was once thought to be a method of cellular waste disposal; EVs are now known to function as vehicles for the transport of bioactive material including miRNAs, proteins, and lipids between cells. Exosomes are the subset of EVs that have piqued the most interest because of their highly regulated biogenesis and function (Vechetti Jr. 2019). While microvesicles directly bud off the cell membrane to enter the extracellular space, exosome biogenesis is more complex. Exosome biogenesis begins with an endosome created from the invagination of the cell membrane. Intraluminal vesicles are formed through the inward budding of the endosome containing bioactive material. An endosome with intraluminal vesicles is a multivesicular body. The multivesicular body can fuse with the cell membrane to release intraluminal vesicles that exit the cell as exosomes. Although the term exosome is frequently used to describe small EVs, the broad term "extracellular vesicle" is favored because of limitations in isolating a specific type of EV.

Most alcohol-induced EV pathology studies have focused in the liver. Alcohol exposure leads to an increase in miRNA-122 and miRNA-19b in hepatocyte EVs. These miRNAs can be transferred to monocytes to make them more sensitive to infection or to hepatic stellate cells to increase fibrosis (Brandon-Warner et al. 2016; Cardellach et al. 1992; Momen-Heravi et al. 2014; Song and Rubin 1972). In addition to altering hepatocyte-derived EVs, alcohol exposure has been shown to alter miRNA or protein cargo of EVs from immune cells, pancreatic islet cells, cardiomyocytes, endothelium, and epithelium (Rahman et al. 2020).

Additional studies are required to fill gaps regarding the effect of alcohol on extrahepatic tissue EVs including SKM. It is clear, however, that myotubes secrete EVs that can function in a variety of ways including increasing myoblast differentiation and increasing beta cell proliferation through the transfer of miRNAs (Rome et al. 2019). Additionally, exercise causes an increase in SKM EV release into circulation, and the miRNA cargo likely contributes to neutralizing ROS and increasing pancreatic beta cell function (Vechetti Jr. et al. 2021). SKM is actively involved in cross talk between organs through the release of myokines and EVs. Accordingly, it is expected that alcohol-induced SKM pathology, including alcohol-related myopathy, contributes to impairments in organ to organ communication and can contribute substantially to chronic disease morbidity and mortality (Fig. 4)

Applications to Public Health: The Aging Population

People over the age of 65 are the growing demographic globally and account for more than 20% of the population in 17 countries and will account for 61% of the population by the year 2100 (Department of Economic and Social Affairs 2019). Biologically, aging is due to accumulation of molecular and cellular damage, leading to decreased physical and mental capacity and increased vulnerability to diseases. Though differences in health are partly genetic, psychosocial, and behavioral, environments play a critical role in healthy aging. The prevalence of lifestyle

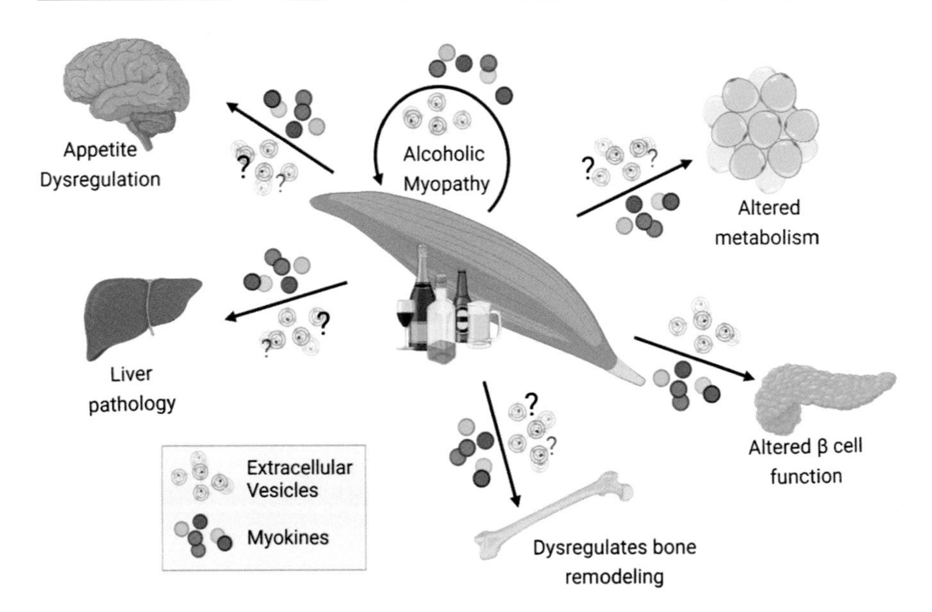

Fig. 4 Alcohol dysregulates muscle-organ cross talk. Alcohol-induced skeletal muscle pathology dysregulates the release of myokines and extracellular vesicles that modulate adipose, pancreas, bone, liver, and brain function and contribute substantially to alcohol-mediated chronic disease burden. Created with BioRender.com

behaviors including at-risk alcohol use is steadily increasing over the past two decades, particularly among women. About 50% of the people over the age of 65 drink alcohol, and approximately 30% of hospitalized older individuals are diagnosed with AUD (Caputo et al. 2012). About 30% of community dwelling and 50% of assisted care facility residents experience falls and fall-related fractures leading to a higher incidence of immobilization, prolonged bed rest, and muscle atrophy and represent the leading cause of injury-related deaths in the aging population (Hartholt et al. 2011; Orces 2013a), with chronic alcohol use representing a significant risk factor (Orces 2013b). Women are at an even higher risk for fractures due to the increased prevalence of osteoporosis, frailty, and decreased muscle strength. There is reduced muscle reserve (Ji et al. 2016), and preinjury functional levels are seldom regained in elderly patients (Wehren et al. 2005). Thus, alcohol use among older individuals exacerbates sarcopenia, and since loss of muscle mass and function is a significant predictor of morbidity and mortality (Volaklis et al. 2015; Wang et al. 2019), it signifies the public health relevance of this problem. Research has shown that alcohol exacerbates biological aging. Mechanisms discussed in this chapter demonstrate an aging muscle phenotype with a shift in anabolic signaling and reduced regenerative capacity ultimately leading to muscle loss. Thus, not only does alcohol induce muscle pathologies but additively adversely affects age-related changes in the muscle, compounding effects and increasing morbidity and mortality among aging individuals.

Key Facts

1. Alcohol's effects on muscle regenerative capacity
2. Alcohol's effect on muscle protein synthesis and breakdown
3. Alcohol's modulation of mitochondrial function
4. Epigenomic adaptations in the muscle due to alcohol
5. Alcohol's effects on exercise adaptations

Mini-dictionary

Alcohol use disorder (AUD) – it is a medical condition in which an individual has impaired ability to stop or control alcohol use despite adverse social, occupational, or health consequences. To be diagnosed with AUD, an individual should have two or more symptoms as outlined in the fifth edition of the *Diagnostic and Statistical Manual of Mental Disorders* (DSM-5).

At-risk alcohol use – it is alcohol use that can have biological and social consequences including heavy episodic drinking, binge drinking, or increased frequent drinking. Heavy episodic drinking is defined as consuming 60 g of alcohol or more on at least one occasion in the past 30 days. Binge drinking is defined as drinking to elevate blood alcohol concentrations to 0.08% (80 mg/dl) or higher and generally occurs with drinking four (women) or five (men) drinks over a 2-h time frame.

Muscle regenerative capacity – it is the ability of muscle stem cells, satellite cells, to commit to the myogenic lineage, proliferate, and differentiate to form myotubes that fuse to existing myofibers or form new myofibers.

Extracellular matrix – it is also defined as the matrisome, the non-cellular component in tissues that provides physical scaffolding for the cells and the critical biochemical and biomechanical cues for tissue morphogenesis, differentiation, homeostasis, and function.

Muscle protein synthesis – the muscle synthesizes protein in response to anabolic stimuli including amino acids, hormones such as insulin and insulin-like growth factor [IGF] 1, and mechanical loading. The major signaling pathway is the mammalian target of rapamycin (mTOR) pathway.

Muscle protein breakdown – it includes two major pathways, ubiquitin proteasome pathway (UPP) system and autophagy. UPP is protein degradation by covalent attachment of multiple ubiquitin molecules to the protein substrate and degradation of the targeted protein by the 26S proteasome complex that releases free and reusable ubiquitin. Autophagy is proteolytic degradation of cytosolic components at the lysosome. In macroautophagy, cytoplasmic cargo is packaged in a double membrane-bound vesicle, the autophagosome, that fuses with the lysosome to form an autolysosome. In microautophagy, cytosolic components are directly taken up by the lysosome by invagination of the lysosomal membrane leading to protein breakdown.

Mitochondrial bioenergetics – it is the production of ATP through oxidative phosphorylation.

Mitochondrial dynamics – it is the joining (fusion) and separation (fission) of components of the mitochondrial network.

Epigenetic changes – these are alterations in gene expression without changes in the DNA sequence. Epigenetic modifications include DNA methylation, histone modifications, and noncoding RNAs that alter the transcription or translation of genes and lead to altered gene expression.

Extracellular vesicles – these are nanometer-sized particles with a lipid bilayer that are released by most cells. They are classified based on the size as exosomes (50–150 nm), microvesicles (100–1000 nm), and apoptotic bodies (50–5000 nm). Exosomes are a subset of EVs that carry functional cargo such as protein, lipids, and microRNAs and can modulate function of other cells in a paracrine or endocrine manner.

Summary Points

1. Mechanisms implicated in alcohol-induced myopathy are multifactorial and interrelated.
2. Alcohol decreases differentiation potential of muscle stem cells and reduces regenerative capacity contributing to delayed or impaired recovery following atrophy, injury, and exercise.
3. Alcohol-induced alterations in host immune function contribute to dysregulation of muscle regenerative mechanisms.
4. Alcohol impairs bioenergetic homeostasis and anabolic/catabolic balance at the cellular and tissue level leading to decreased functional muscle mass and exercise capacity.
5. Alcohol dysregulates muscle mitochondrial function increasing oxidative stress.

Future Issues

1. Evidence indicates that alcohol induces epigenomic adaptations in the muscle. Further research is needed to identify how these adaptations mechanistically contribute to alcohol-related myopathy.
2. Research to identify dynamic interactions of the matrisome and stem cells that are critical for muscle regenerative capacity is warranted to improve muscle recovery strategies following injury or atrophy.
3. The impact of muscle extracellular vesicle cargo on interorgan communication needs to be established and their utility as therapeutic vehicles explored. Whether exercise can modulate alcohol-induced alterations of myokines and extracellular vesicle cargo is merited.

4. Utilizing multiomics technologies and multiscale computational modeling of alcohol-associated muscle changes and their contribution to interorgan communication and pathophysiology must be established.

References

Adler K, Molina PE, Simon L (2019) Epigenomic mechanisms of alcohol-induced impaired differentiation of skeletal muscle stem cells; role of Class IIA histone deacetylases. Physiol Genomics 51:471–479. https://doi.org/10.1152/physiolgenomics.00043.2019

Afshar M et al (2015) Acute immunomodulatory effects of binge alcohol ingestion. Alcohol 49: 57–64. https://doi.org/10.1016/j.alcohol.2014.10.002

Arnold L et al (2007) Inflammatory monocytes recruited after skeletal muscle injury switch into antiinflammatory macrophages to support myogenesis. J Exp Med 204:1057–1069. https://doi.org/10.1084/jem.20070075

Association AP (2013) Diagnostic and statistical manual of mental disorders, 5th edn. American Psychiatric Association

Barnes MJ, Mundel T, Stannard SR (2010) Post-exercise alcohol ingestion exacerbates eccentric-exercise induced losses in performance. Eur J Appl Physiol 108:1009–1014. https://doi.org/10.1007/s00421-009-1311-3

Barnes MJ, Mundel T, Stannard SR (2011) A low dose of alcohol does not impact skeletal muscle performance after exercise-induced muscle damage. Eur J Appl Physiol 111:725–729. https://doi.org/10.1007/s00421-010-1655-8

Barry AE, Piazza-Gardner AK (2012) Drunkorexia: understanding the co-occurrence of alcohol consumption and eating/exercise weight management behaviors. J Am Coll Heal 60:236–243. https://doi.org/10.1080/07448481.2011.587487

Bodine SC (2013) Disuse-induced muscle wasting. Int J Biochem Cell Biol 45:2200–2208. https://doi.org/10.1016/j.biocel.2013.06.011

Bodine SC et al (2001) Akt/mTOR pathway is a crucial regulator of skeletal muscle hypertrophy and can prevent muscle atrophy in vivo. Nat Cell Biol 3:1014–1019. https://doi.org/10.1038/ncb1101-1014

Brandon-Warner E et al (2016) Processing of miR17-92 cluster in hepatic stellate cells promotes hepatic fibrogenesis during alcohol-induced injury. Alcohol Clin Exp Res 40:1430–1442. https://doi.org/10.1111/acer.13116

Caputo F et al (2012) Alcohol use disorders in the elderly: a brief overview from epidemiology to treatment options. Exp Gerontol 47:411–416. https://doi.org/10.1016/j.exger.2012.03.019

Cardellach F et al (1992) Oxidative metabolism in muscle mitochondria from patients with chronic alcoholism. Ann Neurol 31:515–518. https://doi.org/10.1002/ana.410310509

Carvalho AF, Heilig M, Perez A, Probst C, Rehm J (2019) Alcohol use disorders. Lancet 394: 781–792. https://doi.org/10.1016/S0140-6736(19)31775-1

Cederbaum AI (2012) Alcohol metabolism. Clin Liver Dis 16:667–685. https://doi.org/10.1016/j.cld.2012.08.002

Chen GQ et al (2012) Altered microRNA expression in skeletal muscle results from high-fat diet-induced insulin resistance in mice. Mol Med Rep 5:1362–1368. https://doi.org/10.3892/mmr.2012.824

Clary CR, Guidot DM, Bratina MA, Otis JS (2011) Chronic alcohol ingestion exacerbates skeletal muscle myopathy in HIV-1 transgenic rats. AIDS Res Ther 8:30. https://doi.org/10.1186/1742-6405-8-30

Crowell KT, Laufenberg LJ, Lang CH (2019) Chronic alcohol consumption, but not acute intoxication, decreases In Vitro skeletal muscle contractile function. Alcohol Clin Exp Res 43: 2090–2099. https://doi.org/10.1111/acer.14179

Dasarathy J, McCullough AJ, Dasarathy S (2017) Sarcopenia in alcoholic liver disease: clinical and molecular advances. Alcohol Clin Exp Res 41:1419–1431. https://doi.org/10.1111/acer.13425
Davuluri G et al (2021) Activated protein phosphatase 2A disrupts nutrient sensing balance between mechanistic target of Rapamycin Complex 1 and adenosine monophosphate-activated protein kinase, causing Sarcopenia in alcohol-associated liver disease. Hepatology 73:1892–1908. https://doi.org/10.1002/hep.31524
DeFronzo RA, Tripathy D (2009) Skeletal muscle insulin resistance is the primary defect in type 2 diabetes. Diabetes Care 32(Suppl 2):S157–S163. https://doi.org/10.2337/dc09-S302
Dekeyser GJ, Clary CR, Otis JS (2013) Chronic alcohol ingestion delays skeletal muscle regeneration following injury. Regen Med Res 1:2. https://doi.org/10.1186/2050-490X-1-2
Department of Economic and Social Affairs (2019) P. D. World population ageing 2019: highlights (ST/ESA/SER.A/430). Report No. ISBN: 978-92-1-148325-3. United Nations
Dodd T et al (2014) Chronic binge alcohol administration accentuates expression of pro-fibrotic and inflammatory genes in the skeletal muscle of simian immunodeficiency virus-infected macaques. Alcohol Clin Exp Res 38:2697–2706. https://doi.org/10.1111/acer.12545
Dodge T, Clarke P, Dwan R (2017) The relationship between physical activity and alcohol use among adults in the United States. Am J Health Promot 31:97–108. https://doi.org/10.1177/0890117116664710
Dumont NA, Bentzinger CF, Sincennes MC, Rudnicki MA (2015) satellite cells and skeletal muscle regeneration. Compr Physiol 5:1027–1059. https://doi.org/10.1002/cphy.c140068
Duplanty AA, Simon L, Molina PE (2017a) Chronic binge alcohol-induced dysregulation of mitochondrial-related genes in skeletal muscle of simian immunodeficiency virus-infected Rhesus macaques at end-stage disease. Alcohol Alcohol 52:298–304. https://doi.org/10.1093/alcalc/agw107
Duplanty AA et al (2017b) Effect of acute alcohol ingestion on resistance exercise-induced mTORC1 signaling in human muscle. J Strength Cond Res 31:54–61. https://doi.org/10.1519/JSC.0000000000001468
Duplanty AA, Siggins RW, Allerton T, Simon L, Molina PE (2018) Myoblast mitochondrial respiration is decreased in chronic binge alcohol administered simian immunodeficiency virus-infected antiretroviral-treated rhesus macaques. Phys Rep 6. https://doi.org/10.14814/phy2.13625
Eisner V, Lenaers G, Hajnoczky G (2014) Mitochondrial fusion is frequent in skeletal muscle and supports excitation-contraction coupling. J Cell Biol 205:179–195. https://doi.org/10.1083/jcb.201312066
Esteves JV, Enguita FJ, Machado UF (2017) MicroRNAs-mediated regulation of skeletal muscle GLUT4 expression and translocation in insulin resistance. J Diabetes Res 2017:7267910. https://doi.org/10.1155/2017/7267910
Farrar RP, Martin TP, Abraham LD, Erickson CK (1982) The interaction of endurance running and ethanol on skeletal muscle mitochondria. Life Sci 30:67–75. https://doi.org/10.1016/0024-3205(82)90637-3
French MT, Popovici I, Maclean JC (2009) Do alcohol consumers exercise more? Findings from a national survey. Am J Health Promot 24:2–10. https://doi.org/10.4278/ajhp.0801104
Gonzalez-Reimers E et al (2011) Interleukin-15 and other myokines in chronic alcoholics. Alcohol Alcohol 46:529–533. https://doi.org/10.1093/alcalc/agr064
González-Reimers E, Quintero-Platt G, González-Arnay E, Martín-González C, Romero-Acevedo-L, Santolaria-Fernández F (2019) Alcoholic myopathy. Elsevier, pp 529–547
Grant BF et al (2017) Prevalence of 12-month alcohol use, high-risk drinking, and DSM-IV alcohol use disorder in the United States, 2001–2002 to 2012–2013: results from the National Epidemiologic Survey on alcohol and related conditions. JAMA Psychiatry 74:911–923. https://doi.org/10.1001/jamapsychiatry.2017.2161
Grucza RA et al (2018) Trends in adult alcohol use and binge drinking in the early 21st-century United States: a meta-analysis of 6 National Survey Series. Alcohol Clin Exp Res 42:1939–1950. https://doi.org/10.1111/acer.13859

Hartholt KA, Stevens JA, Polinder S, van der Cammen TJ, Patka P (2011) Increase in fall-related hospitalizations in the United States, 2001–2008. J Trauma 71:255–258. https://doi.org/10.1097/TA.0b013e31821c36e7

Hasin DS, Grant BF (2015) The National Epidemiologic Survey on Alcohol and Related Conditions (NESARC) waves 1 and 2: review and summary of findings. Soc Psychiatry Psychiatr Epidemiol 50:1609–1640. https://doi.org/10.1007/s00127-015-1088-0

Haugvad A, Haugvad L, Hamarsland H, Paulsen G (2014) Ethanol does not delay muscle recovery but decreases testosterone/cortisol ratio. Med Sci Sports Exerc 46:2175–2183. https://doi.org/10.1249/MSS.0000000000000339

Hodson N, West DWD, Philp A, Burd NA, Moore DR (2019) Molecular regulation of human skeletal muscle protein synthesis in response to exercise and nutrients: a compass for overcoming age-related anabolic resistance. Am J Phys Cell Phys 317:C1061–C1078. https://doi.org/10.1152/ajpcell.00209.2019

Hong-Brown LQ, Brown CR, Kazi AA, Navaratnarajah M, Lang CH (2012) Rag GTPases and AMPK/TSC2/Rheb mediate the differential regulation of mTORC1 signaling in response to alcohol and leucine. Am J Phys Cell Phys 302:C1557–C1565. https://doi.org/10.1152/ajpcell.00407.2011

Hunter RJ et al (2003) Alcohol affects the skeletal muscle proteins, titin and nebulin in male and female rats. J Nutr 133:1154–1157. https://doi.org/10.1093/jn/133.4.1154

Jewell JL, Russell RC, Guan KL (2013) Amino acid signalling upstream of mTOR. Nat Rev Mol Cell Biol 14:133–139. https://doi.org/10.1038/nrm3522

Ji HM et al (2016) Sarcopenia and sarcopenic obesity in patients undergoing orthopedic surgery. Clin Orthop Surg 8:194–202. https://doi.org/10.4055/cios.2016.8.2.194

Kaji H (2016) Effects of myokines on bone. Bonekey Rep 5:826. https://doi.org/10.1038/bonekey.2016.48

Karvinen E, Miettinen M, Ahlman K (1962) Physical performance during hangover. Q J Stud Alcohol 23:208–215

Khayrullin A et al (2016) Chronic alcohol exposure induces muscle atrophy (myopathy) in zebrafish and alters the expression of microRNAs targeting the Notch pathway in skeletal muscle. Biochem Biophys Res Commun 479:590–595. https://doi.org/10.1016/j.bbrc.2016.09.117

Koh JH, Kim KH, Park SY, Kim YW, Kim JY (2020) PPARdelta attenuates alcohol-mediated insulin resistance by enhancing fatty acid-induced mitochondrial uncoupling and antioxidant defense in skeletal muscle. Front Physiol 11:749. https://doi.org/10.3389/fphys.2020.00749

Korzick DH, Sharda DR, Pruznak AM, Lang CH (2013) Aging accentuates alcohol-induced decrease in protein synthesis in gastrocnemius. Am J Phys Regul Integr Comp Phys 304:R887–R898. https://doi.org/10.1152/ajpregu.00083.2013

Koziris LP, Kraemer WJ, Gordon SE, Incledon T, Knuttgen HG (2000) Effect of acute postexercise ethanol intoxication on the neuroendocrine response to resistance exercise. J Appl Physiol 1985(88):165–172. https://doi.org/10.1152/jappl.2000.88.1.165

Kraemer WJ, Ratamess NA (2005) Hormonal responses and adaptations to resistance exercise and training. Sports Med 35:339–361. https://doi.org/10.2165/00007256-200535040-00004

Kruisselbrink LD, Martin KL, Megeney M, Fowles JR, Murphy RJ (2006) Physical and psychomotor functioning of females the morning after consuming low to moderate quantities of beer. J Stud Alcohol 67:416–420. https://doi.org/10.15288/jsa.2006.67.416

Kumar A et al (2019) Oxidative stress mediates ethanol-induced skeletal muscle mitochondrial dysfunction and dysregulated protein synthesis and autophagy. Free Radic Biol Med 145: 284–299. https://doi.org/10.1016/j.freeradbiomed.2019.09.031

Lakicevic N (2019) The effects of alcohol consumption on recovery following resistance exercise: a systematic review. J Funct Morphol Kinesiol 4. https://doi.org/10.3390/jfmk4030041

Lang CH (2018) Lack of sexual dimorphism on the inhibitory effect of alcohol on muscle protein synthesis in rats under basal conditions and after anabolic stimulation. Phys Rep 6:e13929. https://doi.org/10.14814/phy2.13929

Lang CH et al (2004) Alcohol intoxication impairs phosphorylation of S6K1 and S6 in skeletal muscle independently of ethanol metabolism. Alcohol Clin Exp Res 28:1758–1767. https://doi.org/10.1097/01.alc.0000145787.66405.59

LeCapitaine NJ et al (2011) Disrupted anabolic and catabolic processes may contribute to alcohol-accentuated SAIDS-associated wasting. J Infect Dis 204:1246–1255. https://doi.org/10.1093/infdis/jir508

Lee DE et al (2016) microRNA-16 Is downregulated during insulin resistance and controls skeletal muscle protein accretion. J Cell Biochem 117:1775–1787. https://doi.org/10.1002/jcb.25476

Levitt DE et al (2016) The effect of postresistance exercise alcohol ingestion on lipopolysaccharide-stimulated cytokines. Eur J Appl Physiol 116:311–318. https://doi.org/10.1007/s00421-015-3278-6

Levitt DE et al (2017) Effect of alcohol after muscle-damaging resistance exercise on muscular performance recovery and inflammatory capacity in women. Eur J Appl Physiol 117: 1195–1206. https://doi.org/10.1007/s00421-017-3606-0

Levitt DE et al (2020a) Chronic alcohol dysregulates skeletal muscle myogenic gene expression after hind limb immobilization in female rats. Biomol Ther 10. https://doi.org/10.3390/biom10030441

Levitt DE, Chalapati N, Prendergast MJ, Simon L, Molina PE (2020b) Ethanol-impaired myogenic differentiation is associated with decreased myoblast glycolytic function. Alcohol Clin Exp Res 44:2166–2176. https://doi.org/10.1111/acer.14453

Levitt DE et al (2020c) Alcohol after resistance exercise does not affect muscle power recovery. J Strength Cond Res 34:1938–1944. https://doi.org/10.1519/JSC.0000000000002455

Li Y, Zhang F, Modrak S, Little A, Zhang H (2020) Chronic alcohol consumption enhances skeletal muscle wasting in mice bearing cachectic cancers: the role of TNFalpha/Myostatin Axis. Alcohol Clin Exp Res 44:66–77. https://doi.org/10.1111/acer.14221

Luk HY et al (2019) Resistance exercise-induced hormonal response promotes satellite cell proliferation in untrained men but not in women. Am J Physiol Endocrinol Metab 317: E421–E432. https://doi.org/10.1152/ajpendo.00473.2018

Mahdy MAA (2019) Skeletal muscle fibrosis: an overview. Cell Tissue Res 375:575–588. https://doi.org/10.1007/s00441-018-2955-2

Mandrekar P, Jeliazkova V, Catalano D, Szabo G (2007) Acute alcohol exposure exerts anti-inflammatory effects by inhibiting IkappaB kinase activity and p65 phosphorylation in human monocytes. J Immunol 178:7686–7693. https://doi.org/10.4049/jimmunol.178.12.7686

Mandrekar P, Bala S, Catalano D, Kodys K, Szabo G (2009) The opposite effects of acute and chronic alcohol on lipopolysaccharide-induced inflammation are linked to IRAK-M in human monocytes. J Immunol 183:1320–1327. https://doi.org/10.4049/jimmunol.0803206

McLeay Y, Stannard SR, Mundel T, Foskett A, Barnes M (2017) Effect of alcohol consumption on recovery from eccentric exercise induced muscle damage in females. Int J Sport Nutr Exerc Metab 27:115–121. https://doi.org/10.1123/ijsnem.2016-0171

Minahan C, Joyce S, Bulmer AC, Cronin N, Sabapathy S (2015) The influence of estradiol on muscle damage and leg strength after intense eccentric exercise. Eur J Appl Physiol 115: 1493–1500. https://doi.org/10.1007/s00421-015-3133-9

Molina PE, Lang CH, McNurlan M, Bagby GJ, Nelson S (2008) Chronic alcohol accentuates simian acquired immunodeficiency syndrome-associated wasting. Alcohol Clin Exp Res 32: 138–147. https://doi.org/10.1111/j.1530-0277.2007.00549.x

Molina-Hidalgo C, De-la OA, Jurado-Fasoli L, Amaro-Gahete FJ, Castillo MJ (2019) Beer or ethanol effects on the body composition response to high-intensity interval training. The BEER-HIIT Study. Nutrients 11(4):909. https://doi.org/10.3390/nu11040909

Molina-Hidalgo C, De-la OA, Dote-Montero M, Amaro-Gahete FJ, Castillo MJ (2020) Influence of daily beer or ethanol consumption on physical fitness in response to a high-intensity interval training program. The BEER-HIIT study. J Int Soc Sports Nutr 17:29. https://doi.org/10.1186/s12970-020-00356-7

Momen-Heravi F, Bala S, Bukong T, Szabo G (2014) Exosome-mediated delivery of functionally active miRNA-155 inhibitor to macrophages. Nanomedicine 10:1517–1527. https://doi.org/10.1016/j.nano.2014.03.014

Nguyen VA et al (2012) Impaired insulin/IGF signaling in experimental alcohol-related myopathy. Nutrients 4:1058–1075. https://doi.org/10.3390/nu4081058

Nicolas JM et al (2003) Influence of nutritional status on alcoholic myopathy. Am J Clin Nutr 78: 326–333. https://doi.org/10.1093/ajcn/78.2.326

Oh KH, Sheoran S, Richmond JE, Kim H (2020) Alcohol induces mitochondrial fragmentation and stress responses to maintain normal muscle function in Caenorhabditis elegans. FASEB J 34: 8204–8216. https://doi.org/10.1096/fj.201903166R

Orces CH (2013a) Emergency department visits for fall-related fractures among older adults in the USA: a retrospective cross-sectional analysis of the National Electronic Injury Surveillance System all injury program, 2001–2008. BMJ Open 3. https://doi.org/10.1136/bmjopen-2012-001722

Orces CH (2013b) Prevalence and determinants of falls among older adults in Ecuador: an analysis of the SABE I Survey. Curr Gerontol Geriatr Res 2013:495468. https://doi.org/10.1155/2013/495468

Parr EB et al (2014) Alcohol ingestion impairs maximal post-exercise rates of myofibrillar protein synthesis following a single bout of concurrent training. PLoS One 9:e88384. https://doi.org/10.1371/journal.pone.0088384

Physical Activity Guidelines for Americans (2018) 2nd (sed). Washington, DC. https://health.gov/sites/default/files/2019-09/Physical_Activity_Guidelines_2nd_edition.pdf

Preedy VR et al (2001a) Alcoholic skeletal muscle myopathy: definitions, features, contribution of neuropathy, impact and diagnosis. Eur J Neurol 8:677–687. https://doi.org/10.1046/j.1468-1331.2001.00303.x

Preedy VR et al (2001b) Alcoholic myopathy: biochemical mechanisms. Drug Alcohol Depend 63: 199–205. https://doi.org/10.1016/s0376-8716(00)00219-2

Prentice C, Stannard SR, Barnes MJ (2015) Effects of heavy episodic drinking on physical performance in club level rugby union players. J Sci Med Sport 18:268–271. https://doi.org/10.1016/j.jsams.2014.04.009

Rahman MA, Patters BJ, Kodidela S, Kumar S (2020) Extracellular vesicles: intercellular mediators in alcohol-induced pathologies. J NeuroImmune Pharmacol 15:409–421. https://doi.org/10.1007/s11481-019-09848-z

Rome S, Forterre A, Mizgier ML, Bouzakri K (2019) Skeletal muscle-released extracellular vesicles: state of the art. Front Physiol 10:929. https://doi.org/10.3389/fphys.2019.00929

Ronnestad BR, Nygaard H, Raastad T (2011) Physiological elevation of endogenous hormones results in superior strength training adaptation. Eur J Appl Physiol 111:2249–2259. https://doi.org/10.1007/s00421-011-1860-0

Severinsen MCK, Pedersen BK (2020) Muscle-Organ crosstalk: the emerging roles of myokines. Endocr Rev 41. https://doi.org/10.1210/endrev/bnaa016

Shaw A, Chae S, Levitt DE, Nicholson JL, Vingren JL, Hill DW (2021) Effect of previous day alcohol ingestion on muscle function and performance of severe intensity exercise. Int J Sports Physiol Perform. https://doi.org/10.1123/ijspp.2020-0790

Shukla SD, Zakhari S (2013) Epigenetics–new frontier for alcohol research. Alcohol Res 35:1–2

Simon L et al (2014) Chronic binge alcohol consumption alters myogenic gene expression and reduces in vitro myogenic differentiation potential of myoblasts from rhesus macaques. Am J Phys Regul Integr Comp Phys 306:R837–R844. https://doi.org/10.1152/ajpregu.00502.2013

Simon L, Hollenbach AD, Zabaleta J, Molina PE (2015) Chronic binge alcohol administration dysregulates global regulatory gene networks associated with skeletal muscle wasting in simian immunodeficiency virus-infected macaques. BMC Genomics 16:1097. https://doi.org/10.1186/s12864-015-2329-z

Simon L, Jolley SE, Molina PE (2017a) Alcoholic myopathy: pathophysiologic mechanisms and clinical implications. Alcohol Res 38:207–217

Simon L et al (2017b) Decreased myoblast differentiation in chronic binge alcohol-administered simian immunodeficiency virus-infected male macaques: role of decreased miR-206. Am J Phys Regul Integr Comp Phys 313:R240–R250. https://doi.org/10.1152/ajpregu.00146.2017

Singh SS et al (2021) Multiomics-identified intervention to restore ethanol-induced dysregulated proteostasis and secondary sarcopenia in alcoholic liver disease. Cell Physiol Biochem 55: 91–116. https://doi.org/10.33594/000000327

Song SK, Rubin E (1972) Ethanol produces muscle damage in human volunteers. Science 175: 327–328. https://doi.org/10.1126/science.175.4019.327

Steiner JL, Lang CH (2015) Dysregulation of skeletal muscle protein metabolism by alcohol. Am J Physiol Endocrinol Metab 308:E699–E712. https://doi.org/10.1152/ajpendo.00006.2015

Steiner JL, Lang CH (2019) Ethanol acutely antagonizes the refeeding-induced increase in mTOR-dependent protein synthesis and decrease in autophagy in skeletal muscle. Mol Cell Biochem 456:41–51. https://doi.org/10.1007/s11010-018-3488-4

Steiner JL, Pruznak AM, Navaratnarajah M, Lang CH (2015a) Alcohol differentially alters extracellular matrix and adhesion molecule expression in skeletal muscle and heart. Alcohol Clin Exp Res 39:1330–1340. https://doi.org/10.1111/acer.12771

Steiner JL, Crowell KT, Lang CH (2015b) Impact of alcohol on glycemic control and insulin action. Biomol Ther 5:2223–2246. https://doi.org/10.3390/biom5042223

Szabo G, Mandrekar P, Oak S, Mayerle J (2007) Effect of ethanol on inflammatory responses. Implications Pancreatitis Pancreatol 7:115–123. https://doi.org/10.1159/000104236

Thapaliya S et al (2014) Alcohol-induced autophagy contributes to loss in skeletal muscle mass. Autophagy 10:677–690. https://doi.org/10.4161/auto.27918

Tidball JG (2017) Regulation of muscle growth and regeneration by the immune system. Nat Rev Immunol 17:165–178. https://doi.org/10.1038/nri.2016.150

Vary TC, Frost RA, Lang CH (2008) Acute alcohol intoxication increases atrogin-1 and MuRF1 mRNA without increasing proteolysis in skeletal muscle. Am J Phys Regul Integr Comp Phys 294:R1777–R1789. https://doi.org/10.1152/ajpregu.00056.2008

Vechetti IJ Jr (2019) Emerging role of extracellular vesicles in the regulation of skeletal muscle adaptation. J Appl Physiol 1985(127):645–653. https://doi.org/10.1152/japplphysiol.00914.2018

Vechetti IJ Jr, Valentino T, Mobley CB, McCarthy JJ (2021) The role of extracellular vesicles in skeletal muscle and systematic adaptation to exercise. J Physiol 599:845–861. https://doi.org/10.1113/JP278929

Verster JC, Scholey A, van de Loo A, Benson S, Stock AK (2020) Updating the definition of the alcohol hangover. J Clin Med 9. https://doi.org/10.3390/jcm9030823

Vingren JL, Hill DW, Buddhadev H, Duplanty A (2013) Postresistance exercise ethanol ingestion and acute testosterone bioavailability. Med Sci Sports Exerc 45:1825–1832. https://doi.org/10.1249/MSS.0b013e31828d3767

Volaklis KA, Halle M, Meisinger C (2015) Muscular strength as a strong predictor of mortality: a narrative review. Eur J Intern Med 26:303–310. https://doi.org/10.1016/j.ejim.2015.04.013

Wang H, Hai S, Liu Y, Liu Y, Dong B (2019) skeletal muscle mass as a mortality predictor among nonagenarians and centenarians: a prospective cohort study. Sci Rep 9:2420. https://doi.org/10.1038/s41598-019-38893-0

Wehren LE, Hawkes WG, Hebel JR, Orwig DL, Magaziner J (2005) Bone mineral density, soft tissue body composition, strength, and functioning after hip fracture. J Gerontol A Biol Sci Med Sci 60:80–84

West DW, Phillips SM (2012) Associations of exercise-induced hormone profiles and gains in strength and hypertrophy in a large cohort after weight training. Eur J Appl Physiol 112:2693–2702. https://doi.org/10.1007/s00421-011-2246-z

West DW et al (2010) Elevations in ostensibly anabolic hormones with resistance exercise enhance neither training-induced muscle hypertrophy nor strength of the elbow flexors. J Appl Physiol 1985(108):60–67. https://doi.org/10.1152/japplphysiol.01147.2009

Williams T, Walz E, Lane AR, Pebole M, Hackney AC (2015) The effect of estrogen on muscle damage biomarkers following prolonged aerobic exercise in eumenorrheic women. Biol Sport 32:193–198. https://doi.org/10.5604/20831862.1150300

Wyczechowska D et al (2017) A miRNA signature for cognitive deficits and alcohol use disorder in persons living with HIV/AIDS. Front Mol Neurosci 10:385. https://doi.org/10.3389/fnmol.2017.00385

Yin H, Price F, Rudnicki MA (2013) Satellite cells and the muscle stem cell niche. Physiol Rev 93:23–67. https://doi.org/10.1152/physrev.00043.2011

Yoo JI et al (2017) High prevalence of sarcopenia among binge drinking elderly women: a nationwide population-based study. BMC Geriatr 17:114. https://doi.org/10.1186/s12877-017-0507-3

Neuroimaging and Alcohol-Use Disorder (AUD) 46

Andriana Kakanakova

Contents

Introduction 970
Epidemiology 971
Mechanism of Action 972
Neuroimaging Techniques 972
Computed Tomography (CAT) 973
MRI 973
Functional MRI (fMRI) 974
Additional Functional Methods: PET, SPECT 976
Discussion 976
Applications to Other Areas of Substance-Use Disorders 977
Applications to Public Health 978
Mini-Dictionary of Terms 978
Key Facts of Neuroimaging and Alcohol-Use Disorder 978
Summary Points 979
References 979

Abstract

Alcohol-use disorder (AUD) is one of the most common substance-related disorders, causing significant health and economic consequences. There is race-, gender-, and sex-related differences, as well as different patterns of misuse or "drinking behaviors." Alcohol-use disorder is commonly comorbid to other substance abuses and other psychiatric disorders in general. There is obvious brain "damage" caused by alcohol misuse as found by neuroimaging techniques. Of course, the use of neuroimaging is not widely approved as to confirm AUD in diagnostic plan or as a tool in predicting the course of the disorder, but the contemporary research is focusing on doing so. This short chapter aims at systematizing the general findings via different neuroimaging methods in AUD.

A. Kakanakova (✉)
Department of Psychiatry and Medical Psychology, Medical University Plovdiv, Plovdiv, Bulgaria

V. B. Patel, V. R. Preedy (eds.), *Handbook of Substance Misuse and Addictions*,
https://doi.org/10.1007/978-3-030-92392-1_50

Keywords

Alcohol-use disorder · Neuroimaging · CAT · MRI · Voxel-based morphometry · Diffusion tensor magnetic resonance · fMRI · Magnetic resonance spectroscopy · Positron-emission tomography · Single-photon emission computed tomography

Abbreviations

ACC	Anterior cingulate cortex
AUD	Alcohol-use disorder
BDNF	Brain-derived neurotrophic factor
BOLD	Blood oxygen level dependent (contrast)
CAT	Computed tomography
CSF	Cerebrospinal fluid
DA	Dopamine
DLPFC	Dorsolateral prefrontal cortex
DTI	Diffusion tensor imaging
fMRI	Functional magnetic resonance imaging
GABA	Gamma-aminobutyric acid
LDLPFC	Left dorsolateral prefrontal cortex
MRS	Magnetic resonance spectroscopy
NAA	N-acetylaspartate
NAcc	Nucleus accumbens
OFC	Orbitofrontal cortex
PET	Positron-emission tomography
SPECT	Single-photon emission computed tomography
vmPFC	Ventromedial prefrontal cortex
VS	Ventral striatum
WHO	World Health Organization

Introduction

Alcohol, among all of the substances known to cause significant health (mental and physical) issues, is one of the most commonly misused. Being one of the legal substances, alongside nicotine and caffeine, is one of the major reasons for the free and easy access. In historical and cultural aspects, there has been attempts at making the use of alcohol illegal or at least complicated though with little success in decreasing the alcohol misuse-related consequences. The results of contemporary research on prevalence and mortality impose the urgent need for setting new strategies in limiting alcohol use.

Similar report has been published previously by the WHO in 2018, stating that alcohol misuse has led to three million deaths in 2016 or 5.3% of the world death rate, predominantly among males (Anderson 2018; Poznyak and Rekve 2018).

The financial impact of alcohol misuse has been evaluated by Sacks et al. to be approximately 249 billion USD in 2010 (Sacks et al. 2015), thus making AUD one of the biggest factors in medical economics. Furthermore, AUD is well known to be among the most common comorbidities in psychiatry. In a study on comorbidities, held in the USA in 1994, nearly half of the participants marked down at least one lifetime psychiatric disorder and 30% at least one in the last 12 months, where alcohol misuse, depression, social phobia, and other phobias were the most common (Kessler et al. 1994).

According to Kaplan and Sadock's Synopsis of Psychiatry, psychiatric comorbidities are in general more common in people suffering any substance use-related disorder (Sadock et al. 2015). On the other hand, there are specific psychiatric disorders that often lead to concomitant alcohol and other substance-use disorders, the most prominent one being the borderline personality disorder. In terms of high impulsivity and inability to postpone reward, alcohol and other substance uses are quite common among bipolar patients, especially during a manic state. The other major cause of the significant economic impact of AUD is the serious general medical health-related issues such as significant and often irreversible liver damage, increased blood pressure, and neurological complications like polyneuropathy, causing a real negative economic impact.

There is significant gender-related difference in alcohol misuse in terms of drinking behaviors, psychiatric and somatic comorbidities, impact on social functioning, and stigmatization.

Ever since the 1960s, with the development of CAT (computed tomography), there has been constant attempt in finding a minimally invasive method of studying the live human brain. Although early studies showed little or no diagnostic or prognostic value in brain imaging technique findings, with the development of neuroimaging, more and more possibilities emerged. Nowadays, the most prominent research lays in translational methods and in functional neuroimaging. Accordingly, for those studying the underlying pathological mechanisms in addiction and substance misuse, neuroimaging methods seem to be one of the most promising.

Epidemiology

Alcohol-use disorder is one of the most common substance use-related disorders, with the majority of the population drinking at least at a certain period of life. Usually, alcohol use originates in teenage years, with the quite common experience of intoxication in this period of life. According to Kaplan and Sadock's Synopsis of Psychiatry, the gender-related difference in alcohol consumption is 1.3/1.0 – men/women; in terms of religion, Jews are more likely to consume alcohol and less likely to develop AUD, and Irish are more likely to get in trouble due to alcohol use. AUD is common among Native Americans and Inuits not related to gender. AUD is the leading substance-related disorder in terms of death cause (Sadock et al. 2015).

Asians are producing lower levels of alcohol dehydrogenase and thus are more likely to develop intoxication. In gender-related differences, it is found that females develop earlier (or after shorter exposure) the expected somatic consequences, and they are more likely to develop intoxication with consumption of lesser amounts of alcohol (it is known that levels of alcohol dehydrogenase are lower in females). Males are expected to drink as a sign of "manhood," even in the majority of contemporary societies.

According to a recently published report by the Centers for Disease Control and Prevention, the rate of alcohol-related deaths exceeded 95,000 for the time period 2011–2015 only in the USA, with more than half of them due to chronic liver complications and more than 70% males, with almost half of the deaths in people aged 35–64 (Esser et al. 2020). This only confirms the significance of the alcohol misuse in public health and once again confirms the need for new strategies on decreasing alcohol consumption.

Mechanism of Action

The major mechanism of action of alcohol is linked to GABA, with alcohol known to potentiate the GABA inhibition by increased GABA release via GABA b receptors and acting as a ligand to GABA a receptors, reducing glutamate-mediated excitation by acting directly at presynaptic voltage-sensitive calcium channels or glutamate receptors, and modulating it by NMDA receptors. Alcohol is known to be active at opioid synapses within mesolimbic reward circuitry, leading to increased dopamine release either directly by μ-opioid receptors or by releasing endogenous opioids. Alcohol is also known to be active at cannabinoid receptors with this action not quite clarified yet (Stahl 2013).

Glutamate neurotransmission is the major culprit in alcohol addiction. Alcohol-use disorder (AUD) individuals show significant decrease of glutamate in the cingulate anterior cortex. Glutamate in key areas of the forebrain reward circuit is modulated by alcohol cues in early alcohol dependence (Cheng et al. 2018).

Neuroimaging Techniques

When one has to evaluate different neuroimaging techniques, the most suitable classification would be what exactly different methods measure. Accordingly, we differentiate between methods of structural neuroimaging, including native or contrast CAT scan, structural MRI methods as voxel-based morphometry, and DTI (diffusion tensor magnetic resonance). On top of that, different functional methods of neuroimaging are widely in use in scientific research, promising for future everyday clinical application. The functional methods include fMRI, magnetic resonance spectroscopy (MRS), positron-emission tomography (PET), and single-photon emission computed tomography (SPECT).

Alcohol-use disorder (AUD) is known to cause significant yet not quite specific damage in both the structure and function of the brain (Fauth-Bühler and Mann 2011). It is commonly associated with lower gray matter volume; with negative associations with widespread gray matter volume even among young adults, which has been found to be associated with the severity of the alcohol use in both adults and adolescents; and with lower gray matter volume and white matter integrity only in adults (Thayer et al. 2017).

The gray matter volume is significantly decreased in the mesocorticolimbic system in alcohol-dependent patients, including the dorsal posterior cingulate cortex, dorsal anterior cingulate cortex, medial prefrontal cortex, orbitofrontal cortex, and putamen. There is also decreased fractional anisotropy in the regions connecting the damaged gray matter areas with higher radial diffusivity value in the same areas and decreased resting-state functional connectivity within the reward network as found by Wang et al. (Wang et al. 2016).

Computed Tomography (CAT)

Although CAT is historically the first neuroimaging method, there are repeated findings of general "brain atrophy" presented by increased volumes of cerebrospinal fluid, enlarged brain ventricles especially the third, prefrontal cortical volume decrease, and cerebellum volume decrease as summarized by Fauth-Bühler and Mann in 2011.

More than that, there are some age- and gender-related differences such as faster development of the gray matter volume decrease in females or in older adults as stated in the same meta-analysis by Fauth-Buhler and Mann, 2011. Those findings unfortunately are not disorder specific but at least set the basis for future neuroimaging research in AUD.

MRI

With the development of magnetic resonance imaging, evidence supporting the CAT findings emerged with the early research, which was only providing data on the difference between AUD subjects and healthy controls and only later on being able to evaluate differences between individuals within the group of the AUD patients. The latest magnetic resonance methods include voxel-based morphometry (VBM), deformation-based morphometry, and diffusion tensor magnetic resonance imaging (DTI), all of them being able to study white matter changes as well as gray matter damage and CSF volumes (Table 1).

One recent meta-analysis of voxel-based morphometry(VBM) by Lee (Lee et al. 2014) finds lower gray matter volumes in the right cingulate gyrus, right insula, and left middle frontal gyrus in AUD patients compared to controls.

The most common finding repeats the general finding of earlier CAT studies being decrease in gray as well as white matter volumes and increase of CSF. More to that, it

Table 1 **Structural and functional changes in AUD**. The table summarizes the most common neuroimaging findings in AUD patients, utilizing the different neuroimaging methods

Structural changes in AUD
Increased volumes of cerebrospinal fluid, enlarged brain ventricles especially the third, prefrontal cortical volume decrease, and cerebellum volume decrease (CAT)
Lower gray matter volumes in the right cingulate gyrus, right insula, and left middle frontal gyrus (voxel-based morphometry)
Decrease in volume in the reward system structures (DLPFC–anterior insula–nucleus accumbens–amygdala)
White matter changes in different brain circuits in corpus callosum, medulla oblongata, midbrain, and connections between frontal cortex regions and limbic system (DTI)
Functional changes in AUD
Alcohol cue-related increase in VMPFC, DLPFC, mesolimbic areas, parietal and temporal cortex, precuneus, superior temporal gyrus (BOLD)
Lower glutamate levels in nucleus accumbens and ACC (MRS)
Increased glutamate levels in the hippocamp (MRS)
Greater loss of cortical NAA in frontal brain areas than parietal; increase of Cho/NAA in cerebellar vermis (1H-MRS)
Decreased NAA/Cr and NAA/Cho in cerebellum, frontal lobe, and thalamus
Decreased GABA + homocarnosine in occipital lobe
Increased myoinositol in anterior cingulate cortex, thalamus, and white matter; increased Cr, myoinositol, and Cho in parietal gray matter but not in white matter
Increased GABA and NAA (in the DLPFC, insula, superior corona radiata, and total brain reward system) in nonsmoking compared to smoking alcoholics
Low Cho and Cr, high Glu/Cr, and normal NAA in the anterior cingulate cortex

has linked this increase in CSF volumes to cortical gray matter volume decrease and decrease in volume in the reward system structures (DLPFC–anterior insula–nucleus accumbens–amygdala).

An interesting finding that repeats findings in CAT studies is that with abstinence there is a chance of brain volume recovery (Cardenas et al. 2007).

The MRI method of DTI has been used to observe the changes in the white matter in different brain circuits, and it has been found that in alcoholics, there are such changes in corpus callosum as well as in medulla oblongata and midbrain and in the connections between frontal cortex regions and limbic system. This specific method also confirms the age- and sex-related differences observed in CAT and voxel-based morphometry (Fauth-Bühler and Mann 2011).

Functional MRI (fMRI)

The fMRI is a method using different cues/paradigms to trigger activation in specific brain areas. The typical paradigms used in studying AUD are usually using alcohol versus water cues, including alcohol versus control smells, tastes, and performing neuroimaging before and after exposure. Visual stimuli known to trigger the reward circuits are also used.

Then, the BOLD contrast or glutamate is measured. The typical BOLD contrast findings include alcohol cue-related increase in specific areas of the brain such as VMPFC, DLPFC, mesolimbic areas, parietal and temporal cortex, precuneus, and superior temporal gyrus.

MRS or magnetic resonance spectroscopy measures glutamate levels most commonly, although it can use other metabolites such as N-acetylaspartate (NAA), choline (Cho), creatine (Cr), phosphocreatine, gamma-aminobutyric acid (GABA), and myoinositol (ml).

Usually, 1H is the most commonly used, but other isotopes can also be utilized, such as deuterium (2H), fluorine-19 (19F), phosphorus-31 (31P), and selenium-77 (77Se) (Fauth-Bühler and Mann 2011).

Glutamate metabolism shows promising results in predicting a possible alcohol misuse or relapse in abstinent alcoholics. The findings include lower glutamate levels in nucleus accumbens and ACC not only in individuals with current use but also in acute withdrawal or in abstinent patients (Niciu and Mason 2014).

Glutamate levels in left dorsolateral prefrontal cortex (LDLPFC) are also found to be linked to alcohol craving intensity in patients with AUD (Frye et al. 2016).

There is increased glutamate excitotoxicity in the hippocampus areas visualized by increased glutamate levels in the hippocampus, as studied by Hermens et al., of young adults with depression and risky drinking confirmed in 2015 (Hermens et al. 2015).

Decreased connectivity between the involved gray matter areas and higher radial diffusivity value in those areas are reported. There is decrease in resting-state functional connectivity within the reward network too.

An interesting research on neural correlates of prayer in alcohol use has been performed in Alcoholics Anonymous, where prayers have been associated with reduction in self-reported craving to some extent. Higher activation in left anterior middle frontal gyrus, left superior parietal lobule, bilateral precuneus, and bilateral posterior middle temporal gyrus shows the engagement of neural mechanisms of control of attention and emotion as published by Galanter et al. in 2017 (Galanter et al.).

Proton magnetic resonance spectroscopy ((1) H-MRS) studies have consistently found abnormal brain concentrations of N-acetylaspartate (NAA) and glutamate in individuals with alcohol-use disorders (AUD). There are even inverse associations between recent heavy drinking and dACC glutamate and NAA concentrations as demonstrated by Prisciandaro et al. in a study in 2016 (Prisciandaro et al. 2016).

Meyer (Meyer 2017) summarizes the most common MR spectroscopy findings in AUD in a review, with most consistent of them being greater loss of cortical NAA in frontal brain areas than parietal and increase of Cho/NAA in cerebellar vermis.

Reduced insular glucose concentration was associated with increased alcohol compulsions and, to a lesser extent, with greater alcohol use severity as found by Betka et al. in 2019 (Betka et al. 2019).

Decreased NAA/Cr and NAA/Cho in cerebellum, frontal lobe, and thalamus; decreased GABA + homocarnosine in occipital lobe; increased myoinositol in anterior cingulate cortex, thalamus, and white matter; increased Cr, myoinositol, and Cho in parietal gray matter but not in white matter; increased GABA and NAA (in the DLPFC, insula, superior corona radiata, and total brain reward system) in nonsmoking compared to smoking alcoholics; low Cho and Cr, high Glu/Cr, and normal NAA in the anterior cingulate cortex; and smaller volumes of frontal and temporal gray matter have been found (Meyerhoff 2014).

Proton magnetic resonance spectroscopy ((1) H-MRS) studies have consistently found abnormal brain concentrations of N-acetylaspartate (NAA) and glutamate in individuals with alcohol-use disorders (AUD). There are even inverse associations between recent heavy drinking and dACC glutamate and NAA concentrations as demonstrated by Prisciandaro et al (Prisciandaro et al. 2016).

Additional Functional Methods: PET, SPECT

Proton emission tomography and single proton emission computed tomography are neuroimaging methods using radioactive substances for monitoring the brain function by means of metabolism. Usually, blood flow, oxygen saturation, different enzyme activity, glucose metabolism, and different neurotransmitter activity are measured (Fauth-Bühler and Mann 2011).

In AUD individuals, what is monitored by PET is μ- and Δ-opioid receptor availability in specific brain areas such as nucleus accumbens (NAcc)/ventral striatum (VS), GABA receptor availability, and cannabinoid (CB1) receptors.

Moderate alcohol consumption reduces brain glucose uptake that is detected by PET, probably due to consumption of alcohol metabolites and alcohol itself (Niciu and Mason 2014). The most consistent findings report decreased metabolism in frontal areas of the brain, both cortical and subcortical.

PET and SPECT are used not only to monitor the metabolic changes but also to evaluate receptor densities as well. There is research on different receptor activities, such as GABA, serotonin, dopamine, and opioid receptors. It is found, as summarized by Bühler and Mann in 2011, that in general there is decrease in GABA receptor density, increase in μ-opioid receptor availability, and decrease in the number of serotonin and dopamine transporters and DA receptor density.

Discussion

With the tendency of instrumentalization of medicine and the urge of finding possible biomarkers in psychiatry, thus making it "more medical," the place of neuroimaging as a tool of objectification arouses. Substance-use disorders and AUD in particular should not be an exception. A lot of research has been done in this area with some consistent and as such promising findings, which can be considered as future biomarkers in AUD.

Possible areas of research are those that can be used for predicting which individuals are most likely to switch to misuse or "problem drinking," with studies on teenage or college students, patterns of alcohol use, and imprint on brain structure and function or studies on the impact of sobriety on reducing the brain damage. One such study by Heitzeg et al. (Heitzeg et al. 2015) finds blunted activation in the left middle frontal gyrus to inhibitory errors in a population of children monitored at base pre-teenage, and then only the ones that developed problem drinking have been matched to nondrinking controls. The same study finds increased NAcc activation during reward anticipation associated with higher rate of alcohol problems over 3–5 years of follow-up. Interesting work in this field has been published by Dager et al. in 2014 (Dager et al. 2014), which shows that young adults (age 18–23) who switch to heavy drinking show higher response to alcohol vs. nonalcohol pictures in cue-reactive circuitry (caudate, vmPFC, anterior cingulate, OFC, insula), which more to that predicts more alcohol involvement over 1-year follow-up.

Another emerging neuroimaging method is genotype-linked neuroimaging utilizing different techniques. One such study is that of Dalvie et al. in 2014 (Dalvie et al. 2014), which unfortunately failed to prove statistically significant findings between BDNF gene polymorphism, AUD, and structural brain changes in children with AUD and childhood trauma.

In conclusion, AUD is a disorder with significant impact on public health, there are some consistent findings in neuroimaging in AUD patients, and they deserve further research in order to be standardized as possible biomarkers used for prognostic or diagnostic aims in substance use-related disorders.

Applications to Other Areas of Substance-Use Disorders

In the chapter on neuroimaging and AUD, we have discussed the different neuroimaging techniques available nowadays and the most common findings in individuals with alcohol-use disorder. As AUD is one of the most frequent substance misuses, quite commonly comorbid to other substance use-related disorders, there are two directions to be involved with it. First, all the neuroimaging methods can be used in the evaluation and research on other substance use-related disorders, with the impact on reward system structures supposedly corresponding to those found in AUD patients. Second, other substance misuses need to be implicated as bias in research in cases of alcohol co-misuse. There are some specific correlations already emerging such as cannabinoid receptor activity of alcohol and possible interactions. Another common co-misuse is that of benzodiazepines and alcohol, with both substances sharing the receptor-binding activity at opioid and GABA receptors. Alcohol is a well-known brain depressant and as such is commonly misused simultaneously with other substances in order to relieve withdrawal symptoms or to boost intoxication ones.

Neuroimaging is obviously going to take greater part in contemporary and future clinical practice in order not only to evaluate the present structural damage but also to predict the course or the outcome in substance misuse.

Applications to Public Health

As we have stated in this chapter, AUD is the most common substance misuse, leading to thousands of deaths on a year basis and to common incapacitation. The use of alcohol is widely accepted and legal, and as such nonconsumers are more likely to be socially ostracized, compared to mild users. The easy access and legal status of the substance lead to common use and easier development of substance-related disorders. Alcohol is known to cause significant health (mental and somatic) issues, thus leading to a major impact on public health in medical and economical terms. Being able to predict the possible course and outcome of the disorder by means of neuroimaging techniques might allow for lesser taxing on public health. Another possible path of the impact of AUD on public health is the fact that probably the mostly used method of suicide is the combination of alcohol and benzodiazepines. Possible research using neuroimaging (for example, PET) can show promising findings on the combined effect of those two substances on opioid and GABA receptor density. It can even be speculated as to which individuals are going to have what effect with combined use of benzodiazepines and alcohol, which are known to have an additive effect, potentiating one another in simultaneous use.

Mini-Dictionary of Terms

- Dependence – a pattern of repeated use of a substance, which may include specific withdrawal clinical presentation, commonly labeled physical dependence.
- Abuse–use of a substance (medication, chemical, drug) different than the prescribed way or socially acceptable way.
- Misuse – when it is a matter of a legal substance, such as medication, alcohol, nicotine, and caffeine.
- Addiction – a state in which the individual experiences cravings for the substance and, if not able to use it, gets into a state of distress.
- Intoxication – substance-specific state caused by the intake of a certain substance, usually reversible with the impact on brain function, which results in behavioral changes.
- Withdrawal – substance-specific state caused by usually abrupt cessation of the intake of a certain substance.
- Tolerance – pharmacological phenomenon representing the developing of the need for a higher dose of a specific substance to have the same effect experienced previously with a lower dose of the substance.

Key Facts of Neuroimaging and Alcohol-Use Disorder

Neuroimaging first appeared on the scene in the middle of the twentieth century.
Ever since, it has been developing in order to give more precise picture of what is going on in the substrate of our mind – the brain.

There are quantitative as well as simply qualitative methods in the evaluation of brain structure and function.

Alcohol misuse is found to engage specific brain areas leading to changes in structure, connectivity, and function of the brain.

The effects of substances and alcohol in particular are possible to be observed and monitored by means of neuroimaging.

Summary Points

- Alcohol is one of the most commonly misused substances being legal in the majority of the states.
- It is known to cause significant economical and medical impact on world population.
- There are specific changes in brain areas related especially to reward that can be monitored by means of neuroimaging.
- CAT and MRI find decreased gray matter volumes, increased CSF volumes, and decreased white matter volumes (MRI).
- fMRI and MSI show changes in connectivity and in glutamate levels in DLPFC, VMPFC, precuneus, limbic system, and temporal and parietal cortical areas.
- PET and SPECT use radioactive ligands to mark the specific brain areas involved in different functional activities by nuclear neuroimaging.

References

Anderson P (2018) WHO Reports 3 Million Alcohol-Related Deaths in 2016. Medscape Medical News. Available at https://www.medscape.com/viewarticle/902614. September 27, 2018; Accessed 2 Oct 2018

Betka S, Harris L, Rae C, Palfi B, Pfeifer G, Sequeira H, Duka T, Critchley H (2019) Signatures of alcohol use in the structure and neurochemistry of insular cortex: a correlational study. Psychopharmacology 236:2579–2591. https://doi.org/10.1007/s00213-019-05228-w

Cardenas VA, Studholme C, Gazdzinski S, Durazzo TC, Meyerhoff DJ (2007) Deformation-based morphometry of brain changes in alcohol dependence and abstinence. Neuroimaging 34:879–887

Cheng H, Kellar D, Lake A, Finn P, Rebec GV, Dharmadhikari S, Dydak U, Newman S (2018) Effects of Alcohol Cues on MRS Glutamate Levels in the Anterior Cingulate. Alcohol 53 (3):209–215. https://doi.org/10.1093/alcalc/agx119

Dager AD, Anderson BM, Rosen R, Khadka S, Sawyer B et al (2014) Functional magnetic resonance imaging (fMRI) response to alcohol pictures predicts subsequent transition to heavy drinking in college students. Addiction 109:585–595

Dalvie S, Stein DJ, Koenen K, Cardenas V, Cuzen NL, Ramesar R, Fein G, Brooks SJ (2014) The BDNF p. Val66Met polymorphism, childhood trauma, and brain volumes in adolescents with alcohol abuse

Deaths and years of potential life lost from excessive alcohol use – United States, 2011–2015, Weekly/October 2, 2020/69(39):1428–1433

Esser MB, Sherk A, Yong L, Naimi TS, Stockwell T, Stahre M, Kanny D, Landen M, Saitz R, Brewer RD, Niciu MJ, Mason GF. Neuroimaging in Alcohol and Drug Dependence Published online: 7 January 2014 Springer International Publishing AG 2014

Fauth-Bühler M, Mann KF (2011) Alcohol and the human brain: a systematic review of different neuroimaging methods. Alcoholism Clinical and Experimental Research · July 2011 https://doi.org/10.1111/j.1530-0277.2011.01540.x. Source: PubMed

Frye MA, Hinton DJ, Karpyak VM, Biernacka JM, Gunderson LJ, Geske J, Feeder SE, Choi DS, Port JD (2016) Glutamate levels in the left dorsolateral prefrontal cortex are associated with higher cravings for alcohol. Alcohol Clin Exp Res 40(8):1609–1616. https://doi.org/10.1111/acer.13131. Epub 2016 Jul 20

Galanter M, Josipovic Z, Dermatis H, Weber J, Millard MA (2017) An initial fMRI study on neural correlates of prayer in members of alcoholics anonymous. Am J Drug Alcohol Abuse 43(1):44–54. https://doi.org/10.3109/00952990.2016.1141912. Epub 2016 Mar 25

Heitzeg MM, Nigg JT, Hardee JE, Soules M, Steinberg D, etal. Left middle frontal gyrus response to inhibitory errors in children prospectively predicts early problem substance use. Drug Alcohol Depend 2014; 141:51–57

Heitzeg M, Cope L, Martz M, Hardee J (2015) Neuroimaging Risk Markers for Substance Abuse: Recent Findings on Inhibitory Control and Reward System Functioning. Curr Addict Rep 2:91–103. https://doi.org/10.1007/s40429-015-0048-9

Hermens DF, Chitty KM, Lee RS, Tickell A, Haber PS, Naismith SL, Hickie IB, Lagopoulos J (2015) Hippocampal glutamate is increased and associated with risky drinking in young adults with major depression. J Affect Disord 186:95–98. https://doi.org/10.1016/j.jad.2015.07.009. Epub 2015 Jul 26

Kaplan and Sadock's. Synopsis of Psychiatry, Behavioral Sciences/Clinical Psychiatry 11th edn. Philadelphia: Wolters Kluwer, p

Kessler RC, McGonagle KA, Zhao S, Nelson CB, Hughes M, Eshleman S, Wittchen HU, Kendler KS (1994) Lifetime and 12-month prevalence of DSM-III-R psychiatric disorders in the United States. Results from the National Comorbidity Survey. Arch Gen Psychiatry 51(1):8–19

Lee TS, Quek SY, Krishnan KR (2014) Molecular imaging for depressive disorders. AJNR Am J Neuroradiol 35(6 Suppl):S44-54. https://doi.org/10.3174/ajnr.A3965. Epub 2014 May 15. Review. 17

Li L, Hua Y, Liu Y, Meng Y-j, Li X-j, Zhang C, Liang S, Li M-l, Guo W, Wang Q, Deng W, Ma X, Coid J, Li T (2021) Lower regional grey matter in alcohol use disorders: evidence from a voxel-based meta-analysis. BMC Psychiatry 21:247. https://doi.org/10.1186/s12888-021-03244-9

Meyer JH (2017) Neuroprogression and immune activation in major depressive disorder. Mod Trends Pharmacopsychiatry 31:27–36. https://doi.org/10.1159/000470804. Epub 2017 Jul 24

Meyerhoff DJ (2014) Brain proton magnetic resonance spectroscopy of alcohol use disorders. Handbook of clinical neurology vol 125:313–337. https://doi.org/10.1016/B978-0-444-62619-6.00019-7

Niciu M, Mason G (2014) Neuroimaging in Alcohol and Drug Dependence. Curr Behav Neurosci Rep 1:45–54. https://doi.org/10.1007/s40473-013-0005-7

Poznyak V, Rekve D. Global status report on alcohol and health 2018. World Health Organization. September 21, 2018. Available at http://www.who.int/substance_abuse/publications/global_alcohol_report/gsr_2018/en/

Prisciandaro JJ, Schacht JP, Prescot AP, Renshaw PF, Brown TR, Anton RF (2016) Associations between recent heavy drinking and dorsal anterior cingulate N-Acetylaspartate and glutamate concentrations in non-treatment-seeking individuals with alcohol dependence. Alcohol Clin Exp Res 40(3):491–496. https://doi.org/10.1111/acer.12977. Epub 2016 Feb 8

Sacks JJ, Gonzales KR, Bouchery EE, Tomedi LE, Brewer RD (2015) 2010 National and state costs of excessive alcohol consumption. Am J Prev Med 49(5):e73–e79. [Medline]

Sadock BJ, Sadock VA, Ruiz P (2014) BMC Psychiatry 14:328. https://doi.org/10.1186/s12888-014-0328-2

Sadock BJ, Sadock VA, Ruiz P (2015) Kaplan & Sadock's synopsis of psychiatry behavioral sciences/clinical psychiatry, 11th edn. Wolters Kluwer, Philadelphia, p 621

Stahl SM (2013) Stahl's essential psychopharmacology, neuroscientific basis and practical application, 4th edn. Cambridge University Press, p 649

Thayer RE, YorkWilliams S, Karoly HC, Sabbineni A, Ewing SF, Bryan AD, Hutchison KE (2017) Structural neuroimaging correlates of alcohol and cannabis use in adolescents and adults Addiction. 112(12):2144–2154. https://doi.org/10.1111/add.13923. Epub 2017 Aug 1

Wang J, Fan Y, Dong Y, Ma M, Ma Y, Dong Y, Niu Y, Jiang Y, Wang H, Wang Z, Wu L, Sun H, Cui C (2016) Alterations in brain structure and functional connectivity in alcohol dependent patients and possible association with impulsivity. PLoS One 11(8):e0161956. https://doi.org/10.1371/journal.pone.0161956. eCollection 2016

Wang Y, Chen G, Zhong S, Jia Y, Xia L, Lai S, Zhao L, Huang L, Liu T (2018) Association between resting-state brain functional connectivity and cortisol levels in unmedicated major depressive disorder. J Psychiatr Res 105:55–62. https://doi.org/10.1016/j.jpsychires.2018.08.025. Epub 2018 Sep 1

Alcohol as Prodrug of Salsolinol

47

The Long-Sought Alcohol's Key Mechanism of Action on Dopamine Neurons

Valentina Bassareo, Riccardo Maccioni, Rossana Migheli, Alessandra T. Peana, Pierluigi Caboni, and Elio Acquas

Contents

Mini-Dictionary of Terms 984
Introduction 985
On the Relationship Between Alcohol and the Dopaminergic Mesolimbic System 986
Acetaldehyde, Alcohol's First Metabolite, Comes into Scene 987
On the Role of Acetaldehyde in the Effects of Alcohol on the Dopaminergic Mesolimbic System 988
Salsolinol, Alcohol's Secondary Metabolite, Comes into Scene 990
On the Demonstration that Alcohol Is the Prodrug of Salsolinol for its Actions on the Dopaminergic Mesolimbic System 991

V. Bassareo
Department of Biomedical Sciences and Center of Excellence for the Study of Neurobiology of Addiction, University of Cagliari, Cagliari, Italy
e-mail: bassareo@unica.it

R. Maccioni · P. Caboni
Department of Life and Environmental Sciences, University of Cagliari, Cagliari, Italy
e-mail: caboni@unica.it

R. Migheli
Department of Experimental Medical and Surgical Sciences, University of Sassari, Sassari, Italy
e-mail: rmigheli@uniss.it

A. T. Peana
Department of Chemistry and Pharmacy, University of Sassari, Sassari, Italy
e-mail: apeana@uniss.it

E. Acquas (✉)
Department of Life and Environmental Sciences, Center of Excellence for the Study of Neurobiology of Addiction, University of Cagliari, Cagliari, Italy
e-mail: acquas@unica.it

V. B. Patel, V. R. Preedy (eds.), *Handbook of Substance Misuse and Addictions*,
https://doi.org/10.1007/978-3-030-92392-1_52

Conclusion 994
Applications to Other Areas of Addiction 996
Applications to Other Areas of Public Health 996
Summary Points 999
References 1000

Abstract

Alcohol, the psychopharmacologically active ingredient of alcoholic drinks responsible of their addictive potential, represents a threat to both individual and public health being a risk factor of a number of serious pathological conditions spanning, besides addiction, from liver and cardiovascular diseases to neurological disorders and cancer. The occurrence of altered behaviors toward uncontrolled alcohol intake is a complex and not yet fully understood phenomenon. Notwithstanding, it is unanimously recognized that alcohol's addictive potential resides in its efficiency for activating the mesolimbic dopamine system, an ability that involves several central neurotransmitter systems although the specific mechanism and site of action are still the subject of intense research. In this regard, recent and compelling evidence points to the two-step metabolic conversion, in the posterior ventral tegmental area (pVTA), of alcohol into acetaldehyde and salsolinol, the latter being the product of condensation between acetaldehyde and dopamine, as the key mechanism for eliciting dopamine transmission in the nucleus accumbens and dopamine-mediated behaviors through the involvement of μ opioid receptors. This chapter emphasizes the strategic role of alcohol metabolism and recapitulates the most recent advances in support of the evidence that alcohol is the prodrug of salsolinol for its actions on the dopamine system and hence for its reinforcing effects and addictive liability.

Keywords

Alcohol · Acetaldehyde · Dopamine · Nucleus Accumbens · Salsolinol · μ opioid receptors · pVTA (posterior Ventral Tegmental Area)

Mini-Dictionary of Terms

Addictive liability: Indicates the potential of a substance of triggering addictive behaviors. Alcohol is endowed with addictive liability since it may induce abnormal behaviors toward its excessive intake and eventually toward alcohol-use disorder (AUD). However this is a necessary but not sufficient condition. In other words this is a possibility that does not take place any time a person is exposed to alcohol since a number of other conditions and factors may contribute to translating recreational alcohol intake into alcohol excessive consumption and/or AUD. Among these certainly critical is the genetic vulnerability to it.

Alcohol metabolism: The term metabolism indicates one or more sequential enzymatic reactions (biotransformations) that take place at the cellular level to convert both endobiotics and xenobiotics into molecules that can thus be more easily eliminated from the body. Alcohol metabolism takes place by way of at least three distinct (type 2 alcohol dehydrogenase, CYP2E1, and catalase) and alternative enzymatic mechanisms that yield to alcohol's primary metabolite, acetaldehyde. However, alcohol may also generate secondary metabolites, acetate, the product of further oxidation of acetaldehyde, mediated by type 2 aldehyde dehydrogenase, and salsolinol (1-methyl-6,7-dihydroxy-1,2,3,4-tetrahydroisoquinoline), the product of spontaneous or enzymatic (salsolinol synthase) condensation between acetaldehyde and dopamine.

Mesolimbic system: Anatomically, the mesolimbic system is a neuronal circuit that is made of ascending projections arising from the mesencephalon to the forebrain. Specifically, dopamine cell bodies located bilaterally in the mesencephalic ventral tegmental area (VTA) nucleus send their axons ipsilaterally, for over 95%, and contralaterally, for the remaining 5%, to forebrain target structures such as the nucleus accumbens (in its shell and core subdivisions) and the olfactory bulb. Recent evidence points to the most posterior region of the VTA (pVTA) as the portion of this nucleus mostly involved in the actions of drugs of abuse. Other target structures of VTA dopamine cells' projections also include the bed nucleus of stria terminalis and the central nucleus of the amygdala, part of the extended amygdala complex

Functionally, the mesolimbic system can be defined as the system that plays the pivotal role in the expression of affective reactions and motivated behaviors and whose dysregulation underlies a number of psychiatric morbidities including, besides drug addiction, depression and schizophrenia.

Prodrug: A prodrug (as well as a protoxic) is a molecule that becomes pharmacologically (and toxicologically) active upon biotransformation of its (inactive) parent compound. In the case of alcohol, recent and compelling evidence has demonstrated that this molecule is able, only upon its two-step metabolic conversion into salsolinol, to lead to dopamine release in the nucleus accumbens and activate dopamine neurons in the pVTA.

Reinforcement: The condition, either positive or negative, elicited by a reinforcer by which the possibility of emission of a response is increased (positive reinforcement) or extinguished (negative reinforcement). Alcohol can act as a reinforcer, increasing the probability of responses dependent upon its presentation

Introduction

Alcohol (ethyl alcohol) is an amphipathic molecule not only, in a singular way, in strict chemical terms (since it possesses both *hydrophobic* and *hydrophilic* portions in its structure) but also in terms of its pharmacological and toxicological properties. Thus, alcohol may show both stimulant and sedative central effects (King et al.

2002) and, also, may exert some of its central effects as such or as the prodrug (or protoxic) of other biologically active molecules (Correa et al. 2012; Hipolito et al. 2012). Notably, the serious detrimental effects of excessive alcohol intake on health including, besides addiction (Koob and Volkow 2016), liver and cardiovascular diseases, cancer, and neurological disorders (Axley et al. 2019; Rehm et al. 2017) are the consequence of the chronic exposure to high intoxicating doses of alcohol that are self-administered by some individuals due to the high alcohol's addictive liability. Accordingly, when also other factors and conditions, such as genetic predisposition (Colombo et al. 2006; Dyr and Kostowski 2004; Quintanilla et al. 2006), come into play, alcohol may urge to indulge in its abnormal/heavy intake, thus triggering a loop of compulsive self-intoxication that takes place, up to a certain point, despite the awareness of serious consequences on health (APA, American Psychiatric Association 2013).

On the Relationship Between Alcohol and the Dopaminergic Mesolimbic System

Based on these premises, it is not surprising that to frame the neurobiological basis of abnormal alcohol intake and, hence, of the highly expensive impact on individual and public health (Abrahao et al. 2017) into the proper perspective, one should go back to two early original observations: (i) that monoamines are involved in the reinforcing and euphoriant effects of alcohol (Ahlenius et al. 1973) and (ii) that alcohol preferentially excites mesencephalic dopamine neurons in the ventral tegmental area (VTA) with respect to those in the substantia nigra (Gessa et al. 1985). These observations, inspiring the modern view on the neurobiological bases of abnormal consumption of alcohol, attribute a pivotal role to the mesolimbic dopamine system for mediating alcohol's reinforcing effects (Di Chiara et al. 2004; Volkow et al. 2009; Wise 2009; Bassareo et al. 2017). In particular, according to this view, the acute administration of alcohol results, similarly to the exposure to other addictive substances (Di Chiara et al. 2004), in the phasic stimulation of dopamine neurotransmission preferentially in the shell of the nucleus accumbens (Di Chiara et al. 2004; Di Chiara and Bassareo 2007), a neurochemical event endowed with the significance of (i) mediating the reinforcing properties not only of addictive drugs but also of natural rewards and (ii) supporting the associative learning processes necessary to transfer the affective valence of the substance to the context that may eventually become conditioned to substance's effects (Di Chiara et al. 2004; Di Chiara and Bassareo 2007).

Needless to say in this context, such a pivotal role of the dopamine mesolimbic system, in particular with reference to the acute and chronic effects of alcohol, is supported by the action of many other neurotransmitters and their receptor subtypes such as, among others, GABA (Koob 2004), serotonin (Belmer et al. 2016; Ding et al. 2009, 2012), and opioid peptides (Koob 2014).

Acetaldehyde, Alcohol's First Metabolite, Comes into Scene

Nevertheless, in the last decades, a distinct, complementary and not alternative, perspective on the mechanism by which alcohol excites mesencephalic dopamine neurons and elicits phasic dopamine transmission in the shell of the nucleus accumbens took place after the serendipitous observation published in 1953 by Dr. L.C.F. Chevens (The Hermitage, Twyford, Berks, Australia), member of the council of the Society for the Study of Addiction to Alcohol and Other Drugs (formerly The Society, established in 1884, for the Study of Inebriety) (Fig. 1). In his letter to the Lancet, Dr. Chevens reported that many patients on Antabuse (disulfiram) could feel in a subjective state overall considered desirable and concluded that "*... these patients show the surprising tendency to seek antabuse as an adjunct to their drinking ...*" and, unknowingly, opened the research avenue on the role of acetaldehyde, the main alcohol metabolite, as well as of other alcohol's metabolites in some of the effects of their parent compound. Dr. Chevens' letter to the Lancet reveals, in fact, that "*many ... drinkers ... show a magnificent tolerance for acetaldehyde ... and often claim that a small gin makes them feel like several doubles when on antabuse.*" Antabuse (tetraethyldisulfanedicarbothioamide) is an irreversible inhibitor of aldehyde dehydrogenase exploited since then to discourage people from drinking alcohol being responsible to cause a highly aversive systemic accumulation of acetaldehyde (flushing reaction). However, this observation remained in silence until the 70s of the last century when a surge of studies (Collins 1988; Collins et al. 1979, 1990; Davis and Walsh 1970; Davis et al. 1970) put forward the suggestion of the role of alcohol by-products in its central effects as well

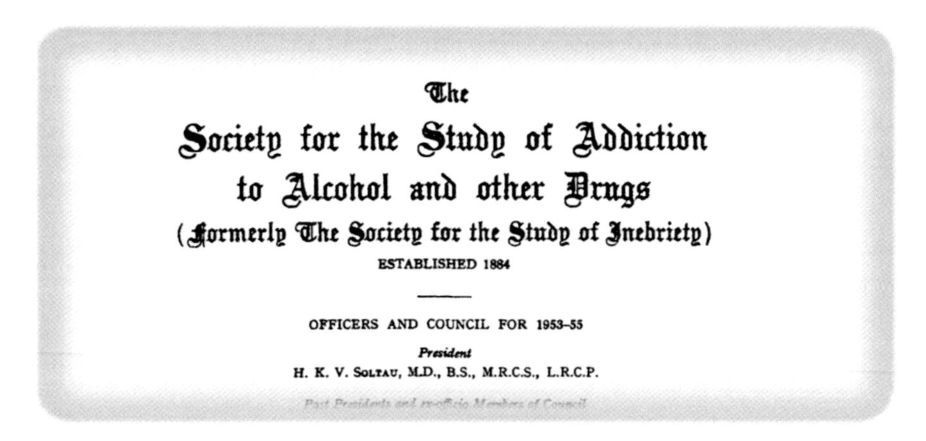
The
Society for the Study of Addiction
to Alcohol and other Drugs
(Formerly The Society for the Study of Inebriety)
ESTABLISHED 1884

OFFICERS AND COUNCIL FOR 1953–55
President
H. K. V. Soltau, M.D., B.S., M.R.C.S., L.R.C.P.

Fig. 1 Title page of the list of members of the council of the ***Society for the Study of Addiction to Alcohol and Other Drugs*** (formerly The Society, established in 1884, for the Study of Inebriety). Dr. L.C.F. Chevens (The Hermitage, Twyford, Berks, Australia), responsible for the serendipitous observation published in 1953 that acetaldehyde may have a role in the addictive properties of its parent compound, was a member of this Society. (Source: https://onlinelibrary.wiley.com/doi/pdf/10.1111/j.1360-0443.1955.tb04674.x)

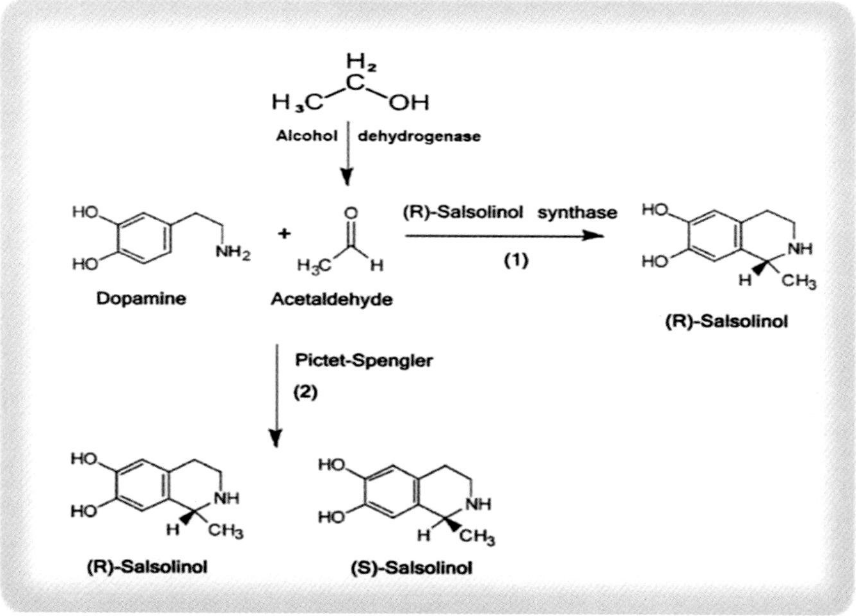

Fig. 2 Schematic and simplified representation of the possible pathways of synthesis of salsolinol

as of their potential responsibility of causing and maintaining abnormal/excessive alcohol intake (Collins 1988; Davis and Walsh 1970; Davis et al. 1970).

The peripheral metabolism of alcohol takes place mainly in the liver by the action of the saturable NAD-dependent alcohol dehydrogenase but also, to a lesser extent, by means of distinct enzymatic systems, the CYP2E1 and the peroxisomal catalase (Cederbaum 2012). On the contrary, alcohol dehydrogenase isoforms expressed centrally do not catalyze alcohol oxidation into acetaldehyde, and hence the main central metabolic pathway is instead represented by peroxisomal H_2O_2-catalase (Aragon et al. 1991; Correa et al. 2009a; Pastor et al. 2002) and secondly by CYP2E1 (Cederbaum 2012; Correa et al. 2009a). Moreover, acetaldehyde can be further oxidized into acetate, a substance with recognized pharmacological properties (Pardo et al. 2013), as well as into salsolinol (1-methyl-6,7-dihydroxy-1,2,3,4-tetrahydroisoquinoline), an intriguing molecule that may be generated upon spontaneous condensation or upon a still-to-be-confirmed enzymatically-mediated reaction (Chen et al. 2018) between acetaldehyde and dopamine (Fig. 2).

On the Role of Acetaldehyde in the Effects of Alcohol on the Dopaminergic Mesolimbic System

Interestingly, despite the fact that acetaldehyde is characterized by a high reactivity with nucleophilic compounds such as monoamines as well as by a very short half-life suggestive of the fact that in the cells this chemical, as such, may last very little, a large body of recent studies also inspired by Chevens' observation (Chevens 1953) suggest that acetaldehyde itself can be responsible for some of the central effects of alcohol (Correa et al. 2012). This evidence, although originally controversial for the uncertainty related to the fact that acetaldehyde produced peripherally could cross the blood–brain barrier (Sippel 1974; Correa et al. 2012), was generated following three main lines of research: the first one based on either the systemic or the local direct administration of acetaldehyde (Brancato et al. 2014; Rodd et al. 2005; Spina et al. 2010; Vinci et al. 2010; Peana et al. 2015); the second one based on the interference, either peripheral or central, with alcohol's oxidative metabolism (Correa et al. 2008; Pastor et al. 2002; Peana et al. 2008; Vinci et al. 2010); and, finally, the third one based on the use, upon alcohol administration, of agents able to control acetaldehyde's bioavailability with acetaldehyde-sequestering agents (Font et al. 2006a, b; Martí-Prats et al. 2010; Orrico et al. 2017). Extensive preclinical studies following the first line of research revealed that similarly to alcohol, but at significantly lower doses (after systemic administration) and concentrations (after local application), acetaldehyde has both sedative (Tambour et al. 2005) and motor stimulant effects (Arizzi-LaFrance et al. 2006; Correa et al. 2009b; Martí-Prats et al. 2013; Sánchez-Catalán et al. 2009; Tambour et al. 2005), activates the dopamine mesolimbic system (Melis et al. 2007), stimulates dopamine transmission (Melis et al. 2007), exerts positive motivational effects (Font et al. 2006a, b; Spina et al. 2010), and is systemically (Brancato et al. 2014; Peana et al. 2010, 2017a) or centrally, in the more posterior region of the VTA (pVTA) (Sanchez-Catalan et al. 2014), self-administered (Rodd et al. 2005). Overall, these experiments point to acetaldehyde as a psychopharmacologically active molecule with a profile of action superimposable, as far as the involvement of the dopamine mesolimbic system is concerned, to that of its parent compound. Moreover, the data collected by the studies that followed this approach also revealed that some common effects between alcohol and acetaldehyde, such as the locomotor stimulation (Sánchez-Catalán et al. 2009) and the oral self-administration (Peana et al. 2011), could similarly be prevented by blockade of opioid receptors (Correa et al. 2012; Font et al. 2013).

On the other hand, the studies generated exploiting the prevention of alcohol metabolism either peripherally (Escarabajal and Aragon 2002a, b; Peana et al. 2008; Vinci et al. 2010) by the alcohol dehydrogenase inhibitor, 4-methylpyrazole, or centrally by the catalase inhibitors, 3-aminotriazole (Aragon and Amit 1985; Aragon et al. 1985; Correa et al. 2008) and cyanamide (Sanchis-Segura et al. 1999a, b, c), disclosed that prevention of alcohol metabolism into acetaldehyde, no matter whether systemically or centrally, could prevent alcohol's effects including its ability of stimulating locomotion (Correa et al. 2001; Escarabajal et al. 2000; Sanchis-Segura et al. 1999a, b, c) and dopamine transmission in the shell of the nucleus accumbens (Melis et al. 2007) and of eliciting conditioned place preference (Peana et al. 2008).

It is critical in the context of the in-depth progression of this description to attract reader's attention to an intrinsic peculiarity of these pharmacological studies: when alcohol is administered systemically, either intraperitoneally or orally, its peripheral metabolism implies that only a fraction of the intact molecule is available for central distribution. On the contrary, due to this metabolism, the increased availability of acetaldehyde may eventually favor its central distribution, thus making this "portion" of acetaldehyde available to contribute indistinguishably to the effects of its parent compound. In other words, since alcohol and acetaldehyde exert similar central effects, in particular with respect to the mesolimbic dopamine system (Correa et al. 2012; Deehan et al. 2013), the experimental approach of inhibiting alcohol metabolism may not allow the direct assessment of the contribution of one or the other molecule to a given effect. Moreover, another case of similar reciprocity concerns the effects of 4-methylpyrazole. In fact, being an irreversible inhibitor of peripheral alcohol dehydrogenase (Di et al. 2021), this compound may promote, for the reasons discussed above, central alcohol availability and therefore may also promote H_2O_2-catalase-mediated alcohol central metabolism. However, 4-methylpyrazole has been reported as also able to inhibit fatty acyl coenzyme synthetase (Bradford et al. 1993), a mechanism by which it may interfere with the cellular availability of H_2O_2, the critical cofactor for the catalase-mediated oxidation of alcohol. Accordingly, it was shown that delivery, at an appropriate concentration, of 4-methylpyrazole in the pVTA could prevent the metabolism of alcohol into acetaldehyde and could also prevent alcohol, but not acetaldehyde, oral self-administration (Peana et al. 2017a).

The third pathway of research based on the rationale of reducing the bioavailability of alcohol-derived and newly formed acetaldehyde, on a similar vein of the two abovementioned strategies, confirmed the critical role of acetaldehyde in some of the effects of alcohol (Font et al. 2006a, b; Martí-Prats et al. 2010; Peana et al. 2008) to the point that acetaldehyde-sequestering agents, such as D-penicillamine and L-cysteine, have been suggested as novel pharmacological tools against the development of AUD (Orrico et al. 2017). Interestingly, in spite of the robustness of the above data, collected along more than two decades of intense research, the lack of a mechanism and of a site of action for acetaldehyde strongly toned down the enthusiasm in support of the suggestion of alcohol as its prodrug (Correa et al. 2012; Deehan et al. 2013; Peana et al. 2016, 2017b; Polache and Granero 2013) and simultaneously revitalized the interest on the secondary by-product of alcohol, salsolinol (Fig. 2). In this context, it is relevant to specify that salsolinol carries in its structure a stereoisomeric center and therefore may exist as (R)- or (L)-enantiomers and that in the progression of the discussion whereby not specified we will refer to the effects of the racemate.

Salsolinol, Alcohol's Secondary Metabolite, Comes into Scene

The suggestion that salsolinol, as well as other tetrahydroisoquinolines, could be involved in the effects of alcohol was originally prompted by the observation that these compounds could be found in the biological fluids of alcoholics (Collins 1988; Davis and Walsh 1970; Davis et al. 1970) in a manner that although controversial (Origitano et al. 1981; Collins et al. 1990) was to some extent related to alcohol consumption (Collins et al. 1979). The original interest in salsolinol and related tetrahydroisoquinolines, which extends also to their potential neuroprotective and neurotoxic properties (Peana et al. 2019; Kurnik-Łucka et al. 2020) as well as to the fact that salsolinol is involved in the hypothalamic secretion of prolactin

(Oláh et al. 2011), was however hampered by the suspect that this molecule, given its structure and relative hydrophilicity, could not cross the blood–brain barrier upon systemic administration (Origitano et al. 1981). This notwithstanding, further experimental evidence sustained the ability of systemically administered salsolinol to elicit conditioned place preference in mildly stressed (Matsuzawa et al. 2000) and in genetically selected alcohol-preferring rats (Quintanilla et al. 2014, 2016) and confirmed that this molecule could exert central reinforcing effects (Hipólito et al. 2012). In fact, the local administration of salsolinol in the pVTA elicits locomotor activity (Hipólito et al. 2010; Quintanilla et al. 2014) and conditioned place preference (Hipólito et al. 2011; Matsuzawa et al. 2000; Quintanilla et al. 2014, 2016) and increases the release of dopamine in the shell of the nucleus accumbens (Hipólito et al. 2009). Also, salsolinol was reported to be contingently self-administered by rats either in the shell of the nucleus accumbens (Rodd et al. 2003) or in the pVTA (Rodd et al. 2008), and the effects of its pVTA delivery on locomotor activity and dopamine transmission in the shell of the nucleus accumbens could be prevented by μ opioid receptor antagonists (Bassareo et al. 2021; Berríos-Cárcamo et al. 2017, 2019; Hipólito et al. 2010, 2011; Xie et al. 2012).

In addition, similarly to acetaldehyde, these effects of salsolinol were also found to take place at doses and concentrations 100 to 1000 times lower than those of alcohol. This observation overall suggests that if there is any relationship between the effects of alcohol and those of acetaldehyde or salsolinol, such ratio indicates that only a significantly smaller fraction of a pharmacologically active dose of alcohol is actually needed, as its by-products, at the target site(s) for eliciting, at high affinity, its specific effects.

On the Demonstration that Alcohol Is the Prodrug of Salsolinol for its Actions on the Dopaminergic Mesolimbic System

The evidence gathered so far stands, therefore, as a strong suggestion toward the possibility that the reinforcing effects of alcohol are mediated by its main metabolites, acetaldehyde, and, being this molecule highly reactive, salsolinol upon its condensation with dopamine. All that being said, the critical steps toward the demonstration that alcohol is indeed the prodrug of salsolinol for its actions on the mesolimbic dopamine system were moved by two studies that firstly by an ex vivo setting and successively by an in vivo design provided the demonstration that to stimulate dopamine neurons in the pVTA alcohol needs to be oxidized into acetaldehyde and this, upon its condensation with dopamine, has to become salsolinol.

In the first of these studies, Melis et al. (2015), making patch-clamp extracellular recordings of dopaminergic cells in mice pVTA, showed that whereas in control animals alcohol, acetaldehyde, and salsolinol could similarly (although at different concentrations) excite dopamine neurons, only salsolinol could do so in mesencephalic slices from mice previously administered α-methyl-p-tyrosine, an agent capable of inhibiting the synthesis of dopamine and of acutely depleting its vesicular stores.

Moreover, whereas this effect of alcohol in slices from control mice was prevented also by the H_2O_2-catalase inhibitor, 3-aminotriazole, in slices from α-methyl-p-tyrosine-treated mice, the lack of effect of alcohol could be restored by the addition of dopamine; however, strikingly, such recovered effect was prevented by 3-aminotriazole (Fig. 3). This ex vivo study, thus, demonstrated that salsolinol plays a key role in the ability of alcohol to stimulate dopamine neurons in the pVTA since alcohol's effects necessitate sequentially of its H_2O_2-catalase-mediated oxidation into acetaldehyde and of acetaldehyde's condensation with dopamine to make salsolinol (Fig. 4). This study also

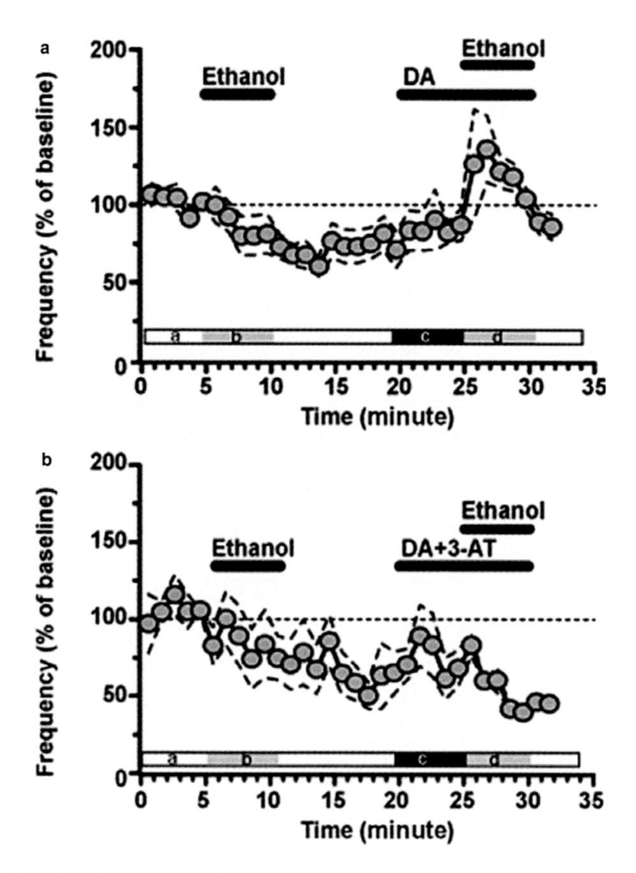

Fig. 3 Alcohol (ethanol)-induced excitation of dopamine neuronal firing rate requires its oxidation into acetaldehyde and the presence of dopamine. (**a**) Time-course graph illustrating the averaged effects of ethanol (100 mM) on the firing rate of dopamine cells of the pVTA in mice pretreated with α-methyl-p-tyrosine (αMpT). Note that the effect of ethanol is restored in the presence of exogenous dopamine (10 nM). (**b**) Time-course graph illustrating the averaged effects of ethanol (100 mM) on the firing rate of dopamine cells of the pVTA in mice pretreated with αMpT. The effect of ethanol is abolished in the presence of dopamine (10 nM) when acetaldehyde formation is prevented by 3-AT application (1 mM). (Reproduced with minor modifications under permission (5114291121565 – CCC RightsLink) from Melis et al. 2015)

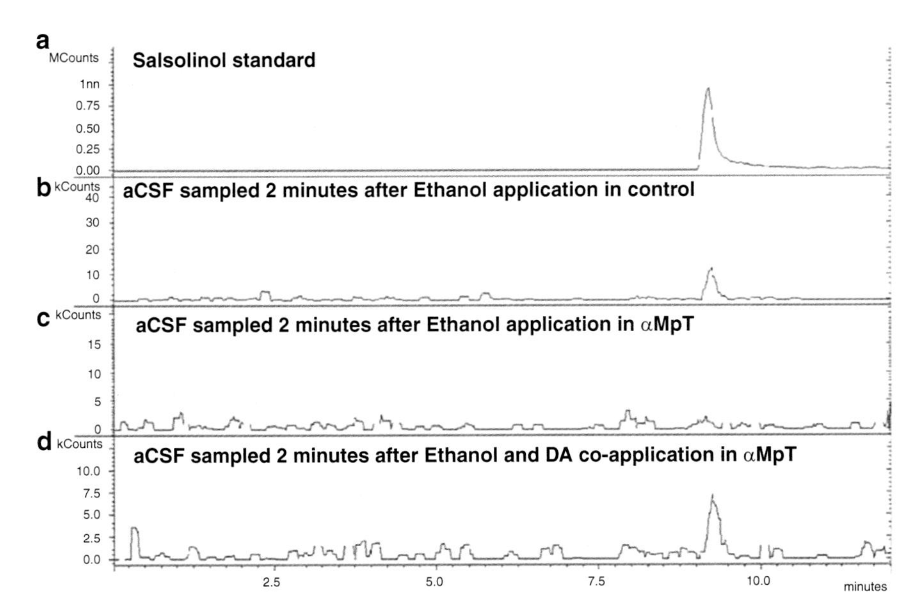

Fig. 4 HPLC-MS/MS detects salsolinol in aCSF after co-application of alcohol (ethanol) and dopamine to slices from αMpT-treated mice. Representative HPLC-MS/MS ion chromatograms (mass transition: 180.1 > 117.1; collision energy −22 V) of (**a**) standard of salsolinol (56 nM) in aCSF; (**b**) aCSF from recording chamber at second-minute application of ethanol (100 mM) in control mouse; (**c**) aCSF from recording chamber at second-minute application of ethanol (100 mM) in αMpT-treated mouse; (**d**) aCSF from recording chamber at second-minute co-application of ethanol (100 mM) and dopamine (10 nM) in α-methyl-p-tyrosine (αMpT)-treated mouse. (Reproduced without modification under permission (5114291121565 – CCC RightsLink) from Melis et al. 2015)

strongly posed the grounds to support the long-standing suggestion of the conversion of alcohol into salsolinol, but, being performed ex vivo in mesencephalic, pVTA-containing, blocks of tissue, it could not allow any further interpretation of the functional significance of this two-step mechanism.

Thus, the questions (Polache and Granero 2013; Peana et al. 2016) compulsory to resolve, i.e., (i) whether there is the formation of salsolinol in the pVTA after systemic administration of alcohol and (ii) whether there is, in vivo, a clear functional relationship between systemic alcohol administration, salsolinol formation in the pVTA, and stimulation of dopamine transmission in the shell of nucleus accumbens, were still unanswered.

A convincing response to such questions and to the search of the long-sought alcohol's key mechanism of action on mesencephalic dopamine neurons was provided recently by an elegant in vivo brain microdialysis study. In this study, Bassareo and colleagues (Bassareo et al. 2021) planned to exploit the possibility of sampling both salsolinol and dopamine, after the systemic administration of a dose of alcohol capable of producing a pharmacologically and clinically relevant alcoholaemia (Gill et al. 1986; Majchrowicz 1975; Nurmi et al. 1994). This sampling was done in brain dialysates collected simultaneously from the pVTA and from the shell of the nucleus accumbens of the same or of the opposite side in order to exploit the peculiarity that the projections from the pVTA to the shell of the nucleus accumbens (and the other target areas) are almost (~95%) ipsilateral while only 5% of these projections are aimed at the contralateral telencephalic target structures (Geisler and Zahm 2005; Ikemoto 2007; Breton et al. 2019). This anatomical peculiarity allowed to establish whether the expected detection of alcohol-dependent newly formed salsolinol in the pVTA could be causally- and temporally-related to the increases of dopamine transmission in the shell of the nucleus accumbens. The results of this study convincingly demonstrated that, upon the systemic administration of alcohol, salsolinol, otherwise undetectable in the pVTA, is synthesized in this area (Fig. 5) and that this synthesis was prevented either by blocking the metabolism of alcohol into acetaldehyde (with 3-aminotriazole) (Fig. 6) or by preventing the availability of either acetaldehyde (with D-penicillamine) (Fig. 6) or dopamine (with the dopamine D_2/D_3 agonist, quinpirole) (Fig. 7). Moreover, the study demonstrated that preventing the formation of salsolinol in the pVTA of one side resulted in the inhibition of the ability of alcohol to stimulate dopamine release in the shell of the nucleus accumbens of the same, but not of the opposite, side. Finally, based on the wealth of experimental evidence in support of the tenet that the effects of salsolinol (similarly to those of acetaldehyde and alcohol) are mediated by μ opioid receptors, Bassareo et al. (2021) also tested the possibility that this alcohol-dependent newly formed salsolinol in the pVTA could be responsible for stimulating dopamine transmission in the shell of the ipsilateral, but not contralateral, nucleus accumbens through the stimulation of these receptors. Indeed, the application in the pVTA of the μ opioid receptor antagonist, naltrexone, fails to affect the synthesis of salsolinol, but, in spite of the presence of salsolinol in pVTA dialysate samples, μ opioid receptor blockade results in the prevention of the alcohol-mediated stimulation of dopamine transmission in the shell of the ipsilateral, but not contralateral, nucleus accumbens (Fig. 8).

Conclusion

The present review of the literature on the role of alcohol's metabolism in its acute reinforcing properties was made under a historical perspective and aimed at summarizing and discussing an over 70-year-long fascinating path of research. Along this dissertation were mostly mentioned the studies that positively contributed to disclosing the described role of metabolism in the effects of alcohol, a topic that at a certain point has been quite debated. This was done mainly because, as far as the acute action of alcohol on the mesolimbic dopamine system is concerned, there is presently a general consensus on the conclusions reached. However, as also already mentioned in this chapter, the evidence here discussed

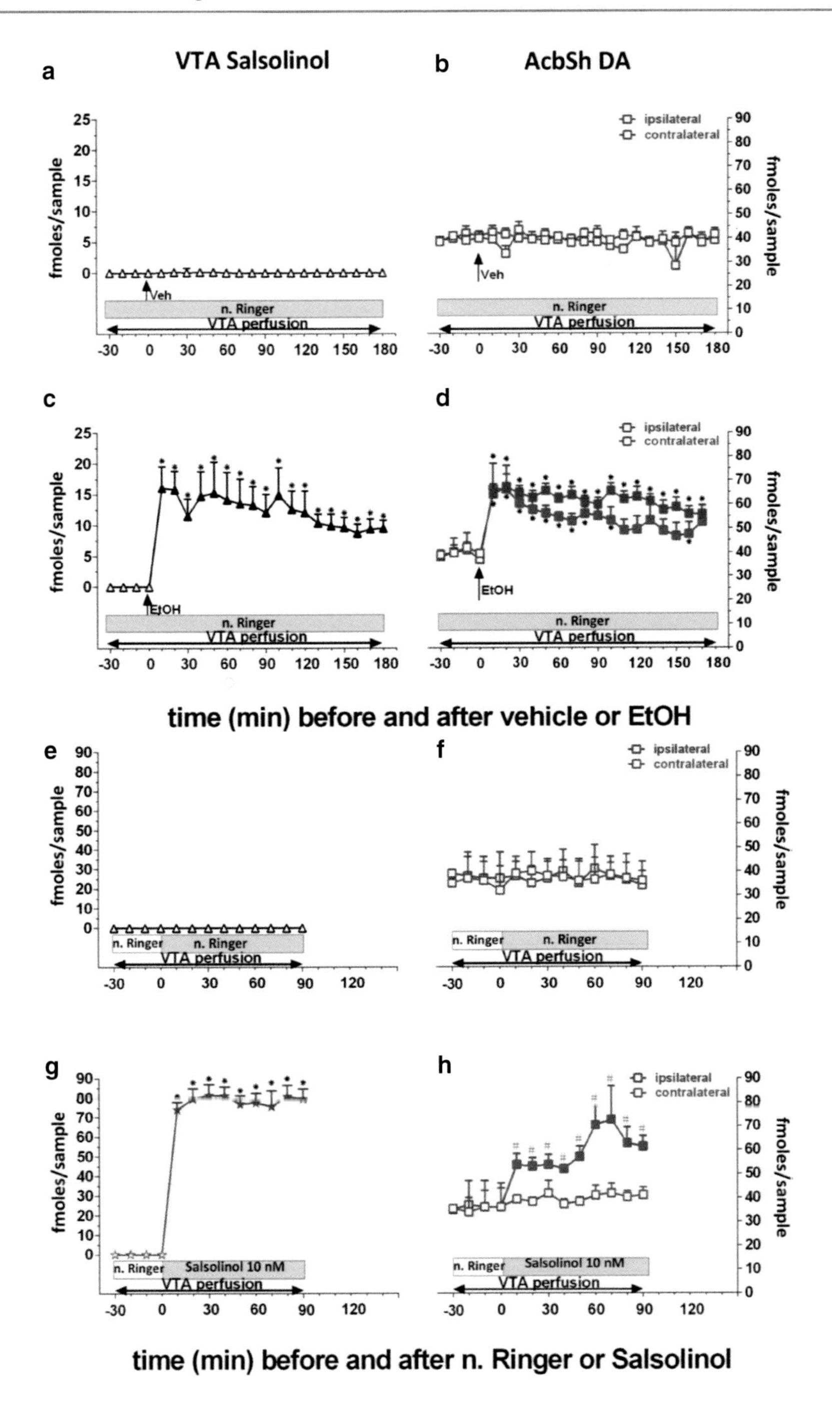

Fig. 5 Effects of intragastric administration of vehicle (tap water, 10 ml/kg) (**a**) (**b**) or alcohol (EtOH) (1 g/kg, 20% v/v) (**c**) (**d**) or of reverse dialysis application in the pVTA of normal Ringer's

refers to the data gathered focusing on the acute action of alcohol and its metabolites, acetaldehyde and salsolinol, on a specific neural circuit, highly relevant for the development of drug-mediated behavioral alterations toward either the substance or the stimuli related to it. In addition, other limitations have to be acknowledged as well, the main of which refers to the fact that the role of salsolinol in the effects of alcohol has yet to be fully determined upon either acute or chronic voluntary consumption. This notwithstanding, the disclosure of the role of metabolic conversion of alcohol in the pVTA as the mechanism potentially responsible for triggering addictive behaviors may represent, given the tremendously high impact that AUD exerts on public health, an innovative strategy toward a better understanding of alcohol consumption as a risk factor or threat for individual and public health.

Applications to Other Areas of Addiction

The topic treated in this chapter can also be viewed in the general perspective of the role and significance of the metabolic manipulation to which all molecules introduced in the body, and therefore also addictive drugs, may potentially undergo. In fact, cases of addictive compounds that act as prodrugs or protoxics may refer to heroin (as the prodrug of morphine), to morphine itself (as the prodrug of morphine-6-glucuronide), to cocaine (as the prodrug of cocaethylene), and to MDMA (as the prodrug of MDA). We overall believe that the topic covered in this chapter represents an excellent example of the critical role that metabolic transformations play in the pharmacological and toxicological consequences of drugs' consumption.

Applications to Other Areas of Public Health

Acetaldehyde, alcohol's main metabolite, is a group 1 human carcinogen responsible for upper gastrointestinal tract cancer (Nieminen and Salaspuro 2018). The reviewed literature on the potential role of alcohol's metabolites offers an interesting perspective on the potential role of acetaldehyde in further public health concerns besides the addiction field. In this regard, reducing the exposure to carcinogenic

Fig. 5 (continued) (n. Ringer's) (**e**) (**f**)] or salsolinol (10 nM) (**g**) (**h**), on pVTA salsolinol (**a**, **c**, **e**, **g**) and on ipsilateral and contralateral AcbSh dopamine (**b**, **d**, **f**, **h**) dialysates. The purple color was used here to highlight the fact that indeed these concentrations of salsolinol were from the reverse dialysis application of salsolinol (10 nM)-enriched n. Ringer's. Horizontal bars depict the contents of the pVTA perfusion fluid along the experiments. Vertical arrows indicate the last pVTA or AcbSh sample before vehicle or EtOH administration. Filled symbols indicate samples representing $p < 0.001$ vs. basal; $p < 0.01$ vs. vehicle administration; $^{\#}p < 0.01$ vs. contralateral area. (Reproduced under a Creative Commons CC-BY license from Bassareo et al. 2021)

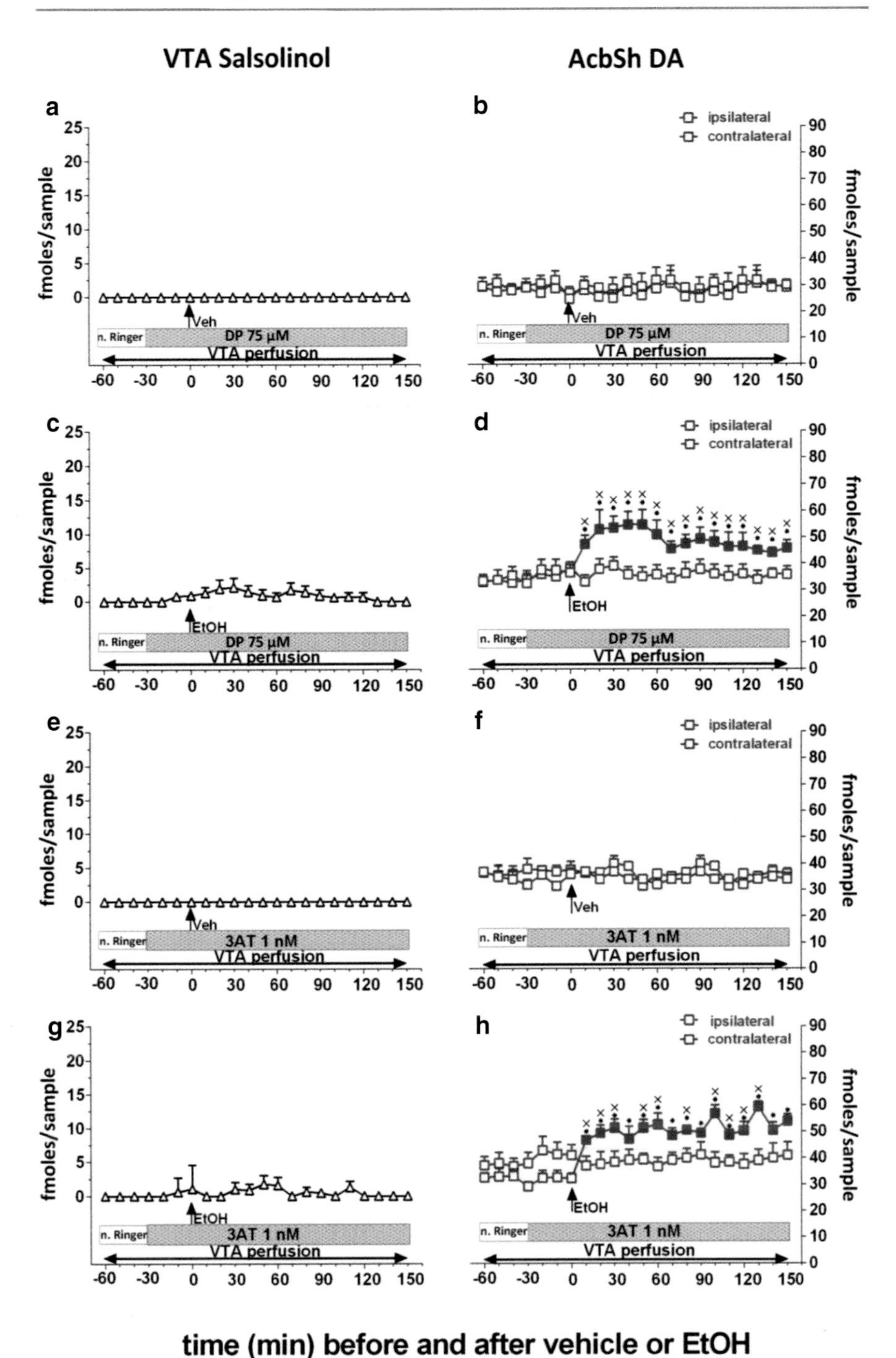

Fig. 6 Effects of intragastric administration of vehicle (tap water, 10 ml/kg) (**a**) (**b**) (**e**) (**f**) or alcohol (EtOH) (1 g/kg, 20% v/v) (**c**) (**d**) (**g**) (**h**) in the presence of reverse dialysis application in the

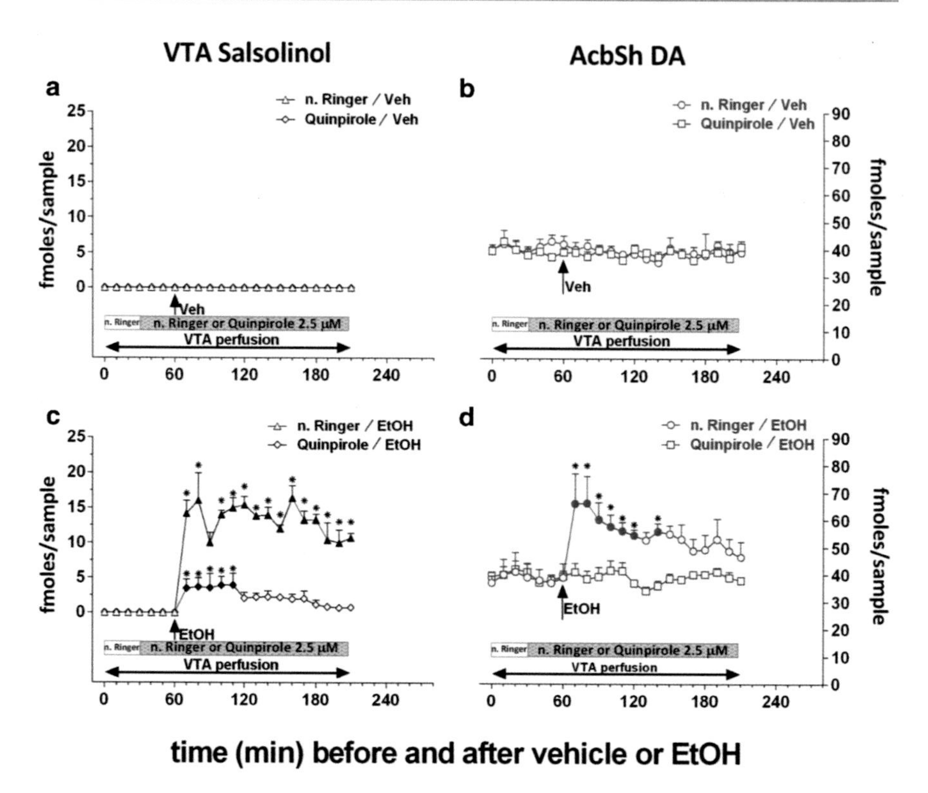

Fig. 7 Effects of intragastric administration of vehicle (tap water, 10 ml/kg) [(**a**), (**b**)] or alcohol (EtOH) (1 g/kg, 20% v/v) [(**c**), (**d**)] in the presence of reverse dialysis application in the pVTA, beginning 30 min before vehicle or EtOH administration, of normal Ringer's (n. Ringer) or quinpirole (2.5 mM) on pVTA salsolinol [(**a**, **c**); triangles: n. Ringer's; lozenges: quinpirole] and on ipsilateral AcbSh DA dialysates [(B,D); circles: n. Ringer's; squares: quinpirole]. Horizontal bars depict the contents of the pVTA perfusion fluid along the experiment. Vertical arrows indicate the last pVTA or AcbSh microdialysis sample before vehicle or EtOH administration. Filled symbols indicate samples representing $p < 0.001$ vs. basal; $*p < 0.05$ vs. vehicle. (Reproduced under a Creative Commons CC-BY license from Bassareo et al. 2021)

acetaldehyde, as discussed above, either by decreasing its production or by sequestering it locally, might represent a prophylactic strategy against acetaldehyde-dependent gastrointestinal cancers (Salaspuro 2007).

Fig. 6 (continued) pVTA, beginning 30 min before EtOH administration, of D-penicillamine (DP) (75 mM) (**a**–**d**) or 3-amino-1,2,4-triazole (3AT) (1 nM) (**e**–**h**) on pVTA salsolinol (**a**, **c**, **e**, **g**) and on ipsilateral and contralateral AcbSh dopamine (**b**, **d**, **f**, **h**) dialysates. Horizontal bars depict the contents of the pVTA perfusion fluid along the experiments. Vertical arrows indicate the last pVTA or AcbSh microdialysis sample before vehicle or EtOH administration. Filled symbols indicate samples representing $p < 0.001$ vs. basal; $p < 0.01$ vs. vehicle administration; $^{x}p < 0.01$ vs. ipsilateral area. (Reproduced under a Creative Commons CC-BY license from Bassareo et al. 2021)

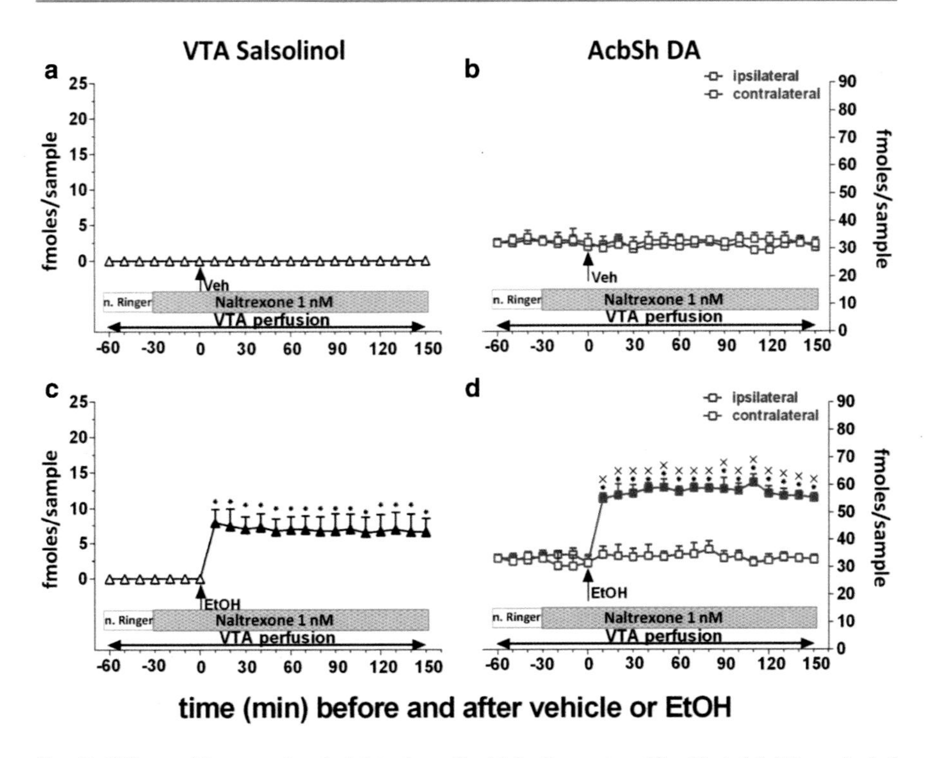

Fig. 8 Effects of intragastric administration of vehicle (tap water, 10 ml/kg) (**a**) (**b**) or alcohol (EtOH) (1 g/kg, 20% v/v) (**c**) (**d**) in the presence of reverse dialysis application in the pVTA, beginning 30 min before EtOH administration, of naltrexone (1 nM) on VTA salsolinol (**a**, **c**) and on ipsilateral and contralateral AcbSh dopamine (**b**, **d**) dialysates. Horizontal bars depict the contents of the pVTA perfusion fluid along the experiment. Vertical arrows indicate the last pVTA or AcbSh microdialysis sample before vehicle or EtOH administration. Filled symbols indicate samples representing $p < 0.001$ vs. basal; $^{*}p < 0.01$ vs. vehicle administration; $^{x}p < 0.01$ vs. ipsilateral area. (Reproduced under a Creative Commons CC-BY license from Bassareo et al. 2021)

Summary Points

- Alcohol is the psychopharmacologically active ingredient of alcoholic drinks.
- As a consequence of its abnormal/excessive consumption, alcohol is a chemical potentially responsible for serious health problems both at the individual and at the societal level.
- Alcohol owns its potential of triggering abnormal behaviors toward its excessive consumption to its ability to activate dopaminergic neurons in the pVTA and stimulate dopamine neurotransmission in the nucleus accumbens.
- The mechanism of alcohol's actions in the activation of pVTA neurons and stimulation of dopamine transmission has long been the subject of intense research, and in spite of the involvement of many neurotransmitter systems, only recently has it been shown that prevention of its metabolic conversion into

salsolinol results in alcohol's failure to activate pVTA dopamine neurons and stimulate nucleus accumbens shell dopamine transmission.

- The above-summarized compelling evidence strongly points to alcohol as the prodrug of salsolinol for its actions on the mesolimbic dopamine system and for its ability to exert its addictive liability.

References

Abrahao KP, Salinas AG, Lovinger DM (2017) Alcohol and the brain: neuronal molecular targets, synapses, and circuits. Neuron 96(6):1223–1238. https://doi.org/10.1016/j.neuron.2017.10.032

Ahlenius S, Carlsson A, Engel J, Svensson T, Södersten P (1973) Antagonism by alpha methyltyrosine of the ethanol-induced stimulation and euphoria in man. Clin Pharmacol Ther 14(4):586–591. https://doi.org/10.1002/cpt1973144part1586

American Psychiatric Association (2013) Diagnostic and statistical manual of mental disorders, 5th edn. American Psychiatric Publishing, Washington, DC

Aragon CM, Amit Z (1985) A two dimensional model of alcohol consumption: possible interaction of brain catalase and aldehyde dehydrogenase. Alcohol 2(2):357–360. https://doi.org/10.1016/0741-8329(85)90075-8

Aragon CM, Spivak K, Amit Z (1985) Blockade of ethanol induced conditioned taste aversion by 3-amino-1,2,4-triazole: evidence for catalase mediated synthesis of acetaldehyde in rat brain. Life Sci 37(22):2077–2084. https://doi.org/10.1016/0024-3205(85)90579-x

Aragon CM, Stotland LM, Amit Z (1991) Studies on ethanol-brain catalase interaction: evidence for central ethanol oxidation. Alcohol Clin Exp Res 15(2):165–169. https://doi.org/10.1111/j.1530-0277.1991.tb01848.x

Arizzi-LaFrance MN, Correa M, Aragon CM, Salamone JD (2006) Motor stimulant effects of ethanol injected into the substantia nigra pars reticulata: importance of catalase-mediated metabolism and the role of acetaldehyde. Neuropsychopharmacology 31(5):997–1008. https://doi.org/10.1038/sj.npp.1300849

Axley PD, Richardson CT, Singal AK (2019) Epidemiology of alcohol consumption and societal burden of alcoholism and alcoholic liver disease. Clin Liver Dis 23(1):39–50. https://doi.org/10.1016/j.cld.2018.09.011

Bassareo V, Cucca F, Frau R, Di Chiara G (2017) Changes in dopamine transmission in the nucleus accumbens shell and core during ethanol and sucrose self-administration. Front Behav Neurosci 11:71. https://doi.org/10.3389/fnbeh.2017.00071

Bassareo V, Frau R, Maccioni R, Caboni P, Manis C, Peana AT, Migheli R, Porru S, Acquas E (2021) Ethanol-dependent synthesis of Salsolinol in the posterior ventral tegmental area as key mechanism of ethanol's action on mesolimbic dopamine. Front Neurosci 15:675061. https://doi.org/10.3389/fnins.2021.675061

Belmer A, Patkar OL, Pitman KM, Bartlett SE (2016) Serotonergic neuroplasticity in alcohol addiction. Brain Plast 1(2):177–206. https://doi.org/10.3233/bpl-150022

Berríos-Cárcamo P, Quintanilla ME, Herrera-Marschitz M, Vasiliou V, Zapata-Torres G, Rivera-Meza M (2017) Racemic salsolinol and its enantiomers act as agonists of the μ-opioid receptor by activating the Gi protein-adenylate cyclase pathway. Front Behav Neurosci 10:253. https://doi.org/10.3389/fnbeh.2016.00253

Berríos-Cárcamo P, Rivera-Meza M, Herrera-Marschitz M, Zapata-Torres G (2019) Molecular modeling of salsolinol, a full G_i protein agonist of the μ-opioid receptor, within the receptor binding site. Chem Biol Drug Des 94(2):1467–1477. https://doi.org/10.1111/cbdd.13523

Bradford BU, Forman DT, Thurman RG (1993) 4-Methylpyrazole inhibits fatty acyl coenzyme synthetase and diminishes catalase-dependent alcohol metabolism: has the contribution of alcohol dehydrogenase to alcohol metabolism been previously overestimated? Mol Pharmacol 43(1):115–119

Brancato A, Plescia F, Marino RA, Maniaci G, Navarra M, Cannizzaro C (2014) Involvement of dopamine D2 receptors in addictive-like behaviour for acetaldehyde. PLoS One 9(6):e99454. https://doi.org/10.1371/journal.pone.0099454

Breton JM, Charbit AR, Snyder BJ, Fong PTK, Dias EV, Himmels P, Lock H, Margolis EB (2019) Relative contributions and mapping of ventral tegmental area dopamine and GABA neurons by projection target in the rat. J Comp Neurol 527(5):916–941. https://doi.org/10.1002/cne.24572

Cederbaum AI (2012) Alcohol metabolism. Clin Liver Dis 16(4):667–685. https://doi.org/10.1016/j.cld.2012.08.002

Chen X, Zheng X, Ali S, Guo M, Zhong R, Chen Z, Zhang Y, Qing H, Deng Y (2018) Isolation and sequencing of salsolinol synthase, an enzyme catalyzing salsolinol biosynthesis. ACS Chem Neurosci 9(6):1388–1398. https://doi.org/10.1021/acschemneuro.8b00023

Chevens LC (1953) Antabuse addiction. Br Med J 1(4825):1450–1451. https://doi.org/10.1136/bmj.1.4825.1450-c

Collins MA (1988) Acetaldehyde and its condensation products as markers in alcoholism. Recent Dev Alcohol 6:387–403. https://doi.org/10.1007/978-1-4615-7718-8_22

Collins MA, Nijm WP, Borge GF, Teas G, Goldfarb C (1979) Dopamine-related tetrahydroisoquinolines: significant urinary excretion by alcoholics after alcohol consumption. Science 206(4423):1184–1186. https://doi.org/10.1126/science.505002

Collins MA, Ung-Chhun N, Cheng BY, Pronger D (1990) Brain and plasma tetrahydroisoquinolines in rats: effects of chronic ethanol intake and diet. J Neurochem 55(5):1507–1514. https://doi.org/10.1111/j.1471-4159.1990.tb04932.x

Colombo G, Lobina C, Carai MA, Gessa GL (2006) Phenotypic characterization of genetically selected Sardinian alcohol-preferring (sP) and -non-preferring (sNP) rats. Addict Biol 11(3–4, 324):–38. https://doi.org/10.1111/j.1369-1600.2006.00031.x

Correa M, Sanchis-Segura C, Aragon CM (2001) Brain catalase activity is highly correlated with ethanol-induced locomotor activity in mice. Physiol Behav 73(4):641–647. https://doi.org/10.1016/s0031-9384(01)00511-x

Correa M, Manrique HM, Font L, Escrig MA, Aragon CM (2008) Reduction in the anxiolytic effects of ethanol by centrally formed acetaldehyde: the role of catalase inhibitors and acetaldehyde-sequestering agents. Psychopharmacology 200(4):455–464. https://doi.org/10.1007/s00213-008-1219-3

Correa M, Viaggi C, Escrig MA, Pascual M, Guerri C, Vaglini F, Aragon CM, Corsini GU (2009a) Ethanol intake and ethanol-induced locomotion and locomotor sensitization in Cyp2e1 knockout mice. Pharmacogenet Genomics 19(3):217–225. https://doi.org/10.1097/fpc.0b013e328324e726

Correa M, Arizzi-Lafrance MN, Salamone JD (2009b) Infusions of acetaldehyde into the arcuate nucleus of the hypothalamus induce motor activity in rats. Life Sci 84(11–12):321–327. https://doi.org/10.1016/j.lfs.2008.12.013

Correa M, Salamone JD, Segovia KN, Pardo M, Longoni R, Spina L, Peana AT, Vinci S, Acquas E (2012) Piecing together the puzzle of acetaldehyde as a neuroactive agent. Neurosci Biobehav Rev 36(1):404–430. https://doi.org/10.1016/j.neubiorev.2011.07.009

Davis VE, Walsh MJ (1970) Alcohol, amines, and alkaloids: a possible biochemical basis for alcohol addiction. Science 167(3920):1005–1007. https://doi.org/10.1126/science.167.3920.1005

Davis VE, Walsh MJ, Yamanaka Y (1970) Augmentation of alkaloid formation from dopamine by alcohol and acetaldehyde in vitro. J Pharmacol Exp Ther 174(3):401–412

Deehan GA Jr, Brodie MS, Rodd ZA (2013) What is in that drink: the biological actions of ethanol, acetaldehyde, and salsolinol. Curr Top Behav Neurosci 13:163–184. https://doi.org/10.1007/7854_2011_198

Di Chiara G, Bassareo V (2007) Reward system and addiction: what dopamine does and doesn't do. Curr Opin Pharmacol 7(1):69–76. https://doi.org/10.1016/j.coph.2006.11.003

Di Chiara G, Bassareo V, Fenu S, De Luca MA, Spina L, Cadoni C, Acquas E, Carboni E, Valentini V, Lecca D (2004) Dopamine and drug addiction: the nucleus accumbens shell connection. Neuropharmacology 47(Suppl 1):227–241. https://doi.org/10.1016/j.neuropharm.2004.06.032

Di L, Balesano A, Jordan S, Shi SM (2021) The role of alcohol dehydrogenase in drug metabolism: beyond ethanol oxidation. AAPS J 23(1):20. https://doi.org/10.1208/s12248-020-00536-y

Ding ZM, Toalston JE, Oster SM, McBride WJ, Rodd ZA (2009) Involvement of local serotonin-2A but not serotonin-1B receptors in the reinforcing effects of ethanol within the posterior ventral tegmental area of female Wistar rats. Psychopharmacology 204(3):381–390. https://doi.org/10.1007/s00213-009-1468-9

Ding ZM, Oster SM, Hauser SR, Toalston JE, Bell RL, McBride WJ, Rodd ZA (2012) Synergistic self-administration of ethanol and cocaine directly into the posterior ventral tegmental area: involvement of serotonin-3 receptors. J Pharmacol Exp Ther 340(1):202–209. https://doi.org/10.1124/jpet.111.187245

Dyr W, Kostowski W (2004) Preliminary phenotypic characterization of the Warsaw High Preferring (WHP) and Warsaw Low Preferring (WLP) lines of rats selectively bred for high and low ethanol consumption. Pol J Pharmacol 56(3):359–365

Escarabajal MD, Aragon CM (2002a) Concurrent administration of diethyldithiocarbamate and 4-methylpyrazole enhances ethanol-induced locomotor activity: the role of brain ALDH. Psychopharmacology 160(4):339–343. https://doi.org/10.1007/s00213-001-0991-0

Escarabajal MD, Aragon CM (2002b) The effect of cyanamide and 4-methylpyrazole on the ethanol-induced locomotor activity in mice. Pharmacol Biochem Behav 72(1–2):389–395. https://doi.org/10.1016/s0091-3057(01)00762-6

Escarabajal D, Miquel M, Aragon CM (2000) A psychopharmacological study of the relationship between brain catalase activity and ethanol-induced locomotor activity in mice. J Stud Alcohol 61(4):493–498. https://doi.org/10.15288/jsa.2000.61.493

Font L, Aragon CM, Miquel M (2006a) Voluntary ethanol consumption decreases after the inactivation of central acetaldehyde by d-penicillamine. Behav Brain Res 171(1):78–86. https://doi.org/10.1016/j.bbr.2006.03.020

Font L, Aragon CM, Miquel M (2006b) Ethanol-induced conditioned place preference, but not aversion, is blocked by treatment with D -penicillamine, an inactivation agent for acetaldehyde. Psychopharmacology 184(1):56–64. https://doi.org/10.1007/s00213-005-0224-z

Font L, Luján MÁ, Pastor R (2013) Involvement of the endogenous opioid system in the psychopharmacological actions of ethanol: the role of acetaldehyde. Front Behav Neurosci 7:93. https://doi.org/10.3389/fnbeh.2013.00093

Geisler S, Zahm DS (2005) Afferents of the ventral tegmental area in the rat-anatomical substratum for integrative functions. J Comp Neurol 490(3):270–294. https://doi.org/10.1002/cne.20668

Gessa GL, Muntoni F, Collu M, Vargiu L, Mereu G (1985) Low doses of ethanol activate dopaminergic neurons in the ventral tegmental area. Brain Res 348(1):201–203. https://doi.org/10.1016/0006-8993(85)90381-6

Gill K, France C, Amit Z (1986) Voluntary ethanol consumption in rats: an examination of blood/brain ethanol levels and behavior. Alcohol Clin Exp Res 4:457–462. https://doi.org/10.1111/j.1530-0277.1986.tb05124.x

Hipólito L, Sánchez-Catalán MJ, Granero L, Polache A (2009) Local salsolinol modulates dopamine extracellular levels from rat nucleus accumbens: shell/core differences. Neurochem Int 55(4):187–192. https://doi.org/10.1016/j.neuint.2009.02.014

Hipólito L, Sánchez-Catalán MJ, Zornoza T, Polache A, Granero L (2010) Locomotor stimulant effects of acute and repeated intrategmental injections of salsolinol in rats: role of mu-opioid receptors. Psychopharmacology 209(1):1–11. https://doi.org/10.1007/s00213-009-1751-9

Hipólito L, Martí-Prats L, Sánchez-Catalán MJ, Polache A, Granero L (2011) Induction of conditioned place preference and dopamine release by salsolinol in posterior VTA of rats: involvement of μ-opioid receptors. Neurochem Int 59(5):559–562. https://doi.org/10.1016/j.neuint.2011.04.014

Hipólito L, Sánchez-Catalán MJ, Martí-Prats L, Granero L, Polache A (2012) Revisiting the controversial role of salsolinol in the neurobiological effects of ethanol: old and new vistas. Neurosci Biobehav Rev 36(1):362–378. https://doi.org/10.1016/j.neubiorev.2011.07.007

Ikemoto S (2007) Dopamine reward circuitry: two projection systems from the ventral midbrain to the nucleus accumbens-olfactory tubercle complex. Brain Res Rev 56(1):27–78. https://doi.org/10.1016/j.brainresrev.2007.05.004
King AC, Houle T, de Wit H, Holdstock L, Schuster A (2002) Biphasic alcohol response differs in heavy versus light drinkers. Alcohol Clin Exp Res 26(6):827–835
Koob GF (2004) A role for GABA mechanisms in the motivational effects of alcohol. Biochem Pharmacol 68(8):1515–1525. https://doi.org/10.1016/j.bcp.2004.07.031
Koob GF (2014) Neurocircuitry of alcohol addiction: synthesis from animal models. Handb Clin Neurol 125:33–54. https://doi.org/10.1016/b978-0-444-62619-6.00003-3
Koob GF, Volkow ND (2016) Neurobiology of addiction: a neurocircuitry analysis. Lancet Psychiatry 3(8):760–773. https://doi.org/10.1016/s2215-0366(16)00104-8
Kurnik-Łucka M, Latacz G, Martyniak A, Bugajski A, Kieć-Kononowicz K, Gil K (2020) Salsolinol-neurotoxic or neuroprotective? Neurotox Res 37(2):286–297. https://doi.org/10.1007/s12640-019-00118-7
Majchrowicz E (1975) Effect of peripheral ethanol metabolism on the central nervous system. Fed Proc 34(10):1948–1952
Martí-Prats L, Sánchez-Catalán MJ, Hipólito L, Orrico A, Zornoza T, Polache A, Granero L (2010) Systemic administration of D-penicillamine prevents the locomotor activation after intra-VTA ethanol administration in rats. Neurosci Lett 483(2):143–147. https://doi.org/10.1016/j.neulet.2010.07.081
Martí-Prats L, Sánchez-Catalán MJ, Orrico A, Zornoza T, Polache A, Granero L (2013) Opposite motor responses elicited by ethanol in the posterior VTA: the role of acetaldehyde and the non-metabolized fraction of ethanol. Neuropharmacology 72:204–214. https://doi.org/10.1016/j.neuropharm.2013.04.047
Matsuzawa S, Suzuki T, Misawa M (2000) Involvement of mu-opioid receptor in the salsolinol-associated place preference in rats exposed to conditioned fear stress. Alcohol Clin Exp Res 24 (3):366–372
Melis M, Enrico P, Peana AT, Diana M (2007) Acetaldehyde mediates alcohol activation of the mesolimbic dopamine system. Eur J Neurosci 26(10):2824–2833. https://doi.org/10.1111/j.1460-9568.2007.05887.x
Melis M, Carboni E, Caboni P, Acquas E (2015) Key role of salsolinol in ethanol actions on dopamine neuronal activity of the posterior ventral tegmental area. Addict Biol 20(1):182–193. https://doi.org/10.1111/adb.12097
Nieminen MT, Salaspuro M (2018) Local acetaldehyde-an essential role in alcohol-related upper gastrointestinal tract carcinogenesis. Cancers (Basel) 10(1):11. https://doi.org/10.3390/cancers10010011
Nurmi M, Kiianmaa K, Sinclair JD (1994) Brain ethanol in AA, ANA, and Wistar rats monitored with one-minute microdialysis. Alcohol 11(4):315–321. https://doi.org/10.1016/0741-8329(94)90098-1
Oláh M, Bodnár I, Daniel G, Tóth BE, Vecsernyés M, Nagy GM (2011) Role of salsolinol in the regulation of pituitary prolactin and peripheral dopamine release. Reprod Med Biol 10(3):143–151. https://doi.org/10.1007/s12522-011-0086-5
Origitano T, Hannigan J, Collins MA (1981) Rat brain salsolinol and blood-brain barrier. Brain Res 224(2):446–451. https://doi.org/10.1016/0006-8993(81)90876-3
Orrico A, Martí-Prats L, Cano-Cebrián MJ, Granero L, Polache A, Zornoza T (2017) Pre-clinical studies with D-Penicillamine as a novel pharmacological strategy to treat alcoholism: updated evidences. Front Behav Neurosci 11:37. https://doi.org/10.3389/fnbeh.2017.00037
Pardo M, Betz AJ, San Miguel N, López-Cruz L, Salamone JD, Correa M (2013) Acetate as an active metabolite of ethanol: studies of locomotion, loss of righting reflex, and anxiety in rodents. Front Behav Neurosci 7:81. https://doi.org/10.3389/fnbeh.2013.00081
Pastor R, Sanchis-Segura C, Aragon CM (2002) Ethanol-stimulated behaviour in mice is modulated by brain catalase activity and H2O2 rate of production. Psychopharmacology 165(1):51–59. https://doi.org/10.1007/s00213-002-1241-9

Peana AT, Enrico P, Assaretti AR, Pulighe E, Muggironi G, Nieddu M, Piga A, Lintas A, Diana M (2008) Key role of ethanol-derived acetaldehyde in the motivational properties induced by intragastric ethanol: a conditioned place preference study in the rat. Alcohol Clin Exp Res 32(2): 249–258. https://doi.org/10.1111/j.1530-0277.2007.00574.x

Peana AT, Muggironi G, Diana M (2010) acetaldehyde-reinforcing effects: a study on oral self-administration behavior. Front Psych 2010 16;1:23. https://doi.org/10.3389/fpsyt.2010.00023

Peana AT, Porcheddu V, Bennardini F, Carta A, Rosas M, Acquas E (2015) Role of ethanol-derived acetaldehyde in operant oral self-administration of ethanol in rats. Psychopharmacology 232 (23):4269–4276. https://doi.org/10.1007/s00213-015-4049-0

Peana AT, Rosas M, Porru S, Acquas E (2016) From ethanol to Salsolinol: role of ethanol metabolites in the effects of ethanol. J Exp Neurosci 10:137–146. https://doi.org/10.4137/jen.s25099

Peana AT, Pintus FA, Bennardini F, Rocchitta G, Bazzu G, Serra PA, Porru S, Rosas M, Acquas E (2017a) Is catalase involved in the effects of systemic and pVTA administration of 4-methylpyrazole on ethanol self-administration? Alcohol 63:61–73. https://doi.org/10.1016/j.alcohol.2017.04.001

Peana AT, Sánchez-Catalán MJ, Hipólito L, Rosas M, Porru S, Bennardini F, Romualdi P, Caputi FF, Candeletti S, Polache A, Granero L, Acquas E (2017b) Mystic acetaldehyde: the never-ending story on alcoholism. Front Behav Neurosci 11:81

Peana AT, Bassareo V, Acquas E (2019) Not just from ethanol. Tetrahydroisoquinolinic (TIQ) derivatives: from neurotoxicity to neuroprotection. Neurotox Res 36(4):653–668. https://doi.org/10.1007/s12640-019-00051-9

Peana AT, Muggironi G, Fois GR, Zinellu M, Vinci S and Acquas E (2011) Effect of opioid receptor blockade on acetaldehyde self-administrationand ERK phosphorylation in the rat nucleus accumbens. Alcohol (45):773–783. https://doi.org/10.1016/j.alcohol.2011.06.003

Polache A, Granero L (2013) Salsolinol and ethanol-derived excitation of dopamine mesolimbic neurons: new insights. Front Behav Neurosci 7:74

Quintanilla ME, Israel Y, Sapag A, Tampier L (2006) The UChA and UChB rat lines: metabolic and genetic differences influencing ethanol intake. Addict Biol 11(3–4):310–323. https://doi.org/10.1111/j.1369-1600.2006.00030.x

Quintanilla ME, Rivera-Meza M, Berrios-Cárcamo PA, Bustamante D, Buscaglia M, Morales P, Karahanian E, Herrera-Marschitz M, Israel Y (2014) Salsolinol, free of isosalsolinol, exerts ethanol-like motivational/sensitization effects leading to increases in ethanol intake. Alcohol 48 (6):551–559. https://doi.org/10.1016/j.alcohol.2014.07.003

Quintanilla ME, Rivera-Meza M, Berríos-Cárcamo P, Cassels BK, Herrera-Marschitz M, Israel Y (2016) (R)-Salsolinol, a product of ethanol metabolism, stereospecifically induces behavioral sensitization and leads to excessive alcohol intake. Addict Biol 21(6):1063–1071. https://doi.org/10.1111/adb.12268

Rehm J, Gmel GE Sr, Gmel G, Hasan OSM, Imtiaz S, Popova S, Probst C, Roerecke M, Room R, Samokhvalov AV, Shield KD, Shuper PA (2017) The relationship between different dimensions of alcohol use and the burden of disease-an update. Addiction 112(6):968–1001. https://doi.org/10.1111/add.13757

Rodd ZA, Bell RL, Zhang Y, Goldstein A, Zaffaroni A, McBride WJ, Li TK (2003) Salsolinol produces reinforcing effects in the nucleus accumbens shell of alcohol-preferring (P) rats. Alcohol Clin Exp Res 27(3):440–449. https://doi.org/10.1097/01.ALC.0000056612.89957.B4

Rodd ZA, Bell RL, Zhang Y, Murphy JM, Goldstein A, Zaffaroni A, Li TK, McBride WJ (2005) Regional heterogeneity for the intracranial self-administration of ethanol and acetaldehyde within the ventral tegmental area of alcohol-preferring (P) rats: involvement of dopamine and serotonin. Neuropsychopharmacology 30(2):330–338. https://doi.org/10.1038/sj.npp.1300561

Rodd ZA, Oster SM, Ding ZM, Toalston JE, Deehan G, Bell RL, Li TK, McBride WJ (2008) The reinforcing properties of salsolinol in the ventral tegmental area: evidence for regional heterogeneity and the involvement of serotonin and dopamine. Alcohol Clin Exp Res 32(2):230–239. https://doi.org/10.1111/j.1530-0277.2007.00572.x

Salaspuro V (2007) Pharmacological treatments and strategies for reducing oral and intestinal acetaldehyde. Novartis Found Symp 285(145–53):discussion 153-7,198-9. https://doi.org/10.1002/9780470511848.ch11

Sánchez-Catalán MJ, Hipólito L, Zornoza T, Polache A, Granero L (2009) Motor stimulant effects of ethanol and acetaldehyde injected into the posterior ventral tegmental area of rats: role of opioid receptors. Psychopharmacology 204(4):641–653. https://doi.org/10.1007/s00213-009-1495-6

Sanchez-Catalan MJ, Kaufling J, Georges F, Veinante P, Barrot M (2014) The antero-posterior heterogeneity of the ventral tegmental area. Neuroscience 282:198–216. https://doi.org/10.1016/j.neuroscience.2014.09.025

Sanchis-Segura C, Miquel M, Correa M, Aragon CM (1999a) The catalase inhibitor sodium azide reduces ethanol-induced locomotor activity. Alcohol 19(1):37–42. https://doi.org/10.1016/s0741-8329(99)00016-6

Sanchis-Segura C, Miquel M, Correa M, Aragon CM (1999b) Cyanamide reduces brain catalase and ethanol-induced locomotor activity: is there a functional link? Psychopharmacology 144(1): 83–89. https://doi.org/10.1007/s002130050980

Sanchis-Segura C, Miquel M, Correa M, Aragon CM (1999c) Daily injections of cyanamide enhance both ethanol-induced locomotion and brain catalase activity. Behav Pharmacol 10(5): 459–465. https://doi.org/10.1097/00008877-199909000-00004

Sippel HW (1974) The acetaldehyde content in rat brain during ethanol metabolism. J Neurochem 23(2):451–452. https://doi.org/10.1111/j.1471-4159.1974.tb04380.x

Spina L, Longoni R, Vinci S, Ibba F, Peana AT, Muggironi G, Spiga S, Acquas E (2010) Role of dopamine D1 receptors and extracellular signal regulated kinase in the motivational properties of acetaldehyde as assessed by place preference conditioning. Alcohol Clin Exp Res 34(4):607–616. https://doi.org/10.1111/j.1530-0277.2009.01129.x

Tambour S, Didone V, Tirelli E, Quertemont E (2005) Dissociation between the locomotor and anxiolytic effects of acetaldehyde in the elevated plus-maze: evidence that acetaldehyde is not involved in the anxiolytic effects of ethanol in mice. Eur Neuropsychopharmacol 15(6):655–662. https://doi.org/10.1016/j.euroneuro.2005.04.014

Vinci S, Ibba F, Longoni R, Spina L, Spiga S, Acquas E (2010) Acetaldehyde elicits ERK phosphorylation in the rat nucleus accumbens and extended amygdala. Synapse 64(12):916–927. https://doi.org/10.1002/syn.20811

Volkow ND, Fowler JS, Wang GJ, Baler R, Telang F (2009) Imaging dopamine's role in drug abuse and addiction. Neuropharmacology 56(Suppl 1):3–8. https://doi.org/10.1016/j.neuropharm.2008.05.022

Wise RA (2009) Roles for nigrostriatal – not just mesocorticolimbic – dopamine in reward and addiction. Trends Neurosci 32(10):517–524. https://doi.org/10.1016/j.tins.2009.06.004

Xie G, Hipólito L, Zuo W, Polache A, Granero L, Krnjevic K, Ye JH (2012) Salsolinol stimulates dopamine neurons in slices of posterior ventral tegmental area indirectly by activating μ-opioid receptors. J Pharmacol Exp Ther 341(1):43–50. https://doi.org/10.1124/jpet.111.186833

Linking Stress, Depression, and Alcohol Use 48

Beata Gavurova, Viera Ivankova, and Martin Rigelsky

Contents

Introduction 1008
Knowledge About Alcohol Use 1009
Alcohol Use and Its Effects on Health 1011
Harmful Alcohol Use Leading to Mental Disorders 1012
Alcohol Addiction as a Mental Disorder 1013
Mental Disorders Associated with Alcohol Use 1014
Schizophrenia 1017
Anxiety 1017
Bipolar Disorder 1017
Obsessive-Compulsive Disorder 1018
Other Mental Disorders 1018
Alcohol and Depression 1018
The Path Between Depression and Alcohol Abuse 1019
The Role of Gender 1020
The Role of Stress 1020
Alcohol and Stress 1020
The Path Between Stress and Alcohol Abuse 1021
Comorbidity Between Alcohol Use Disorder, Stress, and Depression 1022
Applications to Other Areas of Substance Use Disorders 1024
Applications to Areas of Public Health 1025

B. Gavurova (✉)
Department of Addictology, First Faculty of Medicine, Charles University and General University Hospital in Prague, Prague, Czechia
e-mail: beata.gavurova@lf1.cuni.cz

V. Ivankova
Institute of Earth Resources, Faculty of Mining, Ecology, Process Control and Geotechnologies, Technical University of Košice, Košice, Slovakia Republic
e-mail: viera.ivankova@tuke.sk

M. Rigelsky
Faculty of Management and Business, University of Prešov, Prešov, Slovakia
e-mail: martin.rigelsky@unipo.sk

V. B. Patel, V. R. Preedy (eds.), *Handbook of Substance Misuse and Addictions*,
https://doi.org/10.1007/978-3-030-92392-1_53

Mini-Dictionary of Terms 1026
Key Facts of Comorbidity Between Substance Use Disorders and Mental Disorders 1026
Summary Points 1027
References 1027

Abstract

Alcohol is an easily available legal substance that has the most significant negative consequences of all substances due to its frequent occurrence in society, as well as due to social acceptance. It is well-known that alcohol use reduces cognition and is harmful to mental health. This underlines the importance of addressing the link between mental discomfort and alcohol use. Depression and stress often go hand in hand with increased alcohol use. It is possible to talk about alcohol abuse as a consequence of stressful life situations and depressive symptoms. On the other hand, drinking alcohol can lead to stressful situations in the lives of individuals and mental disorders such as depression. Stress may be a critical driver of comorbidity between mental disorders and alcohol use disorder. Educating society about the negatives and risks of alcohol plays an important role in achieving mental health objectives.

Keywords

Alcohol consumption · Problematic drinking · Dependence · Unhealthy pattern · Risk factor · Health burden · Mental discomfort · Mental illness · Disorder · Stress · Depression · Coping strategy · Substance abuse

Abbreviations

COVID-19	Coronavirus disease 2019
EU	European Union
GBD	Global Burden of Disease
GHO	The Global Health Observatory
ICD-10	International Classification of Diseases, Tenth Revision
SIRC	Social Issues Research Centre
WHO	World Health Organization

Introduction

Many international studies point to a relatively strong link between various forms of risky behavior, including alcohol use, and mental discomfort. However, the direction of this relationship is still not entirely clear. As this chapter suggests, the relationship between stress, depression, and alcohol use can be viewed in the same way. On the one hand, it may seem that stress and depression lead to a greater tendency to drink alcohol, but on the other hand, alcohol use can also lead to greater mental discomfort. In other words, alcohol is an addictive substance that affects people's nervous system and their emotions, and, at the same time, emotions affect alcohol use. In addition, this relationship can be mediated by different factors in different areas, making the whole area of research a multifactorial and complex matter.

Problematic drinking and alcohol addiction are a significant health and socioeconomic problem. Its high prevalence is related to its relatively low price and its easy availability of alcohol. There are many ways in which alcohol affects cognitive functions, and they can be combined in different ways (Režnáková 2018). All these facts underline the importance of addressing the issue of linking mental discomfort and alcohol use as one of the most common addictive patterns of behavior. The presented chapter focuses on stress and depression across the population and on the role of alcohol drinking in this problem.

Knowledge About Alcohol Use

Alcohol is an easily available legal social drug that is tolerated, although it is one of the riskiest factors for the health of the population. The importance of this issue is underlined by the fact that alcohol has played a central role in almost all cultures since the Neolithic period (about 4000 before Christ). All societies, without exception, use intoxicating substances, while alcohol is one of the most common (SIRC 1998). In other words, alcohol goes deep into human history; it has found a firm position in society, from which it is not easy to exclude it. For a closer look at the issue of alcohol consumption, Fig. 1 shows the patterns of alcohol use in European countries.

Figure 1 shows the attitudes of the European population toward alcohol use in four variants (in percentages). The countries with the highest proportion of abstainers included Turkey, Tajikistan, or Uzbekistan. On the contrary, the lowest proportion of abstainers was found in Luxembourg. The highest proportion of former alcohol drinkers was observed in Georgia, while the lowest proportion was identified in Turkey, Luxembourg, or Italy. The highest proportion of alcohol consumers were in Luxembourg and the lowest proportion in Turkey. Lithuania, Luxembourg, and Latvia were among the three countries with the highest proportion of heavy episodic drinkers. On the other hand, the lowest proportion of heavy episodic drinkers was found in countries such as Turkey, Uzbekistan, Tajikistan, or Azerbaijan. These findings suggest a drinking culture in individual countries.

Across cultures and nations, alcohol use can be viewed differently. Palm (2006) and Ronzani (2018) presented the following models of alcohol use:

- Moral model: Use of alcohol and other drugs is a sign of weakness and lack of character, whereas abstinence is seen as a sign of virtue. Addiction is seen by society as a crime and therefore should be treated.
- Medical or disease model: There is still a remnant of moralization regarding use, but addiction is no longer seen as a moral issue, but rather as a disease. Addiction is perceived as a problem of the individual and not of the drug itself.
- Rationalist model: Influenced by capitalism, with the normative idea that addiction is the result of a failure in self-control, an irrational act.

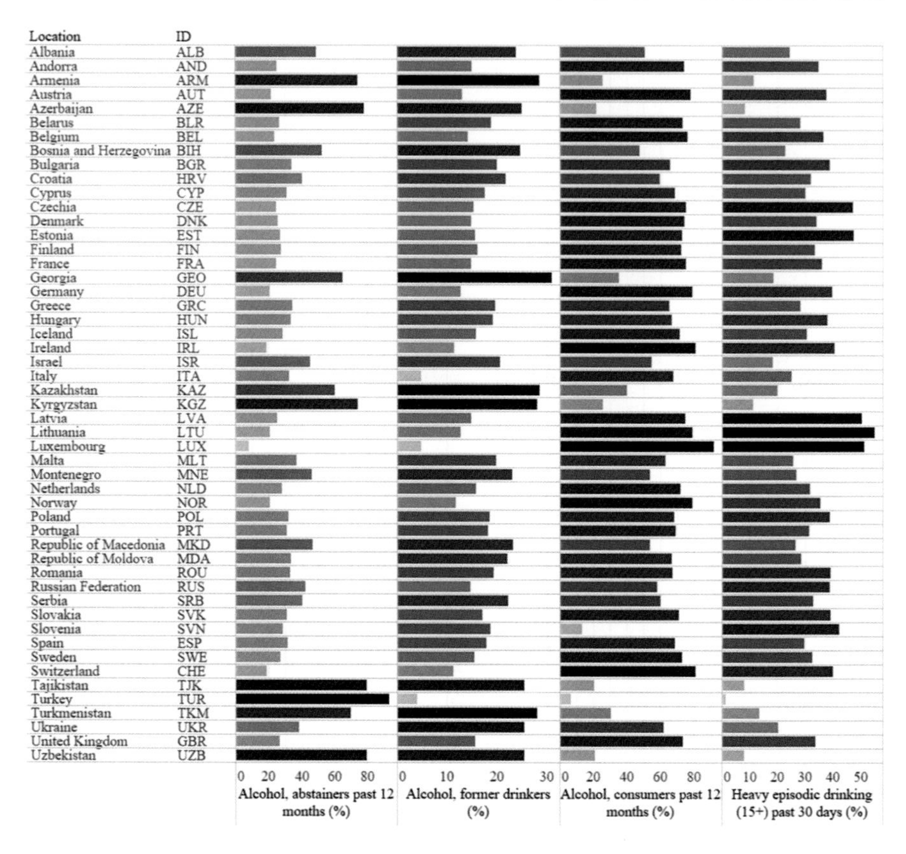

Fig. 1 Patterns of alcohol use in European countries (2016). (Source: Own processing based on data from GHO 2021)

- Public health model: The focus is not the user individually, but the environment and all users and the problems associated with use. Actions are viewed collectively, based on different usage patterns and general health policies. The main concern is to reduce consumption and the overall consequences.
- Social model: Addiction is seen as a consequence of misery and social injustice and therefore should be seen as a problem of society. The core of this subchapter is focused on the area of interconnection of medical or disease model and public health model.

To better understand alcohol use, it is very important to take into account the phenomenon of habit, which is also emphasized by Nieto et al. (2021), who revealed that lifetime years of alcohol abuse were positively associated with lifetime regular drinking years, current alcohol use, alcohol problems, tonic alcohol craving, drinking for the enhancing effects of alcohol, and drinking to cope. Therefore, it is desirable to address the problem of alcohol use, especially in the most vulnerable groups.

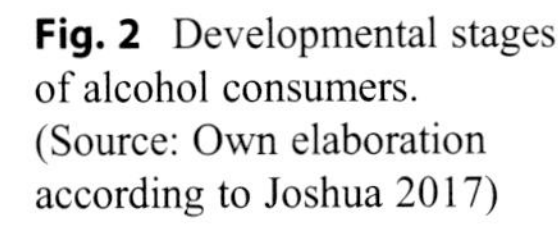

Fig. 2 Developmental stages of alcohol consumers. (Source: Own elaboration according to Joshua 2017)

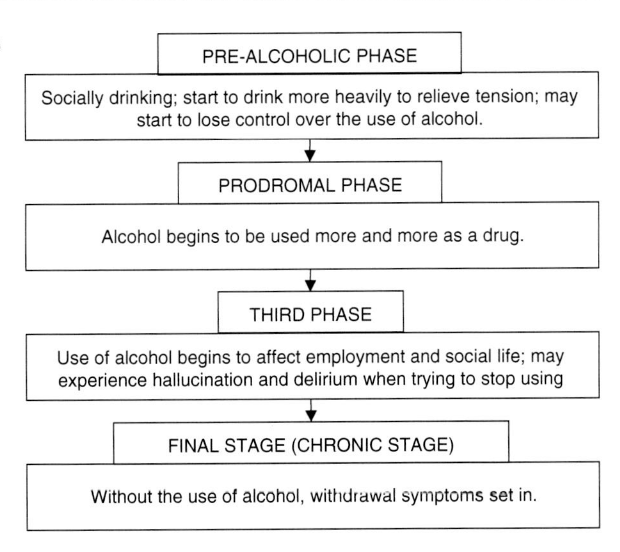

Figure 2 presents the development of alcohol addiction from the perspective of consumers themselves. As can be seen, the first phase seems to be relatively harmless, but even in this phase it is appropriate to be aware of the risk. In each subsequent phase, the risk increases, the negative consequences of increased alcohol consumption also increase, and the positives practically disappear.

Alcohol Use and Its Effects on Health

From a public health perspective, it should be noted that alcohol use can lead to various health problems across the population. Nelson and Kolls (2002) argued that in the past, alcohol use was associated primarily with bacterial pneumonia, but at the present time, chronic drinking as well as acute drinking is associated with specific defects in innate and adaptive immunity.

In any case, alcohol use is considered to be a significant risk factor for health in terms of serious diseases, disabilities, but also deaths (Rehm et al. 2003; Smyth et al. 2015). Evidence showed that alcohol consumption can lead to a higher risk of cancer (Connor et al. 2017; Scoccianti et al. 2013), but also liver cirrhosis (Roerecke et al. 2019), pneumonia (Simou et al. 2018a), tuberculosis (Simou et al. 2018b), or injuries (Cherpitel et al. 2019). The effects of alcohol consumption on public health have been well examined, but the vast majority of studies have looked at registered alcohol in their research. Lachenmeier et al. (2021) pointed out that 25% of the total amount of alcohol consumed is unrecorded alcohol, the consumption of which may also be related to other health problems (e.g., methanol poisoning). Negative effects on mental health are no exception, while Hufford (2001) revealed that alcohol use reduces cognition, increases mental distress and aggression, and promotes suicidal thoughts. In this regard, the findings showed that alcohol use as such, but also alcohol use disorders, is considered a predictor of suicidal behavior, self-harm, and suicidal deaths (Darvishi et al. 2015; Hufford 2001). The role of stress and depression in this mental health problem is also addressed in this chapter.

It can be concluded that alcohol consumption leads to higher mortality, which may result in a reduction in life expectancy (Ranabhat et al. 2020). At the same time, alcohol creates differences in health between individual countries, as evidenced by findings showing that alcohol-related mortality rates are higher in the new Member States of the European Union (EU) (Czech Republic, Hungary, Lithuania, Poland) than in the old EU Member States (France, Sweden, the United Kingdom) (Rehm et al. 2007). This may also be related to the differences in levels of alcohol consumption between individual countries and to the patterns of alcohol use indicated in Fig. 1.

All of the abovementioned facts confirm that alcohol poses a threat to public health in many countries. Public health institutions are responsible for addressing this problem in society, with an emphasis on the specifics of alcohol use across the population (Megyesiova and Gavurova 2019).

Harmful Alcohol Use Leading to Mental Disorders

Regarding harmful alcohol use, it is possible to speak of acute intoxication, which is a transient condition following the administration of alcohol, resulting in disturbances in the level of consciousness, cognition, perception, affect, behavior, or other psychophysiological functions and responses (WHO 1992). From a quantitative point of view, there are four stages of intoxication (Kalina et al. 2015; Režňáková 2018):

1. Mild intoxication – an excitation stage in which unbraked behavior, slow reaction time, or attention deficit disorders predominate (alcoholaemia up to 1.5‰, i.e., 1.5 g/kg)
2. Moderate intoxication – a hypnotic stage in which there are obvious neurological symptoms, memory disorders, and depression (alcoholaemia 1.5–2.5‰)
3. Severe intoxication – a narcotic stage characterized by drowsiness to unconsciousness (alcoholaemia 2.5–3.0‰)
4. Acute alcohol poisoning – an asphyxic stage in which severe intoxication with loss of consciousness, immediate respiratory arrest, or circulatory arrest is identified (alcoholaemia over 3.0‰)

Withdrawal intoxication (also called hangover) is characterized by mood swings (dysphoric, anxiety, or depressive), memory disorders may be present, but vegetative manifestations are also common (headaches, nausea, sweating) (Režňáková 2018). These withdrawal signs are one of the indicators of dependence syndrome, and this latter diagnosis should also be considered.

Based on the abovementioned, it is possible to speak of harmful alcohol use as a pattern that leads to damage to health. The damage may be physical or mental (e.g., episodes of depressive disorder secondary to heavy alcohol consumption). This harmful behavior may lead to alcohol addiction, that is, alcoholism, but harmful use should not be diagnosed if a psychotic disorder, a dependence syndrome, or other specific alcohol-related disorder occurs (WHO 1992).

Alcohol Addiction as a Mental Disorder

Alcoholism is considered a mental disease, when an individual is dependent on alcohol. Dependence syndrome is accompanied by physiological, behavioral, and cognitive phenomena in which alcohol use has a much higher priority for the dependent individual than other activities. The uncontrollable, overwhelming, and irresistible desire for alcohol was first described in 1784 by Benjamin Rush, while Elvin Morton Jellinek described alcoholism as a chronic disease in 1960 and thus fundamentally entered the process of shaping a scientific and medical approach to alcoholism. The current disease concept includes the psychosocial and neurobiological foundations and consequences of alcoholism. This definition continues to this day. Until then, it was considered a behavioral disorder that was directly related to the character of a particular person. Not only alcohol addiction but also other addictions are defined according to the World Health Organization (WHO) as mental diseases; therefore it is necessary to approach and treat them in this way (Mann et al. 2000; WHO 1992). It is hazardous drinking that poses a serious risk for the development of alcohol addiction.

Figure 3 shows the proportions of hazardous alcohol consumption in the classification of population specifics. In general, it can be concluded that women reported a lower proportion of hazardous alcohol consumption compared to men. In this context, it is possible to mention the exception, which is the Nordic countries such as Denmark and Sweden. Some country specificity can also be observed in age groups and educational groups, but the pattern of hazardous alcohol consumption cannot be clearly identified, as it is formed by the specificity of the countries as such.

In terms of drinking patterns, motivation, the presence of pathological features, and the overall course, five types of alcohol abuse can be identified. The alpha type is characterized by problem drinking (often drinking alone), when alcohol abuse is used as a "self-medication" to eliminate dysphoria and suppress tension, anxiety, or depressive feelings. For the beta type, occasional abuse is typical, when alcohol drinking is strongly characterized as a sociocultural habit and norm. Despite the development of serious somatic complications, there are no signs of addiction. In the gamma type (with a preference for beer and spirits), alcohol addiction is characterized by impaired drinking control, a gradual increase in alcohol tolerance with a typical progression of consumption, followed by somatic and psychological impairment, but also more pronounced psychological addiction. Regarding the delta type (with a preference for wine), there is a typical chronic (daily) consumption of alcohol, permanent maintenance of the level without significant signs of intoxication

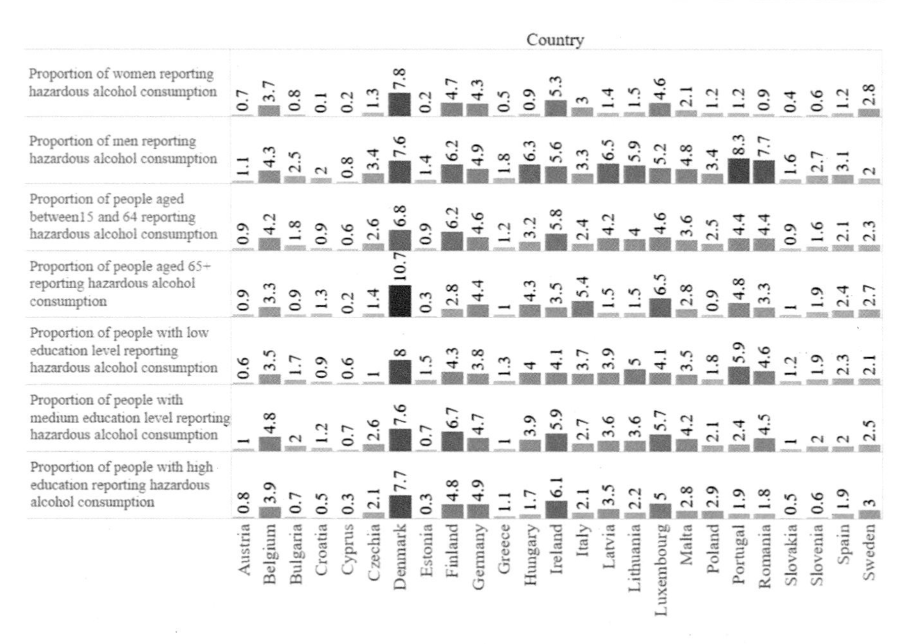

Fig. 3 Proportions of hazardous alcohol drinkers in EU countries (2014). (Source: Own processing based on data from the European Commission 2021)

and loss of control, while more pronounced somatic addiction and damage is evident. The gamma and delta types are often combined with the predominance of one of them. The epsilon type corresponds to periodic drinking, that is, episodic abuse (dipsomania, "quarterly drinking") with longer periods, sometimes with complete abstinence. This is not a common variant of addiction, which is sometimes accompanied by affective disorders (Kalina et al. 2015).

Thus, alcohol use can lead to an onset of alcoholism as a mental disease, but alcohol use is also associated with various other mental diseases, which are addressed in the following subchapters.

Mental Disorders Associated with Alcohol Use

More than 100 years ago, Regier et al. (1900) presented to the world a study in which they emphasized mental and psychological disorders associated with alcohol use and compared these problems with other addictive substances. The mentioned authors focused on the prevalence of disorders such as schizophrenia, antisocial personality, anxiety, panic, or obsessive-compulsive disorder when using alcohol, while their lower prevalence could be observed compared to other substances.

Figure 4 shows the prevalence of selected disorders in EU countries as a percentage of the total population; while the first column includes alcohol use disorders, the

	AUD	AD	ADHD	AN	BD	BN	DYS	MDD	SCZ
Austria	3.04 %	6.60 %	1.21 %	0.12 %	1.10 %	0.39 %	1.44 %	2.57 %	0.36 %
Belgium	2.62 %	5.60 %	1.01 %	0.12 %	1.07 %	0.27 %	1.29 %	3.15 %	0.35 %
Bulgaria	2.07 %	4.04 %	0.75 %	0.03 %	0.56 %	0.10 %	1.47 %	2.30 %	0.37 %
Croatia	2.71 %	4.27 %	0.79 %	0.04 %	0.65 %	0.11 %	1.46 %	2.74 %	0.37 %
Cyprus	1.95 %	7.26 %	1.06 %	0.13 %	1.11 %	0.31 %	1.42 %	2.36 %	0.36 %
Czechia	2.75 %	3.71 %	0.79 %	0.04 %	0.65 %	0.12 %	1.46 %	2.45 %	0.38 %
Denmark	3.46 %	5.47 %	0.71 %	0.12 %	1.13 %	0.30 %	1.41 %	3.08 %	0.31 %
Estonia	2.35 %	3.91 %	0.81 %	0.04 %	0.62 %	0.11 %	1.44 %	3.75 %	0.36 %
Finland	2.46 %	4.38 %	1.25 %	0.13 %	1.07 %	0.28 %	1.64 %	3.40 %	0.33 %
France	2.26 %	6.98 %	1.18 %	0.12 %	1.06 %	0.29 %	1.39 %	3.44 %	0.33 %
Germany	2.33 %	7.09 %	0.43 %	0.13 %	0.91 %	0.23 %	1.35 %	3.11 %	0.34 %
Greece	1.67 %	6.44 %	0.92 %	0.11 %	1.10 %	0.26 %	1.44 %	4.99 %	0.36 %
Hungary	2.80 %	4.07 %	0.79 %	0.04 %	0.64 %	0.12 %	1.47 %	2.48 %	0.37 %
Ireland	3.68 %	7.77 %	1.49 %	0.12 %	0.82 %	0.31 %	1.40 %	3.64 %	0.45 %
Italy	1.52 %	6.15 %	0.76 %	0.10 %	1.09 %	0.34 %	1.37 %	3.29 %	0.38 %
Latvia	2.86 %	4.39 %	0.78 %	0.04 %	0.62 %	0.10 %	1.46 %	3.78 %	0.36 %
Lithuania	2.70 %	5.00 %	0.79 %	0.04 %	0.62 %	0.11 %	1.45 %	4.09 %	0.36 %
Luxembourg	2.74 %	5.91 %	1.05 %	0.17 %	1.09 %	0.40 %	1.42 %	2.65 %	0.37 %
Malta	1.85 %	7.00 %	0.95 %	0.11 %	1.12 %	0.26 %	1.44 %	2.48 %	0.36 %
Netherlands	1.79 %	7.68 %	1.16 %	0.13 %	0.94 %	0.21 %	1.35 %	3.10 %	0.48 %
Poland	3.89 %	3.67 %	0.84 %	0.05 %	0.67 %	0.13 %	1.45 %	1.39 %	0.38 %
Portugal	3.40 %	9.01 %	0.92 %	0.10 %	1.05 %	0.26 %	1.45 %	4.48 %	0.35 %
Romania	2.46 %	3.85 %	0.82 %	0.04 %	0.75 %	0.10 %	1.45 %	2.10 %	0.36 %
Slovakia	2.83 %	4.03 %	0.84 %	0.04 %	0.66 %	0.13 %	1.46 %	2.15 %	0.39 %
Slovenia	3.14 %	4.00 %	0.77 %	0.04 %	0.66 %	0.12 %	1.47 %	2.90 %	0.39 %
Spain	1.78 %	5.85 %	2.08 %	0.14 %	1.12 %	0.37 %	1.47 %	4.61 %	0.35 %
Sweden	2.70 %	5.28 %	0.94 %	0.11 %	1.15 %	0.34 %	1.46 %	3.67 %	0.35 %

Fig. 4 Prevalence of selected psychological disorders in EU countries: mean of prevalence in population (2015–2019). (Source: Own processing based on data from GBD 2019)

other columns show the prevalence of psychological disorders. It is presented mainly because it is a comorbidity with drinking alcohol. The more intense the shade, the higher the prevalence of the disorder, and, as can be seen, the highest values were measured for anxiety disorder.

Alcohol use is a predictor of a wide range of diseases, where mental disorders form a significant part. Jane-Llopis and Matytsina (2006) have undoubtedly confirmed this idea in their research. The authors also pointed to the existence of some comorbidity of alcohol-related mental disorders in higher-income countries, pointing to the prevalence of depressive disorder. Table 1. provides mental and behavioral disorders due to use of alcohol, which are classified into diagnosis groups based on International Classification of Diseases and its tenth revision (ICD-10).

Probst et al. (2020) also agreed with these disorders and their full association with alcohol use. However, the nature of these disorders is mainly related to the high level of alcohol consumption. Also, when assessing the link between alcohol use and mental disorders, it is also appropriate to consider the direction of the interaction, as mental disorders may lead to increased drinking levels and vice versa.

Thus, alcohol abuse is a mental disorder in itself, but it can lead to more serious mental illness or a deepening of poor mental status. The following subchapters are devoted to the description of selected mental disorders associated with alcohol use.

Table 1 Mental and behavioral disorders due to alcohol use

Disorder	Code
Acute intoxication	**F10.0**
Uncomplicated	F10.00
With trauma or other bodily injury	F10.01
With other medical complications (complications such as hematemesis, inhalation of vomitus)	F10.02
With delirium	F10.03
With perceptual distortions	F10.04
With coma	F10.05
With convulsions	F10.06
Pathological intoxication	F10.07
Harmful use	**F10.1**
Dependence syndrome	**F10.2**
Currently abstinent	F10.20
Currently abstinent, but in a protected environment	F10.21
Currently on a clinically supervised maintenance or replacement regime [controlled dependence]	F10.22
Currently abstinent, but receiving treatment with aversive or blocking drugs	F10.23
Currently using the substance (active dependence)	F10.24
Continuous use	F10.25
Episodic use (dipsomania)	F10.26
Withdrawal state	**F10.3**
Uncomplicated	F10.30
With convulsions	F10.31
Withdrawal state with delirium	**F10.4**
Without convulsions	F10.40
With convulsions	F10.41
Psychotic disorder	**F10.5**
Schizophrenia-like	F10.50
Predominantly delusional	F10.51
Predominantly hallucinatory	F10.52
Predominantly polymorphic	F10.53
Predominantly depressive symptoms	F10.54
Predominantly manic symptoms	F10.55
Mixed	F10.56
Amnesic syndrome	**F10.6**
Residual and late-onset psychotic disorder	**F10.7**
Flashbacks	F10.70
Personality or behavioral disorder	F10.71
Residual affective disorder	F10.72
Dementia	F10.73
Other persisting cognitive impairment	F10.74
Late-onset psychotic disorder	F10.75
Other mental and behavioral disorders	**F10.8**
Unspecified mental and behavioral disorder	**F10.9**

Source: own processing based on WHO (1992)

Schizophrenia

As described by Dragoi and Vladuti (2020), the comorbidity of schizophrenia and problematic alcohol use is one of the most common comorbidities reported in patients with these diagnoses. Similar findings were revealed by Ahn et al. (2021), who, based on quantitative examination in a large sample of patients, confirmed the apparent comorbidity of alcohol use and the first episode of schizophrenia. At the same time, the authors in both studies pointed to the relatively low level of scientific knowledge and the need for deeper research in the area of psychological comorbidities associated with alcohol use.

Anxiety

Morris et al. (2005) clearly confirmed the comorbidity between anxiety disorder and alcohol use disorders and pointed to inconsistencies in demonstrating causality or even directionality of the relationship. As a possible explanation of the direction, they mentioned the specific characteristics of the patient (gender, tendency to drink, and others), which can be used to improve treatment processes. In general, there are three opinions in this area:

- Anxiety disorder is a predictor of increased alcohol use.
- Alcohol use is a predictor of anxiety disorder.
- A combination of the above options, anxiety disorder increases alcohol use, while alcohol use aggravates anxiety disorder.

Based on the results of the research, Kushner et al. (2000) agreed on the direction of the trajectory from alcohol use to anxiety disorder, especially in the identified alcohol addiction. At this point, it should be noted that the categories of anxiety disorders also include social phobia, and Mellentin et al. (2018) considered this disorder to be one of the most common anxiety disorders associated with alcohol use.

Bipolar Disorder

Another of the mental disorders that requires special attention is bipolar disorder. Regarding the link with problematic alcohol use, bipolar disorder is insufficiently examined compared to other mental disorders. In this sense, Grunze et al. (2021) emphasized the comorbidity with alcohol disorders occurs in 40–70% of patients with bipolar disorder, with a significant predominance in men. Also, Lagerberg et al. (2017) revealed some links between alcohol use disorders and inter-episodic affective lability in bipolar disorder. In fact, there are currently challenges to expand scientific knowledge in this area, as the absence of specific clinical research undoubtedly complicates the process of selecting and implementing appropriate treatment.

Obsessive-Compulsive Disorder

In the case of problematic drinking, it is also possible to focus on obsessive-compulsive disorder. According to earlier research, there is an apparent comorbidity between obsessive-compulsive disorder and alcohol use disorder. For instance, Dimitriou et al. (1993) presented the findings that 26.4% of patients with obsessive-compulsive disorder also suffer from alcohol disorder. Gungor et al. (2014) reported 13.5% based on the results of their research on obsessive-compulsive disorder in patients with alcohol abuse.

Other Mental Disorders

There are many other mental disorders that may be associated with alcohol use disorders. Bulik et al. (2004) emphasized the comorbidity of alcohol use disorder and eating disorder, and they also pointed to the later onset and presence of major depressive disorder. Other authors have revealed a link between alcohol use and impulsive disorders (Gungor et al. 2014), antisocial personality disorder or borderline personality disorder (Helle et al. 2019), attention-deficit/hyperactivity disorder (Lundervold et al. 2020), and many others. In the case of mental health, it should be borne in mind that the presence of drinking problems as well as other mental disorders can greatly complicate the treatment of patients.

Last but not least, second-hand patients and their poor mental health due to problematic alcohol use by a family member should not be forgotten. In this context, the aspect of an individual's alcohol abuse is expected to translate into the negative consequences experienced by the family. Dostanic et al. (2021) examined the association between alcohol use in men and the mental health of women who shared a household with these men. The results indicated that the mental health of women living with alcohol-dependent partners is seriously endangered, while the authors emphasized the factor of domestic violence (Dostanic et al. 2021). Chinnusamy et al. (2021) described very clearly the negative effects of alcohol consumption on the family and its members, and they associated these negative consequences with conflicts, domestic violence, financial problems, or mental disorders.

The findings presented in this subchapter underline the importance of focusing on mental health in alcohol use problems. As a result, drinking alcohol can lead to mental disorders and exacerbate them, while poor mental health can lead to increased alcohol consumption and the risk of alcohol addiction in individuals. This interaction highlights the need for further investigation of the problem. Depression and stress also play an important role in this area. The following subchapters pay special and detailed attention to these two mental difficulties that may be associated with alcohol use.

Alcohol and Depression

Depression is a mental illness manifested by a persistent feeling of sadness, negative thoughts, and loss of interest in once favorite activities and is accompanied by a variety of somatic problems. In terms of serious consequences, depression is associated with never entering a partner relationship or lower relationship support and higher conflict in the partnership (Leach and Butterworth 2020), suicidality, or social and occupational dysfunction (Adams et al. 2016).

Depression is often accompanied by substance abuse problems. Several studies have shown that alcoholics are likely to suffer from depression; in addition, alcoholics usually suffer from treatment-resistant depression. Alcohol is supposed to help mask discomfort, a strategy used by many people instead of seeking health care. These are prejudices that often prevent people from asking for help, and they suffer from depression and the consequences of problematic alcohol use (Alsheikh et al. 2020). Critical situations that burden mental health require even more attention in terms of the addictive behavior of individuals. Evidence showed that during the coronavirus disease 2019 (COVID-19) pandemic, daily alcohol use was associated with depression and financial concerns (Bonsaksen et al. 2021).

The Path Between Depression and Alcohol Abuse

In some cases, depression occurs first and then alcohol use disorder, and gradually both of these disorders deepen and escalate. There are findings that alcohol use problems can be predicted by individual and intrapersonal factors, including mental discomfort and depressive symptoms. According to Eastman et al. (2021), people with mental discomfort such as depression, anxiety, and loneliness were significantly more likely to report increased alcohol use. In this sense, depression is considered a risk factor as well as a unique predictor for alcohol use, while the younger generation appears to be a population with a high level of vulnerability (Hussong et al. 2017; Isaksson et al. 2020).

However, the opposite situation also happens, when alcohol drinking leads to self-pity, a feeling of inferiority, and depressive thoughts. Onaemo et al. (2020) pointed to the fact that alcohol use disorder is significantly associated with a persistence and recurrence of major depression. According to the authors, alcohol use disorder can be considered a strong risk factor for the persistence or recurrence of major depression. Other factors include female aspect, childhood traumatic events, chronic pain restricting activities, daily smoking, and low self-esteem (Onaemo et al. 2020). Following these findings, it can be noted that when an alcohol use disorder is comorbid with other substance use disorders, it is associated with more severe symptoms of alcohol use disorder as well as higher levels of depressive symptoms (Howe et al. 2021). In addition, the fact that prenatal alcohol use increases a risk of depressive symptoms in early adulthood should not be overlooked in this problem (Duko et al. 2021). There are also conflicting findings, as some studies showed that regular alcohol use is causally associated with a lower risk of depression, but further research is needed to clarify the mechanisms of this causal link (Zhu et al. 2020).

The complexity of the alcohol-depression link is evidenced by the findings of Briere et al. (2014), who examined the comorbidity between major depression and alcohol use disorder from adolescence to adulthood. Their results revealed that most individuals with a history of major depression and/or alcohol use disorder had the second other disorder. Also, adolescent alcohol use disorder predicted early adult major depression, while early adult major depression predicted adult alcohol use disorder. Thus, alcohol use disorder is highly comorbid with psychiatric disorders, such as depression, and the age of individuals also plays an important role in this issue.

The Role of Gender

The symptoms that are diagnosed with depression are the same regardless of the patient's gender. However, the major difficulties may differ between men and women. From a gender perspective, Danzo et al. (2017) revealed that the relationship between depression and alcohol use varies according to gender characteristics. Namely, depression and alcohol use were independent in young men, and no significant mediators were observed. On the contrary, bidirectional effects between depression and alcohol use were identified in young women, while an indirect effect from depression to alcohol use was confirmed through peer deviance. This may be related to the lifestyle of men and the vulnerability of women, as men are generally more characterized by days intoxicated by alcohol and women are significantly more characterized by symptoms of depression (Skaff et al. 1999).

The Role of Stress

Stress should not be forgotten. However, it is difficult to describe the relationship between stress, depression, and alcohol use. Stress can be a symptom of depression and problematic drinking, but also one of the predictors of depression and alcohol use disorder. In fact, depression as well as alcohol use can be attributed to social stress. Some findings suggest that depression and alcohol use may be perceived as controllable and influenced by personal weakness and lifestyle choices (Knettel et al. 2021). In stress and depression, it is possible to talk about the structure of the personality tending to problems with alcohol use, when alcohol can be sought for protection or escape from a certain situation. Perez et al. (2020) examined the relationships between stressful life events, alcohol abuse, and depression and revealed that the combined presence of depression with alcohol abuse can increase suicide risk. Compared to suicidal individuals with depression only, individuals with both depression and alcohol use disorder tended to be younger and experienced higher rates of stressful life events during the 6 months before death. Alcohol abuse is likely to influence interpersonal conflicts, financial difficulties, and legal problems. Thus, programs aimed at coping with life's problems can help reduce the risk of suicide.

Alcohol and Stress

Stress is a situation in which the human organism is exposed to unusual (nonstandard) living conditions. Stress is caused by stressors, which deviate the organism from the norm and force it to take a defensive reaction used to restore balance. Stress is a known risk factor for a number of mental disorders and for this reason is characterized by a common neurobiological link between the disease processes of substance use disorders and mental disorders (National Institute on Drug Abuse 2021). In today's times, people face exposure to critical incidents capable of creating both stress and aversive reactions to stress. Men and women experience these types of stressors, but not necessarily at the same rate, and they may respond differently to them (Goncharenko et al. 2019; Lehavot et al. 2014; Menard and Arter 2014).

The Path Between Stress and Alcohol Abuse

Stress may be one of the significant factors that lead individuals to use alcohol and weaken their inhibitions. In this context, it is possible to talk about the use of alcohol with the function of coping with many difficult and stressful situations in life (social conflicts, financial problems, sexual harassment, racism, stigmatization and abuse from the public or superiors, rejection by friends, problematic family relationships, critical incidents, workload, but also symptoms of physical illness and pain). When an individual is overwhelmed by a large number of urgent tasks, a situation can easily arise in which the available solutions appear to be insufficient, resulting in developmental stress, which can lead to alcohol use. These stressful aspects can lead not only to repeated alcohol use but also to addiction with other health risks (Hupková and Liberčanová 2012). Thus, alcohol use disorders appear to be influenced by stress as such. Increased attention should be paid to the role of various stressors in alcohol consumption and alcohol use disorders, as well as to potential risk moderators when individuals are exposed to stressors (Obeid et al. 2020; Perez et al. 2020). Drinking in response to stress can be risky especially for those who have experienced problematic alcohol use in the past (Cooper et al. 2016; Keyes et al. 2011).

It is necessary to be careful in today's fast and modern times, as people are sensitive to a number of negative stimuli that reduce resistance to stress. In this sense, the findings of several studies indicate that stressors are involved in problematic alcohol use, including its onset, maintenance, and relapse (Keyes et al. 2011; Pilowsky et al. 2013). Problematic alcohol use is strongly influenced by interpersonal- and achievement-related events that can be very stressful for individuals (Pilowsky et al. 2013). Menard and Arter (2014) revealed that critical incidents and their interaction with negative coping, posttraumatic stress disorder, and social stressors are positively associated with drinking problems in men, but are negatively associated with this unhealthy behavior in women. On this basis, gender specificities should also be taken into account, as gender differences are more pronounced in models of alcohol use disorders.

The fact remains that compared to the prevalence in the general population, heavy drinkers have a significantly higher prevalence of posttraumatic stress disorder, while Samala et al. (2018) also confirmed the association between the prevalence of posttraumatic stress disorder and higher alcohol consumption. In terms of causation, posttraumatic stress disorder has a potential causal effect on alcohol use disorder, but not on alcohol consumption as such. Simultaneously, alcohol consumption and alcohol use disorder have no causal effect on posttraumatic stress disorder. In fact, women with posttraumatic stress disorder may be at greater risk for alcohol misuse than men with posttraumatic stress disorder. This evidence agrees with a self-medication model in which individuals misuse alcohol to cope with aversive symptoms associated with stress trauma (Bountress et al. 2021; Goncharenko et al. 2019). Also, Lehavot et al. (2014) confirmed that in individuals with comorbid alcohol addiction and posttraumatic stress disorder, interventions to reduce the symptoms of posttraumatic stress disorder are likely to lower coping motives for men and women, while focusing on coping motives is likely to result in reduced alcohol consumption for women but not for men. It is possible that alcohol use is an indicator of stress in women, for whom drinking alcohol is less of a normative activity, but it is rather an indicator of men's lifestyle. On the other hand, days intoxicated by alcohol may be a better indicator of stress-related drinking for men, as they may be more likely to binge when under stress (Skaff et al. 1999).

The abovementioned findings suggest that alcohol is considered one of the coping strategies in people experiencing stressors. Problematic drinking is not usually included in stress generation research, but there is a presumption that problematic alcohol use can lead to stressful life events. Alcohol use can predict stressful life events in general (Hart and Fazaa 2004), but also specific stressful difficulties such as divorce (Collins et al. 2007), absence from work or school (French et al. 2011), interpersonal conflicts, financial distress, and legal problems (Perez et al. 2020). Thus, as a result of problematic alcohol use, all of these life situations can cause stress. In contrast, several studies have not confirmed that stressful life events often result from alcohol use (Goldstein et al. 2021). This fact proves that views and discussions are still different.

Last but not least, from the point of view on prenatal alcohol consumption and preschool child stress system disturbance, there is the biological association between intrauterine alcohol exposure and the cortisol stress system, partly dose-dependent (Grimm et al. 2021). All this evidence should not be overlooked when addressing alcohol-stress issue.

Comorbidity Between Alcohol Use Disorder, Stress, and Depression

As indicated in the previous subchapters, the simultaneous presence of substance use disorder, mental disorder, and stress is not an exceptional condition in the patient. In this sense, it is possible to state the path leading to the comorbidity (Santucci 2012):

- Stress as a common risk factor can contribute to depression as well as alcohol use and addiction.
- Depression can contribute to alcohol use and addiction as a result of self-medication strategy.
- Alcohol use and addiction can contribute to the development of depression.

Figure 5 shows a scheme indicating that stress at various stages of life can induce changes, which, especially in older age, are reflected in an increased likelihood of alcohol abuse. This causes further stress and the patient enters a vicious circle with an increased risk of alcohol addiction. In addition to increased alcohol use, stress can

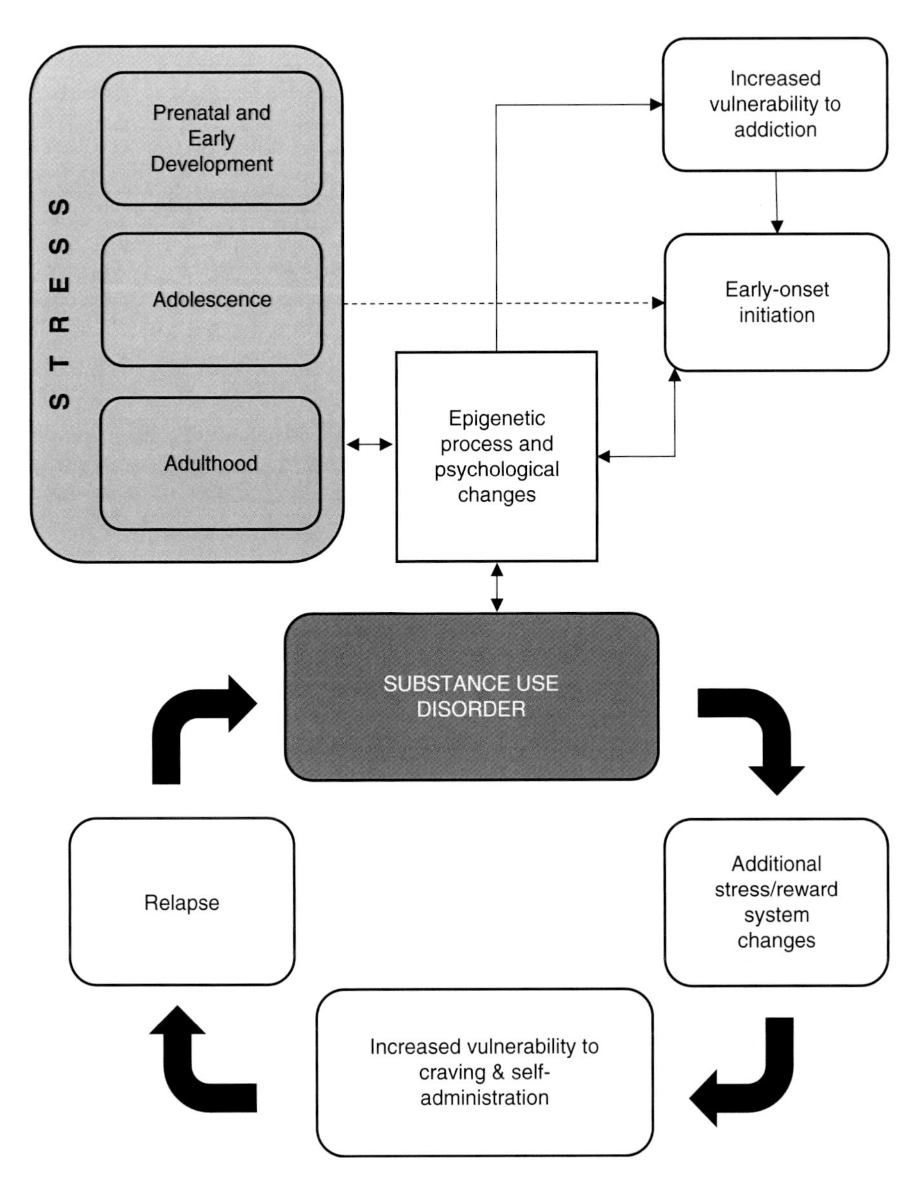

Fig. 5 Interaction of stress exposure with substance use and abuse. (Source: Own elaboration according to Duffing et al. 2014)

increase the likelihood of other mental disorders, which also increase the likelihood of vulnerability to problematic drinking.

However, many other factors contributing to comorbidity need to be considered, as this relationship is complex and it is not easy to clearly define the role of individual factors. For this reason, genetic vulnerabilities, epigenetic influences, environmental influences, and brain region involvement should also be taken into account (National Institute on Drug Abuse 2021). The fact remains that this frequent problem in society should be addressed, given the serious consequences of co-occurrence of mental discomfort and alcohol use disorder.

Applications to Other Areas of Substance Use Disorders

Kalina et al. (2015) emphasized that alcohol has the most significant negative consequences of all addictive substances due to its frequent occurrence in society, as well as social acceptance. Alcohol abuse is a serious but misunderstood disorder; therefore, it should be viewed from several perspectives, for example, from a mental health perspective. This chapter provides support in reconsidering people's vulnerability to stress, depression, and alcohol abuse, which affects not only mental well-being but also quality of life.

Several approaches are used in the treatment of alcohol addiction through drug use, therapies, and combinations of drugs and therapies. Many studies offer different views and recommendations, while Balldin et al. (2003) highlighted the positive effect of naltrexone in the outpatient treatment of alcohol addiction, as well as the effects of cognitive-behavioral therapy. Rupp et al. (2012) pointed to the effects of cognitive remediation therapy during treatment, or Huhne et al. (2021) emphasized the effects of personalized circadian Zeitgeber therapy and stated that treatment should be accompanied by easy-to-apply therapies. At the same time, it should be noted that alcohol addiction is accompanied by many other mental disorders, such as depression and anxiety, or stressful life events. Combination with drug therapy is therefore justified for these reasons as well.

Modern treatment concepts recognize the interaction between these disorders through an integrated therapy approach in which these disorders are addressed together under the same conditions. Motivational interviews, cognitive-behavioral therapies, and socio-therapy involving the family and social environment are the fundamental pillars of psychotherapy, while complementary pharmacological treatment is aimed at reducing desire and optimizing mood stability (Grunze et al. 2021). Accordingly, it is appropriate to highlight family support and family participation in treatment counselling as very important factor, as emphasized by Rowe and Liddle (2008) in the context of multidimensional family therapy. The fact remains that wives, children, and other members of the household shared with people with alcohol use disorders suffer from the negative consequences of alcohol consumption, but it is the family that plays an important role in the treatment of alcoholism (Copello et al. 2005).

Mental discomfort, such as depression and stressful mood, occurs in other addictions including heroin addiction (Moustafa et al. 2020), tobacco addiction, cocaine addiction (Winhusen et al. 2019), or others. It is possible to speculate that the innovative protocols could also help with addictions to other substances. In fact, research in this area is lacking; therefore, further research is needed to develop evidence-based approaches to the treatment of comorbidities of substance use disorders and depression, respecting stressful life events.

Applications to Areas of Public Health

Educating society about the negatives and risks of alcohol plays an important role in achieving health objectives, for which public health professionals are also responsible. Their efforts could highlight the risk and negative consequences of problematic alcohol use. Monitoring and creating the basis for the proper direction of public policies is a very important task that should not be overlooked, as it is gaining in importance in the current pandemic period. Addictology will face a difficult challenge due to long-term social isolation during the COVID-19 pandemic. The pandemic has caused a sudden change in the patterns of behavior and mental health of the population; society and addictology will therefore have to deal with increased substance use and poor mental health in the near future due to the COVID-19 outbreak and social distance (Bonsaksen et al. 2021; Fendrich et al. 2021). These facts should not be ignored even at a time of pandemic, in which the primary focus is on overcoming COVID-19. In order to reduce alcohol use, higher taxes appear to be effective tools for reducing alcohol consumption (Horakova et al. 2020). On the other hand, it is necessary to take into account the fact that restaurants, pubs, nightclubs, or other businesses focused on gastronomic services were closed during this period. Simultaneously, people were detached from social life. For these reasons, it is necessary to take into account great resistance. For illegal substances that are not covered by tax policies, other strategies should be considered.

Country leaders should realize that prevention through successful public policies, programs, and public education is the most effective solution. Public policies on substance use and mental health play a key role, while their approaches should focus on promoting public education about the risks between substance use and mental health, reducing the risk of addictions through evidence-based strategies that prevent mental discomfort, and identifying the necessary areas for research into substance misuse and mental health (Orte et al. 2020). Promoting a healthy lifestyle and sports, as well as increasing health literacy in the population, seem to be a suitable application in the coming period in the position of competitive activities compared to substance use (Rolova 2020).

It should be borne in mind that stress is a common factor that can contribute to mental disorders as well as the use of addictive substances at risk of addiction. The greater severity attributable to comorbidity indicates that tackling mental discomfort and substance use problems is complex and poses a major challenge for treatment, recovery, and abstinence (National Institute on Drug Abuse 2021). Both prevention and treatment of mental and substance disorders should be based on gender-specific analysis.

Mini-Dictionary of Terms

- **Alcohol Addiction.** A disease, also called alcoholism, in which a person has a tireless desire for alcoholic beverages but does not have the ability to stop or control drinking despite adverse social, occupational, or health consequences. A person with this disease needs to drink more to have the same effect, while his or her behavior is accompanied by withdrawal symptoms after stopping alcohol use.
- **Alcohol Use.** It is also called alcohol consumption or drinking. The act of ingesting a beverage containing ethyl alcohol or ethanol. Alcoholic beverages include wine, beer, and spirits.
- **Cognitive-Behavioral Therapy.** Cognitive-behavioral therapy can be performed individually with a therapist or in small groups. This form of therapy aims to identify feelings and situations that lead to substance abuse and to manage stress that can lead to relapse. Emphasis is placed on changing thought processes leading to substance abuse and on developing the skills needed to cope with everyday situations that could encourage problematic behavior.
- **Comorbidity.** Comorbidity means a condition in which two or more disorders (or diseases) occur in the same patient simultaneously or one after the other. For instance, a specific mental disorder and a substance use disorder. Comorbidity also describes interactions between disorders (diseases) that can worsen the course of both.
- **Mental Discomfort.** An unpleasant feeling of a psychological (nonphysical) origin. A set of painful mental symptoms that are associated with functioning and mood.
- **Relapse.** Relapse is a return to substance use after a period of abstinence that is common in people treated for substance use disorder. People with substance problems are most likely to relapse when they experience stress or when they are exposed to people or places associated with past use.

Key Facts of Comorbidity Between Substance Use Disorders and Mental Disorders

- In some cases, an acute psychotic episode may occur in response to substance intoxication or withdrawal.
- People with severe depression are more prone to developing substance use disorders, and, conversely, substance users are vulnerable to major depression.
- Depression, schizophrenia, and bipolar disorder are the most common types of mental disorders in substance users.
- It is not possible to speak of the efficacy of selective serotonin reuptake inhibitors in the treatment of mental disorders where comorbid use disorders also occur.

- There is a little effect of antidepressants on maintaining abstinence. Although the antidepressants are effective in treating depression, only a relative reduction in psychoactive substance use can be observed.
- Integrated treatment is effective in terms of improving psychotic symptoms as well as substance use.

Summary Points

- Alcohol is an easily available legal drug that has the most significant negative consequences of all drugs due to its frequent occurrence in society, as well as due to social acceptance.
- Problematic drinking affects individuals, families, and society as a whole.
- Alcohol use reduces cognition, increases mental distress and aggression, and promotes suicidal thoughts.
- Depression and stress often go hand in hand with increased alcohol use.
- Stress may be a critical driver of comorbidity between mental disorders and alcohol use disorder.
- Educating society about the negatives and risks of alcohol plays an important role in achieving mental health objectives.
- Behavioral therapies can help people develop the ability to prevent and overcome mental and substance problems.
- Both prevention and treatment of mental and substance disorders should be based on gender-specific analysis.

References

Adams GC, Balbuena L, Meng X, Asmundson GJG (2016) When social anxiety and depression go together: a population study of comorbidity and associated consequences. J Affect Disord 206: 48–54. https://doi.org/10.1016/j.jad.2016.07.031

Ahn S, Choi Y, Choi W, Jo YT, Kim H, Lee J, Joo SW (2021) Effects of comorbid alcohol use disorder on the clinical outcomes of first-episode schizophrenia: a nationwide population-based study. Ann General Psychiatry 20(1):32. https://doi.org/10.1186/s12991-021-00353-3

Alsheikh AM, Elemam MO, El-Bahnasawi M (2020) Treatment of depression with alcohol and substance dependence: a systematic review. Cureus 12(10):e11168. https://doi.org/10.7759/cureus.11168

Balldin J, Berglund M, Borg S, Månsson M, Bendtsen P, Franck J, Gustafsson L, Halldin J, Nilsson LH, Stolt G, Willander A (2003) A 6-month controlled naltrexone study: combined effect with cognitive behavioral therapy in outpatient treatment of alcohol dependence. Alcohol Clin Exp Res 27(7):1142–1149. https://doi.org/10.1097/01.ALC.0000075548.83053.A9

Bonsaksen T, Ekeberg Ø, Schou-Bredal I, Skogstad L, Heir T, Grimholt TK (2021) Use of alcohol and addictive drugs during the COVID-19 outbreak in Norway: associations with mental health and pandemic-related problems. Front Public Health 9:667729. https://doi.org/10.3389/fpubh.2021.667729

Bountress KE, Wendt F, Bustamante D, Agrawal A, Webb B, Gillespie N, Edenberg H, Sheerin C, Johnson E, Polimanti R, Amstadter A (2021) Potential causal effect of post-traumatic stress disorder on alcohol use disorder and alcohol consumption in individuals of

European descent: a Mendelian randomization study. Alcohol Clin Exp Res:1–8. https://doi.org/10.1111/acer.14649

Briere FN, Rohde P, Seeley JR, Klein D, Lewinsohn PM (2014) Comorbidity between major depression and alcohol use disorder from adolescence to adulthood. Compr Psychiatry 55(3): 526–533. https://doi.org/10.1016/j.comppsych.2013.10.007

Bulik CM, Klump KL, Thornton L, Kaplan AS, Devlin B, Fichter MM, Halmi KA, Strober M, Woodside DB, Crow S, Mitchell JE, Rotondo A, Mauri M, Cassano GB, Keel PK, Berrettini WH, Kaye WH (2004) Alcohol use disorder comorbidity in eating disorders: a multicenter study. J Clin Psychiatry 65(7):1000–1006. https://doi.org/10.4088/jcp.v65n0718

Cherpitel CJ, Ye Y, Monteiro MG (2019) Dose-response relative risk of injury from acute alcohol consumption in 22 countries: are women at higher risk than men? Alcohol Alcohol 54(4): 396–401. https://doi.org/10.1093/alcalc/agz018

Chinnusamy M, Eugin PR, Janakiraman S (2021) A study on the effect of alcoholism on the family members of alcoholic patients. J Health Allied Sci 11(2):66–72. https://doi.org/10.1055/s-0040-1722426

Collins RL, Ellickson PL, Klein DJ (2007) The role of substance use in young adult divorce. Addiction 102(5):786–794. https://doi.org/10.1111/j.1360-0443.2007.01803.x

Connor J, Kydd R, Maclennan B, Shield K, Rehm J (2017) Alcohol-attributable cancer deaths under 80 years of age in New Zealand. Drug Alcohol Rev 36(3):415–423. https://doi.org/10.1111/dar.12443

Cooper ML, Kuntsche E, Levitt A, Barber LL, Wolf S (2016) Motivational models of substance use: a review of theory and research on motives for using alcohol, marijuana, and tobacco. In: Sher KJ (ed) The Oxford handbook of substance use and substance use disorders. Oxford University Press, New York, pp 375–421

Copello AG, Velleman RDB, Templeton LJ (2005) Family interventions in the treatment of alcohol and drug problems. Drug Alcohol Rev 24(4):369–385. https://doi.org/10.1080/09595230500302356

Danzo S, Connell AM, Stormshak EA (2017) Associations between alcohol-use and depression symptoms in adolescence: examining gender differences and pathways over time. J Adolesc 56: 64–74. https://doi.org/10.1016/j.adolescence.2017.01.007

Darvishi N, Farhadi M, Haghtalab T, Poorolajal J (2015) Alcohol-related risk of suicidal ideation, suicide attempt, and completed suicide: a meta-analysis. PLoS One 10(5):e0126870. https://doi.org/10.1371/journal.pone.0126870

Dimitriou EC, Lavrentiadis G, Dimitriou CE (1993) Obsessive-compulsive disorder and alcohol abuse. Eur J Psychiatry 7(4):244–248

Dostanic N, Djikanovic B, Jovanovic M, Stamenkovic Z, Đeric A (2021) The association between family violence, depression and anxiety among women whose partners have been treated for alcohol dependence. J Fam Violence 2:1–12. https://doi.org/10.1007/s10896-020-00238-1

Dragoi AM, Vladuti A (2020) The comorbidity between schizophrenia and alcohol. Substance addiction and alcohol use link to schizophrenia. Educ Sci Psychol 10(1):141–148

Duffing TM, Greiner SG, Mathias CW, Dougherty DM (2014) Stress, substance abuse, and addiction. Curr Top Behav Neurosci 18:237–263. https://doi.org/10.1007/7854_2014_276

Duko B, Pereira G, Betts K, Tait RJ, Newnham J, Alati R (2021) Prenatal alcohol and tobacco use and the risk of depression in offspring at age of 17 years: findings from the Raine Study. J Affect Disord 279:426–433. https://doi.org/10.1016/j.jad.2020.10.030

Eastman MR, Finlay JM, Kobayashi LC (2021) Alcohol use and mental health among older American adults during the early months of the COVID-19 pandemic. Int J Environ Res Public Health 18(8):4222. https://doi.org/10.3390/ijerph18084222

European Commission (2021) Alcohol. Available at: https://ec.europa.eu/health/alcohol/indicators_en

Fendrich M, Becker J, Park C, Russell B, Finkelstein-Fox L, Hutchison M (2021) Associations of alcohol, marijuana, and polysubstance use with non-adherence to COVID-19 public health guidelines in a US sample. Subst Abus 42(2):220–226. https://doi.org/10.1080/08897077.2021.1891603

French MT, Maclean JC, Sindelar JL, Fang H (2011) The morning after: alcohol misuse and employment problems. Appl Econ 43(21):2705–2720. https://doi.org/10.1080/00036840903357421

GBD (2019) Global burden of disease study. Results. Institute for Health Metrics and Evaluation, Seattle

GHO (2021) World Health Organization databases – Global Health Observatory data repository. Available at: https://www.who.int/data/gho/data/themes/global-information-system-on-alcohol-and-health

Goldstein BL, Armeli S, Adams RL, Florimon MA, Hammen C, Tennen H (2021) Patterns of stress generation differ depending on internalizing symptoms, alcohol use, and personality traits in early adulthood: a five year longitudinal study. Anxiety Stress Coping. https://doi.org/10.1080/10615806.2021.1910677

Goncharenko S, Weiss NH, Contractor AA, Dixon-Gordon KL, Forkus SR (2019) The role of gender in the associations among posttraumatic stress disorder symptom, severity, difficulties regulating emotions, and alcohol misuse. Addict Behav 99:106086. https://doi.org/10.1016/j.addbeh.2019.106086

Grimm J, Stemmler M, Golub Y, Schwenke E, Goecke TW, Fasching PA, Beckmann MW, Kratz O, Moll GH, Kornhuber J, Eichler A (2021) The association between prenatal alcohol consumption and preschool child stress system disturbance. Dev Psychobiol 64:687–697. https://doi.org/10.1002/dev.22038

Grunze H, Schaefer M, Scherk H, Born C, Preuss UW (2021) Comorbid bipolar and alcohol use disorder-A therapeutic challenge. Front Psych 12:660432. https://doi.org/10.3389/fpsyt.2021.660432

Gungor BB, Askin R, Taymur I, Sari S (2014) Obsessive compulsive disorder and impulse control disorder comorbidity and evaluation of impulsivity and compulsivity in alcohol dependent patients. Düşünen Adam 27(3):233–241. https://doi.org/10.5350/DAJPN2014270306

Hart KE, Fazaa N (2004) Life stress events and alcohol misuse: distinguishing contributing stress events from consequential stress events. Subst Use Misuse 39(9):1319–1339. https://doi.org/10.1081/JA-120039390

Helle AC, Watts AL, Trull TJ, Sher KJ (2019) Alcohol use disorder and antisocial and borderline personality disorders. Alcohol Res 40(1):05. https://doi.org/10.35946/arcr.v40.1.05

Horakova M, Bejtkovsky J, Baresova P, Urbanek T (2020) Alcohol consumption among the Member States of the European Union in relationship to taxation. Adiktologie 20(1–2):47–56

Howe LK, Fisher LR, Atkinson EA, Finn PR (2021) Symptoms of anxiety, depression, and borderline personality in alcohol use disorder with and without comorbid substance use disorder. Alcohol 90:19–25. https://doi.org/10.1016/j.alcohol.2020.11.002

Hufford MR (2001) Alcohol and suicidal behavior. Clin Psychol Rev 21(5):797–811. https://doi.org/10.1016/S0272-7358(00)00070-2

Huhne A, Hoch E, Landgraf D (2021) DAILY-A personalized circadian Zeitgeber therapy as an adjunctive treatment for alcohol use disorder patients: study protocol for a randomized controlled trial. Front Psych 11:569864. https://doi.org/10.3389/fpsyt.2020.569864

Hupková I, Liberčanová K (2012) Drogové závislosti a ich prevencia. Trnavská univerzita v Trnave, Trnava

Hussong AM, Ennett ST, Cox MJ, Haroon M (2017) A systematic review of the unique prospective association of negative affect symptoms and adolescent substance use controlling for externalizing symptoms. Psychol Addict Behav 31:137–147. https://doi.org/10.1037/adb0000247

Isaksson J, Schwab-Stone M, Stickley A, Ruchkin V (2020) Risk and protective factors for problematic drinking in early adolescence: a systematic approach. Child Psychiatry Hum Dev 51:231–238. https://doi.org/10.1007/s10578-019-00925-1

Jane-Llopis E, Matytsina I (2006) Mental health and alcohol, drugs and tobacco: a review of the comorbidity between mental disorders and the use of alcohol, tobacco and illicit drugs. Drug Alcohol Rev 25(6):515–536. https://doi.org/10.1080/09595230600944461

Joshua J (2017) The causes and stages of alcohol abuse: from initiation to alcohol dependence. In: Joshua J (ed) The economics of addictive behaviours, vol II. Springer International Publishing, Cham, pp 11–18. https://doi.org/10.1007/978-3-319-54425-0_3

Kalina K et al (2015) Klinická adiktologie. Grada, Prague

Keyes KM, Hatzenbuehler ML, Hasin DS (2011) Stressful life experiences, alcohol consumption, and alcohol use disorders: the epidemiologic evidence for four main types of stressors. Psychopharmacology 218(1):1–17. https://doi.org/10.1007/s00213-011-2236-1

Knettel BA, Cherenack EM, Friis EA (2021) Examining causal attributions for depression, alcohol use disorder, and schizophrenia in a diverse sample of international students at U.S. universities. J Am Coll Heal. https://doi.org/10.1080/07448481.2020.1846046

Kushner MG, Abrams K, Borchardt C (2000) The relationship between anxiety disorders and alcohol use disorders: a review of major perspectives and findings. Clin Psychol Rev 20(2):149–171. https://doi.org/10.1016/s0272-7358(99)00027-6

Lachenmeier DW, Neufeld M, Rehm J (2021) The impact of unrecorded alcohol use on health: what do we know in 2020? J Stud Alcohol Drugs 82(1):28–41. https://doi.org/10.15288/jsad.2021.82.28

Lagerberg TV, Aminoff SR, Aas M, Bjella T, Henry C, Leboyer M, Pedersen G, Bellivier F, Icick R, Andreassen OA, Etain B, Melle I (2017) Alcohol use disorders are associated with increased affective lability in bipolar disorder. J Affect Disord 208:316–324. https://doi.org/10.1016/j.jad.2016.09.062

Leach LS, Butterworth P (2020) Depression and anxiety in early adulthood: consequences for finding a partner, and relationship support and conflict. Epidemiol Psychiatr Sci 29:e141. https://doi.org/10.1017/S2045796020000530

Lehavot K, Stappenbeck CA, Luterek JA, Kaysen D, Simpson TL (2014) Gender differences in relationships among PTSD severity, drinking motives, and alcohol use in a comorbid alcohol dependence and PTSD sample. Psychol Addict Behav 28(1):42–52. https://doi.org/10.1037/a0032266

Lundervold AJ, Jensen DA, Haavik J (2020) Insomnia, alcohol consumption and ADHD symptoms in adults. Front Psychol 11:1150. https://doi.org/10.3389/fpsyg.2020.01150

Mann K, Hermann D, Heinz A (2000) One hundred years of alcoholism: the twentieth century. Alcohol Alcohol 35(1):10–15. https://doi.org/10.1093/alcalc/35.1.10

Megyesiova S, Gavurova B (2019) Analysis of alcohol consumption and death rates resulting from alcohol consumption in EU and OECD countries. Adiktologie 19(4):179–187

Mellentin AI, Mejldal A, Nielsen B, Søgaard Nielsen A (2018) Comorbid social phobia does not predict the outcome in alcohol use disorder outpatient treatment. Drug Alcohol Depend 193:148–153. https://doi.org/10.1016/j.drugalcdep.2018.09.004

Menard KS, Arter ML (2014) Stress, coping, alcohol use, and posttraumatic stress disorder among an international sample of police officers: does gender matter? Police Q 17(4):307–327. https://doi.org/10.1177/1098611114548097

Morris EP, Stewart SH, Ham LS (2005) The relationship between social anxiety disorder and alcohol use disorders: a critical review. Clin Psychol 25(6):734–760. https://doi.org/10.1016/j.cpr.2005.05.004

Moustafa AA, Tindle R, Cashel S, Parkes D, Mohamed E, Abo Hamza E (2020) Bidirectional relationship between heroin addiction and depression: behavioural and neural studies. Curr Psychol. https://doi.org/10.1007/s12144-020-01032-4

National Institute on Drug Abuse (2021) Common comorbidities with substance use disorders research report. Available at: https://www.drugabuse.gov/publications/research-reports/common-comorbidities-substance-use-disorders

Nelson S, Kolls J (2002) Alcohol, host defence and society. Nat Rev Immunol 2:205–209. https://doi.org/10.1038/nri744

Nieto SJ, Baskerville W, Donato S, Bujarski S, Ray L (2021) Lifetime heavy drinking years predict alcohol use disorder severity over and above current alcohol use. Am J Drug Alcohol Abuse. https://doi.org/10.1080/00952990.2021.1938100

Obeid S, Akel M, Haddad C, Fares K, Sacre H, Salameh P, Hallit S (2020) Factors associated with alcohol use disorder: the role of depression, anxiety, stress, alexithymia and work fatigue – a population study in Lebanon. BMC Public Health 20(1):245. https://doi.org/10.1186/s12889-020-8345-1

Onaemo VN, Fawehinmi TO, D'Arcy C (2020) Alcohol use disorder and the persistence/recurrence of major depression. Can J Psychiatr 65(9):652–663. https://doi.org/10.1177/0706743720923065

Orte C, Coone A, Amer J, Gomila MA, Pascual B (2020) Evidence-based practice and training needs in drug prevention: the interest and viability of the European prevention curriculum in prevention training in Spain. Adiktologie 20(1–2):37–46

Palm J (2006) Moral concerns: treatment staff and users perspectives on alcohol and other problems (PhD. thesis). University of Stockholm, Stockholm

Perez J, Beale E, Overholser J, Athey A, Stockmeier C (2020) Depression and alcohol use disorders as precursors to death by suicide. Death Stud. https://doi.org/10.1080/07481187.2020.1745954

Pilowsky DJ, Keyes KM, Geier TJ, Grant BF, Hasin DS (2013) Stressful life events and relapse among formerly alcohol dependent adults. Soc Work Ment Health 11(2):184–197. https://doi.org/10.1080/15332985.2012.711278

Probst C, Kilian C, Sanchez S, Lange S, Rehm J (2020) The role of alcohol use and drinking patterns in socioeconomic inequalities in mortality: a systematic review. Lancet Public Health 5(6):e324–e332. https://doi.org/10.1016/s2468-2667(20)30052-9

Ranabhat CL, Park MB, Kim CB (2020) Influence of alcohol and red meat consumption on life expectancy: results of 164 countries from 1992 to 2013. Nutrients 12(2):459. https://doi.org/10.3390/nu12020459

Regier DA, Farmer ME, Rae DS, Locke BZ, Keith SJ, Judd LL, Goodwin FK (1900) Comorbidity of mental disorders with alcohol and other drug abuse. Results from the Epidemiologic Catchment Area (ECA) Study. JAMA 264(19):2511–2518

Rehm J, Gmel G, Sempos CT, Trevisan M (2003) Alcohol-related morbidity and mortality. Alcohol Res Health 27(1):39–51

Rehm J, Sulkowska U, Manczuk M, Boffetta P, Powles J, Popova S, Zatonski W (2007) Alcohol accounts for a high proportion of premature mortality in Central and Eastern Europe. Int J Epidemiol 36(2):458–467. https://doi.org/10.1093/ije/dyl294

Režňáková V (2018) Kapitoly modernej psychiatrie. Alkoholová demencia. Slovak Psychiatric Association, Bratislava. Available at: http://www.psychiatry.sk/cms/File/kapitoly-modernej-psychiatrie/reznakova-2018.pdf

Roerecke M, Vafaei A, Hasan OSM, Chrystoja BR, Cruz M, Lee R, Neuman MG, Rehm J (2019) Alcohol consumption and risk of liver cirrhosis: a systematic review and meta-analysis. Am J Gastroenterol 114(10):1574–1586. https://doi.org/10.14309/ajg.0000000000000340

Rolova G (2020) Health literacy in residential addiction treatment programs: study protocol of a cross-sectional study in people with substance use disorders. Adiktologie 20(3–4):145–150

Ronzani TM (2018) The context of drug use in the consumer society. In: Ronzani TM (ed) Drugs and social context. Social perspectives on the use of alcohol and other drugs. Springer International Publishing, Cham, pp 3–13. https://doi.org/10.1007/978-3-319-72446-1

Rowe CL, Liddle HA (2008) Multidimensional family therapy for adolescent alcohol abusers. Alcohol Treat Q 26(1–2):105–123. https://doi.org/10.1300/J020v26n01_06

Rupp CI, Kemmler G, Kurz M, Hinterhuber H, Fleischhacker WW (2012) Cognitive remediation therapy during treatment for alcohol dependence. J Stud Alcohol Drugs 73(4):625–634. https://doi.org/10.15288/jsad.2012.73.625

Samala N, Lourens SG, Shah VH, Kamath PS, Sanyal AJ, Crabb DW, Tang Q, Radaeva S, Liangpunsakul S, Chalasani N (2018) Posttraumatic stress disorder in patients with heavy alcohol consumption and alcoholic hepatitis. Alcohol Clin Exp Res 42:1933–1938. https://doi.org/10.1111/acer.13862

Santucci K (2012) Psychiatric disease and drug abuse. Curr Opin Pediatr 24(2):233–237. https://doi.org/10.1097/mop.0b013e3283504fbf

Scoccianti C, Straif K, Romieu I (2013) Recent evidence on alcohol and cancer epidemiology. Future Oncol 9(9):1315–1322. https://doi.org/10.2217/fon.13.94

Simou E, Britton J, Leonardi-Bee J (2018a) Alcohol and the risk of pneumonia: a systematic review and meta-analysis. BMJ Open 8(8):e022344. https://doi.org/10.1136/bmjopen-2018-022344

Simou E, Britton J, Leonardi-Bee J (2018b) Alcohol consumption and risk of tuberculosis: a systematic review and meta-analysis. Int J Tuberc Lung Dis 22(11):1277–1285. https://doi.org/10.5588/ijtld.18.0092

SIRC (1998) Social and cultural aspects of drinking. Available at: http://www.sirc.org/publik/social_drinking.pdf

Skaff MM, Finney JW, Moos RH (1999) Gender differences in problem drinking and depression: different "vulnerabilities?". Am J Community Psychol 27(1):25–54. https://doi.org/10.1023/a:1022813727823

Smyth A, Teo KK, Rangarajan S, O'Donnell M, Zhang X, Rana P, Leong DP, Dagenais G, Seron P, Rosengren A, Schutte AE, Lopez-Jaramillo P, Oguz A, Chifamba J, Diaz R, Lear S, Avezum A, Kumar R, Mohan V, Szuba A, Wei L, Yang W, Jian B, McKee M, Yusuf S (2015) Alcohol consumption and cardiovascular disease, cancer, injury, admission to hospital, and mortality: a prospective cohort study. Lancet 386(10007):1945–1954. https://doi.org/10.1016/S0140-6736(15)00235-4

WHO (1992) The ICD-10 classification of mental and behavioural disorders: clinical descriptions and diagnostic guidelines. World Health Organization, Geneva. https://apps.who.int/iris/handle/10665/37958

Winhusen TM, Theobald J, Lewis DF (2019) Substance use outcomes in cocaine-dependent tobacco smokers: a mediation analysis exploring the role of sleep disturbance, craving, anxiety, and depression. J Subst Abus Treat 96:53–57. https://doi.org/10.1016/j.jsat.2018.10.011

Zhu C, Chen Q, Si W, Li Y, Chen G, Zhao Q (2020) Alcohol use and depression: a mendelian randomization study from China. Front Genet 11:585351. https://doi.org/10.3389/fgene.2020.585351

Alcohol and Disease

49

A Focus on Tuberculosis and Implications for Public Health and Policy

Mihir P. Rupani

Contents

Introduction 1035
Understanding Alcohol-related Terms 1035
Understanding "Standard" Alcohol Drinks and Low-Risk Drinking 1036
Burden of Alcohol Consumption 1036
Burden of Alcohol-Use Disorders 1036
Alcohol and Disease: A Focus on Tuberculosis 1037
Alcohol and Tuberculosis: Implications for Public Health and Policy 1038
Tuberculosis and Alcohol Collaborative Framework 1038
Implementation of Bidirectional Activities for TB–alcohol 1039
Screening for Alcohol Abuse Under the National TB Program (NTP) 1039
Alcohol de-Addiction Clinics/Centers and Screening for TB 1047
Training 1047
Demand Generation 1047
Record Keeping and Reporting 1048
Monitoring Indicators 1048
Supervision 1048
Private sector and Nongovernmental Organization (NGO) Involvement: 1048
Implementation Plan 1049
Applications to Other Areas of Substance-Use Disorders 1050
Applications to Other Areas of Public Health 1051
Mini-Dictionary of Terms 1052

M. P. Rupani (✉)
Department of Clinical Epidemiology, Division of Health Sciences, ICMR – National Institute of Occupational Health (ICMR-NIOH), Ahmedabad, Gujarat, India

Department of Community Medicine, Government Medical College Bhavnagar (Maharaja Krishnakumarsinhji Bhavnagar University), Bhavnagar, Gujarat, India
e-mail: mihir.rupani@icmr.gov.in; mihirrupani@gmail.com

V. B. Patel, V. R. Preedy (eds.), *Handbook of Substance Misuse and Addictions*,
https://doi.org/10.1007/978-3-030-92392-1_54

Key Facts ... 1052
Summary Points ... 1052
References ... 1053

Abstract

Harmful use of alcohol is an established risk factor for tuberculosis (TB). Patients with TB fail to complete their treatment if they continue consumption of alcohol during the course of their treatment. The harms related to excessive consumption of alcohol are multitude – physical, mental, social, vocational, and financial. Focused efforts are required to address the dual burden of TB and alcohol. Validated screening tools are available for early identification of the interventions required for patients depending on the level of their alcohol abuse. Brief interventions are proven counselling tools for helping patients quit their drinking habits. Collaborative activities between the national TB program and the alcohol de-addiction program would help address the dual burden effectively. This chapter reviews the bidirectional collaborative activities for TB-alcohol and suggests the roadmap for implementation in programmatic settings.

Keywords

Alcohol use · Tuberculosis · Policy · Integration · Collaborative framework · Substance abuse · National TB program · De-addiction · Brief interventions · AUDIT · Screening · Mental health · Bidirectional activities · National mental health program · TB elimination

Abbreviations

AUDIT	Alcohol Use Identification Test
BI	Brief interventions
DALY	Disability-adjusted life years
HIV/ AIDS	Human immunodeficiency virus/acquired immune deficiency syndrome
IT	Information technology
MDR-TB	Multidrug-resistant tuberculosis
NGO	Nongovernmental organization
NTP	National Tuberculosis Program
PHI	Public Health Institution
SBI	Screening and brief interventions
TB	Tuberculosis
TB-HIV	Tuberculosis–human immunodeficiency virus
UK	United Kingdom
UNODC	United Nations Office on Drugs and Crime
USA	United States of America
WHO	World Health Organization

Introduction

In the year 2016, alcohol was being consumed by approximately two billion people globally (Griswold et al. 2018). In many countries, it is being consumed during social gatherings as a cultural norm and has become an adjunct to their daily food habits (Griswold et al. 2018; World Health Organization 2018). Alcohol has been implicated as a major risk factor in the causation of many diseases and deaths while offering protection in cardiovascular diseases at low doses (Rehm and Imtiaz 2016; Griswold et al. 2018). However, alcohol being toxic and due to its addiction liability, it is recommended not to start or reduce/stop its consumption among its regular drinkers as a public health measure.

Harmful use of alcohol has been strikingly associated with the risk of developing tuberculosis (TB) (Simou et al. 2018). The prevalence of harmful use of alcohol among people with TB varies across countries (Necho et al. 2021); however, it has been reported to be 30% (95% confidence interval 24–35%) globally (Necho et al. 2021). Apart from the risk of failing to complete treatment (Ragan et al. 2020), it also potentially adds to the burden of costs incurred among people with TB (Rehm et al. 2009a).

A few interventions have been tried to reduce the prevalence of harmful use of alcohol among people with TB (Greenfield et al. 2010; Shin et al. 2013); however, systematic efforts towards implementation of a TB–alcohol collaborative policy are scarce (Viiklepp et al. 2013). With the increasing realization of harmful use of alcohol as a "comorbidity," akin to tobacco, there is a need for the development and implementation of a TB–alcohol collaborative policy envisioned through a comprehensive alcohol policy (Jernigan et al. 2000; Raviglione and Poznyak 2017; World Health Organization 2018). This chapter aims to highlight the global burden of harmful use of alcohol, its implications on tuberculosis, and the development and implementation roadmap of a TB–alcohol collaborative policy.

Understanding Alcohol-related Terms

Harmful use of alcohol: This refers to the consumption of alcohol up to a level that causes adverse physical health (for example, liver damage from chronic drinking) and mental health (for example, depressive episodes after drinking) (World Health Organization 1993; Babor et al. 1994; Babor and Higgins-Biddle 2001).

Hazardous use of alcohol: It refers to the consumption of alcohol, which increases the risk of harmful effects for the user. These effects include not only harm to the user's physical and mental health, but also social impact for the drinker or others (Babor et al. 1994; Babor and Higgins-Biddle 2001).

Alcohol dependence: This refers to at least three or more of the following for at least 1 month or repeatedly in the previous 12 months: a strong desire to consume alcohol, impaired control over its use, persistent use despite adverse consequences, a higher priority given to alcohol than to other activities/obligations, increased tolerance, and a physical withdrawal reaction when alcohol is not consumed (World Health Organization 1993; Babor et al. 1994; Babor and Higgins-Biddle 2001).

Understanding "Standard" Alcohol Drinks and Low-Risk Drinking

The definition of a "standard" alcohol drink may vary from country to country depending on the content and weight of pure alcohol in each drink. To screen people for the level of risk, a standard alcohol drink is assumed to be equal to 10 g of pure alcohol (Babor and Higgins-Biddle 2001; Babor et al. 2001). Low-risk drinking level has been recommended as $\leq$20 g of pure alcohol per day with two nondrinking days in a week (Babor and Higgins-Biddle 2001; Babor et al. 2001).

Burden of Alcohol Consumption

Alcohol was being consumed by 43% of the world's population >15 years of age according to recent estimates (World Health Organization 2018). An increase in the income of countries has been associated with an increase in the consumption of alcohol, with high-income countries also reporting the lowest abstention rates (World Health Organization 2018). The highest alcohol consumption per capita ($\geq$10 l per year $\approx$22 g per day) has been reported from the European region, while the lowest from Muslim-majority countries (World Health Organization 2018). Alcohol consumption beyond 10 g per day increases the absolute risk of dying from alcohol-attributable deaths (Rehm et al. 2011). The consumption is projected to increase worldwide, with the highest increase expected in the Southeast Asia region (major contribution by India) (World Health Organization 2018).

Burden of Alcohol-Use Disorders

Alcohol-use disorders were the 20th leading cause of disability-adjusted life years (DALYs) among people in the age group of 25–49 years in the year 2019 (Vos et al. 2020), while it was the 7th leading cause of premature death and DALYs in 2016 (Griswold et al. 2018). Alcohol use was attributed to causing three million deaths (5.3% of all deaths) and 131 million DALYs (5% of all DALYs) globally in the year 2016 (Shield et al. 2020). It has been incriminated as the most important risk factor for 3.3% of communicable and nutritional diseases, 4.3% of noncommunicable diseases, and 17.7% of injury-related deaths (Shield et al. 2020). It is premature mortality, rather than morbidity, which contributes to the global burden attributable to alcohol use (Shield et al. 2020). Globally, in 2016, alcohol use accounted for 6.8% of male deaths and 2.2% of female deaths among all age groups, which increased to 12.2% and 3.8%, respectively, for the age group of 15–49 years (Griswold et al. 2018). Out of the three million deaths attributable to alcohol, digestive diseases (21.3%), unintentional injuries (20.9%), and cardiovascular diseases and diabetes

(19%) were the major contributors, whereas out of the 133 million DALYs attributable to alcohol, unintentional injuries (30%), digestive diseases (17.6%), and alcohol-use disorders (13.9%) were the major contributors (World Health Organization 2018).

Alcohol has been said to have caused 0.25 million deaths due to TB, 33,000 deaths from HIV/AIDS, and 99,000 deaths from lower respiratory infections in 2016 (World Health Organization 2018). Evidence suggests causal associations between alcohol and development of TB, pneumonia, and HIV/AIDS (Rehm et al. 2009b; Samokhvalov et al. 2010; Gmel et al. 2011; World Health Organization 2018). The association of alcohol in causing TB and lower respiratory infections is mainly due to mechanisms involving lowering of the immunity (Rehm et al. 2009b); however, there is the increased likelihood of indulging in unsafe sex due to alcohol consumption, causing HIV/AIDS (Scott-Sheldon et al. 2016). With an exception of ischemic heart disease (minimal amounts of alcohol found to be protective) (Griswold et al. 2018; World Health Organization 2018), for all the other alcohol-attributable diseases, stopping the consumption of alcohol minimized the risk across the health outcomes (Griswold et al. 2018).

Alcohol and Disease: A Focus on Tuberculosis

Alcohol use has been proven to be the most important risk factor attributable for the development of and death due to TB (Volkmann et al. 2015; Imtiaz et al. 2017; Duarte et al. 2018; Ogbo et al. 2018; Simou et al. 2018). Worldwide, the prevalence of alcohol-use disorder among people with TB has been estimated to be 30%, with the prevalence being higher in Asia and Europe as compared to the USA and Africa (Necho et al. 2021). The burden of tuberculosis attributable to alcohol has been estimated to be 10 million DALYs and 0.24 million deaths (Shield et al. 2020). Among all the communicable diseases, alcohol use has the highest (18.3%) population-attributable fraction of mortality due to tuberculosis (Shield et al. 2020).

The association between alcohol and TB is well established; however, there are gaps in the exact mechanism due to which this association exists (Silva et al. 2018), as the association is confounded by the development of alcohol-use disorders and other social factors. Generally, those who consume alcohol develop nutritional deficiencies due to liver damage, and also social factors like overcrowding and malnutrition play a role in the development of TB. However, it cannot be argued that alcohol consumption significantly increases susceptibility to respiratory diseases, such as TB, by dysregulation of the immune response (Cook 1998; Molina et al. 2010). A meta-analysis showed that alcohol-use disorders (defined as consumption of $\geq$40 g alcohol per day) were associated with a 3.5 times higher risk for TB (Lönnroth et al. 2008).

The use of alcohol has been associated with severe TB in the form of cavitary lesions and higher sputum positivity (Fiske et al. 2009; Hermosilla et al. 2017). Alcohol use has also been demonstrated to lead to poor treatment outcomes, including deaths, among patients with both drug-sensitive as well as drug-resistant

TB, with both categories of patients being at twice the risk for failure in completing the treatment (Ragan et al. 2020). A strong association between alcohol consumption and development of multidrug-resistant TB (MDR-TB) has also been reported (Rajendran et al. 2020). Two addictions among patients with TB are becoming a cause of concern – tobacco smoking and alcohol. The risk of poor treatment outcomes among patients with this dual comorbidity is said to be 4–5 times higher (Soh et al. 2017; Thomas et al. 2019).

The known risk of hepatic injury due to the use of alcohol is aggravated by the hepatotoxicity of the antituberculosis drugs – the first-line drugs like isoniazid, rifampicin, and pyrazinamide are most commonly implicated (Pande et al. 1996; Moreno et al. 2001; Prasad et al. 2019). Acute alcohol intake does not change the pharmacokinetics of the isoniazid drug (Dattani et al. 2004; Wilcke et al. 2004); however, patients with tuberculosis are found to metabolize isoniazid more slowly than healthy subjects (Khalili et al. 2010). It is presumed that chronic alcohol consumption might alter the pharmacokinetics of various antituberculosis drugs in the long run (Thummar and Rupani 2020), and future research may throw some light on the same (Myers et al. 2018). In all possibilities, patients on antituberculosis treatment need to be advised a total abstinence of alcohol to allay any possible aggravation of toxicities caused by the medicines itself.

Alcohol and Tuberculosis: Implications for Public Health and Policy

Collaborative activities are being implemented for addressing the dual burden of TB–tobacco (WHO Country Office for India 2017b; Goel et al. 2018), TB–HIV (Fujiwara et al. 2012; Central TB Division and Department of AIDS Control (Government of India) 2013), and TB–diabetes (World Health Organization and The Union 2011; WHO Country Office for India 2017a) in many countries (Jeon et al. 2010; Creswell et al. 2011; Marais et al. 2013; Gupta et al. 2014). A few countries are also exploring addressing of the burden of TB–alcohol through collaborative activities (Viiklepp et al. 2013; Navya et al. 2019; Thummar and Rupani 2020). However, studies have highlighted the need for a policy on paper and stricter implementation of such a framework (Navya et al. 2019).

Tuberculosis and Alcohol Collaborative Framework

Purpose

The purpose of the TB–alcohol framework is to design and implement collaborative activities between the National TB Programs (NTP) of various countries and the alcohol de-addiction clinics or clinical departments catering to patients with harmful use of alcohol in the respective countries.

Objectives

- To establish mechanisms of collaboration between NTP and de-addiction clinics/ clinics managing patients with harmful use of alcohol

- To screen patients diagnosed with TB under the NTP for harmful alcohol use through Alcohol Use Identification Test – AUDIT (Babor et al. 2001)
- To provide "brief intervention" to all patients diagnosed with TB under the NTP and found to be using alcohol – on the first day of diagnosis
- To refer patients diagnosed with TB and found to be alcohol dependent (using AUDIT) to de-addiction clinics
- To ensure completely free diagnostic and treatment services at the alcohol de-addiction clinics for the referred TB patients
- To screen people with harmful/hazardous use of alcohol at de-addiction clinics for active TB symptoms and refer such patients to health facilities under the NTP for diagnosis
- To generate awareness among the community regarding the TB–alcohol collaborative activities
- To ensure availability of logistics/medicines required for collaborative efforts
- To train TB counsellors on screening through AUDIT and "brief intervention"
- To establish supportive supervision mechanisms through government authorities for on-site corrections and monitoring
- To establish mechanisms for reporting/integration into existing reporting mechanisms for generating data on outcome indicators
- To involve the private health sector and not-for-profit organizations in the bidirectional activities for TB–alcohol

Implementation of Bidirectional Activities for TB–alcohol

Screening for Alcohol Abuse Under the National TB Program (NTP)

Under the NTP, there is a decentralized network of public health institutions (PHIs), which diagnose and treat patients with TB, with referral mechanisms to higher centers when necessary. A patient with TB is counselled on the importance of maintaining nutrition, treatment duration, adherence to the treatment, and others as soon as diagnosed under the NTP. The details of the addiction habits of the patients, like tobacco and alcohol consumption, are also elicited on the first day of diagnosis.

To implement the bidirectional screening of TB–alcohol, the TB health visitors should screen all such patients using AUDIT (Babor et al. 2001). The AUDIT is a 10-item screening tool for assessing the level of drinking problem among routine alcohol consumers with final scores ranging from 0 to 40 (Table 1) (Babor et al. 2001). The health workers should use this interview version to record the responses of the patients. Each question is scored from 0 to 4, and the scores of each question are mentioned before the responses in brackets. After entering the scores of each item in the AUDIT tool, the health worker should then add it up to reach the final score. The first three questions assess hazardous alcohol use, the next three questions assess dependence, and the last four questions assess harmful alcohol use (Table 2) (Babor et al. 2001).

On the AUDIT assessment, those patients with TB who score ≤ 7 should be given education related to the hazards of alcohol consumption; those scoring between 8 and

Table 1 Alcohol Use Disorders Identification Test (AUDIT) – interview version. (From Babor et al. 2001, with permission)

Read questions as written. Record answers carefully. Begin the AUDIT by saying "Now I am going to ask you some questions about your use of alcoholic beverages during this past year." Explain what is meant by "alcoholic beverages" by using local examples of beer, wine, vodka, etc. Code answers in terms of "standard drinks." Place the correct answer number in the box at the right.	
1. How often do you have a drink containing alcohol? 0. Never [Skip to Qs 9–10] 1. Monthly or less 2. 2 to 4 times a month 3. 2 to 3 times a week 4. 4 or more times a week ☐	6. How often during the last year have you needed a first drink in the morning to get yourself going after a heavy drinking session? 0. Never 1. Less than monthly 2. Monthly 3. Weekly 4. Daily or almost daily ☐
2. How many drinks containing alcohol do you have on a typical day when you are drinking? 0. 1 or 2 1. 3 or 4 2. 5 or 6 3. 7, 8, or 9 4. 10 or more ☐	7. How often during the last year have you had a feeling of guilt or remorse after drinking? 0. Never 1. Less than monthly 2. Monthly 3. Weekly 4. Daily or almost daily ☐
3. How often do you have six or more drinks on one occasion? 0. Never 1. Less than monthly 2. Monthly 3. Weekly 4. Daily or almost daily *Skip to Questions 9 and 10 if Total Score for Questions 2 and 3 = 0* ☐	8. How often during the last year have you been unable to remember what happened the night before because you had been drinking? 0. Never 1. Less than monthly 2. Monthly 3. Weekly 4. Daily or almost daily ☐
4. How often during the last year have you found that you were not able to stop drinking once you had started? 0. Never 1. Less than monthly 2. Monthly 3. Weekly 4. Daily or almost daily ☐	9. Have you or someone else been injured as a result of your drinking? (0) No (2) Yes, but not in the last year (4) Yes, during the last year ☐
5. How often during the last year have you failed to do what was normally expected from you because of drinking? 0. Never 1. Less than monthly 2. Monthly 3. Weekly 4. Daily or almost daily ☐	10. Has a relative or friend or a doctor or another health worker been concerned about your drinking or suggested you cut down? (0) No (2) Yes, but not in the last year (4) Yes, during the last year ☐
Record total of specific items here ☐	

15 should be given simple advice on quitting; those scoring between 16 and 19 should be given simple advice and brief counselling; and those scoring ≥20 should be referred to a de-addiction treatment center for further management (Table 3) (Babor et al. 2001).

Table 2 AUDIT questions representing different domains of alcohol use. (From Babor et al. 2001 with permission)

Domains	Question number	Item content
Hazardous alcohol use	1	Frequency of drinking
	2	Typical quantity
	3	Frequency of heavy drinking
Dependence symptoms	4	Impaired control over drinking
	5	Increased salience of drinking
	6	Morning drinking
Harmful alcohol use	7	Guilt after drinking
	8	Blackouts
	9	Alcohol-related injuries
	10	Others concerned about drinking

Table 3 Interventions based on AUDIT score. (From Babor et al. 2001, with permission)

AUDIT score	Risk level	Intervention
0–7	I	Alcohol education
8–15	II	Simple advice
16–19	III	Simple advice plus brief counselling, and continued monitoring
20–40	IV	Referral to specialist for diagnostic evaluation and treatment

Screening and Brief Interventions (SBI) for Hazardous and Harmful Use of Alcohol

Screening and brief interventions (SBI) are an easy-to-use, cost-effective, and evidence-based method of informing the risks of alcohol consumption for low-risk drinkers (Babor, Grant and World Health Organization 1992; Babor 1996; Babor and Higgins-Biddle 2000, 2001). Screening, using AUDIT, is the first step to be undertaken by the TB health visitor/counsellor at the diagnostic center for TB. Since many patients are likely to conceal their drinking habits, it is recommended to screen all patients with TB in the first instance. Future follow-up screenings using AUDIT can be decided as per the feasibility of the healthcare workers and their workload.

Alcohol Education for Risk Level I

Patients with TB scoring $\leq$7 are termed as low-risk drinkers (those who score 0 are considered as abstainers) (Babor et al. 2001). Such patients should be appreciated for their controlled drinking. However, they should also be counselled on the possibility and hazards of their habits turning into harmful use or dependence. Since such counselling takes place at a time when the patient is newly diagnosed with TB, it is important to ask the patients to stop drinking (at least during the course of the treatment as it would affect the pharmacokinetics of antituberculosis drugs). Patients should be further asked to maintain lifelong abstinence from consumption of alcohol during the follow-up visits. It is to be emphasized here that they should be made aware of the hazards of drinking using a pamphlet (Fig. 1) (Babor and Higgins-Biddle 2001).

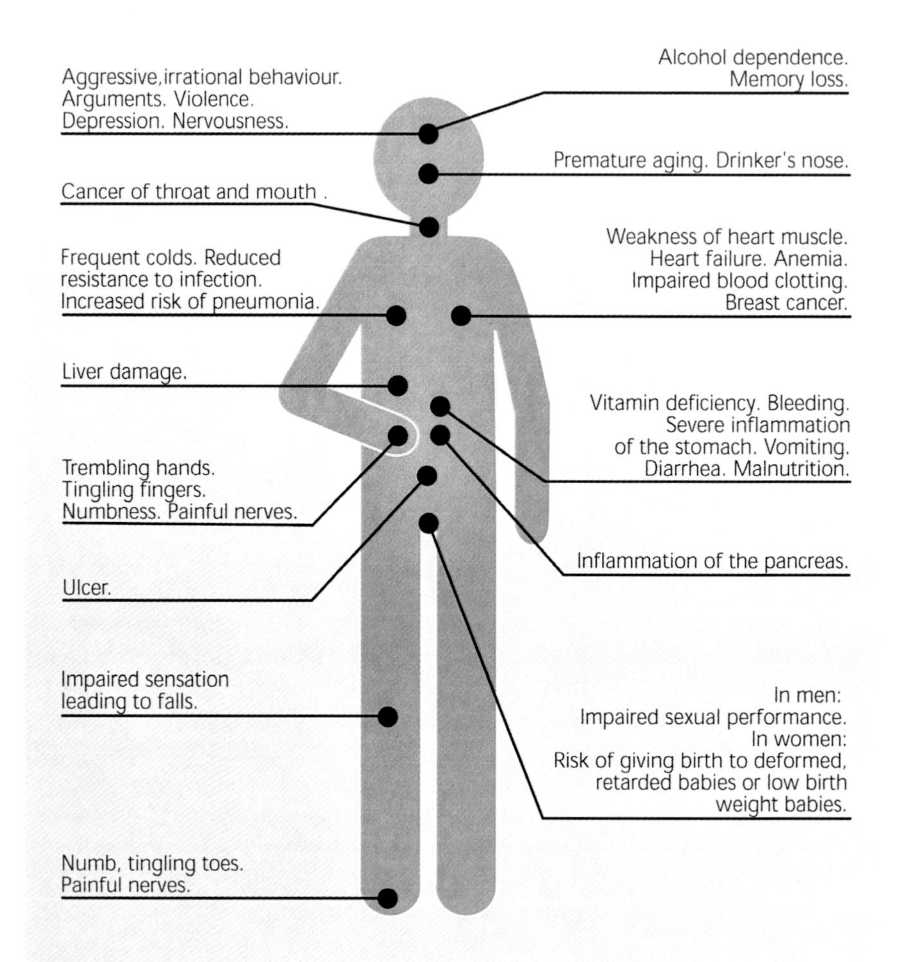

Fig. 1 Pamphlet to be distributed to patients with TB who use alcohol on the first day of treatment initiation. (Figure showing the hazards of alcohol drinking, from Babor and Higgins-Biddle 2001, with permission)

Simple Advice for Risk Level II

A "simple advice" is suitable for patients with TB scoring between 8 and 15 on the AUDIT as any physical harm among them may not be evident yet – hazardous use of alcohol (Babor and Higgins-Biddle 2001; Babor et al. 2001). However, since the amount of alcohol consumed is above the recommended low-risk drinking among patients at this risk level, they are prone to develop chronic alcohol-attributable conditions.

The following steps should be followed for giving simple advice to the patients with TB in the risk level II (Babor and Higgins-Biddle 2001):

Communicate the AUDIT score: The brief intervention of simple advice will start with communicating the AUDIT score to the patients. Generally, it is advisable to start with the fact that the patient's drinking falls into the *risky* category and that they should reduce or stop their alcohol consumption.

Provide information: Fig. 1 should be used to provide information on the hazards of high-risk drinking to the patients, thereby motivating them to reduce or stop their current drinking habits.

Goal setting: The TB health visitors/counsellors need to advise patients with TB to abstain from any form of alcohol drinking as they would be initiating their antituberculosis therapy. The counsellors may consider brief counselling for patients who are not willing to set a goal of total abstinence.

Advice on safe limits and quantity of "standard drinks": The concept of low-risk drinking, as defined by the consumption of ≤20 g of pure alcohol per day with two nondrinking days in a week, should be explained to the patients refusing to abstain from total drinking. The patients also need to be explained about what constitutes a "standard drink" (generally, 10 g of pure alcohol). The best advice for patients with TB would be to reduce their existing number of drinks, gradually reducing to zero drinks on most days, ultimately stopping their drinking completely.

Motivate: Encourage the patients to reinforce the goals they have set for reducing or stopping their regular drinking habits. The patients may complain of the urge to start drinking again, if they stopped once, or may fail to adhere to their set goals. The TB counsellors need to motivate such patients to reflect on the reasons for failing to adhere to their set goals and keep working on them. Again, it is important to emphasize the benefits of total abstinence and the hazards of drinking while they are on their anti-TB drugs.

Be compassionate: The health workers/counsellors need to be empathetic and nonjudgmental to the drinking habits of the patients. A compassionate dialogue and body language during the counselling process are critical.

Follow-up: Frequent follow-up of the patients through home visits by the TB health visitors or during the routine patient visits to the clinics would indicate the adherence of the patients to their goals. Patients denying to set a goal should be followed up more frequently with consideration of brief counselling or referral on a case-to-case basis.

Brief Counselling for Risk Level III

A brief counselling session is recommended for patients with TB who score between 16 and 19 on the AUDIT – harmful use of alcohol – and for those hazardous drinkers among whom drinking is contraindicated (Babor and Higgins-Biddle 2001; Babor et al. 2001). These are the patients among whom the level of drinking is above low risk and the physical/mental harms of high-risk drinking are evident on their health.

The primary goal of brief counselling is to make the patient immediately implement certain change strategies using basic attitudinal approaches.

The steps of providing brief counselling are as follows (Babor and Higgins-Biddle 2001):

Brief advice: Inform the patients about their AUDIT score and that they fall into the high-risk drinking category. The health workers should correlate the score with the physical/mental harms or the indirect effects, which the patients might be experiencing. The patients need to be elaborated on the call for action using Fig. 1.

Assessing Stages of Change: The TB health workers need to assess the stage of motivational change in which the patients are currently in – precontemplation (no change in drinking habits being considered shortly), contemplation (not sure about changing drinking habits, but aware about its harmful effects), preparation (planning to take action on changing drinking habits), action (started cutting down or total abstinence from drinking, but change is temporary), and maintenance (reduced significantly or stopped drinking relatively for longer duration) (Prochaska and DiClemente 1983; Babor and Higgins-Biddle 2001). The health workers can perform this assessment through a simple question, "How willing are they to change their current drinking habits on a scale of 1-10?" (Babor and Higgins-Biddle 2001). Scores ranging from 1 to 3 can be considered as precontemplation, 4 to 6 as contemplation, and 7 to 10 as preparation/action stages (Miller 1999).

Brief intervention based on the stage of change: Depending on the patient's willingness to change their drinking habits, the focus of the brief counselling session can be directed towards the same (Table 4) (Babor and Higgins-Biddle 2001).

Table 4 Brief intervention to be advised as per the stages of change. (From Babor and Higgins-Biddle 2001, with permission)

Stage	Description of stage	Brief intervention
Precontemplation	No change in drinking habits being considered shortly	Communicate the AUDIT score and provide information about the harms of drinking while affected with TB
Contemplation	Not sure about changing drinking habits, but aware of its harmful effects	Provide information about the harms of drinking while affected with TB and help to choose a goal (preferably total abstinence)
Preparation	Planning to take action on changing drinking habits	Explain the importance of total abstinence, advise on safe limits, explain "standard drink" quantity, motivate to reinforce their goal to total abstinence
Action	Started cutting down or total abstinence from drinking, but change is temporary	Reinforce advice on safe limits, motivate to reinforce their goal to total abstinence
Maintenance	Reduced significantly or stopped drinking relatively for a longer duration	Continue motivating for their efforts towards total abstinence

Changing the drinking habits: Try seeking the help of a colleague, friend, family member, relative, or a person who also wishes to change his/her drinking habits. Although total abstinence is recommended for patients with TB, for heavy drinkers, it would be highly beneficial to change the habits to low-risk drinking and ultimately totally abstaining from any kind of drinking. Apart from the fact that stopping the drinking of alcohol would improve the treatment outcomes of the patients with TB, explain the other benefits of total abstinence like longevity, better sleep, feeling happy, cutting down on expenditure, improved relationships, better work performance, body weight maintenance, less likelihood of feeling depressed/suicidal, less likelihood of heart disease/cancer/premature brain damage, less likelihood of dying by drowning/car accident/liver disease, less legal issues, respectful behavior from others, improved sexual performance (for men), and fewer chances of unplanned pregnancy/fetal complications (for women) (Babor and Higgins-Biddle 2001). The health workers should ask the patients to list down the important benefits, which the patients perceive as beneficial for them, and should reinforce the need for total abstinence to get these benefits.

Dealing with "tricky" situations: It is the situation that triggers someone to get the urge to drink alcohol. Arguments, bad mood, boredom, feeling lonely, parties, festival celebrations, failure, weekends, credit of salary, sleeplessness, peer pressure, tension, a long day of work, etc. are situations when this urge takes a rebirth. These "tricky" situations can be dealt with gradually by giving various options to the patients. There are many options, such as engaging in religious activities, helping out in daily chores, helping children at home with their homework, joining not-for-profit organizations such as helping the handicapped, socializing with people who do not drink, visiting friends/family/relatives, finding rewarding activities such as exercise, working till late night, changing friends who are habitual drinkers, and indulging in activities patients can do at home – playing indoor games and playing with their children/grandchildren. Ask the patients to list down what they would do when they encounter tricky situations and reinforce the activities which they enjoy doing it.

Sticking to a plan: Based on the answers given by the patients to the stage of change, benefits of stopping alcohol drinking, and ways to dealing with the tricky situations, help the patients to chalk out a plan to be followed over the next few weeks. Talking to a helper, colleague, or fellow person who also wishes to quit will help stick to the plan. Keep updating this "friend" about the adherence and success achieved each week with this plan. The TB health workers may also play an important role in being this "friend."

Follow-up: It is important to take regular follow-up of the patients in achieving the maintenance stage of the motivational change and adhering to total abstinence. The routine home visits by the health workers should include eliciting the adherence to the plans prepared by the patients for achieving total abstinence.

Referral for Risk Level IV

Those patients with TB scoring $\geq$20 are likely to be dependent on alcohol and thus require referral to a specialized treatment facility for alcohol de-addiction. Patients scoring <20 who are showing symptoms of alcohol dependence, or are not able to achieve their goals of total abstinence despite counselling, should also be considered for such a referral. In the absence of such a treatment facility, the patients should be referred to a psychiatrist for further management in a nearby public health facility. Such a referral should be facilitated by the TB health workers by establishing contacts at such identified facilities in the vicinity. It would be the responsibility of the NTP program staff to identify and prepare a list of such referral facilities, district hospitals, nongovernmental organizations, peer-help groups, and others, who provide services for diagnosis and treatment of patients dependent on alcohol. All efforts should also be made to rehabilitate the patient – physical, mental, social, and vocational rehabilitation.

The patients in this risk level need to be given a modified form of simple advice for facilitating their referral to a specialized center (Babor and Higgins-Biddle 2001):

Communicate the AUDIT score: Communicate clearly to the patients that the level of drinking is far more than limits considered to be safe, possibly being dependent on alcohol. This level of drinking would lead to adverse treatment outcomes of tuberculosis with higher chances of adverse drug reactions during the course of their treatment.

Advice on the condition: The TB health worker needs to emphasize the seriousness of the medical condition of the patient. Any recent/old history of attempts to reduce/quit drinking should be discussed in light of the potential threats to the physical harms to the patients and the social harms to the families of the patients.

Patient's feedback: Patients' response to the above two advice would be critical in deciding the next steps of counselling for a referral. If the patient is willing for a referral, the next advice of providing information and motivation should be followed. The patient should be explained the importance of adhering to the treatments given by the specialists at the referral centers. However, if the patient is unwilling for a referral, subsequent home visits by the TB health worker should be used as an opportunity for the same.

Provide information: Provide information on the different facilities, which would manage them for their drinking problem. It would be prudent to book an appointment on behalf of the patients at the referral centers as it would ease the process. A referral chit mentioning that the patient is on anti-TB drugs would also be helpful to the specialists at the referral centers to provide appropriate care and treatment.

Motivate: Motivation and encouragement to continue the anti-TB drugs along with treatment for their alcohol dependence would be highly beneficial for the patients. Seeking family's, friends', or relatives' support would also help them see through such difficult times.

Follow-up: The TB health workers should follow up with the patients regularly through home visits for their drinking problem as it is likely that the problem relapses after a while. Follow-up via telephone calls to the patients can be considered for reaching out to the maximum number of patients.

Alcohol de-Addiction Clinics/Centers and Screening for TB

For early case finding of TB at the specialized centers dealing with alcohol de-addiction, a list of facilities providing services related to alcohol-related problems needs to be identified. It has to be ensured that organizations/centers providing any services – care, support, diagnosis, treatment, rehabilitation, and palliative – should be identified and enlisted. Countries with well-established national programs on substance abuse or national mental health programs would already be having such a list of facilities.

People who come to avail of any kind of services at all such identified facilities should be screened for symptoms of TB. The four primary symptoms of TB include cough persisting for >2 weeks, fever for >2 weeks, significant weight loss, and hemoptysis. A short questionnaire for "TB screen" with these four symptoms should be added to the routine history-taking sheets being used by the facilities. The presence of any one of the four aforementioned symptoms should be considered a suspect for TB and should be referred to the nearest health facility, which provides services under the NTP.

A psychologist/counsellor at the identified alcohol abuse treatment facilities would be responsible for referring the suspected TB patients using appropriate referral chits and request forms for managing the referred patients. The health facility would test the sputum of the patients using appropriate tests as per the country's TB policy. Further management and course of action would be based on the results of the tests.

Training

"National tuberculosis–alcohol collaborative activities: operational guidelines and implementation plan" can be developed using pointers from this chapter. Relevant training modules based on these guidelines can be designed and can be incorporated with the routine training programs. A national task force group can oversee the training and implementation of such a program. The national team will need to roll out a cascade training starting from state-level program managers of TB and down up to the frontline health workers. A chapter on identifying suspected patients with TB should be added for those working in the alcohol de-addiction centers.

Demand Generation

Use of information technology (IT)-based solutions, social media, local television advertisements, radio jingles, posters, banners, etc. can be utilized for generating awareness on TB–alcohol collaborative initiative. For patients, sending text messages as reminders for abstaining from alcohol consumption or for awareness generation on hazards of harmful use of alcohol can be thought of. National helpline numbers or existing hotlines for alcohol counselling can also be utilized for spreading messages on alcohol cessation, the four main symptoms of TB, when to consult a doctor, and other

TB–alcohol collaborative activities. Job aids for healthcare workers also need to be prepared, which would help them in counselling the patients.

Record Keeping and Reporting

The TB treatment cards and registers will need to be modified to include the AUDIT scores of the patients, the status of the patient in terms of the "stage of change," and the brief intervention given at each visit through the health visitors. This information needs to be entered and reflected on any Web-based interfaces as well (if being maintained under the NTP of that country). On the other side, the alcohol de-addiction centers should also maintain the relevant information on the number of patients screened and referred.

Monitoring Indicators

Indicators for National TB Program: A few indicators given in Table 5 would be useful in monitoring the progress towards the screening using AUDIT at health facilities providing services for TB (Table 5) (WHO Country Office for India 2017b).

Indicators for alcohol de-addiction centers: Similar to the indicators for NTP, a few indicators have been given in Table 6 for the alcohol de-addiction centers for monitoring progress towards TB–alcohol collaborative activities (Table 6) (WHO Country Office for India 2017b).

Supervision

The nodal officers of the national TB program and substance/alcohol abuse treatment program (or mental health program, as applicable) will ensure that adequate human resources, training, logistics, budgetary approvals, and cross-referral for the successful implementation of bidirectional TB–alcohol collaborative activities are available. Regular review and coordination meetings should be planned between the stakeholders of the two programs. Joint monitoring visits can check the changes in treatment cards, review the reporting of the last quarter, evaluate brief interventions, assess the quality of counselling, check the understanding of "TB screen" among alcohol program staff, check referrals, etc.

Private sector and Nongovernmental Organization (NGO) Involvement:

In the highest TB-burden country (India), the private practitioners manage nearly 50–80% of the patients, and yet many are not reported to the national TB program (Central TB Division (Government of India) and WHO Country Office for India 2014; Central TB Division (Government of India) 2017; Rupani et al. 2021).

Table 5 Indicators for monitoring progress under National TB Program for TB–alcohol collaborative activities. (Adapted from the WHO Country Office for India 2017b)

Indicator	Numerator	Denominator
Proportion of registered TB patients screened for alcohol use using AUDIT	No. of patients with TB screened for alcohol use using AUDIT in the reporting period	No. of patients with TB registered in the reporting period
Proportion of screened TB patients identified as hazardous alcohol user (AUDIT score 8–15)	No. of patients with TB identified as hazardous alcohol user (AUDIT score 8–15) in the reporting period	No. of patients with TB screened using AUDIT in the reporting period
Proportion of hazardous alcohol user given simple advice	No. of patients with TB, identified as hazardous alcohol user, given simple advice in the reporting period	No. of patients with TB identified as hazardous alcohol user in the reporting period
Proportion of screened TB patients identified as harmful alcohol user (AUDIT score 16–19)	No. of patients with TB identified as harmful alcohol user (AUDIT score 16–19) in the reporting period	No. of patients with TB screened using AUDIT in the reporting period
Proportion of harmful alcohol user given brief counselling	No. of patients with TB, identified as harmful alcohol user, given brief counselling in the reporting period	No. of patients with TB identified as harmful alcohol user in the reporting period
Proportion of screened TB patients identified as "possible" alcohol dependence (AUDIT score 20–40)	No. of patients with TB identified as "possible" alcohol dependence (AUDIT score 20–40) in the reporting period	No. of patients with TB screened using AUDIT in the reporting period
Proportion of "possible" alcohol dependence referred to specialist for diagnostic evaluation and treatment	No. of patients with TB, identified as "possible" alcohol dependence, referred to specialist in the reporting period	No. of patients with TB identified as "possible" alcohol dependence in the reporting period
Proportion of patients with TB who were alcohol users successfully observed total abstinence post-counselling during the course of treatment	No. of patients with TB who were alcohol users successfully observed total abstinence post-counselling in the reporting period	No. of patients with TB who were alcohol users and received counselling in the reporting period

On the other hand, the role of not-for-profit organizations in substance/alcohol abuse has been noteworthy too (Eriksson et al. 2011). The private practitioners and NGOs involved in managing patients with TB or with alcohol-related problems should be sensitized on the TB–alcohol collaborative activities initiative.

Implementation Plan

A national substance abuse program or national mental health program with a focus on addressing the burden of harmful use of alcohol would be critical for a successful implementation of the TB–alcohol collaborative initiative. Bidirectional activities

Table 6 Indicators for monitoring progress under alcohol de-addiction centers for TB–alcohol collaborative activities. (Adapted from the WHO Country Office for India 2017b)

Indicator	Numerator	Denominator
Proportion of registered clients at alcohol de-addiction center and screened for TB	No. of clients at alcohol de-addiction center screened for four symptoms of TB in the reporting period	No. of clients registered at alcohol de-addiction center in the reporting period
Proportion of screened clients at alcohol de-addiction center found positive for symptoms of TB	No. of screened clients at alcohol de-addiction center found positive for symptoms of TB in the reporting period	No. of clients screened for symptoms of TB at alcohol de-addiction center in the reporting period
Proportion of clients with symptoms of TB referred to a facility under National TB Program for diagnostic evaluation and treatment	No. of clients with symptoms of TB referred to a facility under National TB Program for diagnostic evaluation and treatment in the reporting period	No. of clients with symptoms of TB at alcohol de-addiction center in the reporting period
Proportion of clients referred to NTP and diagnosed positive for TB using standard tests	No. of clients referred to NTP and diagnosed positive for TB using standard tests in the reporting period	No. of clients referred to NTP from alcohol de-addiction center in the reporting period
Proportion of clients referred to NTP and diagnosed with TB, completing the full course of anti-TB treatment	No. of clients referred to NTP and completing the full course of anti-TB treatment in the reporting period	No. of clients referred to NTP from alcohol de-addiction center and diagnosed with TB in the reporting period

with national TB programs would be highly rewarding in addressing the dual burden of TB and the harmful use of alcohol. The implementation of the TB–alcohol collaborative framework can be planned in a phase-wise manner starting with a few demonstration districts initially. With the demonstration of success in such districts, the states can then plan to roll out the program at scale, ultimately covering the entire country. The demonstration districts can plan to roll out the TB–alcohol collaborative framework as discussed in Table 7.

Applications to Other Areas of Substance-Use Disorders

In this chapter, a review exploring collaborative activities between two programs – the national program for tuberculosis and alcohol de-addiction program – was presented. Bidirectional screening and management were well established for tuberculosis and tobacco, but only in India (Hyder et al. 2018). Apart from tobacco and alcohol, other forms of substance abuse like opium are not yet established as direct risk factors for tuberculosis (Safari et al. 2016). However, the increased risk of TB due to injection drug use cannot be ruled out due to coinfection with HIV (Perlman et al. 1995; Armenta et al. 2017). As suggested in this chapter, tri-directional integration between TB, HIV, and injection drug abuse is the need of the hour in high-burden countries for early identification and appropriate management of such

Table 7 Activities and responsibilities of stakeholders for a successful implementation of TB–alcohol collaborative framework. (Adapted from the WHO Country Office for India 2017b)

Activities	Responsibility
Country-level stakeholders of both the programs to send operational guidelines to state-level stakeholders/program managers for implementation of TB–alcohol collaborative activities	National nodal officers (TB and substance abuse programs), Ministry of Health (respective governments)
Finalization of an action plan for TB–alcohol collaborative activities by state with modifications as felt necessary by individual states	State nodal officers and other state-level program managers, program officers, consultants
Cascade training starting with district-level program managers/district-level nodal officers (including training for simple advice, brief interventions, TB screening)	State nodal officers and other state-level program managers, program officers, consultants
Training/sensitization of staff working in national TB program and alcohol de-addiction treatment centers (sub-district/primary care level) – along with other routine program training	District-level nodal officers, district-level program managers, program officers, consultants
Training/sensitization of frontline workers working in other national health programs (to be integrated with weekly/monthly review meetings)	Primary care physicians
Implementation of TB–alcohol collaborative activities	TB health workers, counsellors, alcohol de-addiction centers' staff
Collaborative visits for supportive supervision and monitoring	District-level program managers, program officers, consultants

patients (Haverkos 1991; Sylla et al. 2007; WHO, UNODC and United Nations 2008). Brief interventions are successful in substance-abuse disorders, other than alcohol as well, and it is recommended to implement them at the de-addiction treatment centers (Babor et al. 2007; Wamsley et al. 2018).

Applications to Other Areas of Public Health

In this review, the feasibility and implementation plans of a collaborative approach to public health programs were discussed. It was seen that the concept of bidirectional and collaborative activities was duly utilized by various countries for successful implementation and follow-up of the patients with various diseases/conditions. This was especially true for comorbid conditions, coinfections, or coexisting diseases. As far as reaching the goal of elimination of TB is concerned, countries are exploring as many internal collaborations as possible (Ministry of Health and Family Welfare (Government of India) 2021). Although evidence is uncertain on reducing the costs incurred by the patients/health facilities, the collaborative approach to the public health programs does improve patient satisfaction, perceived quality of care, and access to services (Baxter et al. 2018). It is recommended that governments explore the possibility of implementing such collaborative approaches to public health programs.

Mini-Dictionary of Terms

- Abstainers: People who do not consume alcohol or any other addictive substances such as tobacco, opium, and cocaine.
- Abstinence: The practice of not consuming or using any addictive substances.
- Brief interventions: These are short-timed counselling interventions for people affected by substance abuse, usually directed towards making them quit their addictive habits.
- Counselling: The process of making people understand the importance of a subject or intervention or change, to make their lives better.
- Substance abuse: The use of addictive substances, such as tobacco, alcohol, opium, and cocaine, in quantities which are more than the prescribed limits, generally harming its users physically, mentally, socially, vocationally, and/or economically.

Key Facts

Key facts of alcohol

- Consuming alcohol beyond recommended limits increases the absolute risk of dying from alcohol-attributable causes.
- Alcohol leads to over three million deaths globally every year.

Key facts of alcohol and tuberculosis

- The prevalence of alcohol consumption among people with tuberculosis is estimated to be 30% globally.
- Among all the communicable diseases, alcohol use has the highest (18.3%) population-attributable fraction on mortality due to tuberculosis.

Key facts of policy for alcohol and tuberculosis

- Estonia is one of the first countries to demonstrate the possibility of bidirectional collaborative activities for alcohol and tuberculosis.
- High-burden countries like India have started eliciting the history of alcohol use among patients being diagnosed with tuberculosis.

Summary Points

- Nearly half of the world's population above 15 years of age consumes alcohol in some form.
- One in every three patients with tuberculosis (TB) is an alcohol user.

- Harmful use of alcohol is an established risk factor for the development of TB.
- Patients with TB fail to complete their treatment if they continue consumption of alcohol.
- Focused efforts are required to address the dual burden of TB and alcohol.
- A validated screening tool "AUDIT" is widely in use for early identification of the level of alcohol drinking.
- Brief interventions (BI) are proven counselling tools for helping patients reduce/quit alcohol drinking.
- Collaborative activities between the national TB program and alcohol de-addiction clinics would help address the dual burden effectively.
- All patients with TB should be screened using AUDIT and given appropriate BI, and referral to alcohol de-addiction clinics in case of alcohol dependence.
- All patients presenting at alcohol de-addiction clinics are to be screened for symptoms of TB and are to be referred to the national TB program if found symptomatic.

References

Armenta RF et al (2017) Mycobacterium tuberculosis infection among persons who inject drugs in San Diego, California. Int J Tuberc Lung Dis 21(4):425–431. https://doi.org/10.5588/ijtld.16.0434

Babor T et al (1994) Lexicon of Alcohol and Drug Terms, World Health Organization. https://apps.who.int/iris/bitstream/handle/10665/39461/9241544686_eng.pdf?sequence=1. Accessed 31 May 2021

Babor TF (1996) A cross-national trial of brief interventions with heavy drinkers. Am J Public Health. American Public Health Association Inc 86(7):948–955. https://doi.org/10.2105/AJPH.86.7.948

Babor TF et al (2001) The alcohol use disorders identification test: guidelines for use in primary care. World Health Organization. WHO Press, Geneva. https://doi.org/10.1177/0269881110393051

Babor TF et al (2007) Screening, brief intervention, and referral to treatment (SBIRT): toward a public health approach to the management of substance abuse. Subst Abus 28(3):7–30. https://doi.org/10.1300/J465v28n03_03

Babor TF, Grant M, World Health Organization (1992) Programme on substance abuse : project on identification and management of alcohol-related problems. Report on phase II, an randomized clinical trial of brief interventions in primary health care, World Health Organization. Edited by T. F. Babor and M. Grant World Health Organization. https://apps.who.int/iris/handle/10665/61637. Accessed 17 June 2021

Babor TF, Higgins-Biddle JC (2000) Alcohol screening and brief intervention: dissemination strategies for medical practice and public health. Addiction 95(5):677–686. https://doi.org/10.1046/j.1360-0443.2000.9556773.x

Babor TF, Higgins-Biddle JC (2001) Brief intervention for hazardous and harmful drinking: a manual for use in primary care. World Health Organization

Baxter S et al (2018) The effects of integrated care: a systematic review of UK and international evidence. BMC Health Serv Res 18(1):350. https://doi.org/10.1186/s12913-018-3161-3

Central TB Division (Government of India) (2017) National strategic plan for tuberculosis elimination 2017–2025. Ministry of Health & Family Welfare, Government of India, New Delhi. https://tbcindia.gov.in/WriteReadData/National Strategic Plan 2017-25.pdf. Accessed 24 June 2021

Central TB Division (Government of India) and WHO Country Office for India (2014) Standards for TB care in India. World Health Organization, New Delhi. https://tbcindia.gov.in/showfile.php?lid=3061. Accessed 12 Dec 2018

Central TB Division and Department of AIDS Control (Government of India) (2013) National Framework for Joint HIV/TB Collaborative Activities. Ministry of Health & Family Welfare, Government of India, New Delhi. http://www.naco.gov.in/sites/default/files/National Frame work for Joint HIV TB Collaborative Activities November 2... %281%29.pdf. Accessed 22 June 2021

Cook RT (1998) Alcohol abuse, alcoholism, and damage to the immune system – a review. Alcohol Clin Exp Res 22(9):1927–1942. https://doi.org/10.1097/00000374-199812000-00007

Creswell J et al (2011) Tuberculosis and noncommunicable diseases: neglected links and missed opportunities. Eur Respir J 37(5):1269–1282. https://doi.org/10.1183/09031936.00084310

Dattani RG et al (2004) The effects of acute ethanol intake on isoniazid pharmacokinetics. Eur J Clin Pharmacol 60(9):679–682. https://doi.org/10.1007/s00228-004-0828-y

Duarte R et al (2018) Tuberculosis, social determinants and co-morbidities (including HIV). Pulmonology 24(2):115–119. https://doi.org/10.1016/j.rppnen.2017.11.003

Eriksson C et al (2011) A research strategy case study of alcohol and drug prevention by non-governmental organizations in Sweden 2003–2009. Subst Abuse Treat Prev Policy. https://doi.org/10.1186/1747-597X-6-8

Fiske CT, Hamilton CD, Stout JE (2009) Alcohol use and clinical manifestations of tuberculosis. J Infect Elsevier Ltd 58(5):395–401. https://doi.org/10.1016/j.jinf.2009.02.015

Fujiwara P et al (2012) Implementing collaborative TB-HIV activities: a programmatic guide. International Union against Tuberculosis and Lung Disease (The Union), Paris. https://theunion.org/sites/default/files/2020-08/pub_tb-hivguide_eng_web-1.pdf. Accessed 23 June 2021

Gmel G, Shield KD, Rehm J (2011) Developing a method to derive alcohol-attributable fractions for HIV/AIDS mortality based on alcohol's impact on adherence to antiretroviral medication. Popul Health Metrics 9(1):5. https://doi.org/10.1186/1478-7954-9-5

Goel S et al (2018) Integrating tobacco and tuberculosis control programs in India: a win–win situation. Int J Noncommun Dis Medknow 3(5):9. https://doi.org/10.4103/jncd.jncd_15_18

Greenfield SF et al (2010) Integrated management of physician-delivered alcohol care for tuberculosis patients: design and implementation. Alcohol Clin Exp Res 34(2):317–330. https://doi.org/10.1111/j.1530-0277.2009.01094.x

Griswold MG et al (2018) Alcohol use and burden for 195 countries and territories, 1990–2016: a systematic analysis for the Global Burden of Disease Study 2016. Lancet 392(10152):1015–1035. https://doi.org/10.1016/S0140-6736(18)31310-2

Gupta S et al (2014) Review of policy and status of implementation of collaborative HIV-TB activities in 23 high-burden countries. Int J Tuberc Lung Dis:1149–1158. https://doi.org/10.5588/ijtld.13.0889

Haverkos HW (1991) Infectious diseases and drug abuse. J Subst Abus Treat 8(4):269–275. https://doi.org/10.1016/0740-5472(91)90050-K

Hermosilla S et al (2017) Identifying risk factors associated with smear positivity of pulmonary tuberculosis in Kazakhstan. Plos One. Edited by A Odoi 12(3):e0172942. https://doi.org/10.1371/journal.pone.0172942

Hyder MKA et al (2018) Tuberculosis-tobacco integration in the South-East Asia region: policy analysis and implementation framework. Int J Tuberc Lung Dis 22(7):807–812. https://doi.org/10.5588/ijtld.17.0796

Imtiaz S et al (2017) Alcohol consumption as a risk factor for tuberculosis: meta-analyses and burden of disease. Eur Respir J 50(1):1700216. https://doi.org/10.1183/13993003.00216-2017

Jeon CY et al (2010) Bi-directional screening for tuberculosis and diabetes: a systematic review. Trop Med Int Health 15:1300–1314. https://doi.org/10.1111/j.1365-3156.2010.02632.x

Jernigan DH et al (2000) Towards a global alcohol policy: alcohol, public health and the role of WHO. Bull World Health Organ 78(4):491–499. https://www.ncbi.nlm.nih.gov/pmc/articles/PMC2560748/. Accessed 10 Mar 2021

Khalili H et al (2010) Is there any difference between acetylator phenotypes in tuberculosis patients and healthy subjects? Eur J Clin Pharmacol 66(3):261–267. https://doi.org/10.1007/s00228-009-0745-1

Lönnroth K et al (2008) Alcohol use as a risk factor for tuberculosis – a systematic review. BMC Public Health 8:289. https://doi.org/10.1186/1471-2458-8-289

Marais BJ et al (2013) Tuberculosis comorbidity with communicable and non-communicable diseases: integrating health services and control efforts. Lancet Infect Dis 13(5):436–448. https://doi.org/10.1016/S1473-3099(13)70015-X

Miller WR (1999) TIP 35: enhancing motivation for change in substance abuse treatment: Treatment Improvement Protocol (TIP) series 35, Health San Francisco. CDM Group, Inc. https://www.ncbi.nlm.nih.gov/books/NBK64967/. Accessed 18 June 2021

Ministry of Health and Family Welfare (Government of India) (2021) Collaborative framework for management of tuberculosis in pregnant women, Central TB Division. Ministry of Health and Family Welfare, New Delhi. https://tbcindia.gov.in/WriteReadData/180320_DRAFT_FrameworkforManagementofTBinPregnantWomen.pdf. Accessed 23 June 2021

Molina PE et al (2010) Focus on: alcohol and the immune system. Alcohol Res Health 33(1–2):97–108

Moreno S et al (2001) Treatment of tuberculosis in HIV-infected patients: safety and antiretroviral efficacy of the concomitant use of ritonavir and rifampin. AIDS 15(9):1185–1187. https://doi.org/10.1097/00002030-200106150-00018

Myers B et al (2018) Impact of alcohol consumption on tuberculosis treatment outcomes: a prospective longitudinal cohort study protocol. BMC Infect Dis 18(1):1–9. https://doi.org/10.1186/s12879-018-3396-y

Navya N et al (2019) Are they there yet? Linkage of patients with tuberculosis to services for tobacco cessation and alcohol abuse – a mixed methods study from Karnataka, India. BMC Health Serv Res 19(1):90. https://doi.org/10.1186/s12913-019-3913-8

Necho M et al (2021) Prevalence and associated factors for alcohol use disorder among tuberculosis patients: a systematic review and meta-analysis study. Subst Abuse Treat Prev Policy 16(1):2. https://doi.org/10.1186/s13011-020-00335-w

Ogbo FA et al (2018) 'Tuberculosis disease burden and attributable risk factors in Nigeria, 1990–2016. Trop Med Health 46(1):34. https://doi.org/10.1186/s41182-018-0114-9

Pande JN et al (1996) Risk factors for hepatotoxicity from antituberculosis drugs: a case-control study. Thorax 51(2):132–136. https://doi.org/10.1136/thx.51.2.132

Perlman DC et al (1995) Tuberculosis in drug users. Clin Infect Dis 21(5):1253–1264. https://doi.org/10.1093/clinids/21.5.1253

Prasad R, Singh A, Gupta N (2019) Adverse drug reactions in tuberculosis and management. Indian J Tuberc Elsevier Ltd 66(4):520–532. https://doi.org/10.1016/j.ijtb.2019.11.005

Prochaska JO, DiClemente CC (1983) Stages and processes of self-change of smoking: toward an integrative model of change. J Consult Clin Psychol United States 51(3):390–395. https://doi.org/10.1037/0022-006X.51.3.390

Ragan EJ et al (2020) The impact of alcohol use on tuberculosis treatment outcomes: a systematic review and meta-analysis. Int J Tuberc Lung Dis 24(1):73–82. https://doi.org/10.5588/ijtld.19.0080

Rajendran M, Zaki RA, Aghamohammadi N (2020) Contributing risk factors towards the prevalence of multidrug-resistant tuberculosis in Malaysia: a systematic review. Tuberculosis 122:101925. https://doi.org/10.1016/j.tube.2020.101925

Raviglione M, Poznyak V (2017) Targeting harmful use of alcohol for prevention and treatment of tuberculosis: a call for action. Eur Respir J 50(1):1700946. https://doi.org/10.1183/13993003.00946-2017

Rehm J, Mathers C et al (2009a) Global burden of disease and injury and economic cost attributable to alcohol use and alcohol-use disorders. Lancet 373(9682):2223–2233. https://doi.org/10.1016/S0140-6736(09)60746-7

Rehm J, Samokhvalov AV et al (2009b) The association between alcohol use, alcohol use disorders and tuberculosis (TB). A systematic review. BMC Public Health 9(1):450. https://doi.org/10.1186/1471-2458-9-450

Rehm J et al (2011) Epidemiology and alcohol policy in Europe. Addiction 106:11–19. https://doi.org/10.1111/j.1360-0443.2010.03326.x

Rehm J, Imtiaz S (2016) A narrative review of alcohol consumption as a risk factor for global burden of disease. Subst Abuse Treat Prev Policy 11(1):37. https://doi.org/10.1186/s13011-016-0081-2

Rupani MP et al (2021) “We are not aware of notification of tuberculosis”: a mixed-methods study among private practitioners from western India. Int J Health Plann Manag 36(4):1052–1068. https://doi.org/10.1002/hpm.3151

Safari A et al (2016) Opium consumption: a potential risk factor for lung cancer and pulmonary tuberculosis. Indian J Cancer 53(4):587. https://doi.org/10.4103/0019-509X.204755

Samokhvalov AV, Irving HM, Rehm J (2010) Alcohol consumption as a risk factor for pneumonia: a systematic review and meta-analysis. Epidemiol Infect 138(12):1789–1795. https://doi.org/10.1017/S0950268810000774

Scott-Sheldon LAJ et al (2016) Alcohol use predicts sexual decision-making: a systematic review and meta-analysis of the experimental literature. AIDS Behav 20(S1):19–39. https://doi.org/10.1007/s10461-015-1108-9

Shield K et al (2020) National, regional, and global burdens of disease from 2000 to 2016 attributable to alcohol use: a comparative risk assessment study. Lancet Public Health 5(1):e51–e61. https://doi.org/10.1016/S2468-2667(19)30231-2

Shin S et al (2013) Effectiveness of alcohol treatment interventions integrated into routine tuberculosis care in Tomsk, Russia. Addiction 108(8):1387–1396. https://doi.org/10.1111/add.12148

Silva DR et al (2018) Risk factors for tuberculosis: diabetes, smoking, alcohol use, and the use of other drugs. J Bras Pneumol 44(2):145–152. https://doi.org/10.1590/s1806-37562017000000443

Simou E, Britton J, Leonardi-Bee J (2018) Alcohol consumption and risk of tuberculosis: a systematic review and meta-analysis. Int J Tuberc Lung Dis 22(11):1277–1285. https://doi.org/10.5588/ijtld.18.0092

Soh AZ et al (2017) Alcohol drinking and cigarette smoking in relation to risk of active tuberculosis: prospective cohort study. BMJ Open Respir Res 4(1):e000247. https://doi.org/10.1136/bmjresp-2017-000247

Sylla L et al (2007) Integration and co-location of HIV/AIDS, tuberculosis and drug treatment services. Int J Drug Policy. NIH Public Access 18(4):306–312. https://doi.org/10.1016/j.drugpo.2007.03.001

Thomas BE et al (2019) Smoking, alcohol use disorder and tuberculosis treatment outcomes: a dual co-morbidity burden that cannot be ignored. PLoS One 14(7):e0220507. https://doi.org/10.1371/journal.pone.0220507

Thummar PD, Rupani MP (2020) Prevalence and predictors of hazardous alcohol use among tuberculosis patients: the need for a policy on joint tuberculosis-alcohol collaborative activities in India. Alcohol 86:113–119. https://doi.org/10.1016/j.alcohol.2020.03.006

Viiklepp P et al (2013) A collaborative action on tuberculosis and alcohol abuse in Estonia: first report of a demonstration project, WHO Regional Office for Europe. http://www.euro.who.int/__data/assets/pdf_file/0006/237516/WHO-AUD-TB-project-report_10-final-edited-with-PCO_5Dec-2013_NS_kujundatud_koos_TjaK_2.pdf?ua=1. Accessed 5 Feb 2021

Volkmann T et al (2015) Tuberculosis and excess alcohol use in the United States, 1997–2012. Int J Tuberc Lung Dis 19(1):111–119. https://doi.org/10.5588/ijtld.14.0516

Vos T et al (2020) Global burden of 369 diseases and injuries in 204 countries and territories, 1990–2019: a systematic analysis for the Global Burden of Disease Study 2019. Lancet 396 (10258):1204–1222. https://doi.org/10.1016/S0140-6736(20)30925-9

Wamsley M et al (2018) Alcohol and drug screening, brief intervention, and referral to treatment (SBIRT) training and implementation: perspectives from 4 health professions. J Addict Med 12 (4):262–272. https://doi.org/10.1097/ADM.0000000000000410

WHO Country Office for India (2017a) National framework for joint TB-Diabetes collaborative activities. Ministry of Health & Family Welfare, Government of India, New Delhi. https://tbcindia.gov.in/WriteReadData/National framework for joint TB diabetes 23 Aug 2017.pdf. Accessed 20 June 2021)

WHO Country Office for India (2017b) National framework for joint TB-tobacco collaborative activities. Ministry of Health & Family Welfare, Government of India, New Delhi. https://tbcindia.gov.in/WriteReadData/TB-Tobacco.pdf. Accessed 20 June 2021

WHO, UNODC and United Nations (2008) Policy guidelines for collaborative TB and HIV services for injecting and other drug users, evidence for action technical papers. World Health Organization, Geneva. http://whqlibdoc.who.int/publications/2008/9789241596930_eng.pdf. Accessed 23 June 2021

Wilcke JTR et al (2004) Unchanged acetylation of isoniazid by alcohol intake. Int J Tuberc Lung Dis 8(11):1373–1376

World Health Organization (1993) The ICD-10 classification of mental and behavioural disorders: diagnostic criteria for research. World Health Organization, Geneva. https://apps.who.int/iris/bitstream/handle/10665/37108/9241544554.pdf?sequence=1&isAllowed=y. Accessed 16 June 2021

World Health Organization (2018) Global status report on alcohol and health 2018. World Health Organization, Geneva. https://apps.who.int/iris/rest/bitstreams/1151838/retrieve. Accessed 12 Sept 2020

World Health Organization and The Union (2011) Collaborative framework for care and control of tuberculosis and diabetes. World Health Organization. https://theunion.org/sites/default/files/2020-08/collaborative-framework_tb-diabetes.pdf. Accessed 23 June 2021

Using New Technology and Concepts on the Oldest Addiction on Earth, Alcoholism

50

Features, Applications, and Public Health Implications

Eric Merrell and Brian Johnson

Contents

Introduction ... 1060
The Cost of Alcohol-Related Harm ... 1062
Identification and Interception of AUD ... 1064
Barriers to Treatment of AUD ... 1065
A Tale of Two Drinkers ... 1066
The Economics of Alcohol Consumption Deterrence ... 1066
The Harm Principle ... 1066
A Model for Improvement: Australia's Banned Drinkers Registrar ... 1067
A Proposal for an Alcohol Purchase License ... 1068
Application of an Alcohol Purchase License ... 1068
Features of an Alcohol Purchase License ... 1069
Duration and Adjudication ... 1070
How to Implement ... 1071
Potential Pitfalls of an Alcohol Purchase License ... 1071
Additional Considerations ... 1071
Applications to Other Areas of Addiction ... 1071
Applications to Other Areas of Public Health ... 1072
Mini-dictionary of Terms ... 1072
Key Facts About Alcohol Use ... 1072
Summary Points ... 1073
References ... 1073

E. Merrell
Department of Medicine, SUNY Upstate Medical University, Syracuse, NY, USA

B. Johnson (✉)
Department of Psychiatry, State University of New York (SUNY) Upstate Medical University, Syracuse, NY, USA
e-mail: johnsonb@upstate.edu

V. B. Patel, V. R. Preedy (eds.), *Handbook of Substance Misuse and Addictions*,
https://doi.org/10.1007/978-3-030-92392-1_57

Abstract

Alcohol is the world's most harmful drug. Its effects are felt collectively throughout the fabric of society. Its insidious toxicity can affect all organs of the body and permanently alter brain pathways. For some, it is enjoyed with no repercussion. This is recreational drinking. Most drinkers use alcohol in a way that is always pleasant. In others, alcohol becomes a metaphorical parasite leading to uncontrolled desire, harm, and self-destruction. The definition of alcoholism is most parsimoniously "Repeated harm from use." This distinction has eluded policy makers. The concept of an alcohol purchase license is proposed to make a relatively simple fix to a huge public health issue. Many attempts have been made to control consumption and curb high-risk and heavy use with variable success. In a world of emerging technology, new possibilities for the prevention of serious harm and rehabilitation are possible. In this chapter, the landscape of alcohol policy is reviewed, and a proposal is made for a twenty-first-century solution involving the creation of a licensing system for alcohol use to combat one of the world's most dangerous problems.

Keywords

Public health · Alcohol · Alcohol use disorder · Binge drinking · Public policy · Banned Drinkers Registrar · Alcohol restriction · Addiction · Addiction medicine · Harm reduction

List of Abbreviations

APL	Alcohol purchase license
AUD	Alcohol use disorder
BAC	Blood alcohol content
BDO	Banned Drinkers Order
BDR	Banned Drinkers Register
ICD-10	International Classification of Diseases-10
ID	Identification
USA	United States

Introduction

Alcohol is one of the most destructive drugs on earth. Excessive use is associated with substantial loss of life and monetary cost to society. In 2012, 3.3 million deaths or 5.9% of global deaths were estimated to be attributable to alcohol use (World Health Organization 2014), yet alcohol remains ubiquitous and underregulated with few exceptions globally. In terms of cost to society in monetary expenditure for all drugs, tobacco and alcohol use far exceed all other drugs (Fig. 1). In 2010, tobacco and alcohol were estimated to cost the United States $300 and $249 billion dollars, respectively (U.S. Department of Health and Human Services 2014; Sacks et al. 2015; Xu et al. 2015).

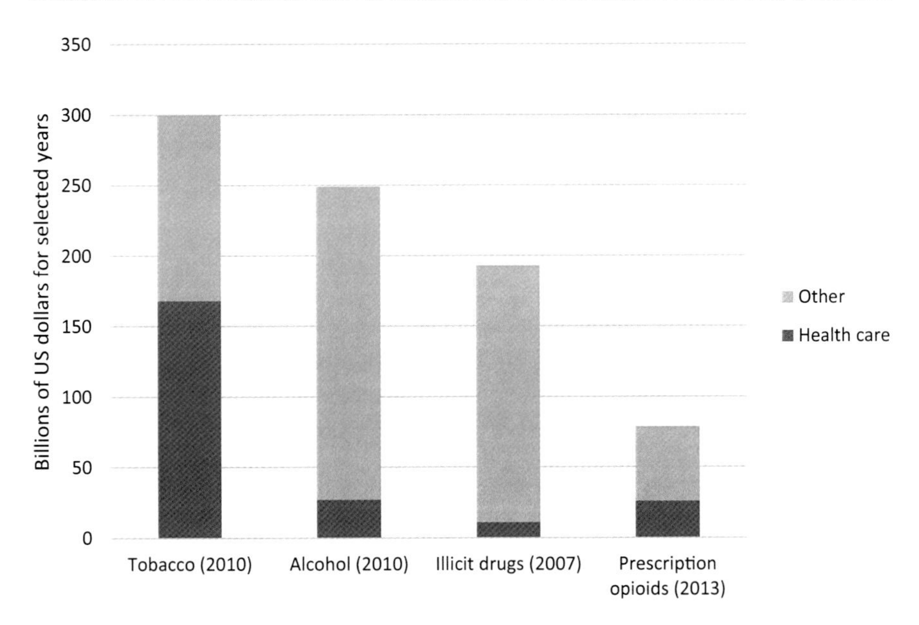

Fig. 1 The cost of drug use in the United States for different drugs in selected years
Data presented as drug (year of available data). "Other" refers to all other harm-related costs involved with drug use including but not limited to loss of productivity, criminal justice, and property damage. Tobacco: (U.S. Department of Health and Human Services 2014) and (Xu et al. 2015). Alcohol: (Sacks et al. 2015). Illicit drug: (National Drug Intelligence Center 2011). Prescription opioids: (Florence et al. 2016)

This chapter will focus on alcohol harm reduction. Tobacco use and its associated sequelae are difficult to compare with alcohol use. Alcohol use is complicated and non-homogenous. Most alcohol users drink recreationally. Even among those who drink excessively (defined as 4 or more drinks for women and 5 or more drinks for men in a single occasion, 8 or more drinks for women or 15 or more drinks a week for men, or any alcohol use for minors or pregnant women), only 10% could be classified as alcohol dependent (Esser et al. 2014). Compare this with tobacco use where around 50% of users meet Diagnostic and Statistical Manual of Mental Disorders (DSM) criteria for dependence (Baker et al. 2012).

Alcoholism is most parsimoniously described as "Repeated harm from use." Persistent heavy alcohol use begets addiction, and drinking becomes a literal horror. Once consistent use is established, the ventral tegmental dopaminergic seeking system is permanently changed resulting in craving, an unquenchable seeking feedback loop that may never disappear (Johnson 2013). The affected person often wakes up in withdrawal and must drink immediately. Social, occupational, legal, and medical consequences ensue.

In 2010, the Independent Scientific Committee on Drugs, a UK-based drugs advisory committee, met to review and appraise drug-related societal and self-harm. A variety of legal and illicit drugs were discussed and assigned a score from 0 (no harm) to 100 (the most harm) for a multitude of factors: physical, psychological, and social harms in two general categories – harms to users and others. The score from these categories was added to form a composite harm score. Alcohol was appraised to cause the most harm with a total score of 72 followed by heroin (55) and crack cocaine (54), methamphetamine (33), cocaine (27), and tobacco (26) (Nutt et al. 2010).

In the United States, alcohol use, particularly high-risk use, is highly prevalent. In 2019, a national survey on drug use and health reported that 56% of respondents 21 years of age and older had used alcohol at least one in the past month, 26% reported binge alcohol use, and 6% reported heavy alcohol use defined as binge drinking on 5 or more days in the past 30 days (SAHMSA 2019). Alcohol use disorder (AUD) as defined by the DSM-5 is highly prevalent as well and grossly undertreated. The National Epidemiologic Survey on Alcohol and Related Conditions III found the 12-month and lifetime prevalence of AUD to be 14% and 29%, respectively (Grant et al. 2015). Among those with lifetime AUD, only 20% were found to have sought treatment.

Binge drinking and heavy alcohol use are associated with innumerable harms at all levels of society and will be further elaborated in the sections to follow. The Gordian knot of alcohol public health policy is the recreational/addiction dichotomy. Increasing the price of alcohol with taxation is the most common intervention. Efficacy is weak. As a political matter, the price of alcohol is paid by all users. Increasing taxes is unlikely to get one elected.

Raising the minimum age to purchase, restrictions on time of sale, and limiting sales outlets, all have been tried with minimal effect. These interventions affect all who drink alcohol, conflating restrictions on recreational users with addicted users. Prohibition has not worked. The seemingly Sisyphean task of creation and implementation of effective public health interventions with a drug that is used both recreationally and addictively requires conceptual clarity and bold action (Table 1).

This chapter will provide a brief review of harm related to alcohol use and the public health tactics employed to reduce it. In an era of emerging technology, new lines of action are possible. A proposal for alcohol use licensing in the United States, an alcohol purchase license, and the means of implementing such a program will be discussed.

The Cost of Alcohol-Related Harm

Harm related to alcohol use penetrates all aspects of society and often causes unnecessary premature loss of life and expenditure of money. As described in the introduction, the cost of alcohol use to society, specifically in the United States, is estimated upward of $249 billion dollars per year (Sacks et al. 2015). This estimation is a composite of several categories of cost including but not limited to healthcare, lost productivity (i.e., impaired productivity at work, incarceration, and absenteeism), criminal justice, property damage, and motor vehicle crashes (Fig. 2). Among this cost is an estimated $100 billion direct cost to the US government. In the setting of an industry that is estimated to have a direct economic impact of $122 billion annually (American Beverage Licensees 2018), what is the true value of alcohol use in America?

Table 1 Logic model of selected alcohol control policies and their proposed impact on drinker groups

Intervention	Drinker Group	Drinker group explicitly targeted?
Advertising restrictions	Heavy	-
	Binge	x
	Low-risk	x
	Youth	x
	Secondary suppliers	x
Minimun age requirement	Heavy	-
	Binge	-
	Low-risk	-
	Youth	x
	Secondary suppliers	x
Minumum price requirement and taxation	Heavy	x
	Binge	x
	Low-risk	x
	Youth	x
	Secondary suppliers	x
Legal BAC limits and penalities for drunk driving	Heavy	x
	Binge	x
	Low-risk	x
	Youth	x
	Secondary suppliers	-
Government monopoly of production, import, export and retail sales	Heavy	x
	Binge	x
	Low-risk	x
	Youth	x
	Secondary suppliers	x
Alcohol purchase license	Heavy	x
	Binge	x
	Low-risk	-
	Youth	x
	Secondary suppliers	x

Groups defined as follows: secondary suppliers, distributors of alcohol; youth, 21 years and younger; low risk, alcohol use below the Dietary Guidelines for Americans alcohol intake recommendations; and binge and heavy, binge drinking on 5 or more days in the past 30 days. “x” denotes a targeted group; “-“ denotes unaffected. BAC, blood alcohol content

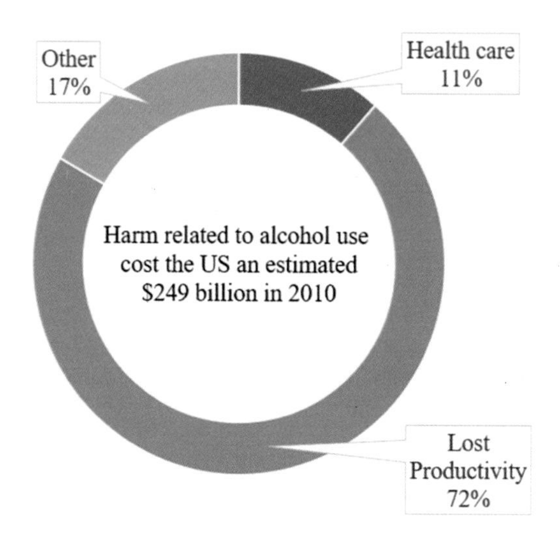

Fig. 2 Percentage breakdown of estimated cost related to harm from alcohol use in the United States in 2010
Sections are labeled as title of category and percentage of total cost. "Other" category includes criminal justice costs, crime-related property damage, motor vehicle crashes, fire losses, and fetal alcohol syndrome. Graph adapted from data presented in Sacks et al. (2015)

Years of alcoholic drinking cause chronic diseases and conditions. Shield et al. (2013) identified 25 chronic diseases and conditions listed in the International Classification of Disease (ICD)-10 that are attributable to alcohol use alone (Shield et al. 2013). These diseases and conditions affect all areas of the body including the neuropsychiatric, gastrointestinal, and cardiovascular systems. Additionally, alcohol has been implicated as a key contributor to as many as 200 other diseases and conditions including a variety of malignant neoplasms, degenerative neurologic condition, diabetes, heart disease, and stroke. In 2010, alcohol-attributable injury, cancer, and liver cirrhosis were estimated to have caused 1,500,000 deaths and 51,898,400 potential years of life lost globally (Rehm and Shield 2013). This loss of life is unacceptable and frequently preventable.

The hostile side of alcoholism is traumatic by imposing harm to others. There is repeated demonstration of associations between alcohol use and violent crimes (~ 40% of cases (Greenfeld and Henneberg 2001)), family and domestic violence (24% to 54% (Mayshak et al. 2020)), suicide attempts (22% (Parks et al. 2014)), traffic-related deaths (28% (National Highway Traffic Safety Administration 2017)), and innumerable other events. The loss of life, psychologic impact, and monetary loss are often priceless and irreplaceable.

Identification and Interception of AUD

The burden of identification and treatment has traditionally fallen on the primary healthcare system as the self-injurious parts of heavy alcohol use, namely, liver cirrhosis, hypertension, sleep, and mood disorders, are commonly screened for and tended to. Unfortunately, the above-listed complications tend to present after the establishment of AUD and would be better treated with prevention than penance. AUD should be identified and treated as a chronic disease. Failure to identify and treat is no different than any other disease and can lead to serious and often fatal outcomes down the line. Reasonable standardized screening should be started early, and initiation of therapy, pharmacologic or elsewise, should be explored as soon as concern is raised.

Unfortunately, this not frequently the case. In a 2013 cross-sectional analysis of ambulatory care users, only 71.1% received alcohol use assessment. Of those who were identified as high risk or dependent, only 2.9% and 7.0%, respectively, were offered further information or intervention (Glass et al. 2016). We cannot depend on primary care alone to identify and proscribe harmful alcohol use.

Barriers to Treatment of AUD

A 2019 systematic review of barriers to treatment for alcohol dependence defined several significant contributors including shame and stigma, the need to continue drinking, lack of perception for treatment need, and a variety of structural barriers (Fig. 3). To effectively reduce harm related to alcohol use, policies will need to transcend these barriers.

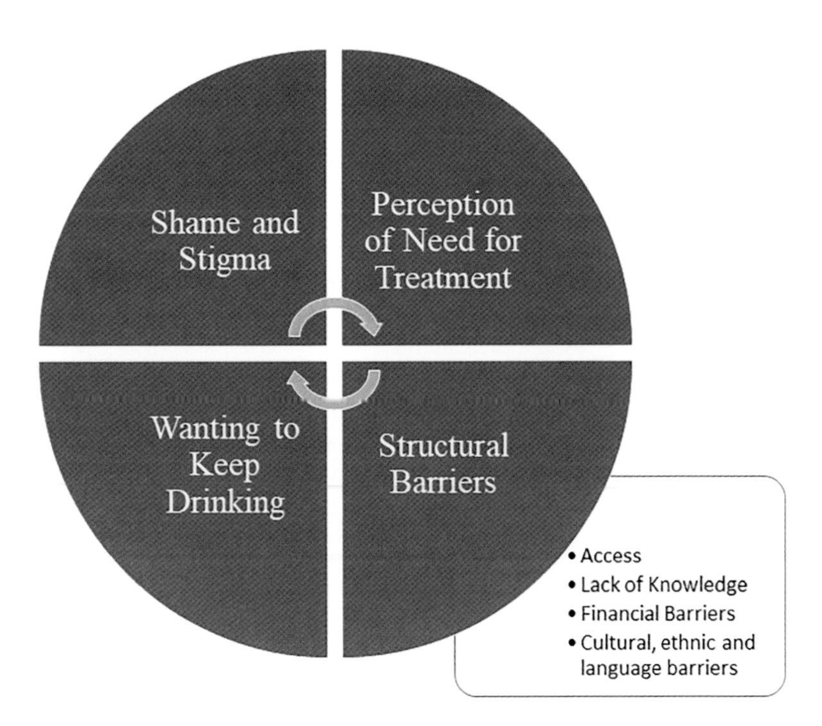

Fig. 3 Common barriers to treatment of alcohol dependence
Adapted from Barriers to Treatment for Alcohol Dependence in the *Journal of Drug and Alcohol Research by* May et al. (2019)

A Tale of Two Drinkers

The distribution of alcohol consumption is preposterously skewed in the United States. The top 10% of drinkers in the United States drink over half of the alcohol consumed per year, while those in the next 60% drink less than one drink per week. The lower 30% consume none at all (Cook 2007). Which group of drinkers would alcohol producers and distributors prefer to be impacted?

The Economics of Alcohol Consumption Deterrence

Most historic alcohol harm minimization policies focus one of two models: total consumption and full-cost models. Both affect the entire population. The total consumption model, supported by Lederman's single distribution theory, proposes that alcohol usage by quantity per capita follows a log-normal curve (Schaffer and Lederman 1965). Therefore, by reducing the average amount of alcohol consumed per capita, binge drinking, heavy alcohol use, and its sequelae would be reduced as well. Several policies have been implemented based on this proposition and have seen variable success - e.g., minimum price requirements (O'Donnell et al. 2019) and increased taxation (Elder et al. 2010; Gehrsitz et al. 2020), advertising restrictions (Anderson et al. 2009), government alcohol monopolies (Nelson 1990), and prohibition (Blocker Jr 2006).

The full-cost model of alcohol consumption uses a different approach (Gruenewald 2011). The full cost of alcohol is defined as convenience of purchase plus monetary cost. Therefore, by reducing availability, or convenience, through tactics such as employing a paternalistic minimum age requirement, restricting places and times of sale, or raising prices through various policies mentioned above, the overall use of alcohol should decrease.

What each of these models fail to consider is the individual nature of alcohol addiction and the context of alcohol use and its by-products (i.e., domestic violence, impaired driving, property damage, etc.). There is no use of the difference with this approach between recreational and addictive use.

With alcohol now more accessible than ever, alcohol policy needs to improve. The advent of new and emerging technologies allows for exciting opportunities in the realm of harm minimization. Careful consideration of the moral implications of harm minimization techniques, such as restriction of liberties, should be reviewed carefully as to not slide into authoritarianism under the guise of utilitarianism.

The Harm Principle

Justifying the restriction of liberties, such as drinking alcohol, is not an easy task. John Stuart Mill approached a framework for moralistic, as opposed to paternalistic, restriction of liberties in his philosophical essay *On Liberty* (Mill 1869; Brink 2018). He proposed that, in the spirit of harm reduction, restriction of personal liberties is justifiable if it will prevent someone from acting immorally or prevent someone from risking non-consensual harm to someone else. The dilemma of implementation is defining genuine harm versus simple offense. Mill described harm as an action capable of causing injury or one which poses a threat to protected liberties. Mill described three basic liberties in this work that should be protected including freedom of thought and emotion, freedom to pursue tastes, and freedom to unite.

For the sake of simplification, let's take the case of alcohol. If a person were to drink too much and make gaudy disrespectful jokes, this may be merely offensive which Mill may argue you have the right to offend and be offended (although there could be a case to be made for psychological harm). If this same person were to then assault a non-consenting person physically or get behind the wheel and drive away while impaired, Mill may support a case for government intervention.

A Model for Improvement: Australia's Banned Drinkers Registrar

The Banned Drinkers Registrar (BDR) is an alcohol supply reduction measure first implemented in 2011 in the Northern Territory of Australia. The aim of the measure was to reduce the harm associated with binge and heavy alcohol use though the implementation of a registry, or official list, of banned drinkers. Those placed on the BDR would be banned from purchase, possession, or consumption of alcohol for the duration of their "Banned Drinker Order" (BDO).

A BDO can be obtained through police referral, court order, other qualified personnel such as social works or child protection workers, or self-application. A BDO can be issued for any of the following concerns:

- Apprehension by police for alcohol-related offences
- Three alcohol-related protective custodies or alcohol infringement notices in 2 years
- Alcohol-related domestic violence
- Court order
- Referral by authorized personnel such as a doctor, nurse, family member, or child protection worker
- Self-referral

Once served a BDO, a duration of 3, 6, or 12 months is assigned. The duration is dependent on offence or self-preference and can be extended at any time for violation of the order. At the time of sale, individuals are verified against the list and if identified as having a BDO are prevented from sale (Smith 2018).

At the recent 24-month evaluation, outcomes appear favorable. Noticeable reductions in contact with the justice system (down-trending since inception), improved health outcomes (as evidenced by increased admission to sobering up shelters, self-referrals, and admission to rehab facilities), and reduced harm for problem drinkers (including reduction in violence surrounding take-away outlets) are evident (Ernst and Young Oceania Evaluation Practice Network 2020).

A Proposal for an Alcohol Purchase License

Licensing for public health safety is not a new idea. Mandatory licensing for motor vehicle drivers in the United Kingdom can be traced back to as early as 1903 (Northcliffe 1906). Features of this license included a minimum age limit, stipulations for suspension in the setting of provable or potential harm (i.e., speeding or dangerous driving), and regulations regarding motor car use. Licensing is now commonplace in many aspects of society and is used to prove qualifications through appropriate regulatory services for a variety of recreations (i.e., hunting, fishing, and motor vehicle operation) and occupations (i.e., medical, legal, cosmetology, and construction). The implementation of an alcohol purchase license could provide an opportunity for alcohol education and awareness, rehabilitation services, and individualized repercussions for alcohol-related harm which is a unique feature of this proposal.

If this same concept for alcohol were to be implemented, the basis would be similar to that of driving and guns. Most users are safe and responsible. We don't want to impinge on responsible alcohol users any more than on responsible drivers or responsible gun users. We need to target those whose drinking is dangerous.

The license concept is related to the nature of alcohol addiction. The addicted person urgently wants the drug even as they know it is harming them. At times, the person with alcohol addiction is hospitalized for complications of drinking – withdrawal seizures, delirium tremens, alcoholic pancreatitis, hepatitis, myopathy, neuropathy, cognitive impairment, cerebellar degeneration, and car crashes – and buys alcohol on the way home. The nature of progression is that the worse the complications, the more ferocious the denial. As people get sicker from alcoholism, their prognosis worsens. The return to drinking becomes more certain.

Often the harms from alcoholism are experienced in the social surround. Partners are abused in drunken rages. Children are mistreated and neglected. Pedestrians and motorists are injured and killed by drunk drivers. Crimes are committed while intoxicated.

General consumption of alcohol is not a concern. The individual and social costs of alcoholism are. The license concept honors autonomy but proscribes hostile and dangerous intoxicated behaviors.

Application of an Alcohol Purchase License

The first step to establish a licensing system is to identify a regulating agency. In the case of the alcohol purchase license in the United States, County Health Departments would be most appropriate as certain aspects of licensing will require legal intervention and would be an unnecessary burden for the state or federal court system. A system such as this would require a central database to be created and maintained.

The next step is establishing a reliable and accessible form of identification (ID). For the sake of convenience and lack of redundancy, IDs could be linked to already existing state-issued ID cards. For example, in New York State, any resident of any age can receive a non-driver's ID, and any resident above the age of 16 can apply for a

New York driver license if desired. At the age of 21, the legal minimum drinking age in the United States, individuals could apply for alcohol purchase licensure. The New York State license is already used by other agencies for licensing, credentialing, and designations, for example, hunting and fishing, passports, boating, and organ donor status. After issuance and at the time of sale, an active alcohol license would need to be verified. To encourage compliance, an easily accessible scanner, via phone applications or state-provided device, could offer an efficient confirmation or denial process.

Features of an Alcohol Purchase License

At the time of issuance, a "drinkers" safety course could be required and offer important information for new alcohol users regarding the short-term and long-term effects of alcohol use, local and state alcohol laws and regulations, alcohol addiction, and information regarding resources for rehabilitation. In a sense, the APL is the inverse of the BDR. All interested individuals would start on the database and be removed as deemed necessary after qualifiable offenses.

In practice, all distributors of alcohol would be required to scan the patrons ID at the time of sale. Current law in New York State does not require mandatory identification at the time of sale; however, it is highly encouraged as the burden of selling to minors, a misdemeanor, falls on the seller. For this reason, it is common practice for most establishments to blanket ID all customers. This means liquor stores, grocery stores, and bars and restaurants would have to scan the ID to see if the customer is eligible to buy.

A key feature of the alcohol purchase license is not its distribution but rather its ability to make privilege tangible and the opportunity for revocation explicit. In other words, if one is a bad driver, one can lose their driver's license. If one is a bad drunk, one can lose their alcohol purchase license. In the setting of immoral behavior or harm to self or others, through a legal process, the alcohol purchase license could be revoked. The dilemma becomes, what constitutes immoral behavior or harm to self or others?

Example criteria for loss of alcohol purchase license:

- Hospital visits for alcohol-related illnesses that indicate that alcohol use cannot be resumed safely: withdrawal seizures, delirium tremens, severe alcohol-related disease such as cirrhosis, alcoholic pancreatitis, alcoholic myopathy, and severe alcohol-related cognitive disorder. Physicians would be mandated reporters to the Banned Drinkers Register.
- Two convictions for driving while intoxicated.
- Alcohol-related family or domestic partner abuse.
- Alcohol-related felony conviction.
- Self-referral.

The process for revocation would require legal or medical involvement. In the setting of driving while intoxicated, domestic violence, and felonies, a qualified officer of the law or legal professional could testify for license suspension at the time of initial court hearing. In the case of medical indications, such as a hospitalization for alcohol-

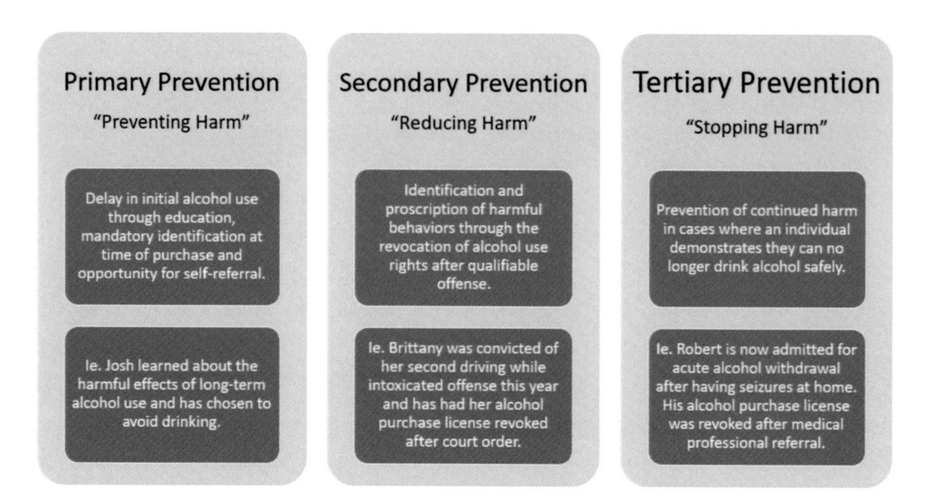

Fig. 4 The interception between prevention and harm reduction in the implementation of an alcohol purchase license with accompanying theoretical examples

related disease that demonstrates the person cannot safely consume alcohol, a referral would be made to the court system for revocation. Physicians and medical facilities would be "mandated reporters," similar to the process for observed child abuse where if one sees hostile, dangerous behavior, it must be reported to a social service agency.

Following revocation of the alcohol purchase license, appropriate information and medical referral could be made for treatment initiation. Refining strict harm-based criteria will allow for targeted harm reduction for those most affected by the alcohol use, the perpetrator and those around them.

In the setting of self-referral, an individual may desire, for any reason, to have their APL revoked. The most common reason would be that an individual decides that they have alcoholism and that they would like to stop drinking. In the setting of addiction, this offers an amazing opportunity to keep recovery honest and promotes accountability. Revocation of APL voluntarily could be reversed without adjudication at the discretion of the individual.

In summary, the implementation of an alcohol purchase license system provides opportunities for primary, secondary, and tertiary prevention of alcohol use and its sequelae (Fig. 4).

Duration and Adjudication

At baseline, the duration of APL revocation would remain 5 years. While it is understood alcohol use disorder is a chronic relapsing disorder, a period of this duration should allow enough time to explore treatment options if desired and reestablish healthy habits. At the end of this period, the individual would be free to reapply for license renewal after appropriate drinker's safety remediation and formal social work evaluation to assess for resolution of harm-inciting behaviors.

In the case of chronic and terminal medical conditions such as decompensated liver cirrhosis and alcohol-related neurocognitive decline, that day may never come. In the event an individual would like to challenge initial APL revocation, they may appear before a judge for hearing regarding their dispute.

How to Implement

Implementation starts through community education, engagement, and organization. Buy-in from strong organizations with similar missions such as Mothers Against Drunk Driving and Alcoholics Anonymous would be key to the success program funding, creation, and implementation.

Potential Pitfalls of an Alcohol Purchase License

The alcohol purchase license will not end alcoholism. It is a concept that falls under harm reduction. It puts a speed bump on the road to relapse. Instead of buying a quart of vodka after hospital discharge for withdrawal seizures, because the alcohol purchase license has been revoked, finding someone else to buy is required, or one has to travel to another state where one can buy without a state license. This means that liabilities include drunk driving back from the other state. Additionally, straw purchases, or illegal alcohol purchase on behalf of another, homebrew, and adherence to strict identification guidelines are loopholes that could be exploited and should be addressed separately through legal involvement and/or heavy fines for offending individuals.

Additional Considerations

There are several elements of a program such as the APL that should be carefully monitored. First, quantity and frequency of alcohol purchase should not be monitored with this system; while a key component of this proposal is harm reduction, it cannot be reliably estimated based on quantity or frequency alone especially in the setting of no appreciable harm. Second, the APL database should not be linked to medical records in order to protect patient privacy. Lastly, the APL database should be stored in an encrypted, Health Insurance Portability and Accountability Act of 1996-compliant database for the sake of confidentiality and should be secured with distributive database technology such as blockchain to mitigate risk for tampering.

Applications to Other Areas of Addiction

The alcohol purchase license, as described, would be of help to other areas of addiction. Alcohol addiction is frequently comorbid with other drug addictions. Removing the harm from alcohol may reduce deaths from other addictive drugs such as alcohol/benzodiazepine overdoses or alcohol/opioid overdoses. Identifying alcohol addiction and facilitating treatment at a specialty service may allow all addictions present to be addressed.

Applications to Other Areas of Public Health

There are many prime examples of harm minimalization through licensing as discussed in the main text (driver's license, gun license, hunting and fishing permits). Not all harm reduction should be approached though means of credentialing or licenses. Unique to alcohol use in the United States is its ubiquitous use and delayed minimum purchase age (21). With new legal drinkers entering the alcohol economic sphere each year, a golden opportunity for primary prevention through means of education is presented. Drinking, as with driving and gun ownership, is a privilege; when abused, they can incite serious and sometimes fatal harm to users and those around them. In an age of emerging technology, new approaches to harm reduction should be explored and employed.

Mini-dictionary of Terms

- **Gordian knot.** A metaphor originating from the life of Alexander the Great. It is meant reflect a problem of impossible difficulty that is solved easily by bold and decisive action.
- **Health Insurance Portability and Accountability Act of 1996.** A US statute created to ensure the confidentiality, integrity, and security of health information in the modern age of electronic health records.
- **John Stuart Mill.** A nineteenth-century English philosopher, economist, and politician.
- **Sisyphean task.** A metaphor based in Greek mythology meant to represent a laborious and futile task.
- **Ventral tegmental dopaminergic seeking system.** Also known as the mesolimbic dopamine pathway, it provokes exploratory behaviors. It is a contributor to the experience of "cravings" and the promotion of drug seeking behavior in alcoholism. It is also the pathway for drinking dreams that show seeking alcohol even when asleep.

Key Facts About Alcohol Use

- Most alcohol use is recreational; this means that there is no harm from use.
- Ten percent of alcohol users drink half of the alcohol.
- Alcoholism or addiction to alcohol is most parsimoniously defined as "repeated harm from use" and affects all aspects of society including social, occupational, legal, and medical.

- Recreational use hurts no one. Alcoholism not only hurts the person who drinks but is hostile toward those in the social environment. The family of the person with alcoholism suffers daily. Persons with alcoholism miss work or work while drinking. The legal system is impacted via arrests for drunken behavior. These behaviors are both symptoms of a disease and at the same time crimes. As the condition progresses, medical complications ensue in the context of ever-denser denial complicated by cognitive impairment.
- At an extreme, one is hopelessly addicted when cognitive impairment makes using interpersonal interventions impossible. The person with alcoholism then drinks themselves to death unless they become so impaired that they can no longer obtain the drug.

Summary Points

- Alcohol presents significant harm to self and others and was evaluated to be the most harmful drug in the world.
- Harm related to alcohol use is financially costly, ~ $249 billion per year in the United States, and at the same time costly to persons with alcoholism, ~ 3.3 million deaths per year around the globe.
- Screening for and treatment of alcohol use disorder are often overlooked and incomplete.
- Harm reduction strategies have been attempted with variable success, but all employ similar strategies which tend to punish those who use responsibly.
- New technologic advances allow for new techniques and an exciting opportunity to individualize harm reduction for those who need it most. This is the concept of the alcohol purchase license.

References

American Beverage Licensees (2018) America's beer, wine & spirits retailers create 2.03 Million Jobs & $122.63 Billion in direct economic impact, 2018 economic impact study of America's beer, wine & spirits retailers. Available at: https://ablusa.org/americas-beer-wine-spirits-retailers-create-2-03-million-jobs-122-63-billion-in-direct-economic-impact/ Accessed 6 Jan 2021.

Anderson P et al (2009) Impact of alcohol advertising and media exposure on adolescent alcohol use: a systematic review of longitudinal studies. Alcohol Alcohol 44(3):229–243. https://doi.org/10.1093/alcalc/agn115

Baker TB et al (2012) DSM criteria for tobacco use disorder and tobacco withdrawal: a critique and proposed revisions for DSM-5. Addiction 107(2):263–275. https://doi.org/10.1111/j.1360-0443.2011.03657.x

Blocker JS Jr (2006) Did prohibition really work? Alcohol prohibition as a public health innovation. Am J Public Health 96(2):233–243. https://doi.org/10.2105/AJPH.2005.065409

Brink DO (2018) Partial responsibility and excuse in moral puzzles and legal perplexities, ed. H. Hurd (New York: Cambridge University Press).

Cook PJ (2007) Paying the tab. Princeton University Press. Available at: http://www.jstor.org/stable/j.ctt7shzt

Elder RW et al (2010) The effectiveness of tax policy interventions for reducing excessive alcohol consumption and related harms. Am J Prev Med 38(2):217–229. https://doi.org/10.1016/j.amepre.2009.11.005

Ernst & Young Oceania Evaluation Practice Network (2020) Medium term outcomes evaluation of the banned drinker register. Available at: https://digitallibrary.health.nt.gov.au/prodjspui/handle/10137/8556.

Esser MB et al (2014) Prevalence of alcohol dependence among US adult drinkers, 2009–2011. Prev Chronic Dis 11:140329. https://doi.org/10.5888/pcd11.140329

Florence CS et al (2016) The economic burden of prescription opioid overdose, abuse, and dependence in the United States, 2013. Med Care 54(10):901–906. https://doi.org/10.1097/MLR.0000000000000625

Gehrsitz M, Saffer H, Grossman M (2020) 'IZA DP No. 13198: The effect of changes in alcohol tax differentials on alcohol consumption'. IZA Institute of Labor and Economics. Available at: http://ftp.iza.org/dp13198.pdf.

Glass JE, Bohnert KM, Brown RL (2016) Alcohol screening and intervention among United States adults who attend ambulatory healthcare. *J Gen Intern Med* 31(7):739–745. https://doi.org/10.1007/s11606-016-3614-5

Grant BF et al (2015) Epidemiology of DSM-5 alcohol use disorder: results from the national epidemiologic survey on alcohol and related conditions III. *JAMA psychiatry* 72(8):757–766. https://doi.org/10.1001/jamapsychiatry.2015.0584

Greenfeld LA, Henneberg MA (2001) Victim and offender self-reports of alcohol involvement in crime. Alcohol Res Health : J National Institute Alcohol Abuse Alcoholism 25(1):20–31. Available at: https://pubmed.ncbi.nlm.nih.gov/11496963

Gruenewald PJ (2011) Regulating availability: how access to alcohol affects drinking and problems in youth and adults. Alcohol Res Health : J National Institute Alcohol Abuse Alcoholism 34(2): 248–256. SPS-AR&H-39

Johnson B (2013) Addiction and will. Front Hum Neurosci. Frontiers Media S.A. 7:545. https://doi.org/10.3389/fnhum.2013.00545

May C, Nielsen AS, Bilberg R (2019) Barriers to treatment for alcohol dependence. J Drug Alcohol Res 8(2). https://doi.org/10.4303/jdar/236083

Mayshak R et al (2020) Alcohol-involved family and domestic violence reported to police in Australia. J Interpers Violence United States:886260520928633. https://doi.org/10.1177/0886260520928633

Mill JS (1869) On liberty. 4th ed. London: Longman, Roberts & Green. www.bartleby.com/130/

National Drug Intelligence Center (2011) National drug threat assessment 2011. National Drug Intelligence Center, pp 1–72. https://doi.org/10.1037/e618352012-001

National Highway Traffic Safety Administration (2017) Traffic safety facts 2016 data: alcohol-impaired driving, Washington, DC. Available at: https://crashstats.nhtsa.dot.gov/Api/Public/ViewPublication/812450

Nelson JP (1990) State monopolies and alcoholic beverage consumption. J Regul Econ 2(1):83–98. https://doi.org/10.1007/BF00139364

Northcliffe AH (1906) Motors and motor-driving, 4th edn. Longmans, Green, and Company (Badminton Library), London. Available at: https://books.google.com/books?id=xKsEAAAAMAAJ

Nutt DJ et al (2010) Drug harms in the UK: a multicriteria decision analysis. Lancet (London, England). Elsevier 376(9752):1558–1565. https://doi.org/10.1016/S0140-6736(10)61462-6

O'Donnell A et al (2019) Immediate impact of minimum unit pricing on alcohol purchases in Scotland: controlled interrupted time series analysis for 2015–18. *BMJ* 366:l5274. https://doi.org/10.1136/bmj.l5274

Parks SE et al. (2014) 'Surveillance for violent deaths – National Violent Death Reporting System, 16 states, 2010.' Morbidity and mortality weekly report. Surveillance summaries (Washington, D.C.: 2002). United States, 63(1), pp. 1–33.

Rehm J, Shield KD (2013) Global alcohol-attributable deaths from cancer, liver cirrhosis, and injury in 2010. Alcohol Res : Curr Rev. National Institute Alcohol Abuse Alcoholism 35(2):174–183. Available at: https://pubmed.ncbi.nlm.nih.gov/24881325

Sacks JJ et al (2015) 2010 National and state costs of excessive alcohol consumption. Am J Prev Med. Elsevier 49(5):e73–e79. https://doi.org/10.1016/j.amepre.2015.05.031

SAHMSA (2019) 'The national survey on drug use and health : 2019 National Survey on Drug Use and Health (NSDUH)', SAMHSA – Substance Abuse and Mental Health Services Administration, (September).

Schaffer HE, Lederman S (1965) Alcool Alcoolisme Alcoolisation. Biometrics 21(4):1018. https://doi.org/10.2307/2528268

Shield KD, Parry C, Rehm J (2013) Chronic diseases and conditions related to alcohol use. Alcohol Res: Curr Rev 35(2):155–173

Smith J (2018) Twelve-month evaluation of the banned drinker register in the northern territory: Part 1 – descriptive analysis of administrative data. Menzies School of Health Research, Darwin

U.S. Department of Health and Human Services (2014) National center for chronic disease prevention and health promotion (US) office on smoking and health. The health consequences of smoking—50 years of progress: a report of the surgeon general., Atlanta (GA): Centers for Disease Control and Prevention (US). Available at: https://www.ncbi.nlm.nih.gov/books/NBK179276/.

World Health Organization (2014) Global Status Report on Alcohol and Health, 2014. Available at: https://books.google.com/books?id=HbQXDAAAQBAJ&pg=PA48&lpg=PA48&dq=In+2012,+about+3.3+million+net+deaths,+or+5.9%25+of+all+global+deaths,+were+attributable+to+alcohol+consumption&source=bl&ots=PcpyEcO_sF&sig=ACfU3U1x7kRMVY0BbSlTBtBT_ZoQrsqDwg&hl=en&sa=X&v.

Xu X et al (2015) Annual healthcare spending attributable to cigarette smoking: an update. *Am J Prev Med* 48(3):326–333. https://doi.org/10.1016/j.amepre.2014.10.012

Google, Public Health, and Alcohol and Drug Policy

51

Abhishek Ghosh, Shinjini Choudhury, and Venkata Lakshmi Narasimha

Contents

Introduction 1079
  Introduction to Various Google Tools 1079
Analysis of Google Trends (GT) Dataset 1080
How Do These Google Trends-Based Data Differ from Traditional Methods of Data Collection? 1081
Use of Google Data in Health Research 1083
Google Trends in Substance Misuse Research 1084
  Alcohol 1084
  New Psychoactive Substances (NPS) and Other Drugs 1085
  Tobacco and Other Nicotine Delivery Systems 1088
Use of Google News in Substance Use Research 1095
Substance Misuse Research Using Other Google Applications 1095
Public Health Implications 1102
Critique of Google Trends and Other Google Tool-Based Research 1103
Conclusion 1104
Key Facts 1104
Mini-Dictionary of Terms 1105
Summary Points 1106
References 1107

A. Ghosh (✉)
Department of Psychiatry & Drug De-addiction and Treatment Centre, Postgraduate Institute of Medical Education and Research, Chandigarh, India

S. Choudhury
Department of Psychiatry, All India Institute of Medical Sciences, Rishikesh, India

V. L. Narasimha
Department of Psychiatry, All India Institute of Medical Sciences (AIIMS), Panchayat Training Institute, Daburgram Jasidih, Deoghar, Jharkhand, India

V. B. Patel, V. R. Preedy (eds.), *Handbook of Substance Misuse and Addictions*,
https://doi.org/10.1007/978-3-030-92392-1_58

Abstract

Ubiquitous use, systematic organization, availability, and access to data have made it possible to utilize the various Google products for public health purposes. Google Trends (GT) is the most commonly utilized tool; Google Earth and News are two other potential candidates. Researchers have used GT to track and forecast infectious diseases, especially influenza-like illness. The use of GT in substance misuse research is a relatively novel phenomenon. Google tool-based research in substance misuse is primarily focused on (a) visualization of trends of use of alcohol, drugs, new psychoactive substance, and electronic nicotine delivery systems and (b) correlation of GT dataset with the existing national or regional data, to show the reliability of GT to measure the use, availability, and consequences of substance misuse. Preliminary research indicates a potential for GT-based forecasting and surveillance for drug and alcohol use. Lack of standardized methods of data capture and analysis, limited research from non-English-speaking countries, and from countries and territories with restricted internet access are a few of the many caveats in any Google tool-based analysis. Future research should address these limitations.

Keywords

Alcohol · Tobacco · Opioids · Electronic nicotine delivery systems (ENDS) · New psychoactive substances (NPS) · Google Trends · Public health · Relative search volume (RSV) · Google News · Google Earth · Google Maps

Abbreviations

API	Application programming interface
ENDS	Electronic nicotine delivery systems
EVALI	E-cigarette or vaping product use-associated lung injury
GE	Google Earth
GETH	Google extended trends API for health
GFT	Google Flu Trends
GIS	Geographic information system
GT	Google Trends
HNB	Heat-not-burn
ILI	Influenza-like illness
ITU	International Telecommunication Union
LLC	Limited liability corporation
LOWESS	Locally weighted scatterplot smoothing
MDMA	3,4-Methylenedioxymethamphetamine
NPS	New psychoactive substances
NRT	Nicotine replacement therapy
RSV	Relative search volume

UK	United Kingdom
UN	United Nations
USA	United States of America
WTS	Waterpipe tobacco smoking

Introduction

Google is a US-based multinational technology company and it is one of the five Big Tech companies in the globe. The primary purpose of Google LLC is to provide internet-based services and products; among these services, the single most popular service is possibly the Google Search engine. The Google Search engine has several components, such as videos, news, shops, maps, images, finances, and others. One can search all these options at one go or search for a specific option. It is also possible to restrict the search to definite time points, languages, and to search verbatim. According to StatCounter, worldwide (https://gs.statcounter.com/search-engine-market-share), Google has the largest market share (92%) of the existing search engines. The market share increases to 95% for searching through mobile devices. The Google search engine usage is more than 90% for all continents. Google LLC's motto reads "Our mission is to organize the world's information and make it universally accessible and useful" (https://about.google/). Ubiquitous use, systematic organization, availability, and access to data have made it possible to utilize the various Google products for public health purposes.

Introduction to Various Google Tools

Google Trends (GT) is an online tool developed by Google. Inc. It helps visualize and discover trends in people's search behavior within Google Search, Google News, Google Images, Google Shopping, and YouTube. GT datasets are anonymized (no one is personally identified), categorized (determining the topic for a search query), and aggregated (grouped together). One can enter a search topic or query to examine the distribution of the search volume of that particular term over a period of time (trends) and within a geographic region. There are several options of customizing the search according to the country of origin (of searches), time range (of performing such searches), categories, and type of searches. The results are displayed as "interest over time" (time-series data) and "interest over subregion" (spatial distribution). The dataset can be downloaded as .csv files for analysis. The unit of analysis is the search volume. GT does not give away an absolute search volume of a user-specified search term but provides a relative search volume (RSV): that is the query share of a user-specified search term, normalized by the highest query share of that term over the time series, for a specific location and period (Choi and Varian 2012). Estimation of RSV is a two-stage process. The first stage estimates the relative popularity, i.e., the ratio of a query's search volume to the sum of the search volumes of all possible queries of the geography and time range. In the second stage, the resulting numbers are scaled on a range of 0–100 based on a topic's proportion to all searches. To illustrate this further the Google Trends website mentions "*A value of 100 is the peak popularity for the term. A value of 50 means that the term is half as popular. A score of 0 means there was not enough data for this term.*" (Google Trends n.d.). The first stage ensures the popularity of the search term should be independent of internet traffic. Moreover, this also eliminates repeated searches by the same person over a short period of time, and it shows only data for popular terms. These prevent spurious inflation of search volume by a single user and ensure the user-specified search terms are searched enough to generate a time-series trend (Ghosh et al. 2021a). Besides, GT gives a list of related topics and queries. These can be either arranged as a list of "top" topics/queries, i.e., the most commonly searched terms, or categorized as the list of "rising" topics/queries, i.e., those terms that have seen the highest increase in recent times (also known as *Breakout*). GT also gives an option of comparing five search queries (or topics) together. GT has a few excellent brief training modules for data visualization and usage, improving search results, and understanding the trends data (Google News Initiative Training Center n.d.). We would like to implore the interested readers to take these lessons before undertaking research on Google Trends. In the end, it should be noted that GT is a potential marker of population-level interest and behavior but does not always reflect actual intent (of search) and behavior.

The images from the Google Earth™ (GE) database are a usable alternative for providing a snapshot of the spatial pattern of a territory. The images displayed by the software come from both satellite and aerial photography. The repeatability update ranges between 6 months and 5 years. Google Earth Pro is free for users with advanced features. One can import and export Geographic Information System (GIS) data and retrieve historical imagery. However, GE has a low spatial data processing capability and no spatial analysis and modeling capability (Lozano-Fuentes et al. 2008).

Analysis of Google Trends (GT) Dataset

Broadly the GT output can be analyzed as a time series or a cross-sectional comparison of various geographical locations at a single point in time. The authors have utilized the GT dataset for (a) visualization: simple visualization of the trends as a screenshot from the website or visualization of smoothed graphs; the change of trends can either be seen and inferred by bare-eyes or authors could perform a change-point analysis to examine the statistical significance of such visual trends, (b) correlations: Correlations may be between Google Trends data and official data, among Google Trends time series, or between Google Trends and other Web-based sources' time series, (c) forecasting: forecasting of either Google Trends time series or diseases, outbreaks, etc., using GT data, independent of the method used, (d) modeling: performed some form of modeling using GT data (Mavragani et al. 2018). GT researchers have performed the following statistical analysis to accomplish the afore-mentioned objectives: simple and cross-correlation, continuous density hidden Markov models, locally weighted scatterplot

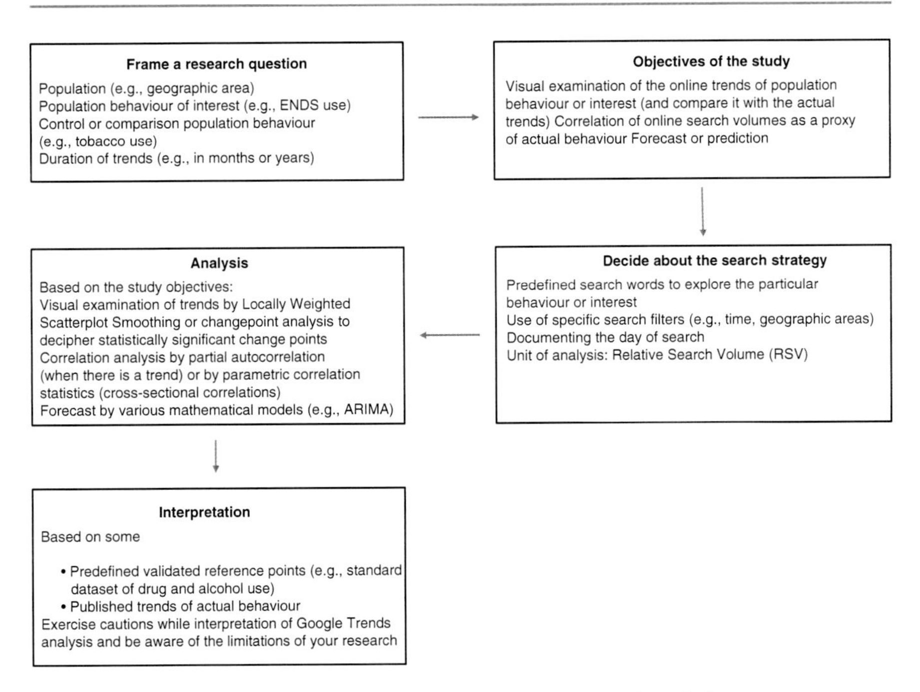

Fig. 1 Flow chart depicting the steps in performing a Google Trends analysis

smoothing, change-point analysis, Box–Jenkins transfer function models, t tests and Mann–Whitney tests, analysis of variance, autocorrelation, multivariable linear regression, time series analyses, wavelet power spectrum analysis, and Cosinor analysis (Nuti et al. 2014; Ghosh et al. 2021a, b, c). GT also provides Application Programming Interface (API), which enables researchers to use statistical models on the output data. However, this is limited to only Google Extended Trends API for Health (GETH) (the newer avatar of the Google Flu Trends API). Google also supplies some elementary Python code samples for accessing the API (Raubenheimer 2021) (Fig. 1).

How Do These Google Trends-Based Data Differ from Traditional Methods of Data Collection?

Google Trends (GT) dataset, which gives outputs for specific search queries, is a marker of population-level interest; however, it neither directly identifies the intent of the searcher nor indicates population behavior. The data is anonymized; hence, it is not possible to assess the social and demographic characteristics of the searchers. Because of the absence of individual-level sampling, no definite sampling frame, and sampling procedure, it is difficult to replicate GT-based results. The analysis of GT output is still evolving and researchers are not yet sure about the best method of analysis or the best model to understand GT dataset (Mavragani et al. 2018). In sum, GT analysis can give signals for change, forecast an epidemic with some degree of accuracy, and can be correlated with the existing official datasets but it cannot

Table 1 Differences between Google Trends-based studies and Standard observational studies

	Google Trends-based data and its analysis	Epidemiological data in observational studies and its analysis
Description	Google trends-based data is obtained based on the online activity on Google search engine	Epidemiological data includes the data collected from a source using a particular method for observational study
Type of studies done using the data	Google Trends analysis	Descriptive studies, case control, cohort studies which explain the relationship between exposure and risk
Setting	A particular region of interest, duration, category, and platform can be selected for inclusion into the study	Setting, locations, and relevant dates, including periods of recruitment, exposure, follow-up, and data collection are described in the study
Variables	In Google Trends analysis only five variables or words of interest can be compared or evaluated and their corresponding relative search volume can be obtained for the study	Multiple variables leading to exposure and its outcomes can be assessed
Data sources/ measurement	Online data provided by Google open-source platform. The data is relative data, absolute numbers are not available	For each variable of interest, required data is obtained from the study populations. Generally, absolute data is obtained
Bias	Bias is generally at the level of selection	Bias includes the selection bias, information bias, and confounding
Study size	Study size includes whole of the population selected	Sample size calculation must be done to achieve adequate power of the study
Statistical analysis	Visualization of trends, time series analysis, correlation, regression can be done using the data and based on available collateral data	Frequency (incidence, mortality) measures, effect measures (relative risk, odds-ratio), regression models, survival analysis
Participants	No direct participants	Participants are selected based on the eligibility of selection and risk of lost to follow-up present
Descriptive data	The relative search volume of the variable of interest is described	Characteristics of study participants (e.g., demographic, clinical, social) and information on exposures and potential confounders. Number of participants with missing data for each variable of interest and the follow-up time (e.g., average and total amount)
Outcome	Changes in RSV with time help in forecasting future events using time series analysis. Association with other RSV and collateral data can be obtained by correlation and regression	Outcomes following the exposure to risk factor of interest are expressed as odds-ratio, relative risk, absolute risk, mortality rate

(continued)

Table 1 (continued)

	Google Trends-based data and its analysis	Epidemiological data in observational studies and its analysis
Other analysis	A range of analysis can be done based on the collateral data/ epidemiological data	Analyses of subgroups and interactions and sensitivity analyses
Limitation	It cannot be a true reflection of the study population, but it gives a proxy indication	Depends on the type of study and the study characteristics
Generalizability of findings	These findings are limited for the search criterion. External validity is significantly low	Has better external validity compared to the google trends and variables under the study
Ethical considerations/ approvals	Not required	Required
Funding	No funding required for the study; it is an open-source platform	Involves funding to conduct these studies

replace traditional methods of data collection. It can only supplement the official data collection by ongoing, real-time (or lag time) monitoring of population-level interest or search behavior. In Table 1 we have enumerated the methodological differences between observational epidemiological studies and research based on Google applications (Table 1).

Use of Google Data in Health Research

Health researchers have worked on several Google products such as Google Trends, News, Maps, Earth, and Street View. However, the use of Google Trends (GT) surpasses others. The most popular and widely studied disease by GT was the influenza-like illness (ILI) (Polgreen et al. 2008; Ginsberg et al. 2009). Most of the other diseases studied by GT are also infectious diseases like gastroenteritis, chickenpox, and others (Pelat et al. 2009; Valdivia and Monge-Corella 2010). Here, researchers have used the GT data for real-time surveillance and to predict disease outbreaks about 7–10 days prior to the conventional Center for Disease Control surveillance system (Carneiro and Mylonakis 2009). The promise of a timely, robust, and sensitive surveillance system encouraged public health researchers to complement the usual data capture strategies with the data generated from GT and other online sources. Google Flu Trends was launched in 2008 (discontinued its service since 2015) with the objectives of estimation of ILI in specific geographic areas and continuous surveillance for an impending epidemic. Over the next few years, GT-based research spread to many different areas. Nuti and coauthors (2014) systematically reviewed GT-based health research published between 2009 and 2013 (Nuti et al. 2014). They identified seventy articles and classified those into four major categories according to the focus on the health condition: infectious diseases, non-communicable diseases, mental health, and substance use, and population behavior. The main purpose of researching GT data has also extended from surveillance to examining causal inference between a widely publicized event and consequent population behavior and descriptive studies such as examining the change of population interest over a period of time (Stein et al. 2013; Ayers et al. 2014). In addition to Google Trends, Google Maps or Google Earth has also been utilized in health research. Google Earth can create a Geographic Information System (GIS) of healthcare facilities, which could aid in healthcare planning at the community level (Richards et al. 1999; Weiss et al. 2020). GIS can also help to investigate the social determinants of health and disease (Lefer et al. 2008). In the subsequent sections of this chapter, the role of Google informatics in substance misuse research will be reviewed.

Google Trends in Substance Misuse Research

Alcohol

While most research using GT analysis was related to illicit substances, the ongoing pandemic led to an increased interest in alcohol. In India, during the lockdown in March 2020, changes in alcohol-related search pre- and post-prohibition were measured using GT (Ghosh et al. 2021c). A significant increase in alcohol-related online search following prohibition was noted. Similarly, another Indian study evaluated changes in alcohol-related searches during lockdown along with three different timelines (pre-lockdown, lockdown 1.0, and lockdown 2.0). Relative search volume (RSV) related to the procurement of alcohol and alcohol withdrawal increased during lockdown 1.0, and RSV related to benzodiazepines increased during lockdown 2.0 (Singh et al. 2020). These two studies underscore the importance of Google data in understanding the sudden policy changes related to alcohol. Another study in the context of the ban on tobacco and alcohol used GT to understand the help-seeking pattern in India. The authors did not find any significant change in the help-seeking patterns during the period of ban on sales (Uvais 2020).

The pandemic also resulted in an association between the (GT) terms related to health, porn, alcohol, economy, news. Such an association was absent before the pandemic. Initially, there was an increase in unemployment-related search with a decrease in health-related search. Later, there was an increase in health-related search, news, alcohol, and porn, along with unemployment. The same pattern has been observed across three states in the USA (Sotis 2021). These findings reflect the socio-economic and health-related changes happening during the pandemic and help policymakers to plan appropriate strategies.

A thematic analysis of GT searches related to antibiotics revealed “whether alcohol can be consumed with antibiotics?” was one of the common questions asked. Further, in this study, an increase in the search for smoking cessation during the month of January every year was highlighted (Hanna and Hanna 2019).

In a worldwide analysis of search related to alcohol, obesity, and smoking (2010–2020), it was observed that alcohol and obesity had higher RSV and were positively correlated (Fabbian et al. 2021). However, tobacco had a lesser RSV and negatively correlated with alcohol. Specifically, in Italy, there was a positive correlation between smoking and alcohol.

GT also helped forecast alcohol-induced deaths, drug-induced deaths, suicides for the upcoming years. Further, the model helped understand the variations across the states (Parker et al. 2017). Forecasting events a priori will have public health impact and help plan interventions appropriately.

In summary, GT reflected the changes in RSV of alcohol and related factors secondary to policy shifts during the pandemic, documenting change in the population-level interest and a potential to forecast alcohol-related health complications and mortality (Table 2).

New Psychoactive Substances (NPS) and Other Drugs

New psychoactive substances (NPS) or legal highs are substances that are not listed on the conventions of the United Nations (UN). Most of them are legally procured through web-based shopping till they are declared illegal.

Mephedrone is a synthetic cathinone, sold on the internet legally till it was banned. GT analysis revealed that the popularity of mephedrone was highly correlated with its legal status (Kapitány-Fövény and Demetrovics 2017). A decrease in web interest is related to mephedrone after changes in legal status to "illegal" and mediated through searches about ecstasy. Further, the persistence of search patterns is related to common drugs like cocaine, MDMA, and heroin.

In Russia, the GT for Krokodil (an injectable drug from codeine) from different regions revealed a significant positive correlation with the legal cases from regions related to the drug (Zheluk et al. 2014). Hence, it serves as a proxy marker for the activities of production, sale of drugs. Further, they observed a consistent pattern of change in the search volumes before and after the ban on the substance across regions.

A common mode of procuring drugs is through the dark web. An association was found between a "dark web" search (assessed using GT analysis) and increased cannabis use in certain states of the USA (assessed using surveys) (Jardine and Lindner 2020). Another study observed a significant increase in cannabis-related searches during US elections, which was found to be more than any other relevant terms like climate change, global warming, etc. This study underscores the importance of cannabis policies to the government, the level of awareness among the public related to cannabis, and the need for physicians to develop appropriate strategies for providing evidence-based support (Torgerson et al. 2020).

GT helps us understand the pattern of the use of drugs. Zhang et al. reported an increase in interest over dabbing from 2004 to 2015, for cannabis use. Additionally, there was a significant correlation between dab and vaping, hash oil, and e-cigarette. In states with legal recreational and medical use, there was an increase in search compared to states with legal medical cannabis use and states without legal approval for either (Zhang et al. 2016).

Table 2 Alcohol misuse research using Google Tools

Author (Year)	Substance focus	Google Tool	Country of origin	Type of study	Analysis methods	Brief findings	Public health implication
Ghosh (2020)	Alcohol	Google Trends	India	Visualization and correlation	Locally weighted scatterplot smoothing Independent sample t-test; linear regression	Post-prohibition, a significant increase in the RSV for searches related to alcohol withdrawal, how to extract alcohol from alternate sources, online and home-delivery of alcohol	Documenting public response following an abrupt change in alcohol policy
Singh (2020)	Alcohol	Google Trends	India	Visualization and comparison of mean RSV between groups	Radar plots; one way ANOVA and Kruskal–Wallis test	Significant interest in procuring alcohol and alcohol withdrawal during lockdown 1; interest in benzodiazepines during lockdown 2	Documenting public response to policy changes over different phases of lockdown
Uvais (2020)	Alcohol and tobacco	Google Trends	India	Visualization	None	No change in search for quitting alcohol and tobacco, but increase in search for sanitizer and COVID-19	Changes in help seeking in pandemic
Sotis (2021)	Alcohol, porn	Google trends	USA	Visualization, interaction	Integrable non-autonomous Lotka–Volterra model	Initial part of pandemic had unemployment-related search and later part had an increase in health-related search, news, alcohol, and porn, along with unemployment	Changes and interactions between different domains during pandemic

Hanna (2019)	Antibiotics, smoking, alcohol	Google Trends and Google	UK	Visualization, average ranking, time series	Seasonal decomposition of time series by Loess	Consumption of alcohol while on antibiotics was one of the common searches. Increased search for smoking cessation during December and January months	Educating the public regarding alcohol and antibiotics. Providing access to services during this period
Fabbian (2021)	Alcohol, smoking, obesity	Google Trends	Worldwide	Visualization and correlation	Pearson or Spearman rank correlation	Alcohol and obesity had higher RSV and positively correlated and tobacco had lesser RSV and negatively correlated with alcohol. Further, varied with region	Understanding area specific search patterns
Parker (2017)	Alcohol, drug, suicide	Google Trends	USA	Predictive modeling	Alternative and L1-regularization	Google Trends could forecast alcohol-induced deaths, drug-induced deaths, and suicide for upcoming years	Forecasting events a priori helps in planning of interventions
Ghosh (2020)	Alcohol	Google News	India	Qualitative study	Thematic analysis	The content analysis of newspaper articles after the sudden policy revealed beneficial, harmful, non-compliance, and popularity as major themes while reporting	Highlighted the media/ public response to policy changes

Table 1: Summary of alcohol misuse research

In Italy, following a change in chronic pain law in 2010, using GT analysis it was observed that there was significant interest in pain-related search, including opioid medications (Miceli et al. 2021). Hence, GT acts as proxy markers for policy changes in the public.

In a study to understand web interest in cannabis as a cure for cancer, the search for cannabis as a cure for cancer was found to be higher than traditional cancer treatments. Interest was observed to be higher in legalized states. Engagement on social media was found to be higher with the false content compared to the accurate content. Hence, it is important for the medical community to communicate accurate content.

In the context of increasing tapentadol misuse in India, using GT data, it was observed an increased RSV for tapentadol compared to omeprazole and the RSV parallels that of tramadol. Additionally, the increase in RSV is correlated to the states with the highest prevalence of opioid use (Mukherjee et al. 2020).

European study observed a correlation between the GT related to "meth" and criminal activities related to methamphetamine crime (Gamma et al. 2016). Hence, GT can be used as a possible predictor of methamphetamine-related crime.

Recently our group has worked on the potential for a GT data output for monitoring the opioid overdose deaths in the USA. We showed that the normalized and regressed trend of "naloxone" was similar to the "opioid overdose" trend published by the National Centre for Health Statistics. The year-wise RSV of "naloxone" and "drug overdose" revealed a significant positive correlation with the yearly age-adjusted overdose mortality rate. Moreover, the state-wise RSV also correlated with the state-wise overdose mortality statistics. GT-based research, therefore, could supplement and strengthen the monitoring of the opioid overdose epidemic (Ghosh et al. n.d.).

In summary, GT appears to be a promising way to study epidemiological trends of NPS and other drugs. Variations in NPS and drug related RSV were associated with policy changes and events like elections. Studies elucidated its potential to act as indicators for production, sale, and availability of drugs, usage patterns, and criminal activities. GT may also help in drug overdose surveillance (Table 3).

Tobacco and Other Nicotine Delivery Systems

In the field of tobacco related research, GT has been used for diverse purposes. As with other substances, search query surveillance using GT has been a valuable and freely accessible tool to study changes in public perceptions of tobacco products as well as near real-time responses to changes in tobacco related policies.

With the advent of Electronic Nicotine Delivery Systems (ENDS), GT has been used to monitor the varying public interest and perceptions of ENDS over time or across various regions. A study estimating the popularity of ENDS across the USA, the UK, Australia, and Canada found that, between 2008 and 2010, Google searches for ENDS were greater than those for nicotine replacement therapies (NRT), varenicline, and snus (Ayers et al. 2011b).

Table 3 Drug misuse research using Google Tools

Author (year)	Substance focus	Google tool	Country of origin	Type of study	Analysis methods	Brief findings	Public health implication
Ghosh (2021)	Opioids	Google Trends	USA	Visualization and correlation	Locally weighted scatterplot smoothing; change-point analysis; cross-correlation function for time-series data	Year-wise and state-wise RSV for "naloxone" and "drug overdose" showed significantly positive correlation with the age-adjusted drug overdose mortality	Google Trends data could supplement and strengthen the monitoring of opioid overdose epidemic
Kapitany-Foveny (2017)	Mephedrone	Google Trends and Google News	Hungary	Visualization, differences between groups and correlation	Independent t-test, ANOVA, Path analysis	Decrease in web interest after legal ban on Mephedrone	Web interest changes secondary to new legal status to the drugs
Zheluk (2014)	Krokodil	Google Trends	Russia	Correlation	Spearman correlation	Positive correlation between the legal cases of Krokodil use and Google search trends of the region	Google Trends can serve as a proxy marker for production and sale of drugs
Jardine (2020)	Cannabis	Google Trends	USA	Visualization and regression	Mixed effects ordinary least squared regression	Dark web interest positively correlates with cannabis consumption pattern across states	Google trends can reflect upon the consumption patterns and policies across the states

(continued)

Table 3 (continued)

Author (year)	Substance focus	Google tool	Country of origin	Type of study	Analysis methods	Brief findings	Public health implication
Torgerson (2020)	Cannabis	Google Trends	USA	Visualization and regression	Autoregressive integrated moving average algorithm for forecasting and linear regression	Increased cannabis-related search during US elections	Importance of cannabis policies to the government
Zhang (2016)	Dabbing	Google Trends	USA	Visualization and correlation	Pearson correlation	Increased dabbing related search in states with legal status for cannabis use	Highlighted the influence of policy on the search related to dabbing
Miceli (2021)	Opioids and pain	Google Trends	Italy	Visualization and regression	Joint point regression analysis	Increased pain-related search following change in legislation (law on chronic pain)	Highlighted the need for scientific community to provide knowledge on the chronic conditions on commonly used search engines
Mukherjee (2020)	Tapentadol	Google Trends	India	Visualization and correlation	Correlation	Association between the states with highest prevalence of opioid use and search for tapentadol	Role of google trends as proxy markers for drug use trends of newer drugs

Gamma (2016)	Methamphetamine	Google Trends	Switzerland, Austria, and Germany	Visualization and correlation	Cross-correlation	Relation between the search of "Meth" and its related crimes	Role of Google Trends to serve as possible predictor for drug related crimes
Forsyth (2012)	Mephedrone	Google News and Google Trends	UK	Visualization and qualitative analysis	Content analysis	News published during the period raised false drug alarms as reflected by Google Trends. Further, resulted in policy changes	Media reporting and its impact on policy changes were highlighted
Bright (2013)	Kronic	Google News and Google Trends	Australia	Qualitative analysis	Content analysis	Media reporting about the Kronic was associated with increased Google Search, further, a "moral panic" leading to ban on the drug	Media reporting and its impact on policy changes highlighted
Jankowski (2016)	Multiple drugs	Google Trends	World	Frequency	Ranking based on the search volume	Popularity and harms related to the drugs changed with the time	Google Trends can help in monitoring the changes in drug popularity
Yin (2012)	Synthetic cathinones (Bath salts)	Google Insights for Search (GIS)	USA	Visualization and correlation	Non-linear regression	Internet search data correlated with the data from poison outbreaks	Google Trends can help in predicting and monitoring drug outbreaks

(continued)

Table 3 (continued)

Author (year)	Substance focus	Google tool	Country of origin	Type of study	Analysis methods	Brief findings	Public health implication
Raubenheimer (2021)	Cannabis	Google Trends	New Zealand	Predictive modeling	–	Google Trend analysis data could broadly predict upcoming cannabis referendum	Google Trends can help in predicting policy decisions
Crawford (2019)	–	Google Street View (GSV)	USA	Descriptive	–	Reliability between the virtual audit and in-person audit was high for health care facilities (83%) and entertainment venues (62%), but low for land use	GSV can be a reliable proxy for monitoring healthcare facilities in rural USA

Online search data trends on smoking cessation related behaviors may provide an estimate of the degree and duration of the effects of various tobacco control measures. In the same study mentioned above, high ENDS popularity correlated with stronger tobacco control measures enforced through clean indoor air laws, cigarette taxes, and anti-smoking populations. This association suggests that ENDS might be used to circumvent or stop smoking as a result of stricter restrictions (Ayers et al. 2011b).

Among newer tobacco products, following the introduction of heat-not-burn (HNB) tobacco products around 2014, GT data was used to examine their rising popularity in the Japanese market from 2015 to 2017 and compared with the Google search query trends for e-cigarettes in the USA. Here, GT data helped make an estimate of the magnitude and potential for growth of HNB tobacco products (Caputi et al. 2017).

Growing popularity of Waterpipe Tobacco Smoking (WTS) was studied in the USA, the UK, Australia, and Canada. The trends in Google search queries related to WTS were compared with those for electronic cigarettes between 2004 and 2013. The long-term national trends in the study showed a consistent increase in online popularity of WTS. The popularity of WTS was comparable to that of e-cigarettes (Salloum et al. 2016).

The impact of tobacco related policies on population-level interests through search trends has been studied across several countries. The changes in Google search volumes between 2004 and 2016 for smoking cessation associated with tobacco control measures were studied in Japan. Higher cigarette price hikes were associated with higher and more long-lasting effects. However, population impact was observed to continue for relatively short periods (Tabuchi et al. 2019). Other studies have shown that tax hikes for tobacco were accompanied by spikes in online searches for cheaper cigarette market alternatives (Ayers et al. 2011a, 2014).

A study in the Netherlands assessed the magnitude and duration of the impact of smoke-free legislation and reimbursement of smoking cessation support on Google searches for quitting smoking. There was an increase in RSV in the first 4 weeks following the introduction of smoking bans in restaurants and bars in 2008. Following the introduction of reimbursement for smoking cessation support in 2011 and 2012, RSV increased significantly during both times (Troelstra et al. 2016). Another GT study detected spikes in interest in cheap cigarettes around the time of tax hikes and suggested online health messaging related to tobacco at such times (Caputi 2018).

GT has also been used to study whether national implementation of pictorial health warnings was associated with an increase in online search queries seeking information on smoking cessation. In this study across six European countries, France and the UK showed a short-term increase in RSV for smoking cessation terms, which however were not significant and were present only during the initial months. Ireland, Norway, Denmark, and Switzerland showed no increase in online searches (Kunst et al. 2019).

A 2015 US study tried to validate the potential utility of GT to supplement traditional surveillance methods. In this study, GT RSV for non-cigarette tobacco products was compared with state-wise prevalence of use of these products. They also assessed whether GT can detect regional trends in non-cigarette tobacco use. Significant correlation was found between state GT cigar RSV and prevalence of cigar use among youth. State GT smokeless tobacco RSV also showed significant positive correlation with prevalence of smokeless tobacco use in both youth and adults. They concluded that GT was a valuable tool which could supplement traditional surveillance methods (Cavazos-Rehg et al. 2015).

In the USA, following the announcement and subsequent ban on flavored cartridge-based e-cigarettes in January of 2020, GT analysis showed declining RSV of search trends for JUUL (pod mod style cartridge based), while the RSV of Puff Bar (a disposable vaping product) kept increasing and surpassed that of JUUL in February 2020. GT provided a real-time online dataset which could be used to monitor rapidly changing products in tandem with changing legislations (Dai and Hao 2020).

Recently our group has examined the validity of GT for assessing the population-level behavior and interest of ENDS from both India and the USA. We have also tested whether the change in the ENDS regulation is reflected by the change of the RSV. Our results showed a strong positive correlation between the geospatial RSV and state-wise prevalence of adult END-switchers in the USA. A complete prohibition of production, sale, and use of ENDS in India was associated with a significant reduction in the relevant search queries; however, the reduction of search behavior was less robust in the USA (Ghosh et al. 2021b).

When there was an outbreak of EVALI cases in the USA, peaking in late 2019, it prompted an increased public interest in vaping cessation, particularly during the initial period. GT analyses showing an increase in search trends for vaping cessation reflected the rapid public response to this news (Leas et al. 2020).

GT has also been used to study the impact of significant days and campaigns related to smoking cessation. A study across the Latin American countries of Mexico, Ecuador, Venezuela, Peru, Chile, Colombia, and Argentina evaluated the potential of online trends surveillance to track population awareness and interest in smoking cessation on *World No Tobacco Day (WNTD)*. The study provided further evidence for the real-time monitoring possible with online search query surveillance as all the countries showed increases in search and news trends for smoking cessation around the time of WNTD (Ayers et al. 2012).

The mass media temporary smoking abstinence campaign during the month of October known as "Stoptober" was started in 2014 in the Netherlands. Using search query data from GT, a significant short-term increase in RSV for search terms associated with smoking cessation was observed during the 2014–2016 Stoptober campaigns in the Netherlands, suggesting possible impact of such intensive media campaigns (Tieks et al. 2019).

Since December 2019, the global pandemic of COVID-19 has been affecting millions across the world. During the initial months of the outbreak, GT was used to examine whether there was any associated increase in interest in smoking cessation. However the study did not find any tendency toward an increase in interest (Heerfordt and Heerfordt 2020).

Altogether, GT analysis has been a free, easily accessible tool for monitoring population response to the introduction of novel nicotine products or novel ways to use tobacco, detect changes in public interest in smoking cessation associated with implementation of tobacco related taxes as well as assess the magnitude and duration of impact of tobacco control policies and smoking regulations. GT appears to have a role in predicting future outbreaks as in the case of electronic cigarettes and potentially for HNB tobacco products (Table 4).

Use of Google News in Substance Use Research

Qualitative (content) and quantitative analyses of google news have provided some insightful results in substance use research. Between 2009 and 2010 in the UK, mephedrone (synthetic cathinones) related deaths resulted in a legal ban within a year. Content analysis of Google News with the later revelations on causes of death identified false alarms (Forsyth 2012). News on the media is correlated with the mephedrone-related search studied using Google Trends analysis. Similar observations were made with the drug Kronic (synthetic cannabis) in Australia using Google News, Trends (Bright et al. 2013). Google News highlighted the "moral panic" from the media outlets that eventually led to an interest in the drug in the public and policy changes from the government.

In India, a qualitative analysis of the 350 newspaper articles published during the initial lockdown (March 2020) reflected the public response related to the sudden alcohol policy changes during lockdown (Ghosh et al. 2020). In this study Google News was used as a search engine to retrieve articles. The authors also underscored the ecological validity of using Google News as a search engine for the study. The thematic analysis of the content revealed four themes related to policy changes: (i) beneficial aspects, (ii) harmful aspects, (iii) non-compliance and attempts to change, and/or subvert (iv) popularity and level of public buy-in. Further, the study also highlighted the ethical aspects and stigmatizing language used while publishing such articles.

Substance Misuse Research Using Other Google Applications

Google Earth is a free, internet-based three-dimensional geographical software program which provides aerial, satellite, and street view images. Virtual walkarounds can be performed using Google Earth and virtual audits of neighborhoods can be done.

Google Street View (GSV) has been used to objectively study particular features of an environment. There have been a few studies which found GSV to be an efficient way to study smoke-free signage in school and hospital grounds (Wilson and Thomson 2015; Wilson et al. 2015, 2018). In another study, GSV was not found to be a sensitive tool for studying smoke-free signage in playgrounds (Thomson and Wilson 2017). However, small sample sizes and limited number and settings of these studies preclude drawing any definite conclusions about the utility and applicability of GSV in assessing smoke-free signage. GSV might be used to assess the locations and density of outlets for sale of alcohol or tobacco.

Table 4 Tobacco and ENDS research by Google Tools

Author (year)	Substance focus	Google tool	Country of origin	Type of study	Analysis methods	Brief findings	Public health implication
Ghosh (2021)	ENDS	Google Trends	USA and India	Visualization and correlation	Locally weighted scatterplot smoothing; change-point analysis; independent-sample t-test; correlation analysis	Visual trends largely mimicked the trend of the National Youth Tobacco Survey in the USA Online search queries correlated strongly with state-wise prevalence of ENDS users in the USA Change in ENDS regulation was associated with significant changes in online search behavior	GT may be a valid tool to examine the population-level behavior and interest of ENDS
Heerfordt (2020)	Tobacco	Google Trends	Denmark	Visualization	None	No change in search queries for smoking cessation	GT can help detect changes in help seeking during a pandemic
Dai (2020)	Juul and Puff Bars	Google Trends	USA	Predictive modeling	ARIMA (autoregressive integrated moving average)	Decreasing RSV for JUUL and increasing trends of online searches for Puff Bar in tandem with changing e-cigarette legislations	GT can help in forecasting effectiveness of policy changes and foresee methods to subvert restrictions
Leas (2020)	Tobacco	Google Trends	USA	Predictive modeling	ARIMA (autoregressive integrated moving average) Piecewise regression	EVALI outbreak generated increased online search for vaping cessation and increased coverage of the harms associated with vaping	GT can help in prioritizing and strategizing resource allocation in response to public interest

Tieks (2019)	Tobacco	Google Trends	Netherlands	Predictive modeling	ARIMA (autoregressive integrated moving average) Box–Jenkins method	The Stoptober program (temporary smoking abstinence campaigns) was associated with a significant increase in RSV from the initial week till 2 weeks after the challenge	GT helped detect the population interest in smoking cessation during a temporary abstinence program. Further plans to effect population-level impact through national policies may thus be guided by these findings
Kunst (2019)	Tobacco	Google Trends	UK, France, Norway, Denmark, Ireland, Switzerland	Predictive modeling	ARIMA (autoregressive integrated moving average) Box–Jenkins method	Only France and the UK showed an increase in quit smoking searches in response to implementation of pictorial health warnings in the initial months None of the countries showed an increase in smoking cessation searches at any other period	GT can be used to assess the magnitude and duration of impact of any policy or legislative changes
Tabuchi (2019)	Tobacco	Google Trends	Japan	Visualization and correlation	Cluster detection test	Larger cigarette price hikes were associated with a greater and more persistent increase in smoking cessation search volumes. The duration of impact though was short	GT data helped examine the population impact of tobacco price hikes on smoking cessation

(continued)

Table 4 (continued)

Author (year)	Substance focus	Google tool	Country of origin	Type of study	Analysis methods	Brief findings	Public health implication
Caputi (2017)	Heat-not-burn (HNB) tobacco products	Google Trends	Japan and USA	Predictive modeling	ARIMA (autoregressive integrated moving average)	Significant increase in HNB searches originating in Japan Online search queries for HNB in Japan were more frequent than those for e-cigarettes in the USA	Use of GT to estimate the growth rate and growth potential of a novel product in a country while comparing with trends of similar product in a different country
Caputi (2017)	Tobacco	Google Trends	USA	Predictive modeling	Anomaly detection with Seasonal Hybrid Extreme Studentized Deviate (SHESD) test and breakout detection with E-Divisive with Means (EDM) test	Spike in online searches for "cheap cigarettes" associated with cigarette tax hikes	GT may be used to monitor online search interests and accordingly tailor an increase in online tobacco related health messaging during such spikes
Ayers (2016)	ENDS	Google Trends	USA	Visualization and predictive modeling	ARIMA (autoregressive integrated moving average)	Rapid rise in ENDS searches Search query terms changing from e-cigarette- to vaping-focused terms in relation to state anti-smoking laws	GT can help in monitoring and predicting changes in popularity of nicotine delivery products

Toelstra (2016)	Tobacco	Google Trends	Netherlands and Belgium	Visualization	Interrupted time series analysis ARIMA (autoregressive integrated moving average)	Both types of policies – smoke-free legislation and reimbursement of smoking cessation support (SCS) – were associated with online search spikes for cessation in the Netherlands. Online search results were inconsistent in Belgium	Effect of tobacco control policies can be examined with the help of GT
Cavazos-Rehg (2015)	Non-cigarette tobacco	Google Trends	USA	Visualization and correlation	Pearson correlation	State GT RSV for cigar positively correlated with prevalence of cigar use among youth Positive and significant correlations between state GT RSV for smokeless tobacco and prevalence of smokeless tobacco use among youth and adults	GT can also be used to detect regional trends in youth and adult tobacco use
Salloum (2016)	Waterpipe tobacco smoking (WTS)	Google Trends	USA, UK, Australia, Canada	Visualization and correlation	Locally weighted scatterplot smoothing Equality-of- means t tests	Steady growth in popularity of WTS in all the countries Online popularity of WTS rivals that of e-cigarettes	GT can compare trends of similar products and predict future growth in popularity

(continued)

Table 4 (continued)

Author (year)	Substance focus	Google tool	Country of origin	Type of study	Analysis methods	Brief findings	Public health implication
Wilson (2015)	Smoking	Google Street View	NZ and USA	Review of 23 articles	Descriptive	GSV is sensitive for smoke-free signages in schools and hospital grounds but not for tobacco litters and tobacco billboards	GSV can be used for surveillance of adherence to some tobacco policy measures
Ayers (2014)	Tobacco	Google Trends	USA	Visualization	Descriptive	The week of the cigarette excise tax hike witnessed a 150% increase in all cigarette avoidance queries and 46% increase in all cessation queries	GT can also detect specific changes in population considerations following legislative changes
Ayers (2012)	Tobacco	Google News and Google Insights for Search	Ecuador, Chile, Venezuela, Perú, Colombia, Argentina, México	Visualization	Descriptive Interrupted time series analysis	World No Tobacco Day (WNTD) was associated with increases in both cessation news trends and cessation query trends across the countries	Feasible to perform digital surveillance for tobacco control and estimate the effectiveness of a program

Ayers (2011a)	Tobacco	Google Insights for Search	USA	Visualization and regression	Least squares regression	Online searches for information on smoking cessation and cheap cigarettes peaked in response to cigarette tax increases	Efforts may be increased to address tax avoidance and support smoking cessation by modifying policies according to the online search trends
Ayers (2011b)	ENDS	Google Insights for Search	USA, UK, Australia, Canada	Visualization and correlation	Locally weighted scatterplot smoothing Equality-of- means t tests	Highest ENDS searches in the USA, closely followed by Canada and the UK, and Australia had the fewest The stronger the tobacco control, the higher the ENDS searches	Online search query surveillance has great potential as a real-time, publicly available means of assessing public interest in new products

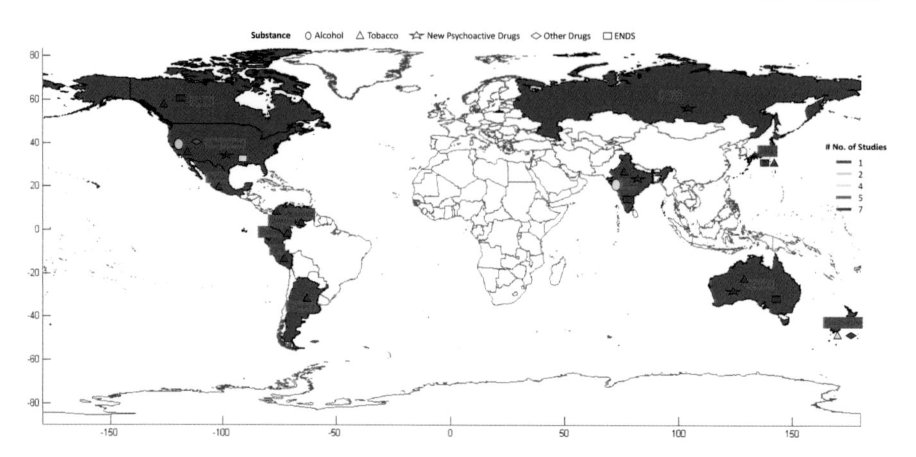

Fig. 2 (**a**) and (**b**) World Map illustrating the Google Trends-based research on substance misuse. The color-coded lines represent the number of studies and symbols depict specific substances; (**b**) zooms out the studies from the European Union

Crawford and his team (2019) studied the reliability of GSV in five counties of rural Kentucky in the USA. His team found that the virtual audit of GSV has good concurrence with the in-person audit for healthcare facilities and entertainment venues, but has little reliability for land use (e.g., dilapidated homes, business, defunct mines, etc.).

Google launched a program initiative named Google Recover Together in September 2019 in the USA during the 30th annual National Recovery Month. Google Recover Tool helps in locating and connecting individuals with substance use disorders in recovery, provides recovery support resources, and may also aid in building up a recovery network through social network groups and the voices project (https://recovertogether.withgoogle.com/#recovery-support-resources). The research application of the Recover tool is not yet known. As part of the program, two new Google Maps locator tools were launched, which would be helpful in connecting to recovery resources. The Recovery Locator Tool maps locations of recovery support meetings and other school based or family support services. The Naloxone Locator Tool provides the nearest pharmacy address where naloxone may be available even without a prescription (https://recovertogether.withgoogle.com/treatment/#naloxone). This tool is intended to help individuals during an overdose emergency. The research application of Naloxone Locator is yet to be known (Fig. 2).

Public Health Implications

Data from the GT analysis can help us understand the popularity and harms of different psychoactive agents (Jankowski and Hoffmann 2016). They act as proxy markers for the drug harms in society as they correlate with data obtained from the other measures. Drug use trends can be monitored using this analysis. Further, it can also help us in predicting and monitoring drug outbreaks, for example, outbreaks related to bath salts correlated significantly with internet search (Yin and Ho 2012). While analysis looked into after effects of policy changes using GT some used it to predict policy change (Ghosh et al. 2021b; Raubenheimer et al. 2021). For example, in New Zealand, GT broadly predicted the upcoming cannabis referendum in 2020 (Raubenheimer et al. 2021).

Critique of Google Trends and Other Google Tool-Based Research

There are several limiting factors in Google's tool-based research. Firstly, the search volume for a specific query/topic in the GT dataset depends on the proportion of internet users in the population studied by the researchers. The figures are widely variable across countries. As per the International Telecommunication Union (ITU) data published in 2019, 87% of the total population in high-income countries use internet-based communications; for low-income countries, the figure is 16% (https://data.worldbank.org/indicator/IT.NET.USER.ZS). Countries with a high proportion of internet users will produce more reliable trends. Hence, all GT-based studies have been conducted in areas with high internet penetration. The latest review by Mavragani and colleagues reported that out of a total of 109 published articles between 2006 and 2016, 60 are from the USA, and the majority of the rest comes from the UK, Australia, Canada, Germany, and Italy (Mavragani et al. 2018). The second limitation of GT research is also related to this data; there is a dominance of research from the English-speaking nations. Third, GT-based research relies on an adequate number of searches made at the population level. Search queries or topics with "insufficient interest" will not generate either a relative search volume or a visual trend. Therefore, the condition studied by the researcher must be either highly prevalent in the community or has become important after a recent change at the policy level or has been widely advertised/reported by the media. These riders will render several health conditions not suitable for GT-based research. Fourth, the search volumes generated by GT are dependent on the search inputs; a slight difference (e.g., adding a punctuation mark, space, changing the spelling) in the search input can give rise to different trends and search volumes. Search inputs are largely based on the researchers' consensus and expertise. The lack of standardization of search queries, therefore, may render GT-based studies less replicable. Fifth, although Google is the preferred search engine in most of the countries (as mentioned in the introduction), search engines like Bing, Yahoo, and Baidu are used by a little more than 5% of the world's population (https://gs.statcounter.com/search-engine-market-share). A GT researcher will not be able to capture the search traffic of these search engines. A point may be important to note here that the Bing search engine by the Microsoft corporation generates absolute search volume; it, therefore, may be suitable for studying even search queries with negligible or "insufficient volumes" that would otherwise not be picked by the GT. Sixth, the original aim of GT research is forecasting or predicting epidemics and outbreaks; however, research done in this area so far focused primarily on the correlation of GT output with the published data from official and other sources. The authors have worked most extensively on Google Flu Trends and designed several forecasting models but are yet to come up with a single-best model to predict influenza-like illness outbreaks before the standard surveillance systems (Cook et al. 2011; Butler 2013). Finally, Nuti and coauthors commented that the absence of a standard guideline for reporting GT-based research has restricted the accuracy, completeness, and transparency of reporting (Nuti et al. 2014; Marušić and Campbell 2016). In fact, they have suggested a checklist for documentation of GT research. Interested authors may like to use it (Nuti et al. 2014). The other Google products-based research is still evolving and insufficient for scientific scrutiny.

Conclusion

Health researchers have been increasingly using Google Trends and other Google Tools because of their ease of access, ability to track public health phenomenon real time, and predict future patterns or both, and potential to signal population response to a recent change in public health policy – all these can be accomplished in a short span of time with minimal requirement for funding and other resources. These characteristics would make GT research a good candidate for health surveillance. Using Google tools in substance misuse research is a relatively recent phenomenon. Most of the research has been conducted on tobacco and alcohol; however, there is also a growing trend of studying the novel psychoactive substances and other drugs through GT. Substance misuse research is largely based on the visual inspection and interpretation of trends and correlation with the available datasets from other sources. Forecasting and predictive modeling have not been tried so far. Despite its potential application in public health, the limitation of Google tool-based research should be kept in mind while conducting and interpreting the results of such studies.

Key Facts

Electronic Nicotine Delivery Systems (ENDS)

- ENDS are non-combustible tobacco products.
- ENDS includes Vapes, vaporizers, vape pens, hookah pens, electronic cigarettes, and e-pipes.
- E-liquid containing nicotine is heated up to generate aerosol (not smoke).
- E-liquid also contains flavorings, propylene glycol, vegetable glycerin, and other ingredients.
- The World Health Organization calls for monitoring and regulation of ENDS at national level.

E-cigarette or Vaping Product Use-Associated Lung Injury (EVALI)

- The term is coined by the Centers for Disease Control and Prevention (CDC), USA.
- The illness was first documented in August 2019.
- EVALI is a lung disease that is linked with vaping.

- Vaping tetrahydrocannabinol or THC may be associated with an increased risk of EVALI.
- Vitamin E acetate has also been implicated for EVALI.
- The treatment is supportive and it may be fatal.

Google Flu Trends (GFT)
- GFT is a forecast model to predict epidemics of influenza-like illness.
- It gathers and analyzes real-time data.
- GFT focuses on a particular geographical area.
- GFT was launched in 2008 by Google.
- GFT failed to predict the 2013 influenza epidemic.
- The model was revised in 2015 and discontinued later.

New Psychoactive Substances (NPS)
- NPS are substances of misuse that are not regulated by international conventions.
- These are also known as designer drugs and synthetic drugs.
- NPS pose significant public health threats.
- NPS misuse has become widespread – 126 countries have reported use of at least one NPS.
- There are around 1047 NPS reported till December 2020.
- Synthetic stimulants are most common NPS, followed by synthetic cannabinoids.

Opioid Overdose
- Opioids are very strong central nervous system depressants.
- High doses may cause respiratory depression, cardiac arrest, and death.
- The triad of opioid overdose is pin-point pupil, shallow and very low respiratory rate, and deep sedation.
- Worldwide more than 30% of all opioid-related deaths are overdose deaths.
- Naloxone (injection or intranasal) can cause rapid reversal of opioid overdose.

Mini-Dictionary of Terms

Juul
- Juul is a popular pod mod brand.
- Pod mods are third generation ENDS.
- These are small, rechargeable devices that aerosolize liquid solutions containing nicotine.
- Pod mods may deliver very high levels of nicotine than the earlier generations of ENDS.
- Juul captured nearly half of the ENDS market in 2019.

Locally Weighted Scatterplot Smoothing (LOWESS)
- LOWESS is a regression analysis.
- It creates a smooth line through a time plot or scatterplot based on noisy or sparse data points.

- LOWESS helps to examine variables of interest.
- It aids in the visualization of trends.
- LOWESS has been used in Google Trends-based analysis.

Meth

- Meth is the street name of methamphetamine.
- Crystal methamphetamine appears as glass fragments or shiny, bluish-white rocks.
- It falls under the central nervous system stimulant category.
- The common modes of intake are smoking, snorting, injecting, and swallowing.
- Methamphetamine is highly addictive and may cause overdose deaths.

Naloxone

- Naloxone is a competitive opioid antagonist.
- It has a high affinity for the mu-opioid receptor.
- It can reverse the opioid overdose rapidly, usually within minutes.
- The half-life of naloxone ranges from 30 to 120 min.
- Naloxone is also combined with buprenorphine to reduce the latter's injection misuse.

Relative Search Volume (RSV)

- RSV indicates relative volumes of a specific search query on the Google search engine.
- RSV is a unit of analysis for Google Trends data.
- It is a product of data normalization.
- Data normalization is performed on the basis of time and location of the search queries.
- Each data point is divided by the total searches of the geography and time range it represents.
- The value ranges from 0 to 100.

Summary Points

- Use of Google Trends to monitor diseases with public health implications started with the launch of Google Flu Trends in 2008.
- Since then, various other Google tools have also been used such as Google News, Google Maps, Google Street View.
- Application of Google tools in substance use research was first published in 2011.
- Till date, most of the Google tool-based substance use research have been conducted on tobacco and electronic nicotine delivery system.
- Other substances that have been targeted in at least three studies are alcohol, cannabis, and the new psychoactive substances.
- Most of the Google tool-based research are from the USA, Canada, Europe, and Australia.

- Substance misuse research is largely based on the visual inspection and interpretation of the trends/street view and correlation with the available datasets from other sources.
- Uses of Google tools for forecasting and predictive modeling are very limited.
- Google tool-based research has limited accuracy, completeness, and transparency of reporting.

References

Ayers JW, Althouse BM, Allem JP et al (2012) A novel evaluation of World No Tobacco day in Latin America. J Med Internet Res 14:e77

Ayers JW, Althouse BM, Allem JP, Leas EC, Dredze M, & Williams RS (2016). Revisiting the Rise of Electronic Nicotine Delivery Systems Using Search Query Surveillance. Am J Prev Med 50(6):e173–e181. https://doi.org/10.1016/j.amepre.2015.12.008

Ayers JW, Althouse BM, Noar SM, Cohen JE (2014) Do celebrity cancer diagnoses promote primary cancer prevention? Prev Med 58:81–84

Ayers JW, Althouse BM, Ribisl KM et al (2014) Digital detection for tobacco control: online reactions to the 2009 US cigarette excise tax increase. Nicotine Tob Res 16:576–583

Ayers JW, Ribisl K, Brownstein JS (2011a) Using search query surveillance to monitor tax avoidance and smoking cessation following the United States' 2009 "SCHIP" cigarette tax increase. PLoS One 6:e16777

Ayers JW, Ribisl KM, Brownstein JS (2011b) Tracking the rise in popularity of electronic nicotine delivery systems (electronic cigarettes) using search query surveillance. Am J Prev Med 40: 448–453

Bright SJ, Bishop B, Kane R et al (2013) Kronic hysteria: exploring the intersection between Australian synthetic cannabis legislation, the media, and drug-related harm. Int J Drug Policy 24:231–237

Butler D (2013) When Google got flu wrong. Nature 494:155

Caputi TL (2018) Google searches for "cheap cigarettes" spike at tax increases: evidence from an algorithm to detect spikes in time series data. Nicotine Tob Res 20:779–783

Caputi TL, Leas E, Dredze M, Cohen JE, Ayers JW (2017) They're heating up: Internet search query trends reveal significant public interest in heat-not-burn tobacco products. PLoS One 12: e0185735

Carneiro HA, Mylonakis E (2009) Google Trends: a web-based tool for real-time surveillance of disease outbreaks. Clin Infect Dis 49:1557–1564

Cavazos-Rehg PA, Krauss MJ, Spitznagel EL et al (2015) Monitoring of non-cigarette tobacco use using Google Trends. Tob Control 24:249–255

Choi H, Varian H (2012) Predicting the present with Google Trends. Econ Rec 88:2–9

Cook S, Conrad C, Fowlkes AL, Mohebbi MH (2011) Assessing Google flu trends performance in the United States during the 2009 influenza virus A (H1N1) pandemic. PLoS One 6:e23610

Crawford ND, Haardöerfer R, Cooper H et al (2019) Characterizing the rural opioid use environment in Kentucky using Google Earth: virtual audit. J Med Internet Res 21:e14923

Dai H, Hao J (2020) Online popularity of JUUL and Puff Bars in the USA: 2019–2020. Tob Control

Fabbian F, Rodríguez-Muñoz PM, López-Carrasco J, Cappadona R, Rodríguez-Borrego MA, López-Soto PJ (2021) Google Trends on obesity, smoking and alcoholism: global and country-specific interest. Healthcare 9:190

Forsyth AJ (2012) Virtually a drug scare: mephedrone and the impact of the Internet on drug news transmission. Int J Drug Policy 23:198–209

Gamma A, Schleifer R, Weinmann W et al (2016) Could Google Trends be used to predict methamphetamine-related crime? An analysis of search volume data in Switzerland, Germany, and Austria. PLoS One 11:e0166566

Ghosh A, Bisaga A, Kaur S, Mahintamani T (2021a) Google Trends data: a potential new tool for monitoring the opioid crisis. European Addict Res. https://doi.org/10.1159/000517302
Ghosh A, Choudhury S, Basu A et al (2020) Extended lockdown and India's alcohol policy: a qualitative analysis of newspaper articles. Int J Drug Policy 85:102940
Ghosh A, Kaur S, Roub F (2021b) Use and interest of Electronic Nicotine Delivery Systems (ENDS): assessing the validity of Google Trends. Am J Drug Alcohol Abuse. https://doi.org/10.1080/00952990.2021.1944171
Ghosh A, Krishnan NC, Choudhury S, Basu A (2021c) Can google trends search inform us about the population response and public health impact of abrupt change in alcohol policy?—a case study from India during the covid-19 pandemic. Int J Drug Policy 87:102984
Ginsberg J, Mohebbi MH, Patel RS, Brammer L, Smolinski MS, Brilliant L (2009) Detecting influenza epidemics using search engine query data. Nature 457:1012–1014
Google Flu Trends (n.d.). Available at: http://datacollaboratives.org/cases/google-flu-trends.html. Accessed 9 June 2021
Google News Initiative Training Center (n.d.). Available at: https://newsinitiative.withgoogle.com/training/lessons?tool=Google%20Trends&image=trends. Accessed 9 June 2021
Google Trends (n.d.). Available at: https://trends.google.com/trends/?geo=IN. Accessed 9 June 2021
Hanna A, Hanna LA (2019) What, where and when? Using Google Trends and Google to investigate patient needs and inform pharmacy practice. Int J Pharm Pract 27:80–87
Heerfordt C, Heerfordt IM (2020) Has there been an increased interest in smoking cessation during the first months of the COVID-19 pandemic? A Google Trends study. Public Health 183:6
Jankowski W, Hoffmann M (2016) Can Google searches predict the popularity and harm of psychoactive agents? J Med Internet Res 18:e38
Jardine E, Lindner AM (2020) The Dark Web and cannabis use in the United States: Evidence from a big data research design. Int J Drug Policy 76:102627. https://doi.org/10.1016/j.drugpo.2019.102627
Kapitány-Fövény M, Demetrovics Z (2017) Utility of Web search query data in testing theoretical assumptions about mephedrone. Hum Psychopharmacol 32:e2620
Kunst AE, van Splunter C, Troelstra SA, Bosdriesz JR (2019) Did the introduction of pictorial health warnings increase information seeking for smoking cessation?: Time-series analysis of Google Trends data in six countries. Tob Prev Cessation 5
Leas EC, Nobles AL, Caputi TL, Dredze M, Zhu SH, Cohen JE, Ayers JW (2020) News coverage of the E-cigarette, or Vaping, product use Associated Lung Injury (EVALI) outbreak and internet searches for vaping cessation. Tob Control
Lefer TB, Anderson MR, Fornari A et al (2008) Using Google Earth as an innovative tool for community mapping. Public Health Rep 123:474–480
Lozano-Fuentes S, Elizondo-Quiroga D, Farfan-Ale JA et al (2008) Use of Google EarthTM to strengthen public health capacity and facilitate management of vector-borne diseases in resource-poor environments. B World Health Organ 86:718–725
Marušić A, Campbell H (2016) Reporting guidelines in global health research. J Glob Health 6
Mavragani A, Ochoa G, Tsagarakis KP (2018) Assessing the methods, tools, and statistical approaches in Google Trends research: systematic review. J Med Internet Res 20:e9366
Miceli L, Bednarova R, Bednarova I, Rizzardo A, Cobianchi L, Dal Mas F, Biancuzzi H, Bove T, Dal Moro F, Zattoni F (2021) What people search for when browsing "Doctor Google." An analysis of search trends in Italy after the Law on Pain. J Pain Palliat Care Pharmacother 35:23–30
Mukherjee D, Shukla L, Saha P, Mahadevan J, Kandasamy A, Chand P, Benegal V, Murthy P (2020) Tapentadol abuse and dependence in India. Asian J Psychiatr 49:101978
Nuti SV, Wayda B, Ranasinghe I et al (2014) The use of Google Trends in health care research: a systematic review. PLoS One 9:e109583
Parker J, Cuthbertson C, Loveridge S, Skidmore M, Dyar W (2017) Forecasting state-level premature deaths from alcohol, drugs, and suicides using Google Trends data. J Affect Disord 213:9–15. https://doi.org/10.1016/j.jad.2016.10.038.
Pelat C, Turbelin C, Bar-Hen A et al (2009) More diseases tracked by using Google Trends. Emerg Infect Dis 15:1327

Polgreen PM, Chen Y, Pennock DM et al (2008) Using internet searches for influenza surveillance. Clin Infect Dis 47:1443–1448

Raubenheimer JE (2021) Google Trends extraction tool for Google Trends extended for health data. J Syst Softw 8:100060

Raubenheimer JE, Riordan BC, Merrill JE, Winter T, Ward RM, Scarf D, Buckley NA (2021) Hey Google! will New Zealand vote to legalise cannabis? Using Google Trends data to predict the outcome of the 2020 New Zealand cannabis referendum. Int J Drug Policy 90:103083

Richards TB, Croner CM, Rushton G, Brown CK, Fowler L (1999) Information technology: Geographic information systems and public health: Mapping the future. Public Health Rep 114:359

Salloum RG, Haider MR, Barnett TE et al (2016) Peer reviewed: waterpipe tobacco smoking and susceptibility to cigarette smoking among young adults in the United States, 2012–2013. Prev Chronic Dis 13

Singh S, Sharma P, Balhara YP (2020) The impact of nationwide alcohol ban during the COVID-19 lockdown on alcohol use-related internet searches and behaviour in India: An infodemiology study. Drug Alcohol Rev

Sotis C (2021) How do Google searches for symptoms, news and unemployment interact during COVID-19? A Lotka–Volterra analysis of Google Trends data. Qual Quant:1–6

Stein JD, Childers DM, Nan B, Mian SI (2013) Gauging interest of the general public in Laser Assisted In Situ Keratomileusis (LASIK) eye surgery. Cornea 32:1015

Tabuchi T, Fukui K, Gallus S (2019) Tobacco price increases and population interest in smoking cessation in Japan between 2004 and 2016: a Google Trends analysis. Nicotine Tob Res 21:475–480

Thomson G, Wilson N (2017) Smokefree signage at children's playgrounds: Field observations and comparison with Google Street View. Tob Induc Dis 15:1–4

Tieks A, Troelstra SA, Hoekstra T, Kunst AE (2019) Associations of the Stoptober smoking cessation program with information seeking for smoking cessation: A Google Trends study. Drug Alcohol Depend 194:97–100

Torgerson T, Roberts W, Lester D, Khojasteh J, Vassar M (2020) Public interest in Cannabis during election season: a Google Trends analysis. J Cannabis Res 2:1–8

Troelstra SA, Bosdriesz JR, De Boer MR et al (2016) Effect of tobacco control policies on information seeking for smoking cessation in the Netherlands: a Google Trends study. PLoS One 11:e0148489

Uvais NA (2020) Interests in quitting smoking and alcohol during COVID-19 pandemic in India: A Google Trends study. Psychiatry Clin Neurosci

Valdivia A, Monge-Corella S (2010) Diseases tracked by using Google Trends, Spain. Emerg Infect Dis 16:168

Weiss DJ, Nelson A, Vargas-Ruiz CA, Gligorić K, Bavadekar S, Gabrilovich E, Bertozzi-Villa A, Rozier J, Gibson HS, Shekel T, Kamath C (2020) Global maps of travel time to healthcare facilities. Nat Med 26:1835–1838

Wilson N, Pearson AL, Thomson G et al (2018) Actual and potential use of Google Street View for studying tobacco issues: a brief review. Tob Control 27:339–340

Wilson N, Thomson G (2015) Suboptimal smokefree signage at some hospitals: field observations and the use of Google Street View. N Z Med J 128:56–59

Wilson N, Thomson G, Edwards R (2015) The potential of Google Street View for studying smokefree signage. Aust N Z J Public Health 39:295–296

Yin S, Ho M (2012) Monitoring a toxicological outbreak using Internet search query data. Clin Toxicol 50:818–822

Zhang Z, Zheng X, Zeng DD, Leischow SJ (2016) Tracking dabbing using search query surveillance: a case study in the United States. J Med Internet Res 18:e252

Zheluk A, Quinn C, Meylakhs P (2014) Internet search and krokodil in the Russian Federation: an infoveillance study. J Med Internet Res 16:e212

Alcohol Consumption in Low- and Middle-Income Settings

52

Jane Brandt Sørensen, Shali Tayebi, Amalie Brokhattingen, and Bishal Gyawali

Contents

Introduction 1112
Types of Alcohol Consumed 1114
Urban and Rural Alcohol Consumption 1115
Alcohol and Poverty 1115
Alcohol as a Social Activity 1116
Gender and Alcohol 1117
Effects on Physical and Mental Health 1117
Alcohol's Harm to Others 1119
The Alcohol Treatment Gap 1120
The Alcohol Industry's Interest in LMICs 1120
Current Alcohol Strategies and Policies 1121
Alcohol Research in an LMIC Context 1122
Applications to Other Areas of Addiction/Applications to Other Areas of Substance Use Disorders 1123
Applications to Other Areas of Public Health/Applications to Public Health/Applications to Areas of Public Health 1124
Key Facts of Alcohol Consumption in Low- and Middle-Income Settings 1124
Summary Points 1124
References 1126

Abstract

Whereas many high-income countries (HICs) have seen a decrease in alcohol consumption in recent years, many low- and middle-income countries (LMICs) have seen an increase. Though these countries experience the highest levels of harm from alcohol, including social, financial, physical, and mental health harms, research on alcohol consumption in LMICs is scarce. While alcohol consumption

J. B. Sørensen (✉) · S. Tayebi · A. Brokhattingen · B. Gyawali
Global Health Section, Department of Public Health, University of Copenhagen, Copenhagen, Denmark
e-mail: janebs@sund.ku.dk; kcw118@alumni.ku.dk; qwx929@alumni.ku.dk; bigyawali@sund.ku.dk

V. B. Patel, V. R. Preedy (eds.), *Handbook of Substance Misuse and Addictions*,
https://doi.org/10.1007/978-3-030-92392-1_59

and cultures are context-specific, patterns of consumption in LMIC contexts can be found. Alcohol is closely linked to poverty, and this association is heavier on poorer countries. In many settings, alcohol consumption is linked to masculine behavior, though women are increasingly consuming alcohol in many settings. Illicit alcohol is common in many LMICs, and in conjunction with oftentimes weak alcohol policies, the control of alcohol is limited. The alcohol industry has a profound interest in LMIC alcohol markets.

Keywords

Alcohol · Low- and middle-income countries · Gender-based violence · Alcohol industry · Alcohol policy · Poverty · Illicit alcohol · Alcohol-based research · Alcohol-related harms · Alcohol-related diseases

Abbreviations

AUD	Alcohol use disorders
FASD	Fetal alcohol spectrum disorders
GBV	Gender-based violence
HED	Heavy episodic drinking
HICs	High-income countries
HIV	Human immunodeficiency viruses
LMICs	Low- and middle-income countries
MICs	Middle-income countries
SDGs	Sustainable Development Goals
SSA	Sub-Saharan Africa
SUD	Substance use disorders
TANU	Traditional alcohol nonusers
TAU	Traditional alcohol users
WHO	World Health Organization

Introduction

Alcohol consumption has reduced in many high-income countries (HICs); however, many low- and middle-income countries (LMICs) have seen an increase (World Health Organization 2018a). For example, a modeling study estimated an increase of alcohol consumption by 46.8% in the World Health Organization's (WHO) South-east Asia region and 33.7% in the Western Pacific region between 2017 and 2030 (Manthey et al. 2019). In El Salvador, Guatemala, and Uruguay, the rate of heavy episodic drinking (HED) is twice the global average (Noel 2020). This increase in alcohol consumption in LMICs is primarily due to growing affluence and increased interest from the alcohol industry in playing a role in LMIC alcohol markets (Connor and Hall 2015). Furthermore, tourists from high-consuming HICs visiting LMICs affect alcohol consumption levels and patterns (Cisneros and Room 2014).

Table 1 Consumption of pure alcohol by type in selected LMICs, 2016 (Population aged 15+)

Per capita consumption of pure alcohol, (in liters)	Sri Lanka	India	Nepal	Tanzania	South Africa	Iran
Male	7.7	9.4	3.6	16.0	16.2	1.9
Female	1.2	1.7	0.6	2.9	2.7	0.1
Average	4.3	5.7	2.0	9.4	9.3	1.0
Types of alcoholic beverage consumption as a percentage to the total alcohol consumption						
Beer	13%	8%	31%	12%	56%	–
Wine	<1%	<1%	49%	<1%	18%	–
Spirits	85%	92%	20%	2%	18%	–
Other[a]	2%	–	–	86%	8%	–

Source: Global status report on alcohol and health 2018 (World Health Organization 2018a)
[a]Other beverages include "informal alcohol" such as fortified wines, rice wine, palm wine, or other fermented beverages made of banana, sorghum, millet, or maize

The proportion of per capita alcohol consumption among adults is increasing in LMICs. For instance, alcohol consumption per capita (aged 15+) (in liters of pure alcohol) in Tanzania has increased by over 18% (from 7.7 to 9.4) between 2010 and 2016. Additionally, in India, the amount of alcohol consumed per capita has risen from 4.3 in 2010 to 5.7 in 2016, a 24% increase (World Health Organization 2014, 2018a) (Table 1).

These trends of increasing alcohol consumption in LMICs have apparent implications for alcohol-related harm, considering that the disease burden per liter of alcohol consumed and the highest levels of harm from alcohol are reported in LMICs (World Health Organization 2018a). In addition, the negative impacts of alcohol tend to affect the poorest of the poor disproportionately in LMICs (Schmidt and Room 2014; Rehm et al. 2009a). These individuals more often drink to intoxication and suffer more social and health harms from alcohol (Schmidt and Room 2014).

Harmful alcohol consumption is a significant contributor to the global burden of disease (World Health Organization 2018a). HED is defined as "drinking at least 60 g or more of pure alcohol on at least one occasion in the past 30 days" and is a major indicator for the acute effects of alcohol consumption. The extent of harmful consumption of alcohol in Tanzania was very high when compared to other selected LMICs (Table 2). A total of 20.3% of the people aged ≥15 years had HED in Tanzania in 2016 (Table 2). The HED was more among males (33.4%) when compared to females (7.7%) in Tanzania.

The distribution of alcohol across LMICs is heterogeneous, and the way alcohol is valued and perceived is context-specific. For instance, alcohol consumption rates are lower in countries adherent to the Islamic faith such as in North Africa and the Middle East. Such contextual differences in alcohol consumption make it difficult to generalize. However, we do see some trends. Whereas alcohol is mostly consumed by middle-aged men and women in HICs, it is consumed by fewer adults in LMICs (Smyth et al. 2015). Furthermore, several factors make it difficult to estimate alcohol consumption rates in many LMICs. First, in many LMIC settings, alcohol

Table 2 Harmful consumption of alcohol in LMICs, 2016

Harmful consumption of alcohol	Sri Lanka	India	Nepal	Tanzania	South Africa	Iran
HED, past 30 days (%)						
Male	16.6	28.4	17.9	33.4	30.6	0.3
Female	2.4	5.4	2.8	7.7	6.5	0.0
Both sexes	9.1	17.2	9.9	20.3	18.3	0.1
AUDs, 12-month prevalence (%)						
Males	5.9	9.1	3.1	11.5	12.4	1.8
Females	0.7	0.5	0.6	2.2	1.8	0.1
Both sexes	3.1	4.9	1.8	6.8	7.0	1.0

Source: Global status report on alcohol and health 2018 (World Health Organization 2018a)

consumption is primarily a male activity, and there are thus much larger gender differences identified in LMICs than in HICs. This also means that statistics based on averages in LMICs underestimate alcohol drinking among men. Second, illicit alcohol is widespread in many LMIC settings. For example, around one-third of the alcohol consumed in Africa is unrecorded, illicit alcohol making it difficult to estimate actual consumption rates (Ferreira-Borges et al. 2017). This also means that initiatives that have proved useful in HICs, such as taxation and pricing of alcohol, cannot stand alone in many LMIC settings. Third, in some LMICs, there is a high abstinence rate overall, so those who do consume alcohol do so at much higher levels than often indicated in numbers (Walls et al. 2020).

Types of Alcohol Consumed

According to the WHO, one-quarter of all alcohol consumed globally is undocumented, informal, and often illicit alcohol (World Health Organization 2018a). Informal alcohol is not recorded under any official statistics as it is produced and distributed outside of formal systems, making actual alcohol consumption estimates difficult to establish as can be documented in Table 1. Both in Sri Lanka and India, industrially produced liquor and artisanal unrecorded beverages are commonly used (Rehm et al. 2014). Though hard to tell from the official numbers in Table 1, in Sri Lanka's rural and poor urban areas, the preferred alcohol is the illicitly produced "kassipu" (Gamburd 2008). A qualitative study of men's alcohol consumption in Sri Lanka found that the availability of financial means influenced the choice of consumption, and kassipu "gave value for money" and was thus the preferred choice when money was low (Sørensen et al. 2019). A nationally representative household survey in Nepal found that the majority of women in Nepal (95.9%) consume home-brewed alcohol (Thapa et al. 2016). In Iran, a civil alcohol policy of prohibition emplaced after the Islamic revolution in 1979 transformed the country from being a well-known producer of alcohol in the Middle East to have a ban on alcohol production, trade, and consumption for the Muslim majority population

(Al-Ansari et al. 2019). Subsequently, alcohol legally produced for medical purposes and homemade, illicit alcohol became a major source of alcohol consumption for leisure (Sanaei-Zadeh et al. 2011). While unrecorded alcohol is widespread in many LMICs, commercially produced alcohol tends to gain a higher status. Thus, illegal alcoholic beverages are often replaced when individuals have the resources to do so (Schmidt and Room 2014). Choices of alcohol thus symbolize social divisions and help create them (Schmidt and Room 2014). Generally, young adult men seem to be most ready to embrace new drinking practices (Schmidt and Room 2014). A qualitative study from Sri Lanka found how symbolic capital was expressed through the choice of alcohol, which was especially important to young, male consumers (Sørensen et al. 2019).

Urban and Rural Alcohol Consumption

Patterns of alcohol consumption seem to differ between urban and rural areas though mechanisms behind such differences may vary between nations and contexts. In Nepal, rural dwellers were more likely to use alcohol than their urban counterparts (World Health Organization 2004). On the contrary, a study exploring alcohol consumption in India found a higher prevalence of alcohol use among older adults in urban areas compared to rural ones (Nadkarni et al. 2013). Likewise, a study examining urban and rural consumption in Mongolia found drinking to be higher in urban dwellers than in rural ones (Demaio et al. 2013). These latter findings were linked to the social and epidemiological transition. As Mongolians become more rich and urbanized and have alcohol more readily available, their consumption rises, even though their knowledge about the harms from alcohol is high (Demaio et al. 2013). The shift of marketing toward Western-style branding of alcohol in the past few decades and its urban association with celebration and social gatherings have also promoted its versatile consumption (Demaio et al. 2013). This is also the case in both Nepal and Sri Lanka where alcohol is often viewed as a status symbol and it is considered incomplete when no alcoholic beverages are served during parties, get-togethers, and festive occasions (Dhital et al. 2001; Sørensen et al. 2019).

Alcohol and Poverty

Alcohol consumption has been found to exacerbate poverty. A persistent pattern of alcohol use and diminished individual and family financial outcomes has been reported across LMICs (Grittner et al. 2012). In Nepal, the use and misuse of alcohol is associated with lower socioeconomic status, placing a financial burden on affected families (Sharma et al. 2020). Alcohol consumption also affects the workforce and economy in LMICs (Laslett et al. 2019). For instance, for heavy drinkers, the drinking may reduce employability and social standing. Unemployment can lead to alcohol abuse, which again can lead to crime, and the combination of crime and alcohol abuse worsens employability chances (Schafer and Koyiet 2018). The

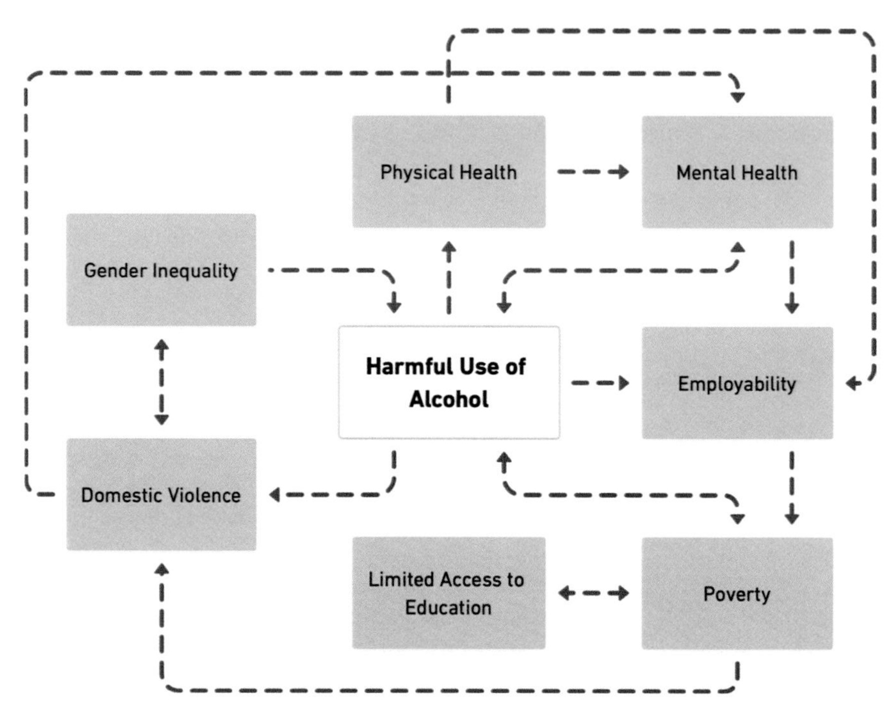

Fig. 1 Conceptual framework of selected dynamics associated with the harmful use of alcohol

burden of this vicious circle of alcohol and poverty as well as other dynamics is visualized in Fig. 1. These consequences are heavier on poorer countries, where families are often faced with challenges in attaining basic needs.

Alcohol as a Social Activity

Alcohol consumption is closely linked to several aspects of social life and is often characterized by intertwined normative codes of conduct that differ according to sociocultural conditions. The social role of alcohol thus differs according to historically embedded culture and traditional social practices, which can be significantly diverse, even within national and local borders. In most LMICs, particularly in rural areas, there is a limited bar and pub culture, and alcohol consumption as a social activity is, therefore, more common within community settings (Walls et al. 2020). In some settings, alcohol consumption is the very center of many social activities and deeply embedded in cultural and social practices, where men often are more likely to engage in drinking than women. For instance, in Sri Lanka, alcohol is often not only used as a stress-releasing substance but also as a means to socialize with other men after long working hours of often hard manual labor (Sørensen et al. 2019). In Nepal, the society can be divided into two ethnic groups, based on their social views on alcohol: traditional alcohol nonusers (TANU) (higher-castes) and traditional alcohol users (TAU) (lower castes and other ethnic and tribal groups) (Parajuli et al. 2015). TAU have traditionally used alcohol as an important part of traditional ceremonies and celebrations, including both consumption and production of alcohol. On the contrary, alcohol consumption has been highly stigmatized and culturally prohibited among the TANU, particularly for women. This categorization is historically embedded and still impacts the views on alcohol as well as the consumption pattern in contemporary Nepal, where alcohol consumption is still significantly more widespread among TAU (Adhikari et al. 2019; Parajuli et al. 2015).

Gender and Alcohol

In LMICs, women tend to consume alcohol less often than men. In settings where patriarchal norms place men in positions of power, higher levels of men's alcohol use have been reported, in conjunction with negative consequences for other men, women, and children (World Health Organization 2007). A difference is often seen between rural and urban areas, where the gender divide is more apparent in rural areas. This gender difference in alcohol consumption is, for instance, seen in Nepal, where men engage more often than women in HED (Adhikari et al. 2019; World Health Organization 2018a). When women do drink alcohol, they drink fewer quantities than men (World Health Organization 2018a). However, while women's drinking went down in most regions in 2018, it went up in Southeast Asia and Western Pacific regions (World Health Organization 2018a). A nationally representative population-based study in Nepal reported that alcohol consumption was a common practice also among Nepalese women, in particular, those from the Janajati ethnic group, who had a primary school education, whose husbands consumed alcohol, and who were from households that produced alcohol (Thapa et al. 2016). Also, the gap between men and women's heavy alcohol consumption is narrowing in sub-Saharan Africa (SSA) due to increased availability of alcohol, changes in women's role in society, and targeted marketing strategies (Ferreira-Borges et al. 2017).

Effects on Physical and Mental Health

Alcohol use is related to a wide variety of negative health outcomes, including morbidity, mortality, and disability. According to the WHO Global Alcohol Report 2018, the alcohol-attributable disease burden was highest in low-income and lower middle-income countries in 2016 when compared to upper middle-income and HICs (World Health Organization 2018a). This report also noted that harmful alcohol use had been linked to mortality from liver cirrhosis, road traffic injuries, and cancer in LMICs. Table 3 shows the age-standardized death rates from liver cirrhosis, road traffic injuries, and cancer in selected LMICs. Indeed, alcohol has become the single largest behavioral risk factor for disease, disability, and mortality in LMICs. The

Table 3 Health consequences by alcohol use in LMICs, 2016

Age-standardized death rates (per 100,000 population)	Sri Lanka	India	Nepal	Tanzania	South Africa	Iran
Males	Liver cirrhosis: 57.4	Liver cirrhosis: 45.8	Liver cirrhosis: 39.9	Liver cirrhosis: 34.7	Liver cirrhosis: 28.9	Liver cirrhosis: 11.4
	Road traffic injuries: 35.4	Road traffic injuries: 50.3	Road traffic injuries: 38.3	Road traffic injuries: 82.7	Road traffic injuries: 42.2	Road traffic injuries: 54.8
	Cancer: 135.4	Cancer: 107.2	Cancer: 107.6	Cancer: 155.8	Cancer: 223.0	Cancer: 153.2
Females	Liver cirrhosis: 9.7	Liver cirrhosis: 14.7	Liver cirrhosis: 15.3	Liver cirrhosis: 27.4	Liver cirrhosis: 9.9	Liver cirrhosis: 7.7
	Road traffic injuries: 9.3	Road traffic injuries: 10.3	Road traffic injuries: 16.0	Road traffic injuries: 33.3	Road traffic injuries: 13.5	Road traffic injuries: 17.7
	Cancer: 99.1	Cancer: 95.3	Cancer: 105.0	Cancer: 136.6	Cancer: 143.8	Cancer: 111.9

Source: Global status report on alcohol and health 2018 (World Health Organization 2018a)

health impact of harmful alcohol use might be different in LMICs compared to HICs since it interacts with other risk factors – for example, alcohol in combination with infectious diseases such as HIV and TB (Imtiaz et al. 2017). One large, prospective cohort study reported that alcohol consumption was associated with a 38% increased risk of a combination of clinical outcomes, including mortality, cardiovascular disease, stroke, heart attack, cancer, injury, and admission to hospital in LMICs (Smyth et al. 2015). Further, heavier drinking patterns, as seen in many LMICs, for example, SSA, are linked with several aspects of HIV, for example, unsafe sex (Rehm et al. 2012; Shuper et al. 2010), reduced adherence to treatment (Imtiaz et al. 2017), immune system impairment, and drug interactions. Gender-specific adverse effects of alcohol, including fetal alcohol spectrum disorders (FASD) resulting from alcohol drinking during pregnancy, are a common issue in some settings (Ferreira-Borges et al. 2017). For example, in South Africa, alcohol use is common during pregnancy where women consider drinking as a coping strategy for their socioeconomic and sociopolitical realities, which may cause a wide range of adverse health effects to the fetus, including FASD (Adebiyi et al. 2019). The prevalence of FASD in South Africa is among the highest in the world, varying from 29 to 290 per 1000 live births (Adebiyi et al. 2019). The consumption of homemade or illicit alcohol can be associated with an increased risk of harm because of potential impurities or contaminants (Ferreira-Borges et al. 2017). For instance, in a study from India, unrecorded alcohol consumption was found to be associated with an increased risk of alcoholic liver disease, in particular, cirrhosis of the liver (Narawane et al. 1998). A number of risks were also identified in consuming illicit alcohol in Sri Lanka, including highly toxic methanol and deliberate adulteration with a number of pesticides in Sri Lanka (Dias 2011). Likewise, alcohol use disorders (AUDs), including alcohol dependence and harmful pattern of alcohol use, are highly prevalent mental health conditions associated with significant morbidity and mortality in LMICs. For instance, South Africa had a significantly higher rate of AUDs in 2016 than that of other selected LMICs, with 12.4% of males and 1.8% of females aged $\geq$15 years having AUDs (Table 2).

As in the rest of the world, alcohol consumption and suicide are closely linked with LMICs (World Health Organization 2018a). A number of studies have emphasized the significance of alcohol's role in self-harm and suicide in Sri Lanka. For instance, studies have documented how a large number of men were intoxicated with alcohol at the time of self-harm (Rajapakse et al. 2013) i.e. a prospective study of 79 patients showed that about 50% of men and a few women were under the influence of alcohol at the time of self-harm (Eddleston et al. 1999). Further, a comparison of nonfatal self-poisoning, using pesticides, among Sri Lankan men and women found hazardous drinking or AUD among more than one-third of 419 men (Rajapakse et al. 2014). This connection has been explained in several ways: (i) the harmful use of alcohol can cause a range of problems to a household; (ii) the harmful use of alcohol has been associated with interpersonal conflict leading up to self-harm (de Alwis 2012; Konradsen et al. 2006; Sørensen et al. 2017), with alcohol exaggerating emotions such as shame and anger, thereby spurring self-harm (Gamburd 2008); (iii) alcohol impairs judgment when self-harming through ingestion of pesticides, making individuals underestimate the amount consumed (Eddleston et al. 1999); and (iv) difficulties in clinically managing individuals intoxicated by both alcohol and pesticides (Eddleston et al. 2009).

Alcohol's Harm to Others

The consequences of alcohol often extend beyond the individual to impact families, friends, and communities. Such harm from alcohol consumption is context-specific and changes over time (Laslett et al. 2019). Harm from alcohol drinking has been found to be more significant for poorer drinkers and their families than for richer drinkers in any given society (Schmidt and Room 2012). Contextual factors likely to disadvantage individuals of lower socioeconomic status regarding alcohol-attributable harm include crowded living arrangements, lack of sanitation, and a higher likelihood of social conflict environment (Rehm et al. 2009b).

Vulnerable population groups are more likely to suffer from others' alcohol consumption, for example, children. A retrospective cross-sectional study including 1501 adults in Vietnam showed that having a heavy drinker in the family was associated with a high risk of reporting at least one specific harm to children (Laslett et al. 2019). The most common harm was verbal abuse, followed by witnessing serious domestic violence. Lower-income families reported more severe negative effects to children from others' drinking than children from high-income families (Laslett et al. 2019).

A strong predictor of experiencing intimate partner violence or gender-based violence is a partner's alcohol abuse (Abrahams et al. 2004). Kenya has one of the highest rates of gender-based violence in the world (Schafer and Koyiet 2018). A study found that 41% of Kenyan women had experienced physical or sexual assault by their intimate partners at least once in their lives (Kenya National Bureau of Statistics and ICF Macro 2010), with alcohol abuse being one of the major contributors (Schafer et al. 2013; Schafer 2014). A cross-sectional study, conducted in the antenatal and postnatal care clinics of a governmental hospital in Kathmandu, in Nepal, found that independently of sociodemographic status, women who were married to men using alcohol were twice as likely to experience domestic violence compared to women who were married to men who did *not* use alcohol (Bhatta et al. 2021). Among the women who suffered from physical, psychological, and sexual violence during the pregnancy and postpartum periods, 70.2%, 67.9%, and 64.2%, respectively, experienced violence due to their husband's drinking habits (Bhatta et al. 2021).

The Alcohol Treatment Gap

Most LMICs have scarce and limited treatment available for alcohol dependence, if at all (World Health Organization 2018a). Service systems for the treatment of AUDs are, when available, mainly located in the tertiary systems in urban areas and usually require high fees. In combination with long waiting times, this means that many individuals go untreated. Nepal's large treatment gap of 94.9% has stemmed from the unaffordability of care, the stigma around being perceived as weak or having mental health problems, or feeling too unwell to seek support (Luitel et al. 2017). Substance use and mental health services can be integrated into primary care to address service needs that emphasizes problem identification, monitoring, short-term interventions, and specialty referrals when needed (Shidhaye et al. 2015). It should be noted, however, that most alcohol-related harm stems from hazardous or harmful drinking, not dependence. Harmful drinking often goes undetected and untreated for long periods in LMICs, though brief and easily delivered interventions exist (Benegal et al. 2009). There is a significant need to implement contextualized community-based interventions targeting moderate alcohol use as well (Walls et al. 2020).

The Alcohol Industry's Interest in LMICs

The alcohol industry is increasingly interested in getting access to markets in LMICs. For instance, South Africa has been a target of the alcohol industry's aim to develop markets in Africa (Ferreira-Borges et al. 2017). Here, international brands are promoted with a message of modernity and prosperity and thus social status.

Further, marketing has focused on encouraging alcohol drinking among women who are typically drinking at relatively low rates in many LMIC settings and young people, with the hope they will adopt heavy drinking patterns (Walls et al. 2020). In India, an alcohol marketing focus has also been on the emerging middle class for growth opportunities (Esser and Jernigan 2015). The industry has been found to tap into contexts where alcohol is most often a male practice related to masculinity. For example, a study by Mager et al. found that the alcohol industry in South Africa focused on masculinity and nationalism to develop a culture where alcohol got even further associated with what it means to be a man (Mager 2005). The alcohol industry is increasingly using digital marketing platforms, such as websites and social media, to reach new markets (Noel et al. 2020).

Current Alcohol Strategies and Policies

There is evidence that alcohol policies related to pricing and availability of alcohol as well as advertising bans are effective strategies to reduce alcohol-related harm. Though large informal alcohol markets exist in many LMICs, such policies have still been linked to lower alcohol consumption (Cook et al. 2014). The number of countries with a written national alcohol policy is steadily increasing, however, primarily among HICs (67%) compared to LMICs (15%) (World Health Organization 2018a). While most countries have some type of restrictions on beer advertising, half of WHO countries reported no restrictions on the Internet and social media. A total of 35 countries had no regulations of any type of media, especially countries in SSA and the Americas.

There are several examples of the alcohol industry seeking to influence national alcohol policymaking, which thus occurs in a context where many LMICs do not have policies to deal with the expansion of the alcohol market. A historical paper on the implementation of an alcohol policy in Thailand showed the continuous, synchronized efforts of the alcohol industry to disable or reduce the strength of a proposed alcohol control law (Sornpaisarn and Rehm 2020). There are also examples of how the alcohol industry promotes partnerships with governments to influence national alcohol policies (Bakke and Endal 2010). Several SSA country alcohol policy documents were, e.g., found to reflect industry interests while they ignored population-based interventions (Bakke and Endal 2010).

Concerted alcohol policy actions are required to reduce alcohol consumption in LMICs (Buse et al. 2017), and it has been noted how effective alcohol control measures are especially important for countries undergoing rapid economic development (Rose et al. 2015). In that connection, the interplay between alcohol and tourism should be considered. Many LMICs are reliant on tourism from HICs with an often wide cultural and financial gap between the visitors and host society. It has been documented how tourists' heavy drinking impacts the host society in a number of ways, including increased consumption levels especially among young people working within the tourism sector (Cisneros and Room 2014). As for the alcohol industry, there are examples of the tourism industry having successfully influenced

LMIC national alcohol policies to become or remain looser (Cisneros and Room 2014).

In some LMIC settings, abolishment of alcohol is high on the agenda, and the policy approach of prohibition has become ingrained in several countries as a social and cultural norm (Sharma et al. 2020). For instance, in Iran, alcohol policy strategies are influenced by treating alcohol consumption as both a public health issue and a criminal act (Al-Ansari et al. 2019). In Sri Lanka, a government aim of eliminating alcohol, drug, and tobacco use (Ministry of Health, Nutrition and Indigenous Medicine, Sri Lanka 2016) is in line with Buddhist and Sinhala values where the aim is to abstain from substances contaminating the mind and body, including meat, tobacco, and alcohol (Gombrich and Obeyesekere 1988). However, such an approach of abolishment of alcohol is complicated by several factors: (i) it does not acknowledge the social components deeply ingrained in many alcohol consumption activities, (ii) it might push individuals into using more illicit alcohol as well as riskier behavior using uncontrolled substances, (iii) and it results in under-reporting of alcohol consumption and associated harms.

While alcohol research in HIC has primarily focused on market-based sources, alcohol policy in LMICs needs to consider a wider context of consumption, including both legal and illegal sources of alcohol. Thus, official alcohol regulation and enforcement typically applied to control alcohol can often not stand alone in LMIC contexts where the majority of what is consumed is illicit (Walls et al. 2020). Culturally appropriate interventions are needed. In Sri Lanka, a setting where illicit alcohol is widespread, a participatory pilot study found that collaboration with communities through an edutainment approach gave them the skills and direction to make sustainable changes in reducing alcohol use and associated harms and improve mental health (Siriwardhana et al. 2012). Instead of focusing on the complete elimination of alcohol drinking through abstinence – a message that is unrealistic to achieve in settings with high alcohol use – a message was given to cut down on harmful and dependent patterns of drinking to gain physical, emotional, and other benefits. Such gain-framed messages led to the overall reduction of consumption (Siriwardhana et al. 2012).

Alcohol Research in an LMIC Context

The research needs associated with alcohol use are large and multidimensional and the complexity of alcohol in many LMICs requires special research attention. So far, much alcohol research has been focused on the relatively stable and formalized alcohol cultures in HICs, including market-based sources (Walls et al. 2020). The context in which people consume alcohol, perceptions of drinking, and problem drinking differ (Savic et al. 2016), and research reflecting this is, therefore, warranted. For example, we know little about the influence of broader ecological factors on alcohol use in LMICs (Giusto and Puffer 2018). Alcohol data in LMICs is more likely than HICs to lack quality and come from small-scale studies. Methods and metrics to obtain knowledge about alcohol environments in HICs need to be developed and tailored to an LMIC setting (Walls et al. 2020) and More epidemiological studies of patterns of alcohol consumption and health outcomes are warranted (Connor and Hall 2015). Further, holistic alcohol research focused on the complex dynamics of alcohol consumption in LMICs is needed, including the diverse range of alcohol sources, the often many distribution channels, and advertising and marketing strategies, while considering the coexistence of both licit and illicit alcohol sources of alcohol (Walls et al. 2020). Similarly, community-based interventions that generally incorporate individual and environmental change strategies have proven to be successful and can result in significant reductions in alcohol consumption and harms regardless of state regulations (Siriwardhana et al. 2012). There is potential for relatively large benefits from such interventions at the population level (Sorensen et al. 1998), and they might be particularly helpful in contexts where there is no specific regulatory framework for alcohol. Finally, more systematic work is needed in regard to tourism's impact on alcohol drinking in LMICs (Cisneros and Room 2014).

Applications to Other Areas of Addiction/Applications to Other Areas of Substance Use Disorders

In this chapter, we have reviewed alcohol consumption in LMICs. While countries experiencing rapid economic development see increased alcohol consumption, they are also increasingly affected by different types of drug use. An Indian study showed that societal changes influenced opportunities and financial resources available to adolescence and thus their consumption patterns (Chowdhury et al. 2006), and a qualitative study of Sri Lankan men's alcohol consumption found that especially young men in semi-urban areas experimented with a range of substances in combination with alcohol (Sørensen et al. 2019). In Nepal, a study reported that young adults from urban areas exhibited significant alcohol consumption and other drug uses that led to mental disorders and substance use disorders (SUDs) (Gyawali et al. 2016). In the study, 51.1% of individuals with SUDs reported high levels of psychological distress. Unfortunately, a number of barriers have limited the existing SUD treatment and prevention services in Nepal, including lack of mental health legislation, insufficient resources, insufficient training, highly expensive treatment, and a shortage of workforce (Rai et al. 2021). Furthermore, underdiagnosed and undertreated SUDs remain salient among those rural residents and those with low income in Nepal. As we have highlighted, many LMICs are challenged by the alcohol industry's interference in government policies. This is similar to the tobacco and unhealthy food industries, using the same tactics to interfere in policies, which is especially effective in contexts of poor governance (Tangcharoensathien et al. 2019). The global community managed to agree on the Framework Convention on Tobacco Control (FCTC), a framework that can be applied to other harmful products, such as alcohol (Tangcharoensathien et al. 2019).

Applications to Other Areas of Public Health/Applications to Public Health/Applications to Areas of Public Health

In this review, we focused on alcohol consumption in LMICs, though it should be highlighted how alcohol is a prime example of a cross-cutting risk factor to global health. The Sustainable Development Goal (SDG) 3, Target 3.5 specifically pertains to alcohol use, in particular to: "strengthen the prevention and treatment of substance abuse, including narcotic drug abuse and harmful use of alcohol" (World Health Organization 2020). The key indicators are 3.5.1, the coverage of treatment interventions (pharmacological, psychosocial, and rehabilitation and aftercare services) for SUDs (including AUDs), and 3.5.2, harmful use of alcohol (per capita consumption of pure alcohol) during a calendar year. Furthermore, alcohol consumption directly relates to a range of health-related indicators, including child health and road injuries. Reducing the harms from alcohol consumption in the LMIC context thus requires a broad focus on a number of other public health issue areas as well. For example, the differences in alcohol consumption and associated harms between settings relate to SDG10, calling for action to reduce inequalities between and within countries. Further, as we have noted, alcohol is closely linked to poverty, and thus SDG1 related to economic and social development (World Health Organization 2020). Similarly, as NCDs are also increasingly becoming a public health concern in LMICs (World Health Organization 2018b), there is a need to take concentrated, inclusive action to address the most prevalent causes of NCDs. Given the overwhelming evidence that alcohol use is linked to major NCDs also in LMICs, it is important to focus on the factors affecting alcohol consumption, especially of heavy and illicit use and particularly those operating on a social and environmental level, using strategies that have been proven to be effective (Parry et al. 2011). An overview of alcohol consumption and the SDGs can be found in Fig. 2.

Key Facts of Alcohol Consumption in Low- and Middle-Income Settings

- Alcohol-attributable disease burden is most prevalent in low-income and lower middle-income countries when compared to upper middle-income and HICs.
- Harmful alcohol consumption is linked to a wide range of health problems, including liver diseases, road accidents and violence, as well as cancers, cardiovascular diseases, suicides, HIV and TB in LMICs.
- The research needs associated with alcohol use are large and multidimensional in LMICs.

Summary Points

- Alcohol consumption differs between LMICs and HICs, and whereas alcohol consumption has reduced in many HICs, many LMICs have seen an increase.

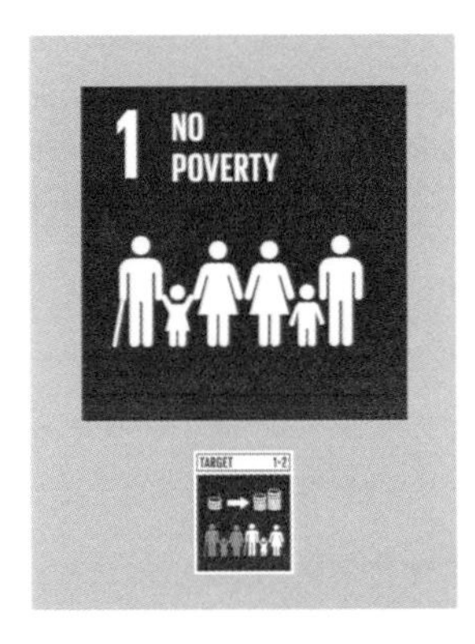

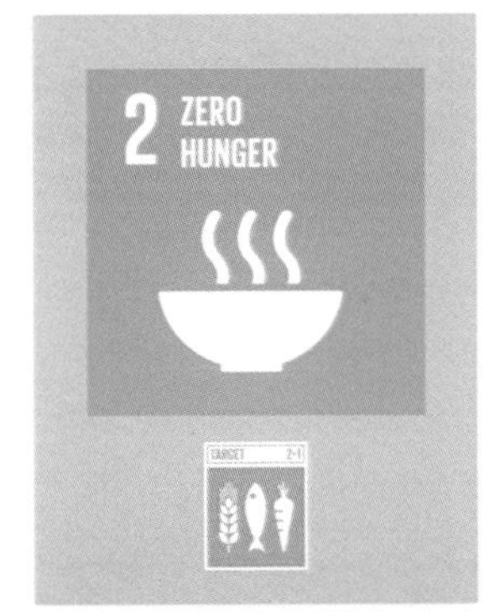

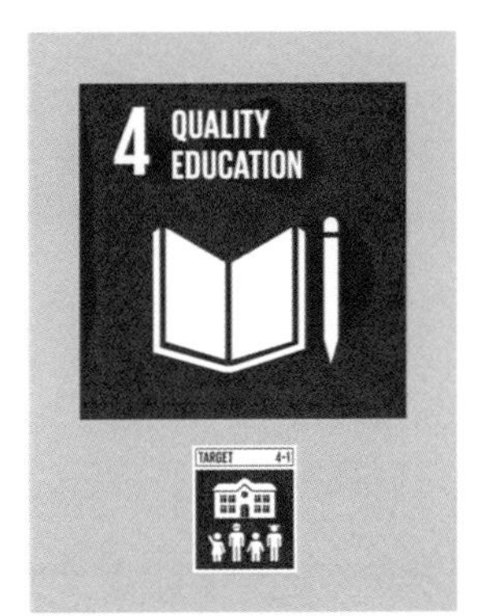

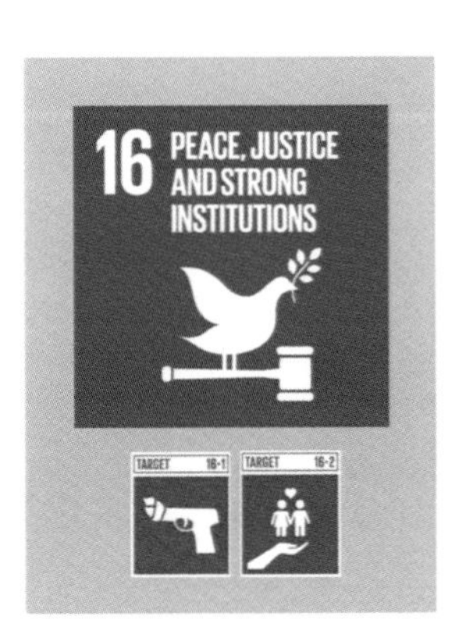

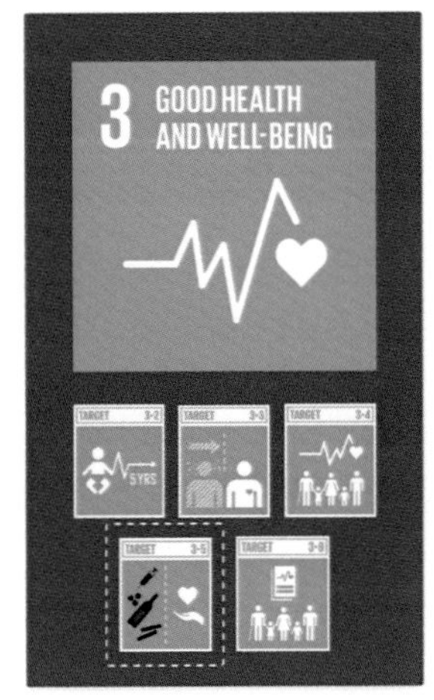

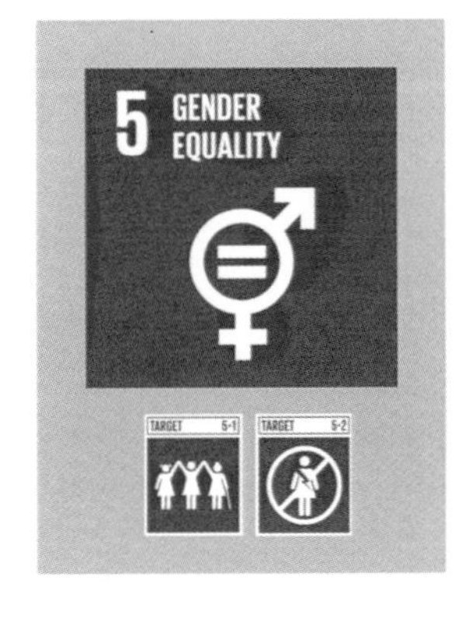

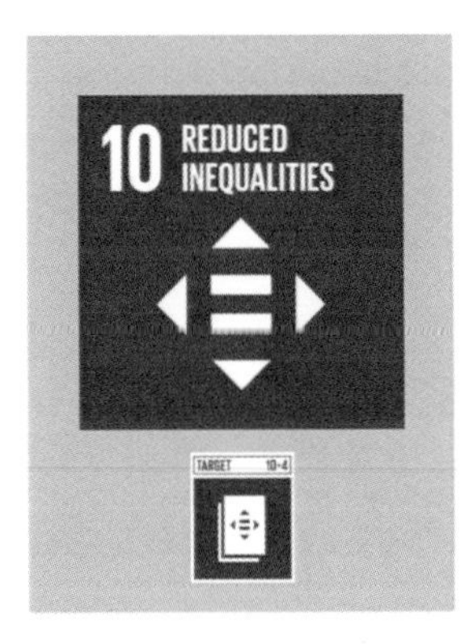

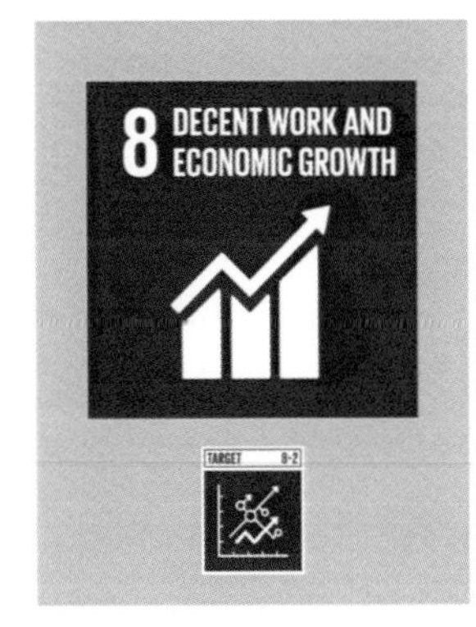

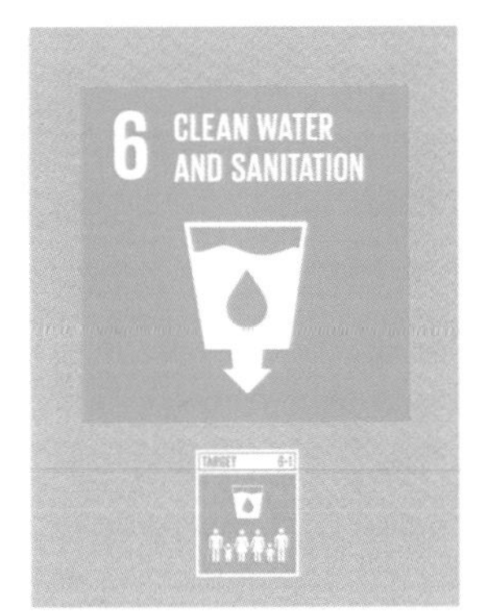

Fig. 2 An overview of alcohol consumption and the sustainable development goals. (Source: World Health Organization 2020)

- LMICs experience the highest levels of harm from alcohol, including social, financial, physical, and mental health harms.
- Research on alcohol consumption in LMICs is scarce.

- Alcohol is closely linked to poverty, and this association is profound in LMICs.
- Illicit alcohol is common in many LMIC settings, and regulation and enforcement typically applied to control alcohol can often not stand alone in LMIC contexts.
- The alcohol industry has a profound interest in getting access to LMIC alcohol markets.
- The oftentimes missing or weak alcohol policies in LMICs make the control of alcohol limited.

References

Abrahams N, Jewkes R, Hoffman M, Laubsher R (2004) Sexual violence against intimate partners in Cape Town: prevalence and risk factors reported by men. Bull World Health Organ 82:330

Adebiyi BO, Mukumbang FC, Beytell A-M (2019) To what extent is fetal alcohol spectrum disorder considered in policy-related documents in South Africa? A document review. Health Res Policy Syst 17(1):46. https://doi.org/10.1186/s12961-019-0447-9

Adhikari TB, Rijal A, Kallestrup P, Neupane D (2019) Alcohol consumption pattern in western Nepal: findings from the COBIN baseline survey. BMC Psychiatry 19:283. https://doi.org/10.1186/s12888-019-2264-7

Al-Ansari B, Thow A-M, Mirzaie M, Day CA, Conigrave KM (2019) Alcohol policy in Iran: policy content analysis. Int J Drug Policy 73:185–198. https://doi.org/10.1016/j.drugpo.2019.07.032

Bakke Ã, Endal D (2010) Vested interests in addiction research and policy alcohol policies out of context: drinks industry supplanting government role in alcohol policies in sub-Saharan Africa: alcohol policies out of context. Addiction 105:22–28. https://doi.org/10.1111/j.1360-0443.2009.02695.x

Benegal V, Chand PK, Obot IS (2009) Packages of care for alcohol use disorders in low- and middle-income countries. PLoS Med 6:e1000170. https://doi.org/10.1371/journal.pmed.1000170

Bhatta N, Assanangkornchai S, Rajbhandari I (2021) Does husband's alcohol consumption increase the risk of domestic violence during the pregnancy and postpartum periods in Nepalese women? BMC Public Health 21:5. https://doi.org/10.1186/s12889-020-10021-y

Buse K, Tanaka S, Hawkes S (2017) Healthy people and healthy profits? Elaborating a conceptual framework for governing the commercial determinants of non-communicable diseases and identifying options for reducing risk exposure. Glob Health 13:34. https://doi.org/10.1186/s12992-017-0255-3

Chowdhury AN, Ramakrishna J, Chakraborty AK, Weiss MG (2006) Cultural context and impact of alcohol use in the Sundarban Delta, West Bengal, India. Soc Sci Med 63(3):722–731. https://doi.org/10.1016/j.socscimed.2006.02.006

Cisneros J, Room R (2014) Impacts of tourism on drinking and alcohol policy in low- and middle-income countries: a selective thematic review. Contempor Drug Probl 41:145–176

Connor JP, Hall W (2015) Alcohol burden in low-income and middle-income countries. Lancet 386:1922–1924. https://doi.org/10.1016/S0140-6736(15)00236-6

Cook WK, Bond J, Greenfield TK (2014) Are alcohol policies associated with alcohol consumption in low- and middle-income countries? Alcohol policies in LAMICs. Addiction 109:1081–1090. https://doi.org/10.1111/add.12571

de Alwis M (2012) 'Girl still burning inside my head': reflections on suicide in Sri Lanka. Contrib Indian Sociol 46:29–51. https://doi.org/10.1177/006996671104600203

Demaio AR, Dugee O, de Courten M, Bygbjerg IC, Enkhtuya P, Meyrowitsch DW (2013) Exploring knowledge, attitudes, and practices related to alcohol in Mongolia: a national population-based survey. BMC Public Health 13:178. https://doi.org/10.1186/1471-2458-13-178

Dhital R, Subedi G, Gurung YB, Hamal P (2001) Alcohol and drug use in Nepal with reference to children. Child Workers in Nepal Concerned Centre (CWIN), Kathmandu

Dias (2011) Paraquat used as a catalyst to increase the percentage of alcohol distillated in illicit brewing industry of Sri Lanka. Advanced Journal of Microbiology Research

Eddleston M, Ariaratnam CA, Meyer WP, Perera G, Kularatne AM, Attapattu S, Sheriff MHR, Warrell DA (1999) Epidemic of self-poisoning with seeds of the yellow oleander tree (Thevetia peruviana) in northern Sri Lanka. Tropical Med Int Health 4:266–273

Eddleston M, Gunnell D, von Meyer L, Eyer P (2009) Relationship between blood alcohol concentration on admission and outcome in dimethoate organophosphorus self-poisoning. Br J Clin Pharmacol 68:916–919. https://doi.org/10.1111/j.1365-2125.2009.03533.x

Esser MB, Jernigan DH (2015) Multinational alcohol market development and public health: Diageo in India. Am J Public Health 105:2220–2227. https://doi.org/10.2105/AJPH.2015.302831

Ferreira-Borges C, Parry C, Babor T (2017) Harmful use of alcohol: a shadow over Sub-Saharan Africa in need of workable solutions. Int J Environ Res Public Health 14:346. https://doi.org/10.3390/ijerph14040346

Gamburd M (2008) Breaking the ashes – the culture of illicit liquor in Sri Lanka. Cornell University Press, Ithaca

Giusto A, Puffer E (2018) A systematic review of interventions targeting men's alcohol use and family relationships in low- and middle-income countries. Glob Ment Health 5:e10. https://doi.org/10.1017/gmh.2017.32

Gombrich R, Obeyesekere G (1988) Buddhism transformed: religious change in Sri Lanka. Motilal Banarsidass, Delhi

Grittner U, Kuntsche S, Graham K, Bloomfield K (2012) Social inequalities and gender differences in the experience of alcohol-related problems. Alcohol Alcohol 47:597–605. https://doi.org/10.1093/alcalc/ags040

Gyawali B, Choulagai BP, Paneru DP, Ahmad M, Leppin A, Kallestrup P (2016) Prevalence and correlates of psychological distress symptoms among patients with substance use disorders in drug rehabilitation centers in urban Nepal: a cross-sectional study. BMC Psychiatry 16(1):314

Imtiaz S, Shield KD, Roerecke M, Samokhvalov AV, Lönnroth K, Rehm J (2017) Alcohol consumption as a risk factor for tuberculosis: meta-analyses and burden of disease. Eur Respir J 50:1700216. https://doi.org/10.1183/13993003.00216-2017

Kenya National Bureau of Statistics (KNBS) and ICF Macro (2010) Kenya demographic and health survey 2008–09. KNBS and ICF Macro, Calverton

Konradsen F, Hoek W, Peiris P (2006) Reaching for the bottle of pesticide – a cry for help. Self-inflicted poisonings in Sri Lanka. Soc Sci Med 2006:1710–1719. https://doi.org/10.1016/j.socscimed.2005.08.020

Laslett A-M, Room R, Waleewong O, Stanesby O, Callinan S, World Health Organization, Department of Mental Health and Substance Abuse (2019) Harm to others from drinking: patterns in nine societies. World Health Organization, Department of Mental Health and Substance Abuse, Geneva

Leo Burnett Bangkok and Thai Health Promotion Foundation (2020) Thai health promotion foundation: replacing alcohol bottle. https://www.bestadsontv.com/ad/117404/Thai-Health-Promotion-Foundation-Replacing-Alcohol-Bottle

Luitel NP, Jordans MJD, Kohrt BA, Rathod SD, Komproe IH (2017) Treatment gap and barriers for mental health care: a cross-sectional community survey in Nepal. PLoS One 12:e0183223. https://doi.org/10.1371/journal.pone.0183223

Mager A (2005) 'One beer, one goal, one nation, one soul': south African breweries, heritage, masculinity and nationalism 1960–1999*. Past Present 188:163–194. https://doi.org/10.1093/pastj/gti021

Manthey J, Shield KD, Rylett M, Hasan OSM, Probst C, Rehm J (2019) Global alcohol exposure between 1990 and 2017 and forecasts until 2030: a modelling study. Lancet 393:2493–2502. https://doi.org/10.1016/S0140-6736(18)32744-2

Ministry of Health, Nutrition and Indigenous Medicine, Sri Lanka (2016) National multisectoral action plan for the prevention and control of noncommunicable diseases 2016–2020. Ministry of Health, Nutrition and Indigenous Medicine

Nadkarni A, Dabholkar H, McCambridge J, Bhat B, Kumar S, Mohanraj R, Murthy P, Patel V (2013) The explanatory models and coping strategies for alcohol use disorders: an exploratory qualitative study from India. Asian J Psychiatry 6:521

Narawane NM, Bhatia S, Abraham P, Sanghani S, Sawant SS (1998) Consumption of 'country liquor' and its relation to alcoholic liver disease in Mumbai. J Assoc Physicians India 46(6): 510–513

Noel JK (2020) Alcohol marketing policy and advertising exposure in low and middle income Latin American countries. Drugs Educ Prev Policy 27:479–487. https://doi.org/10.1080/09687637.2020.1733931

Parajuli VJ, Macdonald S, Jimba M (2015) Social–contextual factors associated with alcohol use among adolescents of traditional alcohol user and nonuser ethnic groups of Nepal. J Ethn Subst Abus 14:151–165. https://doi.org/10.1080/15332640.2014.973624

Parry CD, Patra J, Rehm J (2011) Alcohol consumption and non-communicable diseases: epidemiology and policy implications. Addiction 106(10):1718–1724. https://doi.org/10.1111/j.1360-0443.2011.03605.x

Rai Y, Gurung D, Gautam K (2021) Insight and challenges: mental health services in Nepal. BJPsych Int 18(2):E5. https://doi.org/10.1192/bji.2020.58

Rajapakse T, Griffiths K, Christensen H (2013) Characteristics of non-fatal self-poisoning in Sri Lanka: a systematic review. BMC Public Health 13:331

Rajapakse T, Griffiths KM, Christensen H, Cotton S (2014) A comparison of non-fatal self-poisoning among males and females, in Sri Lanka. BMC Psychiatry 14:221. https://doi.org/10.1186/s12888-014-0221-z

Rehm J, Mathers C, Popova S, Thavorncharoensap M, Teerawattananon Y et al (2009a) Global burden of disease and injury and economic cost attributable to alcohol use and alcohol-use disorders. Lancet 373:2223–2233

Rehm J, Samokhvalov AV, Neuman MG, Room R, Parry C et al (2009b) The association between alcohol use, alcohol use disorders and tuberculosis (TB). A systematic review. BMC Public Health 9:450

Rehm J, Shield KD, Joharchi N, Shuper PA (2012) Alcohol consumption and the intention to engage in unprotected sex: systematic review and meta-analysis of experimental studies: alcohol and intention for unprotected sex. Addiction 107:51–59. https://doi.org/10.1111/j.1360-0443.2011.03621.x

Rehm J, Kailasapillai S, Larsen E, Rehm MX, Samokhvalov AV, Shield KD . . . Lachenmeier DW (2014) A systematic review of the epidemiology of unrecorded alcohol consumption and the chemical composition of unrecorded alcohol. Addiction 109(6):880–893. https://doi.org/10.1111/add.12498

Rose A, Arun R, Minz S, Manohari GP, Vinodh A, George K et al (2015) Community perspectives on alcohol use among a tribal population in rural southern India. Natl Med J India 28:117

Sanaei-Zadeh H, Zamani N, Shadnia S (2011) Outcomes of visual disturbances after methanol poisoning. Clin Toxicol (Phila) 49(2):102–107. https://doi.org/10.3109/15563650.2011.556642

Savic M, Room R, Mugavin J, Pennay A, Livingston M (2016) Defining "drinking culture": a critical review of its meaning and connotation in social research on alcohol problems. Drugs Educ Prev Policy 23:270–282. https://doi.org/10.3109/09687637.2016.1153602

Schafer A (2014) Pilot process evaluation in preparation for the randomized control trial (RCT) for Grand Challenges Canada research initiative, in partnership with University of NSW, World Health Organization, and Kenya Ministry of Health. Unpublished, World Vision Kenya

Schafer A, Koyiet P (2018) Exploring links between common mental health problems, alcohol/substance use and perpetration of intimate partner violence: a rapid ethnographic assessment with men in urban Kenya. Glob Ment Health 5:e3. https://doi.org/10.1017/gmh.2017.25

Schafer A, Anjuri D, Ndogoni L (2013) Kenya community stakeholder consultations in preparation for the Grand Challenges Canada research initiative, in partnership with University of NSW, World Health Organization, and Kenya Ministry of Health. Unpublished, World Vision Kenya

Schmidt LA, Room R (2012) Alcohol and inequity in the process of development: contributions from ethnographic research. Int J Alcohol Drug Res 1:41

Sharma SR, Matheson A, Lambrick D, Faulkner J, Lounsbury DW, Vaidya A, Page R (2020) The role of tobacco and alcohol use in the interaction of social determinants of non-communicable diseases in Nepal: a systems perspective. BMC Public Health 20:1368. https://doi.org/10.1186/s12889-020-09446-2

Shidhaye R, Lund C, Chisholm D (2015) Closing the treatment gap for mental, neurological and substance use disorders by strengthening existing health care platforms: strategies for delivery and integration of evidence-based interventions. Int J Ment Health Syst 9:40. https://doi.org/10.1186/s13033-015-0031-9

Shuper PA, Neuman M, Kanteres F, Baliunas D, Joharchi N, Rehm J (2010) Causal considerations on alcohol and HIV/AIDS – a systematic review. Alcohol Alcohol 45:159–166. https://doi.org/10.1093/alcalc/agp091

Siriwardhana P, Dawson AH, Abeyasinge R (2012) Acceptability and effect of a community-based alcohol education program in rural Sri Lanka. Alcohol Alcohol 48:250–256. https://doi.org/10.1093/alcalc/ags116

Smyth A, Teo KK, Rangarajan S, O'Donnell M, Zhang X, Rana P, Leong DP, Dagenais G, Seron P, Rosengren A, Schutte AE, Lopez-Jaramillo P, Oguz A, Chifamba J, Diaz R, Lear S, Avezum A, Kumar R, Mohan V, Szuba A, Wei L, Yang W, Jian B, McKee M, Yusuf S (2015) Alcohol consumption and cardiovascular disease, cancer, injury, admission to hospital, and mortality: a prospective cohort study. Lancet 386:1945–1954. https://doi.org/10.1016/S0140-6736(15)00235-4

Sorensen G, Emmons K, Hunt MK, Johnston D (1998) Implications of the results of community intervention trials. Annu Rev Public Health 19:379–416. https://doi.org/10.1146/annurev.publhealth.19.1.379

Sørensen JB, Agampodi T, Sørensen BR, Siribaddana S, Konradsen F, Rheinländer T (2017) "We lost because of his drunkenness" – the social processes linking alcohol use to self-harm in the context of daily life stress in marriages and intimate relationships in rural Sri Lanka. BMJ Glob Health. https://doi.org/10.1136/bmjgh-2017-000462

Sørensen JB, Konradsen F, Agampodi T, Sørensen BR, Pearson M, Siribaddana S, Rheinländer T (2019) A qualitative exploration of rural and semi-urban Sri Lankan men's alcohol consumption. Glob Public Health 1–13. https://doi.org/10.1080/17441692.2019.1642366

Sornpaisarn B, Rehm J (2020) Strategies used to initiate the first alcohol control law in Thailand: lessons learned for other low- and middle-income countries. Int J Drug Policy 86:102975. https://doi.org/10.1016/j.drugpo.2020.102975

Tangcharoensathien V, Chandrasiri O, Kunpeuk W, Markchang K, Pangkariya N (2019) Addressing NCDs: challenges from industry market promotion and interferences. Int J Health Policy Manag 8:256–260. https://doi.org/10.15171/ijhpm.2019.02

Thapa N, Aryal KK, Puri R, Shrestha S, Shrestha S, Thapa P . . . Stray-Pedersen B (2016) Alcohol consumption practices among married women of reproductive age in Nepal: a population based household survey. PLoS One 11(4):e0152535. https://doi.org/10.1371/journal.pone.0152535

Walls H, Cook S, Matzopoulos R, London L (2020) Advancing alcohol research in low-income and middle-income countries: a global alcohol environment framework. BMJ Glob Health 5: e001958. https://doi.org/10.1136/bmjgh-2019-001958

World Health Organization (2004) WHO global status report on alcohol. World Health Organization, Geneva

World Health Organization (2007) Engaging men and boys in changing gender-based inequity in health: evidence from programme interventions. World Health Organization, Geneva

World Health Organization (2014) Global status report on alcohol and health 2014. World Health Organization, Geneva

World Health Organization (2018a) Global status report on alcohol and health 2018. World Health Organization, Geneva

World Health Organization (2018b) Noncommunicable diseases country profiles 2018. World Health Organization, Geneva

World Health Organization (2020) Alcohol – sustainable development goals: health targets. Alcohol consumption and sustainable development. World Health Organization, Regional Office for Europe

Metals in Alcoholic Beverages and Public Health Implications

53

Yasir A. Shah and Dirk W. Lachenmeier

Contents

Introduction 1132
Alcoholic Beverages in Human Health 1132
Unrecorded Alcohol 1135
Heavy Metals in Alcoholic Beverages 1137
Arsenic (As) 1137
Cadmium (Cd) 1138
Lead 1139
Copper 1140
Other Metals 1141
Application to Other Areas 1142
Applications to Other Areas of Addiction 1142
Applications to Other Areas of Public Health 1142
Key Facts of the World Health Organization on Unrecorded Alcohol (World Health Organization 2018a) 1143
Mini-Dictionary of Terms 1144
Summary Points 1144
References 1144

Abstract

The consumption of alcoholic beverages is a lifestyle factor with worldwide prevalence that is associated with a number of adverse health outcomes. While most of the effects, including the carcinogenicity of alcoholic beverages, are caused by ethanol and its metabolite acetaldehyde, other compounds were implicated as causing harms beyond ethanol. A common group among these is metals, many of which have toxic including carcinogenic effects. This chapter reviews the occurrence of metals in alcoholic beverages, summarizes their toxic effects,

Y. A. Shah
Department of Food Sciences, Government College University Faisalabad, Faisalabad, Pakistan

D. W. Lachenmeier (✉)
Chemisches und Veterinäruntersuchungsamt Karlsruhe, Karlsruhe, Germany

V. B. Patel, V. R. Preedy (eds.), *Handbook of Substance Misuse and Addictions*,
https://doi.org/10.1007/978-3-030-92392-1_60

and provides evidence that several of them such as arsenic, cadmium, copper, and lead can be regularly detected in alcoholic beverages. However, the typical occurrence is only at trace levels, which according to quantitative risk assessments would not cause any harms for the consumer, as it is, for example, below acceptable levels set for drinking water. Still, quality control should include these contaminants for precautionary public health protection. In other addictions, such as cannabis and tobacco, levels of metal contamination were similarly described to occur, as it is the case in the larger public health area, e.g., in foods and drinking water.

Keywords

Unrecorded alcohol · Risk assessment · Health policy · Metals · Contamination

Abbreviations

AMPHORA	Alcohol Measures for Public Health Research Alliance
EFSA	European Food Safety Authority
IARC	International Agency for Research on Cancer
MOE	margin of exposure
NCD	non-communicable disease
WHO	World Health Organization

Introduction

Alcohols are among the most common organic compounds. They are used as solvents in making perfumes and are valuable intermediates in the synthesis of other compounds. Alcohols are among the most abundantly produced organic chemicals in industry. Perhaps the two best-known alcohols are ethanol and methanol. Ethanol is used in toiletries, pharmaceuticals, and fuels, and it is also used to sterilize hospital instruments (Roehr et al. 2001). Moreover, it is also used in alcoholic beverages.

Methanol is used as a solvent or raw material to manufacture formaldehyde, special resins, special fuels, and antifreeze and for cleaning metals (Dalena et al. 2018). Most of the common alcohols are colorless liquids at room temperature. Methyl alcohol, ethyl alcohol, and isopropyl alcohol are free-flowing liquids with fruity odors (Ali et al. 2001). Metal contamination of alcohol is a problem with potential public health impact (Fig. 1) (Table 1).

Alcoholic Beverages in Human Health

An alcoholic beverage is any product, such as wine, beer, or distilled spirit, containing ethyl alcohol or ethanol (CH_3CH_2OH) as an intoxicating agent. In general, alcoholic beverage consumption is common in most countries worldwide.

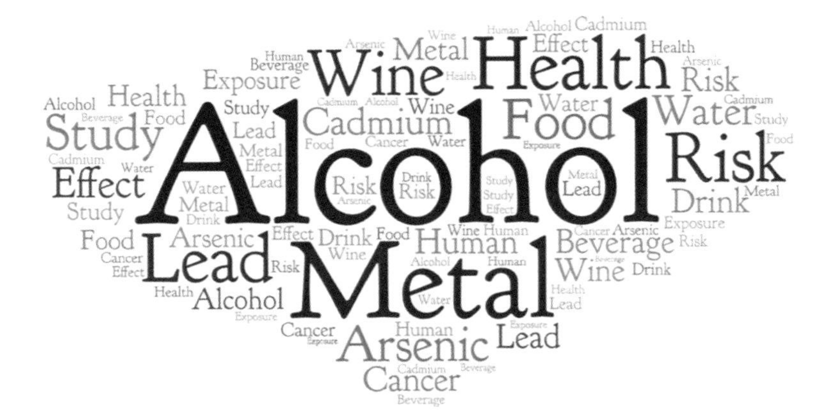

Fig. 1 Word cloud of major terms in the context of metals in alcoholic beverages

Table 1 Overview of metals in alcoholic beverages (data summarized from (IARC Working Group on the Evaluation of Carcinogenic Risks to Humans 2010))

Metal	Average range (μg/L)	Minimum/maximum range (μg/L)
Arsenic (As)	0.8–13	0–102
Cadmium (Cd)	0.3–6	0–40
Lead (Pb)	4–2680	0–11,800
Copper (Cu)	0.25–2.6	0–14.3

For several decades, the carcinogenicity of alcoholic beverages seems to have been a "trending topic." The earliest epidemiological findings were given in 1910 in France when 80% of patients diagnosed with esophageal cancer were heavy users of absinthe, a spirit of strong alcoholic strength (Pflaum et al. 2016). According to the World Health Organization, illicitly distilled drinks and otherwise unrecorded alcohols account for 28.6% of the total alcohol intake worldwide. Alcoholic beverages can be classified into several different types that vary from nation to nation or region wise. Some major classes of alcoholic beverages are fermented beverages, distilled beverages and spirits, fortified beverages and liquor wines, and liqueurs and creams.

Excessive alcohol intake has been identified as one of the leading risk factors contributing to disease burden, associated with more than 60 acute and chronic diseases (Griswold et al. 2018). Globally, alcohol use by people between the ages of 15 and 49 is the fifth leading cause of premature death and disabilities (Fihn et al. 2012). Epidemiological studies have shown that the burden of the alcohol-related disease depends on both the volume of alcohol consumed and the drinking pattern (Horváth et al. 2019). Alcohol is a major disease burden risk factor with a particularly high effect in Central and Eastern Europe. In 2002, Rehm and his colleagues calculated the alcohol-attributable mortality rate in many European countries (Rehm et al. 2006). This study demonstrated different harmful effects of overconsumption of alcohol, including high blood pressure, breast cancer, mental illness, and gastrointestinal problems (alters gut microbiota). Some of the major human disorders associated with alcohol consumption are discussed in the following.

High Blood Pressure

High blood pressure, which accounted for 10·7 million deaths and 211·8 million disability-adjusted life-years worldwide in 2015, is the leading single risk factor for morbidity and mortality (GBD Risk Factors Collaborators 2015). Similarly, despite the often-considered possible beneficial correlation of low alcohol intake with ischemic heart disease, excessive alcohol consumption creates an immense and increasing global disease and economic burden. Thus, alcohol intake and elevated blood pressure are among the leading five risk indicators responsible for the increasing incidence of global non-communicable diseases (NCDs). They are core components of the WHO aiming to reduce NCD mortality by 25% by 2025 (Alwan 2011). Owing to variations in body fat distribution, body size, and alcohol solubility, women and men metabolize alcohol differently. Various studies have demonstrated that excessive alcohol consumption is associated with high blood pressure (Miller et al. 2005; Santana et al. 2018).

Breast Cancer

Among other cancer sites, alcohol is known to be causally linked to breast cancer risk according to the International Agency for Research on Cancer (IARC Working Group on the Evaluation of Carcinogenic Risks to Humans 2010), with a 7–10% rise in risk for every 10 g (1 drink) of alcohol consumed daily by adult women. In both premenopausal and postmenopausal people, this correlation is observed. The breast tends to be more vulnerable to the carcinogenic effects of alcohol compared to other organs. The risk of breast cancer is substantially increased by 4–15% for light intake of alcohol (almost 1 drink/day or 12.5 g/day), which does not significantly raise cancer risk in other women's organs (Bagnardi et al. 2013). As almost half of women of child-bearing age drink alcohol and 15% of drinkers at this age have four or more drinks at a time, this poses a clinical and public health concern. For the advancement of breast cancer prevention strategies, a better understanding of how alcohol intake raises the risk of breast cancer is also important.

Gut Microbiota Dysbiosis

The intestinal microbiota is known within the gastrointestinal tract as the complete set of microbial species. It comprises tens of trillions of microorganisms, including at least 1000 species of recognized bacteria. Microbiota contributes to food energy extraction and vitamin and amino acid synthesis and helps to form barriers to pathogens. Inflammatory bowel disease (IBD) has been associated with the disturbance of intestinal microbiota homeostasis called dysbiosis (Louis et al. 2014), irritable bowel syndrome, celiac disease, food allergies, type 1 diabetes, type 2 diabetes, cancer (Schwabe and Jobin 2013), and obesity (Biasini et al. 2012). While it is uncertain if dysbiosis is the cause or outcome of these diseases, the gut intestinal microbiota is affected by factors that contribute to the development and progression of many of these diseases.

Studies showed that bacterial outgrowth and dysbiosis are also caused by chronic alcohol intake in humans (Akerboom et al. 2012). In another study conducted in a subgroup of alcohol-dependent drinkers with and without liver disease, the microbial population was substantially changed, containing a lower abundance of *Bacteroidetes* and a greater abundance of *Proteobacteria* (Das et al. 2011). Various studies have reported the dysbiosis of gut microbiota associated with alcohol intake (Bajaj 2019; Canesso et al. 2014).

Neural and Cognitive Effects

Studies have shown that several cognitive and other functional deficiencies are associated with adolescent alcohol exposure (Burden et al. 2005; Golub et al. 2015; Lees et al. 2020). The results of human longitudinal work involve deficiencies in verbal comprehension, attention, and visuospatial and memory tasks. In contrast, research using animal models of adolescent alcohol consumption has shown that such exposure is correlated with declines in cognitive flexibility, behavioral inefficiencies, anxiety-like behavior increases, disinhibition, and elevated risk-taking. Repeated exposure to alcohol throughout adolescence in rodent studies causes consistent and precise neural alterations that involve decreases in basal forebrain cholinergic sound, neuroinflammation, neurogenesis disturbances, epigenetic alterations, and persistence adulthood of some adolescent-like neural characteristics (Mattson et al. 2019). Using human longitudinal designs and studies in laboratory animals, there are several critical areas for potential research in this field, which may benefit from a growing emphasis on comparing comparable measures across species. To date, researchers investigating the functional effects of adolescent alcohol consumption have used mainly various approaches, with a focus on neuropsychological or cognitive assessments in humans compared with an emphasis on improvements in risk-taking, anxiety, subsequent alcohol motivation, and sensitivity in rodent studies (Spear 2018).

Unrecorded Alcohol

All forms of alcohol that are not registered in the authority where they are consumed are unrecorded alcohol. This may be due to illicit or informal processing, cross-border shopping, as well as the use of surrogate alcohol not originally intended for human consumption (e.g., automobile goods, cosmetic or pharmaceutical alcohol) (Okaru et al. 2019; World Health Organization 2018b). The bulk of unrecorded alcohol intake in some countries in Central and Eastern Europe, as well as in the Balkans, may be derived from the domestic production of spirits from sugar-containing fruit products, such as cherries, plums, apples, pears, or grapes, which are abundant in these countries (Bujdosó et al. 2019; Marjanovic et al. 2019). In the WHO European Area, the amount of unrecorded consumption ranges from 3% (Austria) to 75% (Azerbaijan) (21% on average) of total alcohol consumption (calculated based on WHO data for 2016 (World Health Organization 2016)). The health effects of unrecorded alcohol consumption thus form a large part of the harm associated with alcohol; however, this portion of alcohol consumption has generally been understudied (Lachenmeier et al. 2017). However, unrecorded alcohol effects beyond recorded alcoholic beverages are an essential subject of investigation. It has been proposed, for example, that variations in the incidence of liver disease between countries that the volume of consumption cannot explain could be due to alcohol-related impacts caused by unrecorded intake of alcohol. There are numerous theories, such as that its major effects could be causally linked to several chemicals in unrecorded alcohol.

Some European countries, such as Hungary, Slovenia, and Romania, have abnormally high liver cirrhosis-related death rates, which are among the highest in the world. Although these high rates have not yet been fully explained, some research suggests that hepatotoxic compounds in illegally produced spirits may be partially responsible, as they have been identified as having very high levels of unrecorded consumption in these countries. This raises the question of the extent to which unrecorded alcohol contains potentially health-threatening properties, including contaminants and high alcoholic strengths (e.g., surrogate, home, and illegally produced alcohol) (Lachenmeier et al. 2009). Most chemical-toxicological studies on unrecorded alcohol in Europe have so far been unable to detect levels of compounds that may cause increased health effects, including liver cirrhosis. The studies, however, usually found higher ethanol levels (i.e., alcoholic strength) in unrecorded alcohols, and epidemiological evidence suggests that unrecorded alcohols are typically consumed in more detrimental drinking patterns. Statistical evidence has shown that the incidence of liver cirrhosis can be explained by variations in drinking habits alone (Lachenmeier et al. 2014). The preference for unrecorded alcohol consumption by people of lower socioeconomic status may be one confounding factor (Kotelnikova 2017). However, the hypothesis that compounds other than ethanol may contribute to the health risks of unrecorded alcohol is worthy of investigation based on the typical low sample sizes in previous chemical studies on unrecorded alcohol.

Two studies on the chemical makeup of unrecorded alcohol were released in 2019, namely, a pilot study from the Slovak Republic on lead contamination of fruit spirits and research on cadmium contaminants in unrecorded plum spirits from Hungary. An exceptionally higher frequency of the two metals was observed in the studies (lead 100%, $n = 18$; cadmium 97%, $n = 35$). The prevalence was far higher than in the Alcohol Measures for Public Health Research Alliance (AMPHORA) project's sample of unrecorded European alcohol ($n = 115$, prevalence lead: 53%; cadmium: 1%) (Lachenmeier and Rehm 2012; Leitz et al. 2011). However, the recent studies have not provided a quantitative risk assessment for metals, using the technique for the margin of exposure (MOE). In a MOE modeling by Lachenmeier (2020), it was found that ethanol itself comprises by far the highest risk of all compounds in alcoholic beverages. Regarding metal contaminants, the risk of cadmium appears negligible; however, lead may pose an additional health risk in heavy drinking circumstances (Table 2).

Table 2 The margin of exposure (MOE)[a] of ethanol, lead, and cadmium in alcoholic beverages calculated for different drinking and contamination scenarios (summarized from Lachenmeier (2020).)

	Scenario 1: One standard drink per day		Scenario 2: Heavy drinker (four standard drinks per day)	
Agent	MOE for average concentration	MOE for maximum concentration	MOE for average concentration	MOE for maximum concentration (worst case)
Ethanol	3	–	0.8	–
Lead	13–70	2–4	3–17	0.4–0.9
Cadmium	1982 - ∞[b]	349–453	496 - ∞[b]	87–113

[a]MOE = BMDL or NOAEL/Exposure. Ethanol, $BMDL_{10}$ = 700 mg/kg bodyweight (bw)/day; lead, $BMDL_{01}$ = 0.0015 mg/kg bw/day; cadmium, NOAEL = 0.01 mg/kg bw/day. Exposure data based on literature sources

[b]The lemniscate symbol indicates that the MOE was not calculable as the average exposure was zero (i.e., below the detection limit of the applied analytical methodology)

Heavy Metals in Alcoholic Beverages

Among the most important environmental contaminations in recent years is the pollution of heavy metals that contributes to food, soil, and water supplies being contaminated. At certain amounts, heavy metal concentration in the human body was associated with severe and even fatal diseases and disorders such as respiratory and digestive issues, cancer, neurological problems (such as Alzheimer's, Parkinson's, and anxiety), and heart disease (Feist and Sitko 2018; Zuberbier et al. 2018). While copper is a crucial element of the body, it can be toxic at high levels. Arsenic, lead, and cadmium are listed as toxic and carcinogenic elements in the body (Tuzen et al. 2016). Continuous food exposure to elevated levels of arsenic (As), lead (Pb), and cadmium (Cd) heavy metals poses a public health risk, and different foods have regularly shown these metals to be present (Redan et al. 2019). A variety of metalloids and metals have been detected in alcoholic beverages such as arsenic (As), cadmium (Cd), chromium (Cr), cobalt (Co), copper (Cu), iron (Fe), manganese (Mn), nickel (Ni), tin (Sn), lead (Pb), and zinc (Zn) (Pál et al. 2020). The most significant metals found in alcoholic beverages are discussed below.

Arsenic (As)

Arsenic pollution may come from a variety of sources, including geological and anthropogenic activities (Abdul et al. 2015). Arsenic is released into the atmosphere as a consequence of volcanic and industrial activity. It can be found in water, air, and living organisms. Arsenic is a metal ion found in the earth's atmosphere and is recognized as a global health threat. Arsenic accumulates in the earth's crust and bedrocks, slowly leaching into drinking water (Vahter 2009). Arsenic enters the human body through various pathways, including ingestion, inhalation, and absorption through the skin. The critical absorption pathway for the general public to arsenic is through polluted food and water. Arsenic has traditionally been used in a wide variety of applications such as in insecticide sprays.

Chronic dietary exposure to high levels of heavy metals such as arsenic (As) presents a health risk (Hettick et al. 2015; Lewchalermvong et al. 2018; Satarug et al. 2017), and these elements have been consistently detected in a variety of foods (Redan et al. 2019). Low concentrations and long-term arsenic susceptibility cause various medical illnesses known as "arsenicosis" (McCarty et al. 2011). Arsenic exposure, primarily by drinking water, has been linked to several complications in adults and infants, including dermatological effects, cardiovascular effects, respiratory disorders, reproductive effects, and neurological effects (Ahsan et al. 2006; Argos et al. 2010; Chen et al. 2004, 2011; Ferreccio et al. 2013; Smith et al. 1998; Sohel et al. 2010; Vahter et al. 2006; Wasserman et al. 2004). Various studies have found a considerable quantity of arsenic in alcoholic beverages.

Beer (0–102.4 g/L), spirits (0–27 g/L), and wine (0–14.6 g/L) have all been found to occasionally contain arsenic (International Agency for Research on Cancer 2010). The total arsenic in red wines was substantially lower than in rosé and white wines (Barbaste et al. 2003). These variations may be attributed to various vinification methods (Aguilar et al. 1987). Some studies observed impaired arsenic metabolism among alcohol drinkers (Huang et al. 2008). The IARC categorizes the known human carcinogens as the semimetal arsenic and inorganic arsenic compounds in group 1. Inorganic arsenic compounds can cause lung, skin, and urinary tract cancer. Moreover, a positive association between arsenic toxicity and inorganic arsenic molecules and liver, kidney, and prostate cancer has been observed (IARC Working Group on the Evaluation of Carcinogenic Risks to Humans 2012). As a secondary effect of genomic instability, long-term, low-dose exposure to inorganic arsenic compounds is likely to cause increased mutagenesis. Rapid induction of oxidative DNA damage and DNA repair inhibition, as well as slower changes in DNA methylation patterns, aneuploidy, and gene amplification, which lead to altered gene expression and genomic instability, are the underlying mechanisms observed at low concentrations (IARC Working Group on the Evaluation of Carcinogenic Risks to Humans 2012). Various studies reported the possible presence of arsenic concentrations in alcoholic beverages, which are summarized in Table 1.

Cadmium (Cd)

Cadmium and cadmium molecules are categorized into IARC group 1 based on "sufficient evidence" for carcinogenic effects (Pflaum et al. 2016). Cadmium (Cd) is a highly toxic heavy metal that builds up in living organisms. Cadmium has been classified as a human carcinogen, based mostly on occupational reports of lung cancer (Nordberg et al. 2018). The IARC assessment is based on the fact that cadmium and its derivatives cause lung cancer and the association between exposure and cancer of the kidneys and prostate. Recent research has shown that cadmium triggers numerous epigenetic changes in human cells, both in vivo and in vitro, contributing to risks of the progression of numerous cancers (Genchi et al. 2020). Dietary sources of cadmium are known to be the most critical route of cadmium exposure in the general population. Several animal studies have shown that alcohol consumption and cadmium exposure have a combined effect on hypertension. Heavy alcohol consumption was found to increase the risk of hypertension when combined with cadmium exposure (Choi et al. 2021).

An overview of the levels of cadmium in different food categories was presented in an EFSA scientific report (Arcella et al. 2012). The median bound mean (MB) occurrence results varied between 0.5 μg/kg for fortified and liqueur wines and 6.0 μg/kg for liqueur in the category of alcoholic beverages. An MB of 1.2 μg/kg was observed for wines including white and red varieties, an MB of 1.8 μg/kg for beer and similar products. The cadmium content in red and white wines is identical to that already reported by Kim (2004) (Kim 2004), where values ranged from <0.1 to 3 μg/L, in line with those previously reported. There was also no significant difference in the content of cadmium in wines with different origins (Kim 2004). These variations may be associated with the wine-making method as well as with both natural and exogenous factors. Grape variety and soil composition are biological factors. The wine-making process and fermentation processing also aid in various types of contamination.

The use of toxic pesticides or fertilizers with this metal could be a cause for the high concentration of cadmium found in wine samples reported by Mena et al. (1996) and Illuminati et al. (2014) (Illuminati et al. 2014; Mena et al. 1996). Canned beers were likely to contain the highest concentrations due to the inadequate quality of containers used, with values ranging from 0.50 to 0.80 μg/l; lower concentrations were found in draught beers with a mean value 0.20 μg/l. Various studies have reported the possible presence of cadmium in alcoholic beverages, which are summarized in Table 1.

Lead

Inorganic lead and lead derivatives are commonly considered "probably carcinogenic to humans" (Group 2A) (IARC Working Group on the Evaluation of Carcinogenic Risks to Humans 1987), whereas organic lead derivatives are "not classifiable as to their human carcinogenicity" (Group 3) (Pflaum et al. 2016). Lead is a bluish-gray metal that naturally occurs in the soil and is widely used due to its physical and chemical properties (Obeng-Gyasi 2019). For a long time, lead has been one of the most harmful environmental toxic compounds in western countries, which is still the case in many parts of the world today. Lead may trigger oxidative stress by releasing reactive oxygen species (ROS), which has been recognized as a critical mechanism in the development of lead toxicity (Farmand et al. 2005; Gurer and Ercal 2000; Kasperczyk et al. 2015; Martinez et al. 2013; Pande and

Flora 2002; Verstraeten et al. 2008; Wang et al. 2007). The International Agency for Research on Cancer has listed lead as a possible human carcinogen (International Agency for Research on Cancer 1980). Lead toxicity has been related to cancers of the stomach, kidney, liver, and brain in epidemiological studies (Boffetta et al. 2011; Kuempel and Sorahan 2010; Liao et al. 2014).

The EFSA study reported that the central nervous system, kidney, and biosynthetic pathways are significantly affected by lead (European Food Safety Authority 2012). A summary of lead dietary exposure from various food categories was seen in the EFSA study. The mean middle bound (MB) incidence for red wine was 22 μg/kg and 29 μg/kg for white wine. Beer and beer-like drinks had an average MB incidence of 12 μg/kg (European Food Safety Authority 2012). Kim's (2004) mean lead concentrations for white and red wines (29 μg/L) are in good agreement with the EFSA report, with no difference in lead concentration between white and red wines (Kim 2004). Tahvonen (1998) found a mean of 33 μg/L in white wines and 34 μg/L in red wines (Tahvonen 1998). Winery systems, lead capsules, and air emissions have been responsible for the critical sources of lead contamination in wine (Lobinski et al. 1994; Medina et al. 2000). The maximum amount of lead in wine recommended by the International Organization of Vine and Wine (OIV) is 150 μg/L (Leitz et al. 2011).

Winery equipment made of brass and alloys that have been commonly used in traditional wine cellars is now replaced by stainless steel products (Illuminati et al. 2014). Before being banned in the 1990s, atmospheric deposition due to leaded gasoline was also a major source of lead in wines. The share of lead pollution today is much lower than in the past (Kim 2004). However, currently produced wines may be not lead-free, so it is necessary to know all the sources of this metal to enable their removal or minimization. The lead concentrations of alcoholic beverages reported by various studies are summarized in Table 1.

Copper

Copper is a valuable metal for both biological and industrial purposes. It's a transition metal with two oxidation states in the first place: copper I (reduced) and copper II (oxidized) (Koch et al. 1997). The oxidation and reduction of these ions are needed for enzyme function in many biological systems. Even though copper is recognized as an essential trace element, there are still questions about Cu reference values for humans, as evidenced by inconsistencies between the recommendations of national authorities (Bost et al. 2016). Although copper is an important nutrient for humans, livestock, and plants, excessive exposure can be harmful to human health. When exposed to high levels of soluble copper salts, susceptible individuals can experience acute gastrointestinal symptoms and, in rare cases, liver toxicity (Taylor et al. 2020). Copper is linked to bone health, immune function, an increased risk of infection, and cardiovascular risk, and cholesterol metabolism changes. Its metabolism is intricately linked to other micro minerals, and a lack of it has been shown to inhibit iron mobilization, resulting in secondary iron deficiency (Araya et al. 2007).

Copper alone or formulated with other agrochemicals is an essential measure in the prevention of fungal disease outbreaks.

Copper can be traced to two important origins in whisky: the copper stills used for distillation and the barley from which the spirit is distilled. The copper content of Brazilian sugarcane spirits was associated with distillate acidity, both present at higher concentrations in the tail fractions. Therefore, if the distillation is stopped at a higher alcoholic grade, the copper content could be decreased (Boza and Horii 2000). Storage in oak barrels is another possibility for reducing the copper levels of Brazilian sugarcane spirits.

Other Metals

Metals including mercury (Hg), nickel (Ni), selenium (Se), zinc (Zn), iron (Fe), thallium (Tl), and antimony were reported in alcoholic beverages by various studies. Dietary exposure is a significant route for trace metals to reach humans, accounting for roughly 90% of all exposure. Long-term metal contamination from food, drinking water, or other occupational sources causes serious problems such as hepatotoxicity, kidney failure, and neurotoxicity (El-Kady and Abdel-Wahhab 2018). Alcohol has been described as a significant risk factor for global disease burden (Rodgers et al. 2004). The determination of wine's elemental composition is intriguing for a variety of reasons. Certain elements can have a major impact on the organoleptic properties of wines, so their concentrations must be controlled at all stages of the process (Pohl 2007; Watson 2003).

A study reported that mercury (Hg) concentrations ranged from 2.6 to 4.9 μg/l for Spanish sweet wines and 1.5 to 2.6 μg/l for Spanish dry wines (Frias et al. 2003). Another study found only 2 out of 100 German beers with concentrations of 0.4 and 0.8 μg/l, mercury (Donhauser et al. 1987). All the samples tested for mercury were below the detection level of 6 μg/l in wine and beer in the Danish market (Pedersen et al. 1994). Nickel (Ni) product concentrations have been registered in the Danish industry. Red wine contained, on average, 49 μg/l of Ni, 42 μg/l of white wine, 93 μg/l of fortified wine, and 23 μg/l of beer (Pedersen et al. 1994). There was a nickel range of 15–210 μg/l for Italian wines (Marengo and Aceto 2003) and a nickel range of 0–0.13 mg/l for Greek wines (Lazos and Alexakis 1989).

In Spain, selenium concentrations ranged from 1.0 to 2.0 μg/l for sweet wines and from 0.6 to 1.6 μg/l for dry wines (Frias et al. 2003). The Spanish beverage survey estimated 0.150–0.375 μg/l of selenium in wine (mean 0.256 μg/l) and 0.885–1.129 μg/l of selenium in beer (mean 1.007 μg/l), respectively (Diaz et al. 1997). For 100 German beers, the mean selenium concentration was 1.2 μg/l (range <0.4–7.2 μg/l) (Donhauser et al. 1987).

Antimony levels in 52 samples of cachaca from Brazil varied from non-detectable to 39 μg/l (Canuto et al. 2003). A study found an antimony range of 0.01–1.00 μg/l in Italian wines (Marengo and Aceto 2003). Zinc (Zn) was calculated in 251 Swiss wine samples with a mean concentration of 614 μg/l (Andrey et al. 1992), Italian wines with a range of concentrations of 0.135–4.80 mg/l (Marengo and Aceto 2003), and Greek wines with a range of concentrations of 0.05–1.80 mg/l (Lazos and Alexakis 1989). Whisky zinc concentrations were in the range of 0.02 to 20 mg/l (Adam et al. 2002). Iron (Fe) concentrations varied between 0.01 and 0.78 mg/l in Brazilian sugarcane spirits with an average of 0.21 mg/l (Bettin et al. 2002). The concentration of iron in whiskey ranged significantly from 0.02 to 28 mg/l of Fe (Adam et al. 2002).

Thallium (Tl) was present frequently in very low wine concentrations, about twice as much in red wines with 0.2 μg/l as in white wines (Eschnauer et al. 1984). With a measurement limit of 10 μg/l, none of the 700 analyzed wines of global origin could find thallium (Kaufmann 1993). For Italian wine, a thallium range of 10–95 ng/l was seen in more sensitive studies (Marengo and Aceto 2003).

Application to Other Areas

Applications to Other Areas of Addiction

Cannabis sativa L. has been used for medicinal purposes and as a recreational psychoactive substance for centuries. Heavy metals (Cr, Pb, Cu, Cd, Ni, and Zn) were assessed in *Cannabis sativa* L. and the soil of the region where the plant was collected in Pakistan. The amount of heavy metals present in plant parts such as roots, stems, and leaves corresponds to their soil contents (Khan et al. 2008).

Tobacco use in different forms, such as cigarettes and hookahs, is one of the world's leading causes of sickness, injury, and premature death (Yousefinejad et al. 2018). Tobacco is a rich source of toxic heavy metals because metals accumulate preferentially in tobacco leaves during plant growth (Golia et al. 2007). Tobacco product use, both smoking and non-smoking, has an impact on smokers' health as well as non-smokers' health through passive smoking and adds metal content to the atmosphere (Galażyn-Sidorczuk et al. 2008). Tobacco smoking is a significant source of toxic metals in humans and the environment (Schneider and Krivna 1993). Tobacco's elemental content is determined by various factors, including soil characteristics, climatic conditions, and plant variety (Musharraf et al. 2012). The tobacco plant, for example, prefers to consume cadmium over lead because cadmium is more mobile and migrates upward (Musharraf et al. 2012), accumulating in the plant in the order of leaves > roots > stems (Clarke and Brennan 1989). Tobacco plants preferentially absorb heavy metals such as Pb, Cd, and Zn (Angelova et al. 2004). The presence/concentration of one element in the soil influences the uptake of another component by plants; for example, in the presence of lead, cadmium absorption or uptake is stimulated.

Applications to Other Areas of Public Health

Human life depends on the availability of safe drinking water, and safe drinking water does not pose a substantial risk to humans (World Health Organization 1993). Metals are found in high concentrations in improperly treated residential, commercial, and agricultural wastewater often discharged into the environment (Chowdhury et al. 2016).

Long-term exposure to trace metal pollution in drinking water presents a danger to human health. Plant waste discharges and widespread use of agrochemicals (Abbas et al. 2014) are two anthropogenic sources of trace metals (Muhammad et al. 2010). Normal occurrences of trace metals as a result of chemical weathering of bed rocks and minerals create metal pollution in water in addition to anthropogenic sources (Krishna et al. 2009). The demand for research into drinking water quality in trace metal delivery, source, and sensitivity to trace metal health risks has increased. It has been recorded that arsenic in drinking water has impacted approximately 150 million people around the world (Ravenscroft et al. 2009). Bangladesh, India, China, Hungary, Pakistan, Argentina, Chile, Mexico, Taiwan, some parts of the USA, and Venezuela are affected (Rahman et al. 2009).

According to many reports, people living in remote settlements who do not have access to filtered drinking water are more likely to use dirty water (Jabeen et al. 2011). Skin diseases, typhoid, dysentery, diarrhea, methemoglobinemia, cancer, and other health problems are often caused by contamination of water supplies reserved for human consumption and domestic usage (Salzman 2017). Heavy metal contamination is currently regarded as one of the most severe risks to water quality (Rezaei et al. 2019). Heavy metals, in particular, are harmful pollutants that have piqued the interest of many researchers in the field of water safety. Heavy metal concentrations in water bodies in urban and suburban areas have increased globally due to the recent rapid rise in industrialization and modernization. Many water bodies in Nigeria's urban and suburban districts have been found to contain moderate to high levels of heavy metals. Edet and Offiong (2002), Egbueri (2018, 2020a, b), and Egbunike (Egbunike 2018) are examples of studies that reported the existence of heavy metals in drinking waters from Nigeria's southeastern region. It is proposed that attempts be made to treat contaminated water bodies before humans ingest them and that more public awareness initiatives be promoted to protect water resources from further depletion.

Key Facts of the World Health Organization on Unrecorded Alcohol (World Health Organization 2018a)

- Unrecorded alcohol refers to alcohol that is not accounted for in official statistics on alcohol taxation or sales in the country where it is consumed because it is usually produced, distributed, and sold outside the formal channels under government control.
- Unrecorded alcohol consumption in a country includes consumption of home-made or informally produced alcohol (legal or illegal), smuggled alcohol, alcohol intended for industrial or medical uses, and alcohol obtained through cross-border shopping (which is recorded in a different jurisdiction).
- Sometimes these alcoholic beverages are traditional drinks that are produced and consumed in the community or in homes.
- Home-made or informally produced alcoholic beverages are mostly fermented products made from sorghum, millet, maize, rice, wheat, or fruits.

- Unrecorded consumption also includes so-called surrogate alcohol, commonly ethanol that was not produced as beverage alcohol but is used as such (e.g., mouthwash, denatured alcohol, medicinal tinctures, aftershaves, and perfumes).

Mini-Dictionary of Terms

- An alcoholic beverage is defined by WHO as any beverage containing ethanol, which is a psychoactive and toxic substance with dependence producing properties.
- A contaminant is defined by the *Codex Alimentarius* as any substance not intentionally added to a food, which is present as the result of the production, manufacture, processing, preparation, treatment, packing, packaging, transport or holding of such food, or environmental contamination.
- Heavy metals are generally defined as metals with high atomic weights, several of which have toxic properties
- The WHO chemicals of public health concern included several metals, namely, arsenic, cadmium, lead, and mercury.
- Unrecorded alcohol is alcohol not registered in the jurisdiction where it is consumed (also see key facts above).

Summary Points

- While most of the effects, including the carcinogenicity of alcoholic beverages, are caused by ethanol and its metabolite acetaldehyde, other compounds were implicated as causing harms beyond ethanol.
- This chapter reviews the occurrence of metals in alcoholic beverages, summarizes their toxic effects, and provides evidence that several of them such as arsenic, cadmium, copper, and lead can be regularly detected in alcoholic beverages.
- Chronic dietary exposure to high levels of heavy metals such as arsenic presents a health risk.
- The typical occurrence of metals in alcoholic beverages is only at trace levels, which according to quantitative risk assessments would not cause any harm for the consumer.
- In other addictions, such as cannabis and tobacco, levels of metal contamination were described to occur, as it is the case in the larger public health area, e.g., in foods and drinking water.

References

Abbas SR, Sabir SM, Ahmad SD et al (2014) Phenolic profile, antioxidant potential and DNA damage protecting activity of sugarcane (*Saccharum officinarum*). Food Chem 147:10–16

Abdul KS, Jayasinghe SS, Chandana EP et al (2015) Arsenic and human health effects: a review. Environ Toxicol Pharmacol 40:828–846

Adam T, Duthie E, Feldmann J (2002) Investigations into the use of copper and other metals as indicators for the authenticity of scotch whiskies. J Inst Brew 108:459–464

Aguilar MV, Martinez MC, Masoud TA (1987) Arsenic content in some Spanish wines influence of the wine-making technique on arsenic content in musts and wines. Z Lebensm Unters Forsch 185:185–187

Ahsan H, Chen Y, Parvez F et al (2006) Arsenic exposure from drinking water and risk of premalignant skin lesions in Bangladesh: baseline results from the health effects of arsenic longitudinal study. Am J Epidemiol 163:1138–1148

Akerboom J, Chen TW, Wardill TJ et al (2012) Optimization of a GCaMP calcium indicator for neural activity imaging. J Neurosci 32:13819–13840

Ali Y, Dolan MJ, Fendler EJ et al (2001) Alcohols. In: Disinfection, sterilization and preservation, 5th edn. Lippincott Williams & Wilkins, Philadelphia, pp 229–253

Alwan A (2011) Global status report on noncommunicable diseases 2010. World Health Organization

Andrey D, Beuggert H, Ceschi M et al (1992) Monitoring-Programm "Schwermetalle in Lebensmitteln". IV: Blei, Cadmium, Kupfer und Zink in Weinen auf dem Schweizer Markt. Teil B: Vorgehen, Resultate und Diskussion. I. Mitt Gebiete Lebensmittelunters Hyg 83:711–736

Angelova V, Ivanov K, Ivanova R (2004) Effect of chemical forms of lead, cadmium, and zinc in polluted soils on their uptake by tobacco. J Plant Nutr 27:757–773

Araya M, Olivares M, Pizarro F (2007) Copper in human health. Int J Environ Health 1:608–620

Arcella D, Cappe S, Fabiansson S et al (2012) Cadmium dietary exposure in the European population. EFSA J 10:2551

Argos M, Kalra T, Rathouz PJ et al (2010) Arsenic exposure from drinking water, and all-cause and chronic-disease mortalities in Bangladesh (HEALS): a prospective cohort study. Lancet 376: 252–258

Bagnardi V, Rota M, Botteri E et al (2013) Light alcohol drinking and cancer: a meta-analysis. Ann Oncol 24:301–308

Bajaj JS (2019) Alcohol, liver disease and the gut microbiota. Nat Rev Gastroenterol Hepatol 16: 235–246

Barbaste M, Medina B, Perez-Trujillo JP (2003) Analysis of arsenic, lead and cadmium in wines from the Canary Islands, Spain, by ICP/MS. Food Addit Contam 20:141–148

Bettin SM, Isique W, Franco DW et al (2002) Phenols and metals in sugar-cane spirits. Quantitative analysis and effect on radical formation and radical scavenging. Eur Food Res Technol 215:169–175

Biasini E, Turnbaugh JA, Unterberger U et al (2012) Prion protein at the crossroads of physiology and disease. Trends Neurosci 35:92–103

Boffetta P, Fontana L, Stewart P et al (2011) Occupational exposure to arsenic, cadmium, chromium, lead and nickel, and renal cell carcinoma: a case-control study from central and Eastern Europe. Occup Environ Med 68:723–728

Bost M, Houdart S, Oberli M et al (2016) Dietary copper and human health: current evidence and unresolved issues. J Trace Elem Med Biol 35:107–115

Boza Y, Horii J (2000) Alcoholic degree and acidity level influence of the distilled product on the copper content in sugar cane based distilled beverage. Food Sci Technol 20:279–284

Bujdosó O, Pál L, Nagy A et al (2019) Is there any difference between the health risk from consumption of recorded and unrecorded spirits containing alcohols other than ethanol? A population-based comparative risk assessment. Regul Toxicol Pharmacol 106:334–345

Burden MJ, Jacobson SW, Jacobson JL (2005) Relation of prenatal alcohol exposure to cognitive processing speed and efficiency in childhood. Alcohol Clin Exp Res 29:1473–1483

Canesso MCC, Lacerda N, Ferreira C et al (2014) Comparing the effects of acute alcohol consumption in germ-free and conventional mice: the role of the gut microbiota. BMC Microbiol 14:1–10

Canuto MH, Siebald HGL, De Lima GM et al (2003) Antimony and chromium determination in Brazilian sugar cane spirit, cachaça, by electrothermal atomic absorption spectrometry using matrix matching calibration and ruthenium as permanent modifier. J Anal At Spectrom 18: 1404–1406

Chen CL, Hsu LI, Chiou HY et al (2004) Ingested arsenic, cigarette smoking, and lung cancer risk: a follow-up study in arseniasis-endemic areas in Taiwan. JAMA 292:2984–2990
Chen Y, Graziano JH, Parvez F et al (2011) Arsenic exposure from drinking water and mortality from cardiovascular disease in Bangladesh: prospective cohort study. BMJ 342:d2431
Choi YH, Huh DA, Moon KW (2021) Joint effect of alcohol drinking and environmental cadmium exposure on hypertension in Korean adults: analysis of data from the Korea National Health and nutrition examination survey, 2008 to 2013. Alcohol Clin Exp Res 45:548–560
Chowdhury S, Mazumder MJ, Al-Attas O et al (2016) Heavy metals in drinking water: occurrences, implications, and future needs in developing countries. Sci Total Environ 569–570: 476–488
Clarke B, Brennan E (1989) Differential cadmium accumulation and phytotoxicity in sixteen tobacco cultivars. JAPCA 39:1319–1322
Gbd Risk Factors Collaborators (2015) Global, regional, and national comparative risk assessment of 79 behavioural, environmental and occupational, and metabolic risks or clusters of risks in 188 countries, 1990–2013: a systematic analysis for the Global Burden of Disease Study 2013. Lancet 386:2287–2323
Dalena F, Senatore A, Marino A et al (2018) Methanol production and applications: an overview. In: Methanol. Elsevier
Das MC, Xu H, Wang Z et al (2011) A Zn 4 O-containing doubly interpenetrated porous metal–organic framework for photocatalytic decomposition of methyl orange. Chem Commun 47:11715–11717
Diaz JP, Navarro M, Lopez H et al (1997) Determination of selenium levels in dairy products and drinks by hydride generation atomic absorption spectrometry: correlation with daily dietary intake. Food Addit Contam 14:109–114
Donhauser S, Wagner D, Jacob F (1987) Critical trace elements in brewing technology. Pt. 2. Occurrence of arsenic, lead, cadmium, chromium, mercury and selenium in beer. Monatsschr Brauwiss 40:328
Edet A, Offiong O (2002) Evaluation of water quality pollution indices for heavy metal contamination monitoring. A study case from Akpabuyo-Odukpani area, Lower Cross River Basin (southeastern Nigeria). GeoJournal 57:295–304
Egbueri JC (2018) Assessment of the quality of groundwaters proximal to dumpsites in Awka and Nnewi metropolises: a comparative approach. Int J Energy Water Resour 2:33–48
Egbueri JC (2020a) Groundwater quality assessment using pollution index of groundwater (PIG), ecological risk index (ERI) and hierarchical cluster analysis (HCA): a case study. Groundwater Sust Develop 10:100292
Egbueri JC (2020b) Heavy metals pollution source identification and probabilistic health risk assessment of shallow groundwater in Onitsha, Nigeria. Anal Lett 53:1620–1638
Egbunike ME (2018) Hydrogeochemical investigation of groundwater resources in Umunya and environs of the Anambra Basin, Nigeria. Pac J Sci Technol 19:351–366
El-Kady AA, Abdel-Wahhab MA (2018) Occurrence of trace metals in foodstuffs and their health impact. Trends Food Sci Technol 75:36–45
Eschnauer H, Gemmer-Čolos V, Neeb R (1984) Thallium in Wein – Spurenelement-Vinogramm des Thalliums. Z Lebensm Unters Forsch 178:453–460
European Food Safety Authority (2012) Lead dietary exposure in the European population. EFSA J 10:2831
Farmand F, Ehdaie A, Roberts CK et al (2005) Lead-induced dysregulation of superoxide dismutases, catalase, glutathione peroxidase, and guanylate cyclase. Environ Res 98:33–39
Feist B, Sitko R (2018) Method for the determination of Pb, Cd, Zn, Mn and Fe in rice samples using carbon nanotubes and cationic complexes of batophenanthroline. Food Chem 249:38–44
Ferreccio C, Smith AH, Duran V et al (2013) Case-control study of arsenic in drinking water and kidney cancer in uniquely exposed Northern Chile. Am J Epidemiol 178:813–818
Fihn SD, Gardin JM, Abrams J et al (2012) 2012 ACCF/AHA/ACP/AATS/PCNA/SCAI/STS guideline for the diagnosis and management of patients with stable ischemic heart disease: executive summary: a report of the American College of Cardiology Foundation/American Heart Association task force on practice guidelines, and the American College of Physicians,

American Association for Thoracic Surgery, Preventive Cardiovascular Nurses Association, Society for Cardiovascular Angiography and Interventions, and Society of Thoracic Surgeons. Circulation 126:3097–3137

Frias S, Diaz C, Conde JE et al (2003) Selenium and mercury concentrations in sweet and dry bottled wines from the Canary Islands, Spain. Food Addit Contam 20:237–240

Galażyn-Sidorczuk M, Brzóska MM, Moniuszko-Jakoniuk J (2008) Estimation of Polish cigarettes contamination with cadmium and lead, and exposure to these metals via smoking. Environ Monit Assess 137:481–493

Genchi G, Sinicropi MS, Lauria G et al (2020) The effects of cadmium toxicity. Int J Environ Res Public Health 17:3782

Golia EE, Dimirkou A, Mitsios IK (2007) Accumulation of metals on tobacco leaves (primings) grown in an agricultural area in relation to soil. Bull Environ Contam Toxicol 79:158–162

Golub HM, Zhou QG, Zucker H et al (2015) Chronic alcohol exposure is associated with decreased neurogenesis, aberrant integration of newborn neurons, and cognitive dysfunction in female mice. Alcohol Clin Exp Res 39:1967–1977

Griswold MG, Fullman N, Hawley C et al (2018) Alcohol use and burden for 195 countries and territories, 1990–2016: a systematic analysis for the Global Burden of Disease Study 2016. Lancet 392:1015–1035

Gurer H, Ercal N (2000) Can antioxidants be beneficial in the treatment of lead poisoning? Free Rad Biol Med 29:927–945

Hettick BE, Canas-Carrell JE, French AD et al (2015) Arsenic: a review of the element's toxicity, plant interactions, and potential methods of remediation. J Agric Food Chem 63:7097–7107

Horváth Z, Paksi B, Felvinczi K et al (2019) An empirically based typology of alcohol users in a community sample using latent class analysis. Eur Addiction Res 25:293–302

Huang YK, Huang YL, Hsueh YM et al (2008) Arsenic exposure, urinary arsenic speciation, and the incidence of urothelial carcinoma: a twelve-year follow-up study. Cancer Causes Control 19: 829–839

Iarc Working Group on the Evaluation of Carcinogenic Risks to Humans (1987) IARC monographs on the evaluation of carcinogenic risks to humans. Supplement 6, genetic and related effects: an updating of selected IARC monographs from volumes 1 to 42. Report of an Ad-hoc IARC Working Group which Met in Lyon, 2–9 December, 1986. International Agency for Research on Cancer

Iarc Working Group on the Evaluation of Carcinogenic Risks to Humans (2010) Alcohol consumption and ethyl carbamate. IARC Monogr Eval Carcinog Risks Hum 96:3

Iarc Working Group on the Evaluation of Carcinogenic Risks to Humans (2012) Pharmaceuticals. Volume 100 A. A review of human carcinogens. IARC Monogr Eval Carcinog Risks Hum 100:1

Illuminati S, Annibaldi A, Truzzi C et al (2014) Recent temporal variations of trace metal content in an Italian white wine. Food Chem 159:493–497

International Agency for Research on Cancer (1980) IARC monographs on the evaluation of the carcinogenic risk of chemicals to humans. vol 22. Some non-nutritive sweetening agents. Distributed for IARC by WHO, Geneva

International Agency for Research on Cancer (2010) Alcohol consumption and ethyl carbamate. IARC Press, International Agency for Research on Cancer

Jabeen S, Mahmood Q, Tariq S et al (2011) Health impact caused by poor water and sanitation in district Abbottabad. J Ayub Med Coll Abbottabad 23:47–50

Kasperczyk S, Slowinska-Lozynska L, Kasperczyk A et al (2015) The effect of occupational lead exposure on lipid peroxidation, protein carbonylation, and plasma viscosity. Toxicol Ind Health 31:1165–1171

Kaufmann A (1993) Schwermetalle in Wein – Vorkommen und Kontaminationsquellen. Mitt Gebiete Lebensmittelunters Hyg 84:88–98

Khan MA, Wajid A, Noor S et al (2008) Effect of soil contamination on some heavy metals content of Cannabis sativa. J Chem Soc Pak 30:805–809

Kim M (2004) Determination of lead and cadmium in wines by graphite furnace atomic absorption spectrometry. Food Addit Contam 21:154–157

Koch KA, Pena MM, Thiele DJ (1997) Copper-binding motifs in catalysis, transport, detoxification and signaling. Chem Biol 4:549–560

Kotelnikova Z (2017) Explaining counterfeit alcohol purchases in Russia. Alcohol Clin Exp Res 41:810–819
Krishna AK, Satyanarayanan M, Govil PK (2009) Assessment of heavy metal pollution in water using multivariate statistical techniques in an industrial area: a case study from Patancheru, Medak District, Andhra Pradesh, India. J Hazard Mater 167:366–373
Kuempel ED, Sorahan T (2010) Identification of research needs to resolve the carcinogenicity of high-priority IARC carcinogens. International Agency for Research on Cancer, pp 61–72
Lachenmeier DW (2020) Is there a need for alcohol policy to mitigate metal contamination in unrecorded fruit spirits? Int J Environ Res Public Health 17:2452
Lachenmeier DW, Rehm J (2012) Unrecorded alcohol–no worries besides ethanol: a population-based probabilistic risk assessment. Alcohol Policy in Europe: Evidence from AMPHORA
Lachenmeier DW, Sarsh B, Rehm J (2009) The composition of alcohol products from markets in Lithuania and Hungary, and potential health consequences: a pilot study. Alcohol Alcoholism 44:93–102
Lachenmeier DW, Monakhova YB, Rehm J (2014) Influence of unrecorded alcohol consumption on liver cirrhosis mortality. World J Gastroenterol: WJG 20:7217
Lachenmeier DW, Walch SG, Commentary on Rehm et al (2017) Composition of alcoholic beverages-an under-researched dimension in the global comparative risk assessment. Addiction 112:1002–1003
Lazos E, Alexakis A (1989) Metal ion content of some Greek wines. Int J Food Sci Technol 24:39–46
Lees B, Mewton L, Jacobus J et al (2020) Association of prenatal alcohol exposure with psychological, behavioral, and neurodevelopmental outcomes in children from the Adolescent Brain Cognitive Development Study. Am J Psychiatr 177:1060–1072
Leitz J, Schoeberl K, Kuballa T et al (2011) Quality of illegally and informally produced alcohol in Europe: results from the AMPHORA project. Adicciones 23:133
Lewchalermvong K, Rangkadilok N, Nookabkaew S et al (2018) Arsenic speciation and accumulation in selected organs after oral administration of rice extracts in Wistar rats. J Agric Food Chem 66:3199–3209
Liao LM, Friesen MC, Xiang Y-B et al (2014) 0346 Occupational exposure to Lead and cancer in two cohort studies of men and women in Shanghai, China. Occup Environ Med 71:A42
Lobinski R, Witte C, Adams FC et al (1994) Organolead in wine. Nature 370:24
Louis P, Hold GL, Flint HJ (2014) The gut microbiota, bacterial metabolites and colorectal cancer. Nat Rev Microbiol 12:661–672
Marengo E, Aceto M (2003) Statistical investigation of the differences in the distribution of metals in Nebbiolo-based wines. Food Chem 81:621–630
Marjanovic A, Omeragic E, Djedjibegovic J et al (2019) Toxic compounds in homemade spirits in Bosnia and Herzegovina: a pilot study. Bull Chem Technol Bosnia Herzeg 53:23–27
Martinez SA, Simonella L, Hansen C et al (2013) Blood lead levels and enzymatic biomarkers of environmental lead exposure in children in Cordoba, Argentina, after the ban of leaded gasoline. Hum Exp Toxicol 32:449–463
Mattson SN, Bernes GA, Doyle LR (2019) Fetal alcohol spectrum disorders: a review of the neurobehavioral deficits associated with prenatal alcohol exposure. Alcohol Clin Exp Res 43:1046–1062
Mccarty KM, Hanh HT, Kim KW (2011) Arsenic geochemistry and human health in South East Asia. Rev Environ Health 26:71–78
Medina B, Augagneur S, Barbaste M et al (2000) Influence of atmospheric pollution on the lead content of wines. Food Addit Contam 17:435–445
Mena C, Cabrera C, Lorenzo ML et al (1996) Cadmium levels in wine, beer and other alcoholic beverages: possible sources of contamination. Sci Total Environ 181:201–208
Miller PM, Anton RF, Egan BM et al (2005) Excessive alcohol consumption and hypertension: clinical implications of current research. J Clin Hypertens 7:346–351
Muhammad S, Shah MT, Khan S (2010) Arsenic health risk assessment in drinking water and source apportionment using multivariate statistical techniques in Kohistan region, northern Pakistan. Food Chem Toxicol 48:2855–2864

Musharraf SG, Shoaib M, Siddiqui AJ et al (2012) Quantitative analysis of some important metals and metalloids in tobacco products by inductively coupled plasma-mass spectrometry (ICP-MS). Chem Cent J 6:1–12
Nordberg GF, Bernard A, Diamond GL et al (2018) Risk assessment of effects of cadmium on human health (IUPAC technical report). Pure Appl Chem 90:755–808
Obeng-Gyasi E (2019) Sources of lead exposure in various countries. Rev Environ Health 34:25–34
Okaru AO, Rehm J, Sommerfeld K et al (2019) The threat to quality of alcoholic beverages by unrecorded consumption. Alcoholic beverages. Elsevier
Pál L, Muhollari T, Bujdosó O et al (2020) Heavy metal contamination in recorded and unrecorded spirits. Should we worry? Regul Toxicol Pharmacol 116:104723
Pande M, Flora SJ (2002) Lead induced oxidative damage and its response to combined administration of alpha-lipoic acid and succimers in rats. Toxicology 177:187–196
Pedersen GA, Mortensen GK, Larsen EH (1994) Beverages as a source of toxic trace element intake. Food Addit Contam 11:351–363
Pflaum T, Hausler T, Baumung C et al (2016) Carcinogenic compounds in alcoholic beverages: an update. Arch Toxicol 90:2349–2367
Pohl P (2007) What do metals tell us about wine? TrAC Trends Anal Chem 26:941–949
Rahman MM, Naidu R, Bhattacharya P (2009) Arsenic contamination in groundwater in the Southeast Asia region. Environ Geochem Health 31:9–21
Ravenscroft P, Brammer H, Richards K (2009) Arsenic in North America and Europe. Arsenic pollution: a global synthesis. Wiley-Blackwell, pp 387–454
Redan BW, Jablonski JE, Halverson C et al (2019) Factors affecting transfer of the heavy metals arsenic, lead, and cadmium from diatomaceous-earth filter aids to alcoholic beverages during laboratory-scale filtration. J Agric Food Chem 67:2670–2678
Rehm J, Taylor B, Patra J (2006) Volume of alcohol consumption, patterns of drinking and burden of disease in the European region 2002. Addiction 101:1086–1095
Rezaei A, Hassani H, Hassani S et al (2019) Evaluation of groundwater quality and heavy metal pollution indices in Bazman basin, southeastern Iran. Groundwater Sust Develop 9:100245
Rodgers A, Ezzati M, Vander Hoorn S et al (2004) Distribution of major health risks: findings from the Global Burden of Disease study. PLoS Med 1:e27
Roehr M, Kosaric N, Vardar-Sukan F et al (2001) The biotechnology of ethanol. Classical and future applications. Molecules 6:1019
Salzman J (2017) Drinking water: a history (Revised edition). Abrams
Santana NMT, Mill JG, Velasquez-Melendez G et al (2018) Consumption of alcohol and blood pressure: results of the ELSA-Brasil study. PLoS One 13:e0190239
Satarug S, Vesey DA, Gobe GC (2017) Current health risk assessment practice for dietary cadmium: data from different countries. Food Chem Toxicol 106:430–445
Schneider G, Krivna V (1993) Multi-element analysis of tobacco and smoke condensate by instrumental neutron activation analysis and atomic absorption spectrometry. Int J Environ Anal Chem 53:87–100
Schwabe RF, Jobin C (2013) The microbiome and cancer. Nat Rev Cancer 13:800–812
Smith AH, Goycolea M, Haque R et al (1998) Marked increase in bladder and lung cancer mortality in a region of Northern Chile due to arsenic in drinking water. Am J Epidemiol 147:660–669
Sohel N, Vahter M, Ali M et al (2010) Spatial patterns of fetal loss and infant death in an arsenic-affected area in Bangladesh. Int J Health Geogr 9:53
Spear LP (2018) Effects of adolescent alcohol consumption on the brain and behaviour. Nat Rev Neurosci 19:197
Tahvonen R (1998) Lead and cadmium in beverages consumed in Finland. Food Addit Contam 15:446–450
Taylor AA, Tsuji JS, Garry MR et al (2020) Critical review of exposure and effects: implications for setting regulatory health criteria for ingested copper. Environ Manag 65:131–159
Tuzen M, Sahiner S, Hazer B (2016) Solid phase extraction of lead, cadmium and zinc on biodegradable polyhydroxybutyrate diethanol amine (PHB-DEA) polymer and their determination in water and food samples. Food Chem 210:115–120
Vahter M (2009) Effects of arsenic on maternal and fetal health. Annu Rev Nutr 29:381–399

Vahter ME, Li L, Nermell B et al (2006) Arsenic exposure in pregnancy: a population-based study in Matlab, Bangladesh. J Health Popul Nutr 24:236–245
Verstraeten SV, Aimo L, Oteiza PI (2008) Aluminium and lead: molecular mechanisms of brain toxicity. Arch Toxicol 82:789–802
Wang C, Liang J, Zhang C et al (2007) Effect of ascorbic acid and thiamine supplementation at different concentrations on lead toxicity in liver. Ann Occupat Hyg 51:563–569
Wasserman GA, Liu X, Parvez F et al (2004) Water arsenic exposure and children's intellectual function in Araihazar, Bangladesh. Environ Health Perspect 112:1329–1333
Watson RR (2003) Reviews in food and nutrition toxicity. CRC Press
World Health Organization (1993) Guidelines for drinking-water quality. World Health Organization
World Health Organization (2016) Global information system on alcohol and health (GISAH). World Health Organization
World Health Organization (2018a) Global status report on alcohol and health 2018. World Health Organization, Geneva
World Health Organization (2018b) WHO recommendations on intrapartum care for a positive childbirth experience. World Health Organization
Yousefinejad V, Mansouri B, Ramezani Z et al (2018) Evaluation of heavy metals in tobacco and hookah water used in coffee houses in Sanandaj city in 2017. Sci J Kurdistan Univ Med Sci 22: 96–106
Zuberbier T, Aberer W, Asero R et al (2018) The EAACI/GA(2)LEN/EDF/WAO guideline for the definition, classification, diagnosis and management of urticaria. Allergy 73:1393–1414

54 Alcohol Consumption and Suicidal Behavior: Current Research Evidence and Potential for Prevention

Kairi Kõlves, Rose Crossin, and Katrina Witt

Contents

Introduction 1152
Overview of Suicidal Behavior and Ideation 1152
The Biopsychosocial Model of Suicide 1154
Alcohol Use and Suicide 1155
Ecological-Level Links 1155
The Distal Relationship Between Alcohol Use and Suicide 1156
Quantifying the Distal Relationship 1156
Potential Mechanisms 1157
The Proximal Relationship Between Alcohol Use and Suicide 1159
Quantifying the Proximal Relationship 1159
Potential Mechanisms and Causality in the Proximal Relationship 1159
Impact of Alcohol-Focused Interventions 1161
Impact of Alcohol Policies on Suicidal Behavior 1162
Summary Points 1167
Applications to Other Areas of Addiction 1168
Mini-dictionary of Terms 1169
Key Facts About Suicide 1169
References 1170

K. Kõlves (✉)
Australian Institute for Suicide Research and Prevention, WHO Collaborating Centre for Research and Training in Suicide Prevention, School of Applied Psychology, Griffith University, Brisbane, QLD, Australia
e-mail: k.kolves@griffith.edu.au

R. Crossin
Department of Population Health, University of Otago, Christchurch, New Zealand
e-mail: rose.crossin@otago.ac.nz

K. Witt
Orygen, Melbourne, VIC, Australia

Centre for Youth Mental Health, The University of Melbourne, Parkville, VIC, Australia
e-mail: katrina.witt@orygen.org.au

V. B. Patel, V. R. Preedy (eds.), *Handbook of Substance Misuse and Addictions*,
https://doi.org/10.1007/978-3-030-92392-1_61

Abstract

Suicide is an ongoing public health issue globally. An individual's risk of suicide is made up of a complex interaction between risk factors that can occur at an ecological (population), distal, or proximal level: "the biopsychosocial model." The World Health Organization identifies alcohol use (including both acute intoxication and chronic use) as a modifiable risk factor for suicide. Globally, it has been estimated that almost one in five suicide deaths is attributable to alcohol use and alcohol can influence suicide risk at all three levels within the biopsychosocial model. This chapter describes the relationship between alcohol use and suicide and outlines potential mechanisms underpinning this relationship. Furthermore, policy and clinical interventions targeted at alcohol use at both the ecological and individual level are presented and discussed, ultimately aimed at preventing suicide.

Keywords

Alcohol · Suicide · Self-harm · Suicidal ideation · Alcohol abuse · Alcohol intoxication · Alcohol interventions · Alcohol policies · Suicide prevention

Abbreviations

AUD Alcohol use disorder
BAC Blood alcohol concentration
HPA Hypothalamic-pituitary-adrenal
WHO World Health Organization

Introduction

Overview of Suicidal Behavior and Ideation

Suicide, the act of intentionally causing one's own death (De Leo et al. 2021), is an important public health issue. Globally, the World Health Organization (WHO) estimates that over 700,000 people die by suicide every year (World Health Organization 2021). Although around three-quarters (77%) of all suicides occur in low- and middle-income countries, suicide rates are generally higher in high-income countries (World Health Organization 2021). In addition to large geographic variation, suicides rates also vary by age and gender. Suicide rates are higher in males than in females in most countries. Suicide is a leading cause of death among males and females aged 15–29 years and represents the leading cause of death for this age group across a number of high-income countries (World Health Organization 2021). Despite a general decline in global age-standardized suicides rates (Naghavi 2019; World Health Organization 2021), there has been an increasing trend in some regions and countries (see Fig. 1 for suicide rates by the WHO regions), particularly in younger people (Glenn et al. 2020). Reducing

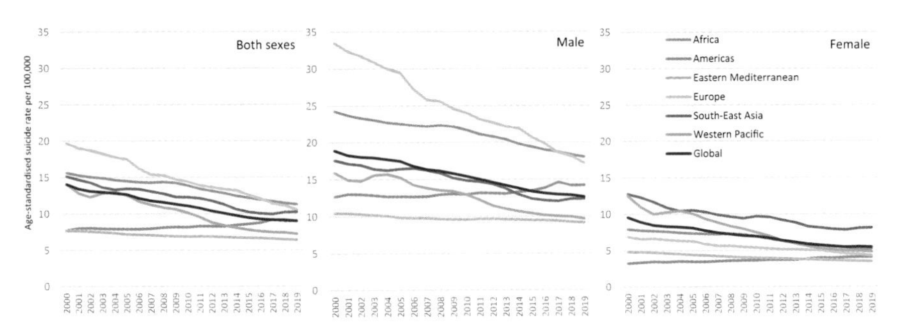

Data source: World Health Organization Global Health Estimates, 2021.

Fig. 1 Age-standardized suicide rates globally and by the World Health Organization regions. (Data source: World Health Organization Global Health Estimates 2021)

suicide is therefore a key indicator for the United Nations' Sustainable Development Goals (United Nations 2015) and the WHO's Mental Health Action Plan 2013–2020 (World Health Organization 2013), which has recently been extended to 2030 (World Health Organization 2021).

In addition to suicide, non-fatal self-harm and suicidal ideation have substantial health and psychological impacts for affected individuals and their families, friends, the healthcare system, and wider society. Non-fatal self-harm, which includes all intentional acts of self-poisoning (such as intentional drug overdoses) or self-injury (such as self-cutting) regardless of degree of suicidal intent or other types of motivation (Hawton et al. 2003; De Leo et al. 2021), is by different estimates at least 20 times more common than suicide (Geulayov et al. 2018; Turecki et al. 2019; Zortea et al. 2020). Many more episodes of self-harm occur in the community and do not necessarily result in presentation to clinical services (Geulayov et al. 2018), with the non-presentation proportion estimated to be as high as 40–50% (Jollant et al. 2020). Prevalence estimates suggest that around one in ten young adults has attempted suicide in their lifetime, with 2.7% making an attempt in the past 12 months (O'Connor et al. 2018b). In contrast to suicide, rates of non-fatal self-harm are typically higher in females (McMahon et al. 2014; Diggins et al. 2017; Griffin et al. 2018) and have been shown to be increasing, particularly for young females (Mercado et al. 2017; Griffin et al. 2018; Kõlves et al. 2018a).

Suicidal ideation, which includes thinking about, considering, or planning suicide, is more widespread than non-fatal self-harm with studies showing 12-month prevalence of between 2% (Borges et al. 2010) and 10% (O'Connor et al. 2018b). Around 1 in 5 (22.8%) young adults reports lifetime suicidal ideation (O'Connor et al. 2018b). Prevalence estimates for both suicidal ideation and self-harm are notably higher for adolescents and young people (Uddin et al. 2019).

Both non-fatal self-harm and suicidal ideation may be linked to subsequent suicide within an ideation-to-action framework (Klonsky et al. 2016). Indeed, a prior suicide attempt is the single largest individual risk factor for subsequent suicide across a range of psychiatric diagnoses (World Health Organization 2014).

The Biopsychosocial Model of Suicide

Suicide is a highly complex multidimensional phenomenon. An individual's risk of suicide is typically the result of a complex interplay between a variety of factors (both risk and protective) at multiple levels. These factors may be biological, psychological, clinical, social or cultural, and environmental (Turecki et al. 2019). They can be categorized as ecological (population)-, distal-, or proximal (individual)-level factors.

Ecological Factors

Ecological factors have an impact at the population level and can provide the context for an individual's risk of suicide. These may include geographic location, socio-economic conditions, social and cultural norms, and policies and systems. Particularly relevant policies and systems include those that impact access to suicide means (e.g., gun control laws or reduced pack sizes of pharmaceuticals (Hawton et al. 2003; Andrés and Hempstead 2011)), access to services that may increase protective factors (e.g., availability of mental health services (Pirkola et al. 2009; Milner et al. 2012)), and alcohol availability.

Distal Factors

Distal factors may predispose an individual to suicide. Early-life distal factors may include genetics and epigenetics, a family history of suicide, and early-life adversities. These factors can act on an individual throughout their life course and may mediate or interact with other factors.

Suicide rates are between four- and sevenfold higher in young people with a first-degree relative (i.e., parent, sibling) who has also died by suicide, even following adjustment for the presence of psychiatric disorders and other relevant factors (Cheng et al. 2014; Lee et al. 2017a). This risk appears to remain elevated even into adulthood (Hua et al. 2019). Despite this, heritability estimates range between 30% and 55% (Voracek and Loibl 2007), suggesting that other factors remain important.

Early-life adversity, which may include exposure to parental interpersonal violence, as well as neglect, maltreatment, and emotional, physical, and/or sexual abuse, may affect the epigenetic regulation of stress-response symptoms that can result in the development of emotional, behavioral, and cognitive phenotypes (Turecki et al. 2012). These, in turn, may influence personality traits (including impulsivity and aggression), cognitive functioning, and psychiatric disorders, which are also associated with chronic substance misuse or substance use disorders; collectively these may all increase predisposed suicide risk in later life (Bolton and Robinson 2010; Turecki et al. 2019).

Proximal Factors

Proximal factors are those that may precipitate an individual to act on suicidal thoughts and indeed may facilitate suicide. These factors may be influenced by both ecological and distal factors. These factors may include adverse life events and stressors such as job loss, financial stress, relationship breakdown, social isolation, illness and pain, or bereavement (Kõlves et al. 2006a; Foster 2011). Other known proximal factors include psychological distress (including feelings of despair or hopelessness), acute symptoms of psychiatric disorders, and substance use or intoxication (Turecki et al. 2019).

Proximal factors are also influenced by access to means. While access to means may be influenced by ecological-level policies (Nordentoft et al. 2007; Andrés and Hempstead 2011), individual risk can also be reduced by restricting access to these means (Yip et al. 2012).

Alcohol Use and Suicide

The WHO identifies alcohol use (including both acute intoxication and chronic use) as a modifiable risk factor for suicide (World Health Organization 2014). Globally, it has been estimated that almost one in five (18%) suicide deaths is attributable to alcohol use (World Health Organization 2019). Alcohol use influences suicide risk at all three levels within the biopsychosocial model (see Fig 2). This chapter will address the relationship between alcohol use and suicide and potential mechanisms underpinning this relationship. Furthermore, policy and clinical opportunities to prevent suicidal behavior and ideation at both the ecological and individual levels by targeting alcohol use will be presented.

Ecological-Level Links

An ecological-level link between alcohol consumption and suicide was analyzed in a systematic review of 16 population-level time-series studies estimating the association between alcohol use per capita and suicide rates (Norström and

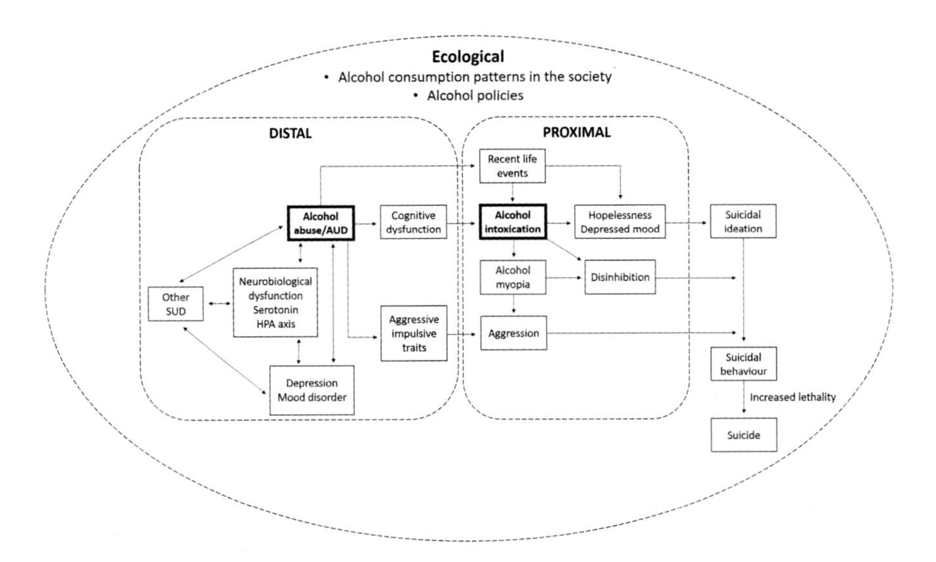

Fig. 2 Different alcohol (ab)use related pathways to suicidal behavior

Rossow 2016). Over half (59%) of the studies reported significant positive associations for males, and 40% reported positive associations for females. The link is likely to depend on the drinking culture, however, with associations appearing to be stronger in countries with so-called "dry" cultures characterized by infrequent but heavier binge drinking and intoxication-oriented drinking patterns, particularly spirits, such as certain Nordic countries and Eastern Europe, as compared to countries from predominately wine-consuming cultures ("wet" cultures) where lower-level and frequent alcohol consumption is more common, such as in Southern Europe (Ramstedt 2001; Landberg 2008; Stickley et al. 2011; Norstrom et al. 2012). Indeed, alcohol consumption measured on a national level is more likely to be associated with national suicide rates in the countries where drinking culture is more detrimental (as defined using a Detrimental Drinking Pattern Score) (Norström and Rossow 2016). However, a subsequent cross-national analysis of 83 countries provided no evidence that drinking cultures were related to suicide rates, though beverage-specific effects were identified (Roche et al. 2018). More specifically, there was a link between spirit and also beer consumption and suicide rates, particularly for males, but not with wine consumption (Roche et al. 2018). Furthermore, the association between alcohol consumption per capita and suicide rates was shown in models even following adjustment for structural confounders such as unemployment, poverty, and urbanicity, leading the authors to conclude that alcohol consumption (and the nature of that consumption) is a key characteristic impacting suicide rates (Roche et al. 2018). Ecological-level links have been explained by alcohol consumption being a socio-cultural factor leading to weakened and deteriorated social integration (Skog 1993), though further research is required to elucidate the mechanisms by which alcohol impacts suicide at an ecological level and how these may interact with other individual-level factors, which will be further discussed.

The Distal Relationship Between Alcohol Use and Suicide

Quantifying the Distal Relationship

Psychological autopsy studies have shown that prevalence of alcohol use disorder (AUD) varies widely in people who died by suicide – from none in Pakistan (Khan et al. 2008) up to 61% in Estonia (Kõlves et al. 2006b). A substantial body of high-quality evidence links AUD with an increased risk of suicidal behavior. A 2015 systematic review and meta-analysis covering 31 studies with 420,372 participants presented a significant association between AUD and suicidal ideation, suicide attempt, and suicide; these results did not appear to be moderated by age or sex (Darvishi et al. 2015).

Roerecke and Rehm (2014) took an alternate approach and conducted a systematic review and meta-analysis on cause-specific mortality among AUD treatment patients that included 17 studies. AUD conferred an additional risk of suicide death in both males and females (Roerecke and Rehm 2014). The authors also highlight that comorbidity in AUD patients who die by suicide was high, particularly for depression (Roerecke and Rehm 2014). In addition, a recent large-scale linkage study analyzed the risk of suicide in those with AUD history in a Swedish birth cohort born in 1950–1970 (Edwards et al. 2020). They found that the risk period was highest in the 5 years following AUD registration; however, the hazard ratio for both males and females remained greater than 2 after 25 or more years. Importantly, this study identified a substantial component of the relationship between AUD and suicide was retained even after adjustment for confounding psychiatric and familial factors, suggestive of a causal relationship (Edwards et al. 2020).

Potential Mechanisms

Norström and Rossow (2016) outline the potential challenges when seeking to understand and quantify the relationship between alcohol abuse and suicide, given that there are potentially direct causal pathways, indirect pathways from alcohol via other risk factors (e.g., depression, impulsivity), and the potential for the drinking of others to impact on suicide risk in their family members. Rather than attempting to make a determination of causality, this chapter will focus on the breadth of potential interactions between alcohol use and distal risk factors for suicide, which enables conceptualization of the scale of the relationship.

Depression and Depressive Disorders

Alcohol abuse has been associated with increases in depressive thoughts (Conner and Duberstein 2004; Jakubczyk et al. 2012). Comorbidity of AUD and depression has been shown to increase the risk of suicidal behavior (Conner et al. 2008). There is evidence that the relationship between alcohol use and major depression is more likely explained by a causal model by which alcohol use led to depression, rather than a self-medication hypothesis from depression to alcohol (Fergusson et al. 2009). Furthermore, the presence of an AUD at least doubles the risk of being diagnosed with major depression via a causal pathway (Boden and Fergusson 2011). Major depressive disorder may also be comorbid with other substance use disorders (SUD) (Currie et al. 2005), with AUD and other SUDs co-occurring in some individuals who die by suicide (Kõlves et al. 2017).

Cognitive Dysfunction

Cognitive functioning, including problem-solving, flexibility, and memory, have all been identified as being associated with suicidal behavior, potentially by impacting how an individual responds to stress or complex problems. Heavy and chronic alcohol use has also been linked to cognitive impairment and reduced executive control via alcohol-related brain damage (Bernardin et al. 2014; Hayes et al. 2016). In addition, cognitive constriction may contribute to increasing suicidal behavior as individuals ruminate on recent adverse events which, in turn, may increase negative affect and depressive thoughts (O'Connell and Lawlor 2005).

Impulsivity and Aggression

There is ongoing research on how impulsivity and aggression are related and if they represent one trait or two (García-Forero et al. 2009); however, both are strongly associated with suicide risk (Conner et al. 2008; Gvion and Apter 2011). It is difficult to disentangle impulsive-aggressive traits, alcohol use, and suicide because of the complex temporal relationship between these factors (Carballo et al. 2006). Impulsivity is associated with the development and maintenance of AUD and other SUDs, particularly the decision-making aspects of impulsivity (Courtney et al. 2012; Coskunpinar et al. 2013). Furthermore, both aggressive and impulsive traits appear to explain the higher incidence of suicide attempts in depressed individuals who have a history of AUD, as compared to depressed individuals without AUD, suggesting these traits may form a common substrate for both AUD and suicide (Sher et al. 2005). However, impulsive-aggressive behaviors may be mediated by the long-term effects of alcohol due to altered serotonin signalling (Volkow et al. 2017), which is also heavily implicated in the impulsive-aggressive trait (Lesch and Merschdorf 2000).

Neurobiological Links Between Alcohol Use and Suicide

While there are different neurobiological mechanisms that plausibly link alcohol use and suicide, two of these have a stronger body of evidence including serotonin dysregulation and effects on stress responsivity via the hypothalamic-pituitary-adrenal (HPA) axis. Dysregulated serotonin function has been associated with increased depression and suicide risk (Turecki et al. 2019). While AUD has also been associated with impaired serotonin transmission (LeMarquand et al. 1994), there is also evidence to suggest that the pathophysiology pathways of serotonin dysregulation differ between AUD and suicide (Underwood et al. 2018).

The HPA axis functions by releasing cortisol in response to a stressor, which triggers a range of physiological responses including increasing blood pressure and cardiac output and decreasing acutely non-essential processes such as the immune system. Cortisol release is controlled via a negative feedback loop, though this regulation can be disrupted by chronic stress. Dysregulation (both hyper- and hypoactivity) of the HPA axis is considered a neurobiological risk factor for suicide (Turecki et al. 2019). HPA axis hyperactivity may be associated with suicidal thoughts and behaviors via the association with major depression and other mood disorders (Pariante and Lightman 2008; Pompili et al. 2010). Conversely, HPA axis hypoactivity has also been associated with increased suicide risk, potentially due to compensatory downregulation following long-term trauma exposure (O'Connor et al. 2018a), which reduces the ability of an individual to adaptively respond to stressors (Pompili et al. 2010; Melhem et al. 2017). While acute alcohol consumption may initially activate the HPA axis, chronic consumption may lead to blunting (hypoactivation) of the HPA axis (Becker 2012).

The Proximal Relationship Between Alcohol Use and Suicide

Quantifying the Proximal Relationship

The acute use of alcohol is frequently identified as a proximal risk factor for suicide. Acute alcohol use has been detected in up to one-third of suicide decedents (Anestis et al. 2014; Conner 2015), although this ranges from between 9.5% in Thailand (Narongchai and Narongchai 2006) to almost three-quarters (74.2%) in Slovenia (Bilban and Škibin 2005). More recent reviews have found a dose-response relationship between the level of acute alcohol use and suicide attempt; higher levels of acute alcohol use were associated with higher odds of suicide attempt (Borges et al. 2017). In addition, the effects of alcohol intoxication may acutely impact suicide risk, and therefore, suicide risk can change dramatically and rapidly while an individual is intoxicated (Hufford 2001).

Some recent studies have provided further understanding of the characteristics of suicide deaths involving acute alcohol use (Lee et al. 2017b; Chong et al. 2020; Kõlves et al. 2020b). In Australia, around one-quarter (26.7%) of suicide decedents had a blood alcohol concentration (BAC) exceeding legal driving limits in Australia of ≥0.05 g/100 mL. Acute alcohol use prior to suicide was associated with acute stress (e.g., separation), particularly in those without known psychiatric diagnoses, except substance use (Kõlves et al. 2020b). Acute alcohol use was also more common in those who died by hanging as compared to those using other methods. An analysis of suicides in South Korea also found that over one-quarter (28.7%) of decedents had a BAC exceeding legal driving limits (≥0.08 g/100 mL) and was also associated with having no underlying medical illness nor psychiatric diagnosis (Lee et al. 2017b). The authors suggest that acute alcohol use may lead to impulsive suicides under stress without pre-existing psychiatric conditions (Lee et al. 2017b; Kõlves et al. 2020b).

Potential Mechanisms and Causality in the Proximal Relationship

There are multiple pathways by which alcohol use may act as a proximal risk factor for suicidal behavior by interacting with other distal or proximal risk factors (Borges et al. 2017). Alcohol can also be a means of suicide (via self-poisoning, with or without concomitant other substance use) or influence other suicide means (Anestis et al. 2014). These pathways may differ in individuals or in population groups or impact on an individual at multiple time points. Thus, these pathways are complex and are likely not mutually exclusive; like the previously discussed distal interactions, these pathways will be discussed, rather than seeking to make conclusions regarding causality.

Recent Life Events

Recent life events may precipitate or trigger suicide. These may include job loss, financial stress, or relationship breakdown (Overholser et al. 2012); these are also typically associated with a sudden change in socioeconomic position or social connectedness. Chronic heavy alcohol use or AUD may contribute to the occurrence of these recent events, and the risk of these stressors is higher in those with alcohol dependence than those without (Conner et al. 2003; Kõlves et al. 2017). Conversely, alcohol use may increase following these events as a coping strategy (Veenstra et al. 2007), ultimately leading to an increasing spiral between adversity and alcohol use.

Acute Effects of Alcohol Intoxication

Aggression

Aggressive behavior can either be self-directed or directed at other individuals. Aggression toward others, however, can also be associated with suicide risk by contributing to acute interpersonal conflict. Alcohol intoxication has a well-established association with aggression (Heinz et al. 2011; Duke et al. 2018), particularly when BAC is in the ascending component of the BAC-time curve (which takes an inverted U shape), which is when alcohol has stimulant effects (Hendler et al. 2011).

Feelings of Depression or Despair

Feelings of despair, hopelessness, or depression are precipitating factors for increased suicide risk, via suicidal ideation. Alcohol may contribute to these feelings at multiple temporal scales (including the distal link between alcohol and depression as previously discussed). Acute alcohol use can induce a depressed mood state, particularly with BACs exceeding 100 mg/mL (Vonghia, Leggio et al. 2008). The depressant effects of alcohol are a function of blood alcohol concentration and metabolism, with negative affect observed predominantly during the descending component of the BAC-time curve (Sutker et al. 1987). However, understanding of the neurobiological underpinnings of this aspect of intoxication is sparse in comparison to understanding the stimulant effects of alcohol on the ascending component of the curve (Hendler et al. 2011).

Disinhibition, Impulsivity, and Impaired Problem-Solving

Acute alcohol use is associated with increased impulsivity (Stamates and Lau-Barraco 2020), which, in turn, has been linked with suicidal behavior (Bagge et al. 2015; Bryan et al. 2016). This may be compounded by the disinhibiting effects of alcohol, which could remove barriers to acting on suicidal ideation. For example, some studies have found that both acute and chronic alcohol use are associated with greater tolerance of pain (Amadi et al. 2020; Jakubczyk et al. 2021), disinhibition of psychological barriers against death (Pompili et al. 2010; Norström and Rossow 2016), and consequently greater risk of using more highly lethal means of suicide. As well as being disinhibiting, alcohol intoxication can create an "alcohol myopia," whereby an individual is less able to perceive or extract meaning from external cues and has a limited focus on instigatory rather than inhibitory cues (Giancola et al. 2010). This limits the capacity to problem-solve or to identify other coping strategies at a time of crisis while having a propensity for impulsive action, which may result in suicidal action (Richardson et al. 2021).

Association with Suicide Means and Lethality

Alcohol as a Means of Suicide

Self-poisoning with drugs and/or medications (also known as "intentional drug overdose" or IDO) is one of the most common suicide means, particularly among females (Värnik et al. 2008; Kõlves et al. 2018b). Alcohol is a central nervous system depressant, which can cause respiratory depression, coma, and death when consumed in high quantities. A potentially lethal BAC can occur above 400 mg/ 100 mL for adults, though this may be lower when complicated by aspiration of vomitus (Heatley and Crane 1990) and will differ for individuals taking into consideration factors like age or comorbidities. Although self-poisoning death by alcohol alone is possible, it is rarely intentional. It is more common for alcohol to be implicated in poly-substance self-poisoning, particularly where other depressant drugs including opioids, benzodiazepines, and gabapentinoids are consumed (Koski et al. 2002; Hickman et al. 2008; Cairns et al. 2019). Thus, the ingestion of multiple depressant drugs, including alcohol, may co-potentiate the effects and result in mortality at lower levels of BAC. In this way, alcohol may act as a facilitator to suicide death by self-poisoning (Hawton et al. 1989). It is also worthwhile noting that alcohol-related liver disease following chronic use may predispose individuals to paracetamol (acetaminophen)-induced hepatotoxicity, thus increasing mortality (Riordan and Williams 2002).

Alcohol Related to Other Means of Suicide

Acute alcohol use has been associated with more lethal suicide means, which are more likely to lead to a fatal outcome (Powell et al. 2001; Sher et al. 2009). In particular, acute alcohol use has been associated with increased gun suicide and death by hanging (Branas et al. 2011; Conner et al. 2014b; Kõlves et al. 2020b), both of which are highly lethal means. Some individuals may use alcohol in order to "numb their fears" or to suppress pain before a suicide attempt (Conner et al. 2014a; Bagge et al. 2015), thus reflecting an aspect of suicide planning. Other individuals may impulsively use a more lethal means while intoxicated, in part due to the disinhibiting effects and impaired decision-making arising from alcohol intoxication (Hufford 2001). It is also possible that this association may reflect overlapping demographics between more lethal suicide means and heavier alcohol use, especially for males.

Impact of Alcohol-Focused Interventions

Given the complex relationship between both acute and chronic alcohol use with suicidal ideation, self-harm, and suicidal behavior, a growing number of studies have included alcohol-focused content into psychological interventions for those at risk of suicide. These studies have used a variety of therapeutic approaches, most commonly cognitive behavioral therapy-based approaches, followed by briefer counselling-based approaches.

While there is still little evidence of an effect for alcohol-focused interventions delivered at the individual level, on suicide deaths either at post-intervention (Gregory et al. 2008; Nadkarni et al. 2017) or at 2–6 months' follow-up (Crawford et al. 2010; Davidson et al. 2014) in four randomized controlled trials (RCTs), few studies have been sufficiently powered to investigate impacts on suicide deaths (Witt et al. 2021). Previous calculations have shown that studies may need to recruit up to a minimum of 8757 participants per treatment arm to detect a clinically significant effect for suicide (Witt et al. 2020).

Alcohol-focused interventions may have some effect in reducing absolute repetition of non-fatal self-harm by the 12-month follow-up assessment in six RCTs (Crawford et al. 2010, Davidson et al. 2014; Gregory et al. 2008; Watt et al. 2008; Nadkarni et al. 2017; McManama-O'Brien et al. 2018). However, there was no apparent difference in effect by therapeutic approach, intervention dose (in hours), or intervention duration (in months) (Witt et al. 2021).

The effect of these approaches on suicidal ideation may be more equivocal. Results from five RCTs investigated effects of these interventions on suicidal ideation scores, measured continuously (Kaminer et al. 2006; Davidson et al. 2014; Morley et al. 2014; McManama-O'Brien et al. 2018; Wilks et al. 2018), finding that these alcohol-focused interventions were not associated with a significant treatment effect. There was some evidence of an effect for an alcohol-focused CBT approach on suicidal ideation scores in some non-RCTs.

The greater effect of alcohol-focused psychological interventions on self-harm and suicide attempts may suggest that alcohol may play an important role in the transition from suicidal ideation to action (Turecki et al. 2019). Differences in the impact of these interventions on self-harm and suicide attempts as compared with suicidal ideation may also reflect differences in outcome measurability (Witt et al. 2021). It is important to note, however, that this chapter excluded studies of pharmacological agents as these do not directly address the psychological factors associated with harmful alcohol use and suicide, self-harm, and/or suicidal ideation (Witt et al. 2021). The effect of pharmacological interventions on these outcomes therefore remains to be determined in future studies, including methods to maintain any effects long term, including via complementing pharmacological interventions with psychological approaches.

Impact of Alcohol Policies on Suicidal Behavior

Considering the links between individual-level suicide risk and ecological-level availability of alcohol as highlighted previously, it is reasonable to assume that national alcohol policies would have an impact on suicide rates. However, it is important to note that alcohol policies are strongly related with the countries' (or territories') political will – alcohol restrictions are traditionally public health measures to reduce alcohol-related harms in the community; however, relaxing alcohol laws often have political or economic motivations (Kõlves et al. 2020a).

A recent systematic review categorized alcohol policies using the WHO's recommended target areas for policy action at the national level (World Health Organization 2018), including alcohol availability (nine studies), alcohol pricing (seven studies), drink-driving countermeasures (three studies), and mixed policies (four studies) to limit alcohol consumption (Kõlves et al. 2020a). Restrictions on alcohol availability, for example, via sales restrictions and/or increased cost via taxation of alcohol, were associated with decreased rates of suicides in this chapter (Kõlves et al. 2020a). Table 1 provides a brief overview of different studies.

Possibly the strictest alcohol restriction policy was the Gorbachev era strict anti-alcohol policy in the former USSR in 1985–1989, which involved multiple measures to reduce alcohol consumption including increases in the prices of alcoholic beverages, decreases in the alcohol production in the country, decreases in the number of retail outlets for alcohol, fines and arrests to people who were drunk in public places, and improvements in alcohol treatment (Värnik et al. 2007). There are several analyses measuring the impact of the policies on mortality, including suicide. Ecological-level analyses showed reduction in suicide rates in Baltic and Slavic republics of the former USSR during those years, where consumption was highest (Wasserman et al. 1994, 1998). Furthermore, there was a decline in the proportion of suicide decedents with positive BAC (Fig. 3; Värnik et al. 2007). This effect was particularly salient for males as compared to females. A less profound effect was measured after a more recent national alcohol policy implemented in March 2003 which established a minimum legal drinking age, tightened liquor licensing laws, and limited sales in Slovenia. Once again, this effect was stronger for males (Pridemore and Snowden 2009).

Similarly, although there was an over 30% decline in male suicide rates in Lithuania (a part of the former USSR) during the Gorbachev era's strict anti-alcohol policy (Wasserman et al. 1994), a more recent anti-alcohol campaign in this country aimed at regulating alcohol advertising, the illegal import of alcohol, time limits on sales, and increase in excise tax found an increase in suicides between 2006 and 2009 (Sauliune et al. 2012). Nevertheless, it must be noted that only a very limited time period (1 year before and 1 year after) was analyzed. In addition, the implementation of this policy coincided with the 2008 Global Financial Crisis, and there was an increase in rates of unemployment, which are also associated with increased suicide rates in some work (Milner et al. 2014), in Lithuania over this period.

Nevertheless, considering different strategies included in national alcohol policies, it is challenging to identify the mechanisms contributing to the changes in suicide rates and to control for all potential confounding factors. Additionally, all studies conducted to date represent "natural experiments" and have measured only changes in suicide rates; only one study to date has analyzed the effect of these policies on rates of non-fatal self-harm admissions to general hospitals (Northridge et al. 1986).

Table 1 A brief description of alcohol policies and main findings of papers analyzing the impact of alcohol policies on suicide

Authors (year)	Alcohol policy	Component (s) of alcohol policy targeted	Main findings
Andreasson et al. (2006)	Abolition of monopolies on the wholesale, import, and export of alcohol, as well as lifting of limits on the private import of alcohol associated with Sweden's entry into the European Union in Jan 1, 1995	Alcohol availability	An increase in alcohol consumption; predicted alcohol-related harm was compared with real alcohol-related harm. Suicides showed a decreasing trend for both sexes
Berman et al. (2000)	State law (Alaska local option law in 1981) which enabled communities to choose between three alcohol availability policies: (1) "dry law," sale and import of alcohol prohibited within the community; (2) "damp law," sale of alcohol prohibited but import for personal use permitted or sale permitted only at one specific store; and (3) "wet law," no prohibition on the sale or import of alcohol within the community	Alcohol availability	The suicide decreased in Alaskan Native communities selecting less restrictive measures – "damp law." There were no reductions in suicide rates in communities selecting more restrictive measures – "dry law"
Birckmayer and Hemenway (1999)	State laws raising the minimum legal drinking age (MLDA) following implementation of the 1986 National Highway Safety Act	Alcohol availability	States with younger MLDAs had 8% higher suicide rates among 18–20-year-olds and 6% higher rates in 21–23-year-olds, even following adjustment for a number of indicators of socioeconomic disparity. No significant effects were found for adolescents below the MLDA
Carpenter (2004)	State zero blood alcohol level (so-called zero tolerance [ZT]) laws for drivers under the age of 21 years following implementation of the 1995 National Highway Systems Designation Act	Drink-driving countermeasures	Reductions in suicide were found for 18–20-year-olds (6.3%), for males between 15 and 17 years old (10.3%), and for males between 18 and 20 years old (7.7%). No meaningful effects were found for females or for older age groups

(continued)

Table 1 (continued)

Authors (year)	Alcohol policy	Component (s) of alcohol policy targeted	Main findings
Joubert (1994)	Legal prohibition of the sale of alcohol from the 1920s, which is still followed by some counties "dry counties," which are not allowing similar sales as "wet counties"	Alcohol availability	Comparison between 41 "wet" and 26 "dry" counties showed higher mean suicide rate in "dry" counties as compared to "wet" counties
Lester (1999)	Removal of state retain monopolies on wine sales in 1971 and 1973	Alcohol pricing (including taxation)	Four states (Idaho, Iowa, Maine, West Virginia) experienced an increase in suicide rates following the removal of monopolies, and two (Montana and New Hampshire) experienced a decrease
Markowitz et al. (2003)	Different state-based laws in the USA: • Excise tax on beer • Outlet density per 1000 population per state • "Dry" counties • Blood alcohol concentration limits for driving across states (0.10, 0.08 g/100 mL, and zero tolerance)	Different laws analyzed separately: • Alcohol pricing (including taxation) • Drink-driving countermeasures • Alcohol availability	Increase in the excise tax on beer was associated with the reduction of suicide numbers in young males, but not for females The number of alcohol outlets increases the number of male suicides. Higher proportion of dry counties is associated with the lower level of suicides in males aged 20–24 Drunk-driving laws had some impact on teenage female suicides
Pridemore and Snowden (2009)	Introduction of a law in Slovenia establishing a MLDA of 18 years for the purchase and consumption of alcohol and tightening of liquor licensing laws governing what type of outlets could sell alcohol, the introduction of time limits on sales, and the prohibition of alcohol distribution from vending machines in 2003	Mixed: • Regulation of alcohol advertising • Alcohol availability	The analyses of the effect of this new alcohol policy showed an immediate reduction in male suicide mortality in Slovenia (period of 1997–2006 was analyzed). There was a significant drop of male suicides, not female suicides
Pridemore et al. (2013)	Introduction of a law regulating the production and sale of ethyl alcohol and alcohol-containing products	Alcohol pricing (including taxation)	There was a drop of 9.2% in monthly male suicide numbers after the introduction of the new

(continued)

Table 1 (continued)

Authors (year)	Alcohol policy	Component (s) of alcohol policy targeted	Main findings
	to control the availability of alcohol and to require registration of alcohol production and distribution facilities on Jan 1, 2006		policy in Russia (period of 2000–2010 was analyzed); the impact was not significant for females
Sauliune et al. (2012)	Introductions of regulations on alcohol advertising, including the introduction of laws against drink driving, the illegal import of alcohol, as well as time limits on sales Jan 1, 2008. Excise taxes were increased by 20% for spirits and 10% for beer/wine	Mixed: • Awareness • Marketing restrictions • Alcohol availability • Alcohol pricing • Drink-driving countermeasures	There was an increase in suicide rates from 2006 to 2009 for males aged 15–64 years; there was no change for females
Skog (1993)	Introduction of taxation on alcohol due to shortages caused by the blockade of Denmark during World War I	Alcohol pricing (including taxation)	With reduction in alcohol consumption, suicide numbers dropped by 19% in 1916–1920 compared to 1911–1915. Decrease was particularly pronounced (over 50%) in alcohol abusers (as defined by the coroner)
Sloan et al. (1994)	Different state-based laws: • Pricing of alcohol • A dram shop laws • Mandatory jail terms for DUI	Different laws: • Alcohol pricing • Alcohol availability • Drink-driving countermeasures	Increase in alcohol price had a significant negative effect on suicide Dram shop laws and mandatory jail terms for DUI did not have impact on suicide
Son and Topyan (2011)	Excise tax on spirits, wine, beer on state level	Alcohol pricing (including taxation)	There was significant negative association between wine tax and suicide rate, but no association with beer or spirits tax
Wasserman et al. (1994, 1998)	Introduction of a very restrictive alcohol policy, *Perestroika* (started June 1985), encompassing anti-alcohol advertising, a decrease in alcohol production, a decrease in the number of retail outlets for the sale of alcohol, time limits on sales, and laws	Mixed: • Alcohol pricing • Alcohol availability • Health services response • Leadership, awareness, and commitment	Aggregate-level alcohol consumption was strongly correlated with a decline in male and female suicide rates in the former USSR from 1984 to 1990. A decline of suicide rates by 31.8% for males and by 19.3% for females was observed

(continued)

Table 1 (continued)

Authors (year)	Alcohol policy	Component (s) of alcohol policy targeted	Main findings
	enabling persons to be arrested for public drunkenness. Taxation also increased alcohol prices by around 80%. Producing home-distilled alcohol was criminalized	• Addressing informal and illicit production	
Wood and Gruenewald (2006)	Alaskan State law (in 1981) which enabled communities to choose between three alcohol availability policies: (1) "dry law," sale and import of alcohol prohibited within the community; (2) "damp law," sale of alcohol prohibited but import for personal use permitted or sale permitted only at one specific store; and (3) "wet law," no prohibition on the sale or import of alcohol within the community	Alcohol availability	Average annual age-adjusted rates per 100,000 population aged 15 and over for total self-harm injuries was 223 in "wet" isolated Alaska Native villages and 245 in "dry" isolated Alaska native villages. Self-harm fatality rates were 77 ("wet" isolated villages) and 76 ("dry" isolated villages)
Yamasaki et al. (2005)	Changes in the taxation on different alcohol products in Switzerland, 1965–1994	Alcohol pricing (including taxation)	The alcohol tax had significant positive correlation to male age-standardized suicide rates, but not for females
Zalcman and Mann (2007)	Three-stage privatization of alcohol retail: (1) the opening of privately owned wine stores (stage 1); (2) the opening of privately owned cold beer stores and sale of spirits and wine in hotels in rural areas (S2); and (3) privatization of all liquor stores (S3)	Alcohol availability	Stages 1 and 2 in 1985 and 1989 were both followed by an increase in suicide rates for both males and females; the stage 3 in 1994 (until 1999) was followed by an increase in suicide rates for males only

Data source: Kolves et al. (2020)

Summary Points

- Growing body of evidence shows ecological- and individual-level associations between alcohol use and suicidal behavior and ideation, which occur across multiple potential pathways.

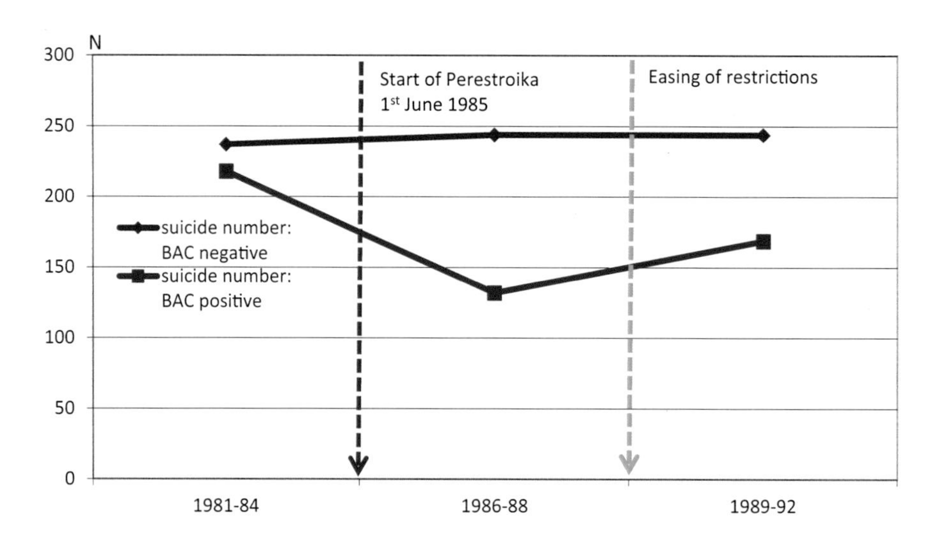

Fig. 3 Changes in average annual suicide numbers (BAC negative and BAC positive) during strict alcohol restrictions at the time of Perestroika in Estonia. (Data source: Värnik et al. 2007)

- Clear causal links are yet to be established, which may reflect the complexity and interactions between multiple risk factors at different time scales.
- There are a limited number of studies measuring the impact of alcohol-related interventions on suicidal behavior and ideation on individual and ecological level.
- Alcohol-focused interventions may have some effect in reducing absolute repetition of non-fatal self-harm by the 12-month follow-up assessment.
- Future studies are encouraged to measure outcomes related to suicidal behavior and ideation and to include a publicly available treatment manual, to clearly establish the alcohol-related therapeutic content of the intervention.
- Restrictions on alcohol availability at a population level, for example, via sales restrictions and/or increased cost via taxation of alcohol, are associated with decreased suicide rates, particularly for males.
- Given the inter-relationship between alcohol and suicide, responses to these issues need to be coordinated and integrated to provide a systems-level response.
- Suicide prevention strategies should include interventions targeted at alcohol use; conversely, changes to alcohol policies should specifically consider potential impacts on suicide.

Applications to Other Areas of Addiction

In this chapter, we focused on links between chronic and acute alcohol use and suicidal behavior. Nevertheless, associations between suicidal behavior and other substances, both chronic and acute use, have been also shown in the literature

(Schneider 2009; Esang and Ahmed 2018). Some reviews have noted particularly the link between suicidality and opioid use disorders (Schneider 2009; Esang and Ahmed 2018), while some others have referred to the association between cocaine and inhalant use (Vijayakumar et al. 2011), especially in young people (Pompili et al. 2012). It could be hypothesized that other central nervous system depressants, such as opioids or inhalants, may share common mechanistic pathways with alcohol, which may contribute to increased suicide risk. Substance use disorders have been found to be linked with suicidality particularly if comorbid with alcohol use disorders and depression as also presented on our visualization of pathways (Fig. 2) contributing factor to suicidal behavior. A recent systematic review and meta-analysis examined the impact of interventions targeting substance use disorders in randomized clinical trials (Padmanathan et al. 2020); however, majority of studies targeted alcohol use disorders. Two studies targeting a combination of alcohol and other substance use (Esposito-Smythers et al. 2011; Morley et al. 2014) and one comorbidity of opioid use disorders and depression (Ahmadi et al. 2018) did not have impact on suicidality.

Mini-dictionary of Terms

Suicide – the act of intentionally causing one's own death.

Non-fatal self-harm – all intentional acts of self-poisoning (such as intentional drug overdoses) or self-injury (such as self-cutting) regardless of the degree of suicidal intent or other types of motivation.

Suicidal ideation – thinking about, considering, or planning suicide.

Distal factors of suicide – individual-level factors that may predispose an individual to suicide throughout their life (e.g., early-life adversities).

Proximal factors of suicide – individual-level factors that may precipitate an individual to act on suicidal thoughts or facilitate suicide (e.g., financial stress, relationship breakdown).

Ecological factors of suicide – population-level factors that can provide the context for an individual's risk of suicide (e.g., gun control laws).

Key Facts About Suicide

- Globally, the World Health Organization (WHO) estimates that over 700,000 people die by suicide every year.
- Around three-quarters (77%) of all suicides occur in low- and middle-income countries.
- Suicide rates are higher in males than in females.
- Suicide is a leading cause of death among males and females aged 15–29 years.
- Global age-standardized suicides rates have been declining in the last two decades.

- Suicide is a complex multidimensional phenomenon involving a contribution of biological, psychological, clinical, social or cultural, and environmental risk factors.

References

Ahmadi J, Jahromi MS, Ehsaei Z (2018) The effectiveness of different singly administered high doses of buprenorphine in reducing suicidal ideation in acutely depressed people with co-morbid opiate dependence: a randomized, double-blind, clinical trial. Trials 19(1):1–8

Amadi S, Berman M, Timmins M, Guillot C, Fanning J, Nadorff M, McCloskey M (2020) Analgesic effect of alcohol mediates the association between alcohol intoxication and deliberate self-harm. Arch Suicide Res. https://doi.org/10.1080/13811118.13812020.11851831

Andreasson S, Holder H, Norström T, Österberg E, Rossow I (2006) Estimates of harm associated with changes in Swedish alcohol policy: results from past and present estimates. Addiction 101: 1096–1105

Andrés AR, Hempstead K (2011) Gun control and suicide: the impact of state firearm regulations in the United States, 1995–2004. Health Policy 101(1):95–103

Anestis MD, Joiner T, Hanson JE, Gutierrez PM (2014) The modal suicide decedent did not consume alcohol just prior to the time of death: an analysis with implications for understanding suicidal behavior. J Abnorm Psychol 123(4):835

Bagge C, Conner K, Reed L, Dawkins M, Murray K (2015) Alcohol use to facilitate a suicide attempt: an event-based examination. J Stud Alcohol Drugs 76:474–481

Becker HC (2012) Effects of alcohol dependence and withdrawal on stress responsiveness and alcohol consumption. Alcohol Res 34(4):448

Berman M, Hull T, May P (2000) Alcohol control and injury death in Alaska Native communities: Wet, damp and dry under Alaska's Local Option Law. J Stud Alcohol 61:311–9

Bernardin F, Maheut-Bosser A, Paille F (2014) Cognitive impairments in alcohol-dependent subjects. Front Psychiatry 5:78

Bilban M, Škibin L (2005) Presence of alcohol in suicide victims. Forensic Sci Int 147:S9–S12

Birckmayer J, Hemenway D (1999) Minimum-age drinking laws and youth suicide, 1970–1990. Am J Public Health 89:1365–8

Boden JM, Fergusson DM (2011) Alcohol and depression. Addiction 106(5):906–914

Bolton JM, Robinson J (2010) Population-attributable fractions of Axis I and Axis II mental disorders for suicide attempts: findings from a representative sample of the adult, non-institutionalized US population. Am J Public Health 100(12):2473–2480

Borges G, Nock MK, Abad JMH, Hwang I, Sampson NA, Alonso J, Andrade LH, Angermeyer MC, Beautrais A, Bromet E (2010) Twelve-month prevalence of and risk factors for suicide attempts in the World Health Organization World Mental Health Surveys. J Clin Psychiatry 71 (12):1617–1628

Borges G, Bagge C, Cherpitel CJ, Conner K, Orozco R, Rossow I (2017) A meta-analysis of acute alcohol use and the risk of suicide attempt. Psychol Med 47(5):949

Branas CC, Richmond TS, Ten Have TR, Wiebe DJ (2011) Acute alcohol consumption, alcohol outlets, and gun suicide. Subst Use Misuse 46(13):1592–1603

Bryan C, Garland E, Rudd M (2016) From impulse to action among military personnel hospitalized for suicide risk: alcohol consumption and the reported transition from suicidal thought to behavior. Gen Hosp Psychiatry 41:13–19

Cairns R, Schaffer AL, Ryan N, Pearson SA, Buckley NA (2019) Rising pregabalin use and misuse in Australia: trends in utilization and intentional poisonings. Addiction 114(6):1026–1034

Carballo JJ, Oquendo MA, Giner L, Zalsman G, Roche AM, Sher L (2006) Impulsive-aggressive traits and suicidal adolescents and young adults with alcoholism. Int J Adolesc Med Health 18 (1):15–19

Carpenter C (2004) Heavy alcohol use and youth suicide: Evidence from tougher drunk driving laws. Policy Anal Manage 23:831–42
Cheng C, Yen W, Chang W, Wu K, Ko M, Li C (2014) Risk of adolescent offspring's completed suicide increases with prior history of their same-sex parents' death by suicide. Psychol Med 44: 1845–1854
Chong D, Buckley N, Schumann J, Chitty K (2020) Acute alcohol use in Australian coronial suicide cases, 2010–2015. Drug Alcohol Depend 212:108066
Conner KR (2015) Commentary on "The modal suicide decedent did not consume alcohol just prior to the time of death: an analysis with implications for understanding suicidal behavior". J Abnorm Psychol 124(2):457–459
Conner KR, Duberstein PR (2004) Predisposing and precipitating factors for suicide among alcoholics: empirical review and conceptual integration. Alcohol Clin Exp Res 28:6S–17S
Conner KR, Beautrais AL, Conwell Y (2003) Risk factors for suicide and medically serious suicide attempts among alcoholics: analyses of Canterbury Suicide Project data. J Stud Alcohol 64(4): 551–554
Conner KR, McCloskey MS, Duberstein PR (2008) Psychiatric risk factors for suicide in the alcohol-dependent patient. Psychiatr Ann 38(11):742–748
Conner KR, Bagge CL, Goldston DB, Ilgen MA (2014a) Alcohol and suicidal behavior: what is known and what can be done. Am J Prev Med 47(3):S204–S208
Conner KR, Huguet N, Caetano R, Giesbrecht N, McFarland BH, Nolte KB, Kaplan MS (2014b) Acute use of alcohol and methods of suicide in a US national sample. Am J Public Health 104 (1):171–178
Coskunpinar A, Dir AL, Cyders MA (2013) Multidimensionality in impulsivity and alcohol use: a meta-analysis using the UPPS model of impulsivity. Alcohol Clin Exp Res 37(9):1441–1450
Courtney KE, Arellano R, Barkley-Levenson E, Gálvan A, Poldrack RA, MacKillop J, David Jentsch J, Ray LA (2012) The relationship between measures of impulsivity and alcohol misuse: an integrative structural equation modeling approach. Alcohol Clin Exp Res 36(6):923–931
Crawford M, Csipke E, Brown A, Reid S, Nilsen K, Redhead J, Touquet R (2010) The effect of referral for brief intervention for alcohol misuse on repetition of deliberate self-harm: an exploratory randomized controlled trial. Psychol Med 40:1821–1828
Currie SR, Patten SB, Williams JV, Wang J, Beck CA, El-Guebaly N, Maxwell C (2005) Comorbidity of major depression with substance use disorders. Can J Psychiatry 50(10):660–666
Darvishi N, Farhadi M, Haghtalab T, Poorolajal J (2015) Alcohol-related risk of suicidal ideation, suicide attempt, and completed suicide: a meta-analysis. PLoS One 10(5):e0126870
Davidson K, Brown T, James V, Kirk J, Richardson J (2014) Manual-assisted cognitive therapy for self-harm in personality disorder and substance misuse: a feasibility trial. Psychiatr Bull 38:108–111
De Leo D, Goodfellow B, Silverman M, Berman A, Mann J, Arensman E, Hawton K, Phillips M, Vijayakumar L, Andriessen K, Kolves K (2021) International study of definitions of English-language terms for suicidal behaviours: a survey exploring preferred terminology. BMJ Open 11(2):e043409
Diggins E, Kelley R, Cottrell D, House A, Owens D (2017) Age-related differences in self-harm presentations and subsequent management of adolescents and young adults at the emergency department. J Adolesc Health 66:470–477
Duke AA, Smith KM, Oberleitner L, Westphal A, McKee SA (2018) Alcohol, drugs, and violence: a meta-meta-analysis. Psychol Violence 8(2):238
Edwards AC, Ohlsson H, Sundquist J, Sundquist K, Kendler KS (2020) Alcohol use disorder and risk of suicide in a Swedish population-based cohort. Am J Psychiatry 177(7):627–634
Esang M, Ahmed S (2018) A closer look at substance use and suicide. Am J Psychiatry Resid J 13:6–8
Esposito-Smythers C, Spirito A, Kahler CW, Hunt J, Monti P (2011) Treatment of co-occurring substance abuse and suicidality among adolescents: a randomized trial. J Consult Clin Psychol 79(6):728
Fergusson DM, Boden JM, Horwood LJ (2009) Tests of causal links between alcohol abuse or dependence and major depression. Arch Gen Psychiatry 66(3):260–266

Foster T (2011) Adverse life events proximal to adult suicide: a synthesis of findings from psychological autopsy studies. Arch Suicide Res 15(1):1–15

García-Forero C, Gallardo-Pujol D, Maydeu-Olivares A, Andrés-Pueyo A (2009) Disentangling impulsiveness, aggressiveness and impulsive aggression: an empirical approach using self-report measures. Psychiatry Res 168(1):40–49

Geulayov G, Casey D, McDonald KC, Foster P, Pritchard K, Wells C, Clements C, Kapur N, Ness J, Waters K (2018) Incidence of suicide, hospital-presenting non-fatal self-harm, and community-occurring non-fatal self-harm in adolescents in England (the iceberg model of self-harm): a retrospective study. Lancet Psychiatry 5(2):167–174

Giancola PR, Josephs RA, Parrott DJ, Duke AA (2010) Alcohol myopia revisited: clarifying aggression and other acts of disinhibition through a distorted lens. Perspect Psychol Sci 5(3): 265–278

Glenn C, Kleiman E, Kellerman J, Pollak O, Cha C, Esposito E, Porter A, Wyman P, Boatman A (2020) Annual research review: a meta-analytic review of worldwide suicide rates in adolescents. J Child Psychol Psychiatry 61:294–308

Gregory R, Chlebowski S, Kang D, Remen A, Soderberg M, Stepkovitch J, Virk S (2008) A controlled trial of psychodynamic psychotherapy for co-occurring borderline personality disorder and alcohol use disorder. Psychotherapy 45(1):28–41

Griffin E, McMahon E, McNicholas F, Corcoran P, Perry IJ, Arensman E (2018) Increasing rates of self-harm among children, adolescents and young adults: a 10-year national registry study 2007–2016. Soc Psychiatry Psychiatr Epidemiol 53(7):663–671

Gvion Y, Apter A (2011) Aggression, impulsivity, and suicide behavior: a review of the literature. Arch Suicide Res 15(2):93–112

Hawton K, Fagg J, McKEOWN SP (1989) Alcoholism, alcohol and attempted suicide. Alcohol Alcohol 24(1):3–9

Hawton K, Harriss L, Hall S, Simkin S, Bale E, Bond A (2003) Deliberate self-harm in Oxford, 1990–2000: a time of change in patient characteristics. Psychol Med 33(6):987

Hayes V, Demirkol A, Ridley N, Withall A, Draper B (2016) Alcohol-related cognitive impairment: current trends and future perspectives. Neurodegener Dis Manag 6(6):509–523

Heatley M, Crane J (1990) The blood alcohol concentration at post-mortem in 175 fatal cases of alcohol intoxication. Med Sci Law 30(2):101–105

Heinz AJ, Beck A, Meyer-Lindenberg A, Sterzer P, Heinz A (2011) Cognitive and neurobiological mechanisms of alcohol-related aggression. Nat Rev Neurosci 12(7):400–413

Hendler RA, Ramchandani VA, Gilman J, Hommer DW (2011) Stimulant and sedative effects of alcohol. Curr Top Behav Neurosci 13:489–509

Hickman M, Lingford-Hughes A, Bailey C, Macleod J, Nutt D, Henderson G (2008) Does alcohol increase the risk of overdose death: the need for a translational approach. Addiction 103(7): 1060–1062

Hua P, Bugeja L, Maple M (2019) A systematic review on the relationship between childhood exposure to external cause parental death, including suicide, on subsequent suicidal behaviour. J Affect Disord 257:723–734

Hufford MR (2001) Alcohol and suicidal behavior. Clin Psychol Rev 21(5):797–811

Jakubczyk A, Klimkiewicz A, Topolewska-Wochowska A, Serafin P, Sadowska-Mazuryk J, Pupek-Pyzioł J, Brower KJ, Wojnar M (2012) Relationships of impulsiveness and depressive symptoms in alcohol dependence. J Affect Disord 136(3):841–847

Jakubczyk A, Wiśniewski P, Trucco E, Kobyliński P, Zaorska J, Skrzeszewski J, Suszek H, Wojnar M, Kopera M (2021) The synergistic effect between interoceptive accuracy and alcohol use disorder status on pain sensitivity. Addict Behav 112:106607

Jollant F, Hawton K, Vaiva G, Chan-Chee C, du Roscoat E, Leon C (2020) Non-presentation at hospital following a suicide attempt: a national survey. Psychol Med 2020:1–8

Joubert C (1994) "Wet" or "dry" county status and its correlates with suicide, homicide, and illegitimacy. Psychol Rep 74:296

Kaminer Y, Burleson J, Goldston D, Burke R (2006) Suicidal ideation among adolescents with alcohol use disorders during treatment and aftercare. Am J Addict 15:43–49
Khan M, Mahmud S, Karim M, Zaman M, Prince M (2008) Case–control study of suicide in Karachi, Pakistan. Br J Psychiatry 193:402–405
Klonsky ED, May AM, Saffer BY (2016) Suicide, suicide attempts, and suicidal ideation. Annu Rev Clin Psychol 12:307–330
Kõlves K, Värnik A, Schneider B, Fritze J, Allik J (2006a) Recent life events and suicide: a case-control study in Tallinn and Frankfurt. Soc Sci Med 62(11):2887–2896
Kõlves K, Värnik A, Tooding LM, Wasserman D (2006b) The role of alcohol in suicide: a case-control psychological autopsy study. Psychol Med 36(7):923–930
Kõlves K, Draper BM, Snowdon J, De Leo D (2017) Alcohol-use disorders and suicide: results from a psychological autopsy study in Australia. Alcohol 64:29–35
Kõlves K, Crompton D, Turner K, Stapelberg NJ, Khan A, Robinson G, De Leo D (2018a) Trends and repetition of non-fatal suicidal behaviour: analyses of the Gold Coast University Hospital's Emergency Department. Australas Psychiatry 26(2):170–175
Kõlves K, McDonough M, Crompton D, De Leo D (2018b) Choice of a suicide method: trends and characteristics. Psychiatry Res 260:67–74
Kõlves K, Chitty KM, Wardhani R, Värnik A, De Leo D, Witt K (2020a) Impact of alcohol policies on suicidal behavior: a systematic literature review. Int J Environ Res Public Health 17(19):7030
Kõlves K, Koo YW, De Leo D (2020b) A drink before suicide: analysis of the Queensland Suicide Register in Australia. Epidemiol Psychiatr Sci 29:e94
Koski A, Ojanperä I, Vuori E (2002) Alcohol and benzodiazepines in fatal poisonings. Alcohol Clin Exp Res 26(7):956–959
Landberg J (2008) Alcohol and suicide in Eastern Europe. Drug Alc Rev 27:361–373
Lee K, Li C, Chang K, Lu T, Chen Y (2017a) Age at exposure to parental suicide and the subsequent risk of suicide in young people. Crisis 39:27–36
Lee JW, Park CHK, Kim EY, Kim SH, Yoo SH, Ahn YM (2017b) Characteristics of completed suicide in different blood alcohol concentrations in Korea. Forensic Sci Int 281:37–43
LeMarquand D, Pihl RO, Benkelfat C (1994) Serotonin and alcohol intake, abuse, and dependence: clinical evidence. Biol Psychiatry 36(5):326–337
Lesch KP, Merschdorf U (2000) Impulsivity, aggression, and serotonin: a molecular psychobiological perspective. Behav Sci Law 18(5):581–604
Lester D (1999) Wine consumption and suicide rates. Psychol Rep 84:1054
Markowitz S, Chatterji P, Kaestner R (2003) Estimating the impact of alcohol policies on youth suicides. J Ment Health Policy Econ 6:37–46
McMahon EM, Keeley H, Cannon M, Arensman E, Perry IJ, Clarke M, Chambers D, Corcoran P (2014) The iceberg of suicide and self-harm in Irish adolescents: a population-based study. Soc Psychiatry Psychiatr Epidemiol 49(12):1929–1935
McManama-O'Brien K, Sellers C, Battalen A, Ryan C, Maneta E, Aguinaldo L, Spirito A (2018) Feasibility, acceptability, and preliminary effects of a brief alcohol intervention for suicidal adolescents in inpatient psychiatric treatment. J Subst Abus Treat 94:105–112
Melhem NM, Munroe S, Marsland A, Gray K, Brent D, Porta G, Douaihy A, Laudenslager ML, DePietro F, Diler R (2017) Blunted HPA axis activity prior to suicide attempt and increased inflammation in attempters. Psychoneuroendocrinology 77:284–294
Mercado MC, Holland K, Leemis RW, Stone DM, Wang J (2017) Trends in emergency department visits for nonfatal self-inflicted injuries among youth aged 10 to 24 years in the United States, 2001–2015. JAMA 318(19):1931–1933
Milner A, McClure R, De Leo D (2012) Socio-economic determinants of suicide: an ecological analysis of 35 countries. Soc Psychiatry Psychiatr Epidemiol 47(1):19–27
Milner A, Morrell S, LaMontagne AD (2014) Economically inactive, unemployed and employed suicides in Australia by age and sex over a 10-year period: what was the impact of the 2007 economic recession? Int J Epidemiol 43(5):1500–1507

Morley K, Sitharthan G, Haber P, Tucker P, Sitharthan T (2014) Efficacy of an opportunistic cognitive behavioral intervention package (OCB) on substance use and comorbid suicide risk: a multisite randomized controlled trial. J Consult Clin Psychol 82(1):130–140

Nadkarni A, Weobong B, Weiss H, McCambridge J, Bhat B, Katti B, Murthy P, King M, McDaid D, Park A-L, Wilson G, Kirkwood B, Fairburn C, Velleman R, Patel V (2017) Counselling for Alcohol Problems (CAP), a lay counsellor-delivered brief psychological treatment for harmful drinking in men, in primary care in India: a randomised controlled trial. Lancet 389:186–195

Naghavi M (2019) Global, regional, and national burden of suicide mortality 1990 to 2016: systematic analysis for the Global Burden of Disease Study 2016. Br Med J 364:l94

Narongchai S, Narongchai P (2006) The prevalence of detectable blood alcohol concentration among unnatural deaths in northern Thailand. J Med Assoc Thai 89(6):809

Nordentoft M, Qin P, Helweg-Larsen K, Juel K (2007) Restrictions in means for suicide: an effective tool in preventing suicide: the Danish experience. Suicide Life Threat Behav 37(6): 688–697

Norström T, Rossow I (2016) Alcohol consumption as a risk factor for suicidal behavior: a systematic review of associations at the individual and at the population level. Arch Suicide Res 20(4):489–506

Norström T, Stickley A, Shibuya K (2012) The importance of alcoholic beverage type for suicide in Japan: A time-series analysis, 1963–2007. Drug Alc Rev 31(3):251–256

Northridge D, McMurray J, Lawson A (1986) Association between liberalization of Scotland's liquor licensing laws and admissions for self poisoning in West Fife. Br Med J (Clin Res Ed) 293 (6560):1466–1468

O'Connell H, Lawlor B (2005) Recent alcohol intake and suicidality – a neuropsychological perspective. Ir J Med Sci 174:51

O'Connor DB, Green JA, Ferguson E, O'Carroll RE, O'Connor RC (2018a) Effects of childhood trauma on cortisol levels in suicide attempters and ideators. Psychoneuroendocrinology 88:9–16

O'Connor RC, Wetherall K, Cleare S, Eschle S, Drummond J, Ferguson E, O'Connor DB, O'Carroll RE (2018b) Suicide attempts and non-suicidal self-harm: national prevalence study of young adults. BJPsych Open 4(3):142–148

Overholser JC, Braden A, Dieter L (2012) Understanding suicide risk: identification of high-risk groups during high-risk times. J Clin Psychol 68(3):349–361

Padmanathan P, Hall K, Moran P, Jones HE, Gunnell D, Carlisle V, Lingford-Hughes A, Hickman M (2020) Prevention of suicide and reduction of self-harm among people with substance use disorder: a systematic review and meta-analysis of randomised controlled trials. Compr Psychiatry 96:152135

Pariante CM, Lightman SL (2008) The HPA axis in major depression: classical theories and new developments. Trends Neurosci 31(9):464–468

Pirkola S, Sund R, Sailas E, Wahlbeck K (2009) Community mental-health services and suicide rate in Finland: a nationwide small-area analysis. Lancet 373(9658):147–153

Pompili M, Serafini G, Innamorati M, Dominici G, Ferracuti S, Kotzalidis GD, Serra G, Girardi P, Janiri L, Tatarelli R (2010) Suicidal behavior and alcohol abuse. Int J Environ Res Public Health 7(4):1392–1431

Pompili M, Serafini G, Innamorati M, Biondi M, Siracusano A, Di Giannantonio M, Giupponi G, Amore M, Lester D, Girardi P (2012) Substance abuse and suicide risk among adolescents. Eur Arch Psychiatry Clin Neurosci 262(6):469–485

Powell KE, Kresnow MJ, Mercy JA, Potter LB, Swann AC, Frankowski RF, Lee RK, Bayer TL (2001) Alcohol consumption and nearly lethal suicide attempts. Suicide Life Threat Behav 32(1 Suppl):30–41

Pridemore WA, Snowden AJ (2009) Reduction in suicide mortality following a new national alcohol policy in Slovenia: an interrupted time-series analysis. Am J Public Health 99(5):915–920

Pridemore W, Chamlin M, Andreev E (2013) Reduction in male suicide mortality following the 2006 Russian alcohol policy: An interrupted time series analysis. Am J Public Health 103:2021–6

Ramstedt M (2001) Alcohol and suicide in 14 European countries. Addiction 96(1s):59–75
Richardson C, Robb KA, O'Connor RC (2021) A systematic review of suicidal behaviour in men: a narrative synthesis of risk factors. Soc Sci Med 2021:113831
Riordan SM, Williams R (2002) Alcohol exposure and paracetamol-induced hepatotoxicity. Addict Biol 7(2):191–206
Roche SP, Rogers ML, Pridemore WA (2018) A cross-national study of the population-level association between alcohol consumption and suicide rates. Drug Alcohol Depend 188:16–23
Roerecke M, Rehm J (2014) Cause-specific mortality risk in alcohol use disorder treatment patients: a systematic review and meta-analysis. Int J Epidemiol 43(3):906–919
Sauliune S, Petrauskiene J, Kalediene R (2012) Alcohol-related injuries and alcohol control policy in Lithuania: effect of the year of sobriety, 2008. Alcohol Alcohol 47:458–463
Schneider B (2009) Substance use disorders and risk for completed suicide. Arch Suicide Res 13(4):303–316
Sher L, Oquendo MA, Galfalvy HC, Grunebaum MF, Burke AK, Zalsman G, Mann JJ (2005) The relationship of aggression to suicidal behavior in depressed patients with a history of alcoholism. Addict Behav 30(6):1144–1153
Sher L, Oquendo MA, Richardson-Vejlgaard R, Makhija NM, Posner K, Mann JJ, Stanley BH (2009) Effect of acute alcohol use on the lethality of suicide attempts in patients with mood disorders. J Psychiatr Res 43(10):901–905
Skog O-J (1993) Alcohol and suicide in Denmark 1911–24 – experiences from a "natural experiment". Addiction 88:1189–1193
Sloan F, Reilly B, Schenzler C (1994) Effect of prices, civil and criminal sanctions, and law-enforcement on alcoholrelated mortality. J Stud Alcohol 55:454–65
Son CH, Topyan K (2011) The effect of alcoholic beverage excise tax on alcohol-attributable injury mortalities. Eur J Health Econ 12(2):103–113
Stamates AL, Lau-Barraco C (2020) Momentary patterns of impulsivity and alcohol use: a cause or consequence? Drug Alcohol Depend 217:108246
Stickley A, Jukkala T, Norström T (2011) Alcohol and suicide in Russia, 1870–1894 and 1956–2005: evidence for the continuation of a harmful drinking culture across time? J Stud Alc Drug 72:341–7
Sutker PB, Goist KC Jr, Allain AN, Bugg F (1987) Acute alcohol intoxication: sex comparisons on pharmacokinetic and mood measures. Alcohol Clin Exp Res 11(6):507–512
Turecki G, Ernst C, Jollant F, Labonté B, Mechawar N (2012) The neurodevelopmental origins of suicidal behavior. Trends Neurosci 35(1):14–23
Turecki G, Brent DA, Gunnell D, O'Connor RC, Oquendo MA, Pirkis J, Stanley BH (2019) Suicide and suicide risk. Nat Rev Dis Primers 5(1):1–22
Uddin R, Burton NW, Maple M, Khan SR, Khan A (2019) Suicidal ideation, suicide planning, and suicide attempts among adolescents in 59 low-income and middle-income countries: a population-based study. Lancet Child Adolesc Health 3(4):223–233
Underwood MD, Kassir SA, Bakalian MJ, Galfalvy H, Dwork AJ, Mann JJ, Arango V (2018) Serotonin receptors and suicide, major depression, alcohol use disorder and reported early life adversity. Transl Psychiatry 8(1):1–15
United Nations (2015) Sustainable development. Retrieved 16 Apr 2021, from https://sdgs.un.org/goals
Värnik A, Kõlves K, Väli M, Tooding LM, Wasserman D (2007) Do alcohol restrictions reduce suicide mortality? Addiction 102(2):251–256
Värnik A, Kõlves K, van der Feltz-Cornelis CM, Marusic A, Oskarsson H, Palmer A, Reisch T, Scheerder G, Arensman E, Aromaa E (2008) Suicide methods in Europe: a gender-specific analysis of countries participating in the "European Alliance Against Depression". J Epidemiol Community Health 62(6):545–551
Veenstra MY, Lemmens PH, Friesema IH, Tan FE, Garretsen HF, Knottnerus JA, Zwietering PJ (2007) Coping style mediates impact of stress on alcohol use: a prospective population-based study. Addiction 102(12):1890–1898

Vijayakumar L, Kumar MS, Vijayakumar V (2011) Substance use and suicide. Curr Opin Psychiatry 24(3):197–202
Volkow ND, Wiers CE, Shokri-Kojori E, Tomasi D, Wang G-J, Baler R (2017) Neurochemical and metabolic effects of acute and chronic alcohol in the human brain: studies with positron emission tomography. Neuropharmacology 122:175–188
Vonghia L, Leggio L, Ferrulli A, Bertini M, Gasbarrini G, Addolorato G, Alcoholism Treatment Study Group (2008) Acute alcohol intoxication. Eur J Intern Med 19(8):561–567
Voracek M, Loibl L (2007) Genetics of suicide: a systematic review of twin studies. Wien Klin Wochenschr 119:463–475
Wasserman D, Värnik A, Eklund G (1994) Male suicides and alcohol consumption in the former USSR. Acta Psychiatr Scand 89(5):306–313
Wasserman D, Värnik A, Eklund G (1998) Female suicides and alcohol consumption during perestroika in the former USSR. Acta Psychiatr Scand 98:26–33
Watt K, Shepherd J, Newcombe R (2008) Drunk and dangerous: a randomised controlled trial of alcohol brief intervention for violent offenders. J Exp Criminol 4:1–19
Wilks C, Lungo A, Ang S, Matsumiya B, Yin Q, Linehan M (2018) A randomized controlled trial of an internet delivered dialectical behavior therapy skills training for suicidal and heavy episodic drinkers. J Affect Disord 232:219–228
Witt K, Townsend E, Arensman E, Gunnell D, Hazell P, Taylor Salisbury T, Van Heeringen K, Hawton K (2020) Psychosocial interventions for people who self-harm: methodological issues involved in trials to evaluate effectiveness. Arch Suicide Res 24(Suppl 2):S32–S93
Witt K, Chitty KM, Wardhani R, Värnik A, De Leo D, Kõlves K (2021) Effect of alcohol interventions on suicidal ideation and behaviour: a systematic review and meta-analysis. Drug Alcohol Depend 226:108885
Wood D, Gruenewald P (2006) Local alcohol prohibition, police presence and serious injury in isolated Alaska Native villages. Addiction 101:393–403
World Health Organization (2013) Mental health action plan 2013–2020. World Health Organization, Geneva
World Health Organization (2014) Preventing suicide: a global imperative. World Health Organization, Geneva
World Health Organization (2018) Global status report on alcohol and health 2018. World Health Organization, Geneva
World Health Organization (2019) Global status report on alcohol and health 2018. World Health Organization, Geneva
World Health Organization (2021) Suicide worldwide in 2019: global health estimates. World Health Organization, Geneva
Yamasaki A, et al (2005) Tobacco and alcohol tax relationships with suicide in Switzerland. Psychol Rep 97:213–6
Yip PS, Caine E, Yousuf S, Chang S-S, Wu KC-C, Chen Y-Y (2012) Means restriction for suicide prevention. Lancet 379(9834):2393–2399
Zalcman RF, Mann RE (2007) The effects of privatization of alcohol sales in Alberta on suicide mortality rates. Contemp Drug Probl 34(4):589–609
Zortea TC, Cleare S, Melson AJ, Wetherall K, O'Connor RC (2020) Understanding and managing suicide risk. Br Med Bull 134(1):73–84

Interventions for Children and Adolescents with Fetal Alcohol Spectrum Disorders (FASD) 55

Gro Christine Christensen Løhaugen, Anne Cecilie Tveiten, and Jon Skranes

Contents

Introduction 1179
Interventions for Cognitive, Neuropsychological, and Adaptive Challenges 1180
Learning Disorders and Intervention 1180
Neuropsychological Deficits and Intervention 1181
ADHD Comorbidity and Treatment 1183
Adaptive Behavior and Interventions 1184
Social Deficits and Intervention 1186
Regulatory Challenges in Children with FASD and Treatment Options 1187
Sleep Disorders in Children with FASD and Intervention 1187
Sleep Hygiene 1188
Melatonin Supplement Therapy 1188
Sensory Processing Deficits and Intervention 1189
Eating Disorders and Intervention 1189
Behavioral Challenges and Intervention 1190
Pharmacological Treatment of Behavioral Disorders 1191
Psychoeducative Interventions for Children and Adolescents with FASD and Behavioral Challenges 1192
Conclusion 1197
Applications to Other Areas of Substance Use Disorder 1197
Applications to Other Areas of Public Health 1198
Mini-Dictionary of Terms 1198

G. Christine Christensen Løhaugen (✉) · A. Cecilie Tveiten
Department of Pediatrics, Sørlandet Hospital, Arendal, Norway
e-mail: gro.lohaugen@sshf.no; anne.cecilie.tveiten@sshf.no

J. Skranes
Department of Pediatrics, Sørlandet Hospital Arendal, Arendal, Norway

Department of Clinical and Molecular Medicine, Faculty of Medicine and Health Sciences, Norwegian University of Science and Technology, Trondheim, Norway
e-mail: jon.skranes@ntnu.no; jon.skranes@sshf.no

V. B. Patel, V. R. Preedy (eds.), *Handbook of Substance Misuse and Addictions*,
https://doi.org/10.1007/978-3-030-92392-1_63

Key Facts of FASD 1198
Summary Points 1199
References 1199

Abstract

Fetal alcohol spectrum disorder (FASD) is an umbrella term for different neurodevelopmental disorders linked to prenatal alcohol exposure (PAE). FASD has a high prevalence, estimated to be 1–3%, but the variance is large between countries (0.1–10%). Early diagnosis and intervention aimed at primary symptoms may prevent secondary disabilities and improve outcome. The complex clinical picture presented in children and adolescents with FASD commands multidisciplinary assessment as basis for intervention planning. The complexity results in high direct and indirect cost for families and society. Interventions discussed in this chapter focus on learning disabilities, low IQ, attention/executive functions, adaptive behavior, and behavioral challenges that have a high prevalence in FASD.

Keywords

FASD · Interventions · Learning disorders · Adaptive behavior · Social challenges · Behavioral disorder · Psychoeducation · Family programs

Abbreviations

ADHD	Attention deficit hyperactivity disorder
ADL	Activity of daily living
ASD	Autism spectrum disorder
BRIEF	Behavioral Rating Inventory for Executive Functions
COS	Circle of Security
CPAT	Computerized Progressive Attention Training
D-Kefs	Delis-Kaplan Executive Function System
EF	Executive functions
FAS	Fetal alcohol syndrome
FASDs	Fetal alcohol spectrum disorders
ID	Intellectual disability
IQ	Intelligence quotient
MILE	Math Interactive Learning Experience
MST	Multisystemic therapy
NEPSY-II	Neuropsychological assessment second edition
NICE	National Institute for Health and Care Excellence
NIPH	Norwegian Institute of Public Health
PAE	Prenatal alcohol exposure
PMTO	Parent management training
RK-MR HSØ	Regional Competence Center for children with prenatal alcohol and/or drug exposure, South-Eastern Norwegian Region of Health

SDSC	Sleep Disturbance Scale for Children
SES	Socioeconomic status
SLD	Specific learning disorder
TDC	Typically developing children
VABS	Vineland Adaptive Behavior Scale
WM	Working memory

Introduction

Fetal alcohol spectrum disorder (FASD) is an umbrella term for different neurodevelopmental disorders caused, at least partially, by prenatal alcohol exposure (PAE). FASD covers one diagnosis, fetal alcohol syndrome (full or partial) (FAS; ICD-10 Q86.0), and a diversity of clinical descriptions (See chapter X by Noble). FASD has common features with other neurodevelopmental disorders like attention deficit hyperactivity disorder (ADHD), autism spectrum disorders (ASD), learning/behavioral disorders, and regulatory challenges. According to Lange et al. (2017), the prevalence of FASD exceeds 1% in 76 countries but ranges from 0.1% to more than 10% (Lange et al. 2017). In special children populations, adoptees from countries with high prevalence of PAE, correctional youth populations, children in an orphanage, and psychiatric care populations, the prevalence may be 10–40 times higher than in the general population (Popova et al. 2019). FASD is one of the most common neurocognitive disorders among children and youth with major challenge for the social, health, and educational system across the world. Estimated yearly cost varies based on educational, correctional, and health system between countries. In Sweden, it was estimated a societal yearly cost of 76,000 euros for children with FAS and 110,000 euros for adults (Ericson et al. 2017). Prevention aimed at women with high risk of having a child with FASD is the most cost-effective intervention (Greenmyer et al. 2020).

During the last 5 years, the Regional Competence Center for children with prenatal alcohol and/or drug exposure in Arendal, Norway (RK-MR HSØ) (Lohaugen et al. 2015), has assessed more than 300 children with prenatal alcohol and/or drug exposure in need of intervention plans. In contrast to the high prevalence, high cost, and complexity of FASD there is limited knowledge regarding effective interventions. A recent systematic review of evidence-based interventions for FASD was only able to include 23 studies (Ordenewitz et al. 2021). In this chapter, we will discuss interventions aimed at children and youth with FASD specifically based on recent research and experience-based knowledge. In addition, interventions aimed at symptoms that are common features of FASD as well as other neurodevelopmental disorders, ASD, ADHD, learning disorders, and behavioral disorders, will be included.

In general, early diagnosis combined with stable living arrangements is regarded as the most important interventions to improve prognosis and long-term outcome (Streissguth et al. 2004). Persons with FASD often experience a range of adverse life outcomes, called secondary disabilities, which include disrupted school experience, troubles with the law, confinement, inappropriate sexual behaviors on repeated occasions, and alcohol–/drug-related problems (Coriale et al. 2013). Early diagnosis and intervention can reduce risk for adverse outcomes by reducing the load of living with FASD. Educating the primary and secondary health services about FASD and how to diagnose it should therefore be a priority.

Petrenko (2015) emphasizes the need for "multicomponent interventions." This encompasses treatment aimed at the child (e.g., medication and self-regulation training) and the family (e.g., by education on FASD and resources and how to access them, improve parental skills, reduce parental stress, and improve parent-child interaction).

Interventions for Cognitive, Neuropsychological, and Adaptive Challenges

Learning Disorders and Intervention

Prevalence of ID in children and youth with FAS is approximately 35%, compared to 2% in the general population (Elgen et al. 2007). Low IQ is more common in children with FASD than in healthy controls (Mattson et al. 2011) and may manifest as learning challenges in mainstream school.

In our experience, the most important intervention would be to conduct a comprehensive cognitive assessment of intelligence using a standardized method like the *Wechsler tests* used in kindergarten throughout adulthood. More important than the total IQ score is the cognitive profile as basis for intervention planning aimed at utilizing the child's strengths and compensating for the weaknesses. For example, if the Wechsler scales identify working memory (WM) challenges often found in children with FASD (Ferreira and Cruz 2017), that would require further neuropsychological assessment and specific interventions in school. Low IQ would indicate the need for special education, reduced/simplified curriculum, and individually tailored teaching as recommended by the school psychologist and/or special educator.

Low IQ, but also low scores on verbal reasoning and WM, may underlay the high prevalence of deficits in mathematical abilities seen in children with FASD (Glass et al. 2017). Randomized controlled trials (RCTs) evaluating the Math Interactive Learning Experience (MILE) program have shown promising results improving math performance. The program is for children 3–10 years of age and lasts for 6 weeks. It includes both parental training and individual training for the child. For the parents, focus will be on improved understanding of FASD as well as how to help the child with math. Results show significant improvement in math skills for the child and parental reports of improved child behavior (Kable et al. 2007, 2015; Coles et al. 2009).

Children with FASD often have sensory processing challenges (>70%) (Jirikowic et al. 2020), and this may affect school functioning if the child is overwhelmed by sensory input. By focusing on environmental adjustments in the classroom, this may be reduced. Keeping the room well organized and making the surroundings calm by minimizing decorations and keep materials out of may be useful. Entering and exiting the room often involves noise and crowding. Also, organizing the students to do so orderly and by a set order reduces sensory input.

A practical guide for teachers and school psychologists is the book *Fetal Alcohol Spectrum Disorders Educational Strategies* that can be downloaded freely at www.usd.edu. It includes suggestions for environmental adjustments and how to reduce sensory load.

Neuropsychological Deficits and Intervention

Neuropsychological deficits are common in children with FASD. The domain most affected seems to be attention/executive functioning (EF), moderated to some extent by IQ and socioeconomic status (SES) (Khoury and Milligan 2019). Executive functions are higher-order functions that we depend on for decision-making in nonroutine cognitive activities. Deficits include fluency, inhibition, problem-solving/planning, concept formation, and set-shifting as well as WM (Mattson et al. 2019), indicating pervasive affection of frontal lobe functioning. EF deficits exceed what would be expected based on intellectual functioning in children with FASD. Deficits in executive functions, especially impulse control, are also observed in other neurodevelopmental disorders (ASD, ADHD) and behavioral disorders (Carter Leno et al. 2018). In FASD, a relationship between deficits in EF is present in children with behavioral disorders even when controlling for ADHD (Doyle et al. 2019). Several studies have focused on improving EF in children with FASD (Ordenewitz et al. 2021).

Executive functioning affects the effectiveness of interventions as shown by Schonfeld et al. (2009); results from the Behavior Rating Inventory for Executive Functions (BRIEF) predicted the outcome of friendship training in children with FASD. We recommend assessment of attention/executive function pretreatment planning. Assessment should include standardized neuropsychological tests; examples would be the developmental neuropsychological assessment (NEPSY-II) and the Delis-Kaplan Executive Function System (D-Kefs).

In addition, the BRIEF questionnaire should be included. Fewer children with FASD obtain impaired scores on neuropsychological testing of executive functions, while a majority is described as impaired on the BRIEF by parents; see Mohamed et al. (2019). As a standardized test situation provides high degree of structure and adult guidance, this may mask EF challenges in daily life situations with higher demand on independence. A combination of parental and teacher evaluation and neuropsychological testing is therefore recommended and intervention adjusted according to function in unstructured situations. Clinically, we often observe improvement in behavior and functioning at home after adjusting demands by increasing adult guidance at school, even if the school did not report any behavioral problems. As demand for independent functioning is reduced, the child is able to function at school using less energy.

Deficits in impulse control may have devastating effects on learning, social functioning, and behavior. Clinically, the child usually presents with a lack of consideration for consequences; there is no "before" or "after," just "here and now," and the child appears "stimulus driven." This also means that "ordinary" strategies for upbringing will not work as providing the child with consequences or punishment will not reduce the problematic behavior. This is due to the child's lack of ability to inhibit behavior (verbal or physical) while evaluating what action would be beneficial. Both in education and within the family, utilizing reinforcement rather than adverse consequences to adhere to the impulse control deficits are indicated. Engle and Kerns (2011) reported that children with FASD improve similar to controls with reinforcement learning if provided with suitable repetitions. However, the FASD group focused on the most recent reinforcement rather than "the whole picture," and this may indicate challenges in transfer effect, impact of WM, and impulse control challenges. Both in school and at home, impaired impulse control represents the need for adult guidance in order to reduce errors and conflicts.

The Alert Program for Self-Regulation is a program for children 8–12 years of age and their parents (Wells et al. 2012). The program develops understanding of arousal/alertness and self-regulation through the analogy of a car engine. Children are thought to recognize level of alertness as being in a "high," "low," or "just right," as finding the right gear in a car engine. In the original program, both the children and their caregivers learn strategies that they can use to self-regulate to maintain or obtain an optimal level of arousal/alertness to the given situation. In order to use this program, there is a course and material to obtain for professionals. Several studies have shown positive effects of this program on executive functions evaluated by the parents (Wells et al. 2012) and on tasks assessing inhibitory control (Nash et al. 2015).

A definition of WM is ability to keep information "online" while manipulating it. The term refers to structures and processes used for temporarily storing and manipulating information (Baddeley 2003). Examples of everyday tasks that require WM are listening to a lecture, doing mental arithmetic, and remembering an instruction or message long enough to act on it. WM is often impaired in ADHD and in children with FASD (Loomes et al. 2008). Interventions toward WM aim to expand the function itself or to improve function through compensatory strategies. WM training is argued to improve the capacity and therefore the function itself. Rehearsal training has shown promising effect on WM capacity in children with FASD (Loomes et al. 2008). Several WM training computer "games" are in existence. One is the "Caribbean Quest," aimed at several attention and executive functions, including the use of meta-cognition strategies for children with FASD or ASD. The program lasts for 8–12 weeks, with training 1 h/week at school to children 6–13 years of age. Results showed improvements in WM, attention, and academic performance, indicating a transfer effect to non-trained tasks (Kerns et al. 2017). The Computerized Progressive Attention Training (CPAT) runs for 4 weeks with a total of 16 h of active intervention training done at school, guided by a teacher or assistant for children with FASD 6–15 years of age. A pilot study showed positive effects on attention and spatial WM (Kerns et al. 2010). See Table 1 for compensatory strategies based on clinical experience that may be useful.

Table 1 Examples of compensatory strategies for children and adolescents with working memory deficits. Practical suggestions to compensate for working memory challenges in kindergarten/schools and at home

1. Provide one message or instruction at a time – KISS: keep it short and sweet
2. Explanations should be clear, brief, and specific
3. Repeat the most important information from instructions/teaching at the end
4. Instruct the child what to do, instead of what not to do. This limits the WM load
5. Provide visual material as support when giving verbal information/teaching (power point, pictures, figures)
6. Multiplication table/alphabet/daily schedule is visible to the child at school/during homework
7. Make rule books for grammar and math with examples and color codes/numbers for where to start and so on
8. Provide a calculator for math
9. Copy of teachers' power point to guide parents in rehearsal of the most important information
10. Teach the child when to ask for repetitions/to check out if they understood correctly
11. Teach and rehearse when and how to make checklists. Having sticky notes and pen available at the counter and desk and in the hallway to ease rehearsal

ADHD Comorbidity and Treatment

Comorbidity in FASD is high, and for a comprehensive overview, we recommend Popova et al. (2016). Relevant for the domain of attention and executive function is ADHD. In children with FASD, the prevalence of ADHD is estimated to be 50%, ten times as high as expected in general population (Weyrauch et al. 2017) all the way up to 89% (Elgen et al. 2007) and 94% (Fryer et al. 2007). The attention deficit in children with FASD is relatively independent of IQ (Fryer et al. 2007).

Differentiating between FASD and ADHD may be possible in research terms but is much more challenging in a clinical setting. Peadon and Elliott (2010) suggested that the four-factor model of attention may be useful: children with ADHD struggle more with focus and sustain, while those with FASD scored lower on encoding and shift; however, the usefulness on an individual, clinical level is unknown.

Common for children with FASD, ASD, and ADHD are impairments in attention and executive functions. One way of talking about this in a clinical setting would be to focus on "the captain of the brain" (frontal lobe) not being present on the bridge. For the child, this may be useful to externalize the "blame" for not remembering, initializing, and fulfilling tasks and so on. For the parents, an explanation based on deviating brain development may be helpful in the day-to-day support of the child.

First choice of intervention is usually environmental modifications and special education interventions. In our opinion, interventions aimed at children with ADHD should also be considered for children with combined ADHD and FASD or FASD with ADHD symptoms. In general, a structured day and emphasis on routines may be beneficial by providing predictability. To compensate for executive deficits, close guidance and monitoring from adults is needed both academically and socially.

There is a lack of studies on medication in children with FASD and ADHD. First choice as medical treatment for ADHD is usually methylphenidate. However, a case series study of 30 children with FASD and comorbid ADHD indicated that only about 22% of the children responded to methylphenidate, while almost 80% had beneficial effects of dexamphetamine (O'Malley et al. 2000).

A recent review of medication in combined FASD and ADHD identified seven animal studies and eight clinical studies. Of the latter, six studied the effect of stimulants, and two of these also included the effect of neuroleptics/mood stabilizers (Ritfeld et al. 2021). In addition, two studies have examined the effect of choline supplement. Choline showed no effect in school-age children (Nguyen et al. 2016b) but may improve memory in preschoolers (Wozniak et al. 2015).

The largest study compared stimulants, no medication, and neuroleptics ($n = 77$). Outcome was effect on social skills (Children's Friendship Training, 12 sessions, each 90 min weekly for 12 weeks). They reported positive effect of social skills training in the group using neuroleptics and no effect of training in the group using stimulants (Frankel et al. 2006).

Given the complexity of FASD and the burden that this disorder places on the individual, we recommend that treatment with stimulants is considered when a diagnosis of ADHD is present. However, any medication will require close surveillance as sleep and nutritional problems may be magnified as side effects of stimulants. In our clinic, the child psychiatrist always recommends to "start low and go slow" regarding dosage for children with FASD. Kodituwakku and Kodituwakku (2011) recommend a combination of behavioral and pharmacological intervention, as is common also in children with ADHD without FASD.

Adaptive Behavior and Interventions

Adaptive behavior denotes how well an individual is able to meet the demands of daily life activity according to age and societal norms. Adaptive behavior assessed by questionnaires or interviews with parents usually covers three domains: communication, activity of daily living, and social functioning. One assessment method is the Vineland Adaptive Behavior Scales, second edition (Sparrow et al. 2011). In children with FASD, adaptive behavior is significantly lower than expected for age. In addition, this discrepancy seems relatively unrelated to IQ, at least in children not intellectually disabled.

Fagerlund et al. (2012) demonstrated this elegantly by comparing children with FASD ($n = 73$), nonexposed controls, and a group matched to those with FASD on verbal IQ, indicating specific learning disorder (SLD). The controls scored within normal limits on all domains. The FASD group scored inferior to the SLD group on all measures. This supports the notion that IQ cannot explain the adaptive challenges in children with FASD.

In our clinical setting, the discrepancy between IQ and Vineland scores often amounts to −3 sd. Clinically, the child's adaptive functioning is the equivalent of children half their age, even if their cognitive function is age-appropriate or only mildly reduced. In practical terms, parents then experience that they care for a very young child for many years. Petrenko et al. (2019) interviewed parents of children, adolescent, and young adults with FASD about the challenges involved in caring for those with FASD. The parents reported a pervasive feeling of worry for the child's adaptive functioning, the need of constant monitoring even at older ages, and worries about what the child may do in unstructured situations that come across.

In addition, the child is often described to function better in kindergarten or school, at least the primary school years, than at home. We believe this is due to the structure that is naturally provided in those settings, compared to free time. In addition, the child has many "models" to imitate/follow in school.

The immaturity in independence in daily life observed in children with FASD is most likely a reflection of an immature central nervous system with delayed development, which seems to be a hallmark of the condition. Looking at other neurodevelopmental disorders like ADHD, the discrepancy between chronological age and independent functioning in daily life is present but seems less pervasive. In high-functioning children with ASD, similar patterns of codependence in daily life as for FASD are observed.

The frustration for many parents is the lack of understanding from the service system around them that does not observe the child's lack of age-appropriate independence. In our experience, this usually changes, as the child gets older. By the fourth or fifth grade, the demands on independence exceed what the child is able to achieve by observing others, and their challenges become more visible in a school setting. At the same time, the curriculum becomes more abstract. Tasks include being able to discuss and present subject summaries. At the same time, focus shifts from becoming a good reader to actually being able to abstract the essence from what you are reading. Suboptimal IQ levels, attention, and EF challenges will have increasingly pervasive effect on learning at this time point and onward resulting in more frustration and less feeling of competence for the child.

Information about the delayed development of independence should be conveyed to kindergartens and schools by professionals that have assessed the child. Even if these challenges still are not visible outside the home environment, access to adequate adult support is needed. By offering more support, the child will use less energy during daytime, and this may improve function at home. Close collaboration between family and kindergarten/school, preferably supported by health professionals, is indicated. This is also in accordance with the proposed model of intervention by Petrenko et al. (2014). Recognition and diagnosis are the basis for any intervention and qualify for services, given that they are available. Implementing services, but also maintaining them over time, may prevent secondary disabilities in children with FASD (Petrenko et al. 2014).

There are some programs aimed at improving aspects of adaptive functioning in children with FASD (see Ordenewitz et al. (2021) for a systematic review of evidence-based interventions):

- The fire and street safety virtual training is a computer game for children aged 4–10 years. The intervention takes about 30 min, guided by an adult. In a small study including 32 children, results showed improved knowledge about safety skills and generalizing occurred (Coles et al. 2007).

- GoFAR aims to improve attention, behavior, and adaptive functioning. This study included 30 children. It has five sessions for the parents and five for the child that teach both children and parents metacognitive strategies to improve impulsive responses and plan future actions. In addition, both child and parent participate together in five training sessions focusing on applying the techniques in daily life activities. Results indicated improved impulse control for the child, and parents rated the child as more independent on the VABS daily living domain (Coles et al. 2018).

Emphasis on functional age will be critical in order to offer enough help and support on a daily basis. In our experience, this is one of the most important interventions to help parents adjust their demands on the child accordingly. By offering appropriate level of support, family stress level may decrease as frustration for both parent and child decreases. The child will have more positive experiences that may encourage proactive behavior.

Social Deficits and Intervention

Deficits in social functioning is common in children and adolescents with FASD (Fagerlund et al. 2012). Rockhold et al. (2021) demonstrated social deficits from preschool age throughout adolescence. In middle childhood and adolescence, social function deficits were related to poorer executive functions, but this relationship was not evident in preschool children, probably due to less demand on EF at this early age. Prevalence of ASD is at least two times higher in FASD than in the general population, adding to the social challenges in this group. Inferior ability to understand social perspective and less empathy have been confirmed by standardized tests (NEPSY-II) and parental reports (Stevens et al. 2015).

Fagerlund et al. (2012) compared social functioning domain on the VABS in children 8–12 years old and adolescents13–20 years of age with FASD to those with SLD matched on SES and IQ (verbal IQ in both groups was 78). The older SLD group obtained better scores in the socialization domain than the younger group, while the opposite was reported in those with FASD. This indicates that while social challenges are present also in children with SLD, this group improves function over time. In contrast, deficits in social functioning seem to increase in the FASD group with age. Increasing challenges in understanding social perspective with age have also been confirmed by Stevens et al. (2015). These results indicate an increasing gap in social skills between adolescents with FASD and typically developing adults over time, and interventions should accommodate this by including a long-term plan for social support. This concurs with our clinical experience and previous literature; children with FASD struggle more in social functioning as they get older, relatively independent of IQ (Kully-Martens et al. 2012). As children grow older, they play less and talk more, and challenges related to WM and pragmatic language will have an increasingly negative impact on functioning. Fagerlund et al. (2012) recommend focusing on diagnosing FASD at an early age to target these challenges within all domains of adaptive behavior but especially within social skills.

Specific programs have been developed to support social skills in children with FASD; one example is the Children's Friendship Training program for children 6–12 years of age. This program lasts for 12 weeks, and children participate in groups focusing on social skills, while parents receive instructions separately. The program has shown positive results regarding social skills and actual social behavior as evaluated by parents, especially in combination with pharmacological treatment (Frankel et al. 2006). Many studies are small, parents are not blinded to group adherence, and participants have not been randomized to the different treatments for natural reasons. Still, these studies do support the notion that adaptive behavior, at least within the socialization domain, improves after training when combined with parental support in utilizing the acquired skills.

A significant problem behavior noted in youth with FASDs is being socially inappropriate and having poor understanding of personal boundaries. An example of this is the unacceptable sexual behavior shown by some individuals with FASD (Streissguth et al. 2004). Findings from Brown et al. (2019) suggest that there is a strong need to develop educational and training programs that better equip professionals with the skills to assist clients with FASD in treatment settings.

Regulatory Challenges in Children with FASD and Treatment Options

Children with FASD have a high prevalence of mental health challenges, with behavioral disorders and affect regulation deficits being among the most frequent (Popova et al. 2016; Temple et al. 2019). In addition, cognitive and ADHD symptoms (impulsivity, attention challenges, and hyperactivity) are frequently coexisting (Elgen et al. 2007). Core symptoms are affected by deficits in basic regulatory autonomic functions: sleep, sensory processing, and feeding. Interventions to optimize sleep and feeding should make up the basis of any intervention plan.

Sleep Disorders in Children with FASD and Intervention

Prevalence of sleep problems in children with FASD varies between studies. Ipsiroglu et al. (2019) reported that 100% of 40 patients with FASD (mean age 9.4 years) had chronic insomnia. Hayes et al. (2020) found that 65% of 107 children aged 5–17 years with FASD had problems with sleeping, including falling asleep (56%), staying asleep (45%), and waking up too early (29%). In comparison, 10% (high-income families) to 28% (low-income families) of normally developing children and adolescents have sleeping problems according to the Norwegian Institute of Public Health (Sleep problems in Norway – NIPH (fhi.no), 2019). Poor sleep quality has been related to increased aggressive behavior in a systematic review by Van Veen et al. (2021).

As basis for intervention planning, a multidisciplinary approach is recommended (Hanlon-Dearman et al. 2018), including medical and neuropsychological assessment as well as evaluation of environmental factors. In our experience, the Sleep Disturbance Scale for Children (SDSC) is useful (Bruni et al. 1996). The scale is relatively short, with 26 questions that make up the following indices: disorders of initiating and maintaining sleep, sleep breathing disorders, disorders of arousal/nightmares, sleep-wake transition disorders, disorders of excessive somnolence, and sleep hyperhidrosis. In addition, assessing family factors like parental stress and strategies used related to sleep routine would provide information to start intervention planning. Knowledge about the neurodevelopmental origin of the child's sleep problems is, in our experience, essential in helping parents to address the problem.

Sleep Hygiene

In our experience, intervention plans have to include practical advice regarding sleep hygiene. Stable day- and nighttime routines are essential. Set daytime routines may reduce dysregulation in the child as well as family stress. In addition, bedtime routines should focus on the child performing the same activities in the same order every evening. A set time for starting the preparation for going to bed should be emphasized, and deviations should be kept to a minimum, even in weekends and holidays (i.e., 1–1.5 h delay). To aid keeping the routines, a physical plan is often helpful. The plan may have pictures/drawings of the activities that are included in the bedtime routine, or be in writing for older children, like a checklist.

In a systematic review by Rigney et al. (2018) of sleep interventions for children with neurodevelopmental disorders, the most used methods were psychoeducation, routines, graduated extinction of sleep problems, and reinforcement. This is in accordance with the advices most often recommended for typically developing children (TDC). Results showed similar effects in clinical groups as in TDC, but none of the studies included children with FASD.

Melatonin Supplement Therapy

One small study ($n = 36$) reported that 79% of children with FASD had an abnormal melatonin profile (Goril et al. 2016). Melatonin supplement may improve sleep in children with FASD and aid in establishing bedtime routines by increasing sleepiness at appropriate time. Treatment should be administered by an experienced medical doctor and only in combination with interventions aimed at improved sleep hygiene. However, studies on the effect of melatonin in children with FASD are lacking. For a comprehensive review and suggestions for interventions, see Hanlon-Dearman et al. (2018).

Sensory Processing Deficits and Intervention

Children with FASD are easily overwhelmed by sensory input but also seek sensory stimulation more than TDC. Sensory processing deficits correlate with sleep problems (Wengel et al. 2011; Jirikowic et al. 2020). Challenges to sensory downregulation at bedtime have also been described by Wengel et al. (2011). To aid downregulating, reducing sensory load at bedtime is recommended. Interventions would be to remove objects that may catch the attention of the child, like toys, computer games, TV, and mobile phone to reduce distractibility. Clear rules regarding the use of these objects as part of the bedtime routine may help. Parents often report to us that setting a time point for when to turn off the Internet, mobile phone, and computer games is essential. Positive reinforcement when adhering to the rules may also help. Evening routines should focus on gradually reducing physical activity, for example, by including a warm bath and reading, or calm conversation. The bedroom should have temperature control and blinders to keep light out during summer months. For some children, a noise-cancelling device (white noise) may be of help.

Eating Disorders and Intervention

Growth restriction at birth is part of the diagnostic criteria in diagnosing FAS. In infancy, feeding problems are common in children with FASD. At later ages, reports are diverse regarding nutrition and weight. Higher prevalence of eating difficulties related to refusal of foods, for example, due to inacceptable texture, poor satiety, and constant snacking, has been reported (Amos-Kroohs et al. 2016). Increased prevalence of overweight is reported among children with partial FAS and of underweight in those with FAS (Fuglestad et al. 2014). Amos-Kroohs et al. (2016) reported lower body mass index (BMI) in males with FASD than TDC at 8 years of age but not in girls. Others have reported significantly poorer nutritional intake in children with FASD (Nguyen et al. 2016a).

Parents often describe challenges related to meals: the child's inability to sit at the table and finishing a meal. Challenges with texture (being a "picky eater") could be related to abnormal oral sensory processing, while hyperactivity and/or attention problems affect ability to share a family meal. At kindergarten and in school, distractibility can affect ability to finish the meals, in combination with hyperactivity challenges.

In the clinic, we recommend accommodating the child regarding both textures and how the meals are organized. At home, bringing an iPad or phone to the meal may help the child to sit still during meals. At kindergarten/schools, we often recommend that the child eat together with an adult before the common meal, for example, in a separate room for 15 min. Afterward, the child eats with the rest of the children. However, then the adult has already ensured that the child has eaten sufficiently and focus may be on the social aspects of sharing a meal.

If the child is not able to eat sufficiently, nutritional drinks may be used as a supplement.

Behavioral Challenges and Intervention

Psychiatric problems are more prevalent in children and adolescents with FASD than in the general population, with externalizing disorders being three to five times more frequent (for review, see Popova et al. (2016) and Lange et al. (2018)). Given the complexity of FASD, this is not surprising. The combination of executive function deficits, dependency of others due to delayed development of adaptive behavior but not mental retardation, places a heavy burden on the individual. Failure to accommodate these challenges sufficiently is likely to result in externalizing problems.

In general, factors that affect the prognosis of children and adolescents with behavioral disorders are:

- Onset before 8 years of age
- Antisocial behavior that is severe, frequent, and variable
- Hyperactivity and attention problems being present
- Low IQ
- Family history of criminal behavior and alcoholism
- Inconsistent parental methods: criticism and lack of warmth, involvement, and supervision
- Low SES, poor living conditions, and ineffective schools (NICE 2013)

Intervention aimed at attention/hyperactivity and improving parental skills and educational services could consequently improve outcome for any child or adolescent with behavior disorder.

The NICE guidelines on recognition, interventions, and management of antisocial behavior and conduct disorders in children and adolescents were published in 2013 (updated in 2018) and may be downloaded free at www.nice.org.uk. The guidelines sum up evidence-based interventions for children and adolescents in general:

- *Children 3–11 years of age*: Parental groups based on social learning theory and positive reinforcement, use of model learning, exercises, and feedback. Interventions should be group-based, 10–16 meeting, each 60–120 min, and manual-based. If challenges are complex, the recommendation is that groups consist of children and parents together, with the same duration. In Norway, Circle of Security (COS) is a commonly used method; however, in our experience, the method is less efficient if used for children with FASD and aggressive behavior. Parent management training (PMT) is an evidence-based method specifically aimed at reducing disruptive behavior in children 3–12 years of age; for a systematic review, see Michelson et al. (2013).
- *Children/adolescents 9–14 years of age*: Intervention should be provided within groups of children focusing on social and cognitive problem-solving, model

learning, exercises, and feedback. Duration should be 10–18 weeks and 120 min for each session.

- *Children/adolescents 11–17 years of age*: Multimodal intervention for the child and parents together, 3–5 months' duration. Multisystemic therapy (MST) is a method with sound evidence base; see Von Sydow et al. (2013) for a systematic review of 47 RCTs.

Challenging behavior causes social exclusion especially if combined with mental disabilities, but still evidence-based interventions are lacking for this group (Ali et al. 2015). NICE guidelines on challenging behavior and learning disabilities: prevention and interventions for people with intellectual impairment whose behavior challenges (NICE 2013) emphasize the points presented in Table 2 to improve understanding and treatment planning.

Pharmacological Treatment of Behavioral Disorders

A recent review of pharmacological treatment in children with FASD and behavioral disorders identified eight clinical studies (Ritfeld et al. 2021). Sample sizes were small, ranging from $n = 4$ to 77. In general, there is a positive effect of stimulants on hyperactivity and less consistent effect regarding attention/impulsivity, all of whom are relevant for behavioral challenges. The authors note in the conclusion that stimulants may not be as effective in children with FASD and ADHD as in idiopathic ADHD. This is in accordance with our clinical experience. According to Ozsarfati and Koren (2015), the most frequently used medication to treat behavioral disorders is risperidone. No studies have evaluated the effect of risperidone in FASD. Ozsarfati and Koren (2015) describe observation from ten children treated during 1 year from a Motherisk FASD diagnostic clinic. They all had FASD, ADHD (medicated with stimulants), and behavioral problems. Reduction in aggressive behavior and impulsivity was observed in eight out of ten children that received risperidone.

Table 2 NICE guideline recommendations for challenging behavior in persons with intellectual impairments. These points should be considered to understand behavioral challenges in persons with intellectual disabilities according to NICE guidelines (2015)

1. Comprehensive assessment to ensure knowledge and understanding related to the condition
2. Medical evaluation
3. Risk assessment (violence, suicide, abuse)
4. Functional behavioral analysis
5. Assessment of psychiatric conditions
6. Defined target behavior and outcome
7. Assessment of and modification of environmental factors
8. Including both professionals and family
9. Plan for when and how to evaluate and make decision to continue or not with intervention
10. Evaluate the need for medication

To sum up, evidence supporting medication in children with FASD and behavioral challenges is in practice lacking. At the same time, symptoms are serious and complex. We would recommend involving an experienced child psychiatrist to consider indication for medication as part of a more comprehensive treatment plan. Mela et al. (2020) developed a treatment algorithm that can aid clinicians in psychopharmacological treatment of children, adolescents, and adults with FASD. In this algorithm, first and second line of treatment is suggested based on four clusters of signs and symptoms: hyperarousal, emotional dysregulation, hyperactivity/reduced neurocognitive, and cognitive flexibility (EF).

Psychoeducative Interventions for Children and Adolescents with FASD and Behavioral Challenges

Few intervention programs aimed at behavioral disorders in FASD exist. To the best of our knowledge, there are only four systematic reviews of interventions for children and adolescents with FASD: Peadon et al. (2009), Reid et al. (2015), Flannigan et al. (2020), and Ordenewitz et al. (2021). There is an urgent need of studies evaluating the effectiveness of intervention on disruptive/externalizing and aggressive behavior in children and adolescents with FASD.

Psychoeducation is an evidence-based treatment approach aimed at empowering both patients and families by providing information about the condition. Several studies have provided psychoeducation about FASD, what services are available, and how to get access to them as well as supporting foster homes. Results include reduced parental stress, fewer moves between foster-home placements, and a tendency toward increased parental confidence (Leenaars et al. 2012; Kable et al. 2012). For examples of programs based on psychoeducation, see Table 3. In our clinic, part of the intervention plan is a feedback session and written reports to parents, kindergarten/schools, and others that work with the family on specific neurodevelopmental profile and intervention suggestions. In addition, two educational lectures on FASD are provided, especially focusing on intervention. The family is offered a home visit for a family network meeting. This lasts for 2 h, and the family invites whoever they want from extended family, friends, neighbors, and so on. The evaluation from these sessions has been overwhelmingly positive. Parents and network report improved understanding and access to more support services in everyday life.

Examples of programs that combine psychoeducation for parents and sessions for children as advised by Petrenko and Alto (2017) are:

Alert Program (Nash et al. 2015; Wells et al. 2012) – improved self-regulation
Families on track (Petrenko et al. 2017) – improved self-regulation
FAR strategy (Coles et al. 2015) – positive effect on metacognitive abilities
GoFAR (Kable et al. 2015) – positive effect on disruptive behavior

The availability of programs like these will vary between countries and even between regions/hospitals. Providing educational lectures aimed at all levels that

Table 3 Programs involving psychoeducation to parents of children with FASD to reduce behavioral challenges. These programs all include psychoeducation to parents of children with FASD, some in combination with sessions for the child

Program name	Content	Age of child	Setting	Format	Frequency/ duration	Outcomes	References
Parent training workshops and psychoeducation	Educate families about FASD, information on effective behavior management strategies, and advocacy tools to access resources	3–10 years	Home or clinic	Information packets or caregiver workshops or web-based programs	Variable	Satisfaction with all intervention formats, increased parent knowledge, and improved behavioral functioning	Coles et al. (2009), Kable et al. (2007, 2012), and Bertrand (2009: Study 4)
Coaching Families (CF) program	Educate families about FASD, helps them access resources, and engages them in successful advocacy	1–23 years	Home	Family goal-based mentoring	Needs basis	Decreased needs, increased goal attainment, and decreased caregiver stress	Leenaars et al. (2012)
Parent-child interaction therapy (PCIT)	Improving the parent-child relationship, increasing appropriate social skills, reducing problem behavior, and creating a positive discipline program	3–7 years	Clinic, home with modifications	Group-based adaptation; parent-child dyad with in vivo coaching	14 weeks, once a week, 90 min	Improved child behavior problems, decreased parent stress; outcomes did not differ from moderate intensity psychoeducation and support group	Gurwitch et al., reported in Bertrand (2009: Study 4)

(continued)

Table 3 (continued)

Program name	Content	Age of child	Setting	Format	Frequency/ duration	Outcomes	References
Families moving forward (FMF)	Modifies specific parenting attitudes and responses toward child problem behavior to reduce challenging behavior and improve family functioning (Bertrand, 2009: Study #5)	5–11 years	Home	Individualized caregiver training	9–11 months, every 2 weeks, 90 min	Improved parent self-care, family needs met, and reduced child problem behavior	Olson et al., reported in Bertrand (2009: Study 5)
Families on track integrated preventive intervention	Based on neuropsychological and diagnostics. Child and families receive a 30-week multicomponent intervention that integrates two existing empirically validated programs:	4–8 years	Home	In-home parent behavioral consultation (FMF) and child skills groups (PATHS)	A single 60-min session (personalized feedback to each caregiver) Weekly groups for the child for 30 weeks	High satisfaction with the program, effects for child emotion regulation, self-esteem, and anxiety. Reduced disruptive behavior. Caregiver outcomes: improved	Petrenko et al. (2017)

	the preschool/ kindergarten Promoting Alternative Thinking Strategies (PATHS) curriculum and Families Moving Forward: modifies specific parenting attitudes and responses toward child problem behavior to reduce challenging behavior and improve family functioning (Bertrand 2009: Study #5)					knowledge and advocacy, attributions of behavior, use of antecedent strategies, parent efficacy, family needs met, social support, and self-care	
GoFAR program ((ii) parent training)	Improve self-regulation and adaptive living skills for children with FASD by increasing metacognitive control of emotions and arousal. The intervention has	5–10 years	Clinic	Individual parent training therapy sessions	Five sessions, 1 h	Significant reductions in parental reports of disruptive behavior, greater improvement in self-regulation skills, and positive treatment effects on	Coles et al. (2015, 2018) and Kable et al. (2016)

(continued)

Table 3 (continued)

Program name	Content	Age of child	Setting	Format	Frequency/duration	Outcomes	References
	three components: (i) GoFAR, a "serious game" designed to teach a metacognitive control strategy in a computer game environment; (ii) parent training on child behavioral regulation; and (iii) behavior analog therapy (BAT) sessions, a practical application of the metacognitive learning methodology by parent and child in the context of learning adaptive skills					attention and adaptive functioning	

work with the child (primary and secondary health care, educational system, family) is a low threshold intervention that are also cost-effective as there is no limit to the number of participants. The family network meeting requires more resources (travelling, only one patient at the time). Given the research support for providing psychoeducation and its potential effect, it could still represent a cost-effective intervention (Leenaars et al. 2012; Kable et al. 2012).

Parental programs aimed at reducing disruptive behavior in general are numerous and have been extensively reviewed compared to programs aimed exclusively at children with FASD. In a recent meta-analysis by Leijten et al. (2019), positive reinforcement, praise, and use of natural/logical consequences were most effective in reducing disruptive behavior. In addition, specific, practical, and concrete techniques had a positive prevention and treatment effect. This is in accordance with Petrenko (2015) focusing on positive behavioral interventions and family support for FASD.

Conclusion

Intervention studies aimed at children and adolescents with FASD are few, and methodological problems, especially related to number of participants, non-randomization, and lack of long-term follow-up, are common. However, there is research support for several types of intervention programs especially developed for children with FASD that should be considered. The availability of these programs varies across countries, languages, and societal resources. Independently of this, any intervention plan should be based on a correct diagnosis and medical, cognitive, neuropsychological, and educational assessments by a multidisciplinary team. FASD usually means complex challenges that are present throughout development and into adulthood. Plans should therefore be long term and also include plans for supporting the parents as well as offering psychoeducation to the child's extended network.

Applications to Other Areas of Substance Use Disorder

Focus of this chapter was interventions for children and adolescents with FASD. There are no diagnostic terms for children with prenatal drug exposure as the clinical manifestations are less studied and more variable. However, the prevalence of attention/executive function deficits is high also in children with prenatal drug exposure, and interventions discussed in this chapter may be useful also for this group. Unfortunately, the prevalence of alcohol and/or drug abuse in adults with FASD is high. The challenges described in this chapter will also be present at later ages (low IQ, attention/executive function deficits, and adaptive behavior impairments) and have to be taken into consideration when planning treatment. Specifically, focus should be on positive reinforcement and activating and educating family and extended network as part of the intervention.

Applications to Other Areas of Public Health

Interventions discussed in this chapter may be applicable to other areas within public health working with families that have children with complex neurodevelopmental disorders. Psychoeducation is a method that can be applied for any diagnosis to provide more knowledge and ownership of the condition in question. Group-based intervention provides a network and support from others in the same situation. Teaching new skills and providing feedback on implementation will probably increase the chance of using the skills after end of intervention. In general, providing specific, practical, and concrete advice and skills is regarded key element to any intervention aimed at children and adolescents with neurodevelopmental challenges.

Mini-Dictionary of Terms

1. FASD is not a diagnosis but an umbrella term that clinically describes outcome after PAE.
2. FAS is a medical diagnosis (Q86.0 in ICD-10) that encompasses growth retardation, specific facial features, affection of the central nervous system, and PAE.
3. Adaptive behavior refers to how well we are able to meet the expectations of society regarding activities of daily living, communication, and social functioning according to the society you live in and your age. Adaptive behavior is modified by guidance, training, and/or time.
4. Executive functions (EF) refer to cognitive functions that are active in situations that are novel or nonroutine. These functions continue to develop throughout young adulthood.
5. Impulse control is a critical EF, enabling us to delay a response or reward. Deficits in impulse control are related to several neurodevelopmental disorders including ADHD.
6. Autism is a neurodevelopmental disorder affecting approximately 2% of the population in the Western world. ASD is an umbrella term that currently encompasses several diagnoses, including Asperger's syndrome and infantile autism. Autism is characterized by impairment in communication, social functioning, and limited, stereotype/rigid behavior. In those with infantile autism, intellectual disability is seen in 80%.

Key Facts of FASD

- FASD affects approximately 1–3% of the population.
- FASD requires a multidisciplinary team to properly assess, diagnose, and plan interventions.
- FASD often includes challenges related to IQ, attention/executive functions, adaptive functioning, and behavior.

- FASD is a lifelong condition in need of multidisciplinary interventions aimed at education, work, living conditions, mental health, and access to guidance.
- FASD diagnosis improves prognosis if assessed at an early age.

Summary Points

- The prevalence of FASD is high, still evidence-based interventions are few, and availability varies across the world.
- Interventions should be aimed at intellectual deficits, including low IQ, SLD, and deficits in executive functions.
- Interventions should be aimed at the individual child, the family, and its network.
- Improving parental understanding of FASD by providing teaching of specific skills and practical guidance improves outcome.
- A diversity of programs for children with FASD exists, and important elements to be included are psychoeducation to parents and network and sessions for parents and children together and separately.

References

Ali A, Hall I, Blickwedel J (2015) Behavioural and cognitive-behavioural interventions for outwardly-directed aggressive behaviour in people with intellectual disabilities. Cochrane Database Syst Rev 2015(4):CD003406. https://doi.org/10.1002/14651858.CD003406.pub4

Amos-Kroohs RM, Fink BA, Smith CJ, Chin L, Van Calcar SC, Wozniak JR, Smith SM (2016) Abnormal eating behaviors are common in children with fetal alcohol Spectrum disorder. J Pediatr 169:194–200.e191. https://doi.org/10.1016/j.jpeds.2015.10.049

Baddeley A (2003) Working memory and language: an overview. J Commun Disord 36(3): 189–208. https://doi.org/10.1016/s0021-9924(03)00019-4

Bertrand J (2009) Interventions for Children with Fetal Alcohol Spectrum Disorders Research Consortium. Res Dev Disabil. 2009 Sep-Oct;30(5):986–1006. https://doi.org/10.1016/j.ridd.2009.02.003. Epub 2009 Mar 26. PMID: 19327965 Review

Brown J, Neal D, Carter MN, Louie J (2019) Sex offender treatment professional perceptions of fetal alcohol spectrum disorder (FASD) in the Midwest. Int J Law Psychiatry 66:101476. https://doi.org/10.1016/j.ijlp.2019.101476

Bruni O, Ottaviano S, Guidetti V, Romoli M, Innocenzi M, Cortesi F, Giannotti F (1996) The Sleep Disturbance Scale for Children (SDSC). Construction and validation of an instrument to evaluate sleep disturbances in childhood and adolescence. J Sleep Res 5(4):251–261. https://doi.org/10.1111/j.1365-2869.1996.00251.x

Carter Leno V, Chandler S, White P, Pickles A, Baird G, Hobson C, Smith AB, Charman T, Rubia K, Simonoff E (2018) Testing the specificity of executive functioning impairments in adolescents with ADHD, ODD/CD and ASD. Eur Child Adolesc Psychiatry 27(7):899–908. https://doi.org/10.1007/s00787-017-1089-5

Coles CD, Strickland DC, Padgett L, Bellmoff L (2007) Games that "work": using computer games to teach alcohol-affected children about fire and street safety. Res Dev Disabil 28(5):518–530. https://doi.org/10.1016/j.ridd.2006.07.001

Coles CD, Kable JA, Taddeo E (2009) Math performance and behavior problems in children affected by prenatal alcohol exposure: intervention and follow-up. J Dev Behav Pediatr 30(1): 7–15. https://doi.org/10.1097/DBP.0b013e3181966780

Coles CD, Kable JA, Taddeo E, Strickland DC (2015) A metacognitive strategy for reducing disruptive behavior in children with fetal alcohol spectrum disorders: GoFAR pilot. Alcohol Clin Exp Res 39(11):2224–2233. https://doi.org/10.1111/acer.12885

Coles CD, Kable JA, Taddeo E, Strickland D (2018) GoFAR: improving attention, behavior and adaptive functioning in children with fetal alcohol spectrum disorders: brief report. Dev Neurorehabil 21(5):345–349. https://doi.org/10.1080/17518423.2018.1424263

Doyle LR, Riley EP, Mattson SN, Glass L, Wozniak JR, Kable JA, Coles CD, Sowell ER, Jones KL (2019) Relation between oppositional/conduct behaviors and executive function among youth with histories of heavy prenatal alcohol exposure. Alcohol Clin Exp Res 43(6):1135–1144

Elgen I, Bruaroy S, Laegreid LM (2007) Lack of recognition and complexity of foetal alcohol neuroimpairments. Acta Paediatr 96(2):237–241. https://doi.org/10.1111/j.1651-2227.2007.00026.x

Engle JA, Kerns KA (2011) Reinforcement learning in children with FASD. J Popul Ther Clin Pharmacol 18(1):e17–e27

Ericson L, Magnusson L, Hovstadius B (2017) Societal costs of fetal alcohol syndrome in Sweden. Eur J Health Econ 18(5):575–585. https://doi.org/10.1007/s10198-016-0811-4

Fagerlund A, Autti-Ramo I, Mirjam K, Pekka S, Eugene H, Sarah M, Marit K (2012) Adaptive behaviour in children and adolescents with foetal alcohol spectrum disorders: a comparison with specific learning disability and typical development. Eur Child Adolesc Psychiatry 21(4): 221–231. [Corrected] [published erratum appears in Eur Child Adolesc Psychiatry 22(2):129, 2013]

Ferreira VKL, Cruz MS (2017) Intelligence and fetal alcohol spectrum disorders: a review. J Popul Ther Clin Pharmacol 24(3):e1–e18. https://doi.org/10.22374/1710-6222.24.3.1

Flannigan K, Coons-Harding KD, Anderson T, Wolfson L, Campbell A, Mela M, Pei J (2020) A systematic review of interventions to improve mental health and substance use outcomes for individuals with prenatal alcohol exposure and fetal alcohol spectrum disorder. Alcohol Clin Exp Res 44(12):2401–2430. https://doi.org/10.1111/acer.14490

Frankel F, Paley B, Marquardt R, O'Connor M (2006) Stimulants, neuroleptics, and children's friendship training for children with fetal alcohol spectrum disorders. J Child Adolesc Psychopharmacol 16(6):777–789. https://doi.org/10.1089/cap.2006.16.777

Fryer SL, McGee CL, Matt GE, Riley EP, Mattson SN (2007) Evaluation of psychopathological conditions in children with heavy prenatal alcohol exposure. Pediatrics 119(3). https://doi.org/10.1542/peds.2006-1606

Fuglestad AJ, Boys CJ, Chang PN, Miller BS, Eckerle JK, Deling L, Fink BA, Hoecker HL, Hickey MK, Jimenez-Vega JM, Wozniak JR (2014) Overweight and obesity among children and adolescents with fetal alcohol spectrum disorders. Alcohol Clin Exp Res 38(9):2502–2508. https://doi.org/10.1111/acer.12516

Coriale G, Fiorentino D, Lauro FD, Marchitelli R, Scalese B, Fiore M, Maviglia M, Ceccanti M (2013) Fetal Alcohol Spectrum Disorder (FASD): neurobehavioral profile, indications for diagnosis and treatment, PMID: 24326748 https://doi.org/10.1708/1356.15062

Glass L, Moore EM, Akshoomoff N, Jones KL, Riley EP, Mattson SN (2017) Academic difficulties in children with prenatal alcohol exposure: presence, profile, and neural correlates. Alcohol Clin Exp Res 41(5):1024–1034. https://doi.org/10.1111/acer.13366

Goril S, Zalai D, Scott L, Shapiro CM (2016) Sleep and melatonin secretion abnormalities in children and adolescents with fetal alcohol spectrum disorders. Sleep Med 23:59–64. https://doi.org/10.1016/j.sleep.2016.06.002

Greenmyer JR, Popova S, Klug MG, Burd L (2020) Fetal alcohol spectrum disorder: a systematic review of the cost of and savings from prevention in the United States and Canada. Addiction 115(3):409–417. https://doi.org/10.1111/add.14841

Hanlon-Dearman A, Chen ML, Olson HC (2018) Understanding and managing sleep disruption in children with fetal alcohol spectrum disorder. Biochem Cell Biol 96(2):267–274. https://doi.org/10.1139/bcb-2017-0064

Hayes N, Moritz KM, Reid N (2020) Parent-reported sleep problems in school-aged children with fetal alcohol spectrum disorder: association with child behaviour, caregiver, and family functioning. Sleep Med 74:307–314. https://doi.org/10.1016/j.sleep.2020.07.022

Ipsiroglu OS, Wind K, Hung Y-H, Berger M, Chan F, Yu W, Stockler S, Weinberg J (2019) Prenatal alcohol exposure and sleep-wake behaviors: exploratory and naturalistic observations in the clinical setting and in an animal model. Sleep Med 54:101–112

Jirikowic TL, Thorne JC, McLaughlin SA, Waddington T, Lee AKC, Astley Hemingway SJ (2020) Prevalence and patterns of sensory processing behaviors in a large clinical sample of children with prenatal alcohol exposure. Res Dev Disabil 100:103617. https://doi.org/10.1016/j.ridd.2020.103617

Kable JA, Coles CD, Taddeo E (2007) Socio-cognitive habilitation using the math interactive learning experience program for alcohol-affected children. Alcohol Clin Exp Res 31(8): 1425–1434. https://doi.org/10.1111/j.1530-0277.2007.00431.x

Kable JA, Coles CD, Strickland D, Taddeo E (2012) Comparing the effectiveness of on-line versus in-person caregiver education and training for behavioral regulation in families of children with FASD. Int J Ment Heal Addict 10(6):791–803. https://doi.org/10.1007/s11469-012-9376-3

Kable JA, Taddeo E, Strickland D, Coles CD (2015) Community translation of the Math Interactive Learning Experience Program for children with FASD. Res Dev Disabil 39:1–11. https://doi.org/10.1016/j.ridd.2014.12.031

Kable JA, Taddeo E, Strickland D, Coles CD (2016) Improving FASD Children's Self-Regulation: Piloting Phase 1 of the GoFAR Intervention. Child Fam Behav Ther 38(2):124–141. https://doi.org/10.1080/07317107.2016.1172880. Epub 2016 May 23. PMID: 29104359

Kerns KA, Macsween J, Vander Wekken S, Gruppuso V (2010) Investigating the efficacy of an attention training programme in children with foetal alcohol spectrum disorder. Dev Neurorehabil 13(6):413–422. https://doi.org/10.3109/17518423.2010.511421

Kerns KA, Macoun S, MacSween J, Pei J, Hutchison M (2017) Attention and working memory training: a feasibility study in children with neurodevelopmental disorders. Appl Neuropsychol Child 6(2):120–137. https://doi.org/10.1080/21622965.2015.1109513

Khoury JE, Milligan K (2019) Comparing executive functioning in children and adolescents with fetal alcohol spectrum disorders and ADHD: a meta-analysis. J Atten Disord 23(14): 1801–1815. https://doi.org/10.1177/1087054715622016

Kodituwakku PW, Kodituwakku EL (2011) From research to practice: an integrative framework for the development of interventions for children with fetal alcohol spectrum disorders. Neuropsychol Rev 21(2):204–223. https://doi.org/10.1007/s11065-011-9170-1

Kully-Martens K, Denys K, Treit S, Tamana S, Rasmussen C (2012) A review of social skills deficits in individuals with fetal alcohol spectrum disorders and prenatal alcohol exposure: profiles, mechanisms, and interventions. Alcohol Clin Exp Res 36(4):568–576. https://doi.org/10.1111/j.1530-0277.2011.01661.x

Lange S, Rovet J, Rehm J, Popova S (2017) Neurodevelopmental profile of fetal alcohol spectrum disorder: a systematic review. BMC Psychol 5(1):22. https://doi.org/10.1186/s40359-017-0191-2

Lange S, Rehm J, Anagnostou E, Popova S (2018) Prevalence of externalizing disorders and autism spectrum disorders among children with fetal alcohol spectrum disorder: systematic review and meta-analysis. Biochem Cell Biol 96(2):241–251. https://doi.org/10.1139/bcb-2017-0014

Leenaars L, Denys K, Henneveld D, Rasmussen C (2012) The impact of fetal alcohol spectrum disorders on families: evaluation of a family intervention program. Community Ment Health J 48(4):431–435. https://doi.org/10.1007/s10597-011-9425-6

Leijten P, Gardner F, Melendez-Torres GJ, van Aar J, Hutchings J, Schulz S, Knerr W, Overbeek G (2019) Meta-analyses: key parenting program components for disruptive child behavior. J Am Acad Child Adolesc Psychiatry 58(2):180–190. https://doi.org/10.1016/j.jaac.2018.07.900

Lohaugen GC, Flak MM, Gerstner T, Sundberg C, Lerdal B, Skranes J (2015) Establishment of the South-Eastern Norway Regional Health Authority resource center for children with prenatal alcohol/drug exposure. Subst Abuse 9(Suppl 2):67–75. https://doi.org/10.4137/SART.S23542

Loomes C, Rasmussen C, Pei J, Manji S, Andrew G (2008) The effect of rehearsal training on working memory span of children with fetal alcohol spectrum disorder. Res Dev Disabil 29(2): 113–124. https://doi.org/10.1016/j.ridd.2007.01.001

Mattson SN, Crocker N, Nguyen TT (2011) Fetal alcohol spectrum disorders: neuropsychological and behavioral features. Neuropsychol Rev 21(2):81–101. https://doi.org/10.1007/s11065-011-9167-9

Mattson SN, Bernes GA, Doyle LR (2019) Fetal alcohol spectrum disorders: a review of the neurobehavioral deficits associated with prenatal alcohol exposure. Alcohol Clin Exp Res 43(6):1046–1062. https://doi.org/10.1111/acer.14040

Mela M, Hanlon-Dearman A, Ahmed AG, Rich SD, Densmore R, Reid D, Barr AM, Osser D, Anderson T, Suberu B, Ipsiroglu O, Rajani H, Loock C (2020) Treatment algorithm for the use of psychopharmacological agents in individuals prenatally exposed to alcohol and/or with diagnosis of fetal alcohol spectrum disorder (FASD). J Popul Ther Clin Pharmacol 27(3):e1–e13. https://doi.org/10.15586/jptcp.v27i3.681

Michelson D, Davenport C, Dretzke J, Barlow J, Day C (2013) Do evidence-based interventions work when tested in the "real world?" A systematic review and meta-analysis of parent management training for the treatment of child disruptive behavior. Clin Child Fam Psychol Rev 16(1):18–34. https://doi.org/10.1007/s10567-013-0128-0

Mohamed Z, Carlisle ACS, Livesey AC, Mukherjee RAS (2019) Comparisons of the BRIEF parental report and neuropsychological clinical tests of executive function in fetal alcohol spectrum disorders: data from the UK national specialist clinic. Child Neuropsychol 25(5): 648–663. https://doi.org/10.1080/09297049.2018.1516202

Nash K, Stevens S, Greenbaum R, Weiner J, Koren G, Rovet J (2015) Improving executive functioning in children with fetal alcohol spectrum disorders. Child Neuropsychol 21(2): 191–209. https://doi.org/10.1080/09297049.2014.889110

Nguyen TT, Risbud RD, Chambers CD, Thomas JD (2016a) Dietary nutrient intake in school-aged children with heavy prenatal alcohol exposure. Alcohol Clin Exp Res 40(5):1075–1082. https://doi.org/10.1111/acer.13035

Nguyen TT, Risbud RD, Mattson SN, Chambers CD, Thomas JD (2016b) Randomized, double-blind, placebo-controlled clinical trial of choline supplementation in school-aged children with fetal alcohol spectrum disorders. Am J Clin Nutr 104(6):1683–1692. https://doi.org/10.3945/ajcn.116.142075

NICE (2013) Antisocial behaviour and conduct disorders in children and young people: recognition and management Clinical guideline Published: 27 March 2013. www.nice.org.uk/guidance/cg158

O'Malley KD, Koplin B, Dohner VA (2000) Psychostimulant clinical response in fetal alcohol syndrome. Can J Psychiatry 45(1):90–91

Ordenewitz LK, Weinmann T, Schluter JA, Moder JE, Jung J, Kerber K, Greif-Kohistani N, Heinen F, Landgraf MN (2021) Evidence-based interventions for children and adolescents with fetal alcohol spectrum disorders – a systematic review. Eur J Paediatr Neurol 33:50–60. https://doi.org/10.1016/j.ejpn.2021.02.001

Ozsarfati J, Koren G (2015) Medications used in the treatment of disruptive behavior in children with FASD – a guide. J Popul Ther Clin Pharmacol 22(1):e59–e67

Peadon E, Elliott EJ (2010) Distinguishing between attention-deficit hyperactivity and fetal alcohol spectrum disorders in children: clinical guidelines. Neuropsychiatr Dis Treat 6:509–515. https://doi.org/10.2147/ndt.s7256

Peadon E, Rhys-Jones B, Bower C, Elliott EJ (2009) Systematic review of interventions for children with fetal alcohol spectrum disorders. BMC Pediatr 9:35. https://doi.org/10.1186/1471-2431-9-35

Petrenko CL (2015) Positive behavioral interventions and family support for fetal alcohol spectrum disorders. Curr Dev Disord Rep 2(3):199–209. https://doi.org/10.1007/s40474-015-0052-8

Petrenko CL, Alto ME (2017) Interventions in fetal alcohol spectrum disorders: an international perspective. Eur J Med Genet 60(1):79–91. https://doi.org/10.1016/j.ejmg.2016.10.005

Petrenko CL, Tahir N, Mahoney EC, Chin NP (2014) Prevention of secondary conditions in fetal alcohol spectrum disorders: identification of systems-level barriers. Matern Child Health J 18(6):1496–1505. https://doi.org/10.1007/s10995-013-1390-y

Petrenko CLM, Pandolfino ME, Robinson LK (2017) Findings from the families on track intervention pilot trial for children with fetal alcohol spectrum disorders and their families. Alcohol Clin Exp Res 41(7):1340–1351. https://doi.org/10.1111/acer.13408

Petrenko CLM, Demeusy EM, Alto ME (2019) Six-month follow-up of the families on track intervention pilot trial for children with fetal alcohol spectrum disorders and their families. Alcohol Clin Exp Res 43(10):2242–2254. https://doi.org/10.1111/acer.14180

Popova S, Lange S, Shield K, Mihic A, Chudley AE, Mukherjee RAS, Bekmuradov D, Rehm J (2016) Comorbidity of fetal alcohol spectrum disorder: a systematic review and meta-analysis. Lancet 387(10022):978–987. https://doi.org/10.1016/S0140-6736(15)01345-8

Popova S, Lange S, Shield K, Burd L, Rehm J (2019) Prevalence of fetal alcohol spectrum disorder among special subpopulations: a systematic review and meta-analysis. Addiction 114(7): 1150–1172. https://doi.org/10.1111/add.14598

Reid N, Dawe S, Shelton D, Harnett P, Warner J, Armstrong E, LeGros K, O'Callaghan F (2015) Systematic review of fetal alcohol spectrum disorder interventions across the life span. Alcohol Clin Exp Res 39(12):2283–2295. https://doi.org/10.1111/acer.12903

Rigney G, Ali NS, Corkum PV, Brown CA, Constantin E, Godbout R, Hanlon-Dearman A, Ipsiroglu O, Reid GJ, Shea S, Smith IM, Van der Loos HFM, Weiss SK (2018) A systematic review to explore the feasibility of a behavioural sleep intervention for insomnia in children with neurodevelopmental disorders: a transdiagnostic approach. Sleep Med Rev 41:244–254. https://doi.org/10.1016/j.smrv.2018.03.008

Ritfeld GJ, Kable JA, Holton JE, Coles CD (2021) Psychopharmacological treatments in children with fetal alcohol spectrum disorders: a review. Child Psychiatry Hum Dev. https://doi.org/10.1007/s10578-021-01124-7

Rockhold MN, Krueger AM, de Water E, Lindgren CW, Sandness KE, Eckerle JK, Schumacher MJ, Fink BA, Boys CJ, Carlson SM, Fuglestad AJ, Mattson SN, Jones KL, Riley EP, Wozniak JR (2021) Executive and social functioning across development in children and adolescents with prenatal alcohol exposure. Alcohol Clin Exp Res 45(2):457–469. https://doi.org/10.1111/acer.14538

Schonfeld AM, Paley B, Frankel F, O'Connor MJ (2009) Behavioral regulation as a predictor of response to Children's Friendship Training in children with fetal alcohol spectrum disorders. Clin Neuropsychol 23(3):428–445. https://doi.org/10.1080/13854040802389177

Sparrow SS, Cicchetti DV, Balla DA (eds) (2011) Vineland-II: Vineland Adaptive Behavior Scales. Manual, 2nd edn. Pearson, Stockholm

Stevens SA, Dudek J, Nash K, Korean G, Rovet J (2015) Social perspective taking and empathy in children with fetal alcohol spectrum disorders. J Int Neuropsychol Soc 21(1):74–84. https://doi.org/10.1017/S1355617714001088

Streissguth AP, Bookstein FL, Barr HM, Sampson PD, O'Malley K, Young JK (2004) Risk factors for adverse life outcomes in fetal alcohol syndrome and fetal alcohol effects. J Dev Behav Pediatr 25(4):228–238. https://doi.org/10.1097/00004703-200408000-00002

Temple VK, Cook JL, Unsworth K, Rajani H, Mela M (2019) Mental health and affect regulation impairment in fetal alcohol spectrum disorder (FASD): results from the Canadian National FASD Database. Alcohol Alcohol 54(5):545–550

Van Veen MM, Lancel M, Beijer E, Remmelzwaal S, Rutters F (2021) The association of sleep quality and aggression: a systematic review and meta-analysis of observational studies. Sleep Med Rev 59:101500. https://doi.org/10.1016/j.smrv.2021.101500

Von Sydow K, Retzlaff R, Beher S, Haun M, Schweitzer J (2013) The efficacy of systemic therapy for childhood and adolescent externalizing disorders: a systematic review of 47 RCT. Fam Process 52(4):576–618. https://doi.org/10.1111/famp.12047

Wells AM, Chasnoff IJ, Schmidt CA, Telford E, Schwartz LD (2012) Neurocognitive habilitation therapy for children with fetal alcohol spectrum disorders: an adaptation of the Alert Program®. Am J Occup Ther 66(1):24–34. https://doi.org/10.5014/ajot.2012.002691

Wengel T, Hanlon-Dearman AC, Fjeldsted B (2011) Sleep and sensory characteristics in young children with fetal alcohol spectrum disorder. J Dev Behav Pediatr 32(5):384–392. https://doi.org/10.1097/DBP.0b013e3182199694

Weyrauch D, Schwartz M, Hart B, Klug MG, Burd L (2017) Comorbid mental disorders in fetal alcohol spectrum disorders: a systematic review. J Dev Behav Pediatr 38(4):283–291. https://doi.org/10.1097/DBP.0000000000000440

Wozniak JR, Fuglestad AJ, Eckerle JK, Fink BA, Hoecker HL, Boys CJ, Radke JP, Kroupina MG, Miller NC, Brearley AM, Zeisel SH, Georgieff MK (2015) Choline supplementation in children with fetal alcohol spectrum disorders: a randomized, double-blind, placebo-controlled trial. Am J Clin Nutr 102(5):1113–1125. https://doi.org/10.3945/ajcn.114.099168

Mothers of Children with Fetal Alcohol Spectrum Disorder

56

Larry Burd and Svetlana Popova

Contents

Introduction 1207
Exposure Assessment 1207
Barriers to Prenatal Screening 1207
Clinical Practice Implications 1209
Prevalence of FASD 1210
If FASD Is So Common Why Don't We See IT? 1210
Benefits of a Diagnosis of FASD 1211
Additional Factors Impacting Diagnosis 1212
FASD a Diagnosis of Exclusion? 1213
The FASD Mortality Effect 1213
Public Policy Implications of FASD 1215
Parenting and FASD 1215
FASD Becomes More Complex Across the Lifespan 1216
Mothers with Current Substance Use Disorders 1216
Applications to Other Areas of Addiction 1218
Applications to Other Areas of Public Health 1218
Mini Dictionary of Terms 1219
Key Facts of Mothers of Children with Fetal Alcohol Spectrum Disorder 1219
Summary Points 1219
References 1220

L. Burd (✉)
Department of Pediatrics, University of North Dakota School of Medicine and Health Sciences, Grand Forks, ND, USA
e-mail: larry.burd@und.edu

S. Popova
Centre for Addiction and Mental Health, Toronto, ON, Canada
e-mail: lana.popova@camh.ca

V. B. Patel, V. R. Preedy (eds.), *Handbook of Substance Misuse and Addictions*,
https://doi.org/10.1007/978-3-030-92392-1_64

Abstract

Among 130 million live births each year globally, approximately 10% are exposed to alcohol during pregnancy, which increases risk of adverse neonatal outcomes and fetal alcohol spectrum disorders (FASD). Current estimates show that 1 of every 13 (7.7%) pregnant women who consumes alcohol during pregnancy delivers a child with FASD. The risk of FASD among infants is individualized and depends on variability of maternal-fetal protective and susceptibility factors for FASD. The factors include environmental risk modifiers such as smoking and other substance use and nutritional status. The role of paternal influences on FASD susceptibility requires additional research.

Globally, prenatal alcohol exposure results in 1.04 million new cases of FASD each year. This equates to 86,000 new cases/month (20,000/week or 2849/day, 118/h or 2/min). It is estimated that less than 1 of every 800 people living with FASD have been diagnosed. The annual cost of care for children with FASD is $23,810 per child, and additional unreimbursed costs of $25,993 to the family (total $53,683). For adults, the annual cost is $49, 077.

The high prevalence rate and costs of care underscores the potential benefits of targeted screening in high-risk populations. These populations include children of women in substance use disorder treatment, and all children entering foster care or juvenile corrections. Further research to improve routine screening in prenatal care, at delivery sites, and neonatal intensive care nurseries is needed. Every mother and child should be provided screening at least once during a well-child visit.

Since FASD is a very common cause of birth defects and developmental disabilities, screening for FASD should be a routine part of the clinical assessment of these children. Importantly, the diagnosis of other chromosomal, metabolic, or syndromal disorders does not reduce the need to investigate both prenatal alcohol exposure and FASD. No known disorder provides protection from prenatal alcohol exposure.

Recurrence among sibships accounts for nearly 20% of all cases of FASD. Identification of these women and intervention to prevent alcohol exposure during a subsequent pregnancy can prevent cases of FASD among younger siblings. Thus, proactive alcohol screenings and FASD diagnosis can be useful in prevention efforts by identification of risky alcohol behavior during pregnancy. Early identification of FASD also allows for early entry into diagnosis-informed care and can reduce excess disability in the future.

Keywords

Mothers · Pregnancy · Mortality · Fetal alcohol spectrum disorder · Prevention · Cost · Recurrence · Dosimetry · Exposure assessment · Screening

Abbreviations

BAC	Blood Alcohol Concentrations
FASD	Fetal alcohol spectrum disorder
NICU	Neonatal Intensive Care

Introduction

Globally, alcohol use among childbearing age women is increasing (WHO 2018). Up to 65% of pregnancies are unplanned (Bearak et al. 2018), placing these fetuses at risk of unintentional prenatal alcohol exposure early in pregnancy. Among pregnant women the global prevalence rate of prenatal alcohol exposure (PAE) is extremely variable with some evidence of increasing alcohol use in pregnancy in some countries during the COVID-19 pandemic (Kar et al. 2021; Rodriguez et al. 2020; Sher 2020; Smith et al. 2021). Despite decades of efforts in raising awareness about the risk of prenatal alcohol use, an astounding 10% of women drink during pregnancy, with the highest prevalence rate (25%) in the European region (Popova et al. 2017).

Exposure Assessment

In a clinical context these drinking days are referred to as exposure episodes. For the typical pregnancy, confirmation of pregnancy occurs around gestational week 6–8. Thus, a typical pregnancy would have multiple episodes of exposure before conformation of pregnancy. The most common pattern of drinking in the preconception period is weekend drinking. A typical drinking day ranges from one to five drinks during a 3–4-h period. Binge drinking during pregnancy (four or more drinks on an occasion) greatly increases risk for adverse outcomes including FASD (May and Gossage 2011). About 10% of pregnancies occur among women who drink at binge levels (four or more drinks per drinking day) (May and Gossage 2011). This pattern of alcohol use could result in 12–16 drinking days with one to five drinks during each episode before confirmation of pregnancy. This could result in 12–80 drinks prior to confirmation of pregnancy. Most of these women would meet criteria for "risky drinking," which if they become pregnant increases the risk of adverse outcomes for the fetus. Routine exposure assessments would demonstrate that: post-conceptual exposure did occur; exposure occurred in the first trimester of pregnancy. This would identify the need for ongoing attention to alcohol and likely other substance use during subsequent prenatal care visits.

Barriers to Prenatal Screening

Unfortunately, routine periconceptional, or prenatal alcohol use assessment appears to be suboptimal. Multiple factors contribute to this problem. One important factor is that many prenatal care providers believe that many women do drink – BUT – just not the women they see. Multiple obstetric societies have issued a position statement on PAE and recommended screening for risk assessment of alcohol use among pregnant women and brief interventions to tackle this major public health issue. For instance, screening for PAE should be an integral component of health supervision visits for newborns and new patients according to the *Bright Futures Guidelines for Health Supervision of Infants, Children, and Adolescents* (4th Edition, page 343).

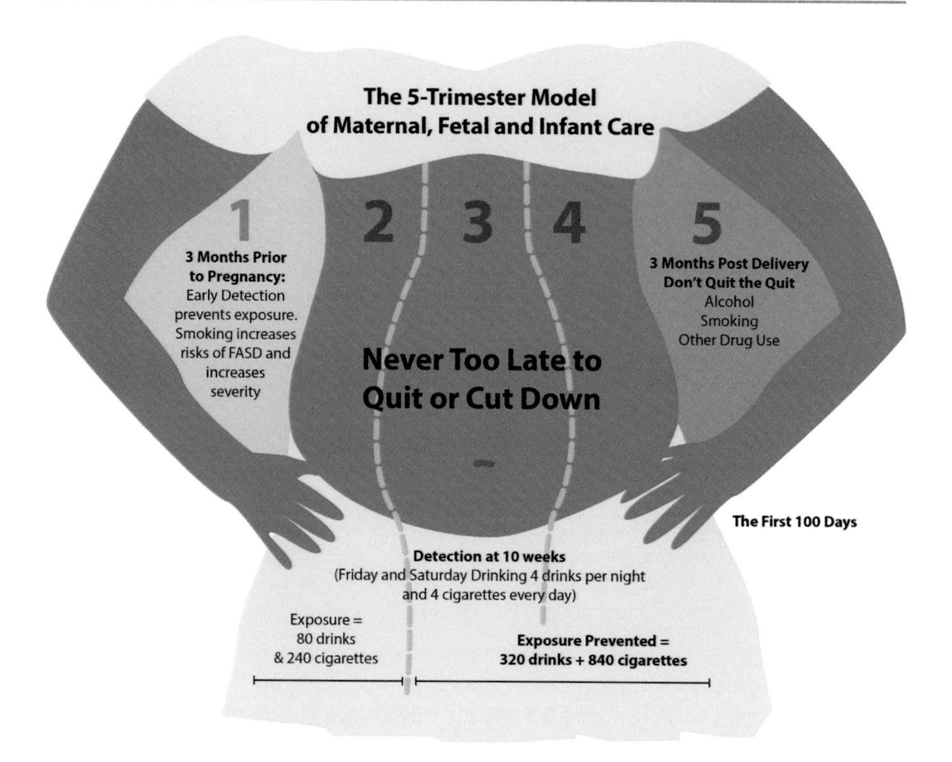

Fig. 1 Don't Quit the Quit. The model depicting the components of the Don't Quit the Quit program over the five trimesters

Nevertheless, most obstetricians, midwives, and other prenatal care providers lack specialized skills and training for screening pregnant patients for PAE and for early and timely diagnosis of FASD, or for FASD diagnosis at all. Virtually no training for use of a continuum of care or population-based intervention like Don't Quit the Quit (Fig. 1) is provided to most health care professionals. Research has illuminated the urgency for both developing and piloting evidence-based brief interventions in office-based settings and training the relevant healthcare staff accordingly (Wouldes et al. 2021).

The issue of exposure detection becomes more problematic as the pregnancy proceeds. For example, pregnant women using the emergency department are screened for substance use about 25% less frequently than nonpregnant women with similar presenting causes who are the same age (Greenmyer et al. 2020b; Moyer et al. 2018).

Recent evidence have detected prenatal alcohol use biomarkers in one of every 12 women in the USA during the last trimester of pregnancy (1 of every 16 pregnant women) (Burd 2020). This underscores the importance of improved alcohol use screening both at the clinical and population level. Interviews with FASD family support groups reported that several (six in our support group) birth mothers have mentioned being intoxicated during labor and delivery. Further investigations of the medical records of these women revealed that medical notes or health records of any of these women had no documentation of alcohol use or intoxication and no evidence of confirmatory lab tests (e.g., blood alcohol concentration (BAC)) were ordered or results found in the woman's medical chart. This problem is far worse in the neonatal intensive care units where over the past 20 years we have discussed this issue with dozens of staff neonatologists, and in several cases they have completed routine chart assessments and have failed to identify a single case of maternal intoxication or an infant with a positive BAC. While this is anecdotal evidence, the conclusions are supported by findings from a comprehensive literature review over the past 40 years using all languages. Over this four decade period the 130,000,000 global births per year (approximately 5.2 billion births) 12 peer reviewed reports found only 16 BAC cases of intoxicated mother and infants with a positive BAC (Schaff et al. 2019). We estimate this to be one report among every 325 million births.

Clinical Practice Implications

The clinical importance of this data is demonstrated by three findings. The mortality proportion for infants with alcohol withdrawal (25% of the infants in the study) was similar to rates for adults undergoing alcohol withdrawal (Schaff et al. 2019). Three symptoms were thought to suggest alcohol not opioid withdrawal (seizures, abdominal dilation, and opisthosomas). Since the onset and recognition of withdrawal can present hours to 1 or 2 days after delivery, clinicians should consider management of infants with a positive BAC in a neonatal intensive care unit for 72 h. Another example is that when the fetal or infant BAC was >200 mg/dL, the mortality rate was 50% (including stillbirths and newborn deaths).

We have demonstrated that use of a one question screen in prenatal care was useful for the recognition of alcohol use during pregnancy (Williams et al. 2013). We also found that very low-cost interventions during routine prenatal care could reduce the risk of exposure for subsequent pregnancies (Williams et al. 2014). In this same series of studies we used a breathalyzer to screen women attending routine prenatal care visits and found that 29% had a positive breathalyzer screen during the first trimester (Greenmyer et al. 2020a). The importance of early recognition of pregnancy is demonstrated by the rate of ongoing alcohol use. Among those women with a positive screen early in pregnancy 69% had second positive at a subsequent prenatal care visit. An additional screen during labor and delivery was again positive for 31% of the women who had a previous positive screen during prenatal care. Among women with a positive screen during pregnancy 19% had a positive breathalyzer screen at all three screens (Greenmyer et al. 2020a). The dosimetry of exposure was assessed in women who had a positive on the first and second assessments. Among these women 30% had a reading that was above 0.07 mg/dl, which is nearly equivalent to alcohol concentrations from binge drinking (four or more standard drinks in about 2 h). While the mean breathalyzer reading decreased as the pregnancy progressed, routine screening demonstrated that multiple opportunities for identification of women who were drinking on the day of a routine prenatal care visit are available. We estimate that every year in the USA alone, 93 newborns are delivered on a day when the mother was drinking.

Improved identification of PAE is not complex. First, we need to acknowledge that the magnitude of PAE is very large. This suggests that we should screen all pregnancies. The burden of screening could be very modest. The One-Question Screen "When was your last drink?" or an equivalent validated screen could be used (Schaff et al. 2019). A routine breathalyzer screen during pregnancy may be another useful, easy to use, inexpensive option for future research.

Prevalence of FASD

Globally, there are 130 million births each year. The global prevalence of FASD is about 0.77%. Recent research has demonstrated that 630,000 children can be expected to be born with FASD each year (Lange et al. 2017). This demonstrates that every month 52,000 new cases are born, that is, 12,100 every week or 1726 every day, 72 per h or 1 per min. This suggests that over 11 million children under the age of 18 years would have FASD. The young adult population is comprised of an additional 14 million individuals between ages 19 and 40 (Popova et al. 2019a). The remaining adult population of people with FASD would be in the tens of millions. It is difficult to imagine that even 100,000 have been diagnosed with FASD. We estimate that 1 in every 187 cases of FASD are diagnosed. Recent prevalence data from the USA, using active case ascertainment methodologies result in prevalence estimates between 3.1% and 9.9% in school-aged children (May et al. 2018). If the actual FASD prevalence rate is in this range then only 1 of every 1170 children are being currently diagnosed. Tens of millions of adults and elderly people also remain undiagnosed. The diagnosis of FASD is of high importance to mothers, families, and to people of all ages with FASD. Parenting children with FASD is complex. In addition to the neurocognitive impairments that characterize FASD, misdiagnosis of the disorder increases complexity of parenting even more, especially for the mothers with substance use disorders who themselves need the support and care that an accurate diagnosis would allow (Richards et al. 2020). This data demonstrates that millions of people around the world have FASD. It is likely that these prevalence estimates are conservative due to challenges related to access to diagnosis.

If FASD Is So Common Why Don't We See IT?

The most often cited reasons for not devoting more resources to FASD are:

1. It's too much stigma for the mothers and the children. This seems unlikely. For instance, Autism spectrum disorders (AUD) are also a congenital and life-long disorder, but we rarely hear these arguments being made for not diagnosing them.

2. Why devote resources to children with a known developmental disability? Almost every state, providence or country has autism-specific services. These services start after the diagnosis is made. These treatments are usually not curative but are designed to decrease future disability and to improve the quality of life for the person. We should have similar services for people with FASD.
3. We are already doing everything we would do if they had a diagnosis of FASD. This is clearly misleading. In FASD, the younger siblings have increasing risk of having an FASD and to have a more severe FASD phenotype compared to their older siblings (Abel 1988). These younger siblings also have greatly increased mortality risk (Burd et al. 2004). Children with FASD have increased mortality risk (Burd et al. 2008), increasing risk for exposure to adverse childhood experiences (Kambeitz et al. 2019), school failure, and increasing risk for mental health impairments (Popova et al. 2019b; Weyrauch et al. 2017), increasing risk for multiple foster home placements, a 19-fold increase in risk for incarceration in juvenile corrections, and increased risk for placement into foster care (Conant et al. 2021).
4. Why diagnose FASD if we don't have specific interventions for the condition? We now have an increasing evidence base demonstrating the value of diagnosis-informed care. FASD has a distinctive developmental course and accurate diagnosis is imperative to meet the unique needs of patients. Children and adolescents with FASD obtain limited benefit from treatment programs that do not accommodate their deficits in adaptive behavior, such as the ability to work independently, meet self-care needs, manage money and time, and adhere to societal rules and expectations (Burd FASD affidavit – available at the National Juvenile Defenders website). Assessment of deficits in adaptive behavior functioning are useful indicators of the future capacity for independent living. This is an area where accurate diagnosis and targeted diagnosis-informed interventions can be life changing. Measures of adaptive behaviors are used with IQ to determine eligibility of services as a person with an intellectual disability.

Benefits of a Diagnosis of FASD

Best practices for treatment of people with FASD include development of a future-oriented prevention plan, prevention of substance use disorders, and risk reduction for further involvement in legal proceedings. Published research has demonstrated the potential benefits from use of these diagnosis-dependent interventions. At two juvenile corrections sites, screening and FASD diagnosis-informed interventions were associated with the following: (Bisgard et al. 2010)

- 74% of youth with FASD had no new offenses and no probation violations in the first 6 months
- 89% had no new probation violations 12 months after implementation of intervention services

- 95% had either no change in placement or were moved to a placement that was equally or more appropriate for their needs, as specified in the diagnostic evaluation report
- 83% showed no or reduced numbers of school suspensions at follow-up, as compared to baseline
- 100% showed no school expulsions at follow-up
- 67% showed increased school attendance levels, and
- 25% showed no or reduced numbers of school incident reports at follow-up, as compared to baseline.

Outcomes from the second site were similar:

- 85% of FASD-diagnosed individuals successfully completed probation and had no further arrests; (baseline recidivism was 50% in the first year).

Outcomes for children with FASD are substantially dependent on the quality of services provided to them. Research identifies several characteristics key to improving interventions:

- Understand FASD
- Treatment often needs to proceed at a slower pace due to impairments, comorbidity, and increased levels of need
- The use of picture schedules can be helpful where needed
- Decrease memory burden by changing the pace, increasing repetition, using multimodal teaching strategies, and changing to positive behavior management strategies
- Manage the effects of anxiety around school and other learning demands, and
- Understanding the effects of comorbidity

Additional Factors Impacting Diagnosis

One factor impacting the low rate of diagnosis in a heightened sense of concern about mis-categorizing unexposed women as having used alcohol during pregnancy or misdiagnosing unexposed children as having FASD. As a result, the general trend is to set the sensitivity for screening or reports of PAE at very high levels. Examples abound, one is requiring "confirmed" PAE. While confirmed is a comforting term asserting etiological validity to the diagnosis it's not at all clear what "confirmed" means. More than once we have had the birth mother denying alcohol use at any point in pregnancy and the father, who lived with her, assuring us she drank a lot and often throughout the entire pregnancy. Both offer confirmation but of what? If we interviewed either without the other, we arrive at a different exposure conclusion and both are confirmed. In our experience misdiagnosis (which nearly always means undiagnosed) of FASD can increase risk for exposure in subsequent pregnancies.

FASD a Diagnosis of Exclusion?

Another example is the often-stated observation that FASD is a diagnosis of exclusion. What should be excluded? In most cases the emphasis is on the exclusion of mostly children with genetic, metabolic, or chromosomal abnormalities (Leibson et al. 2014). This suggests that these conditions either protect the fetus from PAE or so completely capture the abnormalities and predict the developmental course and needed interventions that identifying FASD is not important. However, we wonder if instead that these children may be even more susceptible to PAE/FASD and have even more need for FASD to be identified since it is going to be crucial in determining future concerns, treatment needs, and diagnosis-specific risks (Burd 2016; Popova et al. 2020). Yet another version of this argument is that all children suspected of FASD need thorough clinical evaluation by a physician to rule out other potential causes for the presenting problems. Thus, having no history of PAE is an exclusionary factor, but evidence of "confirmed" exposure is only a conditional inclusionary factor. It has also been suggested that routine testing for chromosomal abnormalities by the use of routine microarrays and more recently whole genome sequencing are needed in the routine diagnostic evaluation of people with FASD. Some authors have even proposed a list of specific conditions that need to be excluded prior to making a diagnosis of FASD (Leibson et al. 2014). Some centers routinely include microarray and whole genome sequencing as a part of the diagnosis of FASD. Perhaps a moment or two of reflection would lead us to rethink this proposition when focusing on the cost-benefit aspect of this technique. Currently a microarray study costs $800–$4000 and whole genome sequencing costs about twice that amount. About 5% of these tests are positive and of these only about one in four has some potential or known influence on the diagnosis. So, in summary for a condition with a prevalence rate of 5% we exclude 30 or more disorders (many are extremely rare) with prevalence rates of only 1 in a million or even 100 million live births (Leibson et al. 2014). Is it reasonable to spend $6000 to $10,000 on tests that infrequently offer an alternative diagnosis to FASD? We argue that these tests should be used when clinically indicated rather than as a part of a routine test battery. Requirements for this testing not only increases costs but results in barriers that reduce accessibly for children who most need evaluations for FASD. Most importantly, currently we have no known rational for assuming that genetic or chromosomal disorders like Fragile X syndrome, Williams's syndrome or deletions, duplication, translocations, other similar findings would exclude FASD as a diagnosis or protect against prenatal alcohol exposure. This strategy would be similar to excluding all cases with a genetic or chromosomal abnormality from access to an autism spectrum disorder diagnostic clinic and a diagnosis of autism. We need to recognize that this was an idea without evidence which became popular.

The FASD Mortality Effect

The association between increased maternal mortality and offspring with FASD has been well-established in two population-based studies which linked FASD registers with their birth mothers and death records (Burd et al. 2008; Li et al. 2012).

These studies utilized linkage of state vital record and cases from a population-based FASD registry. In this methodology each FASD case was used to identify the birth mother. Her data was then used to identify vital records for all births for her. These records were then used to link birth and death certificates for the mother and her children. This data was then used to construct controls based on child's year of birth and mothers age at death. In this study, 87% of birth mothers of a person diagnosed with FASD died by age 50. This represents 31.3 years of productive life lost. We found that 67% of these deaths were attributed to cancer, accidents, or classified as alcohol related. The mortality effect estimated by comparing the mothers of children with FASD to age and year of birth-matched non-FASD control mothers produced an estimate of mortality risk which was (OR = 44) (194). A 44-fold increase in mortality risk should provide a compelling area of interest for efforts to reduce maternal mortality and overall mortality rates among women.

Interestingly, we estimate the disability adjusted life years for these mothers to be 7.8 years. The combined loss of quality-of-life years is 39.1 years. For nearly 10% of these women this alcohol-related disability begins at adolescence and continues until their premature death. Figure 2 presents an example of "Mom's life story."

People with FASD have an increased all-cause mortality rate. The mortality proportion is about 5% (risk ratio of 530%) (Burd et al. 2008). An unexpected finding was that the mortality rate is similar for siblings whether or not they have a

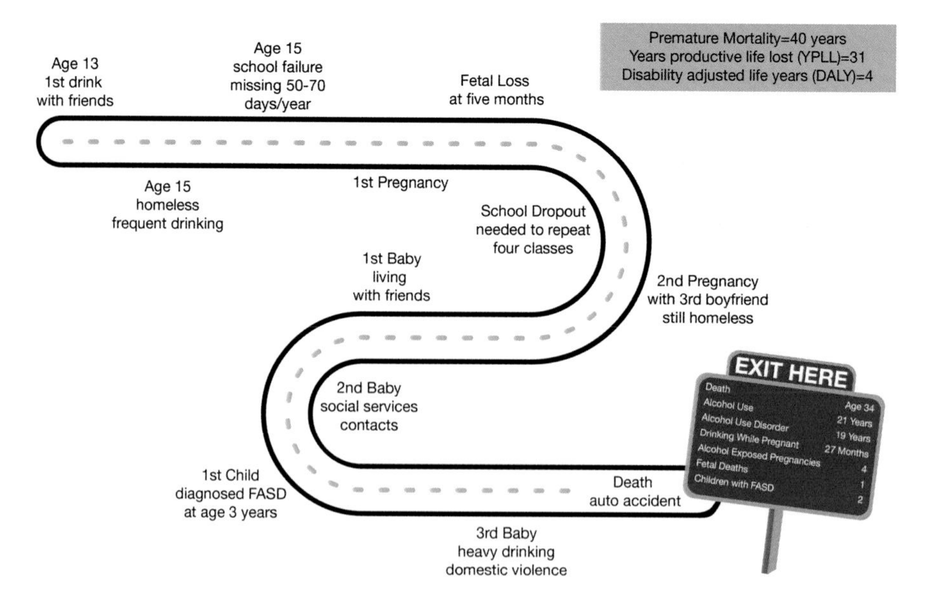

Fig. 2 Mom's Life Story. Example of one "Mom's life story"

diagnosis of FASD (Burd et al. 2008; Burd et al. 2004). One of the complexities of assessment of mortality is that many people with FASD may die before they are diagnosed (Elliott et al. 2020).

A similar mechanism likely is present for the relationship between PAE and stillbirth (Burd et al. 2008; Burd and Wilson 2004; Odendaal et al. 2021). Thus, while it's often noted that fetal alcohol syndrome (FAS) is the most severe manifestation of FASD, mortality may represent a more useful indicator of phenotypic severity. Since nearly all cases of infant and child death would occur before a diagnosis of FASD mortality rates may be underestimated.

Public Policy Implications of FASD

The diagnosis of FASD is often described as a source of stigma for the birth mothers. However, in our experience, we often find multiple benefits from a diagnosis of FASD for both the mother and the child. A diagnosis of FASD had implications for both the mother and her children.

Mothers

- Huge risk for premature mortality
- Greatly increased risk for another alcohol exposed pregnancy
- Since FASD is both generational and familial we have an opportunity to determine if mother or other children have an FASD
- If mother has reduced prenatal exposure we can encourage and assist in maintaining the Quit or reduction (Don't Quit the Quit) especially between pregnancies
- Opportunity to establish an ongoing relationship with a woman needing supportive intervention

Children

- Prevention of exposure to ACEs
- Reduce development of secondary disabilities/adverse outcomes
- Reduce costs of care for children and adolescents
- Begin diagnosis-informed care
- Opportunity to develop a diagnosis-specific long-term plan

Parenting and FASD

Recognition of FASD is of paramount important to improve management of the child, reduce family stress and dysfunction. Parenting a child with FASD is complex due to the wide range of exposure to adversity, increased risk for development of mental disorders, and ongoing risk for secondary disabilities. Many of these secondary disabilities are likely preventable. Among the frequent concerns reported by parents are:

Sleep disorders
Eating disorders
Fine and gross motor delays
Toilet training
Speech and language disorders
Learning and behavior impairments at school
Difficulty completing homework
Social skill deficits
Need for medication(s)
Ongoing travel for therapies
Availability of childcare for children with complex behavioral impairments
Availability of respite care services

FASD Becomes More Complex Across the Lifespan

The complexity of parenting also seems to increase across development. Adolescence and young adult life may be especially complex. Recognition of FASD and early emphasis on prevention of these problems and secondary disabilities can be useful and may decrease long-term demands on parents. A diagnosis of FASD may also indicate a diagnosis-specific need for multiple accommodations, specific interventions, parenting supports (respite care, use of parents support groups, ongoing effort to maintain sobriety, and the need to educate systems of care about people with FASD).

In people with FASD we often observe increasing comorbidities and increasing parental demands across the lifespan. This stresses the need for increased therapy appointments and with providers, need for effective communication among service providers, and the need to be accommodative and mindful of the limited time and resources that these parents have. These demands require additional services especially behavioral support, often in-home services and respite care. Without these, parents can have increasing difficulty in keeping appointments. This can lead to therapists becoming critical and they may even discontinue therapy. Often, they need to meet to determine how to add extra resources to decrease demand on the parents. These might include improving transportation options, and rescheduling therapy to maximize efficiency of time and travel for parents. This is especially problematic for parents with ongoing substance use disorders.

Mothers with Current Substance Use Disorders

Many women go through prenatal care, labor and delivery, a lengthy stay in a neonatal intensive care nursery and begin follow-up visits without detection of

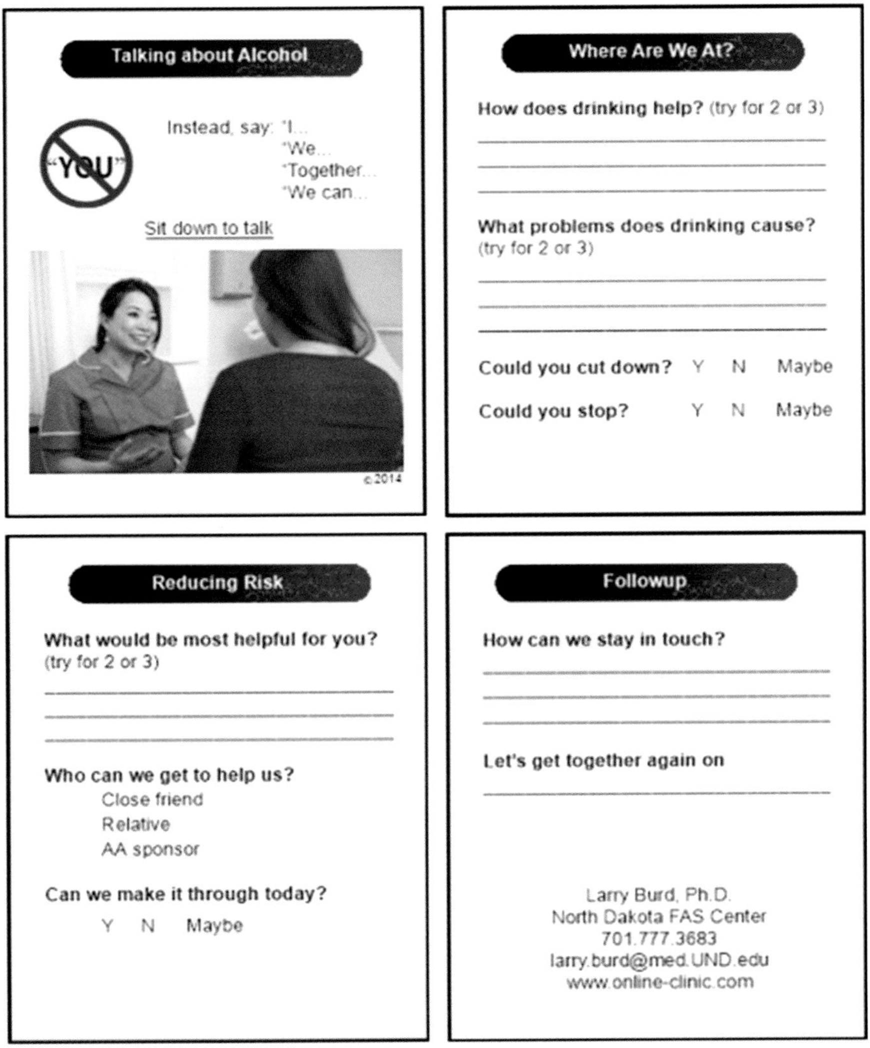

Talking about Alcohol

"YOU"

Instead, say: "I...
"We...
"Together...
"We can...

Sit down to talk

©2014

Where Are We At?

How does drinking help? (try for 2 or 3)

______
______
______

What problems does drinking cause? (try for 2 or 3)

______
______
______

Could you cut down? Y N Maybe

Could you stop? Y N Maybe

Reducing Risk

What would be most helpful for you? (try for 2 or 3)

______
______
______

Who can we get to help us?
Close friend
Relative
AA sponsor

Can we make it through today?
Y N Maybe

Followup

How can we stay in touch?

______
______
______

Let's get together again on

______

Larry Burd, Ph.D.
North Dakota FAS Center
701.777.3683
larry.burd@med.UND.edu
www.online-clinic.com

Fig. 3 Talking about alcohol with women. A brief office-based intervention for women drinking during pregnancy

substance use disorders. Alternatively, others may have these substance use disorders recognized but may not receive adequate interventions. We recommend beginning with a brief office-based intervention as summarized in Fig. 3.

For women in special circumstances, treatment of the substance use disorder should be an immediate priority. This includes those with children in a neonatal intensive care unit: women who are incarcerated; women with involvement in the foster care system; and pregnant women with substance use disorders in corrections systems. Some mothers with children in neonatal intensive care units spend weeks or months with their infants in these stressful clinical settings. These are settings where treatment would be of immediate and future benefit. These services should be offered in easily accessible settings and women should be supported to attend them as a part of the NICU treatment plan. We need to be aware of the outcomes for women who utilize these services since that will impact our expectations for these women. FASD is generational and substance use disorder treatment programs are cognitive interventions. As a result, treatment plans will often need modification to meet the needs of these mothers if they are to be successful. Improving treatment means improving access to treatment and especially improving access to high quality treatment. We recommend the following:

- Develop a Substance Abuse Team at every delivery hospital
- Provide routine referral and easy access to a substance abuse treatment program for women (often for both parents) at all NICU programs.
- Begin treatment immediately (especially for mothers (parents) whose infants who require lengthy hospital stays).
- Develop a follow-up plan for the mother and her children.
- Add substance treatment consultation to early intervention services for infants.

In our experience, many mothers who have children with FASD want and urgently need access to these services. Lastly, we must lead by example and support each other in our efforts to demonstrate our respect, concern, and commitment for these women who have a serious and often life-threatening disease.

Applications to Other Areas of Addiction

This chapter provides information on recent changes to improve screening for prenatal alcohol exposure. These strategies may be useful to develop screening for all women. In addition, this screening strategy may identify women in need of treatment in a variety of settings.

This chapter provides a general rational to support routine screening for alcohol use during well-child visits by pediatricians.

Applications to Other Areas of Public Health

The data also provide an important rationale for screening all children entering foster care, juvenile corrections, and residential care. The complexity and demands of parenting these children may be due in part to the complex phenotype of FASD. Public health programs should become aware of the significant impact of FASD as a potentially preventable cause of morbidity and mortality, especially for the mothers of children with an FASD.

Mini Dictionary of Terms

- **Dosimetry.** The quantification of prenatal alcohol exposure specifying number of days exposed, drinks per drinking day, what is a drink, date of last drink during pregnancy.
- **Exposure assessment.** A multistep strategy to determine if alcohol exposure during pregnancy did occur.
- **Fetal Alcohol Spectrum Disorder.** FASD is a complex disorder with expression over the lifespan. The FASD phenotype is comprised of increased mortality beginning during pregnancy, increased risk for neuropsychiatric disorders and susceptibility to chronic illness. The complexity of the phenotype is increased by delayed diagnosis and accumulating effects from multiple adverse life experiences. The lack of long-term anticipatory planning with an emphasis on risk reduction increases the complexity of care across the lifespan.

Key Facts of Mothers of Children with Fetal Alcohol Spectrum Disorder

- Globally, maternal alcohol use during pregnancy results in 86,000 new cases of FASD each month.
- The annual cost of care for FASD is $23,810 per child.
- FASD is associated with a five-fold increase in mortality risk for children and adolescence.
- Birth mothers of children diagnosed with FASD have a 44-fold increase in mortality risk.
- Early identification of prenatal alcohol exposure could prevent exposure in subsequent pregnancies.

Summary Points

- The global impact of adverse outcomes from prenatal alcohol exposure affects tens of millions of people.
- FASD is a common developmental disorder and most cases of FASD are undiagnosed.
- FASD is associated with increased demands on parents and schools, frequent entry into special education, foster care, juvenile corrections, and residential care for severe mental health conditions.
- FASD is an important marker for increased mortality risk for diagnosed cases, their siblings (even if undiagnosed), and especially the premature death of the mother.
- Diagnosis of FASD and referral for treatment could prevent prenatal alcohol exposure in younger siblings.

References

Abel EL (1988) Fetal alcohol syndrome in families. Neurotoxicol Teratol 10:1–2

Bearak J, Popinchalk A, Alkema L, Sedgh G (2018) Global, regional, and subregional trends in unintended pregnancy and its outcomes from 1990 to 2014: estimates from a Bayesian hierarchical model. Lancet Glob Health 6:e380–e389

Bisgard EB, Fisher S, Adubato S, Louis M (2010) Screening, diagnosis, and intervention with juvenile offenders. J Psychiatry Law 38:475–506

Burd L (2016) Invited commentary: FASD: complexity from comorbidity. Lancet 387:926–927

Burd L (2020) Drinking at the end of pregnancy: why don't we see it? Pediatr Res 88:142

Burd L, Wilson H (2004) Fetal, infant, and child mortality in a context of alcohol use. Am J Med Genet C Semin Med Genet 127:51–58

Burd L, Klug MG, Martsolf J (2004) Increased sibling mortality in children with fetal alcohol syndrome. Addict Biol 9:179–186

Burd L, Klug MG, Bueling R, Martsolf J, Olson M, Kerbeshian J (2008) Mortality rates in subjects with fetal alcohol spectrum disorders and their siblings. Birth Defects Res A Clin Mol Teratol 82:217–223

Conant BJ, Sandstrom A, Jorda M, Klug MG, Burd L (2021) Relationships between fetal alcohol spectrum disorder, adverse childhood experiences, and neurodevelopmental diagnoses. Open J Pediatr 11:580–596

Elliott AJ, Kinney HC, Haynes RL, Dempers JD, Wright C, Fifer WP, Angal J, Boyd TK, Burd L, Burger E, Folkerth RD, Groenewald C, Hankins G, Hereld D, Hoffman HJ, Holm IA, Myers MM, Nelsen LL, Odendaal HJ, Petersen J, Randall BB, Roberts DJ, Robinson F, Schubert P, Sens MA, Sullivan LM, Tripp T, Van Eerden P, Wadee S, Willinger M, Zaharie D, Dukes KA (2020) Concurrent prenatal drinking and smoking increases risk for sids: safe passage study report. EClinicalMedicine 19:100247

Greenmyer JR, Klug MG, Nkodia G, Popova S, Hart B, Burd L (2020a) High prevalence of prenatal alcohol exposure detected by breathalyzer in the Republic of the Congo, Africa. Neurotoxicol Teratol 80:106892

Greenmyer JR, Stacy JM, Klug MG, Foster K, Tiongson C, Burd L (2020b) Pregnancy status is associated with screening for alcohol and other substance use in the emergency department. J Addict Med 14:e64–e69

Kambeitz C, Klug MG, Greenmyer J, Popova S, Burd L (2019) Association of adverse childhood experiences and neurodevelopmental disorders in people with fetal alcohol spectrum disorders (FASD) and non-FASD controls. BMC Pediatr 19:498

Kar P, Tomfohr-Madsen L, Giesbrecht G, Bagshawe M, Lebel C (2021) Alcohol and substance use in pregnancy during the covid-19 pandemic. Drug Alcohol Depend 225:108760

Lange S, Probst C, Gmel G, Rehm J, Burd L, Popova S (2017) Global prevalence of fetal alcohol spectrum disorder among children and youth: a systematic review and meta-analysis. JAMA Pediatr 171:948–956

Leibson T, Neuman G, Chudley AE, Koren G (2014) The differential diagnosis of fetal alcohol spectrum disorder. J Popul Ther Clin Pharmacol 21:e1–e30

Li Q, Fisher WW, Peng CZ, Williams AD, Burd L (2012) Fetal alcohol spectrum disorders: a population based study of premature mortality rates in the mothers. Matern Child Health J 16: 1332–1337

May PA, Gossage JP (2011) Maternal risk factors for fetal alcohol spectrum disorders: not as simple as it might seem. Alcohol Res Health 34:15–26

May PA, Chambers CD, Kalberg WO, Zellner J, Feldman H, Buckley D, Kopald D, Hasken JM, Xu R, Honerkamp-Smith G, Taras H, Manning MA, Robinson LK, Adam MP, Abdul-Rahman-O, Vaux K, Jewett T, Elliott AJ, Kable JA, Akshoomoff N, Falk D, Arroyo JA, Hereld D, Riley EP, Charness ME, Coles CD, Warren KR, Jones KL, Hoyme HE (2018) Prevalence of fetal alcohol spectrum disorders in 4 US communities. JAMA 319:474–482

Moyer CL, Johnson S, Klug MG, Burd L (2018) Substance use in pregnant women using the emergency department: undertested and overlooked? West J Emerg Med 19:579–584
Odendaal H, Dukes KA, Elliott AJ, Willinger M, Sullivan LM, Tripp T, Groenewald C, Myers MM, Fifer WP, Angal J, Boyd TK, Burd L, Cotton JB, Folkerth RD, Hankins G, Haynes RL, Hoffman HJ, Jacobs PK, Petersen J, Pini N, Randall BB, Roberts DJ, Robinson F, Sens MA, Van Eerden P, Wright C, Holm IA, Kinney HC (2021) Association of prenatal exposure to maternal drinking and smoking with the risk of stillbirth. JAMA Netw Open 4:e2121726
Popova S, Lange S, Probst C, Gmel G, Rehm J (2017) Estimation of national, regional, and global prevalence of alcohol use during pregnancy and fetal alcohol syndrome: a systematic review and meta-analysis. Lancet Glob Health [Online] 5. Available: https://doi.org/10.1016/S2214-109X(17)30021-9
Popova S, Lange S, Shield K, Burd L & Rehm J (2019a) Prevalence of fetal alcohol spectrum disorder among special sub-populations: a systematic review and meta-analysis. Addiction [Online] 114. Available: https://onlinelibrary.wiley.com/doi/epdf/10.1111/add.14598
Popova S, Lange S, Shield K, Burd L, Rehm J (2019b) Prevalence of fetal alcohol spectrum disorder among special subpopulations: a systematic review and meta-analysis. Addiction 114: 1150–1172
Popova S, Dozet D, Burd L (2020) Fetal alcohol spectrum disorder: can we change the future? Alcohol Clin Exp Res. https://doi.org/10.1111/acer.14317
Richards T, Bertrand J, Newburg-Rinn S, Mccann H, Morehouse E, Ingoldsby E (2020) Children prenatally exposed to alcohol and other drugs: what the literature tells us about child welfare information sources, policies, and practices to identify and care for children. J Public Child Welf 16(1):71–94
Rodriguez LM, Litt DM, Stewart SH (2020) Drinking to cope with the pandemic: the unique associations of covid-19-related perceived threat and psychological distress to drinking behaviors in American men and women. Addict Behav 110:106532
Schaff E, Moreno M, Foster K, Klug MG, Burd La-OHOO (2019) What do we know about prevalence and management of intoxicated women during labor and delivery? Glob Pediatr Health 6:2333794X19894799
Sher J (2020) Fetal alcohol spectrum disorders: preventing collateral damage from covid-19. Lancet Public Health 5:e424
Smith CL, Waters SF, Spellacy D, Burduli E, Brooks O, Carty CL, Ranjo S, Mcpherson S, Barbosa-Leiker C (2021) Substance use and mental health in pregnant women during the covid-19 pandemic. J Reprod Infant Psychol:1–14
Weyrauch D, Schwartz M, Hart B, Klug MG, Burd L (2017) Comorbid mental disorders in fetal alcohol spectrum disorders: a systematic review. J Dev Behav Pediatr 38:283–291
WHO (2018) Global status report on alcohol and health, 2018. World Health Organization, Geneva
Williams AD, Nkombo Y, Nkodia G, Leonardson G, Burd L (2013) Prenatal alcohol exposure in the Republic of the Congo: prevalence and screening strategies. Birth Defects Res A Clin Mol Teratol 97:489–496
Williams AD, Nkombo Y, Nkodia G, Martsolf K, Burd L (2014) Effectiveness of a novel low cost intervention to reduce prenatal alcohol exposure in the Congo. Open J Pediatr 4:84–92
Wouldes TA, Crawford A, Stevens S, Stasiak K (2021) Evidence for the effectiveness and acceptability of e-SBI or e-SBIRT in the management of alcohol and illicit substance use in pregnant and post-partum women. Front Psych 12:469

Childhood Alcohol Use: Global Insights 57

Ingunn Marie Stadskleiv Engebretsen and Vilde Skylstad

Contents

Introduction 1224
Childhood Alcohol Use: Variations Over Child Age, Place, and Time 1225
Genetic Factors of Early Alcohol Use 1228
Mental Health: Vulnerability and Resilience 1231
Family and Friends 1233
Culture and the Community 1236
Policy for Protection Against Alcohol 1237
Summary 1240
Applications to Other Areas of Addiction 1240
Applications to Other Areas of Public Health 1241
Mini-Dictionary of Terms (5–15 Terms) 1241
Key Facts of Childhood Alcohol Use 1242
Summary Points 1242
References 1242

Abstract

This chapter presents an overview of childhood alcohol use, including global patterns, trends, and systems surrounding the child, based on current theoretical understanding of child development. Key areas are discussed regarding patterns and trends, including age of initiation, and current use related to children's age and sex. Data and findings from large international surveys are presented and limitations are herein mentioned. In short, varying trends on current alcohol use are seen globally, and large European and North American regional surveys point toward slowly declining trends, although for certain regions, such as the Balkans, the opposite is seen. Also, disparities are observed within the varying regions, exemplified as past-30-days alcohol use among 12–15-year-olds spanning from

I. M. S. Engebretsen (✉) · V. Skylstad
Centre for International Health, Department of Global Public Health and Primary Care, Medical Faculty, University of Bergen, Bergen, Norway
e-mail: ingunn.engebretsen@uib.no; vilde.skylstad@uib.no

V. B. Patel, V. R. Preedy (eds.), *Handbook of Substance Misuse and Addictions*,
https://doi.org/10.1007/978-3-030-92392-1_65

5–60% in African countries. Alcohol use is discussed in relation to both genetic and mental health-related factors, as well as environmental factors, such as parents and peers. The chapter finally discusses cultural influence and the potential for modulating child environment and cultural influence through policy, such as regulating advertisement, product placement, and access.

Keywords

Childhood · Alcohol · Substance · Drinking · Use · Abuse · Dependence · Parent · Upbringing · Environment · Trends · Prevalence · Social influence · Mental health · Policy

Abbreviations

ACE	Adverse Childhood Experiences
ADHD	Attention-Deficit/Hyperactivity Disorders
APA	American Psychiatric Association
API	Alcohol Policy Index
AUD	Alcohol Use Disorder
CDC	Centers for Disease Control and Prevention
COGA	The Collaborative Studies on the Genetics of Alcoholism
DSM	Diagnostic and Statistical Manual of Mental Disorders
EMCDDA	European Monitoring Centre for Drugs and Drug Addiction
ESPAD	The European School Survey Project on Alcohol and Other Drugs
GISAH	Global Information System on Alcohol and Health
GSHS	Global School Based Health Survey
GxE	Gene and Environment Interaction
HBSC	Health Behavior in School-Aged Children
LMIC	Low- and Middle-Income Countries
SDG	Sustainable Development Goals
US	United States
WHO	World Health Organization
YRBSS	The Youth Risk Behavior Surveillance System

Introduction

Substance use is a leading contributor to the burden of disease among youth worldwide (Lim et al. 2012; Erskine et al. 2015). The importance of tackling substance use is emphasized in target 3.5 of the Sustainable Development Goals (SDG), which aims to "Strengthen the prevention and treatment of substance abuse, including narcotic drug abuse and harmful use of alcohol" (United Nations 2017). One of the indicators of SDG 3.5 is to track harmful use of alcohol among the population aged 15 years and older. The reality is that alcohol use often starts earlier, even in early childhood. While the SDG 3.5 use the term "abuse," this chapter deliberately uses the term "alcohol use" to include any use in childhood. This is

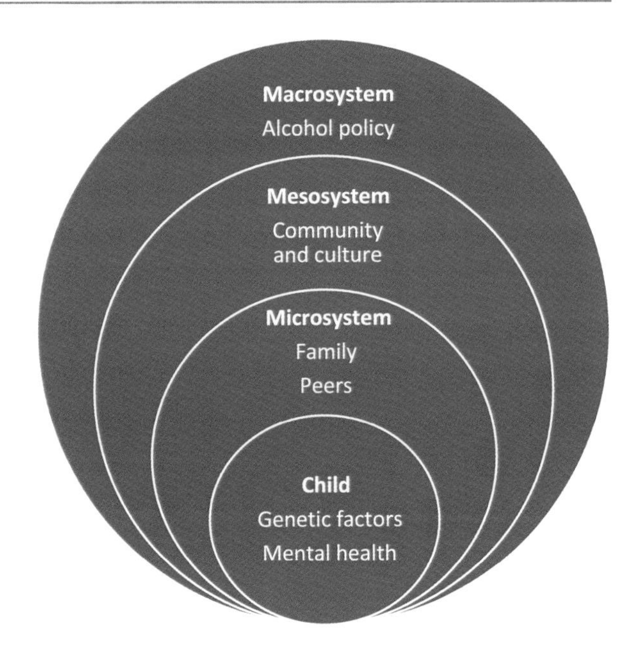

Fig. 1 Adapted version of Bronfenbrenner's socioecological systems theory with factors raised in this chapter

because "abuse" is often related to clinical criteria developed for adults and any use in children is necessary to understand. Also, we consider children aged 0–18 years, and any age group within this range will be specified. This chapter will, in line with the title of this book, address childhood onset of alcohol intake from "biology to public health." Inspired by Bronfenbrenner's socioecological theory (Bronfenbrenner 1979), the chapter investigates childhood onset alcohol from different systems surrounding the child, as well as the complex interplay between these, spanning factors from the individual child, their families, community, and governmental policy (Fig. 1). The chapter starts with exploring the current global situation and historical trends of childhood alcohol use. It then continues to examine individual factors, such as genetic factors and mental health, before it moves on to environmental factors, including family, peers, culture, and community. Finally, we address policy and interventions for harmful alcohol use. Research from low- and middle-income countries (LMIC) is often absent in book chapters on substance use and has intentionally been included.

Childhood Alcohol Use: Variations Over Child Age, Place, and Time

The prevalence of early alcohol use has varied around the globe, at different child ages and at different times. To monitor this, large collaborations have been established between the World Health Organization (WHO), the Centers for Disease Control and Prevention (CDC), European Monitoring Centre for Drugs and Drug Addiction (EMCDDA), and independent research teams to undertake large school-based surveys. This section reviews global prevalence estimates and trends from the Global School Based Health Survey (GSHS), Health Behavior in School-Aged Children (HBSC), the Youth Risk Behavior Surveillance System (YRBSS), and the European School Survey Project on Alcohol and Other Drugs (ESPAD). Among large data sets and a range of indicators, we focus on age of initiation and current use.

Measuring the Age of Initiation and Current Use

When measuring early and childhood alcohol use, different studies use different definitions and indicators. For example, in the HSBS, ESPAD, YRBSS, and GSHS, the specifications of what qualifies as a drink vary from "a drink other than a few sips" in the GSHS and YRBSS (CDC 2021; WHO and CDC 2021), "more than a small amount" in the HBSC (Currie et al. 2014), and "at least one glass" in the ESPAD (ESPAD 2019). Further, when measuring the age of initiation of alcohol intake, the lowest age possible varies between "7 years old or younger" in the GSHS and "11 years old or less" in the HSBC. When measuring current use, the surveys include different measures on weekly, monthly, and yearly frequency. Further, at the stage of analysis, the cut-off for early use also varies, where some place it at use before age 10 (Chan et al. 2018), while the ESPAD and YRBSS place it at use before age 13 (CDC 2019; ESPAD Group 2020). Further, the age of participants varies in the surveys, as does the length of recall for age of initiation. These inconsistencies complicate the comparability of the results and interpretation of analyses. Childhood and adolescence are characterized by rapid changes, including in alcohol use (Erskine et al. 2015), and small variations in indicators and measurements can introduce substantial variation in outcomes, requiring cautious interpretation. An important limitation is that these surveys do not capture children who are out of school, which is not an insignificant proportion of children worldwide and an important risk factor for alcohol use (Embleton et al. 2013). Before the Covid-19 pandemic, the out-of-school population counted around 260 million children worldwide, with the majority living in LMICs and belonging to older age groups (The UNESCO Institute for Statistics 2018). While 90% start primary school globally, the dropout is gradual, and by the time of upper secondary school level, only one third remain. These numbers have been exacerbated by the pandemic, resulting in 214 million children from pre-primary to upper secondary having lost 3/4th of classroom instruction time since March 2020 in 23 countries (UNICEF 2021). In addition, the countries that practiced school closing most had the least internet coverage and availability, thus interrupting structured learning, and leaving more children at risk for abuse and neglect, including child labor, domestic violence, and teenage pregnancies. The full overview of the effect on children, including a possible increase in alcohol use, is not yet established.

Early use of alcohol is an established risk factor for later life alcohol dependency and a range of adverse social and health-related outcomes, including unemployment and injuries (Donovan 2014). There is, however, some discussion about the relative importance of the different indicators (e.g., age of first use, age of first drunkenness, or pattern of drinking) as predictors for later harmful use. In a study using data from the HBSC in 38 European and North American countries, Kuntsche and colleagues argued that early drunkenness, and not age of first drink, was a risk factor for problem behavior at age 15 (Kuntsche et al. 2013).

However, using cross-sectional data, a causal inference could not be made, and in large prospective cohort studies from Australia (Aiken et al. 2018) and Canada (Holligan et al. 2019), a different conclusion was made. In both studies, lower age of alcohol initiation was a risk factor for higher level and more harmful pattern of drinking in later adolescence. Moreover, in Australia, no significant association was found between the age of first drunkenness and harmful pattern of drinking in later adolescence (Aiken et al. 2018). This section will not try to disentangle all the relations between the indicators and their causal contribution but review the variation in global prevalence and trends.

Global Patterns and Trends of Childhood Alcohol Use

The patterns of alcohol initiation and use vary substantially across the globe. In a study using GSHS data from 45 LMICs, the prevalence of early alcohol onset (defined as "10 or 11 years old or earlier") ranged from 4.1% in Cambodia to 52.1% in Dominica. Within-continent differences ranged from 13.4% in Mauritius to 15.5% in Benin for Africa, 8.7% in Bolivia and 52.1% in Dominica for the Americas, 4.1% in Cambodia and 23.7% in Lebanon for Asia, and 6.0% in Vanuatu and 38.8% in Samoa in Oceania (Chan et al. 2018). In the European 2019 ESPAD survey, defining early alcohol use as before age 13, Georgia had the highest rate of early use at 60%, while Iceland had the lowest rate at 7.1%. On average, among all participating countries, 6.7% of students had experienced alcohol intoxication before age 13, ranging from 1.8% in Iceland to 25% in Georgia (ESPAD Group 2020). We also note that research done outside these large global surveys have identified alcohol abuse and dependence (according to the American Psychiatric Association (APA) Diagnostic and Statistical Manual of Mental Disorders (DSM) version IV criteria) as early as age 5–8-years in Uganda (Engebretsen et al. 2020), and alcohol use among 8-year-olds in Argentina (Pilatti et al. 2013) and among elementary school students in the United States (US) (Donovan 2007).

The available trends on early alcohol use are uplifting. Most European countries have observed a halving of early alcohol initiation (from 46% to 28% on average) and drunkenness at age 13 (from 17% to 8% on average) from 2002 to 2014. There are large regional variations, and Slovenia observed an increase in early initiation (before age 13) in both genders, whereas Greece saw an increase in girls only (WHO 2018a). In the US, the onset of alcohol use before age 13 has fallen steadily from 32.7% in 1991 to 15.0% in 2019 (CDC 2019). Similar overviews of trends in LMIC have not been identified.

As with age of initiation, there is a great variation in the levels of current use. The within-region variation of GSHS prevalence estimates of past-30-day alcohol use among 12–15-year-olds from 68 LMIC is summarized in Table 1. A wide range was observed from the lowest to the highest prevalence within and between regions, but boys consistently drank more than girls (Leung et al. 2019).

Numbers were captured from the article by Leung and colleagues (Leung et al. 2019)

As with early initiation of alcohol intake, a declining trend for weekly drinking among 15-year-olds has been observed from 2002–2014 in HBSC data from Europe (WHO 2018a) (Fig. 2).

Table 1 The table shows the included countries with the highest and lowest reported prevalence of past 30-day alcohol intake among 12-15-year-olds within each region, and the respective prevalence estimates for boys and girls within these countries

Region	Prevalence range	Country	Boys %	Girls %
Africa	Lowest	Senegal	5.8	1.7
	Highest	Seychelles	59.7	56.2
Americas	Lowest	Honduras	14.5	16.9
	Highest boys	Saint Lucia	58.8	52.3
	Highest girls	Colombia	53.2	56.1
Eastern Mediterranean Region	Lowest	Morocco	10.5	3.36
	Highest	Lebanon	29.3	14.0
Europe	Lowest	Tajikistan	1.0	0.4
	Highest	Macedonia	47.3	37.7
Asia	Lowest	Myanmar	3.0	0.6
	Highest	Thailand	21.0	9.2
Western Pacific Region	Lowest	Brunei	5.7	2.7
	Highest boys	Kiribati	46.9	19.9
	Highest girls	Samoa	45.3	27.6

Data from the ESPAD survey among 15–16-year-old adolescents show similar findings. Trends from 1999 to 2015 in Northern, Southern, Western, and Eastern Europe and the Balkans showed a consistent decline in weekly drinking for both genders in all regions except for the Balkans. However, for girls, there was an increase in monthly heavy episodic drinking in all regions, except for the Northern region. For boys, there was a decrease in monthly heavy episodic drinking in the north, west, and east, while it increased in the Southern region and the Balkans (Kraus et al. 2018). A similar declining trend has been observed for past-month use in the US (CDC 2019). There are few reports on trends from LMIC in GSHS data, but one study showed that past-month alcohol use in Lebanon increased from 19.5% to 27.4% between 2005 and 2011 (Ghandour et al. 2015).

Childhood alcohol use patterns vary across child age, place, and time, and monitoring these indicators is important. The data show that prevalence estimates vary greatly, and while the trends are declining in most of Europe and North America, it is increasing in the Balkans and in Lebanon. These disparities demand further exploration. The remaining sections of this chapter seek to explore evidence related to associated factors that can help us understand these prevalence estimates and trends, from biology to public health policy.

Genetic Factors of Early Alcohol Use

Genetic factors relevant for early-onset substance use have been investigated in a range of family studies, adoption and twin studies, and studies on candidate gene and environment interaction (GxE). It is known that there is a correlation between parent and child alcohol use, but the challenge is to separate out what is shared genetic

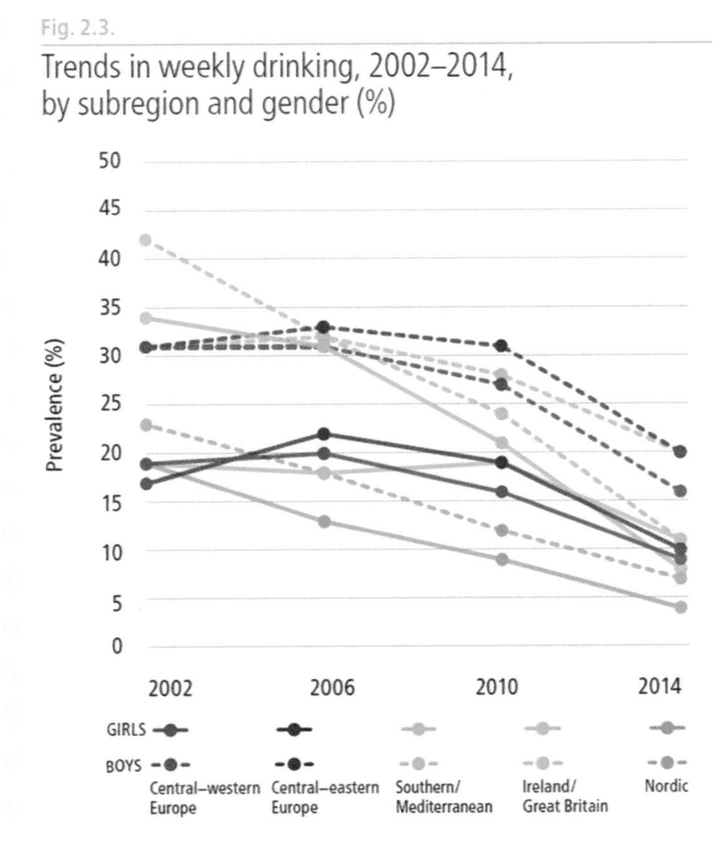

Fig. 2 Trend curve of weekly drinking from HBSC survey reprinted from Adolescent alcohol-related behaviours: trends and inequalities in the WHO European Region, 2002–2014, Editors Inchley J, Currie D et al., figure 2.3, page 12, World Health Organization 2018, reprinted with permission

makeup and what is a shared environment. Establishing a clear causal heritability of substance use has proven difficult, as many factors play a simultaneous role in child development. A recurring finding is that the genetic influence on the variance in drinking initiation and drinking patterns is lower in childhood and early adolescence and increases steadily into adulthood (Hopfer et al. 2003). Despite this, and without contributing to a dichotomized discussion on whether it is nature or nurture, this section reviews some of the findings related to genetic explanations for early alcohol use. The field is large and complex, and this chapter will not be exhaustive, but refer to more comprehensive sources for interested readers. Studies on genetic factors from low- and middle-income countries are scarce, and the implications of this is unknown.

Family, Adoption and Twin Studies

With an aim to investigate genetic factors of alcohol use and dependence, the Collaborative Studies on the Genetics of Alcoholism (COGA) (cogastudy.org) was launched in 1989 (Begleiter et al. 1995). This large family study has investigated 1300 participants recruited from addiction treatment centers in seven locations in the US, their families, and randomly selected control families, including all first-grade relatives aged 7 years or older (Bucholz et al. 2017). A review of the identified genes and findings related to the heritability of alcohol dependence, severity, and co-occurrence of alcohol use disorder and affective disorders from the COGA study can be found in a review by Edenberg and Foroud (2006). Relevant to the focus of this chapter is the Prospective Study of the Collaborative Study on the Genetics of Alcoholism launched in 2004, investigating the trajectory of alcohol involvement across stages of development with biennial assessments from age 12 (Bucholz et al. 2017). At wave 1, the sample included 3573 children from 2147 nuclear families, of which 75% were genotyped, and by wave 5 in 2016, 1197 children remained in the study. The study investigated four alcohol use transitions from time to first drink to first diagnosis. The study found that the risk of onset before age 16 was 22% higher among those with a parent with alcohol use disorder (AUD), and maternal AUD increased the risk of the child alcohol use developing into an alcohol use problem by 27% (Bucholz et al. 2017). Similarly, a systematic review of longitudinal studies on the influence of parental drinking on child drinking found a consistent positive association, but that the included studies had insufficient capacity to establish a causal inference (Rossow et al. 2016).

Adoption studies and twin studies compare biologic vs adoptive parents and monozygotic vs dizygotic twins, respectively. The general hypothesis postulates that if there is a genetic causal component, the biologic child-parent dyads and monozygotic twins should be more likely to have the same alcohol use phenotype compared to adoptive child-parent dyads and dizygotic twins, who share less genetic material. In a review, Stickel and colleagues found that in large twin studies, heritability estimates for alcohol dependence ranged from 16% to 72%, while adoption studies of alcohol use phenotypes identified a rage of 2–52% heritability (Stickel et al. 2017). A meta-analysis of twin and adoption studies found an overall estimated 49% heritability of alcohol use disorder (Verhulst et al. 2015). Interestingly, a systematic review of twin and adoption studies found that the genetic component explained more of the variance in later ages, while factors related to the environment, including parents and siblings, explained more of the variance in earlier ages (Hopfer et al. 2003). One example was a longitudinal study on Finnish twins that found a small genetic effect for girls drinking at age 14 and a nonsignificant association for boys (Rose et al. 2001a), while in the same cohort, the proportion of variance attributable to genetic factors increased to 33% at age 16 and further to 50% at age 18 (Rose et al. 2001b).

Candidate Genes and Gene-Environment Interaction

In addition to the genetic components alone, large studies have investigated specific genes and how they interact with environmental factors. Identified genes are related to the dopamine system, the serotonin system, the opioid system, glucocorticoids, alcohol metabolism, and more. Each of these genes account for a small portion of variance of the alcohol use phenotype, and studies on gene-environment interaction (GxE) show that the effect of genetic predisposition can change as a function of the environment in which it exists (Kim and Park 2018). While a full review of the genes and their effects is beyond the scope of this chapter (for further reading, consult reviews of GxE (Dick and Kendler 2012; Kim and Park 2018)), some examples are relevant for childhood alcohol use. An example is a GxE study that showed the relative importance of a gene, depending on the exposure to different levels of social control. More parental control and religiosity reduced the effect of genetic predispositions for alcohol use, while more permissive environments allowed for a stronger expression of genetic predispositions (Dick and Kendler 2012). Findings related to the GABRA2 gene has illustrated how the genetic influences on onset of early alcohol use are complex, vary across developmental stages, and co-occur with other psychiatric phenotypes. While the gene has been associated with alcohol and other drug dependence in adulthood, the same was not found in a sample of children ages 7–17. In childhood, the gene was strongly associated with childhood conduct disorder, but the association to alcohol dependence symptoms was not evident until the mid-20s (Dick et al. 2006).

In summary, the individual contribution of a gene to alcohol use is relatively small, often insignificant, in early childhood and adolescence, but increases with age. Further, the importance can change in different environments, which will be investigated in the coming sections of this chapter, including mental health, near family, peers, and the wider community.

Mental Health: Vulnerability and Resilience

Mental health embraces neurological, psychiatric, psychological, social, and substance use conditions, and the old slogan "No health without mental health" (Prince et al. 2007) acknowledges the WHO understanding of health as "a state of complete physical, mental and social well-being and not merely the absence of disease or infirmity." (Larsen 2021). Alcohol use by children has been found to be associated with various mental health conditions. A study on GSHS data, which included more than 20,000 adolescents from Kenya, Namibia, Swaziland, Uganda, Zambia, and Zimbabwe, found that school truancy, loneliness, sleeping problems, sadness, suicidal ideation, suicide plans, and poverty were associated with substance use including tobacco, alcohol, and illicit drugs (Peltzer 2009). A similar assessment was published in 2021 looking at 41 LMICs, where substance use was associated with psychological distress in the African, American, Southeast region, and Western Pacific regions (Tian et al. 2021). Although strong linkages have been described between mental health conditions and substance use in various studies that have used observational designs, no causal relationship can be drawn. Mental health conditions may exist without substance use and vice versa.

Mental Health and Alcohol Use: Common Risk Factors

Mental illness and alcohol use share many risk factors. Parental alcohol use, including prenatal exposure, or family factors, such as being permissive of alcohol use, may create both developmental challenges due to neurodevelopmental effects and adverse upbringing conditions (Gardiner et al. 2021; Roos et al. 2021). Other overlapping risk factors include oppression, conflict and poverty, adverse upbringing conditions including abuse and neglect, peer and familial substance use, and intergenerational poor socioeconomic development.

Thus, a psychiatric disease focus may seem reductionistic when discussing vulnerability and resilience for child alcohol drinking. Morover, some of the conditions described may be inherently related to substance use, such as conduct disorders, which are characterized by "breaking social norms." Still there may be room for looking at some of the bold categories of disorders in the DSM-5 psychiatric classification system released in 2013 (APA 2013). Neurodevelopmental disorders are mentioned first, disorders that often become prominent during childhood. These include intellectual disabilities, communication disorders, autism spectrum disorders, attention-deficit/hyperactivity disorders (ADHD), specific learning disorder, motor disorders, and other neurodevelopmental disorders. The DSM-5 classifies other bold domains of disorders, of which substance use is a separate disorder group. Not all disorder groups in the DSM-5 are relevant in childhood, but in addition to the neurodevelopmental disorders, the following are of high relevance: depressive and anxiety disorders, obsessive-and related disorders, trauma-, stressor-, and dissociative disorders, feeding-, eating- and sleep disorders and conduct disorders (APA 2013).

Symptom Interplay

Rutter described 20 years ago that psychiatric conditions were overlapping and each condition often extended broadly but were also distinct, i.e., clear and identifiable (Rutter 2003). Therefore, there is no surprise that substance dependence may overlap with other mental health conditions. A clinical study in Uganda, using DSM-IV criteria, found psychiatric comorbidities in 10 out of 11 children that were diagnosed with alcohol dependence and abuse and had a high psychiatric symptom score at screening. These are presented in Table 2 (Engebretsen et al. 2020).

For a number of the conditions, alcohol use may have a medicating effect. Both mental health conditions and substance use disorders affect the dopaminergic and serotonergic circuits in the brain. For depression and anxiety, alcohol may serve as a tranquillizer and may be taken as self-medication. When children with anxiety or depression drink alcohol, it may be part of complex mechanisms, including context and conditions, that make drinking an option. For psychiatric conditions characterized by reduced control of impulsivity and hyperactivity, an increased risk for illicit substance use has been described, as well as later dependence, the latter including alcohol (Lee et al. 2011). Alcohol use is not a unidimensional response to

Table 2 Conditions found among 10 children aged 5–8 years old in Eastern Uganda with moderate and high symptom scores (≥14) on the Strengths and Difficulties Questionnaire, diagnosed with alcohol abuse and dependence according to the DSM-IV criteria using MINI International Neuropsychiatric Interview for Children and Adolescents (MINI-KID) (Sheehan et al. 1998)

Alcohol abuse and/or dependence last 12 months	SDQ ≥14 *N* = 10* *N*, %
Major depressive episode	
Current	1 (10.0)
Past	1 (10.0)
Recurrent	1 (10.0)
Suicidality	3 (30%)
Panic disorder	1 (10.0)
Separation anxiety disorder	5 (50.0)
Specific phobia	1 (10.0)
Post-traumatic disorder	1 (10.0)
ADHD, inattentive	1 (10.0)
Conduct disorders	1 (10.0)

cope with mental health suffering, but one option in complex pathways that link mental health conditions to substances use and potential dependence. Within this, there is an interplay of peer and family use and hereditability and risk of parental mental health disorders (Ossola et al. 2020). Gender differences may also come into play where boys seem more susceptible when having a drinking father, and measures are needed for early identication and support for families that are struggling with adversities, including parental drinking.

There are multiple pathways between parental substance use, mental health conditions, and child alcohol use, the relationship is complex and not causal, indicating the opportunity for multiple other outcomes (Almquist et al. 2020). Strong narratives have shown that supportive communities, such as religious groups and sports and school participation, can promote resilience in adverse situations. A recent study from Brazil, which measured resilience (Neto et al. 2020) using the Resilience Scale (a scale that measures 25 positive issues on personal competence, acceptance of self, and life), found that social project participation was favorable but not strongly associated with alcohol or drug intake. Similarly, a Swedish cohort study, with more than 14,000 participants, found that school performance interacted with intergenerational transmission of alcohol misuse. Those with higher perfor mances had a lower likelihood of next-generation drinking (Almquist et al. 2020).

Building on knowledge of prenatal and alcohol use in pregnancy as risk factors for mental health conditions in childhood, risks of adverse upbringing conditions and the mechanisms supporting resilience during adversities, investment in pregnancy and early childcare, supportive school and social environments seem to be favorable policy directions.

Family and Friends

The complexity of a childhood in all its dimensions of development, interaction, stimulation, relations, upbringing, and safety, nurturing, and care can hardly be given justice in a book chapter. However, John E. Donovan has given a strong overview of socialization into substance use in the Oxford Handbook for Adolescent Substance Abuse (Donovan 2019). Donovan sketches out relevant socialization theories, placing both pathways of control, identification, and bonding into a network involving the child, their friends, and significant adults' alcohol use, as well as child and adult cognition, relational quality, and measures of controls as confounding factors – all hard to measure in their complexity. The chapter further describes how socialization is not an outcome in and of itself but a lifelong process initiated in childhood involving the individual, with its personality, attitudes, and behavior, and their environment, including a range of mechanisms, processes, and social agents. Such agents can be immediate family, typically parents, guardians, and siblings; extended family; close friends; less close friends, such as classmates or schoolmates; various subcultures through sports and ideological or religious communities; and online closer mates or friends, such as gaming fellows, and people in wider interactive and media circles. However, this interplay between social agents is often reduced to a two-dimensional influence, the family environment mostly represented by parents and peers that could be represented by primarily closer friends or peers, but in the absence of school or age mates with weaker bonding. This reductionistic dichotomization may be useful for research purposes, sketching out bold influences on the child.

Parents and Early Alcohol Use

Parental drinking may influence drinking among children through various pathways, and elements of parental drinking may have both a catalytic and inhibiting effect on children. Donovan's review summarized that parental drinking is associated with child tasting and sipping, modest increase in adolescent drinking frequency, initiation of drinking, and drinking in younger ages (Donovan 2019). Parental, and in particular paternal, alcoholism tends to be associated with more severe child and adolescent drinking patterns. Regarding this, Donovan discriminates general parenting from alcohol specific parenting, where the latter considers parental beliefs and rules related to child alcohol use.

One obvious pathway through which parental drinking may enhance childhood drinking includes availability and access to alcohol. Donovan further mentions that just as important is the fact that parenting styles and strategies, such as quality of relationship and authority, are affected by the drinking habits of these significant adults. Parenting may be impaired by relational tension, fewer family activities, greater discipline, and less warmth, closeness, and bonding. As pointed toward below, these factors may also aggregate emotional suffering, development of conduct issues, and various mental health conditions in the child. The heavy alcohol drinking or alcohol dependent parent may be inconsistent in boundaries and setting rules compared to a nondrinking parent, and in addition, alcoholism can in and of itself impair parenting and be related to child abuse and neglect, which may induce both behavioral and emotional effects in the child (Haugland et al. 2021). Further, parental alcohol drinking may be associated with being permissive of alcohol drinking, which has been shown to be associated both with smoking, alcohol use, and illicit drug use by children. A recent publication that used data from the European Drug Addiction Prevention trial from 7 European countries (including more than 7000 students) identified a strong relationship between permissiveness and adolescent alcohol use (Mehanović et al. 2021).

Parents' drinking habits, drinking permissiveness, and parenting styles are related to a web of factors, including characteristics of culture, socioeconomic class and economic ability, educational background, and own mental health. These factors may lay the foundation for children's upbringing conditions, and it is becoming more common to look at an index or a cluster of factors as risks, rather than individual risk factors. A recent study from the British Avon Longitudinal Study of Parents and Children (ALSPAC) cohort from 1992 addressed adverse childhood experiences (ACEs) on educational attainment and adolescent health up to 17 years (Houtepen et al. 2020). ACEs included sexual, physical, or emotional abuse, emotional neglect, parental substance abuse, parental mental illness or suicide attempt, violence between parents, parental separation, bullying, and parental criminal conviction. Health at age 17 years included depression, obesity, harmful alcohol use, smoking, and illicit drug use. This study found that four or more ACEs were only weakly associated with harmful alcohol use at age 17 but more strongly associated with lower educational attainment and higher risk of depression, drug use, and smoking. It is hard to disentangle the reasons why some relationships are stronger and weaker, and the role of peers and a rapidly shifting culture may also be mediating factors.

Family or Peers?

The interplay between child and parent does, as stated, not happen in a vacuum. Peers and other behavioral risk factors have simultaneous impacts and synergies, and it is difficult to tease out the individual impact of each actor. A recent publication of a Finish cohort found that parental alcohol use, including prenatal drinking and parental drinking when the child was 16 years old, was associated with a higher risk for adolescent heavy drinking, which was further interrelated with childhood externalizing behaviors and contact with deviant peers. Sex differences were also seen in this study indicating a higher risk for later life alcohol use disorder among males (Parra et al. 2020). This study clearly described pathways via maternal prenatal drinking to childhood externalizing behavior and later influence from deviant peers. The latter had a direct relationship with adolescent drinking. These behaviors can in turn affect parenting strategies, where more deviant behaviors may result in more punishment and reduced warmth, leading to a vicious cycle.

As mentioned, a decline in adolescent alcohol use has been observed. Caluzzi and colleagues have argued that a denormalization of drinking and a normalization of nondrinking has been observed (Caluzzi et al. 2021). Normalization of nondrinking could include alternative child reactions toward alcohol use such as disgust and non-association with parental drinking behaviors; a competitive youth culture on multiple arenas including school, sports, and culture; preventive youth work; lack of connection with parental expressed and practiced norms; and effects of a globalized social media network. All in all, although parental drinking early and later in children's lives constitute major risks, both via access, norms, permissiveness and boundaries, and relations that may lead to adverse health effects and socioeconomic immobility, there is no absolute causality between parental drinking and drinking in children. Children's norms and culture are also changing, and wider influences are steering toward a decline in adolescent drinking.

Culture and the Community

To understand why some children start earlier and drink more or more often than others, we have to look beyond individual health, family, and peers and explore the context and conditions in which they grow up. In accordance with Bronfenbrenner's socioecological systems theory, the levels of influence on child development are in constant interplay with each other, meaning that that microsystem of the family and peers interacts with the mesosystem of community and culture, and vice versa.

A large multicountry comparison study from 2019, comparing GSHS data from 68 LMICs, found that boys had a more than twice as high odds ratio of alcohol use compared to girls in the pooled estimates (Leung et al. 2019). There were some regional and country differences, indicating that gender norms and culture were influencing practices. Globally and historically, psychoactive substances have been part of traditional and cultural practices connected to religion, social connection, and coping (Westermeyer 2016). One example is in Uganda, where alcohol use has been reported to be widely acceptable, including introducing it to children at an early age (Ssebunnya et al. 2020).

While recovery and sobriety movement embedded in various religious and ideologic, including feministic, movements are on the rise, the opposite is also seen. Through commercial, political, religious, cultural and regular media channels, as well as social media (Harding et al. 2021), there is a vast potential for advertisement, product placement, and social influence. For example, through social media, celebrities and role models may promote alcohol drinking among youth. A follow-up study among 15-year-old children from the ALSPAC cohort in the UK found that alcohol use in films was related to problematic and frequent drinking but had a smaller effect on trying out alcohol (Waylen et al. 2015). Another study from six European countries showed that increased visual film exposure was related to increased experimenting and binge drinking, although the risk was small (Hanewinkel et al. 2014). Relatively few studies have looked at the influences of social media on these behaviors, despite the large potential for influence, especially among youth. To which degree manufacturers' promotions or nonregulations are involved in promoting alcohol supportive trends goes beyond the scope of this chapter. However, where regulations of advertisements for children and youth are weak and alcohol use is culturally associated with wealth and status, one can imagine that the potential for alcohol promotion can have detrimental effects on children. Culture and community factors influence the perceived needs and opportunities for interventions and laws, and thus the possibility for effective implementation thereof.

Policy for Protection Against Alcohol

Protecting children from alcohol-related harm requires political priority and implementation of preventive policies. To help countries navigate the myriad of suggested interventions to prevent and reduce the harmful effects of alcohol, the WHO published a Global Strategy to Reduce the Harmful Use of Alcohol (WHO 2010), as well as "best buys" for tackling noncommunicable diseases, including the harmful use of alcohol (WHO 2017). The WHO "best buys" were developed to inform member states of the interventions that are most effective, cost-effective, and feasible to implement, including in LMICs (WHO 2017). The WHO's Global Information System on Alcohol and Health (GISAH) contains information on national-level alcohol-related health indicators and alcohol policy status and forms the basis for the WHO Global Status Report on Alcohol and Health (WHO 2018b). The report includes a global situation analysis of alcohol policy and interventions in addition to individual country profiles, summarizing alcohol-related statistics for 218 countries. The report shows large discrepancies between the WHO regions, where Africa and the Americas held the largest proportion of countries with no national policy on alcohol, a weakness the alcohol industry has been reported to exploit (Jernigan and Babor 2015). In this section, we will review the alcohol policies related to preventing early alcohol use in different continents, and their effect, focusing on the "best buys" relevant for childhood alcohol use; minimum legal drinking age; restricting access (hours, days, and places for sales); and regulating marketing and prices.

Protecting Children From Access to Alcohol

Albeit large discrepancies, most countries regulate alcohol access to some extent. According to the WHO report, 93% of the responding nations had implemented a minimum age limit for on-premises purchase (e.g., in bars) of alcoholic beverages. Note that while the most common age limit was 18 years, some countries had age limits as low as 13, 14, and 15 years of age. LMICs and countries from the African region included the most countries without an age limit (WHO 2018b). A study that used GSHS and ESPAD data to estimate the association between adolescent drinking and alcohol restricting policies found that implementing a minimum legal purchasing age of 21 years could reduce the odds of adolescent lifetime drinking by 21.6% (Noel 2019).

Further, there are policies regulating the availability of alcohol through hours and places for sale with for example monopolies (WHO 2018b). Eighty-six percent of the countries included in the WHO report had national licensing for at least part of the alcohol production and distribution, indicating that a large share of the market was unregulated. While licensing is intended to regulate alcohol sales, the increase in licensing of alcohol production may paradoxically also result in increased alcohol availability. Low-income countries in Africa and Southeast Asia have had the largest increase in licensing as well as the largest use of unrecorded alcohol, such as homebrewing (Picture 1).

According to the same WHO report, regulation of hours and days of sales and alcohol outlet density was not as common. Less than a third of responding countries

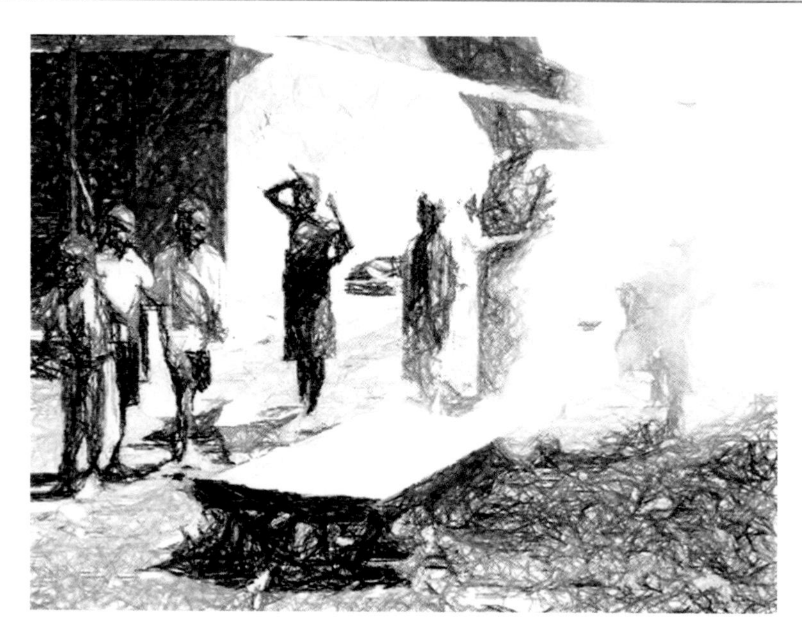

Picture 1 Illustration photo: brewing of millet in a Ugandan village exposing children to available brew. (Photo: IMS Engebretsen)

reported regulations on days of sale and alcohol density, while hours of sale were more commonly regulated. Restrictions on drinking in public and in specific places varied, but relevant for children, many had a total ban on intake in educational buildings (60%) and sporting events (30%) (WHO 2018b). Moreover, the WHO has stated that increasing the price of alcohol is among the most effective measures to reduce the access to and use of alcohol by youth and heavy drinkers, but implementation of price-related interventions has varied across WHO regions (WHO 2010). In the afore mentioned study, estimating the association between adolescent drinking in GSHS and ESPAD data and alcohol restricting policies, found that implementing excise taxes on alcoholic products for the first time had a theoretical opportunity to reduce the odds of adolescent lifetime drinking by 54% (Noel 2019). Further, increased pricing has been found to increase the likelihood of enrolment and graduation in secondary and post-secondary school, improve school performance, and reduce sexual transmitted diseases and teen pregnancy (Xu and Chaloupka 2011).

Laws that regulate alcohol marketing vary and the alcohol industry plays different roles in societies across the globe. Policies that regulate alcohol marketing are especially geared toward protecting youth against exposure to advertising and promotions through social media, television, and cinema, which can potentially nudge them into early initiation. It is noteworthy that social media and internet regulations were among the least commonly reported interventions in the WHO report, a platform where youth are especially active. Again, having no restrictions across media platforms was mostly reported from countries in the African region and in the Americas (WHO 2018b). In a systematic review, Jernigan and colleagues identified 12 longitudinal studies investigating the impact of marketing on youth drinking behavior. They found that marketing was significantly associated with the initiation of alcohol use in some studies (OR 1.00–1.7) while all studies found a one-and-a-half to twofold increase in marketing on hazardous drinking. These effects had been observed in children as young as 10 years and were significant after adjusting for family and peer drinking behavior (Jernigan et al. 2017).

Policy Synergy and Context

While it is important to investigate the effect of each policy to make sure interventions are as effective as possible, it is also important to keep in mind that these policies work in synergy. In one study, Pachall and colleagues investigated the association between adolescent drinking habits and an Alcohol Policy Index (API) score based on five policy domains (physical availability, drinking context, price, advertising, and motor vehicles). Using ESPAD data and other national school surveys from 26 countries, they found that a higher API score (indicating more comprehensive policies) was inversely correlated with any past 30-day alcohol intake and with reporting three or more drinking occasions in the past month (Paschall et al. 2009). Further, for an alcohol policy to be effective, it must be successfully implemented and enforced (Jones-Webb et al. 2014). The culture and context have a reciprocal relationship with local practices, where higher access can reinforce a culture for high intake. Further, different policies can have different effects in different contexts. While reducing alcohol-related harm will have a long-term benefit for the society, it is costly, both directly and indirectly, to implement policy recommendations and monitoring systems. When resources are scare, priority for alcohol restricting measures may have to yield for more acute and pressing matters, such as famine or insurgency. When evaluating the global developments in alcohol policies since the launch of the WHO Global Strategy to Reduce the Harmful Use of Alcohol, the WHO found that no low-income country reported having increased their resource allocation for implementing alcohol policies, including those that would protect children against exposure to alcohol and drinking (Jernigan and Trangenstein 2017). Moreover, economic development may have conflicting interests with restriction of access to alcohol since production of alcoholic beverages may offer employment and tax income. Regulating the sales of alcohol may have direct implications for the possible earnings of the individuals that depend on sales. In places where unregulated production of alcoholic brews are prevalent, alternative ways to generate income must be put in place before people's livelihood is removed. The complex effort to protect children from harmful substances must be a concerted effort from the international community, national governments, and local communities. In short, childhood drinking must not be neglected, it must be investigated, and when identified, necessary actions are needed.

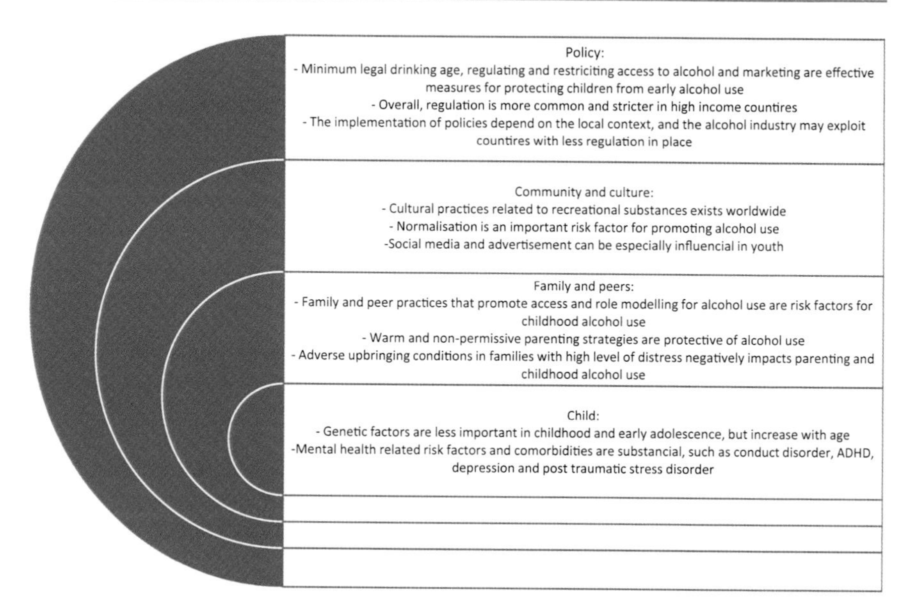

Fig. 3 Summary of points from each level of Bronfenbrenner's socioecological systems covered in this chapter

Summary

This chapter has sought to explore and review factors related to childhood alcohol use, spanning all levels of Bronfenbrenner's socioecological systems theory (Fig. 3). Individual, family, and community factors, and the complex interplay between them, make childhood substance use an interesting but complicated field, with many actors in play. Childhood alcohol use varies between different contexts, with changing prevalence estimates, risk profile, and outcomes. It is therefore crucial that the context is investigated and considered when planning and implementing interventions. While much has been done, vast amounts of work remain.

Applications to Other Areas of Addiction

The topics raised in this chapter has clear relevance for other addictive substances, such as marijuana, opioids, benzodiazepines, and stimulants. The difference in legality is clear – while alcohol is illegal to sell to minors, it is readily available in the community. Moreover, the use of multiple substances often happens simultaneously, and many of the same mechanisms for risk factors and outcomes are at play. In one paper from the COGA Prospective Study, Bucholz and colleagues found that ever use of cannabis increased with age and was associated with an 85% increase in early alcohol use before age 13 (Bucholz et al. 2017). As with alcohol, genetic components have been investigated for many substances, and family correlations, associations with other mental health issues, community factors, and policy are all relevant. The debate on legalization and decriminalization of addictive substances is ongoing in many countries and is not possible to justifiably recount here. However, for many, the main concern is related to youth and harmful impacts over their life course (Ladegard et al. 2020). Without taking a stance in the debate on decriminalization, it is of outmost importance to protect children from drugs and addiction, regardless of the substance. Effective implementation of policies and building safe drug-free environments are important factors for the future generations to thrive.

Applications to Other Areas of Public Health

Childhood alcohol and other substance use have wide-ranging implications. Alcohol is one of the leading drivers of the burden of disease among youth (Erskine et al. 2015), and the WHO acknowledges that alcohol use is a risk factor for a range of diseases, including cancer, infections, and injuries, through its effect on the immune system, risky behavior, and poor adherence to therapy (WHO 2018b). Further, alcohol use and alcohol use disorders have implications on other social determinants of health, such as teen pregnancies and education (Xu and Chaloupka 2011; Donovan 2014). Moreover, early alcohol use directly affects the developing brain, with consequences for cognitive development and skills necessary to thrive throughout the life course (Squeglia and Gray 2016). As stated in this chapter, mental health and substance use are closely related, and a study on young users of a mental health facility in Australia showed that early onset (mean 13.6 years) compared to later onset (mean 16.9 years) had poorer outcomes on the Social and Occupational Functioning Assessment Scale (SOFAS) at all follow-up times (Crouse et al. 2019). Further, among healthy adolescents, followed-up to young adulthood, earlier onset of drinking was associated with poorer psychomotor speed and visual attention, and an earlier onset of weekly drinking predicted poorer working memory and cognitive inhibition (Nguyen-Louie et al. 2017). These outcomes can impact later life education and employment opportunities, which are important social determinants of health. It is imperative that we address early alcohol use as an important public health issue, with its direct impact on children throughout their life course.

Mini-Dictionary of Terms (5–15 Terms)

- Alcohol use: Intentional alcohol drinking, regardless of amount, for recreational or other purposes.
- Alcohol abuse and dependence and alcohol disorder: Clinical terms from DSM-IV and DSM-5 that describe a patterns of symptoms related to the diagnosis of pathological alcohol use.
- Bronfenbrenner's ecological systems theory: Explores child development as influenced by multiple systems that interact, spanning the immediate microsystem of family and peers, mesosystem of community and culture, and macrosystem of policy and governance.
- Childhood: Developmental period that spans ages 0–18 years.

- Sustainable Development Goals: 17 goals adopted by United Nations Member States in 2015 to improve development indicators up to year 2030. SDG 3 describes the global goals for health and well-being.

Key Facts of Childhood Alcohol Use

- Children are drinking alcohol at very young ages in some parts of the world.
- Clinically verified alcohol abuse and dependence (DSM-IV) has been described in children as young as 5–8 years of age living under adult care in some communities in Uganda.
- Alcohol abuse and dependence (DSM-IV) has been found to be associated with other psychiatric comorbidities.
- Alcohol is a neurotoxic substance which is harmful to children.
- Monitoring, assessment, and follow-up are needed where alcohol drinking among children is found. This must be anchored in policies implemented into education and health systems.

Summary Points

- Age and sex stratified early exposure and current use of alcohol are useful indicators for comparison across groups.
- There are large variations in prevalence estimates of alcohol use among children across the globe, spanning from a few percent to more than half of the children.
- Environmental factors seem to be more important than genetic explanations for alcohol use among the young.
- Parents, peers, and culture may promote childhood alcohol use through permissive attitudes and norms.
- Risk factors for childhood alcohol use are multiple and often interconnected.
- Cultures are changing, and declining trends in alcohol use among children and adolescents are seen in many parts of the world.
- Many risk factors for childhood alcohol drinking are modifiable through policies and regulations.
- Most of the literature on childhood alcohol use include adolescents and come from high income countries, and more research from LMICs and earlier childhood is needed.

References

Aiken A et al (2018) Age of alcohol initiation and progression to binge drinking in adolescence: a prospective Cohort Study. Alcohol Clin Exp Res 42(1). https://doi.org/10.1111/acer.13525

Almquist YB et al (2020) Intergenerational transmission of alcohol misuse: mediation and interaction by school performance in a Swedish birth cohort. J Epidemiol Community Health 74(7). https://doi.org/10.1136/jech-2019-213523

APA (2013) Diagnostic and statistical manual of mental disorders: DSM-5. American Psychiatric Association, Washington, DC
Begleiter H et al (1995) The collaborative study on the genetics of alcoholism. Alcohol Health Res World 19(3):228–236. Available at: https://pubmed.ncbi.nlm.nih.gov/31798102
Bronfenbrenner U (1979) The ecology of human development. Harvard University Press
Bucholz KK et al (2017) Comparison of parent, peer, psychiatric, and cannabis use influences across stages of offspring alcohol involvement: evidence from the COGA Prospective Study. Alcohol Clin Exp Res 41(2). https://doi.org/10.1111/acer.13293
Caluzzi G et al (2021) Declining drinking among adolescents: are we seeing a denormalisation of drinking and a normalisation of non-drinking? Addiction. https://doi.org/10.1111/add.15611
CDC (2019) Trends in the prevalence of alcohol use national YRBS: 1991–2019. Centers for Disease Control and Prevention (CDC). Available at: https://www.cdc.gov/healthyyouth/data/yrbs/factsheets/2019_alcohol_trend_yrbs.htm
CDC (2021) Middle school youth risk behavior survey. CDC.. Available at: https://www.cdc.gov/healthyyouth/data/yrbs/pdf/2021/2021-YRBS-Standard-MS-Questionnaire.pdf
Chan GCK et al (2018) Familial alcohol supply, adolescent drinking and early alcohol onset in 45 low and middle income countries. Addict Behav 84:178–185. https://doi.org/10.1016/j.addbeh.2018.04.014
Crouse JJ et al (2019) Exploring associations between early substance use and longitudinal socio-occupational functioning in young people engaged in a mental health service. PLoS One 14(1). https://doi.org/10.1371/journal.pone.0210877
Currie C, Inchley J, Molcho M, Lenzi M, Veselska Z, Wild F (eds) (2014) Health Behaviour in School-aged Children (HBSC) study protocol: background, methodology and mandatory items for the 2013/14 survey. CAHRU, St Andrews. Available at: http://www.hbsc.org
Dick DM, Kendler KS (2012) The impact of gene-environment interaction on alcohol use disorders. Alcohol Res Curr Rev
Dick DM et al (2006) The role of GABRA2 in risk for conduct disorder and alcohol and drug dependence across developmental stages. Behav Genet 36(4). https://doi.org/10.1007/s10519-005-9041-8
Donovan JE (2007) Really underage drinkers: the epidemiology of children's alcohol use in the united states. Prev Sci 8(3):192–205. https://doi.org/10.1007/s11121-007-0072-7
Donovan JE (2014) The burden of alcohol use: focus on children and preadolescents. Alcohol Res Curr Rev 35(2):186–192. Available at: http://www.ncbi.nlm.nih.gov/pmc/articles/PMC3908710/
Donovan JE (2019) Child and adolescent socialization into substance use. Oxford Hand Adolesc Subst Abuse. https://doi.org/10.1093/oxfordhb/9780199735662.013.018
Edenberg HJ, Foroud T (2006) The genetics of alcoholism: identifying specific genes through family studies. Addict Biol. https://doi.org/10.1111/j.1369-1600.2006.00035.x
Embleton L et al (2013) The epidemiology of substance use among street children in resource-constrained settings: a systematic review and meta-analysis. Addiction 108(10):1722–1733. https://doi.org/10.1111/add.12252
Engebretsen IMS et al (2020) "I feel good when I drink"—detecting childhood-onset alcohol abuse and dependence in a Ugandan community trial cohort. Child Adolesc Psychiatry Ment Health 14, 42 (2020). https://doi.org/10.1186/s13034-020-00349-z
Erskine HE et al (2015) A heavy burden on young minds: the global burden of mental and substance use disorders in children and youth. Psychol Med 45(7):1551–1563. https://doi.org/10.1017/S0033291714002888
ESPAD (2019) ESPAD report 2019 master questionnaire. ESPAD. Available at: http://espad.org/sites/espad.org/files/espad-2019-Student-Master-Questionnaire.pdf
ESPAD Group (2020) ESPAD report 2019: results from the European School Survey Project on alcohol and other drugs. EMCDDA Joint Publications, Publications Office of the European Union, Luxembourg
Gardiner E et al (2021) Behavior regulation skills are associated with adaptive functioning in children and adolescents with prenatal alcohol exposure. Appl Neuropsychol Child. https://doi.org/10.1080/21622965.2021.1936528

Ghandour L et al (2015) Time trends and policy gaps: the case of alcohol misuse among adolescents in Lebanon. Subst Use Misuse 50(14). https://doi.org/10.3109/10826084.2015.1073320

Hanewinkel R et al (2014) Portrayal of alcohol consumption in movies and drinking initiation in low-risk adolescents. Pediatrics 133(6). https://doi.org/10.1542/peds.2013-3880

Harding KD, Whittingham L, McGannon KR (2021) #sendwine: an analysis of motherhood, alcohol use and #winemom culture on instagram. Subst Abuse Res Treat 15. https://doi.org/10.1177/11782218211015195

Haugland SH et al (2021) Associations between parental alcohol problems in childhood and adversities during childhood and later adulthood: a cross-sectional study of 28047 adults from the general population. Subst Abuse Treat Prevent Policy 16(1). https://doi.org/10.1186/s13011-021-00384-9

Holligan SD et al (2019) Age at first alcohol use predicts current alcohol use, binge drinking and mixing of alcohol with energy drinks among Ontario grade 12 students in the COMPASS study. Health Promot Chronic Dis Prev Can 39(11). https://doi.org/10.24095/hpcdp.39.11.02

Hopfer CJ, Crowley TJ, Hewitt JK (2003) Review of twin and adoption studies of adolescent substance use. J Am Acad Child Adolesc Psychiatry 42(6). https://doi.org/10.1097/01.CHI.0000046848.56865.54

Houtepen LC et al (2020) Associations of adverse childhood experiences with educational attainment and adolescent health and the role of family and socioeconomic factors: a prospective cohort study in the UK. PLoS Med 17(3). https://doi.org/10.1371/journal.pmed.1003031

Jernigan DH, Babor TF (2015) The concentration of the global alcohol industry and its penetration in the African region. Addiction 110(4). https://doi.org/10.1111/add.12468

Jernigan D, Trangenstein P (2017) Global developments in alcohol policies: progress in implementation of the WHO global strategy to reduce the harmful use of alcohol since 2010. In: Background paper developed for the WHO Forum on alcohol, drugs and addictive behaviours, pp 26–28

Jernigan D et al (2017) Alcohol marketing and youth alcohol consumption: a systematic review of longitudinal studies published since 2008. Addiction. https://doi.org/10.1111/add.13591

Jones-Webb R et al (2014) An implementation model to increase the effectiveness of alcohol control policies. Am J Health Promot 28(5). https://doi.org/10.4278/ajhp.121001-QUAL-478

Kim J, Park A (2018) A systematic review: Candidate gene and environment interaction on alcohol use and misuse among adolescents and young adults. Am J Addict. https://doi.org/10.1111/ajad.12755

Kraus L et al (2018) “Are The Times A-Changin”? Trends in adolescent substance use in Europe. Addiction 113(7). https://doi.org/10.1111/add.14201

Kuntsche E et al (2013) Not early drinking but early drunkenness is a risk factor for problem behaviors among adolescents from 38 European and North American countries. Alcohol Clin Exp Res 37(2). https://doi.org/10.1111/j.1530-0277.2012.01895.x

Ladegard K, Thurstone C, Rylander M (2020) Marijuana legalization and youth. Pediatrics 145(2). https://doi.org/10.1542/PEDS.2019-2056D

Larsen LT (2021) Not merely the absence of disease: a genealogy of the WHO’s positive health definition. Hist Hum Sci. https://doi.org/10.1177/0952695121995355

Lee SS et al (2011) Prospective association of childhood attention-deficit/hyperactivity disorder (ADHD) and substance use and abuse/dependence: a meta-analytic review. Clin Psychol Rev. https://doi.org/10.1016/j.cpr.2011.01.006

Leung J et al (2019) Alcohol consumption and consequences in adolescents in 68 low and middle-income countries – a multi-country comparison of risks by sex. Drug Alcohol Depend 205. https://doi.org/10.1016/j.drugalcdep.2019.06.022

Lim SS et al (2012) A comparative risk assessment of burden of disease and injury attributable to 67 risk factors and risk factor clusters in 21 regions, 1990-2010: a systematic analysis for the Global Burden of Disease Study 2010. Lancet (London, England) 380(9859):2224–2260. https://doi.org/10.1016/S0140-6736(12)61766-8

Mehanović E et al (2021) Does parental permissiveness toward cigarette smoking and alcohol use influence illicit drug use among adolescents? A longitudinal study in seven European countries. Soc Psychiatry Psychiatr Epidemiol 1:3. https://doi.org/10.1007/s00127-021-02118-5

Neto EDC et al (2020) The resilience of adolescent participants in social projects for sport. Ciencia e Saude Coletiva 25(3). https://doi.org/10.1590/1413-81232020253.18362018

Nguyen-Louie TT et al (2017) Earlier alcohol use onset predicts poorer neuropsychological functioning in young adults. Alcohol Clin Exp Res 41(12). https://doi.org/10.1111/acer.13503

Noel JK (2019) Associations between alcohol policies and adolescent alcohol use: a pooled analysis of GSHS and ESPAD data. Alcohol Alcohol 54(6). https://doi.org/10.1093/alcalc/agz068

Ossola P et al (2020) Alcohol use disorders among adult children of alcoholics (ACOAs): gene-environment resilience factors. Prog Neuro-Psychopharmacol Biol Psychiatry. https://doi.org/10.1016/j.pnpbp.2020.110167

Parra GR et al (2020) Parental alcohol use and the alcohol misuse of their offspring in a Finnish Birth Cohort: investigation of developmental timing. J Youth Adolesc 49(8). https://doi.org/10.1007/s10964-020-01239-5

Paschall MJ, Grube JW, Kypri K (2009) Alcohol control policies and alcohol consumption by youth: a multi-national study. Addiction 104(11). https://doi.org/10.1111/j.1360-0443.2009.02698.x

Peltzer K (2009) Prevalence and correlates of substance use among school children in six African countries. Int J Psychol 44(5). https://doi.org/10.1080/00207590802511742

Pilatti A et al (2013) Underage drinking: Prevalence and risk factors associated with drinking experiences among Argentinean children. Alcohol 47(4):323–331. https://doi.org/10.1016/j.alcohol.2013.02.001

Prince M et al (2007) No health without mental health. Lancet. https://doi.org/10.1016/S0140-6736(07)61238-0

Roos A et al (2021) Central white matter integrity alterations in 2-3-year-old children following prenatal alcohol exposure. Drug Alcohol Depend 225:108826. https://doi.org/10.1016/J.DRUGALCDEP.2021.108826

Rose RJ, Dick DM, Viken RJ, Pulkkinen L et al (2001a) Drinking or abstaining at age 14? A genetic epidemiological study. Alcohol Clin Exp Res 25(11). https://doi.org/10.1111/j.1530-0277.2001.tb02166.x

Rose RJ, Dick DM, Viken RJ, Kaprio J (2001b) Gene-environment interaction in patterns of adolescent drinking: regional residency moderates longitudinal influences on alcohol use. Alcohol Clin Exp Res 25(5). https://doi.org/10.1111/j.1530-0277.2001.tb02261.x

Rossow I et al (2016) Does parental drinking influence children's drinking? A systematic review of prospective cohort studies. Addiction 111(2). https://doi.org/10.1111/add.13097

Rutter M (2003) Categories, dimensions, and the mental health of children and adolescents: keynote address. Ann N Y Acad Sci. https://doi.org/10.1196/annals.1301.002

Sheehan DV et al (1998) The Mini-International Neuropsychiatric Interview (M.I.N.I.): the development and validation of a structured diagnostic psychiatric interview for DSM-IV and ICD-10. J Clin Psychiatry

Squeglia LM, Gray KM (2016) Alcohol and drug use and the developing brain. Curr Psychiatry Rep. https://doi.org/10.1007/s11920-016-0689-y

Ssebunnya J et al (2020) Social acceptance of alcohol use in Uganda. BMC Psychiatry 20(1):52. https://doi.org/10.1186/s12888-020-2471-2

Stickel F et al (2017) The genetics of alcohol dependence and alcohol-related liver disease. J Hepatol. https://doi.org/10.1016/j.jhep.2016.08.011

The UNESCO Institute for Statistics (2018) One in five children, adolescents and youth is out of school - UIS fact sheet no. 48. The UNESCO Institute for Statistics (UIS)

Tian S et al (2021) Substance use and psychological distress among school-going adolescents in 41 low-income and middle-income countries. J Affect Disord 291. https://doi.org/10.1016/j.jad.2021.05.024

UNICEF (2021) COVID-19 and school closures: one year of education disruption

United Nations (2017) Progress towards the Sustainable Development Goals E/2017/66, Economic and environmental questions: sustainable development. United Nations

Verhulst B, Neale MC, Kendler KS (2015) The heritability of alcohol use disorders: a meta-analysis of twin and adoption studies. Psychol Med 45(5). https://doi.org/10.1017/S0033291714002165

Waylen A et al (2015) Alcohol use in films and adolescent alcohol use. Pediatrics 135(5). https://doi.org/10.1542/peds.2014-2978

Westermeyer J (2016) Historical and social context of psychoactive substance use disorders. Clin Textb Addict Disord:22–40

WHO (2010) Global strategy to reduce the harmful use of alcohol. World Health Organization

WHO (2017) Tackling NCDs: 'best buys' and other recommended interventions for the prevention and control of noncommunicable diseases. World Health Organization

WHO (2018a) Adolescent alcohol-related behaviours: trends and inequalities in the WHO European region, 2002–2014. World Health Organization

WHO (2018b) Global status report on alcohol and health. World Health Organization

WHO and CDC (2021) GSHS questionnaire – core questionnaire modules. Available at: https://www.who.int/teams/noncommunicable-diseases/surveillance/systems-tools/global-school-based-student-health-survey/questionnaire

Xu X, Chaloupka FJ (2011) The effects of prices on alcohol use and its consequences. Alcohol Res Health 34(2)

Alcohol Use Disorders and Neurological Illnesses

58

Lekhansh Shukla, Venkata Lakshmi Narasimha, and
Arun Kandasamy

Contents

Introduction 1249
Encephalopathies Associated with Alcohol Use 1249
  Acute Encephalopathies 1249
Neuropathies Associated with AUD 1260
  Alcohol-Related Peripheral Neuropathies 1260
  Toxic Nutritional Optic Neuropathy 1263
Movement Disorders and AUD 1264
  Cerebellar Dysfunction in AUD 1264
  Tremors and AUD 1265
  Essential Tremors and AUD 1268
Application to Other Substance Use Disorders 1269
Application to Other Areas of Public Health 1269
Mini-Dictionary of Terms 1269
Key Facts 1270
  Key Facts of Encephalopathies Associated with Alcohol Use 1270
Summary Points 1270
References 1271

Abstract

Alcohol use disorder (AUD) is associated with numerous neurological syndromes. In this chapter, we focus on conditions causing acute encephalopathy, neuropathy, and movement disorders.

L. Shukla (✉)
Centre for Addiction Medicine Office, Female Wing, NIMHANS Campus, Bangalore, India

V. L. Narasimha
Department of Psychiatry, All India Institute of Medical Sciences (AIIMS), Panchayat Training Institute, Daburgram Jasidih, Deoghar, Jharkhand, India

A. Kandasamy
Centre for Addiction Medicine, Department of Psychiatry, National Institute of Mental Health and Neurosciences, Bangalore, India

V. B. Patel, V. R. Preedy (eds.), *Handbook of Substance Misuse and Addictions*,
https://doi.org/10.1007/978-3-030-92392-1_66

A combination of nutritional deficiencies and direct neurotoxicity can lead to demyelination and neuronal apoptosis, causing acute encephalopathy. Pathophysiology, clinical features, and management of these presentations are discussed with a focus on nutritional supplementation.

A similar mechanism can lead to neuronal death in the peripheral nerves and cerebellum. This chapter discusses diagnostic workup and management of alcohol-related neuropathies and cerebellar degeneration. Finally, we discuss the clinical conundrums involved in the diagnosis and management of tremors in AUD patients.

Keywords

Alcohol use disorder · Wernicke's encephalopathy · Marchiafava-Bignami disease · Osmotic demyelination syndrome · Extra-pontine myelinolysis · Peripheral neuropathy · Toxic optic neuropathy · Nutritional optic neuropathy · Cerebellar degeneration · Alcohol withdrawal syndrome · Essential tremors

Abbreviations

AIDS	Acquired immune deficiency syndrome
AUD	Alcohol use disorders
CMAP	Compound muscle action potential
CNS	Central nervous system
CPM	Central pontine myelinolysis
CT	Computed tomography
DNA	Deoxyribonucleic acid
DWI	Diffusion-weighted imaging
EPM	Extra-pontine myelinolysis
ET	Essential tremors
GGT	Gamma-glutamyl transferase
Hz	Hertz
KGDH	Alpha-ketoglutarate dehydrogenase complex
LHON	Leber's hereditary optic neuropathy
MBD	Marchiafava-Bignami disease
MDMA	3,4-Methylenedioxymethamphetamine
mEq/L	Milliequivalents per liter
mg	Milligram
MRI	Magnetic resonance imaging
NCS	Nerve conduction study
NINDS	National Institute of Neurological Disorders and Stroke
ODS	Osmotic demyelination syndromes
PDHC	Pyruvate dehydrogenase complex
ROS	Reactive oxygen species
SNAP	Sensory nerve action potentials
SUD	Substance use disorders
TON-NON	Toxic-nutritional optic neuropathy
TPP	Thiamine pyrophosphate
WE	Wernicke's encephalopathy

Introduction

As seen in alcohol use disorders (AUD), excessive and chronic alcohol exposure is associated with numerous neurological syndromes. There are three broad mechanisms of alcohol-related neurological illnesses. First, alcohol has a direct neurotoxic effect, as seen in alcohol-related peripheral neuropathies. Second, alcohol use is associated with micronutrient deficiencies that cause neurological syndromes, for example, Wernicke's encephalopathy. Third, alcohol use is a risk factor for vascular diseases like atherosclerosis leading to stroke.

We can broadly classify neurological illnesses associated with alcohol use into encephalopathies, seizure disorders, movement disorders, neuropathies, and long-term neurocognitive sequelae of alcohol use. In this chapter, we discuss acute encephalopathies and neuropathies associated with AUD in detail.

Encephalopathies Associated with Alcohol Use

Various terms like "encephalopathy," "acute confusional state," "delirium," and "organic brain syndrome" are used interchangeably (and confusingly) to describe an altered mental state. We use this term as defined by the National Institute of Neurological Disorders and Stroke (NINDS) to denote "a diffuse disease of the brain that alters brain function or structure and has a hallmark of altered mental state." Encephalopathies can be divided into two types – acute and chronic. Acute encephalopathies develop rapidly (hours to days) and are frequently reversible, for example, post-concussion syndrome and hypoglycemic encephalopathy. On the other hand, chronic encephalopathies develop over weeks to months and are rarely wholly reversible, for example, heavy metal poisoning. Both types of encephalopathies can be seen in AUD patients. An example of chronic encephalopathy due to AUD is Korsakoff psychosis which has substantial overlap with alcohol-related dementia.

Acute Encephalopathies

By definition, a heavy bout of alcohol use produces a reversible alteration of mental state; an extreme form of the same is seen in blackouts. Similarly, delirium tremens is an apt example of acute encephalopathy. However, we wish to focus on conditions that represent a more profound alteration in brain functioning.

Wernicke's Encephalopathy

Wernicke's encephalopathy (WE) is a potentially reversible confusional state seen in patients with severe thiamine deficiency. The high-risk groups include patients undergoing starvation due to confinement, malabsorption syndromes, malignancies or anorexia nervosa, and malnourished AUD cases.

Epidemiology

The true incidence of WE is unknown as only 30–40% of cases are diagnosed premortem. Postmortem studies have shown characteristic lesions in 1–3% of adults. Regional prevalence of WE depends on dietary, socioeconomic, and cultural characteristics. In developed countries, AUD patients represent most cases of WE in recent times. Systematic studies have shown a shockingly high incidence (12.5–35%) of WE-related lesions in AUD patients (Sechi and Serra 2007; Harper et al. 1986).

Clinical Features

WE is characterized by acute onset of confusion, ataxia, and abnormalities of extraocular muscles (nystagmus or diplopia). Caine, Harper, and Halliday have shown that the complete triad is rare, and the presence of a single sign is the most common presentation (Harper et al. 1986). Therefore, a presumptive diagnosis of WE should be considered in any patient at risk of thiamine deficiency who presents with one or more of the following signs:

1. Oculomotor abnormalities like lateral rectus palsy, nystagmus, or diplopia.
2. Cerebellar dysfunction in the form of ataxia, dysmetria, or dysdiadochokinesia.
3. Altered mental state including mild memory impairment, inattention, or frank disorientation.

Furthermore, symptoms are fluctuating and transient. Thus, a high risk of suspicion is needed to diagnose.

Laboratory Investigations

Thiamine Deficiency Markers

Chemical (blood thiamine diphosphate levels) and functional (erythrocyte transketolase activity) thiamine assays have limited utility in diagnosing WE. Peripheral levels of thiamine are poorly correlated with brain levels.

Neuroimaging

Magnetic resonance imaging (MRI) is preferable over computed tomography (CT) as the aim is to find signal changes in small soft-tissue structures. Contrast-enhanced CT may reveal disruption of the blood-brain barrier in late stages. MRI typically shows symmetrically increased T2 signal in bilateral medial thalami and paraventricular region (80%), periaqueductal region (55%), mammillary bodies (40%), and tectal plate (35%) (Zuccoli and Pipitone 2009). We must note that MRI may be normal in almost half of the patients. MRI has a low sensitivity of 53% compared to the 85% sensitivity of the clinical criterion mentioned above (Sechi and Serra 2007).

In addition to the typical lesions noted above, lesions of the caudate nucleus, pons, and cerebellar nuclei may be seen in some patients. The significance of these atypical lesions is twofold. Involvement of these regions in addition to the typical brain regions portends a poor prognosis in WE. However, in the absence of typical lesions, they indicate a pathology other than thiamine deficiency.

Pathophysiology

An absolute deficiency of biologically functional thiamine in the brain is the ultimate cause of WE.

Thiamine Homeostasis

Thiamine exists in mono-, di-, and triphosphate forms. Thiamine diphosphate is called thiamine pyrophosphate (TPP) and is the storage and biologically active form. The triphosphate form may be specific to neuronal processes (Bettendorff 2014).

An adult must consume 1–2 mg of thiamine every day to maintain homeostasis. Total body stores are 30–40 mg in an adult, and thus deficiency starts developing within a fortnight of restricted intake.

Thiamine is absorbed in the duodenum and jejunum via an active process that is saturated at 1.5 mg/day. Passive diffusion can occur at doses several times higher than the usual diet, such as 100–600 mg. However, it is possible that oral absorption cannot exceed 10–20 mg per day even if both absorption mechanisms are working optimally.

Thiamine levels in the brain depend on an active transport process operating at its maximal even in normal physiological states. The daily turnover of thiamine in the brain is approximately 0.3 mg per hour per gram of brain tissue, and active transport is 0.3–0.5 mg per hour per gram. Thus, thiamine homeostasis in the brain is precarious and easily disturbed due to low intake or increased demand (Bettendorff 2014; Thomson et al. 2012).

Biological Role of Thiamine

TPP is a cofactor of pyruvate dehydrogenase complex (PDHC) and alpha-ketoglutarate dehydrogenase complex (KGDH). These enzymes are essential for aerobic respiration, and loss of their activity due to thiamine deficiency causes lactate accumulation. In the brain, there are additional effects like a deficiency of acetyl-choline reserve and synaptic accumulation of glutamate. Figure 1 shows the biochemical changes associated with thiamine deficiency in the brain.

Neuropathology

Within 3–4 days of thiamine deficiency, cytotoxic edema in neurons and proliferation of astrocytes are seen. If the deficiency persists, loss of blood-brain barrier, acidosis, and cell death set in the next 7–10 days.

For unknown reasons, certain brain regions are more susceptible to thiamine deficiency. These areas include periaqueductal and periventricular gray matter, medial nuclei of the thalamus, mammillary bodies, and tectal plate. The symptoms can be understood from the lesion site; periaqueductal gray matter is part of the reticular activating system controlling arousal and consciousness. Therefore, its dysfunction explains acute changes in mental state. Medial nuclei of the thalamus and mammillary bodies are part of the hippocampal network involved in memory

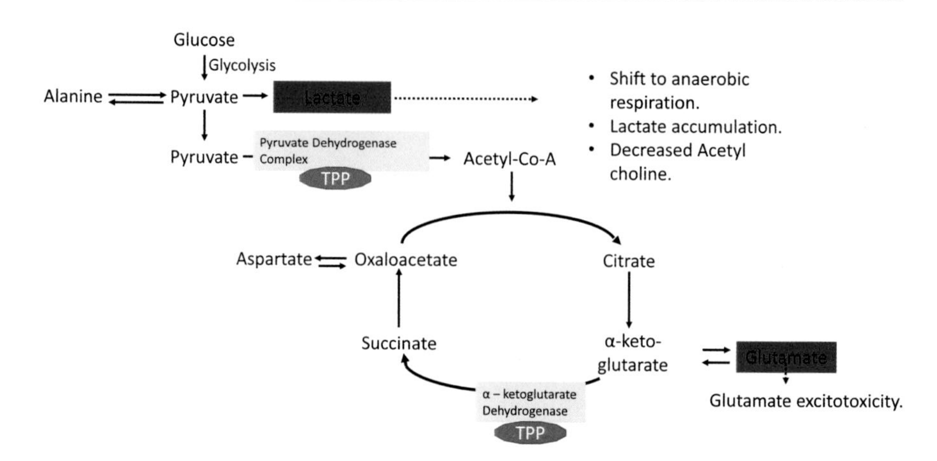

Fig. 1 Pathophysiology of Wernicke's encephalopathy. This figure shows the cellular and neurochemical consequences of thiamine pyrophosphate (TPP) deficiency in the context of Wernicke's encephalopathy

encoding, time stamping, and retrieval. Dysfunction of this network explains the sequel of WE. Finally, the tectal plate containing superior colliculi is part of the network that coordinates extraocular movements to enable fixation, gaze, and visual attention. Therefore, this site may explain the eye abnormalities seen in WE.

Natural History and Course

Even in countries with good nutritional standards, more than half of AUD admissions have severe malnutrition (Thomson et al. 2012). Thus, it is likely that patients suffer multiple episodes of WE, which remain undetected. A typical pattern is to have multiple waves of confusion and ataxia that leave behind permanent neurocognitive deficits. This "burnt-out" phase is called Korsakoff psychosis.

Periods of High Risk of WE

Periods of intercurrent illness and alcohol withdrawal present a high risk of developing WE due to the following reasons:

1. Alcohol withdrawal is a hypermetabolic state with increased brain activity. This hypermetabolic state can precipitate thiamine deficiency.
2. During withdrawal or medical treatment for any illness, the patient's food intake may increase as they are not drinking anymore. This ingestion of carbohydrates increases the cellular demand for thiamine.

Thus, it is not a coincidence that many WE episodes occur in a therapeutic context (Thomson et al. 2012).

Differences Between Alcoholic and Nonalcoholic WE

WE in hyperemesis and anorexia is fundamentally different from that seen in AUD patients.

1. AUD patients have multiple bouts of encephalopathy that leave behind a state of "quiet confusion" in their aftermath. In contrast, nonalcoholic WE presents as a single dramatic episode.
2. It is rare for nonalcoholic WE to progress into a chronic state, whereas more than 80% of untreated alcoholic WE patients progress to Korsakoff psychosis.
3. Nonalcoholic WE patients respond promptly to lower doses of thiamine given orally, whereas AUD patients require high dose intravenous therapy.

Prevention and Management of WE

Following facts are essential for the management of confirmed or presumptive diagnosis of WE:

1. Early administration of adequate doses of thiamine will prevent progression to Korsakoff psychosis, an untreatable condition with high morbidity.
2. Alcoholic WE does not respond to traditional doses of thiamine replacement (100–200 mg per day).
3. A high concentration gradient between the blood and brain is required to supply adequate thiamine using passive diffusion. An intravenous infusion most readily achieves this goal.
4. Thiamine is a nontoxic molecule that is readily excreted via urine.
5. Thiamine replacement must precede refeeding or glucose administration.

Table 1 shows the key features of the management of WE.

Table 1 Management of Wernicke's encephalopathy

Assess individual risk	Poor oral intake Losses: vomiting, diarrhea Increased demand: alcohol withdrawal, intercurrent illness, refeeding Protein energy malnutrition
Make presumptive diagnosis	Any of the above risk factors with one or more of: ataxia, eye signs, or confusion
Avoid:	Dextrose/glucose infusion
Treat with high dose vitamins	Parenteral administration of any preparation that delivers 1500 mg thiamine per day continued for at least 5 days
Consider adjunctive treatments	Consider correction of hypomagnesemia
Continue treatment	Continue parenteral administration of at least 500 mg thiamine per day if symptoms continue to improve
Continue oral supplementation in confirmed cases or patients at high risk	Oral thiamine 100 mg per day

Vitamin Supplementation

As AUD patients have multiple vitamin deficiencies, it is prudent to use a vitamin preparation that supplies folic acid, pyridoxine, and niacin also. However, there is a higher risk of adverse effects with multicomponent preparations; thus, thiamine-only preparations can be preferred for treatment beyond 5 days. Clinicians must acquaint themselves with various components of multivitamin preparations and doses required to provide 1500 mg of thiamine per day. Infusions should be given in 100 ml saline over 30 min, delivering 500 mg of thiamine. Three such infusions will be needed every day to provide 1500 mg of thiamine.

Adjunctive Treatments

Magnesium deficiency is common in AUD patients. Hypomagnesemia causes neuronal hyperexcitability and may contribute to glutamate neurotoxicity. Therefore, there is theoretical merit for magnesium supplementation in patients with confirmed WE. However, there is no evidence that it is effective in the prevention or treatment of this condition. In selected cases, magnesium supplementation can be considered after ruling out renal dysfunction and hypocalcaemia.

Prevention of Further Episodes

Education of the patient and family about nutrient deficiencies and high-risk periods may help in preventing further episodes. If alcohol use is stopped or moderated, the patient will likely absorb adequate thiamine from meals.

We prescribe oral multivitamins to all patients immaterial of their abstinence goals. Although there is no evidence that it will prevent further episodes, we believe it is helpful prevention given the minimal cost and adverse effects.

Marchiafava-Bignami Disease

Marchiafava-Bignami disease (MBD) is a poorly understood, relatively rare (compared to WE) neurological syndrome characterized by injury to the corpus callosum.

Epidemiology

MBD is a rare illness; a study in 2013 could locate a total of 153 confirmed cases in published and indexed literature, i.e., less than five cases per year (Hillbom et al. 2014). After being reported by Marchiafava and Bignami in 1903, it was believed that this illness only occurs in Italian AUD patients who consume a particular beverage. It is now known that MBD can occur with excessive alcohol use and malnutrition immaterial of geographical region or type of beverage. Furthermore, MBD can rarely occur in other conditions like cardiac carcinoma surgery, sickle cell disease, and carbon monoxide poisoning.

Clinical Features

MBD manifests as acute to subacute onset of altered mental state in combination with myriad focal neurological signs. Focal signs distinguish MBD from other causes of confusion in AUD patients like delirium tremens and WE. Pyramidal tract symptoms like paraparesis and tetraparesis, dysarthria, limb dystonias, and incontinence commonly accompany florid confusion. Furthermore, an overall obtunded state like stupor, locked-in syndrome, and dramatic ataxia similar to astasia-abasia should also alert the clinician about the possibility of MBD.

Laboratory Investigations

A definitive antemortem diagnosis cannot be made without a neuroimaging study, preferably MRI. A scan done within 3–5 days of symptom onset shows edema of corpus callosum evidenced by T2 hyperintensities involving the whole corpus callosum. In later stages, T2 hyperintensities revert to isointense signal and may progress to hypointensities due to hemosiderin deposition. Finally, in 2–3 months with cyst formation, T1 hypointensities are seen. Important points that distinguish MBD-related neuroimaging findings from other pathologies that affect corpus callosum are as follows:

1. There are no pressure effects despite edema of the corpus callosum.
2. The middle laminae are affected, leaving a rim of normal signal above and below the T2 hyperintense signal (sandwich sign).
3. The lesions do not show contrast enhancement.

Furthermore, other white matter tracts like anterior and posterior commissures and cortical white matter bundles may also show signal changes.

Pathophysiology

The exact pathophysiology of MBD is not known. Nevertheless, there is enough evidence that vitamin deficiencies, especially thiamine deficiency in patients with AUD, cause MBD. However, it is unclear why none of the reported MBD cases has MRI lesions typical of WE, which is also caused by thiamine deficiency and is much more common than MBD. Furthermore, unlike WE, no relationship with withdrawal states or refeeding has been described in MBD.

Synergism between thiamine deficiency and oxidative stress due to alcohol binge may explain MBD's widespread white matter destruction (Fernandes et al. 2017). Unlike WE, there may be an essential role of inflammation as evidenced by necrosis (as opposed to apoptosis), microbleeds, and edema.

It is interesting to note that MBD symptoms cannot be explained by necrosis of the corpus callosum. We know that congenital agenesis of corpus callosum rarely manifests any symptoms; similarly, surgical resection for epilepsy also does not produce MBD like syndrome.

Natural History and Course

Recent reports have questioned a long-held view that MBD invariably has a poor prognosis. The wider availability of MRI has allowed diagnosis of more cases with varying severity levels, whereas, earlier, mostly the diagnosis was made in autopsy.

Types of MBD Based on Prognosis

It is recently proposed that MBD can be of two types: Type A where the patient presents with profound alteration of consciousness and MRI reveals T2 signal changes involving the whole corpus callosum and Type B in which sensorium is intact and MRI shows sparing of some regions of the corpus. Follow-up has shown that Type A cases have a poor prognosis characterized by high mortality, vegetative state, or severe cognitive deficits. On the other hand, Type B cases have minimal mortality and recover with only persisting deficits characteristic of cerebral disconnection.

Management of MBD

The treatment consists of high dose multivitamin replacement. A protocol similar to WE can be used to replace vitamin B complex and folate. An additional consideration is to start corticosteroids to suppress inflammation, necrosis, and demyelination. The evidence for this strategy is only at the level of case reports. We recommend that a case by case decision be made considering the extent of corpus callosum involvement and the risks associated with steroids. It bears repeating that patients with complete corpus callosal involvement and poor sensorium have a grave prognosis, and thus, reasonably heroic measures can be argued for. Nevertheless, many of these patients are also at risk of gastrointestinal bleeding, infections, and hyperglycemia due to steroids. If corticosteroids are used, doses similar to that used in other demyelinating conditions like prednisolone 40 mg per day (or equivalent dose of other glucocorticoids) can be used.

Osmotic Demyelination Syndromes

Osmotic demyelination syndrome (ODS) refers to two distinct but frequently co-occurring syndromes – central pontine myelinolysis (CPM) and extra-pontine myelinolysis (EPM). We know that CPM is caused by rapid correction of serum sodium levels (more than 6 mEq/L correction in 24 h) in patients with chronic hyponatremia. We believe ODS deserves discussion in the context of this chapter for two reasons. First, an overwhelming majority of ODS cases (70%) are seen in AUD patients. Second, we now know that ODS can occur in AUD cases without the typical sequence of events: chronic severe hyponatremia and rapid overcorrection. Thus, clinicians caring for acutely sick AUD clients must keep the possibility of ODS in mind.

Epidemiology

ODS is a rare condition with a reported incidence of less than 1 per million years in developed countries (Aegisdottir et al. 2019). It is likely to be higher in countries where malnutrition is more common and depends on prevalent protocols for managing severe hyponatremia. However, we may never know the true incidence as premortem diagnosis requires MRI.

Clinical Features

A typically described sequence of events is as follows: A poorly nourished AUD patient develops moderate to severe hyponatremia (serum sodium less than 130, mostly less than 120 mEq/L) due to poor intake or intercurrent illness. Hyponatremia is likely chronic but with further decrease in recent days. The hyponatremia is symptomatic, causing seizures or hypoactive delirium. Therefore, the clinician is justified in promptly correcting the sodium deficit with hypertonic saline. This treatment produces an expected improvement in the clinical condition. However, in 2–5 days, severe neurological dysfunction sets in due to ODS (Martin 2004).

The symptoms range from dysarthria and spastic paresis to a locked-in state in case of CPM. Frequently, EPM co-occurs with CPM, leading to various symptoms ranging from movement disorders to psychiatric manifestations. EPM symptoms can occur in the absence of CPM symptoms also.

In summary, a biphasic course of encephalopathy in AUD patients should alert the clinician to the possibility of ODS.

Laboratory Investigations

Serial serum electrolytes and liver and renal function tests give a clear picture of a patient's risk to develop ODS. In addition to evidence of rapidly corrected hyponatremia, certain other abnormalities increase the risk of ODS. Hypokalemia, hypoalbuminemia, and evidence of free water excess in the form of abnormally low uric acid and urea point toward low reserve of osmolytes in the body and risk of ODS.

MRI gives definitive evidence of ODS but after a gap of 1–2 weeks from the onset of symptoms. Typical findings are diffusion weighted imaging (DWI) abnormalities in the first week followed by contrast non-enhancing T2 hyperintensities with T1 hypointensity in the affected regions. The location of lesions is the basis pontis in CPM and symmetrical bilateral basal ganglia and thalamus in EPM. EPM can also involve the cerebellum, geniculate bodies, cortical white matter, and hippocampus. Frequently the two coexist and are also accompanied by MRI findings typical of MBD and WE.

Pathophysiology

In summary, the inability of oligodendrocytes to rapidly reverse the compensatory changes of hyponatremia in the face of sodium correction leads to their death and demyelinating lesions (Fig. 2). Figure 2 also shows why AUD patients are particularly at risk of demyelination with less dramatic sodium abnormalities.

Natural History and Course

AUD: A Sufficient Cause of ODS

As noted earlier, the risk of ODS due to dramatic changes in serum sodium is much higher in AUD subjects than in those who do not have AUD. It is telling that the initial conceptualization of ODS by Adam was around AUD patients only. There are reasons to believe that ODS can be seen in AUD patients without a clear history of chronic hyponatremia followed by rapid correction (Chatterjee et al. 2015). We must

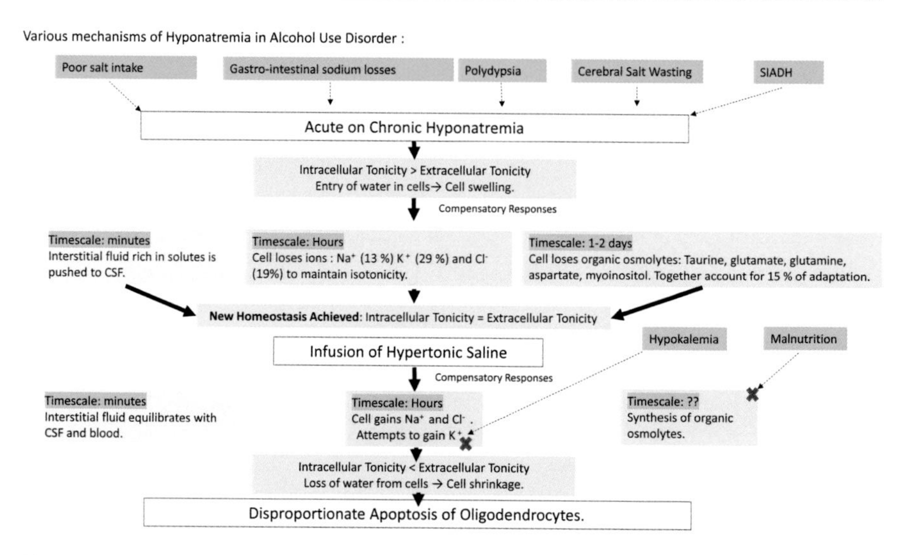

Fig. 2 Pathophysiology of osmotic demyelination in alcohol use disorders. This figure shows a schematic of sequence of events that culminate in osmotic demyelination. Cellular responses are shown in gray boxes. Note that alcohol use disorder impairs the cell's ability to gain back osmotically active ions, i.e., sodium (Na^+), chloride (Cl^-), and potassium (K^+). Most critically due to multiple vitamin deficiencies, cells fail to secrete organic osmolytes, indicated by an unknown timeline for this step

remember that ethanol is osmotically active, and there are substantial changes in serum osmolality and sodium concentrations during binge drinking (Ogata et al. 1968).

ODS and Therapeutic Nihilism

We must dispel the notion that the prognosis of ODS is uniformly poor. Furthermore, the site or extent of demyelination is not a reliable enough prognostic factor (Martin 2004). Therefore, supportive care allowing an adequate duration during which recovery can be observed is necessary.

Nevertheless, ODS can lead to brain death or locked-in state in up to 10% of cases and may leave lasting disabilities in another 20% of cases.

Treatment and Prevention

Admittedly, treating an AUD patient with moderate to severe hyponatremia and symptoms like seizures or coma is delicate. Damned if you do, damned if you do not! A detailed discussion of safe correction of chronic hyponatremia is beyond the scope of this chapter. However, we summarize some fundamental principles concerning AUD patients:

1. Prevention is the key: Clinician must run a risk stratification, adding one point each for AUD, underweight, thiamine deficiency, hypokalemia, hypocalcemia,

hypophosphatemia, and hypoalbuminemia. The higher the number of risk factors, the more brittle is patient's osmotic homeostasis is.

2. Optimize overall metabolic state: Hypokalemia must always be corrected before correcting hyponatremia. Thiamine supplementation at doses for WE should also be started. Hypocalcemia, hypomagnesemia, and hypophosphatemia can be corrected concurrently or immediately after starting correction of sodium deficit.
3. Expect overcorrection: Hypovolemia due to fluid loss or redistribution is a maintaining factor for hyponatremia in most cases. Therefore, even isotonic saline and ringer lactate will produce brisk water diuresis, and the correction will overshoot the expected levels.
4. Be conservative with correction: The clinician must aim to convert severe hyponatremia to moderate hyponatremia and moderate to mild rather than complete correction. In any case, the correction rate must not exceed six to eight points in 24 h.
5. Reactive strategies: If the rate of correction exceeds safe limits, an intensivist must be involved. Depending on the case, available options are an infusion of dextrose or desmopressin administration to lower the serum sodium.

A Note on the Overlap Between Causes of Acute Encephalopathies in AUD

Although we study syndromes of acute encephalopathy in AUD as separate entities, we must not ignore the substantial overlap between them. This overlap is at all levels – risk factors, pathophysiology, clinical presentation, and treatment.

It is difficult to miss how nutritional risk factors, alcohol's direct effects on the brain, and allostatic stress due to an illness or alcohol withdrawal together cause neurological emergencies. Figure 3 shows the interplay between these factors.

In summary, multiple nutritional deficiencies compromise two critical cellular pathways – the three-carbon cycle (Krebs cycle) and the one-carbon cycle. The effect of the first perturbation is decreased energy production and therefore decreased ability of the cell to maintain its size and homeostasis. Decreased one-carbon cycle reactions limit the cells' ability to regulate gene expression in response to stressors. Furthermore, the synthesis of glycine, serine, methionine, and glutamate decreases. These osmotically active molecules need to be synthesized when there is an increase in serum osmolality to prevent the movement of water to the interstitial compartment. Also, these molecules are starting substrates for glutathione which is an essential defense against reactive oxygen species (ROS).

To make matters worse, acetaldehyde is produced by the local metabolism of alcohol by neuronal tissue. This oxidation step uses already scarce reduced substrates and generates acetaldehyde which induces enzymes that themselves generate reactive oxygen species (ROS). ROS can lead to DNA fragmentation triggering apoptosis or can cause lipid peroxidation.

Simplistically, if lipid damage dominates, demyelination is the predominant pathology (as in MBD and ODS), whereas apoptosis in particular regions is seen in WE.

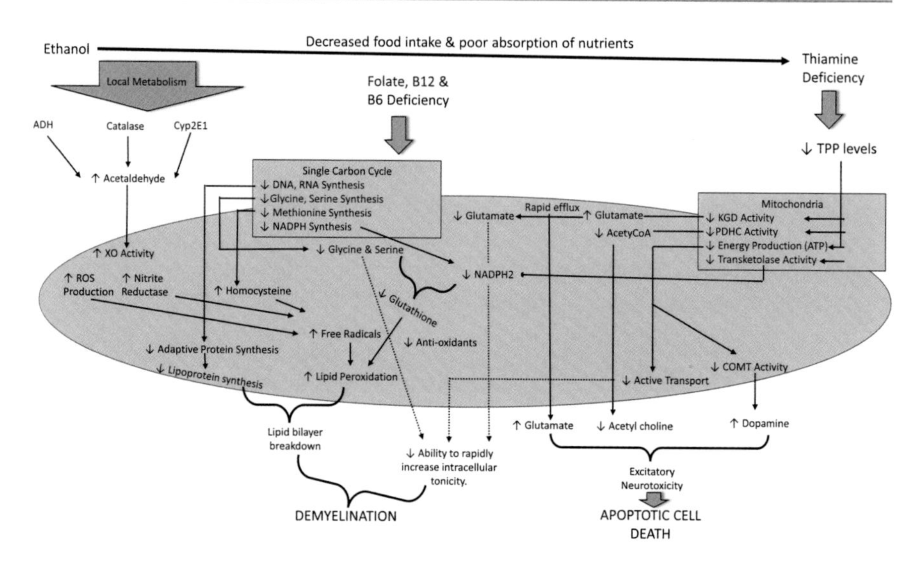

Fig. 3 Shared pathophysiology of acute encephalopathies in alcohol use disorder. This figure shows how the interaction between nutritional deficiencies and excessive alcohol use affects Krebs and one-carbon cycles, causing demyelination and cell death. ADH = alcohol dehydrogenase; Cyp2E1 = cytochrome-P 2E1; TPP = thiamine pyrophosphate; NADPH = nicotinamide adenine dinucleotide phosphate; KGD = keto-glutarate dehydrogenase; PDHC = pyruvate dehydrogenase complex; XO = xanthine oxidase; ROS = reactive oxygen species; COMT – catechol-O-methyltransferase

Neuropathies Associated with AUD

Although alcohol is considered a risk factor for optic neuropathy, an overwhelming majority of "alcohol-induced neuropathies" are peripheral neuropathies.

Alcohol-Related Peripheral Neuropathies

Epidemiology

One-third to half of treatment-seeking AUD patients have clinical symptoms of peripheral neuropathy. If a nerve conduction study (NCS) is used for diagnosis, 35–60% of AUD patients are expected to have peripheral neuropathy (Julian et al. 2018). We suspect that the actual prevalence of neuropathy in AUD patients may be higher than these figures for two reasons. First, approximately one-third of patients may have small fiber neuropathy, which is not detected by NCS (Zambelis et al. 2005). Second, a substantial minority of patients may have isolated autonomic neuropathy that can only be detected with autonomic function tests (Nicolosi et al. 2005). In summary, a conservative estimate is to expect every second patient with chronic AUD also to have peripheral neuropathy.

The total lifetime dose of ethanol is the strongest predictor of neuropathy in AUD patients. Middle-aged AUD patients with a history of daily heavy drinking constitute the majority of cases. Poor nutritional status is a decisive additive risk factor, with two caveats. First, peripheral neuropathy in the absence of any demonstrable nutrient deficiency is well known. Second, there is no consensus about the specific deficiencies that increase the risk of peripheral neuropathy in AUD patients.

Lastly, genetic predisposition to slower clearance of acetaldehyde is also implicated as a risk factor.

Clinical Features

The classically described presentation is of insidious onset, slowly progressive paraesthesia of the lower limbs. Patients describe it as tingling and numbness of soles and edges of the feet. The lower limbs are invariably affected first and remain affected more than the upper limbs. In the initial stages, loss of vibratory sensation may be the only objective finding. However, there are substantial variations to this clinical picture:

1. Superimposed thiamine deficiency can make the onset subacute or acute and cause marked motor deficits (Koike et al. 2003).
2. In our experience, allodynia, electric shock-like sensations, and other painful symptoms are prominent in many patients.
3. A substantial minority of patients have absent ankle and knee-deep tendon reflexes at the time of initial assessment.
4. In long-standing cases, it is common to find autonomic function abnormalities like hyperhidrosis, hyperemia, claudication, and trophic skin changes.

Laboratory Investigations

Nerve Conduction Studies and Electromyography

The typical NCS findings are as follows:

1. More abnormalities in the lower limbs (sural and tibial nerve) than upper limbs (median and radial).
2. Sensory nerves are more frequently involved than motor nerves.
3. Axonopathy pattern as evidenced by reduced amplitudes.

So, the expected findings are the reduced sensory nerve action potentials (SNAP) of the sural nerve and reduced compound muscle action potential (CMAP) of the tibial nerve. Electromyography shows decreased recruitment of motor units in early cases and typical findings of denervation like fibrillation in advanced cases.

There are numerous exceptions to this pattern. Most importantly, NCS may be completely normal in patients who have a small fiber neuropathy. Also, vitamin B12 deficiency can confuse the findings by producing a demyelinating pattern in severe cases.

Nerve Biopsy

In a patient with asymmetric, patchy paraesthesias and numbness, a punch biopsy of the skin is needed to diagnose small fiber neuropathy. Reduced density of epidermal nerve fibers and denervation of sweat glands are the hallmark findings.

Other Investigations

It is crucial to establish micronutrient deficiencies in patients with alcohol-related neuropathy. However, there is no evidence to recommend a battery of tests likely to yield actionable information. Nevertheless, serum folate, vitamin B12, and homocysteine should be considered if available.

Pathophysiology

The exact mechanisms by which alcohol causes axonal injury and neuronal death are not known. However, a clinician must keep the following pathways in mind:

1. Thiamine, folic acid, niacin, and vitamin B12 deficiency have a prominent role in alcohol-related neuropathies. However, we must note that the clinical features may not conform to the typical syndromes associated with these vitamins like dry beri-beri or subacute combined degeneration.
2. In general, inflammation or autoimmunity does not play a key role in alcohol-related neuropathies.
3. Oxidative stress due to acetaldehyde is a significant contributor.

Natural History and Course

The long-term course of alcohol neuropathy is not well-studied. Treatment outcome research (Julian et al. 2018) and our experience with patients allow drawing the following generalizations:

1. In cases with acute onset and short course, abstinence and parenteral multivitamins produce a rapid improvement (within 1–2 weeks).
2. There is some improvement in all patients who maintain abstinence and receive oral multivitamins, but this improvement occurs slowly over 3–6 months.
3. Fixed sensory or motor deficits rarely improve completely; however, subjective distress may decrease.
4. We have seen a slow but steady progression of paraesthesias with involvement of the upper limbs; however, we have never seen motor deficits in the upper limbs, even with continued alcohol use.
5. In our experience, we have not seen relentless progression despite abstinence, and such a course should prompt a workup for other neuropathy causes.

Management of Alcohol-Related Peripheral Neuropathy

Abstinence from alcohol is the primary strategy to prevent further worsening of neuropathic symptoms.

There is good quality evidence that supplementing vitamin B complex and folic acid improves symptoms and objective signs of neuropathy.

Therefore, oral supplements that provide thiamine, vitamin B12, pyridoxine, niacin, and folic acid should be given to all patients. There is no evidence that costly preparations like benfotiamine are superior to generic vitamin supplements.

Standard treatment strategies for neuropathies, including physical rehabilitation, pain management, and control of blood sugars, should be used. Dysesthesias and pain should be promptly treated as chronic pain conditions adversely affect the chances of sustained abstinence. Gabapentin is a particularly suitable choice as it is effective in neuropathic pain and can work as an anti-craving agent in AUD (Anton et al. 2020). Duloxetine can also be used, but it can cause tachycardia and tremors at effective doses. AUD patients have considerable anxiety due to protracted alcohol withdrawal and do not tolerate these side effects well.

Toxic Nutritional Optic Neuropathy

We are mindful that optic neuropathy in patients who drink and smoke excessively is a hotly debated entity. At different times the same clinical syndrome has been called toxic amblyopia, alcohol-tobacco optic neuropathy, and toxic-nutritional optic neuropathy (TON-NON). We discuss this scenario only to highlight some pragmatic considerations.

Clinical Features

Progressive, symmetrical, and painless loss of vision is the expected clinical picture in TON-NON. Loss of visual acuity is preceded by dyschromatopsia, i.e., change in the hue and saturation of colors. Distinctively, peripheral vision is relatively preserved (Grzybowski et al. 2015).

Tobacco: Ethanol Exposure Is Not "Sufficient Cause" for Optic Neuropathy

While some patients who smoke and heavily drink develop a characteristic optic neuropathy, it is essential to realize that "tobacco-alcohol amblyopia" is not an accepted entity anymore (Grzybowski et al. 2015). It is now known that such cases represent an interaction of genetic and environmental factors that causes optic neuropathies. For example, Leber hereditary optic neuropathy [LHON] can interact with environmental toxins like alcohol or nutritional deficiencies to precipitate blindness (Kirkman et al. 2009).

Therefore, it is vital to offer the same workup for optic neuropathy to AUD patients as would be offered to those who do not consume alcohol.

Nutritional Aspects Must Be Addressed

More often than not, deficiency of vitamins B12, thiamine, niacin, riboflavin, and folic acid plays an essential role in TON-NON. Therefore, multivitamin supplementation similar to that in peripheral neuropathy must be given.

Movement Disorders and AUD

Cerebellar Dysfunction in AUD

Alcohol use causes acute, reversible cerebellar dysfunction manifesting as ataxia (drunken gait), slurring of speech, and swaying. However, our focus of discussion is cerebellar dysfunction seen in chronic AUD patients, which is not explained by acute drunkenness.

Epidemiology

The exact prevalence of cerebellar symptoms in AUD patients is not known. Although 20–30% of AUD patients who have been consuming five or more drinks for 10 or more years have cerebellar atrophy, only half of them have clinical symptoms. A conservative estimate is that 10–15% of chronic AUD patients have ataxia (Del Brutto et al. 2016). The risk factors in the order of importance are individual susceptibility, duration of regular drinking, malnutrition, and amount of drinking.

Individual susceptibility plays such a dominant role that patients who developed cerebellar dysfunction with 5 grams ethanol use have been reported (Setta et al. 1998).

Patients with severe thiamine due to causes other than AUD have a cerebellar syndrome indistinguishable from that seen in AUD. Furthermore, repeated episodes of WE can leave behind chronic cerebellar dysfunction. Therefore, malnutrition, especially thiamine deficiency, may be the proximal cause of cerebellar degeneration in AUD.

Pathophysiology and Clinical Features

Chronic alcohol use leads to selective atrophy of midline parts of the cerebellum, specifically the anterior vermis. Autopsy studies have shown loss of Purkinje and molecular cell layers with relative sparing of white matter tracts. Due to the similarity with WE, thiamine deficiency and direct neurotoxicity are speculated to cause cell death. It bears repeating that clinical symptoms do not necessarily accompany atrophy visible in MRI/CT. However, in patients with the cerebellar syndrome, there is always some degree of atrophy visible on imaging.

Patients usually present with slowly progressive (months to years) symptoms of self-perceived gait imbalance. This unsteadiness is followed by a wide-based stance, swaying while walking, a 3-hertz leg tremor, and truncal ataxia that can appear like head bobbing and titubation. Objective examination shows a dramatic imbalance in tandem walking and dysmetria, affecting the lower limbs more than upper limbs (knee shin test). Since cerebellar hemispheres are minimally affected, it is rare to find scanning speech, dysdiadochokinesia, or spontaneous nystagmus.

Natural Course and Outcome

As described above, cerebellar dysfunction in AUD is slowly progressive, and an acute onset should prompt a workup for posterior circulation stroke. However, it is common to have acute worsening during periods of stress like illness, alcohol withdrawal, or exposure to antiepileptics.

Although some authors have reported the onset of cerebellar syndrome in AUD patients who have remained abstinent, such a course is rare. In most cases, there is a very gradual but unmistakable improvement in postural stability with abstinence. The improvement is most marked and sustained with long-term abstinence (18–24 months) (Smith and Fein 2011). There is little literature on the course of illness if abstinence is not achieved. In our experience, the deficits become fixed and can be severe enough to preclude ambulation in some patients.

Treatment

Alcohol abstinence and vitamin supplementation are the main treatments for AUD-related cerebellar degeneration. It is essential to realize that cerebellar lesions seen in these patients are indistinguishable from those seen in WE; thus, similar parenteral doses of multivitamins should be tried for initial treatment. Gait rehabilitation can improve the quality of life of these patients.

Tremors and AUD

Tremors are a common complaint in AUD patients, seen in patients who are drinking and those who have achieved abstinence. We discuss this topic for two reasons. First, it is common to see all sorts of tremors being ascribed to alcohol withdrawal, depriving the patient of a good diagnostic workup. Second, alcohol has a salutary effect on many types of tremors, and therefore patients with these kinds of tremors may feel compelled to drink to make themselves steady.

Clinical Approach to an AUD Patient with Tremors

Tremor is defined as a rhythmic, oscillatory, and involuntary movement of a body part. While it is not our intention to discuss the evaluation of tremors in general, it is essential to review the classification of tremors before discussing differential diagnosis in AUD patients. Figure 4 shows how to classify tremors.

For an accurate etiological diagnosis, it is vital to collect the following information in AUD patients who are being evaluated for tremors:

1. Onset and course with respect to alcohol use disorder.
2. Acute effects of alcohol on tremors.
3. Objective tests for quantity and frequency of alcohol consumption like carbohydrate-deficient transferrin and gamma-glutamyl transferase (GGT).
4. Family history of tremors.
5. A physical examination to identify signs of other neurological and systemic illnesses that can cause tremors, for example, thyroid and liver dysfunction.

Alcohol Withdrawal Tremors

The most common cause of tremors in AUD patients is alcohol withdrawal. However, alcohol withdrawal is also the most common erroneous diagnosis given for tremors in AUD. Therefore, we must know what is and what is not withdrawal tremor.

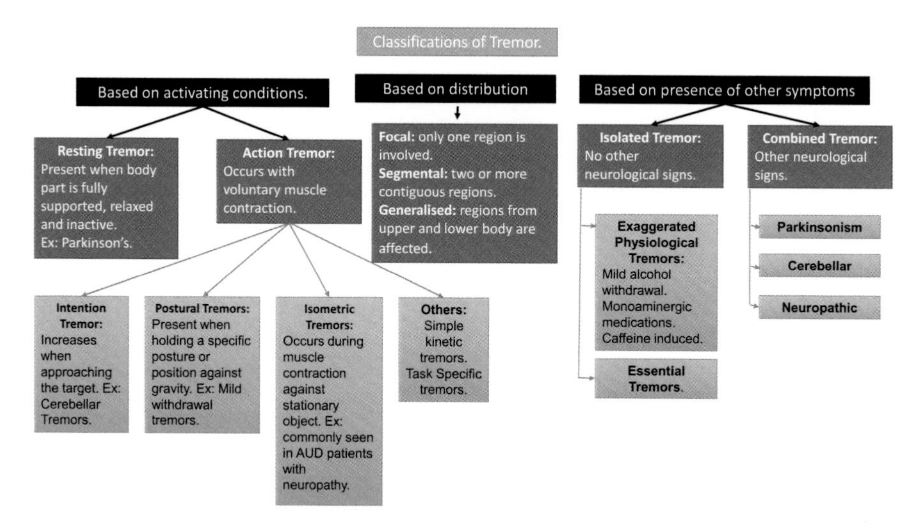

Fig. 4 Clinical classification of tremors

Alcohol Withdrawal Tremors: A Type of Exaggerated Physiological Tremors

Low amplitude, high frequency (above 8 Hz) postural tremors are seen in everyone to varying degrees and are thus called physiological tremors. Adrenergic receptors on muscle fibers significantly contribute to physiological tremors (Deuschl et al. 2001). Stimuli that increase adrenergic activity exaggerate these tremors. These conditions include anxiety, monoaminergic drugs (antidepressants), adrenergic medicines (bronchodilators), hypoglycemia, and alcohol withdrawal syndrome. In summary, we must note that alcohol withdrawal tremors are a manifestation of increased sympathetic activity characteristic of acute alcohol withdrawal. Therefore, it must be accompanied by other markers of increased sympathetic activity like tachycardia and must not last beyond 10–14 days.

Evolution and Course

The evolution and course must be accessed along two axes. First is the appearance and progression of reversible tremors after years of heavy drinking. Second is the evolution of tremors during an acute alcohol withdrawal episode.

Most patients report that they have known for years that they develop tremors when they do not drink. This realization starts as tremors after a heavy binge, which is dismissed as "hangover." It is clear to most patients who take an eye-opener drink that they will have incapacitating tremors if they miss it. With the progression of AUD, patients also notice that tremor has generalized to include almost the whole body except voice.

In an episode of alcohol withdrawal, observable tremors of outstretched hands begin within 8–12 h of the last drink. Depending on the severity and duration of AUD, tremors worsen to include the whole body in the next 24–36 h. Generalized tremulousness is a hallmark of impending delirium tremens. By definition, alcohol withdrawal tremors must improve substantially in 3–4 days and disappear in a week of sustained abstinence.

Clinical Features Suggesting Other Etiologies

The following clinical features must deter a clinician from making a confident diagnosis of alcohol withdrawal tremors:

1. Onset before or within 1–2 years of regular alcohol use. These patients may have tremors due to other etiologies.
2. Tremors that occur in the absence of other signs of alcohol withdrawal like insomnia and tachycardia.
3. Alcohol withdrawal does not cause resting or intention tremors. In patients with chronic severe AUD, there may be multiple types of tremors during acute withdrawal. However, an attempt must be made to rule out parkinsonism and cerebellar syndromes in patients with resting or intention tremors.
4. Alcohol withdrawal tremors do not persist beyond a week to 10 days of alcohol abstinence. Possibilities include ongoing alcohol use, cerebellar degeneration, anxiety disorders, and essential tremors.

Treatment of Alcohol Withdrawal Tremors

Benzodiazepines are the mainstay of treating alcohol withdrawal syndrome. Alcohol withdrawal tremors respond well to benzodiazepines, and no additional treatment is required for them.

Other Alcohol-Related Etiologies Causing Tremors

Table 2 lists some of the etiologies that can lead to tremors in AUD patients.

Table 2 Alcohol-related etiologies of tremors[a]

	Description of tremors	Possible etiologies
1.	Intention tremors with ataxia	Cerebellar degeneration
2.	Postural tremors in the legs with loss of vibration sense	Peripheral neuropathy
3.	Isometric tremors that appear with minimal resistance. The patient may complain of tremors when getting up from a squatting posture or while lifting moderately heavy objects	Myopathy
4.	Low frequency (less than 4 hertz), large-amplitude postural tremor of the upper limbs that worsens with action. These tremors are known as rubral/midbrain/Holmes tremors	Past midbrain lesions due to Wernicke's encephalopathy or osmotic demyelination
5.	Action myoclonus and asterixis (not a tremor in strict sense)	Alcoholic liver disease

[a]Withdrawal tremors are the most common etiology and have been discussed in text

Persistent Exaggerated Physiological Tremors in Detoxified AUD Patients

A sizeable minority of AUD patients continue to have postural tremors despite months of abstinence. The phenomenology of these tremors resembles exaggerated physiological tremors. However, the tremors in these cases are of a lower frequency (less than 8 hertz) and larger amplitude. This condition has been recognized for a long time but subsumed under withdrawal tremors (Koller et al. 1985).

Undiagnosed essential tremors, anxiety disorders, thyrotoxicosis, and ongoing alcohol use may explain tremors in most of these patients. However, if no explanation is found, a trial of sustained-release propranolol (40–160 mg per day) should be considered.

Essential Tremors and AUD

Essential tremors (ET) is the most common cause of action tremors, with a prevalence of 1% in the general population and 5% in adults above 60 years of age. ET has a strong genetic component but also occurs sporadically. In patients who have an onset before 40 years of age, family history is present in 80%.

The usual course is the onset of postural tremors of the hands in the third decade of life, with a gradual increase in amplitude and generalization to the head and voice over the next two decades. Conditions that increase adrenergic tonc like anxiety, hypoglycemia, exhaustion, and alcohol withdrawal worsen ET. We note that ET is not a benign condition; it causes substantial disability. In the late stages, the tremors resemble intention tremors seen in cerebellar degeneration and interfere with writing and other activities.

There is a dramatic decrease in the amplitude of tremors in ET patients when they consume alcohol. Alcohol is superior to propranolol for temporary suppression of ET (Hess and Saunders-Pullman 2006). However, there is a rapid development of tolerance and rebound worsening as blood alcohol levels fall. There is some evidence that patients with ET are likely to drink more frequently than the general population.

More importantly, it is virtually impossible to distinguish alcohol withdrawal tremors from ET without careful longitudinal assessments. Consider this; most AUD patients report the onset of regular heavy drinking in the second decade, and withdrawal tremors start in 5–10 years, i.e., in the third decade. By definition, withdrawal tremors improve dramatically with alcohol use and worsen with stress. Furthermore, both alcohol withdrawal tremors and ET respond to propranolol and benzodiazepines. In the absence of family history, it is impossible to distinguish such a patient from a patient suffering from ET and AUD. Therefore, ET must be considered a differential diagnosis for persistent exaggerated physiological tremors in AUD patients who have undergone detoxification.

Propranolol and primidone are effective treatments for ET. In AUD patients with comorbid ET, gabapentin and topiramate can be considered as anti-craving agents. Both these agents have evidence of efficacy in AUD as well as ET.

Application to Other Substance Use Disorders

Some of the neurological conditions discussed in this chapter are also relevant to other substance use disorders (SUD). Theoretically, nutritional encephalopathies can occur in patients who have poor intake due to any SUD. For example, WE has been reported in stimulant use disorder patients (Sukop et al. 2016). Similarly, ODS is a concern when treating MDMA (ecstasy)-induced hyponatremia. ODS has also been reported in stimulant users, which may be due to direct toxicity to oligodendrocytes (Baker et al. 2021).

Finally, tremors are seen in withdrawal syndromes of all CNS depressants like sedatives, solvents, opioids, and gamma-aminobutyric acid. CNS hyperexcitability and sympathetic overactivity are common to all these withdrawal syndromes. Therefore, tremors in these conditions can also be understood as an exaggeration of physiological tremors. Unsurprisingly, the treatment of tremors in these conditions is the same as in alcohol withdrawal – benzodiazepines and beta-blockers.

Application to Other Areas of Public Health

It is evident that most of the AUD-related neurological complications discussed in this chapter are largely due to malnutrition. This realization has three main implications.

First, clinicians who work with economically disadvantaged populations are likely to see these syndromes more frequently than clinicians working in better-off neighborhoods. On a global scale, these conditions are more common in underdeveloped and developing countries. Nevertheless, clinicians must be made aware of these conditions. Even doctors working with well-nourished populations are likely to see cases of gross undernutrition in situations of mass migration, disasters, and patients with cancer, AIDS, and anorexia nervosa.

Second, nutritional counseling and vitamin supplementation are crucial secondary prevention strategies in AUD patients. We urge the clinician to take a step further and consider vitamin supplementation as a harm reduction measure even for patients who do not seek abstinence.

Finally, we believe a rational discussion about the fortification of alcoholic beverages with vitamins is essential. On the one hand, there is a concern about public messaging when vitamins are added to a harmful edible product. On the other hand, there will be a substantial decrease in most AUD-related neurological complications if alcoholic beverages contain vitamins.

Mini-Dictionary of Terms

1. Alcohol use disorder (AUD) refers to a psychiatric syndrome seen in patients with regular and excessive alcohol consumption. Cardinal symptoms of AUD include the inability to control the quantity and frequency of drinking, irresistible urge to drink, and characteristic withdrawal symptoms if alcohol is not used.

2. Encephalopathy is an umbrella term to describe patients who present with confusion. Careful evaluation of these patients reveals abnormalities in arousal, i.e., patient may be too excited or hypoactive and drowsy. These patients also cannot orient themselves to time and place.
3. Neuropathy is an umbrella term to describe various symptoms and pathological findings seen in patients with injury to the nerves. Neuropathy can involve the nerves that supply the eyes, ears, and facial region, nerves that supply the limbs and trunk, and nerves that control involuntary functions like sweating and blood pressure.
4. Dysmetria: inability to judge the correct range and distance of a motion. This deficit manifests as clumsy and overshooting movements.
5. Dysdiadochokinesia: inability to perform rapidly alternating movements.

Key Facts

Key Facts of Encephalopathies Associated with Alcohol Use

1. Wernicke's encephalopathy has an incidence of 12–35% in AUD patients; it commonly remains undiagnosed.
2. High dose thiamine (1500 mg per day) should be provided parenterally to all AUD patients at risk of Wernicke's encephalopathy.
3. Marchiafava-Bignami disease can occur with excessive alcohol use and malnutrition immaterial of geographical region or type of alcoholic beverage.
4. AUD patients are at high risk of osmotic demyelination syndrome.

Summary Points

1. Acute encephalopathy in AUD patients can be due to Wernicke's encephalopathy, Marchiafava-Bignami disease, and osmotic demyelination syndrome.
2. Vitamin B and folic acid deficiencies play an essential role in causing these encephalopathies.
3. Alcohol-related peripheral neuropathy can present in various patterns. A typical pattern is of a gradually progressive, length-dependent, predominantly sensory axonopathy.
4. Excessive alcohol use should not be considered a sufficient explanation for optic neuropathy. Most of these patients have nutritional or genetic causes, and alcohol use is one of the contributing factors.
5. Alcohol-related cerebellar degeneration preferentially affects the anterior vermis and is gradually progressive.
6. Unlike other neurological complications of AUD, cerebellar degeneration has a poor correlation with the amount of drinking. It is more strongly linked to the duration of alcohol use and individual susceptibility.

7. Alcohol withdrawal is the most common etiology of tremors in AUD patients. However, a careful assessment is needed if tremors persist beyond the usual duration of withdrawal syndrome.
8. Essential tremors and AUD have a bidirectional relationship. Essential tremors may explain the persistence of postural tremors in detoxified AUD patients.

References

Aegisdottir H, Cooray C, Wirdefeldt K, Piehl F, Sveinsson O (2019) Incidence of osmotic demyelination syndrome in Sweden: a nationwide study. Acta Neurol Scand 140:342–349

Anton RF, Latham P, Voronin K, Book S, Hoffman M, Prisciandaro J, Bristol E (2020) Efficacy of Gabapentin for the treatment of alcohol use disorder in patients with alcohol withdrawal symptoms: a randomized clinical trial. JAMA Intern Med 180:728–736

Baker S, Oster J, Liu A (2021) Central pontine myelinolysis in a patient with methamphetamine abuse. Brain, Behav, Immun – Health 10:100166

Bettendorff L (2014) Thiamine. In: Janos Zempleni JWS, Gregory JF, Stover PJ (eds) Handbook of vitamins, 5th edn. CRC Press, Boca Raton

Chatterjee K, Fernandes AB, Goyal S, Shanker S (2015) Central pontine myelinolysis in a case of alcohol dependence syndrome. Ind Psychiatry J 24:198–201

Del Brutto OH, Mera RM, Sullivan LJ, Zambrano M, King NR (2016) Population-based study of alcoholic cerebellar degeneration: the Atahualpa Project. J Neurol Sci 367:356–360

Deuschl G, Raethjen J, Lindemann M, Krack P (2001) The pathophysiology of tremor. Muscle Nerve 24:716–735

Fernandes LMP, Bezerra FR, Monteiro MC, Silva ML, De Oliveira FR, Lima RR, Fontes-Júnior EA, Maia CSF (2017) Thiamine deficiency, oxidative metabolic pathways and ethanol-induced neurotoxicity: how poor nutrition contributes to the alcoholic syndrome, as Marchiafava-Bignami disease. Eur J Clin Nutr 71:580–586

Grzybowski A, Zülsdorff M, Wilhelm H, Tonagel F (2015) Toxic optic neuropathies: an updated review. Acta Ophthalmol 93:402–410

Harper CG, Giles M, Finlay-Jones R (1986) Clinical signs in the Wernicke-Korsakoff complex: a retrospective analysis of 131 cases diagnosed at necropsy. J Neurol Neurosurg Psychiatry 49: 341–345

Hess CW, Saunders-Pullman R (2006) Review: movement disorders and alcohol misuse. Addict Biol 11:117–125

Hillbom M, Saloheimo P, Fujioka S, Wszolek ZK, Juvela S, Leone MA (2014) Diagnosis and management of Marchiafava-Bignami disease: a review of CT/MRI confirmed cases. J Neurol Neurosurg Psychiatry 85:168–173

Julian T, Glascow N, Syeed R, Zis P (2018) Alcohol-related peripheral neuropathy: a systematic review and meta-analysis. J Neurol 2019 Dec;266(12):2907–2919. https://doi.org/10.1007/s00415-018-9123-1. Epub 2018 Nov 22. PMID: 30467601; PMCID: PMC6851213.

Kirkman MA, Yu-Wai-Man P, Korsten A, Leonhardt M, Dimitriadis K, De Coo IF, Klopstock T, Chinnery PF (2009) Gene-environment interactions in Leber hereditary optic neuropathy. Brain J Neurol 132:2317–2326

Koike H, Iijima M, Sugiura M, Mori K, Hattori N, Ito H, Hirayama M, Sobue G (2003) Alcoholic neuropathy is clinicopathologically distinct from thiamine-deficiency neuropathy. Ann Neurol 54:19–29

Koller W, O'Hara R, Dorus W, Bauer J (1985) Tremor in chronic alcoholism. Neurology 35: 1660–1662

Martin RJ (2004) Central pontine and extrapontine myelinolysis: the osmotic demyelination syndromes. J Neurol Neurosurg Psychiatry 75:iii22–iii28

Nicolosi C, Di Leo R, Girlanda P, Messina C, Vita G (2005) Is there a relationship between somatic and autonomic neuropathies in chronic alcoholics? J Neurol Sci 228:15–19

Ogata M, Mendelson JH, Mello NK (1968) Electrolyte and osmolality in alcoholics during experimentally induced intoxication. Psychosom Med 30:463–488

Sechi G, Serra A (2007) Wernicke's encephalopathy: new clinical settings and recent advances in diagnosis and management. Lancet Neurol 6:442–455

Setta F, Jacquy J, Hildebrand J, Manto MU (1998) Ataxia induced by small amounts of alcohol. J Neurol Neurosurg Psychiatry 65:370

Smith S, Fein G (2011) Persistent but less severe ataxia in long-term versus short-term abstinent alcoholic men and women: a cross-sectional analysis. Alcohol Clin Exp Res 35:2184–2192

Sukop PH, Kessler FH, Valerio AG, Escobar M, Castro M, Diemen LV (2016) Wernicke's encephalopathy in crack-cocaine addiction. Med Hypotheses 89:68–71

Thomson AD, Guerrini I, Marshall EJ (2012) The evolution and treatment of Korsakoff's syndrome: out of sight, out of mind? Neuropsychol Rev 22:81–92

Zambelis T, Karandreas N, Tzavellas E, Kokotis P, Liappas J (2005) Large and small fiber neuropathy in chronic alcohol-dependent subjects. J Peripher Nerv Syst 10:375–381

Zuccoli G, Pipitone N (2009) Neuroimaging findings in acute Wernicke's encephalopathy: review of the literature. AJR Am J Roentgenol 192:501–508

Alcohol and Brain-Derived Neurotrophic Factor (BDNF) 59

Candelaria Martín-González, Emilio González-Arnay,
Camino María Fernández-Rodríguez, Alen García-Rodríguez, and
Emilio González-Reimers

Contents

Introduction ... 1275
The Molecule ... 1276
Metabolic Effects ... 1287
Metabolic Effects of BDNF on Neurons ... 1287
Systemic Metabolic Effects of BDNF ... 1288
Applications to Other Areas of Addiction ... 1289
Application to Other Areas of Public Health ... 1291
Mini-Dictionary of Terms ... 1292
Key Facts of Inflammation and BDNF ... 1293
Summary Points ... 1294
References ... 1294

Abstract

Brain-derived neurotrophic factor (BDNF) is a neurotrophin, heavily involved in hippocampal neurogenesis, dendritogenesis, synaptogenesis, and synaptic plasticity and stability, therefore playing a key role in learning process and memory formation. These effects depend on the mature form of the molecule that binds to the TRKB receptor. The pro-molecule, which contains both the mature form and the BDNF prodomain, induces apoptosis and long-term depression after binding to the p75 NTR receptor. Mature BDNF plays major roles in addiction, increasing after acute slight to moderate drinking, but exerting a regulatory effect on alcohol

C. Martín-González (✉) · C. M. Fernández-Rodríguez · A. García-Rodríguez ·
E. González-Reimers
Servicio de Medicina Interna, Universidad de La Laguna. Hospital Universitario de Canarias, Canary Islands, Spain
e-mail: mmartgon@ull.edu.es; egonrey@ull.edu.es

E. González-Arnay
Departamento de Ciencias Básicas, Sección de Anatomía, Universidad de La Laguna, Hospital Universitario de Canarias, Canary Islands, Spain

V. B. Patel, V. R. Preedy (eds.), *Handbook of Substance Misuse and Addictions*,
https://doi.org/10.1007/978-3-030-92392-1_182

drinking. Chronic ingestion and/or inebriation decrease BDNF expression and may disrupt this homeostatic mechanism. In addition to the neurologic effects, BDNF is a major regulator of energy balance, since it decreases appetite and increases thermogenesis, fatty acid oxidation, and glucose uptake. Exercise, learning, episodic fasting, and environmental enrichment increase BDNF expression and secretion, lending support to the beneficial effect of exercise on the maintenance of cognitive functions. It keeps an inverse relationship with inflammation. BDNF muscle expression increases after exercise and optimizes the metabolic status of the muscle fiber. BDNF levels are reduced in various neurodegenerative disorders. The frequently observed brain atrophy, muscle atrophy-impeding exercise, and inflammatory status observed in excessive drinkers may alter BDNF expression and secretion, although some disparate results have been reported. The possible pathogenetic role of BDNF on muscle and/or brain atrophy in these patients needs future research.

Keywords

Brain-derived neurotrophic factor · BDNF · Alcoholism · Alcoholic myopathy · Brain atrophy · Myokines · Synaptic plasticity · Hippocampus · Synaptogenesis · Synaptic plasticity

Abbreviations

Akt	Alpha serine-threonine protein kinase
AMPA	α-Amino-3-hydroxy-5-methyl-4-isoxazolepropionic acid
AMPK	AMP (adenosine monophosphate)-activated protein kinase
Arc	Activity-related cytoskeleton-associated protein
Bcl-2	B-cell lymphoma 2
BDNF	Brain-derived neurotrophic factor
BMI	Body mass index
CaMK	Calcium-calmodulin-dependent protein kinases
CREB	Cyclic AMP response element-binding protein
CRH	Corticotropin-releasing hormone
Elk-1	ETS (erythroblast transformation specific) like 1 transcription factor
ERK	Extracellular signal-regulated kinase
eRNA	Enhancer RNA
FNDP5	Fibronectin type III domain-containing protein 5
FOXO-3	Forkhead box O3 protein
GABA	*Gamma*-aminobutyric acid
GLP-1	Glucagon-like peptide 1
GTPase	Guanosine triphosphate hydrolases
HbA1C	Glycated hemoglobin
IL	Interleukin
JNK	c-Jun amino-terminal kinase
lncRNA	Long noncoding RNA

MAPK	Mitogen-activated protein kinase
MARKCS	Myristoylated alanine-rich C kinase substrate
MBD	Methyl-binding domain
MecbP-2	Methyl CpG-binding protein-2
MEK	Mitogen-activated protein kinase kinase
mRNA	Messenger RNA
mTOR	Mechanistic target of rapamycin
NFκB	Nuclear factor kappa B
NGF	Nerve growth factor
NMDA	N-methyl D-aspartate
NT	Neurotrophins
p75NTR	p75 Neurotrophin receptor
PGC 1-alpha	Peroxisome proliferator-activated receptor-gamma coactivator
PI3K	Phosphatidyl-inositol-3 kinase
PKC	Protein kinase C (PKC)
PLC	Phospholipase C–protein kinase C
Rac 1	Ras-related C3 botulinum toxin substrate 1
Rack 1	Receptor for activated C kinase 1
Rho-A	Ras homologue gene family member A
TNF	Tumor necrosis factor
TRH	Thyrotropin-releasing hormone
TRK	Tropomyosin receptor kinase
UTR	Untranslated region

Introduction

Excessive drinkers develop brain atrophy and a chronic myopathy characterized by atrophy of muscle fibers. Affectation of any of these two organs may have direct consequences, such as disturbed cognition, learning and memory impairment (alcoholic dementia), and also gait disturbance and muscle weakness to such an extent that patients may become bedridden. Although several independent mechanisms triggered by ethanol are involved in muscle or brain alterations, there is growing interest in analyzing the possible links between sarcopenia and brain atrophy mediated by several myokines and other molecules. BDNF is one of these molecules, and exercise is a main factor triggering its brain and muscle expression and secretion. BDNF is mainly involved in brain development, synaptic plasticity, memory and learning, and maintenance of structural neuronal connectivity. BDNF is also a modulator of ethanol intake, strongly involved in addiction and dependence, and a major regulator of energy balance. Moreover, BDNF exerts widespread systemic effects on many remote organs and tissues, such as adipose tissue, pancreatic β cells, prostate, airway smooth muscle, or glomerular podocytes, as well as on systemic alterations associated with chronic pain or inflammation. Detailed analysis of these effects exceeds the purpose and limits of this review, mainly focused on describing the actions of BDNF on muscle, brain, and energy regulation, and the results of some studies performed on chronic excessive drinkers, in whom brain and muscle atrophy and low-grade inflammation are outstanding features.

The Molecule

About 40 years ago, Barde et al. (1982) purified a new neurotrophic factor from pig brain. This new molecule was called BDNF, adding to the neurotrophin family members, which also include NGF, NT-3, and 4 (Noble et al. 2011; Gonzalez et al. 2016) and other similar molecules described in fish. In addition to its neurodevelopmental effects, BDNF is heavily involved in the structural and functional maturation of hippocampus and frontal cortex, in the maintenance of synaptic plasticity and stability, in addiction, and in a variety of systemic metabolic effects.

BDNF Synthesis

Neurons constitute the major source of BDNF, which is secreted both constitutively and in an activity-dependent fashion. Activity in glutamatergic excitatory synapses leads to increased intracellular calcium influx, which activates CAMK, PKC, and MAPK. These kinases activate the transcription factors NFκB and CREB (Steven et al. 2020). CREB, in turn, induces *Bdnf* gene transcription (Chen and Russo-Neustadt 2009; Marosi and Mattson 2014). As commented later, mature BDNF is able to activate MAPK and transcription factors, creating a functional amplification loop (Cheng et al. 2011) (Fig. 1).

Bdnf gene (located on chromosome 11) is relatively complex. BDNF synthesis is controlled by several promoters differently activated in a tissue-specific, activity-dependent, fashion (Timmusk et al. 1993; Bishop et al. 1994). Several exons, each with its own promoter, generate many species of mature transcripts, which may differ according to cell type, brain region, and the kind of stimulus that leads to *Bdnf* expression (physical activity, antidepressant treatment, acute stress, among others). Final *Bdnf* expression is also modulated by antisense *Bdnf* gene transcripts (Pruunsild et al. 2007; Notaras and van den Buuse 2019; Di Liegro et al. 2019).

Transcription of the DNA sequence into mRNA generates two different mRNA transcripts, one with a short UTR and the other with a long UTR. The proportions of both kinds of BDNF mRNA differ according to brain regions. The long UTR mRNA is more abundant in the cortex, and the short UTR mRNA, in the brainstem. As it occurs with other molecules, some mRNA is sorted from the nucleus to dendrites into large ribonucleoprotein particles and transported along microtubules in relation to increased neuronal activity (Cohen-Cory et al. 2010). Therefore, dendrites contain mRNA destined to local BDNF translation upon activation. Long UTR mRNA is more abundant in dendrites than in somata (An et al. 2008). There is evidence that short UTR BDNF may be involved in neuronal survival and maintenance, whereas long UTR BDNF, locally produced in dendrites, and subjected to activity-induced secretion, is important in the regulation of dendrite arborization, synaptic plasticity, and maturation of dendritic spines (Tongiorgi et al. 1997). The importance of dendrite BDNF long UTR mRNA is underscored by the observation that mice

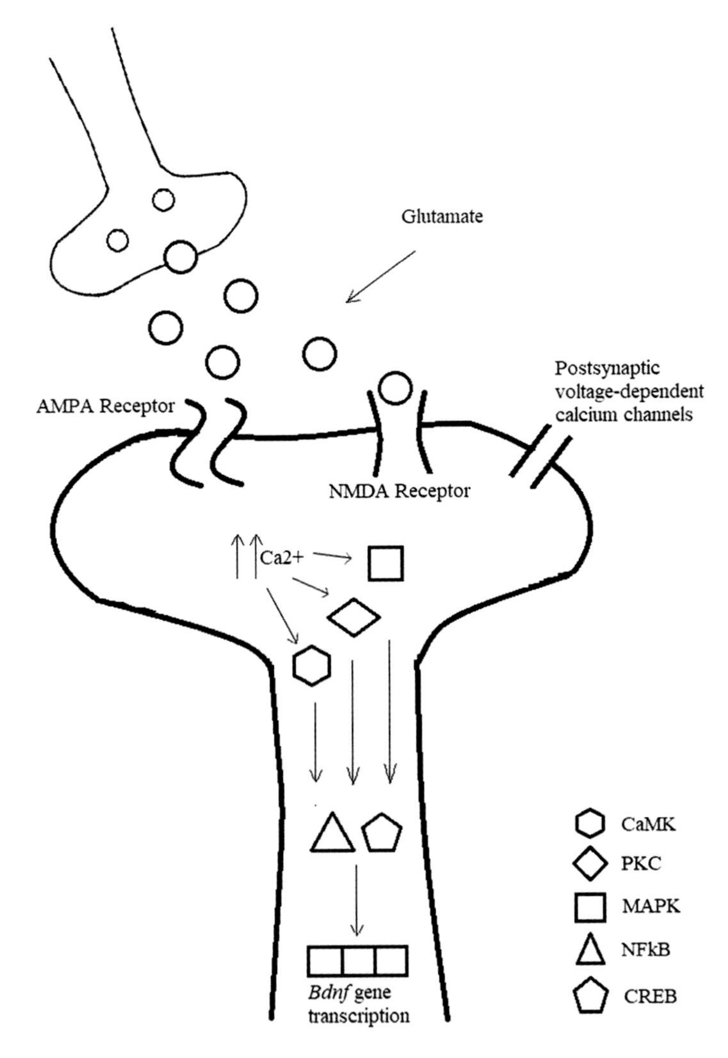

Fig. 1 BDNF secretion. Simplified schematic illustration of BDNF synthesis. Glutamate binds at the postsynaptic membrane to AMPA and NMDA receptors and triggers calcium influx. Increased calcium activates CAMK, PKC, and MAPK. These enzymes activate the transcription factors NFkB and CREB, which induce BDNF gene transcription

with truncated long UTR mRNA show altered maturation of hippocampal dendrite spines, reduced plasticity of dendrite-associated synapses, and impaired long-term potentiation (An et al. 2008).

Adding complexity to this scenario, a frequent polymorphism consisting of the substitution of guanine by adenine at position 196 translates a prodomain (vide infra) in which valine is substituted by methionine at position 66 (Val66Met). This single-nucleotide polymorphism, that affects up to 25% of the population (Anastasia et al.

2013), may alter the binding affinity of the molecule and ultimately reduces BDNF secretion.

BDNF Secretion

After transcription and translation, final secretion of BDNF involves several steps (Kowianski et al. 2018). BDNF is synthesized in the endoplasmic reticulum as a pre-pro-protein. This product is cleaved in the Golgi apparatus to pro-BDNF, a molecule containing a mature domain region (called mature BDNF or m-BDNF) and a prodomain region (Hempstead 2015). Both m-BDNF and pro-BDNF are functionally active molecules. The pro-BDNF molecule is translocated to the trans-Golgi network and later secreted in two kinds of secretory vesicles: constitutive vesicles, which release the molecules in a calcium-independent fashion, and regulated secretory vesicles, which release BDNF in a calcium-dependent fashion, in response to secretory stimuli (Pollock et al. 2001). By binding to BDNF prodomain, sortilin is necessary for the intracellular transport of pro-BDNF to secretory pathways (Chen et al. 2005). During transport, part of the pro-BDNF translocated from the Golgi system suffers a second cleavage either by furin (in the trans-Golgi network) or by other convertases (in the secretory vesicles), being transformed into the mature form. The mature domain of BDNF binds to carboxypeptidase E in the vesicles. These vesicles, if not released in the synaptic cleft, are transported back to the cell body, a process for which binding to carboxypeptidase E is essential (Park et al. 2008).

The vast majority of dendrites lack Golgi-like structures and cleavage enzymes, so most of the long UTR mRNA-derived BDNF is secreted as pro-BDNF and cleaved extracellularly (An et al. 2008).

Therefore, pro-BDNF (as a complete molecule), m-BDNF, and BDNF prodomain are released into the extracellular space, in a proportion that varies according to age (higher pro-BDNF in the postnatal period, higher m-BDNF in adulthood; Yang et al. 2009). Mature BDNF is more dependent upon activity-dependent secretion (Duman et al. 2021).

In the extracellular space, pro-BDNF is also subjected to cleavage by plasmin (derived from tissue plasminogen activator) and matrix metalloproteases 3, 7, and 9 (Vafadari et al. 2016), leading to the formation of more m-BDNF and BDNF prodomain. Therefore, the total pool of m-BDNF is composed of intracellular m-BDNF (the major proportion) and extracellularly generated m-BDNF (Anastasia et al. 2013). m-BDNF and pro-BDNF bind to different receptors and exert specific functions.

Globally, BDNF promotes morphological changes, including axonogenesis, dendritogenesis, synaptogenesis, and hippocampal neurogenesis, and differentiation of neural progenitor cells into mature neurons. Neurogenesis implicates the division of neural stem cells, either to generate two identical undifferentiated stem cells or to generate an identical daughter cell and a second cell that starts to differentiate and must be integrated into the existing hippocampal circuitry. Synaptogenesis and synaptic plasticity promote synapse assembly and disassembly and synaptic stability. This has an effect on learning, memory formation, and increased cognition. It

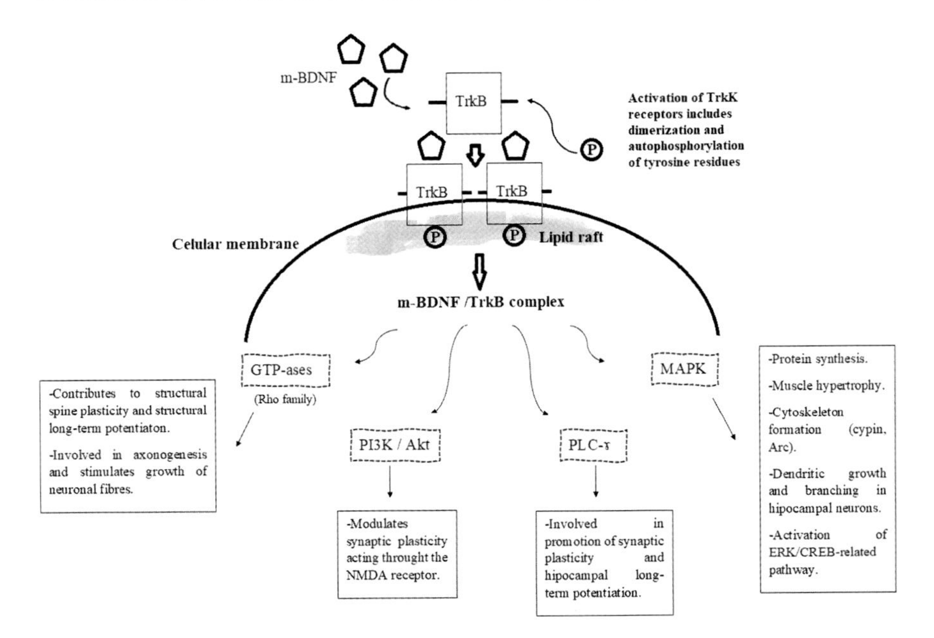

Fig. 2 BDNF signaling pathways. Interaction of mature BDNF with TrkB receptor. M-BDNF binds to TrkB receptor, provoking its dimerization, autophosphorylation, and translocation to cell membrane lipid rafts, triggering activation of downstream signaling pathways

also increases synaptic transmission. Synaptic transmission and firing of action potentials require energy; in this sense, BDNF is also a major regulator of neuronal energetic metabolism. Moreover, by induction of apoptosis of non-connected neurons, or nonsynchronous activated synapses, BDNF also contributes to the so-called brain plasticity All these effects are achieved by BDNF by binding to specific receptors that activate different downstream molecular pathways (Fig. 2).

BDNF Interaction with Receptors and Downstream Effects

m-BDNF effects are strongly related, but not limited, to synaptic plasticity, defined as an activity-dependent modification of the strength of the synaptic transmission. Synaptic plasticity includes short-term facilitation and depression, as well as long-term potentiation and depression. Any of these mechanisms can be elicited by morphological changes (i.e., dendritic spine growth/shrinkage, disassembly of pre-existing synapses) or biochemical changes, both at the transcriptional or posttranscriptional levels (e.g., phosphorylation/dephosphorylation of receptor subunits). Overall, m-BDNF exerts a facilitating (= "positive") or enhancing role at the synaptic level through the interaction of m-BDNF with TRK receptors. Conversely, pro-BDNF tends to exert a "halting" or "negative" influence on synaptic transmission, mostly related to morphological changes, leading to long-term depression, a function related to the interaction of pro-BDNF with p75 NTR receptors.

Pro-BDNF Binding

Pro-BDNF binds to p75NTR, belonging to the TNF family of receptors. This receptor has a cytoplasmic tail involved in apoptosis. p75NTR binds to the mature domain of pro-BDNF, whereas the prodomain region binds to sortilin. Sortilin belongs to the so-called vacuolar protein-10 protein family of receptors, which also include the SorC1, SorCS2, SorCS3, and SorLA or SORL1 receptors (Nyborg et al. 2006). In addition to playing a key role in intracellular trafficking of pro-BDNF from the Golgi apparatus to cell membrane, sortilin also protects the prodomain from proteolytic cleavage, allowing the pro-BDNF molecules to travel to the cell surface (Bronfman and Fainzilber 2004). Sortilin, particularly SorCS-2, acts as a co-receptor of p75NTR, forming a complex that facilitates the interaction of p75NTR with the downstream signaling pathway. The importance of sortilin is underscored by the fact that the Val66Met variant is associated with a reduction in hippocampal volume, an increased risk of depression and anxiety disorders, altered cognition, and extinction learning (Dincheva et al. 2012). This happens because methionine at position 66 impairs the ability of the pro-BDNF molecule to bind sortilin, therefore impairing the trafficking of pro-BDNF and later cleavage by furin or convertases, ultimately altering the secretion of the mature molecule upon excitatory stimuli (Anastasia et al. 2013). This impairs the "positive" effects of m-BDNF. Interestingly, mice carrying the mouse homolog of this polymorphism (Met68BDNF) showed a similar phenotype and an increased propension to alcohol addiction (Warnault et al. 2016).

After binding of pro-BDNF with p75NTR and sortilin/SorCS-2, this receptor complex activates different signaling pathways, including JNK, Rho-A, and NFκB transcription factor. Activation of the JNK signaling pathway induces neuronal apoptosis, and the Rho-A signaling pathway promotes dendritic spine shrinkage and growth cone retraction. As a result, pro-BDNF exerts a halting influence on brain development (Lee et al. 2001; Hempstead 2015), contributing to the elimination of damaged or malfunctioning cells and/or abnormal connections not involved in the acquisition of memory and learning. It was shown that asynchronous or low-frequency electrical stimulation of neurons in hippocampal slices causes a reduction in synaptic transmission efficiency mediated by pro-BDNF release and activation of p75NTR, a potential mechanism of BDNF-mediated long-term depression. Conversely, experimentally increasing local synchronicity by stimulating synapses in response to spontaneous activity at neighboring synapses stabilized synaptic transmission (Winnubst et al. 2015; Tien and Kerschensteiner 2018). High-frequency stimulation facilitates extracellular cleavage of pro-BDNF to m-BDNF by plasmin (Nagappan et al. 2009), leading to a predominance of the m-BDNF-mediated "positive" effects.

M-BDNF Binding

m-BDNF, already cleaved from the complete pro-BDNF molecule, can bind to p75NTR (with very low affinity, Sasi et al. 2017) and, with high affinity, to TRKB. There are three TRK receptors: TRKA, activated by NGF and NT3; TRKB, activated by m-BDNF and NT4; and TRKC, which binds to NT3. Both m-BDNF and TRK receptors are present in presynaptic axon terminals and postsynaptic dendrites. Activation of TRK receptors includes dimerization and autophosphorylation of tyrosine residues. After activation, receptor complex is translocated to membrane lipid rafts.

Binding of m-BDNF to TRKB leads to increased synaptic efficiency and long-term potentiation, which sharply contrast with the effects derived from p75NTR activation (Lu et al. 2005).

There are four versions of TRKB receptors: a full-length version and three truncated versions: TRKB-1, TRKB-2, and TRKB-4 forms, derived from alternative splicing. These truncated forms, especially TRKB-1, inhibit the activity of m-BDNF, interfering with the normal signaling pathway of the complex m-BDNF–full-length TRKB (Braken and Turrigiano 2009).

As just commented, m-BDNF is heavily involved in synaptic plasticity, dendritic spine formation and dendrite branching, and glio- and neurogenesis. Some important signaling pathways become activated after binding of m-BDNF with full-length TRKB:

PI3K–akt-mTOR pathway, which modulates synaptic plasticity acting through the NMDA receptor.

MAPK is a pathway involved in protein synthesis, muscle hypertrophy, cytoskeleton formation, and dendritic growth and branching in hippocampal neurons (Kwon et al. 2011). Many of these effects involve MAPK activation of transcription factors such as CREB. By this way, MAPK activation results in increased cypin mRNA and protein levels. Cypin is a guanine deaminase, which binds to tubulin heterodimers and promotes microtubule assembly, being involved in proximal dendrite branching (Kwon et al. 2011). MAPK also activates other kinases, such as ERK1/2, which in turn activates many transcription factors and regulatory molecules related to the formation and maintenance of axonal branches (Roskoski 2012; Deinhart and Chao 2014). Also, MAPK recruits transcription factors other than CREB, such as Elk-1, which enhance the expression of Arc protein immediate early gene that is related to dendrite spine arborization and long-term potentiation (Palmisano and Pandey 2017).

PCγ-PKC pathway is involved in multiple biochemical pathways. One important function is binding of PKC to the so-called MARKCS-related domain of the protein β-adducin, a protein that controls actin polymerization and integrates actin filaments into the spectrin network. This effect is essential for the maintenance of synaptic stability – a key step in learning process. Learning implies the rapid assembly of new synapses, disassembly of others, and long-term maintenance of a small number of the newly formed synapses. In an experimental model, β-adducin also participates in the rescue and reassemble of labile synapses (Bednarek and Caroni 2011).

BDNF/TRKB pathway also regulates cytoskeletal dynamics, mainly through the GTPase proteins Rac-1 and Cdc42. This pathway induces the formation of axons from immature neurite growth cones, gathering actin filaments and generating the so-called actin waves, which define the first stages of axonal development. TrkB also relocates a master regulator protein, Ankyrin G, in the axon initial segments (Woo et al. 2019). Globally, this pathway contributes to structural spine plasticity and structural long-term potentiation. It is involved in axonogenesis and stimulates the growth of neuronal fibers (Gonzalez et al. 2016).

Therefore, by means of relative activation and secretion of the pro-molecule and the mature molecule, BDNF exerts several actions in brain, which surely play a major role in homeostatic plasticity (Tien and Kerschensteiner 2018), both during growth and in the mature nervous system. In this sense, it is important to note that in the developing cortex and in hippocampus, the activity of neighboring synapses strengthens synaptic connection, whereas deafferented synapses or synapses lacking synchronic stimuli become depressed. Mature BDNF increases synaptic strength and decreases excitability of (inhibitory) hippocampal GABA-ergic neurons, underscoring its role in neurogenesis, enhancement of developmental process, and improved memory and cognition (Kowianski et al. 2018).

Several stimuli contribute to BDNF secretion. It has been observed that environmental enrichment (Nilsson et al. 2020), hippocampus-dependent learning (Epp et al. 2013), and physical exercise (Novkovic et al. 2015) are accompanied by increased BDNF levels. Other well-known factors that stimulate BDNF secretion include seizures, ischemia, osmotic stress, and antidepressant treatment (Cunha et al. 2010). Several molecules, such as flavonoids and quercetin, or neuropeptide Y may upregulate BDNF expression (Numakawa et al. 2018).

Of special interest is the connection between proinflammatory cytokines and BDNF expression. Intraperitoneal injections of IL-1β or lipopolysaccharide – which lead to increased brain production of proinflammatory cytokines (Qin et al. 2007) – significantly decrease BDNF mRNA levels in the rat hippocampus (especially in CA1 and CA3 areas) and several cortical regions, and this is accompanied by sickness behavior in rodents (Zhang et al. 2016). The same reduction in hippocampal BDNF was observed in aged rats (Chapman et al. 2012). In humans, an inverse correlation between C-reactive protein and serum BDNF among 97 excessive drinkers (rho $= -0.27$, $p = 0.007$) was observed (Fig. 3). Overall, the relationship between brain function and inflammatory cytokines is well known: BDNF expression is low in patients affected by depression (Duman et al. 2012), and depression is accompanied by an increase in proinflammatory cytokines such as TNFα or IL-6 (Dowlati et al. 2010). In chronic pain models, several neuropsychological functions become impaired, and hippocampal volume is reduced (Mao et al. 2016). Cytokine release induced by chronic pain leads to impaired memory, and an inverse correlation between proinflammatory cytokines and BDNF was observed (Liu et al. 2017).

BDNF and Alcohol Addiction

Given its outstanding role on synaptic plasticity, learning, and memory, it is not surprising that BDNF levels become altered in various diseases that affect central nervous system, such as depression, degenerative disorders, and drug addiction. In this sense, the role of BDNF changes associated with cocaine and alcohol abuse has been more extensively studied (Ornell et al. 2018).

Ethanol is consumed by human beings either to achieve euphoric effects or to combat dysphoria caused by ethanol withdrawal. Rewarding effects depend on the activation of the mesolimbic dopaminergic pathway, especially dopaminergic

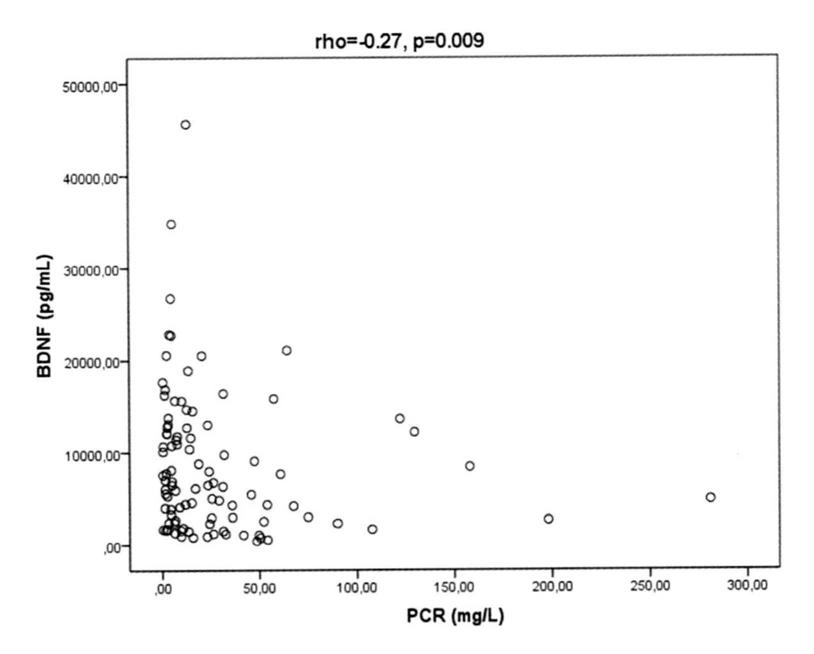

Fig. 3 BDNF and inflammation. Inverse relationship between serum BDNF and C-reactive protein among 97 alcoholics ($\rho = -0.27$; $p = 0.009$)

projections from ventral tegmental areas to *nucleus accumbens* (Koob and Volkow 2016; Fig. 4), whereas activation of the amygdaloid brain regions, especially the central and medial nuclei of amygdala, is involved in dysphoria, depression, and anxiety caused by withdrawal (Fig. 4). Changes in synaptic plasticity play a major role in the regulation of addiction, withdrawal-associated dysphoria, and reward after consumption (Pandey et al. 2017). Previous existence of anxiety and mood disorders or stress can increase susceptibility to the development of alcohol abuse.

In this paragraph, we will discuss the effects of BDNF on alcohol consumption and the alterations that ethanol addiction may cause on *Bdnf* expression and BDNF levels.

Ethanol Consumption, BDNF, and the CREB Pathway

CREB is a major component of a transcription complex able to activate the expression of many genes. CREB deficiency in the amygdala is observed in the so-called P alcohol-preferring rats (innately predisposed to increased ethanol consumption), and a similar reduction in CREB levels in amygdala was observed after withdrawal of ethanol. BDNF/TRKB signaling, via MAPK, activates CREB; in a positive loop, CREB acts as a transcription factor both for BDNF and TRKB genes. In accordance with these observations, together with CREB, BDNF was lower in central and medial amygdala of P rats, and the low BDNF expression in amygdala was accompanied by anxiety and increased ethanol intake. As previously commented, Arc proteins rapidly induce the expansion of actin cytoskeleton in dendrite spines, and

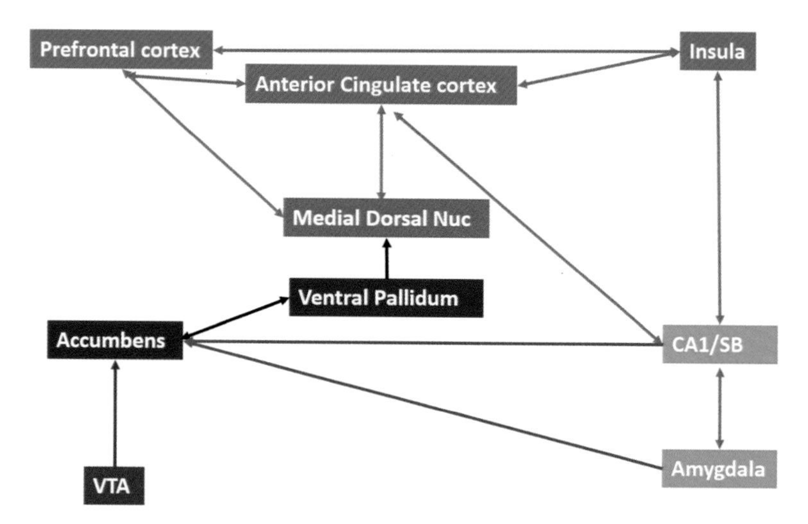

Fig. 4 Mesolimbic reward system. Schematic diagram of some pathways involved in pleasure, reward, and addiction. Pleasurable activities and some chemicals (putative drugs of abuse) elicit dopamine release (golden arrow, which is the main component of the mesocorticolimbic pathway) in the nucleus accumbens, which in turn sends GABAergic projections (black arrows) to the ventral pallidum. The activity of this circuitry produces a thalamic mediated activation (medial dorsal nucleus) of prefrontal cortex, cingulate cortex, and other regions involved in high-order processing. Note the strong interconnections between pathways involved in pleasure/addiction and circuits of memory (CA1/subiculum in the hippocampus), emotional processing (amygdala and CA1/subiculum), pain processing (medial dorsal nucleus, insula), and anxiety (amygdala, and its reciprocal connections with anterior cingulate cortex and insula among others). VTA: ventral tegmental area; SB: subiculum. Purple indicates midbrain structures, red indicates basal ganglia, and green indicates cortical or related structures (including allocortex and basolateral amygdala). Blue arrows indicate excitatory connections

Arc expression is upregulated by BDNF and CREB. Reduced Arc proteins and reduced spine density as a consequence of reduced BDNF and reduced CREB are likely involved in increased anxiety linked to alcohol withdrawal (Moonat et al. 2010). P rats show decreased spine density that increases after alcohol consumption.

Epigenetic Changes of BDNF and Drug Addiction

Epigenetic mechanisms are defined as those that contribute to the regulation of genetic information without modification of the DNA sequence and include chemical modifications of histones (by histone deacetylases) and methylation of DNA (by DNA methyltransferases). Other related factors that change final BDNF expression include the actions of microRNA and long noncoding RNA molecules.

Histones are relatively short-chained basic proteins, rich in arginine and lysine residues, around which DNA is wrapped, forming nucleosomes that become packed together building the chromatin fibers. In addition to providing protection to the DNA chain, histones also regulate transcription machinery and gene expression. Modifications of the histone molecules by methylation and/or acetylation (at specific lysine residues of the histone molecules) change the electrostatic strength by which these molecules are bound to DNA, so that hypoacetylation favors nucleosome condensation, hindering transcription and eventually leading to gene silencing, whereas hyperacetylation causes the opposite effect (Moonat and Pandey 2012).

DNA methylation is mediated by DNA methyltransferases, which act inhibiting transcription. DNA methylation (methylation of cytosine) takes place at the so-called CpG sites, which are DNA regions where a cytosine is followed by a guanine nucleotide. These regions are relatively common along the DNA chain and may be targeted by a group of methyl-CpG-binding proteins such as MeCP2 (especially abundant in the mature central nervous system) among others (Fan and Hutnick 2005). Gene silencing associated with DNA methylation may occur both by direct methylation of cytosine and by binding to MBD proteins recruited by methylated cytosine. In turn, MBD proteins are also able to recruit histone deacetylases and DNA methyltransferases. Other proteins may exert opposite effects. Protein RACK 1 dissociates MeCP2 from the *BDNF* gene, increasing histone acetylation, and therefore increasing BDNF expression.

Drinking during adolescence decreases the activity of the orbitofrontal cortex and increases amygdala activity. This is an important issue, since the structure and connectivity of amygdala suffer important changes during adolescence, which may be disrupted by ethanol consumption. This may explain some behavioral alterations observed in adolescents with alcohol overuse, consisting of loss of executive control and changes in decision-making and emotional impulsivity, alterations that may persist later in life. The so-called long noncoding RNA (lncRNA) sequences, which are molecules longer than 200 base pairs lacking a functional open reading frame, constitute another factor involved in epigenetic BDNF changes, since they may regulate gene expression by inducing changes in chromatin or altering the function of transcription factors. These lncRNA sequences may alter BDNF expression in the amygdala and may be therefore involved in alcohol addiction during adolescence (Bohnsack et al. 2019). Recent research (Kim et al. 2015) led to the discovery of a subclass of lncRNA, the so-called eRNA that may also regulate target gene expression.

Therefore, epigenetic mechanisms are involved in alterations of BDNF expression, and, by this way, they may affect the formation of dendrite spines and synaptic plasticity. These epigenetic mechanisms may be triggered by a variety of situations. For instance, acute stress increased the levels of *BDNF* mRNA in hippocampus (Marmigère et al. 2003), and it was shown that this increase was associated with increased MeCP2 phosphorylation. Chronic stress causes decreased *BDNF* expression in the hippocampus, and this decrease was associated with histone methylation that was reversed by antidepressants (Tsankova et al. 2007). Inhibition of BDNF expression in the amygdala derived from a higher expression of histone deacetylase 2 increases anxiety associated with ethanol withdrawal. Inhibition of deacetylases leads to an increase in BDNF and reduces dysphoria, in a way similar to that exerted by ethanol, whose anxiolytic effects may be associated with an increase in BDNF signaling in central and medial amygdala nuclei in P rats (Moonat et al. 2011). Therefore, histone modifications in the amygdala are related to alcohol exposure

(Starkman et al. 2012), and epigenetic alterations play major roles in addiction (Palmisano and Pandey 2017).

Epigenetic changes also affect the expression of Arc proteins. In an animal (rat) model of adolescent intermittent ethanol exposure, increased anxiety was observed in the adulthood. This was related to long-lasting epigenetic alterations in the amygdala, specifically at the promoter regions of *Bdnf* and *Arc* genes, possibly explaining the decreased dendritic spine density and increased anxiety and alcohol intake seen in these animals. This reduction in *Bdnf* expression depends on the increased activity of histone deacetylase 2, and compulsive alcohol drinking in adulthood may become attenuated by inhibiting histone deacetylase activity (Pandey et al. 2015). Arc gene is subjected to the positive effect of an eRNAm, which function can be epigenetically regulated (Kyzar et al. 2019).

BDNF in Excessive Drinkers

As a consequence of both direct *Bdnf* gene activation and epigenetic changes, BDNF levels are closely related to alcohol addiction. Ethanol exposure in low/moderate dose leads to increased *Bdnf* expression in the dorsal striatum; in a homeostatic fashion, BDNF exerts an inhibitory action on alcohol intake, acting via the signaling pathway TKRB-MAPK/ERK1/2 (Jeanblanc et al. 2013). On the contrary, consumption of ethanol in large amounts to achieve blood ethanol levels over 80 mg/dl, as well as chronic consumption of excessive amounts of ethanol, did not alter BDNF mRNA expression in the dorsal striatum (Logrip et al. 2015), but caused a marked reduction of *BDNF* expression in the medial prefrontal cortex and hippocampus, leading to decreased serum BDNF levels in chronic alcoholics. This reduction in BDNF response is related to an increase in two microRNA molecules, which specifically target *BDNF* mRNA transcripts (Darcq et al. 2015). Assuming the role of BDNF in the dorsal striatum as a negative regulator of ethanol intake, the lack of increase of BDNF production in the dorsal striatum (and possibly in other areas such as hippocampus or medial prefrontal cortex) in chronic drinkers or inebriated individuals disrupts the inhibitory loop that maintains ethanol ingestion in “safe” limits. In accordance with this hypothesis, it was shown that genetically conditioned, alcohol-preferring rats had lower BDNF levels in nucleus accumbens and other areas of the central nervous system (Prakash et al. 2008). All these data strongly suggest that increased BDNF secretion associated with moderate alcohol ingestion protects the individual from ingestion of toxic doses of ethanol. However, consumption of toxic doses disrupts this protective effect, blocking the action of BDNF acting through microRNA that hampers *Bdnf* mRNA transcription.

BDNF levels in alcoholics may differ in situations of chronic active alcohol consumption (decreased plasma levels), acute ethanol administration (increased brain expression and plasma levels), and withdrawal (recovery to normal values). Clinical observations have yielded, however, some controversial results. Some authors failed to find differences with controls (Geisel et al. 2016), and others have reported decreased plasma levels in patients with alcohol dependence

(Joe et al. 2007). Lee et al. (2009) observed higher values among 41 alcohol-dependent individuals (drinkers of >10 standard drinks daily) than among 41 controls (blood extracted the day after admission). On the contrary, Costa et al. found no differences at baseline with controls, although alcoholics that remained abstinent for 6 months showed a significant increase in BDNF values (Costa et al. 2011). Higher levels were also found in dependent patients after 4 weeks of abstinence (D'Sa et al. 2012). Other studies revealed lower BDNF in 30-day abstinent patients (Joe et al. 2007). Huang et al. (2008) found no differences after admission, but an increase in BDNF in alcohol-dependent subjects one week later, and other authors report low BDNF in depressed alcoholic patients (Umene-Nakano et al. 2009). A recent meta-analysis suggests lower serum (but not plasmatic) BDNF levels among excessive drinkers (Ornell et al. 2018).

Alteration of BDNF levels in alcoholics is important for the understanding of the effects of BDNF on addiction. BDNF also exerts systemic effects, which may contribute to some of the systemic alterations observed in alcoholics, and that we summarize below.

Metabolic Effects

Synaptic transmission, neurogenesis, axonogenesis, and maintenance of synaptic stability consume energy by the neurons. BDNF regulates energy supply, both in neurons and peripheral organs.

Metabolic Effects of BDNF on Neurons

Within the neurons, BDNF exerts the following metabolic effects:

- It increases glucose transport via inducing the expression of GLUT3, the main neuronal glucose transporter.
- It increases sodium-dependent amino acid uptake and protein synthesis.
- It upregulates PGC-1α, a master regulator of mitochondrial biogenesis, a necessary step for synaptic plasticity.
- It enhances the respiratory coupling efficiency of mitochondria involving mechanisms associated with MEK and Bcl-2.
- It upregulates mitochondrial superoxide dismutase, via the transcription factor FOXO-3.
- It enhances the utilization of ketones by neurons, upregulating monocarboxylate transporter 2, a protein involved in ketone uptake.

Therefore, BDNF optimizes the neuronal metabolic status favoring fuel uptake and improving mitochondrial efficiency and protects the cell against oxidative damage.

Systemic Metabolic Effects of BDNF

In addition to the central nervous system, BDNF is also expressed in many other organs, especially liver, prostate, lymphocytes, airway smooth muscle, heart, skeletal muscle, and adipose tissue, among others, and it is also stored in platelets (Fujimura et al. 2002); it also freely crosses the blood–brain barrier (Klein et al. 2011).

In peripheral organs, BDNF exerts both systemic and local effects. As a major regulator of energy balance, it controls appetite and governs intermediate metabolism and energy expenditure. Fasting induces BDNF brain expression, but BDNF has anorexigenic activity (Lapchak and Hefti 1992), inducing satiety (Xu and Xie 2016). This seems to be mediated by an effect on hypothalamus.

Inhibition of appetite is the predominant effect of injected BDNF, although response varies according to the specific site of injection (Noble et al. 2011). Overexpression of the *Bdnf* gene in the hypothalamus is associated with increased expression of TRKB, insulin receptor, CRH, and TRH; a sharp decrease in leptin; and increased adiponectin secretion. It also increases thermogenesis, increasing uncoupling protein 1 expression in the brown adipose tissue, and also induces a switch of white adipose tissue to brown adipose tissue in response to environmental stimuli (Cao et al. 2011).

Regarding glucose metabolism, BDNF increases the number of pancreatic β cells, the total area of islets, and the number of secretory granules (Yamanaka et al. 2006). BDNF metabolism is also linked to incretins. In fact, GLP1 induces brain BDNF expression (Spielman et al. 2017), and BDNF shares with GLP-1 the effects on glucose uptake by liver, myocardium, and skeletal muscle (Yamanaka et al. 2007). On the opposite, high glucose levels reduce production and release of BDNF by brain cells (Krabbe et al. 2007), and BDNF haploinsufficient mice develop hyperphagia, obesity, and diabetes (Kernie et al. 2000). BDNF binding to hepatocytes through TRKB receptor decreases fat synthesis, increases fatty acid oxidation, promotes glycogen storage, and decreases gluconeogenesis (Genzer et al. 2017).

Exercise markedly increases BDNF expression and secretion (Cotman and Berchtold 2002; Ferris et al. 2007). This increased expression is mediated by CREB and CMK, a molecule that is able to regulate CREB-dependent transcription (Vaynman et al. 2007; Lonze and Ginty 2002). Importantly, during exercise, peripheral stimuli can also increase BDNF in neurons. Exercise induces muscle production of a protein called FNDC5, which is cleaved and secreted as irisin. Irisin induces the expression of *BDNF gene* in the hippocampus (Wrann et al. 2013). FNDC5 is also expressed in neurons, liver, and other tissues. PGC 1α enhances cortical neuronal FNDC5 expression after endurance exercise.

Given the induction of satiety by BDNF and its metabolic effects increasing energy expenditure, BDNF should ameliorate the metabolic syndrome. However, in humans, the relationship between BDNF and BMI is not consistent; some authors report positive correlations, and others find negative correlations with body fat. This last result was also observed by ourselves in 64 alcoholic patients, in whom there was a lack of relationship with body fat. In a preliminary survey on 85 alcoholic patients, we failed to find differences in BDNF values among diabetics and non-diabetics, but there was a significant, positive correlation between HbA1C levels and BDNF (rho $= 0.27$; $p = 0.0012$), especially in the cirrhotic subgroup (rho $=0.44$; $p = 0.01$; Fig. 5), a result opposed to the hypoglycemic effect of BDNF.

Effects on Muscle

Synthesis of BDNF shows a robust increase after exercise, due to a marked increase of BDNF expression in both muscles and brain. Matthews et al. (2009) showed that muscle contraction enhances muscle cells' BDNF expression, which acts locally in muscle fibers, mostly via the AMPK pathway, increasing fatty acid oxidation. AMPK phosphorylates acetyl coenzyme A carboxylase, and therefore reduces cellular malonyl-coenzyme A levels. The increase in fatty acid oxidation by muscle explains in part the effect of BDNF on body weight, provoking weight loss.

Recent studies have shown that muscle also secretes BDNF, inducing insulin secretion by pancreatic β-cells (Fulgenzi et al. 2020). Muscle-derived BDNF not only prepares the muscle cell metabolically to face an increased activity, but also optimizes the utilization of glucose by the whole body, contributing to the anti-hyperglycemic effect of exercise. As commented previously, muscle activity leads to increased irisin production, and it was also shown that muscle activity releases cathepsin B, which, in turn, increases BDNF secretion by brain, enhancing neurogenesis, memory, and learning (Moon et al. 2016), contributing to the beneficial effects of exercise on brain functions.

Patients with alcohol overuse frequently show brain atrophy. Altered BDNF values are frequently observed in other neurodegenerative conditions (Zuccato and Cattaneo 2009). Given the importance of increased BDNF production as a homeostatic mechanism protecting against excessive drinking, theoretically the BDNF response to alcohol intake in excessive drinkers with already atrophied brains should be suboptimal. The association between BDNF levels and brain atrophy in alcoholics has not been extensively explored. Given the high prevalence of chronic alcoholic myopathy, it is tempting to speculate that perhaps there is a pathogenetic link between (atrophied) muscle and (atrophied) brain (Fig. 6). In a previous study, we showed that BDNF was related more intensely to handgrip strength than to brain atrophy, suggesting a greater importance of muscle wasting (Martín-González et al. 2020).

Applications to Other Areas of Addiction

Studies on BDNF in users of psychoactive substances yield disparate results. In general, there is a trend to lower BDNF values in chronic consumers. These differences may be partly explained by the fact that drug addiction overlaps with several psychiatric disorders that also alter BDNF secretion, such as depression or bipolar disorders. An additional difficulty in the interpretation of BDNF levels in

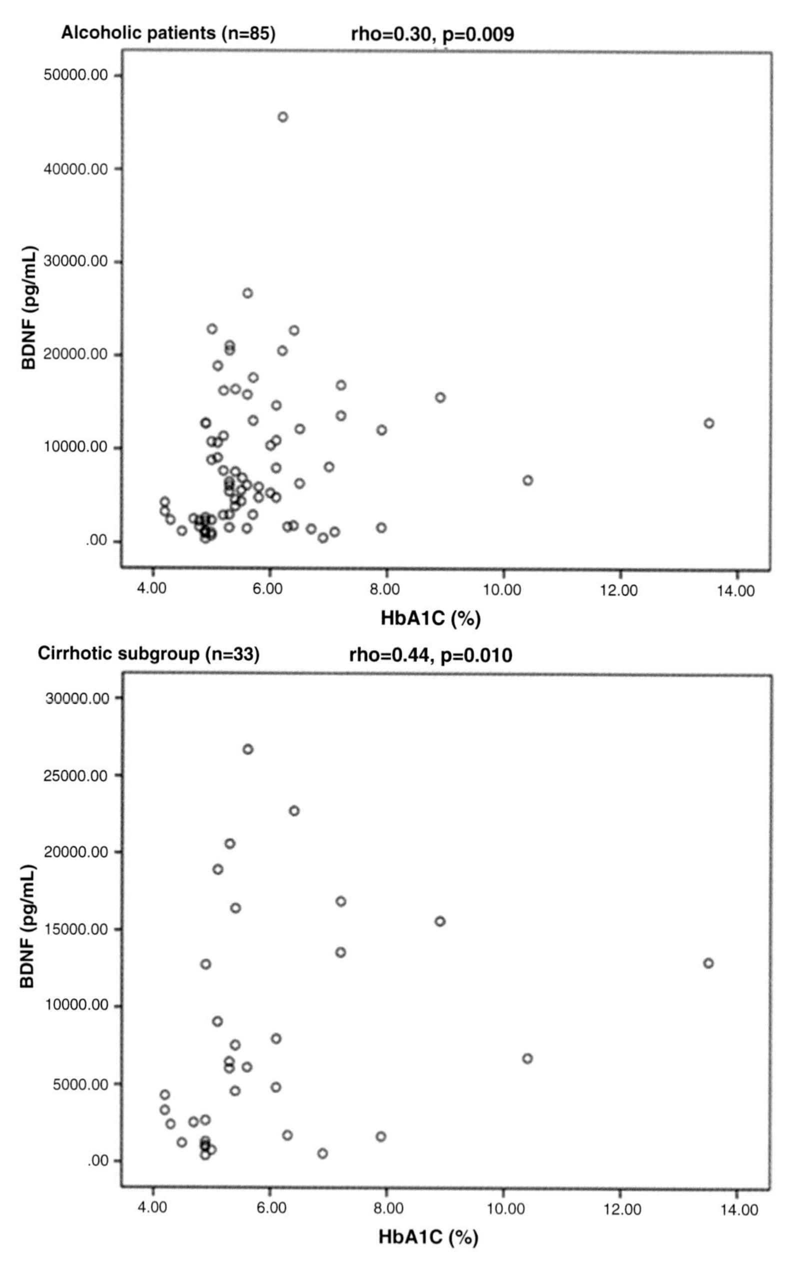

Fig. 5 BDNF and intermediate metabolism. Relationships between serum BDNF and HbA1C levels in alcoholic patients (Fig. 5a, $\rho = 0.30$, $p = 0.009$) and cirrhotics (Fig. 5b, $\rho = 0.44$; $p = 0.010$)

psychiatric conditions resides in the fact that there are marked differences according to the stage of the disease (remission or acute phase). BDNF also varies according to the severity and stage of drug use (e.g., acute, chronic, recovery).

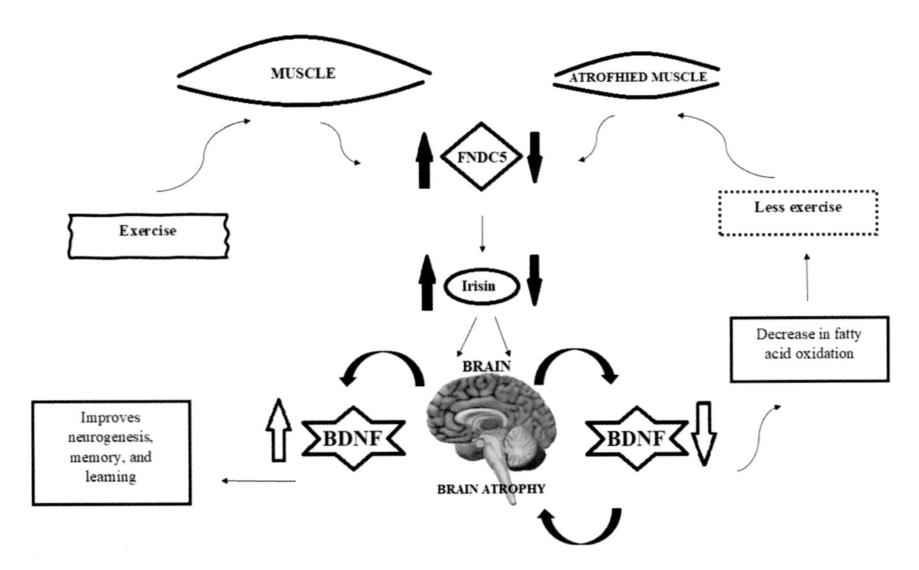

Fig. 6 Hypothetical link between muscle and brain atrophy in excessive drinkers. Hypothetical link between muscle and brain atrophy. Atrophied brain and atrophied muscles produce less BDNF upon stimulation (i.e., exercise). Reduced muscle contraction leads to decreased irisin and cathepsin secretion, which in turn further reduce brain BDNF secretion. Reduced BDNF in muscle reduces fatty acid oxidation, which impairs exercising capacity. Eventually, reduced brain BDNF impairs brain plasticity and may favor persistence in drinking habit

Acute use of alcohol, ecstasy, or cocaine transiently increases brain BDNF levels, but prolonged and excessive use of alcohol or cocaine leads to a robust reduction in BDNF expression. On the other hand, acute administration of benzodiazepine leads to a significant reduction in hippocampal BDNF, but chronic use failed to alter BDNF hippocampal expression. Another factor is whether BDNF levels were determined in plasma or serum, since differences may exist also in relation to conditions of extraction, use of heparin, or EDTA.

Different drugs may cause different alterations in BDNF levels. Concomitant use of different substances (especially tobacco and alcohol with cocaine/crack) also obscures the interpretation of BDNF behavior. Also, in many studies, there is a lack of information about tobacco consumption. Similar to alcohol, initial consumption of cocaine triggers biochemical compensatory mechanisms (involving increased expression of CREB, MeCP2, BDNF, and mRNA in the striatum), which serve to protect against addiction. In chronic alcoholics, homeostatic mechanisms become disrupted.

Epigenetic changes related to histone modifications affecting amygdaloid *BDNF* expression are heavily involved in drug addiction (Renthal and Nestler 2008).

Application to Other Areas of Public Health

The importance of BDNF in alcoholic patients is enormous, as briefly synthesized in this review. Especially interesting fields are those related to the treatment of anxiety and dysphoria associated with ethanol withdrawal in excessive consumers;

the potential use of BDNF as a regulator of metabolic syndrome, insulin sensitivity, and antidiabetic; its role as a therapy for alcoholic and nonalcoholic steatohepatitis; and its behavior in alcohol-mediated brain atrophy and chronic myopathy and the potential connection of BDNF (and other myokines) between these two facts. At this moment, it is difficult to discern whether the decreased BDNF levels are the cause or the consequence of brain atrophy: either atrophied brain produces lower amounts of BDNF or atrophied muscle produces scarce amounts of myokines that affect brain BDNF expression, leading to brain atrophy. Theoretically, an atrophied brain secretes less BDNF, and this effect perhaps impairs the regulatory effect of BDNF on drinking. The importance of endurance exercise and the role of BDNF in this context require future research. Another important field of research in excessive drinkers derives from the association of proinflammatory cytokines and reduced BDNF values. Alcoholism may be viewed as a proinflammatory condition. The potential inhibition exerted by pro-inflammatory cytokines on brain BDNF secretion could theoretically occur, although the true impact of this effect on brain atrophy and/or on addiction is incompletely known.

Given the widespread effects of BDNF, it is not surprising that research on this molecule importantly affects (and will affect) other areas of medicine and public health, far beyond the effects on excessive drinkers. BDNF plays a major role in addiction to other drugs, and it probably serves as a therapeutic tool in the treatment of neurodegenerative conditions, as briefly outlined. But BDNF also affects intermediate metabolism, metabolic syndrome, and its consequences, including diabetes, steatohepatitis, and heart disease; asthma, or prostate cancer, where high BDNF levels may be deleterious; and kidney failure, or glaucoma, as some examples of the many diseases in which BDNF may be involved, a matter subjected to active research, which description and analysis lay far beyond the scope of this review.

Mini-Dictionary of Terms

CA1: Subregion of the cornu ammonis: three-layered cortex in the parahippocampal gyrus and the hippocampal formation, with a loosely packed main layer of glutamatergic pyramidal neurons. It receives connections from the amygdala, entorhinal cortex, and CA3 and projects to the septum, basal prosencephalon, nucleus accumbens, prefrontal cortex, and diencephalon. It is essential for episodic memory formation and emotional responses.

CA3: Subregion of the cornu ammonis with a densely packed main layer of glutamatergic pyramidal neurons. It receives connections from the dentate gyrus and the entorhinal cortex and projects to the septum, basal prosencephalon, and diencephalon. It is essential in pattern completion during episodic memory formation.

Dentate gyrus: Three-layered cortex that forms its own gyrus and is part of the hippocampal formation, with a very densely packed main layer of granular glutamatergic neurons that are involved in adult neurogenesis. It receives connections from the entorhinal cortex and projects to CA3. It is essential in pattern separation during episodic memory formation.

Extinction learning: A behavioral concept related to neuroplasticity, where a behavioral trait acquired through conditioned learning fades and disappears when the conditioning stimulus disappears.

Long-term depression: Long-lasting diminished strength of the synaptic transmission between two neurons based upon the previous activity (or its lack). It is one of the main mechanisms of neuroplasticity along with long-term potentiation.

Long-term potentiation: Long-lasting enhancing of synaptic strength and efficacy based on the previous activity. It is one of the main mechanisms of neuroplasticity and relies upon structural and biochemical changes both at the pre- and posttranscriptional stages.

MicroRNAm are short single-stranded noncoding RNA molecules, which bind to complementary sequences within mRNA molecules, altering their translation.

Neuroplasticity: Structural or functional changes including neuronal remodeling, formation of new synapses, and birth of new neurons that allow the nervous system to adapt to environmental challenges.

Key Facts of Inflammation and BDNF

- The cytokines TNF-α, IL-1β, and IL-6 are major mediators of inflammation. IL-10 exerts an anti-inflammatory function.
- Any systemic illness and psychiatric diseases, such as stress or depression, are accompanied by increased production of proinflammatory cytokines.
- Antidepressant therapy is accompanied by a decrease in cytokine levels.
- Intraperitoneal injection of lipopolysaccharide triggers an increased production of proinflammatory cytokines and the development of the so-called sickness behavior (fever, hypersomnia, anorexia, reduced mobility, and decreased interest in exploration), which is accompanied by reduced hippocampal and prefrontal BDNF expression. This effect can be reproduced by intraperitoneal administration of IL-1β.
- Conversely, BDNF can suppress TNF-α mRNA expression and increases IL-10 mRNA expression.
- In addition to increased cytokine levels, chronic endotoxin administration induces a depressive behavior that may be reverted with antibiotics.
- Proinflammatory cytokines impair neurogenesis: incubation of hippocampal progenitor cells with recombinant IL-6 decreases neurogenesis and reduces neuronal differentiation.
- TNF-α induces oxidative stress and, acting through TNF receptor 1, decreases neural stem cell proliferation and differentiation, induces apoptosis, and decreases synaptic strength and plasticity.
- Neuroinflammation not only reduces neurogenesis, but also impairs the appropriate integration of new neurons into preexisting circuits, probably contributing to the effect of TNF-α impairing memory.

Summary Points

- BDNF is synthesized as a pre-pro-protein, which is first cleaved into a pro-molecule and later into a mature molecule and a prodomain. These transformations occur both in the neuron and in the synaptic cleft.
- Environmental enrichment, exercise, and learning are the main triggers of BDNF expression and secretion.
- Mature BDNF is involved in synaptic plasticity, axonogenesis, dendritogenesis, and neurogenesis.
- The pro-BDNF molecule is involved in neuronal apoptosis.
- BDNF increases neuronal amino acids, glucose, and ketone body uptake.
- BDNF regulates energy balance. It increases thermogenesis, fat oxidation, and glucose uptake by peripheral organs.
- BDNF has an anorexigenic effect.
- Serum BDNF is decreased in alcoholics compared with age-matched controls.
- Inflammation decreases BDNF expression and secretion.
- Moderate alcohol ingestion leads to an increase in BDNF expression and secretion, which downregulates further ingestion. This "homeostatic" loop becomes disrupted in chronic drinkers or after consumption of inebriating doses.
- Chronic alcohol consumption reduces BDNF. This reduction is involved in withdrawal-associated anxiety.

References

An JJ, Gharami K, Liao G-Y et al (2008) Distinct role of long 3' UTR BDNF mRNA in spine morphology and synaptic plasticity in hippocampal neurons. Cell 134:175–187. https://doi.org/10.1016/j.cell.2008.05.045

Anand, Prakash Huaibo, Zhang Subhash C., Pandey (2008) Innate Differences in the Expression of Brain-Derived Neurotrophic Factor in the Regions Within the Extended Amygdala Between Alcohol Preferring and Nonpreferring Rats. Alcoholism: Clinical and Experimental Research 32(6):909–920. https://doi.org/10.1111/j.1530-0277.2008.00650.x

Anastasia A, Deinhardt K, Chao MV et al (2013) Val66Met polymorphism of BDNF alters prodomain structure to induce neuronal growth cone retraction. Nat Commun 4:2490. https://doi.org/10.1038/ncomms3490

Barde YA, Edgar D, Thoenen H (1982) Purification of a new neurotrophic factor from mammalian brain. EMBO J 1:549–553

Bednarek E, Caroni P (2011) β-Adducin is required for stable assembly of new synapses and improved memory upon environmental enrichment. Neuron 69:1132–1146.5

Bohnsack JP, Teppen T, Kyzar EJ, Dzitoyeva S, Pandey SC (2019) The lncRNA BDNF-AS is an epigenetic regulator in the human amygdala in early onset alcohol use disorders. Transl Psychiatry 9:34. https://doi.org/10.1038/s41398-019-0367-z

Braken BK, Turrigiano GG (2009) Experience dependent regulation of TRK-B isoforms in rodent visual cortex. Dev Neurobiol 69:267–278

Bronfman FC, Fainzilber M (2004) Multi-tasking by the p75 neurotrophin receptor: sortilin things out? EMBO Rep 5:867–871

Cao L, Choi EY, Liu X et al (2011) White to brown fat phenotypic switch induced by genetic and environmental activation of a hypothalamic-adipocyte axis. Cell Metab 14:324–338. https://doi.org/10.1016/j.cmet.2011.06.020

Chapman TR, Barrientos RM, Ahrendsen JT et al (2012) Aging and infection reduce expression of specific brain-derived neurotrophic factor mRNAs in hippocampus. Neurobiol Aging 33(832): e1–e14. https://doi.org/10.1016/j.neurobiolaging.2011.07.015

Chen MJ, Russo-Neustadt AA (2009) Running exercise-induced up-regulation of hippocampal brain-derived neurotrophic factor is CREB-dependent. Hippocampus 19:962–972. https://doi.org/10.1002/hipo.20579

Chen ZY, Ieraci A, Teng H et al (2005) Sortilin controls intracellular sorting of brain-derived neurotrophic factor to the regulated secretory pathway. J Neurosci 25:6156–6166. https://doi.org/10.1523/JNEUROSCI.1017-05.2005

Cheng PL, Song A-I, Wong YH, Wang S, Zahng X, Poo MM (2011) Self-amplifying autocrine actions of BDNF in axon development. Proc Natl Acad Sci U S A 108:18430–18435. https://doi.org/10.1073/pnas.1115907108

Cohen-Cory S, Kidane AH, Shirkey NJ, Marshak S (2010) Brain derived neurotrophic factor and the development of structural neuronal connectivity. Dev Neurobiol 70:271–288

Costa MA, Girard M, Dalmay F, Malauzat D (2011) Brain-derived neurotrophic factor serum levels in alcohol-dependent subjects 6 months after alcohol withdrawal. Alcohol Clin Exp Res 35: 1966–1973. https://doi.org/10.1111/j.1530-0277.2011.01548.x

Cotman CW, Berchtold NC (2002) Exercise: a behavioral intervention to enhance brain health and plasticity. Trends Neurosci 25:295–301

Cunha C, Brambilla R, Thomas KL (2010) A simple role for BDNF in learning and memory? Front Mol Neurosci 3:1. https://doi.org/10.3389/neuro.02.001.2010

D'Sa C, Dileone RJ, Anderson GM, Sinha R (2012) Serum and plasma brain-derived neurotrophic factor (BDNF) in abstinent alcoholics and social drinkers. Alcohol 46:253–259. https://doi.org/10.1016/j.alcohol.2011.12.001

Darcq E, Warnault V, Phamluong K, Besserer GM, Liu F, Ron D (2015) MicroRNA-30a-5p in the prefrontal cortex controls the transition from moderate to excessive alcohol consumption. Mol Psychiatry 20:1219–1231. https://doi.org/10.1038/mp.2014.120

Deinhart K, Chao MV (2014) Shaping neurons: long and short range effects of mature and proBDNF signalling upon neuronal structure. Neuropharmacology 76:603–609

Di Liegro CM, Schiera G, Proia P, Di Liegro I (2019) Physical activity and brain health. Genes (Basel) 10(9):720. https://doi.org/10.3390/genes10090720

Dincheva I, Glatt CE, Lee FS (2012) Impact of the BDNF Val66Met polymorphism on cognition: implications for behavior genetics. Neuroscientist 18:439–451

Dowlati Y, Herrmann N, Swardfager W et al (2010) A meta-analysis of cytokines in major depression. Biol Psychiatry 67(5):446–457. https://doi.org/10.1016/j.biopsych.2009.09.033

Duman RS, Deyama S, Fogaça MV (2021) Role of BDNF in the pathophysiology and treatment of depression: activity-dependent effects distinguish rapid-acting antidepressants. Eur J Neurosci 53:126–139. https://doi.org/10.1111/ejn.14630

Epp JR, Chow C, Galea LM (2013) Hippocampus-dependent learning influences hippocampal neurogenesis. Front Neurosci 7. Published: 16 April 2013. https://doi.org/10.3389/fnins.2013.00057

Fan G, Hutnick L (2005) Methyl-CpG binding proteins in the nervous system. Cell Res 15:255–261

Ferris LT, Williams JS, Shen CL (2007) The effect of acute exercise on serum brain-derived neurotrophic factor levels and cognitive function. Med Sci Sports Exerc 39:728–734

Fujimura H, Altar CA, Chen R et al (2002) Brain-derived neurotrophic factor is stored in human platelets and released by agonist stimulation. Thromb Haemost 87:728–734

Fulgenzi G, Hong Z, Tomassoni-Ardori F et al (2020) Novel metabolic role for BDNF in pancreatic β-cell insulin secretion. Nat Commun 11:1950. https://doi.org/10.1038/s41467-020-15833-5

Geisel O, Hellweg R, Müller CA (2016) Serum levels of brain-derived neurotrophic factor in alcohol-dependent patients receiving high-dose baclofen. Psychiatry Res 240:177–180. https://doi.org/10.1016/j.psychres.2016.04.007

Genzer Y, Chapnik N, Froy O (2017) Effect of brain-derived neurotrophic factor (BDNF) on hepatocyte metabolism. Int J Biochem Cell Biol 88:69–74. https://doi.org/10.1016/j.biocel.2017.05.008

Gonzalez A, Moya-Alvarado G, González-Billault C, Bronfman FC (2016) Cellular and molecular mechanisms regulating neuronal growth by brain-derived neurotrophic factor. Cytoskeleton 73: 612–628

Hempstead BL (2015) Brain derived neurotrophic factor: three ligands, many actions. Trans Am Clin Climatol Assoc 126:9–19

Huang M-C, Chen C-H, Chen C-H et al (2008) Alterations of serum brain-derived neurotrophic factor levels in early alcohol withdrawal. Alcohol Alcohol 43:241–245. https://doi.org/10.1093/alcalc/agm172

Jeanblanc J, Logrip ML, Janak PH, Ron D (2013) BDNF-mediated regulation of ethanol consumption requires the activation of the MAP kinase pathway and protein synthesis. Eur J Neurosci 37: 607–612. https://doi.org/10.1111/ejn.12067

Joe K-H, Kim Y-K, Kim T-S et al (2007) Decreased plasma brain-derived neurotrophic factor levels in patients with alcohol dependence. Alcohol Clin Exp Res 31(11):1833–1838. https://doi.org/10.1111/j.1530-0277.2007.00507.x

John F, Bishop Gregory P, Mueller M.Maral, Mouradian (1994) Alternate 5′ exons in the rat brain-derived neurotrophic factor gene: differential patterns of expression across brain regions. Molecular Brain Research 26(1–2):225–232. https://doi.org/10.1016/0169-328X(94)90094-9

Joshua J, Park Niamh X, Cawley Y. Peng, Loh (2008) A bi-directional carboxypeptidase E-driven transport mechanism controls BDNF vesicle homeostasis in hippocampal neurons. Molecular and Cellular Neuroscience 39(1):63–73. https://doi.org/10.1016/j.mcn.2008.05.016

Kernie SG, Liebl DJ, Parada LF (2000) BDNF regulates eating behavior and locomotor activity in mice. EMBO J 19:1290–1300. https://doi.org/10.1093/emboj/19.6.1290

Kim T-K, Hemberg M, Gray JM (2015) Enhancer RNAs: a class of long noncoding RNAs synthesized at enhancers. Cold Spring Harb Perspect Biol 7:a018622. https://doi.org/10.1101/cshperspect.a018622

Klein AB, Williamson R, Santini MA et al (2011) Blood BDNF concentrations reflect brain-tissue BDNF levels across species. Int J Neuropsychopharmacol 14:347–353. https://doi.org/10.1017/S1461145710000738

Koob GF, Volkow ND (2016) Neurobiology of addiction: a neurocircuitry analysis. Lancet Psychiatry 3:760–773. https://doi.org/10.1016/S2215-0366(16)00104-8

Kowianski P, Lietzau G, Czuba E, Waskow M, Steliga A, Morys J (2018) BDNF: a key factor with multipotent impact on brain signaling and synaptic plasticity. Cell Mol Neurobiol 38:579–593

Krabbe KS, Nielsen AR, Krogh-Madsen R et al (2007) Brain-derived neurotrophic factor (BDNF) and type 2 diabetes. Diabetologia 50:431–438

Kwon M, Fernández JR, Zegarek GF, Lo SB, Firestein BL (2011) BDNF-promoted increases in proximal dendrites occur via CREB-dependent transcriptional regulation of cypin. J Neurosci 31:9735–9745

Kyzar EJ, Zhang H, Pandey SC (2019) Adolescent alcohol exposure epigenetically suppresses amygdala arc enhancer RNA expression to confer adult anxiety susceptibility. Biol Psychiatry 85:904–914. https://doi.org/10.1016/j.biopsych.2018.12.021

Lapchak PA, Hefti F (1992) BDNF and NGF treatment in lesioned rats: effects on cholinergic function and weight gain. Neuroreport 3:405–408. https://doi.org/10.1097/00001756-199205000-00007

Lee R, Kermani P, Teng KK, Hempstead BL (2001) Regulation of cell survival by secreted proneurotrophins. Science 294:1945–1948

Lee BC, Choi I-G, Kim Y-K et al (2009) Relation between plasma brain-derived neurotrophic factor and nerve growth factor in the male patients with alcohol dependence. Alcohol 43:265–269. https://doi.org/10.1016/j.alcohol.2009.04.003

Liu Y, Zhou LJ, Wang J et al (2017) TNF-α differentially regulates synaptic plasticity in the hippocampus and spinal cord by microglia-dependent mechanisms after peripheral nerve injury. J Neurosci 37(4):871–881. https://doi.org/10.1523/JNEUROSCI.2235-16.2016

Logrip ML, Barak S, Warnault V, Ron D (2015) Corticostriatal BDNF and alcohol addiction. Brain Res 1628(Pt A):60–67. https://doi.org/10.1016/j.brainres.2015.03.025

Lonze BE, Ginty DD (2002) Function and regulation of CREB family transcription factors in the nervous system. Neuron 35:605–623. https://doi.org/10.1016/s0896-6273(02)00828-0
Lu B, Pand PT, Woo NH (2005) The Yin and Yang of neurotrophin action. Nat Rev Neurosci 6: 603–614
Mao CP, Bai ZL, Zhang XN, Zhang QJ, Zhang L (2016) Abnormal subcortical brain morphology in patients with knee osteoarthritis: a cross-sectional study. Front Aging Neurosci 8:3. https://doi.org/10.3389/fnagi.2016.00003
Marmigère F, Givalois L, Rage F, Arancibia S, Tapia-Arancibia L (2003) Rapid induction of BDNF expression in the hippocampus during immobilization stress challenge in adult rats. Hippocampus 13:646–655. https://doi.org/10.1002/hipo.10109
Marosi K, Mattson MP (2014) DBNF mediates adaptive brain and body responses to energetic challenges. Trends Endocrinol Metab 25:89–98. https://doi.org/10.1016/j.tem.2013.10.006.6
Martín-González C, Romero-Acevedo L, Fernández-Rodríguez CM et al (2020) Brain-derived neurotrophic factor among patients with alcoholism. CNS Spectr 19:1–6. https://doi.org/10.1017/S1092852920001431
Matthews VB, Aström MB, Chan MHS et al (2009) Brain-derived neurotrophic factor is produced by skeletal muscle cells in response to contraction and enhances fat oxidation via activation of AMP-activated protein kinase. Diabetologia 52:1409–1418. https://doi.org/10.1007/s00125-009-1364-1
Moon HY, Becke A, Berron D et al (2016) Running-induced systemic Cathepsin B secretion is associated with memory function. Cell Metab 24:332–340. https://doi.org/10.1016/j.cmet.2016.05.025
Moonat S, Pandey SC (2012) Stress, epigenetics, and alcoholism. Alcohol Res 34(4):495–505
Moonat S, Starkman BG, Sakharkar A, Pandey S (2010) Neuroscience of alcoholism: molecular and cellular mechanisms. Cell Mol Life Sci 67:73–88. https://doi.org/10.1007/s00018-009-0135-y
Moonat S, Sakharkar AJ, Zhang H, Pandey SC (2011) The role of amygdaloid brain-derived neurotrophic factor, activity-regulated cytoskeleton-associated protein and dendritic spines in anxiety and alcoholism. Addict Biol 16:238–250. https://doi.org/10.1111/j.1369-1600.2010.00275.x
Nagappan G, Zaltsev E, Senatorov VV, Yang J, Hempstead BL, Lu B (2009) Control of extracellular claevage of proBDNF by high frequency neuronal activity. Proc Natl Acad Sci 106:1267–1272
Nilsson J, Ekblom O, Ekblom M et al (2020) Acute increases in brain-derived neurotrophic factor in plasma following physical exercise relates to subsequent learning in older adults. Sci Rep 10: 4395. https://doi.org/10.1038/s41598-020-60124-0
Noble EE, Billington CJ, Colz CM, Wang CF (2011) The lighter side of BDNF. Am J Physiol Regul Integr Comp Physiol 300:R1053–R1069
Notaras M, van den Buuse M (2019) Brain-derived neurotrophic factor (BDNF): novel insights into regulation and genetic variation. Neuroscientist 25:434–454. https://doi.org/10.1177/1073858418810142
Novkovic T, Mittmann T, Manahan-Vaughan D (2015) BDNF contributes to the facilitation of hippocampal synaptic plasticity and learning enabled by environmental enrichment. Hippocampus 25:1–15
Numakawa T, Odaka H, Adachi N (2018) Actions of brain-derived neurotrophic factor in the neurogenesis and neuronal function, and its involvement in the pathophysiology of brain diseases. Int J Mol Sci 19:3650. https://doi.org/10.3390/ijms19113650
Nyborg AC, Ladd TB, Zwizinski CW, Lah JJ, Golde TE (2006) Sortilin, SorCS1b, and SorLA Vps10p sorting receptors, are novel gamma-secretase substrates. Mol Neurodegener 1:3. https://doi.org/10.1186/1750-1326-1-3
Ornell F, Hansen F, Schuch FB et al (2018) Brain-derived neurotrophic factor in substance use disorders: a systematic review and meta-analysis. Drug Alcohol Depend 193:91–103. https://doi.org/10.1016/j.drugalcdep.2018.08.036

Palmisano M, Pandey SC (2017) Epigenetic mechanisms of alcoholism and stress-related disorders. Alcohol 60:7–18. https://doi.org/10.1016/j.alcohol.2017.01.001
Pandey SC, Sakharkar AJ, Tang L, Zhang H (2015) Potential role of adolescent alcohol exposure-induced amygdaloid histone modifications in anxiety and alcohol intake during adulthood. Neurobiol Dis 82:607–619
Pandey SC, Kyzar EJ, Zhang H (2017) Epigenetic basis of the dark side of alcohol addiction. Neuropharmacology 122:74–84. https://doi.org/10.1016/j.neuropharm.2017.02.002
Pollock GS, Vernon E, Forbes ME, Yan Q, Ma YT, Hsieh T, Robichon R, Frost DO, Johnson JE (2001) Effects of early visual experience and diurnal rhythms on BDNF mRNA and protein levels in the visual system, hippocampus, and cerebellum. J Neurosci 21(11):3923–3931. https://doi.org/10.1523/JNEUROSCI.21-11-03923.2001
Pruunsild P, Kazantseva A, Aid T, Palm K, Timmusk T (2007) Dissecting the human BDNF locus: bidirectional transcription, complex splicing, and multiple promoters. Genomics 90:397–406. https://doi.org/10.1016/j.ygeno.2007.05.004
Qin L, Wu X, Block ML et al (2007) Systemic LPS causes chronic neuroinflammation and progressive neurodegeneration. Glia 55:453–462. https://doi.org/10.1002/glia.20467
Renthal W, Nestler EJ (2008) Epigenetic mechanisms in drug addiction. Trends Mol Med 14: 341–350. https://doi.org/10.1016/j.molmed.2008.06.004
Ronald S, Duman Nanxin, Li (2012) A neurotrophic hypothesis of depression: role of synaptogenesis in the actions of NMDA receptor antagonists. Philosophical Transactions of the Royal Society B: Biological Sciences 367(1601):2475–2484. https://doi.org/10.1098/rstb.2011.0357
Roskoski R (2012) ERK1/2 MAP kinases: structure, function, and regulation. Pharmacol Res 66(2): 105–143. https://doi.org/10.1016/j.phrs.2012.04.005
Sasi M, Vignoli B, Canossa M, Blum R (2017) Neurobiology of local and intercellular BDNF signaling. Pflugers Arch-Eur J Physiol 469:593–610
Spielman LJ, Gibson DL, Klegeris A, Spielman LJ et al (2017) Incretin hormones regulate microglia oxidative stress, survival and expression of trophic factors. Eur J Cell Biol 96(3): 240–253. https://doi.org/10.1016/j.ejcb.2017.03.004
Starkman BG, Sakharkar AJ, Pandey SC (2012) Epigenetics-beyond the genome in alcoholism. Alcohol Res 34:293–305
Steven A, Friedrich M, ,Jank P, et al What turns CREB on? And off? And why does it matter? Cell Mol Life Sci 2020; 77(20): 4049–4067
Tien NW, Kerschensteiner D (2018) Homeostatic plasticity in neural development. Neural Dev 13: 9. https://doi.org/10.1186/s13064-018-0105-x
Tongiorgi E, Righi M, Cattaneo A (1997) Activity-dependent dendritic targeting of BDNF and TrkB mRNAs in hippocampal neurons. J Neurosci 17:9492–9505. https://doi.org/10.1523/JNEUROSCI.17-24-09492.1997
Tõnis, Timmusk Kaia, Palm Madis, Metsis Tõnu, Reintam Viiu, Paalme Mart, Saarma Håkan, Persson (1993) Multiple promoters direct tissue-specific expression of the rat BDNF gene. Neuron 10(3):475–489. https://doi.org/10.1016/0896-6273(93)90335-O
Tsankova N, Renthal W, Kumar A, Nestler EJ (2007) Epigenetic regulation in psychiatric disorders. Nat Rev Neurosci 8:355–367
Umene-Nakano W, Yoshimura R, Ikenouchi-Sugita A et al (2009) Serum levels of brain-derived neurotrophic factor in comorbidity of depression and alcohol dependence. Hum Psychopharmacol 24:409–413. https://doi.org/10.1002/hup.1035
Vafadari B, Salamian A, Kaezmarek I (2016) MMP-9 in translation: from molecule to brain physiology, pathology and therapy. J Neurochem 139(Suppl 2):91–114
Vaynman S, Ying Z, Gomez-Pinilla F (2007) The select action of hippocampal calcium calmodulin protein kinase II in mediating exercise-enhanced cognitive function. Neuroscience 144: 825–833. https://doi.org/10.1016/j.neuroscience.2006.10.005

Warnault V, Darcq E, Morisot N et al (2016) The BDNF valine 68 to methionine polymorphism increases compulsive alcohol drinking in mice that is reversed by tropomyosin receptor kinase B activation. Biol Psychiatry 79:463–473

Winnubst J, Cheyne JE, Niculescu D, Lohmann C (2015) Spontaneous activity drives local synaptic plasticity in vivo. Neuron 87(2):399–410. https://doi.org/10.1016/j.neuron.2015.06.029

Woo D, Seo Y, Jung H et al (2019) Locally activating TrKB receptor generates actin waves and specific axonal fate. Cell Chem Biol 26:1652–1663

Wrann CD, White JP, Salogiannnis J et al (2013) Exercise induces hippocampal BDNF through a PGC-1α/FNDC5 pathway. Cell Metab 18:649–659. https://doi.org/10.1016/j.cmet.2013.09.008

Xu B, Xie X (2016) Neurotrophic factor control of satiety and body weight. Nat Rev Neurosci 17: 282–292. https://doi.org/10.1038/nrn.2016.24

Yamanaka M, Itakura Y, Inoue T et al (2006) Protective effect of brain-derived neurotrophic factor on pancreatic islets in obese diabetic mice. Metabolism 55:1286–1292. https://doi.org/10.1016/j.metabol.2006.04.017

Yamanaka M, Tsuchida A, Nakagawa T et al (2007) Brain-derived neurotrophic factor enhances glucose utilization in peripheral tissues of diabetic mice. Diabetes Obes Metab 9:59–64. https://doi.org/10.1111/j.1463-1326.2006.00572.x

Yang J, Siao CJ, Nagappan G et al (2009) Neuronal release of proBDNF. Nat Neurosci 12:113–115

Zhang JC, Yao W, Hashimoto K (2016) Brain-derived neurotrophic factor (BDNF)-TrkB signaling in inflammation-related depression and potential therapeutic targets. Curr Neuropharmacol 14: 721–731. https://doi.org/10.2174/1570159x14666160119094646

Zuccato C, Cattaneo E (2009) Brain-derived neurotrophic factor in neurodegenerative diseases. Nat Rev Neurol 5(6):311–322. https://doi.org/10.1038/nrneurol.2009.54

Alcohol and Cirrhosis

60

Beata Gavurova and Viera Ivankova

Contents

Introduction 1302
Liver Cirrhosis 1303
Alcohol as a Risk Factor 1304
Alcohol-Related Liver Cirrhosis 1306
  Diagnosis 1307
  Complications 1307
  Treatment 1308
Abstinence as a Protective Factor 1311
Applications to Other Areas of Addiction 1311
Applications to Public Health 1313
Mini-Dictionary of Terms 1313
Key Facts of Alcohol and Cirrhosis 1314
Summary Points 1314
References 1315

Abstract

Alcohol is one of the main causes of liver disease, as it is in the liver that alcohol is broken down. Excessive alcohol consumption is therefore considered a significant risk factor for liver cirrhosis. The risk increases depending on the amount and total duration of alcohol consumption, with daily heavy drinkers being most at risk. Alcohol is estimated to be responsible for approximately 50% of all liver cirrhosis worldwide. Patients diagnosed with alcohol-related cirrhosis have

B. Gavurova (✉)
Department of Addictology, First Faculty of Medicine, Charles University and General University Hospital in Prague, Prague, Czechia
e-mail: beata.gavurova@lf1.cuni.cz

V. Ivankova
Institute of Earth Resources, Faculty of Mining, Ecology, Process Control and Geotechnologies, Technical University of Košice, Košice, Slovak Republic
e-mail: viera.ivankova@tuke.sk

V. B. Patel, V. R. Preedy (eds.), *Handbook of Substance Misuse and Addictions*,
https://doi.org/10.1007/978-3-030-92392-1_188

poorer health outcomes and higher mortality than those with non-alcohol-related cirrhosis. This indicates that alcohol-related cirrhosis represents a huge health burden. The first prerequisite for the successful treatment of alcohol-related cirrhosis, including the treatment of its complications, is complete abstinence. The co-existence of alcohol-related liver disease and alcohol use disorder in patients requires multidisciplinary care. With regard to cirrhosis, reducing alcohol consumption should be seen as an important health policy objective.

Keywords

Liver · Cirrhosis · Etiology · Alcohol · Drinking · Alcohol use disorder · Risk factor · Diagnosis · Treatment · Symptoms · Complications · Health burden · Hepatologists · Addiction specialists

Abbreviations

ALDH	Aldehyde dehydrogenase
INR	International normalized ratio
MELD	Model for End-stage Liver Disease
NASH	Non-alcoholic steatohepatitis

Introduction

Alcohol is an available and relatively well socially accepted addictive substance. However, alcohol is associated with various health consequences ranging from mental to damage to various parenchymatous organs. In this context, long-term excessive alcohol consumption can lead to severe liver damage such as alcohol-related cirrhosis. Although it does not develop in all alcoholics, the risk of developing it is very high. Therefore, alcohol-related liver cirrhosis is currently considered a huge health burden, to a greater extent than ever before (Tonon and Piano 2021). Global alcohol consumption contributes to this reality and raises further concerns (GBD 2017, Cirrhosis Collaborators 2020; Moon et al. 2020). This is also highlighted by the fact that increasing cirrhosis may be associated with a dramatic increase in harmful alcohol consumption (Pimpin et al. 2018). Heavy daily drinking on a population level significantly influences the weight of alcohol in the cirrhosis burden. Moreover, half of cirrhosis mortality worldwide is attributable to alcohol, approximating 60% in North America and Europe (Stein et al. 2016). The seriousness of the problem lies precisely in premature mortality.

In general, cirrhosis of the liver – a disease known as "hardening of the liver" is a serious condition in which the vital tissue of the liver slowly turns into a stiff and scarred mass. The whole process goes unnoticed for a long time. The liver does not hurt, it works less, but in normal daily activities the individual is not significantly limited by this slight insufficiency. By the time the disease begins to bother them in everyday life, the liver tissue is already largely damaged (Ehrmann et al. 2018). For this reason, there is a need to pay attention to individual factors, and it is evident from the previous paragraph that one such factor is alcohol. The literature deals extensively with the issue of alcohol consumption and liver cirrhosis, but there is still room for in-depth research. At the same time, it is possible to look at this issue in terms of alcohol addiction.

Liver Cirrhosis

The liver is the largest parenchymatous organ of the human body, which plays a central role in maintaining metabolic homeostasis, including protein metabolism, carbohydrate metabolism, fat metabolism, cholesterol metabolism, bile acid metabolism, enterohepatic bile acids circulation, bilirubin metabolism, bile production, and metabolic detoxification. In other words, it is an integrating unit that is involved in all metabolic and other important processes in the human body. Accordingly, the main functions of the liver are:

1. Synthesizes specialized proteins, sugars, and lipids
2. Maintains a stable level of the amino acid glucose in the systemic circulation
3. Provides bile acids and bicarbonates for digestive processes
4. Is the main biotransformation and excretion organ for large and hydrophobic metabolites, contaminants, and drugs (Maasová and Hulín 2013).

The structure of the liver, including the blood and bile ducts, is responsible for the optimal provision of these functions. Normally, the liver is a very resilient organ and is able to regenerate damaged cells. However, if it is damaged, it cannot function properly.

Cirrhosis is a serious disease caused by long-term exposure to toxins, such as alcohol or viral infections. More specifically, liver cirrhosis is defined as the histological development of regenerative nodules surrounded by fibrous bands in response to chronic liver injury leading to portal hypertension and end-stage liver disease (Schuppan and Afdhal 2008). The term cirrhosis was introduced by René Théophile Hyacinthe Laennec in 1826. It comes from the Greek word "scirrhus" – the surface of an orange – referring the brown-yellow surface of the liver, which is seen at autopsy. Chronic disease often persists 10–30 years before the clinical manifestation phase. Liver cirrhosis is the end stage of chronic liver diseases from the functional and morphological point of view. Damage to the liver is characterized by destruction of its architecture and fibrous formations that contain regenerative nodules of hepatocytes. There is compensated (asymptomatic stage) or decompensated (symptomatic stage) cirrhosis (Maasová and Hulín 2013).

The cause of the cirrhotic process is persistent necrosis of hepatocytes. If complications occur, the patient's quality of life as well as the patient's survival is affected. The main complications of cirrhosis include gastrointestinal bleeding, ascites formation, development of hepatorenal syndrome and hepatic encephalopathy, hemocoagulation disorders, hepatocellular carcinoma, acquired immunodeficiency, inflammatory complications, hepatopulmonary syndrome, cholelithiasis

(4–5 times more frequent than in the healthy population), osteopathy (16–23% – reduction of bone density), metabolic and endocrine disorders. Patients with liver cirrhosis have a higher incidence of bacterial bronchopneumonia, uroinfection, pulmonary tuberculosis, and tuberculous peritonitis. The most common etiological agents are Gram-negative rods, in bronchopneumonia Staphylococcus epidermidis, Staphylococcus aureus, Streptococcus viridans, Pseudomonas aeruginosa, and Candida albicans. Fatal infections in patients with liver cirrhosis occur in 7% of cases in the compensated state and in 20% of cases in the decompensated state. Invasive diagnostic and treatment procedures are a frequent source of infection (Maasová and Hulín 2013). Last but not least, acute liver failure should be emphasized, which is a life-threatening complication leading to multisystem failure (Mahl and O'Grady 2014; Piano et al. 2017).

All the above-mentioned complications can contribute to the deterioration of the condition, which can have serious consequences. This is evidenced by the fact that cirrhosis of the liver is the cause of approximately 1.32 million deaths per year worldwide, and ranks 11th in the global mortality rate (Asrani et al. 2019; GBD 2017, Cirrhosis Collaborators 2020). Moreover, patients with cirrhosis clearly have a higher risk of death compared to the general population (Fleming et al. 2012). From an economic point of view, in addition to the increased risk of death associated with lost productivity, cirrhosis of the liver has a significant impact on health systems and on the quality of life of patients, as it is among the top 20 causes of disability-adjusted life years worldwide (Asrani et al. 2019).

Table 1 shows different causes of cirrhosis. In general, the etiology of liver cirrhosis is most often associated with alcohol or arises in patients with metabolic syndrome (non-alcoholic steatohepatitis [NASH]). It can also occur as a consequence of viral hepatitis B and C, autoimmune hepatitis or primary biliary cirrhosis, in metabolic diseases such as hemochromatosis, Wilson's disease or antitrypsin deficiency. In some patients, the etiology cannot be recognized, and then it is possible to speak of cryptogenic cirrhosis of the liver. Cryptogenic forms of cirrhosis are declining due to improvements in diagnostic methods (Bureš et al. 2014).

In more detail, it was confirmed in a recent study with long-term data of 5138 patients that the most common etiology of cirrhosis is alcohol-related liver disease (39.5%), followed by NASH (18.2%) and hepatitis B virus (10.8%) (Jain et al. 2021). The attending physician must always very carefully confirm or exclude an alcoholic origin of liver damage. Possible mistakes can have serious consequences. Bearing in mind that alcohol-related cirrhosis contributes significantly to overall cirrhosis and that it is becoming an increasing part of the total burden of liver disease; there is a continuing need to address this problem (Lucey 2019).

Alcohol as a Risk Factor

Alcohol is a well-known risk factor for liver cirrhosis, with the risk increasing exponentially (Roerecke et al. 2019). Thus, the relative risk of cirrhosis increases rapidly depending on the amount and total duration of alcohol consumption.

Table 1 Etiology of cirrhosis. This table shows the etiology of cirrhosis in the classification of viral/infectious, metabolic, cholestatic, and vascular causes. Alcohol etiology is one of the most common. The table was compiled according to Suva (2014)

Cause of cirrhosis	
Viral/infectious	Hepatitis B
	Hepatitis C
	Schistosomiasis
Metabolic	Alcohol
	Toxins, medications
	Hereditary hemochromatosis
	Wilson's disease
	Non-alcoholic steatohepatitis (NASH)
	Insulin resistance
Cholestatic	Primary biliary cirrhosis
	Primary sclerosing cholangitis
	Biliary atresia
	Secondary biliary cirrhosis
Vascular	Right heart failure
	Bud-Chiari syndrome
	Alpha-1-antitrypsin deficiency
	Sarcoidosis
	Cystic fibrosis

Source: own processing according to Suva (2014)

Compared with 20 grams of alcohol per day for 10 to 12 years, the risk is six times higher with 40–60 grams of alcohol per day and even 14 times higher with 60–80 grams of alcohol per day. Also, 50% of daily consumers of 210 grams of alcohol over 22 years and 80% of those consuming the same amount for 33 years will develop liver cirrhosis. It is generally reported that some cirrhosis will develop with daily alcohol drinking of 180–200 grams in 25 years. For females, the reported values are less by up to half (Ehrmann et al. 2018). This can be explained by the fact that the same amount of average alcohol consumption is related to a higher risk of liver cirrhosis in females than in males (Rehm et al. 2010). Other factors that need to be taken into account include the regularity or frequency of binge drinking and the consumption of alcohol fasting or during meals. Evidence shows that daily alcohol consumption, together with not drinking with meals, can be associated with more than a doubling of cirrhosis incidence (Simpson et al. 2019). In terms of liver damage, binge drinking appears to be less dangerous than less but daily consumption, as the liver has time to regenerate. Several findings also show that liver damage is not related to the type of drink, but only to the amount of alcohol that it contains (Ehrmann et al. 2018; Stein et al. 2016). Klatsky and Armstrong (1992) also pointed out that past and current alcohol drinking is strongly associated with the risk of cirrhosis, but usual choice of alcoholic beverage does not show an independent relationship. Similar results were found by Askgaard et al. (2015), who confirmed that daily alcohol drinking was associated with an increased risk of alcohol-related cirrhosis in males; also, recent alcohol consumption rather than earlier in life was associated with risk of alcohol-related cirrhosis. On the other hand, they confirmed that compared to beer and liquor, wine might be associated with a lower risk of alcohol-related cirrhosis.

Smoking can also be included among the possible factors of alcohol-related cirrhosis. In this context, daily smokers of a pack of cigarettes or more have a threefold higher risk compared to lifelong nonsmokers. On the other hand, coffee drinking is considered a factor, which is inversely associated with the risk of alcohol-related cirrhosis. That is, smoking is risky in terms of alcohol-related cirrhosis, while coffee drinking might be protective (Klatsky and Armstrong 1992).

Alcohol-Related Liver Cirrhosis

When mentioning the adverse effects of alcohol, the lay and often the professional medical community is primarily concerned with liver damage. The cause of alcoholic liver damage is the overuse of the liver's enzymes to break down large amounts of alcohol and its direct toxic effect on liver cells. Worldwide, approximately 2 billion people consume alcohol, with up to 75 million people diagnosed with alcohol-related disorders and at risk of alcohol-related liver disease (Asrani et al. 2019). This fact increases interest in the effects of alcohol on the liver. Alcohol damage to the liver includes many diseases, and one of them is alcohol-related cirrhosis (Liangpunsakul et al. 2016). "Hardening of the liver" is a dreaded disease of excessive drinkers. As early as 1793, Matthew Baillie described the clinical picture of cirrhosis in detail and stated that it often occurs in heavy drinkers. Alcohol damage to the liver was later pointed out (in 1836) by Thomas Addison, who described fatty liver degeneration due to excessive alcohol consumption (Ehrmann et al. 2018).

The fact is that patients with alcohol-related cirrhosis have a worse prognosis than patients with non-alcohol-related cirrhosis (Fleming et al. 2012). They also have significantly higher readmission rates, more complications, a higher risk of mortality, and worse liver function (Jain et al. 2021; Tonon and Piano 2021). According to Rehm et al. (2010), alcohol consumption has a greater impact on mortality from liver cirrhosis compared to morbidity. This is reflected in the fact that alcohol-related cirrhosis contributes significantly to global mortality. Also, it is considered a global health burden (Rehm et al. 2013).

Evidence shows that alcohol-related liver disease is increasingly common in many parts of Asia, but is declining in Western Europe (Liangpunsakul et al. 2016). With regard to alcohol-related cirrhosis, information on prevalence is fairly accurate in developed countries and deaths from alcohol-related cirrhosis are somewhere a measure of alcohol consumption. Globally, alcohol is estimated to be responsible for about 50% of all liver cirrhosis, but with considerable geographical differences (e.g., related to the prevailing religion) (Ehrmann et al. 2018; Masarone et al. 2016). The findings of Lucey (2019) also showed that alcohol-related cirrhosis accounts for up to 50% of the overall cirrhosis burden in the United States. These findings suggest that alcohol-related cirrhosis is a widespread problem across countries and therefore should not be overlooked in public health policies but also in medical practice.

Diagnosis

Although cirrhosis has long been considered an irreversible condition, in the light of new knowledge, the disease is seen as a dynamic and potentially reversible condition in some cases (Ehrmann et al. 2018). Rather than being viewed in terms of its own stages, cirrhosis is often seen as the final stage of liver disease. According to Tsochatzis et al. (2014), cirrhosis can be divided into clinical stages with marked differences in prognosis and in some cases can even be reversed by successful etiological treatment. Early diagnosis and close monitoring of the cirrhotic patient's condition is essential due to the need for treatment and detection of possible complications. As symptoms are variable, medical examination most often focuses on the skin stigmata of liver disease and portal hypertension. Diagnosis of cirrhosis includes serological test, histological test, transient elastography, and radio techniques such as ultrasonography, computerized tomography scan, and magnetic resonance imaging (Suva 2014). Laboratory tests play an important role in the diagnosis and evaluation of patients' conditions and their results mainly show increased prothrombin time, increased bilirubin, increased albumin, and low thrombocyte count (Mahl and O'Grady 2014). According to Whitfield et al. (2018), international normalized ratio (INR) and bilirubin show the best separation of patients with alcohol-related cirrhosis. The severity of the patient's condition can be determined in routine clinical practice according to the Child-Pugh classification shown in Table 2.

Complications

The clinical picture of liver cirrhosis is very varied, ranging from asymptomatic to comatose. Approximately 30–40% of patients with liver cirrhosis are free of

Table 2 Child-Pugh score to assess severity of cirrhosis. This table provides the Child-Pugh classification for assessing the severity of cirrhosis. The higher the Child-Pugh score, the more severe the cirrhosis. In this way, "C" patients represent the highest risk group. The table was compiled according to Joshi and Shriwastav (2016)

	Points assigned		
Parameter	1	2	3
Albumin, g/dL	>3.5	2.8–3.5	<2.8
Bilirubin, mg/dL	<2	2–3	>3
Prothrombin time (second over control) or International normalized ratio (INR)	<4 <1.7	4–6 1.7–2.3	>6 >2.3
Ascites	Absent	Slight	Moderate to severe
Encephalopathy (grade)	0 (none)	I–II (mild to moderate)	III–IV (severe)
Class A = 5–6 points, Class B = 7–9 points, Class C = 10–15 points			

Source: own processing according to Joshi and Shriwastav (2016)

problems for years and the disease first manifests itself only with complications. Sometimes the patient seeks help late, at the moment of liver failure (Ehrmann et al. 2018). Although patients are initially free of complications, they usually develop ascites, variceal bleeding, or hepatic encephalopathy later on. According to Jepsen et al. (2010), the presence and type of complications at diagnosis are predictors of mortality. In their study, one-year mortality was 17% among patients with no initial complications, 20% following variceal bleeding alone, 29% following ascites alone, 49% following ascites and variceal bleeding (from the onset of the later of the two complications), and 64% following hepatic encephalopathy. Table 3 presents the symptoms and objective findings in alcohol-related liver cirrhosis.

In the study by Jain et al. (2021), patients with alcohol-related cirrhosis were more likely to be younger, male, and to have more complications, including sepsis, ascites, spontaneous bacterial peritonitis, acute kidney injury, acute variceal bleeding, and hepatic encephalopathy compared to patients with other etiologies. They also showed worse prognostic scores and higher mortality compared to patients with non-alcohol-related cirrhosis. It is true that patients with cirrhosis of different etiologies have different types of complication, with alcohol-related cirrhotic patients facing a higher risk of hepatic encephalopathy and acute-on-chronic liver failure (Zhuang et al. 2021). In addition, evidence shows that alcohol-related cirrhosis is associated with higher inpatient mortality compared to non-alcohol-related cirrhosis. Fan et al. (2019) found that nutritional deficiency in patients with alcohol-related cirrhosis may cause a higher rate of coagulopathy; also, low thiamine and phosphate depletion in alcohol-related cirrhosis may contribute to hepatic encephalopathy. The authors emphasized that alcohol impairs immune function and may increase the risk of infection, leading to higher complications and poorer outcomes. In fact, alcohol-related cirrhosis requires more aggressive intervention and a systemic approach in the hospital environment.

Treatment

In alcohol-related cirrhosis, treatment is focused primarily on the underlying disease (i.e., alcohol addiction), complications, support measures (regime measures – abstinence from alcohol), as well as liver transplantation. Thus, the first prerequisite for the successful treatment of alcohol-related cirrhosis, including the treatment of its complications, is abstinence, preferably complete. This requires the patient's trust and cooperation with the attending physician, psychologist, or psychiatrist. Also, family help is essential. Often abstinence alone improves clinical and laboratory findings. Pharmacological methods based on the inhibition of aldehyde dehydrogenase (ALDH). After alcohol intake, acetaldehyde levels increase with subsequent nausea, vomiting and headaches. These substances include disulfiram, calcium carbimide, or cyanamide. The disadvantages of this treatment are the side effects, especially neuropathy, heart, and liver damage. Therefore, in addition to judicious selection of patients, regular clinical and laboratory monitoring is required (Ehrmann et al. 2018). In fact, pharmacological treatment of alcohol use disorders is often challenging in patients with liver disease because many drugs are metabolized in the liver or, in

Table 3 Symptoms and objective findings in alcohol-related liver cirrhosis. This table shows the symptoms and objective findings in alcohol-related liver cirrhosis, which are divided into nine medical groups. The table was compiled according to Ehrmann et al. (2018)

Group	Symptoms and findings
General symptoms	Weakness, malaise, fatigue Inappetence, weight loss Subfebrile to fever Hepatic fever Changes on the nails (noticeably large white lunettes) “Varnished” lips Smooth tongue Excoriation due to scratching in cholestasis Hyperpigmentation of the skin
Icterus	Prehepatic (overproduction of bilirubin with increased hemolysis) Hepatic (impaired bilirubin conjugation in hepatocellular injury) Cholestatic (impaired secretion of conjugated bilirubin by the liver cell)
Gastrointestinal symptoms and findings	Bleeding (esophageal, gastric, rectal varices) Hypertensive portal gastropathy and colopathy Peptic ulcer lesions Diarrhea, flatulence Hepatomegaly, splenomegaly Ascites Caput medusae
Hematological symptoms and findings	Anemia (from folate deficiency – macrocytic, hemolytic, Zieve’s syndrome, due to hypersplenism) Thrombocytopenia Leukopenia Petechiae, ecchymoses Coagulopathies (hematomas, suffusions) Disseminated intravascular coagulation Hemosiderosis
Endocrine symptoms and findings	Hypogonadism: Men – loss of libido, testicular atrophy, impotence Women – dysmenorrhea, loss of secondary sexual characteristics, infertility Symptoms from increased estrogen levels (spider nevi, palmar erythema, gynecomastia, loss of axillary and pubic hair) Impaired carbohydrate metabolism Hyperparathyroidism
Renal symptoms and findings	Secondary hyperaldosteronism Hepatorenal syndrome Renal tubular acidosis
Cardiac symptoms and findings	Hypercirculatory state
Pulmonary symptoms and findings	Shortness of breath (but also due to ascites) Hydrothorax Hepatopulmonary syndrome Primary pulmonary hypertension

(continued)

Table 3 (continued)

Group	Symptoms and findings
	Hyperventilation Hypoxemia Mallet fingers
Neurological, psychiatric and musculoskeletal symptoms and findings	Hepatic encephalopathy (disorders of consciousness, behavior and intellect) Peripheral neuropathy (“flapping tremor”) Nystagmus Ataxia Changes in speech Hyper- or hyporeflexia Reduction in muscle mass Dupuytren’s contracture Umbilical hernia Osteodystrophy

Source: own processing according to Ehrmann et al. (2018)

some cases, can cause liver toxicity (Young et al. 2016). The second prerequisite for improving the quality and prolonging the life of patients is the management of complications of cirrhosis, i.e., liver failure, portal hypertension and their consequences, ascites, hepatic encephalopathy, cholestasis, and hepatorenal syndrome. However, this also includes the early diagnosis and treatment of hepatocellular carcinoma, as well as Zieve’s syndrome and Mallory-Weiss syndrome. The third factor affecting the quality and length of life of patients with alcohol-related cirrhosis is the medical treatment of the fibrotic process (Ehrmann et al. 2018).

Liver transplantation has become an important treatment procedure for patients with cirrhosis. Asrani et al. (2019) emphasized that the second most common solid organ transplantation is liver transplantation. Nevertheless, with the current number of transplants, less than 10% of global needs are met. An indicative consideration of the appropriateness of liver transplantation addresses two basic questions. First, is the patient’s disease severe enough that liver transplantation, despite its risks, offers a higher probability of survival than other treatments? Second, will liver transplantation really bring the expected benefit to the patient and is the patient capable of the demanding procedure as well as capable of lifelong continued cooperation? (Ehrmann et al. 2020) The need and indication for liver transplantation in relation to the progress and severity of the patient’s condition is determined by the specialist using the MELD (Model for End-stage Liver Disease) classification (Belovičová 2009). According to the European Association for the Study of the Liver (2018), liver transplantation should be considered in patients with alcohol-related liver disease (classified as Child-Pugh “C” or MELD $\geq$15), as it can improve their survival. The main problem is finding patients who can be expected to be abstinent. Therefore, psychosocial assessment is necessary to determine the likelihood of long-term abstinence (Ehrmann et al. 2020). In fact, severe relapse causes a significant reduction in survival after transplantation (Donnadieu-Rigole et al. 2015). The three main risk factors for alcohol relapse are length of abstinence before transplantation, poor social background and family history of alcoholism. Most programs require a

6-month period of abstinence for patients. It is hypothesized that a 6-month period of abstinence will allow some patients to recover from their liver disease and eliminate the need for liver transplantation, and also identify subgroups of patients who are likely to maintain abstinence for liver transplantation. Although only a minority of patients with alcohol use disorder meet the strict criteria required for liver transplantation, the number of transplantations performed for patients with alcohol-related liver disease has increased over the past two decades (Ehrmann et al. 2020). For example, in France, the leading cause of liver transplantation is alcohol-related cirrhosis (Donnadieu-Rigole et al. 2015).

Abstinence as a Protective Factor

Any drinking of alcohol by patients with cirrhosis is considered inappropriate and harmful. Therefore, abstinence plays an important role in the management of pre-existing alcohol-related cirrhosis (Arab et al. 2019; European Association for the Study of the Liver 2018). Alcohol abstinence improves the prognosis of alcohol-related cirrhosis in both compensated and decompensated patients (Marot et al. 2016). Verrill et al. (2009) highlighted that abstinence from alcohol 1 month after diagnosis of cirrhosis is an important determinant of survival, with 7-year survival being 72% in abstinent patients compared with 44% in patients who continued to drink. Although it may be easy to stop drinking, it is more difficult to maintain this behavior change. In this context, it is important to approach abstinence in a more constructive and positive way, in the sense that abstinence includes opportunities for a better and higher quality of life. Otherwise, there is a risk of relapse (Pešek 2018). In particular, people with alcohol use disorder are considered a vulnerable group to relapse (National Institute on Alcohol Abuse and Alcoholism 2021).

Studies focus on relapse factors, especially in patients after transplantation. Arab et al. (2018) found that major risks include post-transplant depression, smoking in the 6 months before transplantation, age (older age is protective), and steatohepatitis. In addition, in their study, relapse with high-dose alcohol was associated with death. According to Chuncharunee et al. (2019), psychiatric comorbidities are the strongest predictor of alcohol relapse.

Figure 1 presents an example of the course of relapse, which can be seen as a vicious circle. In general, relapse is most often caused by triggers in the form of unmanaged emotional states, then social pressure (e.g., people offering alcohol) and finally interpersonal conflicts, which are also accompanied by negative emotions and most often occur in partner relationships, family, or at work (Pešek 2018). These aspects should also be kept in mind in the management of alcohol-related cirrhosis.

Applications to Other Areas of Addiction

The issue of alcohol consumption is complex and can be viewed from different perspectives, including alcohol abuse and liver cirrhosis in addition to addiction. This perspective, presented in the chapter, highlights the need for effective health

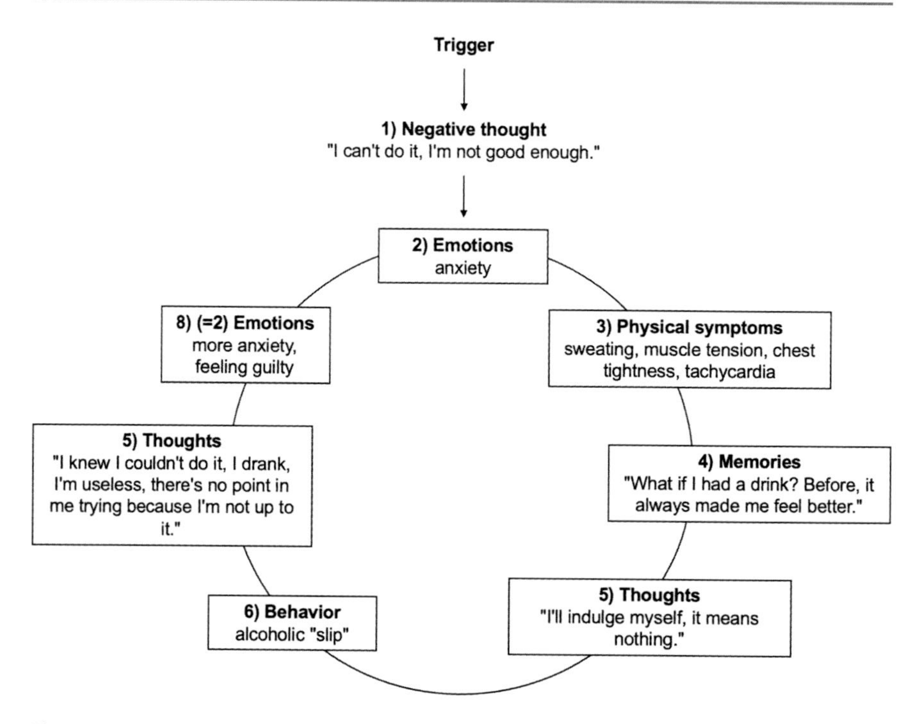

Fig. 1 Example of the course of relapse (vicious circle). This figure shows an example of the course of relapse that poses a risk in abstinence. The course represents a vicious circle. There is a trigger at the beginning that leads to the individual's negative thoughts being reflected in emotions. The figure was processed according to Routhu and Hosák (2018)

policies aimed at reducing alcohol consumption, with a closer focus on the fields of addiction medicine and gastroenterology/hepatology. Alcohol-related cirrhosis is typically a comorbid condition in association with alcohol use disorder, with both conditions needing increased attention and treatment (Lucey 2019). Getting rid of alcohol addiction and maintaining abstinence is crucial (Tonon and Piano 2021), but it is not a simple process. Rather, it is an ongoing process that frustrates primary care providers, family members, and patients themselves (Mahl and O'Grady 2014). On the other hand, abstinence improves the course of pre-existing alcohol-related cirrhosis (Lackner et al. 2017). Today, it is emphasized that it is more effective to focus initially on the patient's motivation for treatment than on his or her will. Motivation must be supported by all, i.e., the general practitioner, hepatologist, gastroenterologist, internist, and others (Ehrmann et al. 2020; Routhu and Hosák 2018).

Interventions and measures should be activated that include early screening for alcohol use disorders (Pimpin et al. 2018; Tonon and Piano 2021). Primary care facilities for the treatment of alcohol use disorders should be widely available. At the same time, screening for alcoholic liver disease should be introduced in these facilities as they concentrate people at high risk. Thus, screening of patients with alcohol use disorder should include liver function tests and measurement of liver fibrosis. Patients detected by screening should undergo a brief intervention and be referred to a multidisciplinary team. Help should also be available in the other direction; therefore, gastroenterology/hepatology departments should have access to services providing effective psychosocial therapy (European Association for the Study of the Liver 2018; Ehrmann et al. 2020). In other words, treatment of alcohol use disorders should be considered in patients with alcohol-related cirrhosis (Haque et al. 2020). The comorbidity of alcohol-related liver disease and alcohol use disorder definitely requires multidisciplinary care provided by hepatologists and addiction specialists. However, this is not well established in practice, and efforts should therefore be focused on removing and overcoming barriers at the patient, clinician, and system levels (DiMartini et al. 2022). A multidisciplinary approach including addiction specialists should also be applied to identify and minimize the risk of serious relapse (Donnadieu-Rigole et al. 2015).

Applications to Public Health

In the context of public health, it is strongly advocated that health policies should focus on preventing complications and further progression of alcohol-related liver disease, which can be supported by targeted interventions. According to Ventura-Cots et al. (2019), the percentage of the population that drinks heavily is a major factor influencing the burden of alcohol-related cirrhosis at the population level. Thus, reducing excessive and harmful drinking should be seen as an important objective of public health policies (Stein et al. 2016; Gavurová et al. 2021). To achieve this objective, alcohol policies should be strict. Policy-makers should also be aware that a stricter environment and a higher number of policies are associated with lower mortality from alcohol-related cirrhosis (Díaz et al. 2021; Hadland et al. 2015). Attention should also focus on health literacy (Rolová 2020). Reducing alcohol abuse in a country requires the "government-wide" and "society-wide" approaches, together with the implementation of evidence-based alcohol control policies, the monitoring of public health priorities, and the adoption of appropriate long-term policies (Park and Kim 2020). This could be addressed by marketing restrictions, increases in minimum alcohol prices, taxation, and regulated alcohol availability (Ehrmann et al. 2020; Horáková et al. 2020; Tonon and Piano 2021; Zhao et al. 2013). Ventura-Cots et al. (2019) consider price regulation and taxation to be the most effective interventions and emphasize that the interaction between pricing policies, other types of policies, and local factors is key in reducing alcohol consumption and the resulting alcohol-related liver disease. Thus, public health policies should involve a multi-component and multi-level approach and take into account a wide range of factors of drinking and harms caused by alcohol.

Mini-Dictionary of Terms

- **Ascites.** Ascites, also known as "fluid in the abdomen," is a condition of unnatural accumulation of fluid in the abdominal cavity. If ascites is severe, it can be painful.

- **Cirrhosis.** A diffuse process of liver parenchyma characterized by the presence of fibrosis, the formation of regenerative nodules, and the destruction of the liver architecture. Etiological factors of this disease include viral hepatitis, excessive alcohol intake, and non-alcoholic steatohepatitis.
- **Hepatic Encephalopathy.** A decline in brain function that occurs as a result of severe liver disease. A condition in which the liver is unable to properly remove toxins and typically occurs in patients with severe liver disease, including cirrhosis. When the liver doesn't work properly, toxins build up in the blood and reach the brain.
- **Hepatocellular Carcinoma.** Hepatocellular carcinoma is the most common type of primary liver cancer.
- **Portal Hypertension**. Portal hypertension is defined as an increase in blood pressure within a system of veins called the portal venous system. The portal vein is a major vein leading to the liver. The most common cause of portal hypertension is liver cirrhosis.

Key Facts of Alcohol and Cirrhosis

Alcohol as a chemical molecule has accompanied mankind for thousands of years. Consumption of ethanol, which is metabolized in all tissues, is ultimately harmful to the organism. In addition to liver damage, ethanol abuse also causes damage to the pancreas, nervous system and muscles, affects the immune system, and can contribute to cancer.

The spectrum of liver damage due to alcohol consumption is wide, and liver cirrhosis is one of them. However, the symptomatology of the condition does not differ in principle from other causes.

Alcohol is estimated to cause up to 50% of all cases of liver cirrhosis worldwide, but the adverse effects of excessive alcohol consumption are also significant in areas other than organic liver damage.

Organ damage, including liver damage, depends not only on the amount but also on the duration of alcohol consumption.

There is no specific treatment for alcohol-related liver cirrhosis. Treatment focuses primarily on the underlying disease (alcohol addiction), complications, supportive measures, as well as liver transplantation. The first prerequisite is complete abstinence. The prognosis of alcohol-related cirrhosis depends on the treatment of its complications and on liver transplantation, if indicated.

Summary Points

- Alcohol is a well-known risk factor for liver cirrhosis, and the relative risk increases depending on the amount and total duration of alcohol consumption.
- It is estimated that alcohol is responsible for approximately 50% of all cases of liver cirrhosis.

- Patients with alcohol-related cirrhosis have a worse prognosis, more complications, worse liver function, and a higher risk of death compared to patients with other etiologies.
- In alcohol-related cirrhosis, treatment focuses primarily on the underlying disease (i.e., alcohol use disorder), complications, support measures, as well as liver transplantation.
- Complete abstinence plays an important role in the management of pre-existing alcohol-related cirrhosis.
- The comorbidity of alcohol-related liver disease and alcohol use disorder definitely requires multidisciplinary care involving hepatologists and addiction specialists.

References

Arab J, Schneekloth T, Niazi S, Simonetto D (2018) Predictors of alcohol relapse after transplant for alcoholic liver disease. Hepatology 68:817–818A

Arab JP, Roblero JP, Altamirano J, Bessone F, Chaves Araujo R, Higuera-De la Tijera F, Restrepo JC, Torre A, Urzua A, Simonetto DA, Abraldes JG, Méndez-Sánchez N, Contreras F, Lucey MR, Shah VH, Cortez-Pinto H, Bataller R (2019) Alcohol-related liver disease: clinical practice guidelines by the Latin American Association for the Study of the Liver (ALEH). Ann Hepatol 18(3):518–535. https://doi.org/10.1016/j.aohep.2019.04.005

Askgaard G, Grønbæk M, Kjær MS, Tjønneland A, Tolstrup JS (2015) Alcohol drinking pattern and risk of alcoholic liver cirrhosis: a prospective cohort study. J Hepatol 62(5):1061–1067. https://doi.org/10.1016/j.jhep.2014.12.005

Asrani SK, Devarbhavi H, Eaton J, Kamath PS (2019) Burden of liver diseases in the world. J Hepatol 70(1):151–171. https://doi.org/10.1016/j.jhep.2018.09.014

Belovičová M (2009) Liver cirrhosis – old but unbeaten disease. Via Pract 6(2):59–62

Bureš J, Horáček J, Malý J et al (2014) Vnitřní lékařství. Galén, Prague

Chuncharunee L, Yamashiki N, Thakkinstian A, Sobhonslidsuk A (2019) Alcohol relapse and its predictors after liver transplantation for alcoholic liver disease: a systematic review and meta-analysis. BMC Gastroenterol 19(1):150. https://doi.org/10.1186/s12876-019-1050-9

Díaz LA, Idalsoaga F, Fuentes-López E, Márquez-Lomas A, Ramírez CA, Roblero JP, Araujo RC, Higuera-de-la-Tijera F, Toro LG, Pazmiño G, Montes P, Hernandez N, Mendizabal M, Corsi O, Ferreccio C, Lazo M, Brahmania M, Singal AK, Bataller R, Arrese M, Arab JP (2021) Impact of public health policies on alcohol-associated liver disease in Latin America: an ecological multinational study. Hepatology 74(5):2478–2490. https://doi.org/10.1002/hep.32016

DiMartini AF, Leggio L, Singal AK (2022) Barriers to the management of alcohol use disorder and alcohol-associated liver disease: strategies to implement integrated care models. Lancet Gastroenterol Hepatol 7(2):186–195. https://doi.org/10.1016/S2468-1253(21)00191-6

Donnadieu-Rigole H, Perney P, Pageaux GP (2015) Consommation d'alcool après greffe de foie chez les patients transplantés pour cirrhose alcoolique [Alcohol consumption after liver transplantation in patients transplanted for alcoholic cirrhosis]. Presse Med 44(5):481–485. https://doi.org/10.1016/j.lpm.2014.09.019

Ehrmann J, Schneiderka P, Ehrmann J Jr, Vitek L, Jirsa M, Zima T, Aiglová K (2018) Alkoholem podmíněné jaterní poškození. In: Hůlek P, Urbánek P et al (eds) Hepatologie, 3rd edn. Grada Publishing, Prague, pp 335–362

Ehrmann J, Aiglová K, Urban O, Cveková S, Dvoran P (2020) Onemocnění jater související s alkoholem (ALD). Vnitř Lék 66(5):e3–e15

European Association for the Study of the Liver (2018) EASL clinical practice guidelines: management of alcohol-related liver disease. J Hepatol 69(1):154–181. https://doi.org/10.1016/j.jhep.2018.03.018

Fan X, Hershman M, Weisberg I (2019) Alcoholic cirrhosis is associated with higher in-patient mortality compared to non-alcoholic cirrhosis. J Hepatol 70(1):e276–e277. https://doi.org/10.1016/S0618-8278(19)30527-4

Fleming KM, Aithal GP, Card TR, West J (2012) All-cause mortality in people with cirrhosis compared with the general population: a population-based cohort study. Liver Int 32(1):79–84. https://doi.org/10.1111/j.1478-3231.2011.02517.x

Gavurová B, Tarhaničová M, Kulhánek A (2021) The regional differences in mortality attributable to alcohol in the Czech Republic in 2017. Adiktologie 21(1):43–50. https://doi.org/10.35198/01-2021-001-0004

GBD 2017 Cirrhosis Collaborators (2020) The global, regional, and national burden of cirrhosis by cause in 195 countries and territories, 1990-2017: a systematic analysis for the Global Burden of Disease Study 2017. Lancet Gastroenterol Hepatol 5(3):245–266. https://doi.org/10.1016/S2468-1253(19)30349-8

Hadland SE, Xuan Z, Blanchette JG, Heeren TC, Swahn MH, Naimi TS (2015) Alcohol policies and alcoholic cirrhosis mortality in the United States. Prev Chronic Dis 12:150200. https://doi.org/10.5888/pcd12.150200

Haque LY, Jakab S, Deng Y, Ciarleglio MM, Tetrault JM (2020) Substance use disorders in recently hospitalized patients with cirrhosis. J Addict Med 14(6):e337–e343. https://doi.org/10.1097/ADM.0000000000000677

Horáková M, Bejtkovský J, Baršová P, Urbánek T (2020) Alcohol consumption among the Member States of the European Union in relationship to taxation. Adiktologie 20(1–2):47–56. https://doi.org/10.35198/01-2020-001-0004

Jain P, Shasthry SM, Choudhury AK, Maiwall R, Kumar G, Bharadwaj A, Arora V, Vijayaraghavan R, Jindal A, Sharma MK, Bhatia V, Sarin SK (2021) Alcohol associated liver cirrhotics have higher mortality after index hospitalization: long-term data of 5,138 patients. Clin Mol Hepatol 27(1):175–185. https://doi.org/10.3350/cmh.2020.0068

Jepsen P, Ott P, Andersen PK, Sørensen HT, Vilstrup H (2010) Clinical course of alcoholic liver cirrhosis: a Danish population-based cohort study. Hepatology 51(5):1675–1682. https://doi.org/10.1002/hep.23500

Joshi KS, Shriwastav RR (2016) Highly active antiretroviral therapy and changing spectrum of liver diseases in HIV infected patients. Int J Res Med Sci 4(8):3125–3129. https://doi.org/10.18203/2320-6012.ijrms20162170

Klatsky AL, Armstrong MA (1992) Alcohol, smoking, coffee, and cirrhosis. Am J Epidemiol 136 (10):1248–1257. https://doi.org/10.1093/oxfordjournals.aje.a116433

Lackner C, Spindelboeck W, Haybaeck J, Douschan P, Rainer F, Terracciano L, Haas J, Berghold A, Bataller R, Stauber RE (2017) Histological parameters and alcohol abstinence determine long-term prognosis in patients with alcoholic liver disease. J Hepatol 66(3):610–618. https://doi.org/10.1016/j.jhep.2016.11.011

Liangpunsakul S, Haber P, McCaughan GW (2016) Alcoholic liver disease in Asia, Europe, and North America. Gastroenterology 150(8):1786–1797. https://doi.org/10.1053/j.gastro.2016.02.043

Lucey MR (2019) Alcohol-associated cirrhosis. Clin Liver Dis 23(1):115–126. https://doi.org/10.1016/j.cld.2018.09.013

Maasová D, Hulín I (2013) Funkčné a morfologické základy porúch pečene. In: Kiňová S, Hulín I et al (eds) Interná medicína. Pro Litera, Bratislava

Mahl T, O'Grady J (2014) Fast facts: liver disorders. Health Press Limited, Abingdon

Marot A, Henrion J, Knebel JF, Doerig C, Moreno C, Deltenre P (2016) Alcohol abstinence improves the prognosis of alcoholic liver disease related cirrhosis in both compensated and decompensated patients. Swiss Med Wkly 146:165–165

Masarone M, Rosato V, Dallio M, Abenavoli L, Federico A, Loguercio C, Persico M (2016) Epidemiology and natural history of alcoholic liver disease. Rev Recent Clin Trials 11(3): 167–174. https://doi.org/10.2174/1574887111666160810101202

Moon AM, Singal AG, Tapper EB (2020) Contemporary epidemiology of chronic liver disease and cirrhosis. Clin Gastroenterol Hepatol 18(12):2650–2666. https://doi.org/10.1016/j.cgh.2019.07.060

National Institute on Alcohol Abuse and Alcoholism (2021) Understanding alcohol Use disorder. https://www.niaaa.nih.gov/alcohol-health/overview-alcohol-consumption/alcohol-use-disorders

Park SH, Kim DJ (2020) Global and regional impacts of alcohol use on public health: emphasis on alcohol policies. Clin Mol Hepatol 26(4):652–661. https://doi.org/10.3350/cmh.2020.0160

Pešek R (2018) Jak se zbavit závislosti na alkoholu. Pasparta Publishing, Prague

Piano S, Tonon M, Vettore E, Stanco M, Pilutti C, Romano A, Mareso S, Gambino C, Brocca A, Sticca A, Fasolato S, Angeli P (2017) Incidence, predictors and outcomes of acute-on-chronic liver failure in outpatients with cirrhosis. J Hepatol 67(6):1177–1184. https://doi.org/10.1016/j.jhep.2017.07.008

Pimpin L, Cortez-Pinto H, Negro F, Corbould E, Lazarus JV, Webber L, Sheron N, EASL HEPAHEALTH Steering Committee (2018) Burden of liver disease in Europe: epidemiology and analysis of risk factors to identify prevention policies. J Hepatol 69(3):718–735. https://doi.org/10.1016/j.jhep.2018.05.011

Rehm J, Taylor B, Mohapatra S, Irving H, Baliunas D, Patra J, Roerecke M (2010) Alcohol as a risk factor for liver cirrhosis: a systematic review and meta-analysis. Drug Alcohol Rev 29(4):437–445. https://doi.org/10.1111/j.1465-3362.2009.00153.x

Rehm J, Samokhvalov AV, Shield KD (2013) Global burden of alcoholic liver diseases. J Hepatol 59(1):160–168. https://doi.org/10.1016/j.jhep.2013.03.007

Roerecke M, Vafaei A, Hasan OSM, Chrystoja BR, Cruz M, Lee R, Neuman MG, Rehm J (2019) Alcohol consumption and risk of liver cirrhosis: a systematic review and meta-analysis. Am J Gastroenterol 114(10):1574–1586. https://doi.org/10.14309/ajg.0000000000000340

Rolová G (2020) Health literacy in residential addiction treatment programs: study protocol of a cross-sectional study in people with substance use disorders. Adiktologie 20(3–4):145–150

Routhu M, Hosák L (2018) Alkoholismus a abúzus alkoholu. In: Hůlek P, Urbánek P et al (eds) Hepatologie, 3rd edn. Grada Publishing, Prague, pp 363–375

Schuppan D, Afdhal NH (2008) Liver cirrhosis. Lancet 371(9615):838–851. https://doi.org/10.1016/S0140-6736(08)60383-9

Simpson RF, Hermon C, Liu B, Green J, Reeves GK, Beral V, Floud S, Million Women Study Collaborators (2019) Alcohol drinking patterns and liver cirrhosis risk: analysis of the prospective UK Million Women Study. Lancet Public Health 4(1):e41–e48. https://doi.org/10.1016/S2468-2667(18)30230-5

Stein E, Cruz-Lemini M, Altamirano J, Ndugga N, Couper D, Abraldes JG, Bataller R (2016) Heavy daily alcohol intake at the population level predicts the weight of alcohol in cirrhosis burden worldwide. J Hepatol 65(5):998–1005. https://doi.org/10.1016/j.jhep.2016.06.018

Suva M (2014) A brief review on liver cirrhosis: epidemiology, etiology, pathophysiology, symptoms, diagnosis and its management. Inventi Rapid Mol Pharmacol 2014(2):1–5

Tonon M, Piano S (2021) Alcohol-related cirrhosis: the most challenging etiology of cirrhosis is more burdensome than ever. Clin Mol Hepatol 27(1):94–96. https://doi.org/10.3350/cmh.2020.0305

Tsochatzis EA, Bosch J, Burroughs AK (2014) Future treatments of cirrhosis. Expert Rev Gastroenterol Hepatol 8(5):571–581. https://doi.org/10.1586/17474124.2014.902303

Ventura-Cots M, Ballester-Ferré MP, Ravi S, Bataller R (2019) Public health policies and alcohol-related liver disease. JHEP Rep 1(5):403–413. https://doi.org/10.1016/j.jhepr.2019.07.009

Verrill C, Markham H, Templeton A, Carr NJ, Sheron N (2009) Alcohol-related cirrhosis - early abstinence is a key factor in prognosis, even in the most severe cases. Addiction 104(5):768–774. https://doi.org/10.1111/j.1360-0443.2009.02521.x

Whitfield JB, Masson S, Liangpunsakul S, Hyman J, Mueller S, Aithal G, Eyer F, Gleeson D, Thompson A, Stickel F, Soyka M, Daly AK, Cordell HJ, Liang T, Foroud T, Lumeng L, Pirmohamed M, Nalpas B, Bence C, Jacquet JM, Louvet A, Moirand R, Nahon P, Naveau S, Perney P, Podevin P, Haber PS, Seitz HK, Day CP, Mathurin P, Morgan TM, Seth D, GenomALC Consortium (2018) Evaluation of laboratory tests for cirrhosis and for alcohol use, in the context of alcoholic cirrhosis. Alcohol 66:1–7. https://doi.org/10.1016/j.alcohol.2017.07.006

Young S, Wood E, Ahamad K (2016) Pharmacotherapy for alcohol addiction in a patient with alcoholic cirrhosis and massive upper gastrointestinal bleed: a case study. Drug Alcohol Rev 35 (2):236–239. https://doi.org/10.1111/dar.12289

Zhao J, Stockwell T, Martin G, Macdonald S, Vallance K, Treno A, Ponicki WR, Tu A, Buxton J (2013) The relationship between minimum alcohol prices, outlet densities and alcohol-attributable deaths in British Columbia, 2002-09. Addiction 108(6):1059–1069. https://doi.org/10.1111/add.12139

Zhuang YP, Wang SQ, Pan ZY, Zhong HJ, He XX (2021) Differences in complications between hepatitis B-related cirrhosis and alcohol-related cirrhosis. Open Med 17(1):46–52. https://doi.org/10.1515/med-2021-0401

Part VI

Cannabinoids

Synthetic Cannabinoids and Neurodevelopment

61

João Pedro Silva, Helena Carmo, and Félix Carvalho

Contents

Introduction 1322
Biological Effects of Synthetic Cannabinoids 1323
Modulation of Neuronal Function by SCs 1324
SC-mediated Dysregulation of Neurotransmission 1327
The Endocannabinoid Signaling in the Regulation of Neurogenesis 1328
The CB1R in SC-mediated Neurogenesis 1329
Role of the CB2R in SC-mediated Neurogenesis 1331
Neurogenesis Control Via SCs' Actions on Glial Cells 1335
Epigenetic Regulation of Neurogenesis by SCs 1335
Applications to Other Areas of Substance Use Disorders 1336
Applications to Public Health 1337
Mini-Dictionary of Terms 1337
Key Facts of Synthetic Cannabinoids 1338
Summary Points 1338
References 1339

Abstract

The recreational use of synthetic cannabinoids (SCs) is increasing worldwide, often associated with reports of acute intoxications and deaths. Adolescents and young adults, including women of childbearing age or even pregnant, stand among the most frequent SC users. The developing brain is especially vulnerable to cannabinoid-elicited effects, due to the key role played by the endocannabinoid system (SCs' main target) in regulating neurogenesis. However, the mechanisms of SC-induced neurotoxicity remain mostly unexplored. In particular, studies on

J. P. Silva (✉) · H. Carmo · F. Carvalho (✉)
Associate Laboratory i4HB – Institute for Health and Bioeconomy, Faculty of Pharmacy, University of Porto, Porto, Portugal

UCIBIO, Laboratory of Toxicology, Department of Biological Sciences, Faculty of Pharmacy, University of Porto, Porto, Portugal
e-mail: jpmsilva@ff.up.pt; felixdc@ff.up.pt

V. B. Patel, V. R. Preedy (eds.), *Handbook of Substance Misuse and Addictions*,
https://doi.org/10.1007/978-3-030-92392-1_67

the mechanisms underlying SC-triggered neurogenic perturbations remain scarce, despite accumulating evidence that SC use may lead to the onset of neurodevelopmental disorders (e.g., psychosis, autism spectrum).

This chapter revises some of the main outcomes and mechanisms underlying the modulation of neurogenic processes by SCs, including the key role played by the endocannabinoid system and the dysregulation of neurotransmitter signaling by these drugs.

Keywords

New psychoactive substances · Drug abuse · Substance use disorders · "Spice" · Endocannabinoid system · Cannabinoid receptors · Central Nervous System · Neuroplasticity · Neurogenesis · Neurodevelopmental disorders · Mental health

Abbreviations

5-HT	5-Hydroxytryptamine
BDNF	Brain-Derived Neurotrophic Factor
cAMP	Cyclic Adenosine Monophosphate
CB1R	Cannabinoid Receptor 1
CB2R	Cannabinoid Receptor 2
CBR	Cannabinoid Receptor
DG	Dentate Gyrus
GABA	Gamma-aminobutyric Acid
GPCR	G protein-coupled Receptor
NMDA	*N*-methyl-D-aspartate
NMDAR	*N*-methyl-D-aspartate Receptor
NPS	New Psychoactive Substances
SC	Synthetic Cannabinoid
SVZ	Subventricular Zone
THC	Tetrahydrocannabinol

Introduction

Synthetic Cannabinoids (SCs) comprise a structurally diverse group of New Psychoactive Substances (NPS) designed to mimic, with stronger potency, the psychoactive effects of tetrahydrocannabinol (THC, the molecule mainly responsible for cannabis' psychoactive action) (Pertwee et al. 2010). These substances were initially developed for research purposes, namely to provide a better characterization and understanding of the endocannabinoid system's function, as well as to explore their therapeutic use (e.g., pain management, nausea, and vomiting prevention) (Pertwee et al. 2010). However, the first evidence of their recreational use was reported in December 2008 by German and Austrian authorities, who detected the presence of the SC JWH-018 in a herbal blend labeled as "Spice" (Auwarter et al. 2009). Since then, several SCs have emerged, prevailing in NPS seizures between 2009 and 2019

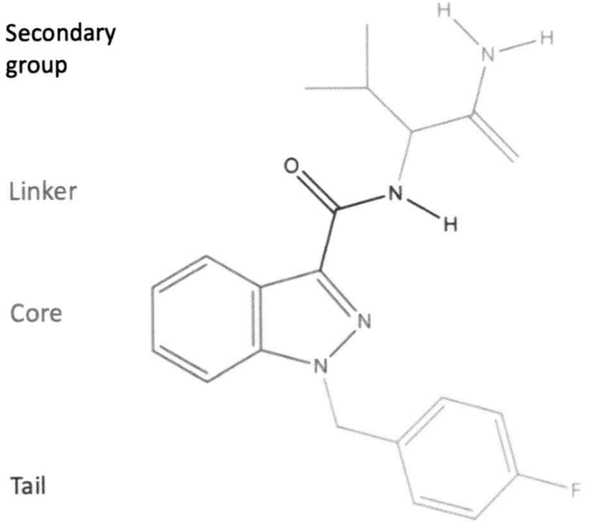

Fig. 1 General structure of synthetic cannabinoids. The structure of synthetic cannabinoids comprises a core and a secondary group connected through a linker and having a tail group attached (AB-FUBINACA is shown as a representative structure)

(EMCDDA 2021; UNODC 2020). These substances have a modular structure usually comprising a core and a secondary group connected through a linker and often having a tail group attached (Fig. 1). The large number of substituents that can replace each of these groups accounts for the plethora of structurally different SCs that reach the drug market. SCs are usually dissolved in organic solvents (e.g., acetone, methanol) and sprayed over plant materials (sometimes mixed with other substances of abuse). This blend is then dried and marketed in appealing packages mostly as "natural products," as these do not mention the presence of SCs in the product information, leading inexperienced users to the misconception that they are "natural" and risk-free (Debruyne and Le Boisselier 2015; Lauritsen and Rosenberg 2016). The number of new SCs reaching the drug market has decreased between 2014 and 2018. However, the increasing correlation of their misuse with acute intoxications and deaths has become a major concern for public health and a challenge for regulatory authorities (EMCDDA 2021; UNODC 2020). Of note, recent changes to the legal status of cannabis and its derivatives may anticipate increased use of cannabinoids (including SCs) (Hall et al. 2019).

Biological Effects of Synthetic Cannabinoids

The search for cannabinoids able to induce psychotropic effects that are similar, but more potent than those of cannabis, has turned common cannabis users into SCs. These users mainly look for effects such as relaxation, mood elevation, euphoria, social disinhibition, and increased sensorial awareness. Such effects often start almost immediately after administration and may last up to 2–6 h (Debruyne and Le Boisselier 2015).

There are accumulating reports of acute intoxications, and even deaths, resulting from SC misuse (Cohen and Weinstein 2018). SC-related intoxications are characterized by a variety of acute adverse effects, often involving neurological and cardiovascular events. Typical acute neurological and mental effects include drowsiness, hallucinations, paranoia, confusion, delusions, vertigo, anxiety, mood changes, panic attacks, agitation, memory impairment, and cognitive deficits, or attention difficulties (Cohen and Weinstein 2018; Debruyne and Le Boisselier 2015). At the cardiovascular level, tachycardia and chest pain are the most commonly reported symptoms, but there are also reports of heart failure, myocardial infarction, cardiac arrest, and acute cerebral ischemia (Ozturk et al. 2019). Other major complications involve severe respiratory depression, acute kidney injury, gastrointestinal problems (e.g., nausea, vomiting, changes in appetite), rhabdomyolysis, and hyperthermia (Cohen and Weinstein 2018).

There is accumulating evidence suggesting that, in the long term, the use of SCs may induce structural and functional changes in the central nervous system (CNS) that may trigger or exacerbate pre-existing psychiatric disorders. In particular, the chronic use of SCs has been reported to induce irritability, persistent anxiety, insomnia, nightmares, depression, and cognitive impairment (e.g., memory and attention deficits) (Cohen and Weinstein 2018; Debruyne and Le Boisselier 2015). Prolonged SC use has also been associated with serious cardiovascular complications, kidney damage, and severe weight loss (Cohen and Weinstein 2018; Ozturk et al. 2019). Moreover, chronic SC use increases the risk of developing dependence and tolerance phenomena (Tai and Fantegrossi 2014). The biological effects induced by SCs are summarized in Fig. 2.

Modulation of Neuronal Function by SCs

Similar to their natural and endogenous counterparts, SCs modulate the endocannabinoid system by binding and activating at least one of the main classical cannabinoid receptors (CBRs), type-1 (CB1R) and type-2 (CB2R), belonging to the G protein-coupled receptor (GPCR) family. CB1R are among the most abundant GPCRs in the brain, being highly expressed in the pre-synaptic terminals of neurons from the hippocampus and prefrontal cortex, although they are also present in basal ganglia and post-synaptic areas (e.g., neurons, astrocytes, and other glial cells, and endothelial brain cells) at a lower density (Howlett and Abood 2017). Activation of CB1R causes the dissociation of the βγ subunits of the G protein ($G_{i/0}$) from the α subunit (Gi_{α}). While the Giα subunit inhibits adenylyl cyclase activity and decreases the formation of cyclic adenosine monophosphate (cAMP), the $Gi_{\beta\gamma}$ subunit inhibits the N- and P/Q-type voltage-gated calcium channels, and triggers the opening of G protein-gated inward rectifying K^+ channels (GIRK) (Cristino et al. 2020; Walsh and Andersen 2020). The combination of these actions induces the hyperpolarization of pre-synaptic terminals that cause the inhibition of neurotransmitter (e.g., dopamine, glutamate, GABA) release (Di Marzo et al. 2015). The mechanisms involved in the modulation of neurotransmitter release upon activation of the endocannabinoid

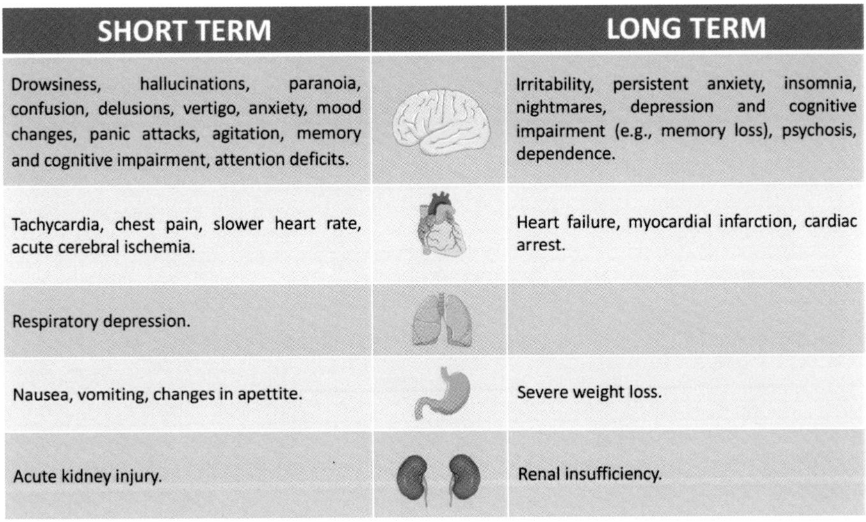

SHORT TERM		LONG TERM
Drowsiness, hallucinations, paranoia, confusion, delusions, vertigo, anxiety, mood changes, panic attacks, agitation, memory and cognitive impairment, attention deficits.		Irritability, persistent anxiety, insomnia, nightmares, depression and cognitive impairment (e.g., memory loss), psychosis, dependence.
Tachycardia, chest pain, slower heart rate, acute cerebral ischemia.		Heart failure, myocardial infarction, cardiac arrest.
Respiratory depression.		
Nausea, vomiting, changes in apettite.		Severe weight loss.
Acute kidney injury.		Renal insufficiency.

Fig. 2 Short- and long-term adverse effects of synthetic cannabinoids use. Synthetic cannabinoid-related intoxications are characterized by a variety of acute adverse effects (left panel), mainly involving neurological and cardiovascular events, but also targeting other biological systems (e.g., respiratory, gastrointestinal, or renal systems). In the long term, the use of these substances may trigger more severe complications at the target organs (right panel)

system are further detailed in Fig. 3. As a result of its involvement in neurotransmission signaling, CB1R mediates most of the psychoactive and behavioral effects of SCs (Cooper 2016). CB2Rs prevail mostly in cells from the immune system, actively participating in the immune response, but are also present in other peripheral organs and tissues (e.g., liver, spleen, kidneys, lungs, tonsils, gastrointestinal tract). CB2Rs have also been detected in the brain, in particular in microglia and post-synaptic terminals of neurons (Howlett and Abood 2017). Notably, up-regulation of CB2R has been observed in some pathological conditions (e.g., anxiety, addiction, inflammation, epilepsy), suggesting the key involvement of these receptors in psychiatric and neurological diseases (Chen et al. 2017). In addition, SCs may also bind and modulate the activity of other receptors, including the G protein-coupled receptors 55 (GPR55) and 18 (GPR18), the receptors from the peroxisome proliferator-activated receptor (PPAR) family, and the transient receptor potential vanilloid 1 (TRPV1) channels (Cristino et al. 2020).

There is accumulating evidence suggesting that SCs activate CBRs, namely CB1Rs, via biased receptor agonism, possibly explaining the different pharmacological actions produced by SCs upon binding to the same GPCR (Walsh and Andersen 2020). Differences in SCs interaction with the CB1R toggle switch (comprising residues F200 and W356 in the TM2/TM6 binding pocket) have been observed using cryoelectron microscopy. For example, the strong aromatic interaction of SCs comprising an indole or indazole ring (e.g., MDMB-FUBINACA, AB-FUBINACA, 5F-MDMB PICA) with this toggle switch has been shown to

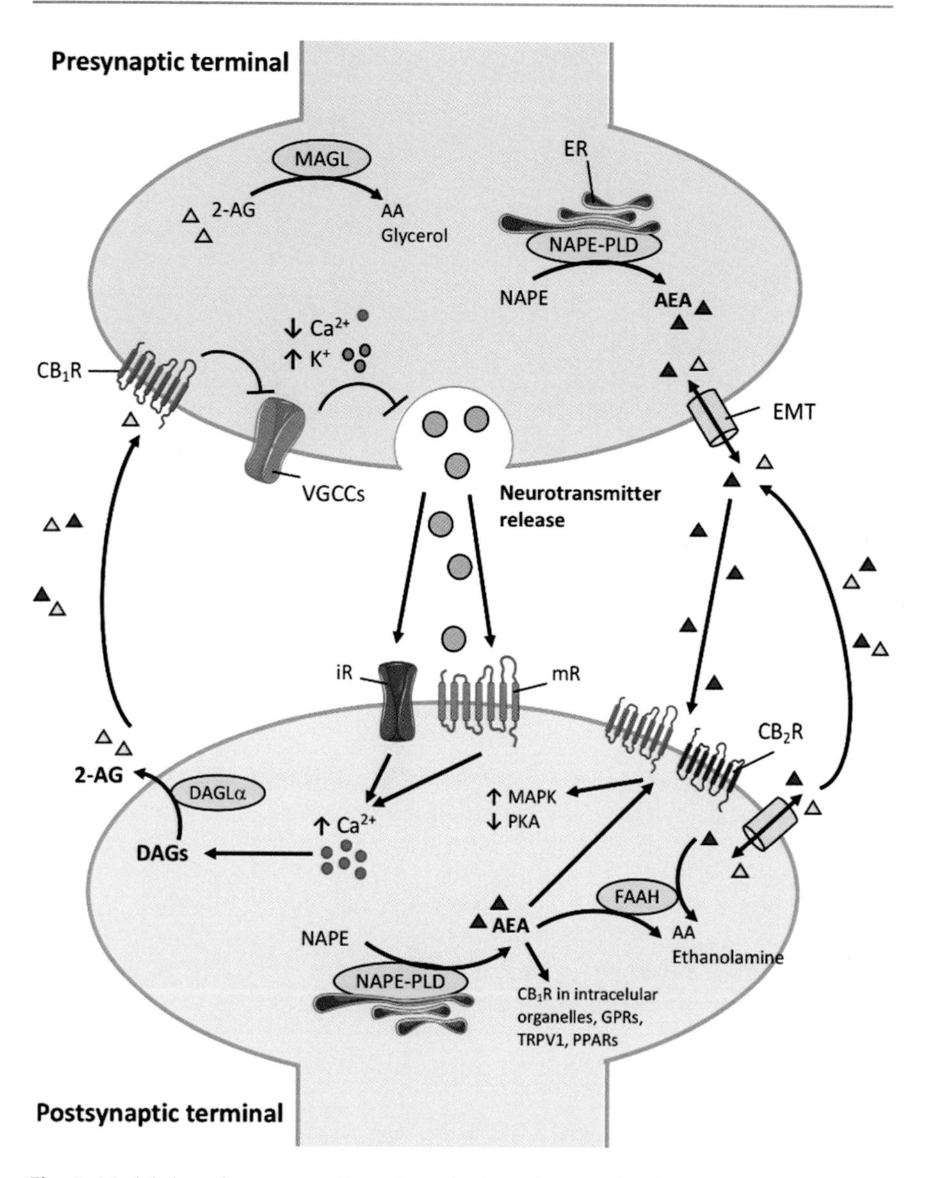

Fig. 3 Modulation of neurotransmitter release by the endocannabinoid system. Neurotransmitter binding to the post-synaptic neuron through ionotropic or metabotropic receptors increases Ca^{2+} levels and the biosynthesis of 2-AG through the action of DAGLα. 2-AG then moves to the pre-synaptic neuron, resulting in the retrograde activation of CB1R, which in turn inhibits neurotransmitter release by suppressing Ca^{2+} and K^{+} influx from voltage-dependent channels. 2-AG may be also degraded in the pre-synaptic neuron by the action of MAGL. AEA is synthesized in the membranes of intracellular organelles at pre- and post-synaptic terminals by NAPE-PLD and degraded by FAAH, which locates in post-synaptic terminals. The distribution of NAPE-PLD and FAAH accounts for the anterograde and intracellular signaling of AEA. Noteworthy, AEA may also bind to other non-cannabinoid receptors, including GPR18, GPR55, TRPV1, or PPARs.

stabilize the active conformation of the receptor, thus increasing these ligands' binding efficacy (Krishna Kumar et al. 2019). While indole/indazole-containing SCs seem to have equal potencies for stimulating Gi and β-arrestin, thus having balanced signaling actions, other SCs (e.g., CP55,940, PNR-420) have reported less activity towards β-arrestin, thus preferably acting on the G_i-mediated pathways (Ford et al. 2017; Walsh and Andersen 2020). Although the CB1R mainly couples to G_i, SCs have also been reported to act via G_s and G_q (Lauckner et al. 2005). For example, WIN55,212-2, CP-55,940, JWH-018, and AB-FUBINACA have been shown to increase cAMP levels above those induced by forskolin in the presence of an inhibitor of $G_{i/0}$ (Patel et al. 2020).

SC-mediated Dysregulation of Neurotransmission

Neurotransmitters such as dopamine, gamma-aminobutyric acid (GABA), serotonin, and glutamate not only mediate neuronal communication but also play a critical role in the neurogenesis modulation in both developing and adult brains (Shohayeb et al. 2018). Considering that the endocannabinoid system regulates the main neurotransmitters' signaling, it is thus reasonable to expect that SC-mediated dysregulation of neurotransmission could affect neurogenesis. Cannabinoid-induced dysregulation of the mesolimbic dopaminergic system, in particular via interference with the dopamine synthesis/metabolism, release, and reuptake, has been pointed out as a risk factor for the onset of several psychiatric disorders (Zou and Kumar 2018). A decrease in dopamine D1 receptor density has been previously observed in the brains of adolescents, but not adult, rats treated with the SC HU-210, further evidencing the vulnerability of the adolescent brain to cannabinoid-mediated effects (Dalton and Zavitsanou 2010). Ma et al. (2019) showed the inhibition of dopamine neuron firing in slices from the ventral tegmental area of adolescent mice treated with different SCs, in a process involving the activation of CB2R. Also, Ossato et al. (2017) reported that the psychostimulant action of two SCs, JWH-018 and AKB48, in mice, was induced by increasing dopamine release in the nucleus accumbens.

GABA acts as an important neurodevelopmental signal, influencing proliferation and migration of neuroblasts, cell fate decision, as well as synaptic formation and

Fig. 3 (continued) The endocannabinoids remaining in the synapse can be transported between pre- and post-synaptic neurons through the EMTs for degradation. 2-AG: 2-arachidonyl glycerol; AA: arachidonic acid; AEA: anandamide; DAGs: diacylglycerols; DAGLα: diacylglycerol lipase alpha; EMT: endocannabinoid membrane transporter; ER: endoplasmic reticulum; FAAH: fatty acid amide hydrolase; GPRs: G protein-coupled receptors; iR: ionotropic receptor; MAGL: monoacylglycerol lipase; MAPK: mitogen-activated protein kinases; mR: metabotropic receptor; NAPE: N-arachidonoyl-phosphatidylethanolamine; NAPE-PLD: N-acylphosphatidylethanolamine (NAPE)-specific phospholipase D; PKA: protein kinase A; PPARs: peroxisome proliferator-activated receptors; TRPV1: Transient Receptor Potential Vanilloid 1 channel; VDCs: voltage-dependent channels. (Reproduced from Alexandre et al. 2019 with permission from John Wiley & Sons – Books)

plasticity (de Oliveira et al. 2019; Pallotto and Deprez 2014). For example, early and mid-adolescence exposure of mice to WIN55,212-2 was shown to cause GABAergic hypofunction, which is often associated with neuropsychiatric traits (de Salas-Quiroga et al. 2020).

In general, SCs binding to CB1Rs triggers the internalization of these receptors, and upon internalization CB1Rs associate with the NR1 subunit of *N*-methyl-D-aspartate (NMDA) receptors (NMDARs). This CB1R-NMDAR association causes the reduction of expression of glutamate receptors, decreased glutamic acid decarboxylase activity, and reduced glutamate outflow, further preventing intracellular Ca^{2+} release or altering synaptic plasticity (Sánchez-Blázquez et al. 2013). Moreover, through the activation of the NMDARs, glutamate regulates the survival of neuroblasts during their migration from the postnatal subventricular zone, while exerting an inhibitory effect on cell proliferation in the dentate gyrus (Platel et al. 2010). WIN55,212-2 has been reported to have a high efficacy to inhibit the glutamatergic synaptic transmission, and MAM-2201 was shown to suppress GABA and glutamate release in mice via activation of pre-synaptic CB1Rs in Purkinje cells. In addition, WIN55,212-2 has been shown to increase glutamate uptake by promoting the overexpression of the glutamate transporter 1 (GLT1) and the excitatory amino acid carrier 1 (EAAC1) in the rat frontal cerebral cortex (Cohen et al. 2019). Sánchez-Zavaleta et al. (2018) further demonstrated the involvement of CB2Rs in the modulation of the glutamatergic system, as three specific CB2R synthetic agonists (GW833972A, GW405833, and JHW-133) inhibited glutamate release via the modulation of P/Q-channels in rat subthalamic-nigral terminals, in a CB2R activation-dependent manner.

Exposure to SCs may also interfere with serotonergic neurotransmission. For example, Bambico et al. (2007) observed decreased firing rates of serotonergic neurons in the dorsal raphe nucleus of rats treated with high WIN55,212-2 doses (> 0.2 mg/ kg), whereas low doses increased serotonergic activity (Cohen et al. 2019). Recently, Yano et al. (2020) reported that SCs comprising an indole group within their structure (e.g., AM-2201, JWH-018) could allosterically modulate the 5-HT_{1A} receptor, thus confirming the ability of such SCs to directly activate the serotonergic receptors. Interestingly, sub-chronic administration of the SC CP55,940 to male rats has been shown to increase the expression of D2 dopaminergic and 5-HT_{2A} receptors, followed by the formation of heteromers between these two types of receptors. Additionally, the dysregulation of the interaction between such receptors has been suggested as a potential mechanism of SC-induced psychosis (Franklin and Carrasco 2012).

The Endocannabinoid Signaling in the Regulation of Neurogenesis

Neurogenesis comprises a complex series of interconnected processes leading to the generation of functional neurons in the nervous system. These processes include the proliferation of neural stem cells, fate specification of neural progenitors, neuronal migration, differentiation and maturation, and ultimately the integration of newly generated neurons into a network of functional synapses (Prenderville et al. 2015). In most brain regions, these processes occur mainly during embryonic and perinatal stages. However, in the hippocampal subgranular of the dentate gyrus and the ventricular–subventricular zone, neurogenesis remains active during the postnatal period and throughout adulthood as part of the brain structural and functional plasticity (Ming and Song 2011). In particular, adult neurogenesis resumes many features of the developmental process of embryonic neurogenesis although the formation and migration of new neurons tend to decline with age (Spalding Kirsty et al. 2013).

Endocannabinoid signaling is ubiquitously involved in the regulation of several neuronal processes during embryonic and adult stages, including neurogenic processes ranging from the generation to migration and survival of neurons (de Oliveira et al. 2019). As depicted in Fig. 4a, CB1R-mediated transactivation of the epidermal growth factor receptor (EGFR) further activates the Raf1-ERK1/2 signaling pathway, promoting neuronal cell proliferation in a distinct process from the one evoked by classical $G\alpha_{i/0}$ protein coupling. In turn, blockade of the Raf1-ERK1/2 pathway or the activation of a $G\alpha_{i/0}$-mediated signaling cascade that leads to the proteasomal degradation of the Rap1/B-Raf pathway result in increased neurite outgrowth (Fig. 4b). Moreover, the association of CB1R with the activation of Src tyrosine kinases triggers the phosphorylation of the Tropomyosin receptor kinase B (TrkB), promoting neuronal migration, as noted in Fig. 4c (Galve-Roperh et al. 2013; Harkany et al. 2007). Notably, while assessing the behavioral neurogenic effects of chronic exposure of adolescent rats to the CBR non-selective agonist WIN55,212-2 (an SC), Abboussi et al. (2014) observed that the animals presented impaired cognition and decreased dorsal hippocampal neurogenesis, whereas no such effects were detected in adult animals, confirming that the rat adolescent brain is more vulnerable to the effects of this SC.

Given its important role in the regulation of neurogenesis, dysregulation of the endocannabinoid system by synthetic (or other exogenous cannabinoids) has been increasingly associated with the onset of neurodevelopmental disorders (e.g., psychosis, autism spectrum, attention deficit, and hyperactivity). For example, epidemiological and preclinical data have already suggested that prenatal cannabinoid (e.g., THC, cannabis) exposure leads to psychotic-like perturbations usually noted during adolescence (Friedrich et al. 2016; Radhakrishnan et al. 2014). However, to the best of our knowledge, the impact of prenatal SC exposure remains equivocal, as data from different studies show distinct effects in neurogenic processes, mostly depending on the cell/animal model, dosage frequency, or SCs tested (Alexandre et al. 2019).

The CB1R in SC-mediated Neurogenesis

Stimulation of pre-synaptic CB1R has been shown to promote neurogenesis and modulate the fate of neural progenitor cells. For example, Jin et al. (2004) observed that CB1R-knockout mice presented a reduced number of 5-bromo-2′-deoxyuridine (BrdU)-positive cells, indicative of lower proliferative ability, compared to wild-type

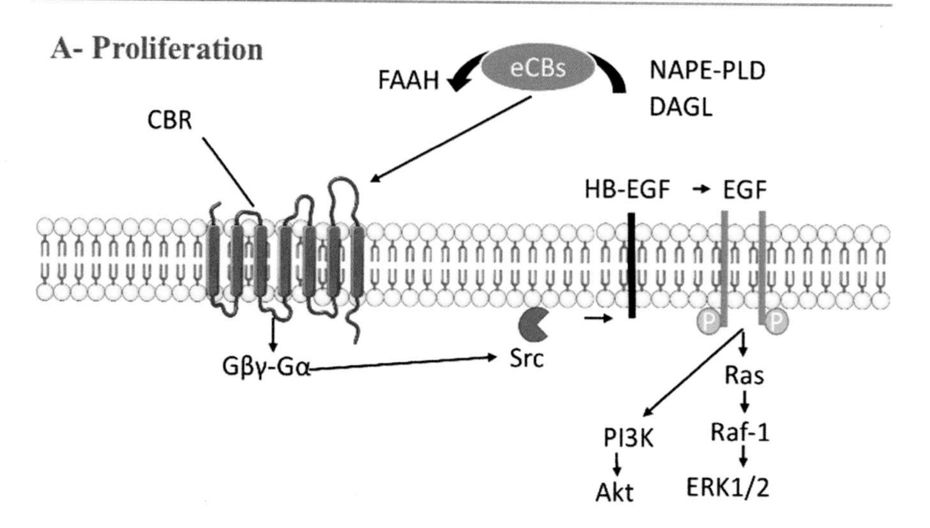

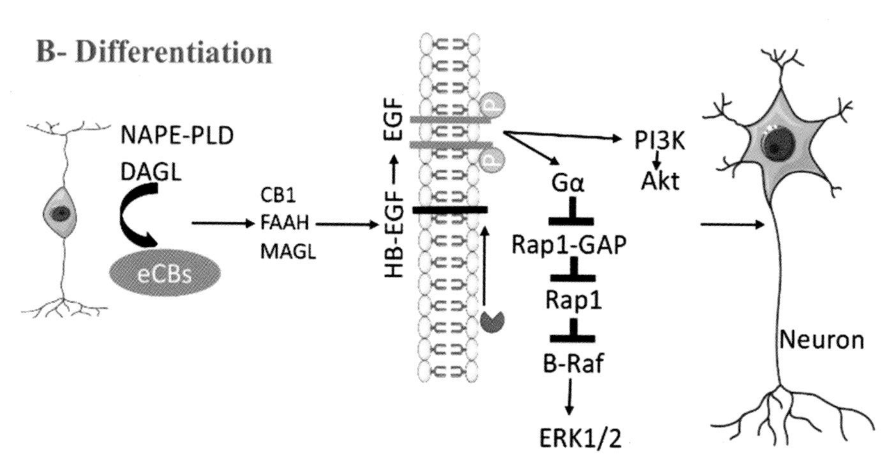

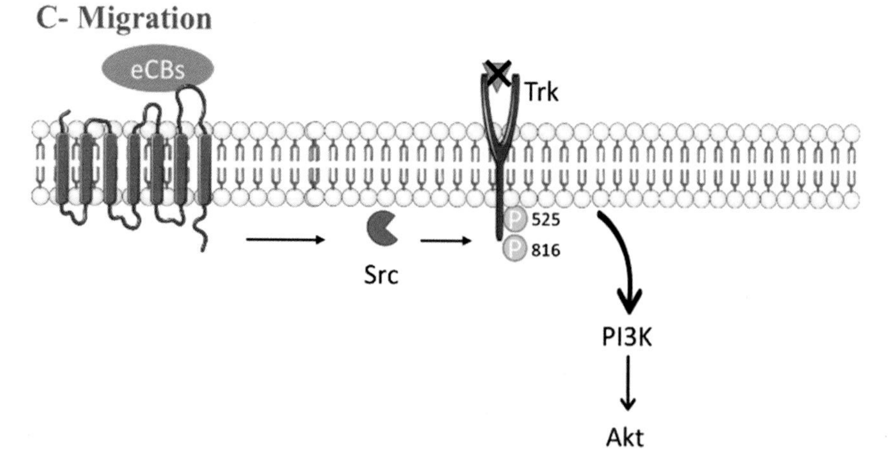

Fig. 4 (continued)

animals, in the dentate gyrus and subventricular zone. Jiang et al. (2005) observed increased proliferation and survival of hippocampal cells in the dentate gyrus of rats via CB1R-mediated signaling, following chronic treatment with HU-210. The SC (R)-(+)-methanandamide (R-m-AEA) has also been reported to increase self-renewal, proliferation, and differentiation of neurons from the mouse neonatal subventricular zone by stimulating CB1Rs, as a specific antagonist of this receptor (AM251) blocked the SC-induced effects (Xapelli et al. 2013). Our research team recently demonstrated an increase in neurite outgrowth in NG108-15 neuroblastoma x glioma hybrid cells (a cell model often used in neurodevelopmental studies) exposed to two synthetic cannabinoids, 5F-PB22 and THJ-2201, at human-relevant concentrations (< 1 μM). This SC-mediated effect was shown to be dependent on the activation of the CB1R, as the cells' incubation with a specific CB1R antagonist, SR141716A, reverted differentiation ratios (calculated as the number of newly formed neurites divided by the total number of cells) to basal levels, as depicted in Fig. 5 (Alexandre et al. 2020).

It is worth noting that activation of CB1R by different SCs may trigger distinct downstream signaling pathways. For example, although JWH-018 and JWH-081, two structurally similar SCs, bind and activate the CB1R, JWH-018 decreases pERK1/2 expression, whereas JWH-081 does not, rather impairing calcium/calmodulin-dependent protein kinase IV (CaMKIV) and Cyclic AMP-responsive element-binding protein 1 (CREB-1) levels. In turn, CaMKIV and CREB are related to the expression of the activity-regulated cytoskeleton-associated (Arc) protein, which is further associated with the regulation of neuronal plasticity (Atwood and Mackie 2010; Uchiyama et al. 2011).

Role of the CB2R in SC-mediated Neurogenesis

The contribution of CB2R to neurogenesis remains equivocal. Palazuelos et al. (2006) observed that the chronic administration of the CB2R selective agonist HU-308 enhanced hippocampal proliferation of adult mice. The same authors further

Fig. 4 Endocannabinoid signaling-mediated actions during neurogenic processes. (**a**) Proliferation: CB1R-mediated transactivation of the EGF-receptor activates the Raf1-ERK1/2 signaling pathway, thus promoting neuronal cell proliferation in a distinct process from the one evoked by classical $G\alpha_{i/0}$ protein coupling. (**b**) Differentiation: the blockade of second messengers' cascades from the Raf1-ERK1/2 pathway (e.g., Rap1, B-Raf) or the activation of a $G\alpha_{i/0}$-mediated signaling cascade that leads to the proteasomal degradation of the Rap1/B-Raf pathway results in increased neurite outgrowth. (**c**) Migration. The association of CB1R with the activation of Src tyrosine kinases triggers the phosphorylation of the Tropomyosin receptor kinase B (TrkB), promoting neuronal migration. Abbreviations: Akt: protein kinase; B: B-Raf, mitogen-activated protein kinase (MAPK) kinase; DAGL: diacylglycerol lipase; eCB: endocannabinoid; FAAH: fatty acid amide hydrolase; GAP: GTPase-activating protein; HB-EGF: heparin-binding EGF-like growth factor; MAGL: monoacylglycerol lipase; NAPE-PLD: N-acyl phosphatidylethanolamine-specific phospholipase D; PI3K: phosphatidylinositol 3-kinase; Raf-1: MEK kinase; Src: non-receptor tyrosine kinases. (Reproduced from Gomes et al. 2020, with permission from Elsevier Ltd.)

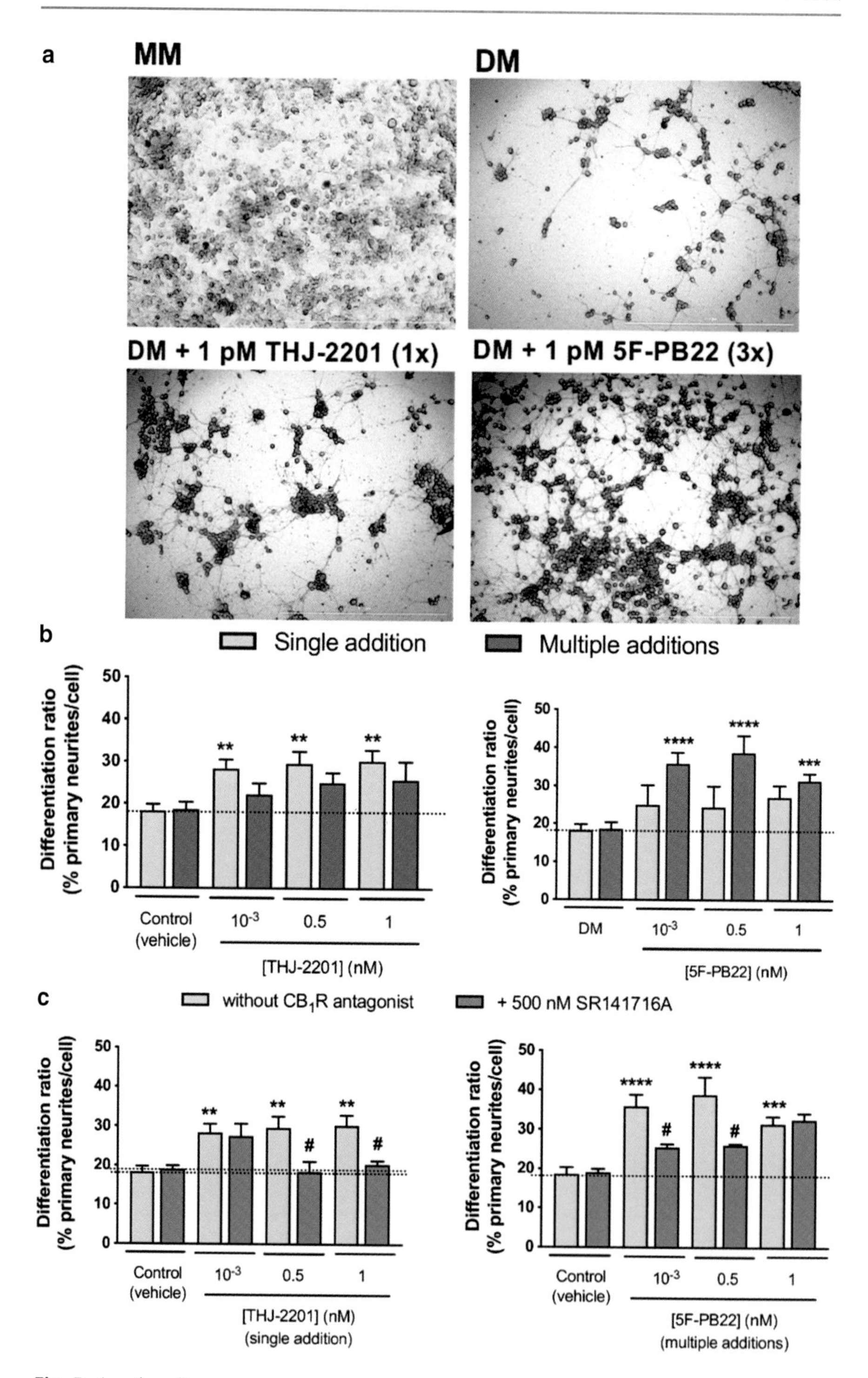

Fig. 5 (continued)

noted a decreased number of proliferative cells in the dentate gyrus of CB2R-deficient mice, suggesting the involvement of this receptor, at least partially, in neurogenic processes. A similar outcome on neuronal proliferation was reported by Rubio-Araiz et al. (2008), as the authors showed that both arachidonyl-2-′-chloroethylamide (ACEA) and JWH-056, selective CB1R and CB2R agonists, respectively, enhanced proliferation of murine cortical neurospheres. In contrast, Compagnucci et al. (2013) observed that while the CB1R selective agonist arachidonyl-2′-chloroethylamide (ACEA) increased differentiation of murine NPCs, the CB2R selective agonist JWH-133 did not affect this parameter.

Postnatal exposure of rats to the CB2R selective agonist JWH-056 for 15 days was shown to increase the expression of polysialylated neural cell adhesion molecule (PSA-NCAM) in the dorsolateral subventricular zone (Arévalo-Martín et al. 2007). Interestingly, these authors noted that only exposure to the non-selective SC WIN55,212-2 increased myelin basic protein expression in the subcortical white matter, suggesting that the activation of both CBRs is required to promote remyelination. Also, Palazuelos et al. (2012) observed that the CB2R selective agonist HU-308 enhanced the proliferation of hippocampal HiB5 NPCs via activation of the phosphatidylinositol 3-kinase (PI3K)/Akt/mammalian target of rapamycin complex 1 (mTORC1) pathway.

Recently, Rodrigues et al. (2017) observed that the non-selective SC WIN55,212-2 promoted neuronal cell proliferation in the dentate gyrus (DG), but not in the subventricular zone (SVZ), of cultured NPCs from early postnatal (P1-3) Sprague-Dawley rats. Nevertheless, cell proliferation in the SVZ was enhanced by a CB1R selective agonist. The authors further showed that WIN55,212-2 increased neuronal differentiation at both DG and SVZ, an effect that was mimicked by either CB1R or CB2R selective agonists and blocked by either CB1R or CB2R selective antagonists, evidencing cross-antagonism and indicating a close interplay between both CBRs in the modulation of neurogenesis. Later data from the same research lab further

Fig. 5 Effects of THJ-2201 and 5F-PB22 on neuronal differentiation. Neuronal differentiation was induced by replacing maintenance medium (MM) with differentiation medium (DM) in the presence of the SC or the vehicle (0.1% DMSO). SCs were added to NG108–15 cells either once (single addition at day 0, in gray) or every 24 h up to 72 h (total of 3 additions, in purple). (**a**) Representative images of NG108–15 cells at 72 h following induction of differentiation, and treated once with 0.1% DMSO (DM) or 1 pM THJ-2201 (single addition) or 1 pM 5F-PB22 (multiple additions). Cells cultured in MM (in the absence of differentiation factors) continued to proliferate, preventing the analysis of neurite outgrowth. Scale bars correspond to 1 mm; (b) Differentiation ratios induced by THJ-2201 (left panel) and 5F-PB22 (right panel), calculated as the number of neurites longer than 20 μm divided by the total number of cells per well. (**c**) Differentiation ratios in the presence of each SC following exposure to 500 nM SR141716A, a selective CB1R antagonist (blue bars). Each bar represents the mean ± SEM, for at least five independent experiments, performed in duplicate. $*p < 0.05$, $**p < 0.01$, $***p < 0.001$, $****p < 0.0001$, compared to vehicle control (one-way ANOVA, followed by Dunnett's post-test). $^{\#}p < 0.05$, compared to the respective SC concentration in the absence of antagonist (one-way ANOVA, followed by Sidak's multiple comparisons test). (Adapted and reproduced from Alexandre et al. 2020, with permission from MDPI)

showed that the presence of BDNF was crucial for CBR-mediated neurogenesis (Ferreira et al. 2018). In fact, not only BDNF promoted an increase in cell proliferation within the DG and SVZ, which was blocked by a CB2R selective antagonist, but CB1R activation-mediated increase in the cell proliferation in both brain areas was dependent on BDNF. Similarly, BDNF enhanced neuronal differentiation in DG and SVZ, in a process prevented by blocking either CB2R (in the DG) or both CBRs (in the SVZ). In turn, CBR-triggered neuronal differentiation was blocked by sequestering endogenous BDNF.

Some of the signaling pathways modulated by SCs upon their binding to cannabinoid receptors are summarized in Fig. 6.

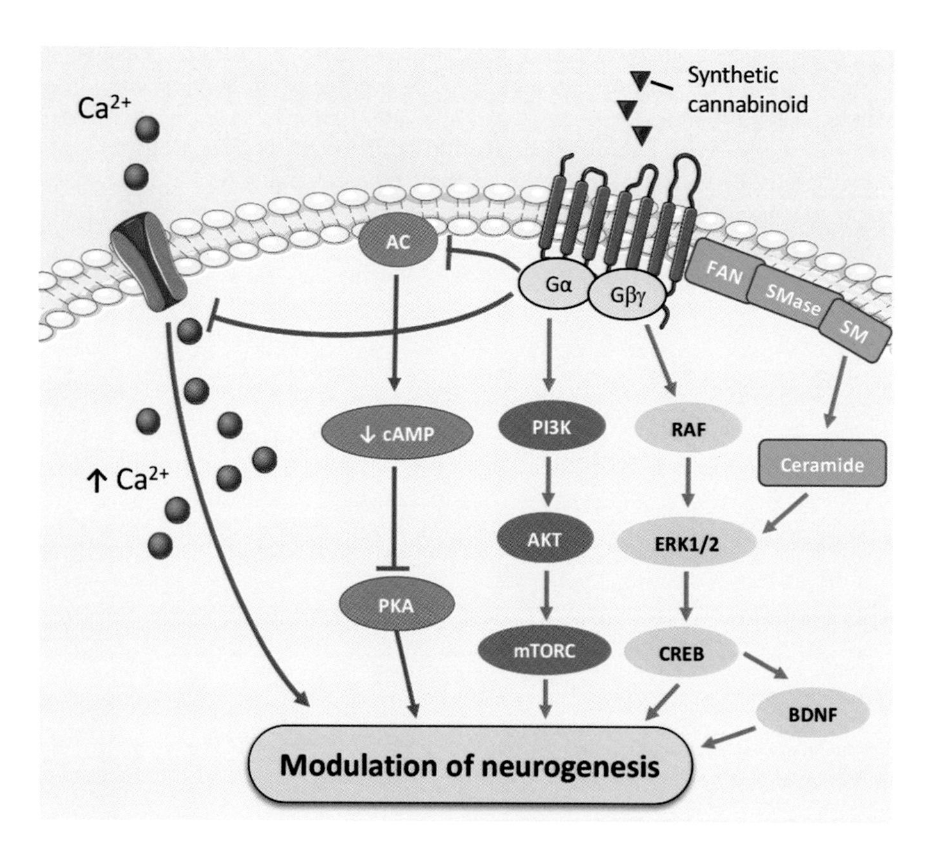

Fig. 6 Downstream mechanisms elicited upon CBR activation by SCs during neurogenesis. The effects of cannabinoid receptor activation by synthetic cannabinoids comprise the inhibition of the adenylyl cyclase (AC)-cyclic AMP (cAMP)-protein kinase A (PKA) pathway, as well as the activation of mitogen-activated protein kinase (MAPK) cascades, such as the phosphoinositide 3-kinase (PI3K)/protein kinase B (Akt) or the extracellular-signal-regulated kinase 1/2 (ERK1/2)-mediated pathways. These effects also include the modulation of the ion mobilization through the inhibition of voltage-sensitive Ca^{2+} channels (VSCC), by the release of Ca^{2+} from intracellular stores, and the production of ceramide through FAN-sphingomyelinase (factor associated with neutral sphingomyelinase activation, SMase). (Adapted from Alexandre et al. 2019)

Neurogenesis Control Via SCs' Actions on Glial Cells

Glial cells present in the CNS play an important role in the modulation of neurotransmission and formation of the neuronal network, besides providing neuronal protection and support. Astrocytes, for example, are essential for neuronal functioning, as well as differentiation and maturation of synapses, mostly due to their expression of gliotransmitters, which comprise a range of chemicals (e.g., homocysteic acid, taurine) released from glial cells that facilitate neurotransmission (Klapper et al. 2019; Santello et al. 2019).

While addressing the dynamics of different cell populations during the differentiation of neural progenitor cells (NPCs) derived from the cortices of 2-day old rat pups, Aguado et al. (2006) observed that NPCs exposure to WIN-55,212-2 increased the differentiation of glial cells, as indicated by the increased number of glial fibrillary acidic protein (GFAP), and reduced neuronal differentiation (decreased number of b-tubulin-III cells), pointing out the role of glial cells during neurogenesis. Activation of CB1R in hippocampal or spinal astrocytes triggers endocannabinoid signaling, increasing intracellular Ca^{2+} levels, which in turn stimulate glutamate release and further activate NMDA receptors in neurons (Hegyi et al. 2018; Navarrete and Araque 2008). Hablitz et al. (2020) further showed that activation of CB1R by WIN55,212-2 reduced the GABA receptor-mediated postsynaptic current frequency by a mechanism involving astrocytes, and decreased adenosine-1 receptors' activation on the pre-synaptic axon terminals.

Epigenetic Regulation of Neurogenesis by SCs

The interplay between the endocannabinoid system and the epigenetic machinery has already been shown to play a key role in modulating neurogenesis, as we recently reviewed (Gomes et al. 2020). On the one hand, the genes coding for some of the endocannabinoid system elements, like CBRs (*cnr1* and *cnr2*, for CB1R and CB2R, respectively) may undergo epigenetic changes (e.g., DNA methylation, histone modifications), thus altering their function (Börner et al. 2012). For example, hypermethylation of the *cnr1* promoter by histone methyltransferases downregulates CB1R transcription (D'Addario et al. 2013). On the other hand, the endocannabinoid system's elements may regulate epigenetic mechanisms by acting as epigenetic factors. For example, endocannabinoids may induce transcriptional changes in the enzymes related to histone modifications (e.g., histone deacetylases, acetyltransferases, methylases) (Stein and Stein 1984). Moreover, anandamide has been shown to protect neurons from inflammatory damage by promoting the histone H3 phosphorylation of *mpk-1* (the gene encoding for MAPK phosphatase-1) in activated microglial cells, resulting in the dephosphorylation of ERK1/2 (Upham et al. 2003).

There is accumulating evidence that the prenatal and adolescent use of phytocannabinoids (e.g., THC) causes epigenetic changes that may impair neurogenic processes, or affect the parental germline (Szutorisz and Hurd 2018). For example, the offspring of animals treated with cannabinoids have been shown to develop a drug-seeking behavior during adulthood (DiNieri et al. 2011). Nevertheless, although chronic SC exposure has been increasingly associated with epigenetic modifications that may ultimately impact neurogenesis, their epigenetic imprint remains sparsely explored. For example, administration of WIN55,212-2 to adolescent rats increased adult hippocampal anandamide levels and promoted DNA hypermethylation of the intracellular signaling modulator Rgs7, which acts as an antagonist of GPCR signaling by facilitating the GTP hydrolysis of G protein (Tomas-Roig et al. 2017).

Specific CBR agonists HU-210 (for CB1R) and JWH-133 (for CB2R) have already been reported to modulate the differentiation of glioma cells derived from a human brain tumor by increasing H3K9me3 levels in a CB1R- and CB2R-dependent manner (Aguado et al. 2007).

Večeřa et al. (2018) observed in a rat model of schizophrenia that treatment with the specific inverse antagonist of CB1R, AM-251, restored H3K9ac levels in the hippocampi to those of normal brains demonstrating the relevance of CB1R in the regulation of epigenetic mechanisms during neurodevelopment. Treatment of female rats with HU-210 after postnatal day 35 was shown to modify the expression of miRNA in the left hemisphere of the entorhinal cortex, a brain area often associated with schizophrenia (Hollins et al. 2014).

Moreover, daily exposure of adolescent male rats to WIN55,212-2 for 1 week was reported to increase global DNA methylation, accompanied by an altered transcription of DNA methyltransferases 1 (DNMT1) and 3 (DNMT3) in the prefrontal cortex (Ibn Lahmar Andaloussi et al. 2019). Notably, the authors further associated these alterations with anxiogenic-like effects, which were not limited to the exposed individuals, but also passed on to their offspring. Recently, exposure of adolescent (but not adult) rats to WIN55,212-2 was also found to induce histone hyperacetylation and reduce histone deacetylase 6 (HDAC6) levels in the prefrontal cortex (Scherma et al. 2020).

Applications to Other Areas of Substance Use Disorders

In this chapter we reviewed the potential consequences of SC misuse to the developing brain, summarizing some of the main mechanisms underlying neurogenesis that have been reported to be disrupted upon exposure to SCs. As noted, many studies described an increased neuronal differentiation induced by SCs. Similarly, other psychoactive substances, including lysergic acid diethylamide (LSD), N-dimethyltryptamine (DMT), 2,5-dimethoxy-4-iodoamphetamine (DOI), or ketamine, have been reported to increase neurogenesis and synaptogenesis, subsequently enhancing neuroplasticity (Ly et al. 2018). Whether these substances could have disruptive effects on perinatal and adolescent neurodevelopment is a subject that requires due attention in the near future.

Moreover, SC misuse has been increasingly associated with the onset of neuropsychiatric perturbations that have already been correlated to dysregulation of neurogenic processes. For example, psychosis is often described as a side effect of

SC use, but psychotic events have also been reported following the use of other new psychoactive substances, including cathinone and cocaine derivatives, benzodiazepines, or arylcyclohexylamines. Putative common mechanisms, involving defined adverse outcome pathways are also a matter of interest to develop therapies that may contribute to risk reduction.

Applications to Public Health

The impact of SC exposure on neurodevelopment represents a core issue, as adolescents and young adults, which include women of childbearing age/pregnant women, stand among the main SC users (EMCDDA 2021). Most important, impaired neuronal development may lead to the onset of neurodevelopment-related disorders (e.g., psychoses, autism spectrum). SCs have prevailed in NPS seizures between 2009 and 2019. A total of 209 new SCs have been detected in Europe since 2008, including 11 reported for the first time in 2020, and along with synthetic cathinones, SCs accounted for near 60% of total NPS seizures reported by European Union Member States. Although the number of emerging SCs has decreased between 2014 and 2018, the increasing association of these substances with intoxications and deaths, particularly compared to cannabis, has turned their use into a major public health concern and a challenge for regulatory agencies. Of note, an outbreak of 21 deaths related to the use of an SC, 4F-MDMB-BICA, occurred in Hungary in 2020 (EMCDDA 2021; UNODC 2020). Moreover, due to the recent changes regarding the legal status of cannabis and its synthetic derivatives' use, it is reasonable to expect an increase in recreational SC use (Hall et al. 2019).

The latest European Drug Report further noted the European Union's concern regarding the presence on the market of cannabis products adulterated with potent SCs, evidencing the need to provide policy-makers with updated and scientifically robust data that can help regulatory authorities design effective policies to prevent SC use. The unintentional consumption of SCs in such adulterated cannabis products is worrisome, considering the scarce information on the toxicity of these substances (EMCDDA 2021).

Mini-Dictionary of Terms

- **Endocannabinoid system.** *A complex cell signaling network comprising endogenous cannabinoids, enzymes responsible for the synthesis and degradation of endocannabinoids, and cannabinoid receptors that help regulate several functions within the organism.*
- **New Psychoactive Substances.** *Conventionally defined as "substances of abuse, either in a pure form or a preparation, that are not controlled by the 1961 Single Convention on Narcotic Drugs or the 1971 Convention on Psychotropic Substances, but that may pose a public health threat."*

- **Synthetic cannabinoids**. *A diverse group of man-made new psychoactive substances designed to mimic, with higher potency, the psychotropic effects of tetrahydrocannabinol (THC).*
- **Neurodevelopment disorders**. *A group of disorders in which the development of the central nervous system is disturbed, possibly manifesting in neuropsychiatric perturbations (*e.g.*, psychosis, autism spectrum) or impaired motor function, learning, language, or non-verbal communication.*
- **Neurogenesis**. *The process by which new neurons are formed in the brain.*

Key Facts of Synthetic Cannabinoids

209 new Synthetic Cannabinoids have been detected in the European Union since 2008.

Together with synthetic cathinones, synthetic cannabinoids account for 60% of the total New Psychoactive Substances' seizures in the European Union.

SCs are full agonists of cannabinoid receptors, contrasting endo- and phytocannabinoids, which are partial agonists of the same receptors.

These drugs are most commonly looked for causing relaxation, mood elevation, euphoria, social disinhibition, and increased sensorial awareness.

Chronic SC use induces serious adverse effects, including persistent anxiety, depression, and cognitive impairment, as well as cardiovascular and kidney complications.

Summary Points

- Recreational SC use is increasing worldwide, being often associated with reports of acute intoxications and deaths.
- Adolescents and young adults (a group that includes women of childbearing age/pregnant) stand among the most common SC users.
- The developing brain is especially vulnerable to SC-elicited effects.
- Information on the impact of SCs on neurogenesis remains scarce.
- There is accumulating evidence that SC use may lead to the onset of neurodevelopmental disorders (e.g., psychosis, autism spectrum).
- SCs target the endocannabinoid system, which in turn modulates several biological processes, including neurogenesis.
- SC-mediated activation of CB1R and CB2R particularly seems to interfere with neurotransmission and neuroplasticity, through an intricate network of signaling pathways.
- Long-term SC exposure has been increasingly associated with epigenetic changes (e.g., DNA methylation, histone modifications) that may impact neurogenesis.
- Further research is required to clarify the main mechanisms underlying SC-mediated effects on neurogenesis and their impact on neurodevelopment, thus expectedly contributing to reducing SC misuse by high-risk groups.

Acknowledgments This work was financed by: FEDER – Fundo Europeu de Desenvolvimento Regional funds through the COMPETE 2020 – Operational Programme for Competitiveness and Internationalisation (POCI), and by Portuguese funds through FCT – Fundação para a Ciência e a Tecnologia, I.P., in the framework of the project POCI-01-0145-FEDER-029584; and by national funds from FCT in the scope of the projects UIDP/04378/2020 and UIDB/04378/2020 of the Research Unit on Applied Molecular Biosciences (UCIBIO) and the project LA/P/0140/2020 of the Associate Laboratory Institute for Health and Bioeconomy (i4HB).

References

Abboussi O, Tazi A, Paizanis E et al (2014) Chronic exposure to WIN55,212-2 affects more potently spatial learning and memory in adolescents than in adult rats via a negative action on dorsal hippocampal neurogenesis. Pharmacol Biochem Behav 120:95–102

Aguado T, Palazuelos J, Monory K et al (2006) The endocannabinoid system promotes astroglial differentiation by acting on neural progenitor cells. J Neurosci 26:1551–1561

Aguado T, Carracedo A, Julien B et al (2007) Cannabinoids induce glioma stem-like cell differentiation and inhibit gliomagenesis. J Biol Chem 282:6854–6862

Alexandre J, Carmo H, Carvalho F et al (2019) Synthetic cannabinoids and their impact on neurodevelopmental processes. Addict Biol 25:e12824

Alexandre J, Malheiro R, Dias da Silva D et al (2020) The synthetic cannabinoids THJ-2201 and 5F-PB22 enhance in vitro CB1 receptor-mediated neuronal differentiation at biologically relevant concentrations. Int J Mol Sci 21:6277

Arévalo-Martín Á, García-Ovejero D, Rubio-Araiz A et al (2007) Cannabinoids modulate Olig2 and polysialylated neural cell adhesion molecule expression in the subventricular zone of postnatal rats through cannabinoid receptor 1 and cannabinoid receptor 2. Eur J Neurosci 26: 1548–1559

Atwood BK, Mackie K (2010) CB2: a cannabinoid receptor with an identity crisis. Br J Pharmacol 160:467–479

Auwarter V, Dresen S, Weinmann W et al (2009) 'Spice' and other herbal blends: harmless incense or cannabinoid designer drugs? J Mass Spectrom 44:832–837

Bambico FR, Katz N, Debonnel G et al (2007) Cannabinoids elicit antidepressant-like behavior and activate serotonergic neurons through the medial prefrontal cortex. J Neurosci 27:11700–11711

Börner C, Martella E, Höllt V et al (2012) Regulation of opioid and cannabinoid receptor genes in human neuroblastoma and T cells by the epigenetic modifiers trichostatin A and 5-aza-2-′-deoxycytidine. Neuroimmunomodulation 19:180–186

Chen D-J, Gao M, Gao F-F et al (2017) Brain cannabinoid receptor 2: expression, function and modulation. Acta Pharmacol Sin 38:312–316

Cohen K, Weinstein AM (2018) Synthetic and non-synthetic cannabinoid drugs and their adverse effects – a review from public health prospective. Front Public Health 6:162–162

Cohen K, Weizman A, Weinstein A (2019) Modulatory effects of cannabinoids on brain neurotransmission. Eur J Neurosci 50:2322–2345

Compagnucci C, Di Siena S, Bustamante MB et al (2013) Type-1 (CB1) cannabinoid receptor promotes neuronal differentiation and maturation of neural stem cells. PLoS One 8:e54271

Cooper ZD (2016) Adverse effects of synthetic cannabinoids: management of acute toxicity and withdrawal. Curr Psychiatry Rep 18:52

Cristino L, Bisogno T, Di Marzo V (2020) Cannabinoids and the expanded endocannabinoid system in neurological disorders. Nat Rev Neurol 16:9–29

D'Addario C, Di Francesco A, Pucci M et al (2013) Epigenetic mechanisms and endocannabinoid signalling. FEBS J 280:1905–1917

Dalton VS, Zavitsanou K (2010) Differential treatment regimen-related effects of cannabinoids on D1 and D2 receptors in adolescent and adult rat brain. J Chem Neuroanat 40:272–280 de Oliveira RW, Oliveira CL, Guimaraes FS et al (2019) Cannabinoid signalling in embryonic and adult neurogenesis: possible implications for psychiatric and neurological disorders. Acta Neuropsychiatr 31:1–16

de Salas-Quiroga A, García-Rincón D, Gómez-Domínguez D et al (2020) Long-term hippocampal interneuronopathy drives sex-dimorphic spatial memory impairment induced by prenatal THC exposure. Neuropsychopharmacology 45:877–886

Debruyne D, Le Boisselier R (2015) Emerging drugs of abuse: current perspectives on synthetic cannabinoids. Subst Abus Rehabil 6:113–129

Di Marzo V, Stella N, Zimmer A (2015) Endocannabinoid signalling and the deteriorating brain. Nat Rev Neurosci 16:30–42

DiNieri JA, Wang X, Szutorisz H et al (2011) Maternal cannabis use alters ventral striatal dopamine D2 gene regulation in the offspring. Biol Psychiatry 70:763–769

EMCDDA – European Monitoring Center for Drugs and Drug Addiction (2021) European drug report 2021: trends and developments. Publications Office of the European Union, Luxembourg

Ferreira FF, Ribeiro FF, Rodrigues RS et al (2018) Brain-derived neurotrophic factor (BDNF) role in cannabinoid-mediated neurogenesis. Front Cell Neurosci 12:441

Ford BM, Franks LN, Tai S et al (2017) Characterization of structurally novel G protein biased CB1 agonists: implications for drug development. Pharmacol Res 125:161–177

Franklin JM, Carrasco GA (2012) Cannabinoid-induced enhanced interaction and protein levels of serotonin 5-HT(2A) and dopamine D_2 receptors in rat prefrontal cortex. J Psychopharmacol 26: 1333–1347

Friedrich J, Khatib D, Parsa K et al (2016) The grass isn't always greener: the effects of cannabis on embryological development. BMC Pharmacol Toxicol 17:45–57

Galve-Roperh I, Chiurchiù V, Díaz-Alonso J et al (2013) Cannabinoid receptor signaling in progenitor/stem cell proliferation and differentiation. Prog Lipid Res 52:633–650

Gomes TM, Dias da Silva D, Carmo H et al (2020) Epigenetics and the endocannabinoid system signaling: an intricate interplay modulating neurodevelopment. Pharmacol Res 162:105237

Hablitz LM, Gunesch AN, Cravetchi O et al (2020) Cannabinoid signaling recruits astrocytes to modulate presynaptic function in the suprachiasmatic nucleus. eNeuro 7(1):1–19

Hall W, Stjepanović D, Caulkins J et al (2019) Public health implications of legalising the production and sale of cannabis for medicinal and recreational use. Lancet 394:1580–1590

Harkany T, Guzman M, Galve-Roperh I et al (2007) The emerging functions of endocannabinoid signaling during CNS development. Trends Pharmacol Sci 28:83–92

Hegyi Z, Olah T, Koszeghy A et al (2018) CB1 receptor activation induces intracellular Ca(2+) mobilization and 2-arachidonoylglycerol release in rodent spinal cord astrocytes. Sci Rep 8: 10562

Hollins SL, Zavitsanou K, Walker FR et al (2014) Alteration of imprinted Dlk1-Dio3 miRNA cluster expression in the entorhinal cortex induced by maternal immune activation and adolescent cannabinoid exposure. Transl Psychiatry 4:e452

Howlett AC, Abood ME (2017) CB(1) and CB(2) receptor pharmacology. Adv Pharmacol 80: 169–206

Ibn Lahmar Andaloussi Z, Taghzouti K, Abboussi O (2019) Behavioural and epigenetic effects of paternal exposure to cannabinoids during adolescence on offspring vulnerability to stress. Int J Dev Neurosci 72:48–54

Jiang W, Zhang Y, Xiao L et al (2005) Cannabinoids promote embryonic and adult hippocampus neurogenesis and produce anxiolytic- and antidepressant-like effects. J Clin Invest 115: 3104–3116

Jin K, Xie L, Kim SH et al (2004) Defective adult neurogenesis in CB1 cannabinoid receptor knockout mice. Mol Pharmacol 66:204–208

Klapper SD, Garg P, Dagar S et al (2019) Astrocyte lineage cells are essential for functional neuronal differentiation and synapse maturation in human iPSC-derived neural networks. Glia 67:1893–1909

Krishna Kumar K, Shalev-Benami M, Robertson MJ et al (2019) Structure of a signaling cannabinoid receptor 1 – G protein complex. Cell 176:448–458
Lauckner JE, Hille B, Mackie K (2005) The cannabinoid agonist WIN55,212-2 increases intracellular calcium via CB(1) receptor coupling to G(q/11) G proteins. Proc Natl Acad Sci U S A 102: 19144–19149
Lauritsen KJ, Rosenberg H (2016) Comparison of outcome expectancies for synthetic cannabinoids and botanical marijuana. Am J Drug Alcohol Abuse 42:377–384
Ly C, Greb AC, Cameron LP et al (2018) Psychedelics promote structural and functional neural plasticity. Cell Rep 23:3170–3182
Ma Z, Gao F, Larsen B et al (2019) Mechanisms of cannabinoid CB2 receptor-mediated reduction of dopamine neuronal excitability in mouse ventral tegmental area. EBioMedicine 42:225–237
Ming G-L, Song H (2011) Adult neurogenesis in the mammalian brain: significant answers and significant questions. Neuron 70:687–702
Navarrete M, Araque A (2008) Endocannabinoids mediate neuron-astrocyte communication. Neuron 57:883–893
Ossato A, Uccelli L, Bilel S et al (2017) Psychostimulant effect of the synthetic cannabinoid JWH-018 and AKB48: behavioral, neurochemical, and dopamine transporter scan imaging studies in mice. Front Psych 8:130
Ozturk HM, Yetkin E, Ozturk S (2019) Synthetic cannabinoids and cardiac arrhythmia risk: review of the literature. Cardiovasc Toxicol 19:191–197
Palazuelos J, Aguado T, Egia A et al (2006) Non-psychoactive CB2 cannabinoid agonists stimulate neural progenitor proliferation. FASEB J 20:2405–2407
Palazuelos J, Ortega Z, Díaz-Alonso J et al (2012) CB2 Cannabinoid receptors promote neural progenitor cell proliferation via mTORC1 signaling. J Biol Chem 287:1198–1209
Pallotto M, Deprez F (2014) Regulation of adult neurogenesis by GABAergic transmission: signaling beyond GABAA-receptors. Front Cell Neurosci 8:166
Patel M, Manning JJ, Finlay DB et al (2020) Signalling profiles of a structurally diverse panel of synthetic cannabinoid receptor agonists. Biochem Pharmacol 175:113871
Pertwee RG, Howlett AC, Abood ME et al (2010) International union of basic and clinical pharmacology. LXXIX. Cannabinoid receptors and their ligands: beyond CB1 and CB2. Pharmacol Rev 62:588–631
Platel J-C, Dave KA, Gordon V et al (2010) NMDA receptors activated by subventricular zone astrocytic glutamate are critical for neuroblast survival prior to entering a synaptic network. Neuron 65:859–872
Prenderville JA, Kelly ÁM, Downer EJ (2015) The role of cannabinoids in adult neurogenesis. Brit J Pharmacol 172:3950–3963
Radhakrishnan R, Wilkinson ST, D'Souza DC (2014) Gone to pot – a review of the association between cannabis and psychosis. Front Psychiatry 5:54
Rodrigues RS, Ribeiro FF, Ferreira F et al (2017) Interaction between cannabinoid type 1 and type 2 receptors in the modulation of subventricular zone and dentate gyrus neurogenesis. Front Pharmacol 8:516
Rubio-Araiz A, Arévalo-Martín Á, Gómez-Torres O et al (2008) The endocannabinoid system modulates a transient TNF pathway that induces neural stem cell proliferation. Mol Cell Neurosci 38:374–380
Sánchez-Blázquez P, Rodríguez-Muñoz M, Garzón J (2013) The cannabinoid receptor 1 associates with NMDA receptors to produce glutamatergic hypofunction: implications in psychosis and schizophrenia. Front Pharmacol 4:169
Sánchez-Zavaleta R, Cortés H, Avalos-Fuentes JA et al (2018) Presynaptic cannabinoid CB2 receptors modulate [3H]-glutamate release at subthalamo-nigral terminals of the rat. Synapse 72:e22061
Santello M, Toni N, Volterra A (2019) Astrocyte function from information processing to cognition and cognitive impairment. Nat Neurosci 22:154–166

Scherma M, Qvist JS, Asok A et al (2020) Cannabinoid exposure in rat adolescence reprograms the initial behavioral, molecular, and epigenetic response to cocaine. Proc Natl Acad Sci U S A 117: 9991–10002

Shohayeb B, Diab M, Ahmed M et al (2018) Factors that influence adult neurogenesis as potential therapy. Transl Neurodegener 7:4

Spalding Kirsty L, Bergmann O, Alkass K et al (2013) Dynamics of hippocampal neurogenesis in adult humans. Cell 153:1219–1227

Stein GS, Stein JL (1984) Is human histone gene expression autogenously regulated? Mol Cell Biochem 64:105–110

Szutorisz H, Hurd YL (2018) High times for cannabis: epigenetic imprint and its legacy on brain and behavior. Neurosci Biobehav Rev 85:93–101

Tai S, Fantegrossi WE (2014) Synthetic cannabinoids: pharmacology, behavioral effects, and abuse potential. Curr Addict Rep 1:129–136

Tomas-Roig J, Benito E, Agis-Balboa R et al (2017) Chronic exposure to cannabinoids during adolescence causes long-lasting behavioral deficits in adult mice. Addict Biol 22:1778–1789

Uchiyama N, Kikura-Hanajiri R, Goda Y (2011) Identification of a novel cannabimimetic phenylacetylindole, cannabipiperidiethanone, as a designer drug in a herbal product and its affinity for cannabinoid CB1 and CB2 receptors. Chem Pharm Bull 59:1203–1205

UNODC – United Nations Office on Drugs and Crime (2020) World drug report 2020. United Nations Publications, Vienna, Austria

Upham BL, Rummel AM, Carbone JM et al (2003) Cannabinoids inhibit gap junctional intercellular communication and activate ERK in a rat liver epithelial cell line. Int J Cancer 104:12–18

Večeřa J, Bártová E, Krejčí J et al (2018) HDAC1 and HDAC3 underlie dynamic H3K9 acetylation during embryonic neurogenesis and in schizophrenia-like animals. J Cell Physiol 233:530–548

Walsh KB, Andersen HK (2020) Molecular pharmacology of synthetic cannabinoids: delineating CB1 receptor-mediated cell signaling. Int J Mol Sci 21:6115

Xapelli S, Agasse F, Sardà-Arroyo L et al (2013) Activation of type 1 cannabinoid receptor (CB1R) promotes neurogenesis in murine subventricular zone cell cultures. PLoS One 8:e63529

Yano H, Adhikari P, Naing S et al (2020) Positive allosteric modulation of the 5-HT1A receptor by indole-based synthetic cannabinoids abused by humans. ACS Chem Neurosci 11:1400–1405

Zou S, Kumar U (2018) Cannabinoid receptors and the endocannabinoid system: signaling and function in the central nervous system. Int J Mol Sci 19:833

Cannabis and Organ Damage: A Focus on Pancreatitis (to Include Different Scenarios)

62

Angela Saviano

Contents

Introduction 1344
Pancreas and Cannabinoids Receptors 1345
Acute Pancreatitis and Cannabis 1346
Chronic Pancreatitis and Cannabis 1347
Applications to Public Health 1348
Mini-Dictionary of Terms 1349
Key Facts 1350
Summary Points 1350
References 1351

Abstract

Cannabis is a widely and commonly used illicit drug. The regular use of cannabis has revealed numerous side effects on different body sites. From 2004 (Grant and Gandhi 2004) to now, literature data have been reporting an increased number of acute pancreatitis related to cannabis use and/or abuse. The mechanism by which cannabis induces acute pancreatitis has not been fully understood and recent researches are still underway to determine the exact pathophysiology. It is known that cannabinoids receptors named cannabinoids receptor type 1 (CB1) and type 2 (CB2) are sited in the pancreatic islets of Langerhans. So, the active cannabinoids compounds may "influence" the pancreatic activity through the binding with these receptors, with effects "dose-related," according to the recent evidence. This review aims to summarize the current knowledge regarding the effects of cannabis and cannabinoids derivatives on pancreas, since its use and/or abuse is progressively increasing and a large widely legalization is achieving.

A. Saviano (✉)
Department of Emergency Medicine, Catholic University of the Sacred Heart, Rome, Italy

V. B. Patel, V. R. Preedy (eds.), *Handbook of Substance Misuse and Addictions*,
https://doi.org/10.1007/978-3-030-92392-1_68

Keywords

Cannabis · Acute pancreatitis · Chronic pancreatitis · THC · Marijuana · Psychotropic drugs · Lipase · Pain · Pancreatic stellate cells · CBN · Cannabinoid's receptor type 1 · Cannabinoid's receptor type 2 · Addiction · Cannabinoids · Dependence

Abbreviations

AP	Acute pancreatitis
CB1	Cannabinoid's receptor type 1
CB2	Cannabinoid's receptor type 2
CBD	Cannabidiol
CBN	Cannabinol
CP	Chronic pancreatitis
THC	Delta-9-tetrahydrocannabinol

Introduction

Cannabis is one of the most cultivated and trafficked Asian plant (*Cannabis sativa*) (Pollio 2016; Cerino et al. 2021; Echeverry et al. 2021; Andre et al. 2016). It is used both for recreational purposes and, in some cases, for therapeutic ones (Grotenhermen and Müller-Vahl 2012). It belongs to the family of Cannabaceae (Pollio 2016) and contains three different bioactive molecules known as flavonoids, terpenoids, and cannabinoids (Andre et al. 2016). The primary active compound of cannabis is delta-9-tetrahydrocannabinol (THC), but to date about 113 cannabinoids have been documented, besides other 500 substances contained in it (Adams and Martin 1996; Grotenhermen 2003; Grotenhermen and Müller-Vahl 2012; Karila 2017). Cannabinoids bind two specific G-protein-linked receptors of the endogenous cannabinoid system, the cannabinoids receptor type 1 (CB1) and type 2 (CB2) (Mackie 2007, 2008; Pacher et al. 2020). CB1 receptors are sited prevalently in the central and peripheral nervous system (brain cortex, hippocampus, basal ganglia, etc.), while CB2 receptors are found mainly in immune tissues (such as lymphocytes and macrophages) and in the gastrointestinal tract (Grotenhermen 2003; Bátkai 2006). Cannabinoids, both endogenous and exogenous, can mediate many functions acting on CB1 and CB2 receptors.

These receptors are able to modulate the release of neurotransmitters, acting on presynaptic sites. Their activation opens the potassium channels and closes the calcium channels, with the subsequent effect of hyperpolarization of the presynaptic site and the inhibition of release of some neurotransmitters such as acetylcholine glutamate, dopamine, etc. (Baron 2015). Moreover, the activation of CB1 receptors leads to the inhibition of GABA, serotonin, and noradrenaline release. The CB1 receptor is a G-protein receptor located in the peripheral and central nervous system. In particular, some cerebral areas such as cerebral cortex, hippocampus, amygdala, basal ganglia, cerebellum, periaqueductal gray matter, spinal interneurons, etc. are populated by CB1 receptors which mediate pain-related and cardiopulmonary functions, providing also the substrate for potential therapeutic targets (Baron 2015). Furthermore, CB1 receptors mediate anti-inflammatory effects through the inhibition of enzymes that are engaged in the conversion of arachidonic acid.

The CB2 receptors are mainly located in the peripheral tissues, especially in the immune system, with low concentrations in some cerebral regions as periaqueductal gray matter, astrocytes, oligodendrocytes, etc. (Baron 2015). They show inhibitory effects on some serotonin receptors, and act on endocannabinoid pathways, playing analgesics, anti-inflammatory, and antiemetic roles (Baron 2015). Furthermore, CB2 receptors can influence the release of different cytokines and induce immune cells migration. These actions are mediated by some ligands of endocannabinoids receptors such as anandamide, 2-arachidonoylglycerol, *N*-arachidonoylphosphatidylethanolamine, *N*-acylamides, etc. (Baron 2015; Hourani and Alexander 2018).

So, endocannabinoids effects (Pacher et al. 2006, 2020) range from cognitive, emotional, psychoactive, and behavioral to anti-inflammatory, immunosuppressive, antispastic, and metabolic disorders (Huestis 2002; Reyes-Parada 2021). Cannabis and its derivatives have been legalized in many states of America and Europe. Literature data underline that about 4% of the world's population make use of marijuana per year (Sly et al. 2021). In addition to the recreational use, synthetic cannabinoids have also emerged today in the treatments for pain (as in cancer) (Lafaye et al. 2017). Synthetic cannabinoids differ from cannabis due to the fact they are full agonists of CB1 and CB2 receptors. They have a binding affinity stronger than THC or endogenous cannabinoids molecules, thus provoking much more marked psychoactive effects (Lafaye et al. 2017). Different synthetic cannabinoids may have variable compositions, even if they belong to the same brand; so, their effects depend on the dosage and on the type of product taken (Lafaye et al. 2017). In addition, their pharmacokinetics depend on the route of administration. Numerous effects have been observed in cannabis users, such as agitation, anxiety, irritability, delirious symptoms, sleep disorders, hallucinations, and panic attacks, but also cardiovascular, pulmonary, renal, intestinal, and pancreatic disorders (Lafaye et al. 2017).

Pancreas and Cannabinoids Receptors

The pancreatic tissue has an exocrine and endocrine function and it expresses CB1 and CB2 receptors. Bermudez-Silva et al. (2008) detected these receptors in the islets of Langerhans, with a possible role on insulin sensitivity, feeding, and obesity (Pagliari et al. 2019). Goyal and Singla (2018) described the presence of these receptors in the area of pancreatic inflammation with a high concentration of macrophages and pancreatic stellate cells. Pancreatic stellate cells are still under investigation, but literature data recognized that they have a pivotal role in inflammatory processes, as described by Masamune et al. (2009), too.

Yang et al. (2020) in their experimental models of AP (Yang et al. 2021) showed that pancreatic stellate cells contributed to pancreatic fibrosis. Interestingly,

Michalski et al. (2007, 2008), analyzing the effects of cannabinoids on pancreatic tissue, revealed that CB1 receptors are involved in pancreatic fibrosis while CB2 receptors may be responsible of antifibrotic effects (Michalski et al. 2007). The expression of these receptors and their activation usually increases when the pancreas is inflamed as in case of AP (Goyal and Singla 2018). So, cannabis-active compounds can modulate the pancreatic inflammation. THC, one of the most studied active cannabis compound, acts as partial agonist of CB1 and CB2 receptors with higher affinity for CB1 receptors mediating many of the toxic psychoactive effects of cannabis, and with activity on CB2 receptors mediating many immunosuppression and anti-inflammatory activities. CBD, another well-studied cannabis derivative, may decrease inflammation-binding cannabis receptors CB1-CB2, as described by Burstein (2015). In fact, it reduces the pro-inflammatory cytokines, such as IL-6 and IL-10, and increases the anti-inflammatory cytokines, such as IL-10 (Burstein 2015; Pagliari et al. 2019). Cannabinol (CBN) is another minor component derived from the degradation of THC that can regulate the pancreatic enzymes secretion (Laezza et al. 2020), exerting its effects through CB1 and CB2 receptors (Laezza et al. 2020).

Acute Pancreatitis and Cannabis

AP has several etiologies ranging from biliary stones, alcohol, viral infections, congenital malformation, drugs, and toxins to "idiopathic," unknown pancreatitis.

The evaluation of AP should start collecting a detailed history focusing on clinical symptoms and presentation (Mederos et al. 2021). Of course, most common etiologies as gallbladder stones, alcohol use, hypertriglyceridemia, hypercalcemia, and history of autoimmune diseases or trauma have to be ruled out (Mederos et al. 2021). The use of drugs- or toxins-induced AP are a rare entity. In particular, the role of cannabis in AP has not been defined yet, but it has to be considered an important differential diagnosis in cases without a clear etiology (Grant and Gandhi 2004; Herrero et al. 2016). In this case, the urine toxicological screening can be useful in the workup of acute idiopathic pancreatitis.

The diagnosis of AP includes laboratory tests as pancreatic enzymes (amylase and lipase), diagnostic for a value greater than three times the superior normal limit; clinical presentation with mild-severe abdominal pain and tenderness; and imaging examinations as abdominal ultrasound, contrasted computed tomography scan, or abdominal magnetic resonance imaging (after the acute phase) to visualize pancreatic and extra-pancreatic inflammation, duct abnormalities, gallbladder stones, biliary duct obstruction, etc. (Mederos et al. 2021; Chatila et al. 2019). About 15–20% of AP are severe forms (Chatila et al. 2019). Many criteria and score systems assess the severity of AP (Ranson's criteria, APACHE II, and BISAP score), giving important indication on patient's risk and the first management of this condition (Chatila et al. 2019). Medical history remains essential to detect the etiology of AP and target the subsequent therapeutic strategies. Moreover, in order to examine the use of cannabis in the differential diagnosis of AP, it is important to ask patients specific questions regarding its illicit use/abuse of drugs (Sly et al. 2021). From 2004 until now, different case reports have showed the association between cannabis consumption and acute pancreatic inflammation. Barkin et al. (2017) described 26 cases of AP induced by cannabis; Culetto et al. (2017) reported 18 cases of cannabis-associated AP. Simons-Linares et al. (2018) and Barkin (2018) found 9 cases of AP among cannabis users. Chandy et al. (2019) presented a case of a young female with AP, referring a daily use of marijuana from the past 14 months (before AP) and she had a urine drug test positive for THC. Pagliari et al. (2019) reported a case of a young male with three episodes of AP and a daily consumption of cannabis. No evidence of other etiologies of AP were found (as biliary, autoimmune, or genetic). After interrupted cannabis use, no other episodes of AP appeared in the next follow-up time of 12 months. Fatma et al. (2013) described the case of a young male, with regular user of cannabis, who developed AP after 2 days of excessive smoke of cannabis. Herrero et al. (2016) documented cannabis-associated AP in a young male with positive urine test for THC and daily assumption of cannabis.

John et al. (2019) discussed a case of AP in a young patient who assumed 2–3 g of marijuana, daily from many years. Sly et al. reported the case of a 20-year-old male who developed AP secondary to cannabis use (Sly et al. 2021). Studies on animals (mainly, rats' models) underline the possible link between cannabis and AP severity, too (Matsuda et al. 2005; Dembiński et al. 2008). Infact, the administration of anandamide, an endogenous ligand for CB1 receptors, was associated with an increased severity inflammation and pancreatic edema in murine models of cerulein-induced AP (Matsuda et al. 2005; Dembiński et al. 2008). The dosage, the latency time between cannabis intake and development of AP, and the short- and long-term effects of cannabis regular use are not yet well known. More studies are needed to explore these issues.

Chronic Pancreatitis and Cannabis

CP is a progressive and irreversible disorder of the pancreas characterized by inflammation, fibrosis, and sclerosis (Barry2018). Its etiology is multifactorial and includes alcohol use, tobacco smoking, medications or toxins, obstructive etiologies as tumors, pancreas divisum (27%), pancreatitis of unknown origin (17%), autoimmunity (4%), and hereditary and genetic factors, involving some genes as PRSS1, CFTR, and SPINK1 (4%) (Etemad and Whitcomb 2001; Pham and Forsmark 2018). The exocrine and endocrine pancreatic functions are often lost. CP is characterized by variable calcification and pancreatic fibrosis; the pancreatic ducts can be dilatated or present structuring or distortion; often, some pancreatic pseudocysts can appear with a narrowing effect on the duodenum. CP can be characterized by thrombosis of superior mesenteric vein, and/or portal and/or splenic vein (Singh et al. 2019). There are some criteria for diagnosing CP by endoscopic ultrasound that consider pancreatic hyperechoic aspects with/without shadowing; calcifications of main pancreatic duct, pancreatic lobularity with honeycombing features, or pseudocysts; dilatation or irregularity of the main pancreatic duct; and dilatation of ≥ 3 duct branches

(Beyer et al. 2020). The pathogenesis of pancreatic fibrosis identifies a key factor in pancreatic stellate cells. These last synthetized an increased amounts of collagen and other extracellular proteins when activated by proinflammatory cytokines and oxidant stress mediators (Apte et al. 2015). Literature researches have showed that cannabis can induce a functionally and metabolically quiescence of pancreatic stellate cells, contributing to treat inflammation and fibrosis in CP (Michalski et al. 2008; Masamune and Shimosegawa 2009). To date, data about the role of cannabis in CP and in the pathophysiology of this disease are still lacking. On the contrary, more literature evidences assessed the analgesic role of cannabis in CP pain (De Vries et al. 2016; Romero-Sandoval et al. 2017; Barlowe et al. 2019). The role of cannabis in pain for the treatment of pain has been studied for many years (Hill et al. 2017). In the past, it was used as a medicine to treat articular pain, constipation, female reproductive discomfort, and pain related to surgical procedures (Hill et al. 2017). To date, it has been studied for the treatment of cancer-related pain and CP, too (Hill et al. 2017; Barlowe et al. 2019). Pain is a subjective complex experience including physiological, cognitive, affective, and motivational components (Hill et al. 2017). Chronic pain is the main clinical presentation of CP (Beyer et al. 2020). The lack of strong safety profile of cannabis and trials to support its efficacy do not approve the standardized use of it in the treatment of chronic pancreatic pain and more researches are required to investigate this topic. In summary, treatment options of CP include a multidisciplinary approach with medical, endoscopic, or surgical treatments (Singh et al. 2019), but to date more studies are needed to understand whether cannabis compounds can be used as a medical treatment for pain in patients with CP (Barlowe et al. 2019).

Applications to Public Health

Pancreatitis is a critical public health issue, with an increasing incidence in the last years. It is a common gastrointestinal cause for hospital admission. AP, in its severe forms, is a medical emergency with high mortality risk of complications and death and high public health costs. Toxic causes, as prolonged and heavy use of cannabis and cannabinoids compounds, have been identified among risk factors. Repetitive episodes of AP with tissue inflammation led to fibrosis and sclerosis, typical of CP. This last is a medical condition characterized by chronic pain, exocrine and endocrine pancreatic failure, a reduced patients' quality of life, and the need of continuous follow-up due to the risk of cancer. Cannabis has been proposed as an analgesic treatment for chronic pain, but strong data on CP are still lacking. In these different scenarios, the knowledge of cannabis effects on pancreas, both positive and negative, could add medical information to decide if its use is legalized or not, for therapeutic purposes. The concern about the use of cannabis, also for therapeutic purposes, is related to the variety of health side effects that range from cognitive and respiratory impairment to psychotic, anxiety episodes, addiction, car crashes, and crime's risk. Moreover, more evidences regarding the effectiveness of cannabinoids compounds and safety profile are needed to modify the current jurisdictions and regulate cannabis' commercialization (Figs. 1, 2, and Table 1).

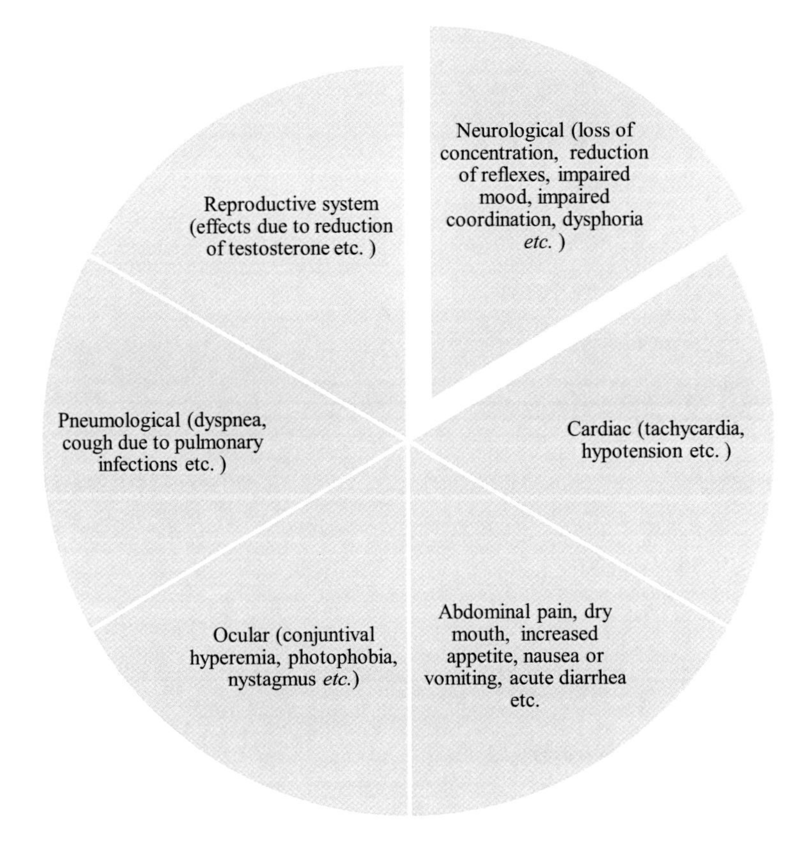

Fig. 1 Main clinical effects of cannabis use

Fig. 2 Report of cannabis-related acute pancreatitis

Mini-Dictionary of Terms

Cerulein: This is an oligopeptide that stimulates digestive secretions (as pancreatic ones). In experimental studies, it is used to induce acute pancreatitis in animals.

Endocrine function: This function consists in the secretion of hormones, enzymes, and other substances directly into interstitial spaces and then in blood rather than using a duct.

Exocrine function: This function consists in the secretion of hormones, enzymes, and other substances on an epithelial surface using a duct.

Pancreas *divisum*: It is a congenital anatomical anomaly in which pancreas has not a single normal pancreatic duct but the main pancreatic duct remains divided into two distinct dorsal and ventral ducts.

Table 1 Cannabinoids, cannabinoids receptors, and pancreas

	CB1 receptors	CB2 receptors
Site	Pancreas Immune system Brain Gastrointestinal tract Liver Bone and bone marrow Muscles Cardiovascular systems Lungs Reproductive organs	Pancreas Immune system Spleen Liver Bone and bone marrow Skin
Effects on pancreas	Fibrotic effects Modulation of pain	Antifibrotic effects Modulation of pain A possible role in "*insulin resistance*"
Site on pancreas	Area of pancreatic inflammation with macrophages and pancreatic stellate cells	Area of pancreatic inflammation islets of Langerhans
Ligands	Endogenous cannabinoids: anandamide and 2-arachidonoylglycerol Exogenous cannabinoids: THC, CBN, and cannabidiol (CBD)	Endogenous cannabinoids: anandamide and 2-arachidonoylglycerol Exogenous cannabinoids: THC, CBN, and cannabidiol (CBD)

Receptors: These are chemical structures, made up of protein, that receive and transduce signals in biological systems.

Key Facts

- Cannabis is an illegal drug responsible of different health effects, both positive and negative ones, opening different scenarios.
- The pancreatic tissue expresses both CB1 and CB2 receptors.
- The cannabis-active compounds, in particular THC, can modulate the pancreatic inflammation.
- The heavy and prolonged use of cannabis can induce AP with an important tissue damage.
- As regards therapeutic effects, cannabis can give relief from chronic pain, thus improving symptoms of CP.

Summary Points

- Cannabis is a widely and commonly used illicit drug.
- The regular or heavy use of cannabis can be responsible of AP and of severity of clinical manifestations.
- Data about cannabis dosage and the latency time between cannabis intake and AP development are still lacking.

- As regards CP, cannabis could play a role in the management of chronic pancreatic pain and in the reduction of pancreatic fibrosis.
- Many researches and well-conducted trials are needed to better identify cannabis' effects on acute and chronic pancreatitis.

References

Adams IB, Martin BR (1996) Cannabis: pharmacology and toxicology in animals and humans. Addiction 91:1585–1614

Andre CM, Hausman JF, Guerriero G (2016) Cannabis sativa: the plant of the thousand and one molecules. Front Plant Sci 7:19

Apte M, Pirola RC, Wilson JS (2015) Pancreatic stellate cell: physiologic role, role in fibrosis and cancer. Curr Opin Gastroenterol 31:416–423

Barkin JA, Nemeth Z, Saluja AK et al (2017) Cannabis-induced acute pancreatitis: a systematic review. Pancreas 46:1035–1038

Barlowe TS, Koliani-Pace JL, Smith KD et al (2019) Effects of medical cannabis on use of opioids and hospital visits by patients with painful chronic pancreatitis. Clin Gastroenterol Hepatol 17: 2608–2609.e1

Baron EP (2015) Comprehensive review of medicinal marijuana, cannabinoids, and therapeutic implications in medicine. Headache 55:885–916

Barry K (2018) Chronic pancreatitis: diagnosis and treatment. Am Fam Physician 97:385–393

Bermúdez-Silva FJ, Suárez J, Baixeras E et al (2008) Presence of functional cannabinoid receptors in human endocrine pancreas. Diabetologia 51:476–487

Beyer G, Habtezion A, Werner J et al (2020) Chronic pancreatitis. Lancet 396:499–512

Burstein S (2015) Cannabidiol (CBD) and its analogs: a review of their effects on inflammation. Bioorg Med Chem 23:1377–1385

Cerino P, Buonerba C, Cannazza G et al (2021) A review of hemp as food and nutritional supplement. Cannabis Cannabinoid Res 6:19–27

Chandy J, Hassan A, Sciarra M (2019) "HASH"ing out pancreatitis: the new increasingly common culprit. J Community Hosp Intern Med Perspect 9:360–361

Chatila AT, Bilal M, Guturu P (2019) Evaluation and management of acute pancreatitis. World J Clin Cases 7:1006–1020

Culetto A, Bournet B, Buscail L (2017) Clinical profile of cannabis-associated acute pancreatitis. Dig Liver Dis 49:1284–1285

De Vries M, Van Rijckevorsel DC, Vissers KC et al (2016) Single dose delta-9-tetrahydrocannabinol in chronic pancreatitis patients: analgesic efficacy, pharmacokinetics and tolerability. Br J Clin Pharmacol 81:525–537

Dembiński A, Warzecha Z, Ceranowicz P et al (2008) Dual, time-dependent deleterious and protective effect of anandamide on the course of cerulein-induced acute pancreatitis. Role of sensory nerves. Eur J Pharmacol 591:284–292

Echeverry C, Reyes-Parada M, Scorza C (2021) Constituents of Cannabis sativa. Adv Exp Med Biol 1297:1–9

Etemad B, Whitcomb DC (2001) Chronic pancreatitis: diagnosis, classification, and new genetic developments. Gastroenterology 120:682–707

Fatma H, Mouna B, Leila M et al (2013) Cannabis: a rare cause of acute pancreatitis. Clin Res Hepatol Gastroenterol 37:e24–e25

Goyal H, Singla U (2018) Cannabis and acute pancreatitis. Pancreas 47:e32–e33

Grant P, Gandhi P (2004) A case of cannabis-induced pancreatitis. JOP 5:41–43

Grotenhermen F (2003) Pharmacokinetics and pharmacodynamics of cannabinoids. Clin Pharmacokinet 42:327–360

Grotenhermen F, Müller-Vahl K (2012) The therapeutic potential of cannabis and cannabinoids. Dtsch Arztebl Int 109:495–501

Hill KP, Palastro MD, Johnson B et al (2017) Cannabis and pain: a clinical review. Cannabis Cannabinoid Res 2:96–104
Hourani W, Alexander SP (2018) Cannabinoid ligands, receptors and enzymes: pharmacological tools and therapeutic potential. Brain Neurosci Adv 2:2398212818783908
Huestis MA (2002) Cannabis (marijuana) – effects on human performance and behavior. Forensic Sci Rev 14:15–60
John J, Gandhi S, Nam D, Niakan L (2019) A case of cannabis-induced acute pancreatitis. Cureus 11:e5754
Laezza C, Pagano C, Navarra G et al (2020) The endocannabinoid system: a target for cancer treatment. Int J Mol Sci 21:747
Lafaye G, Karila L, Blecha L et al (2017) Cannabis, cannabinoids, and health. Dialogues Clin Neurosci 19:309–316. https://doi.org/10.31887/DCNS.2017.19.3/glafaye
Laura Nunez Herrero BC, Singh S, Deshpande V, Patel SH (2016) Acute pancreatitis secondary to marijuana consumption. https://www.primescholars.com/articles/acute-pancreatitis-secondary-to-marijuana-consumption-99006.html
Mackie K (2007) From active ingredients to the discovery of the targets: the cannabinoid receptors. Chem Biodivers 4:1693–1706
Mackie K (2008) Cannabinoid receptors: where they are and what they do. J Neuroendocrinol 20 (Suppl 1):10–14
Masamune A, Shimosegawa T (2009) Signal transduction in pancreatic stellate cells. J Gastroenterol 44:249–260
Masamune A, Watanabe T, Kikuta K et al (2009) Roles of pancreatic stellate cells in pancreatic inflammation and fibrosis. Clin Gastroenterol Hepatol 7:S48–S54
Matsuda K, Mikami Y, Takeda K et al (2005) The cannabinoid 1 receptor antagonist, AM251, prolongs the survival of rats with severe acute pancreatitis. Tohoku J Exp Med 207:99–107
Mederos MA, Reber HA, Girgis MD (2021) Acute pancreatitis: a review. JAMA 325:382–390
Michalski CW, Laukert T, Sauliunaite D et al (2007) Cannabinoids ameliorate pain and reduce disease pathology in cerulein-induced acute pancreatitis. Gastroenterology 132:1968–1978
Michalski CW, Maier M, Erkan M et al (2008) Cannabinoids reduce markers of inflammation and fibrosis in pancreatic stellate cells. PLoS One 3:e1701
Pacher P, Bátkai S, Kunos G (2006) The endocannabinoid system as an emerging target of pharmacotherapy. Pharmacol Rev 58:389–462
Pacher P, Kogan NM, Mechoulam R (2020) Beyond THC and endocannabinoids. Annu Rev Pharmacol Toxicol 60:637–659
Pagliari D, Saviano A, Brizi MG et al (2019) Cannabis-induced acute pancreatitis: a case report with comprehensive literature review. Eur Rev Med Pharmacol Sci 23:8625–8629
Pham A, Forsmark C (2018) Chronic pancreatitis: review and update of etiology, risk factors, and management. F1000Res 7:607
Pollio A (2016) The name of. Cannabis Cannabinoid Res 1:234–238
Romero-Sandoval EA, Kolano AL, Alvarado-Vázquez PA (2017) Cannabis and cannabinoids for chronic pain. Curr Rheumatol Rep 19:67
Simons-Linares CR, Barkin JA, Wang Y et al (2018) Is there an effect of cannabis consumption on acute pancreatitis? Dig Dis Sci 63:2786–2791
Singh VK, Yadav D, Garg PK (2019) Diagnosis and management of chronic pancreatitis: a review. JAMA 322:2422–2434
Sly M, Clark K, Karaghossian G et al (2021) Cannabis-induced pancreatitis in a young adult male. J Investig Med High Impact Case Rep 9:23247096211035238
Yang X, Yao L, Fu X et al (2020) Experimental acute pancreatitis models: history, current status, and role in translational research. Front Physiol 11:614591
Yang B, Davis JM, Gomez TH et al (2021) Characteristic pancreatic and splenic immune cell infiltration patterns in mouse acute pancreatitis. Cell Biosci 11:28

Cannabidiol (CBD) and Its Biological Toxicity

63

Modelling Preclinical Studies

M. M. Dziwenka and R. W. Coppock

Contents

Introduction 1354
Applicable Acts, Regulations, and Research Standards 1355
Hemp Production Act 1355
USFDA Botanical Drug Development Guidance for Industry 1355
New Dietary Ingredient Notification (NDIN) 1355
European Regulations 1356
Toxicologic Evaluation 1356
Research Standards 1356
In Vitro Toxicology 1356
In Vivo Toxicology 1357
Available Forms of CBD 1360
Standards for Enabling Applications to Humans 1361
Potential Future Direction with Preclinical Studies 1363
Applications to Other Areas of Addiction 1363
Key Points 1364
Dictionary of Terms 1364
Summary Points 1365
References 1365

Abstract

There is a significant growing interest in the consumption of CBD for its potential health benefits in both humans and companion animals. The regulatory framework for CBD and CBD-containing products around the world is complex and ever changing as is the evaluation of the safety of these products. A broad summary of considerations for the selection and design of both in vitro and

M. M. Dziwenka (✉)
Toxalta Consulting Ltd., Vegreville, AB, Canada

R. W. Coppock
DVM, Toxicologist and Associates Ltd., Vegreville, AB, Canada
e-mail: r.coppock@toxicologist.ca

V. B. Patel, V. R. Preedy (eds.), *Handbook of Substance Misuse and Addictions*,
https://doi.org/10.1007/978-3-030-92392-1_69

in vivo toxicity studies is reviewed. The importance of considering the reproducibility of the results from preclinical in vitro and in vivo toxicology studies and the translation of those results to be applicable to humans is introduced. This chapter also includes a brief overview of current preclinical research with CBD and CBD-containing extracts and the importance of thoroughly characterizing the test material prior to conducting any studies. A discussion of information gaps in the knowledge of CBD and CBD-containing products is included as well as recommendations for future studies.

Keywords

Toxicology · CBD · Cannabidiol · Regulations · Preclinical studies · Hemp

Abbreviations

ARRIVE	Animal Research: Reporting of In Vivo Experiments
CBD	Cannabidiol
DFRs	Acute dose range finding studies
DNA	Deoxyribonucleic acid
EMA	European Medicines Agency
EU	European Union
GLPs	Good laboratory practices
GRAS	Generally regarded as safe
NDIN	New dietary ingredient notification
NOAEL	No observed adverse effect level
OECD	Organization for Economic Co-operation and Development
THC	Δ9-tetrahydrocannabinol
UGTs	UDP-glucuronosyltransferases
US	United States of America
USFDA	United States Food and Drug administration

Introduction

There is increasing interest in the general health benefits from hemp (*Cannabis sativa*) phytochemicals that lack psychotropic activity (Andre et al. 2016; Britch et al. 2021; Martin et al. 2021). The interest in CBD products rapidly increased after the US Congress passed the 2018 Farm Bill (US Government 2018). Since then, CBD-rich extracts have received considerable praise in the scientific literature for improving health. CBD has been approved as a drug (Epidiolex® (Greenwich Biosciences, Inc., Carlsbad, CA)) by the US Food and Drug Administration (USFDA) and the European Union (EU). The indication for Epidiolex® is the treatment of seizures associated with Lennox-Gastaut and Dravet syndromes (Abu-Sawwa et al. 2020). With approval of purified CBD as a drug, the chemistry of the phytochemicals in hemp are being more clearly defined. Crude hemp extracts, as with other extracts of phytochemicals, vary in composition due to differing manufacturing methods and plant strain variation (Pellati et al. 2018; Dziwenka et al. 2020; Nuapia et al. 2020). Toxicity testing may be required because of differing phytochemical composition and product formulation (Dziwenka et al. 2020). The type of regulatory testing for CBD will vary depending on the intended market and if efficacy claims are made for the product.

Applicable Acts, Regulations, and Research Standards

Hemp Production Act

Congress, in response to pressures to exclude CBD and other nonpsychotropic hemp phytochemicals from the Controlled Substance Act, passed the Hemp Production Act (US Government 2018). This act, also known as the 2018 Farm Bill, included changes to the production and marketing of hemp and derivatives of cannabis that have less than 0.3% delta9-tetrahydrocannabinol (THC). This act also removed hemp products with <0.3% THC from the Controlled Substances Act. The Hemp Farm Act did not change the responsibility of the USFDA in protecting the US public from detrimental health effects of the nonpsychotropic hemp phytochemicals. The general position of the USFDA is drug regulations are applied when a CBD product is claimed to have therapeutic benefit because it is classified as a drug.

USFDA Botanical Drug Development Guidance for Industry

The USFDA guidance documents do not establish legally enforceable responsibilities. Instead, they describe FDA's current thinking and should be viewed as recommendations. The USFDA requires a pure CBD product with medical claims to be tested as a drug. The USFDA, in 2016, published the Botanical Drug Development Guidance for Industry (USFDA 2016). This document, considering the uniqueness of botanical drugs, outlines the current thinking of the USFDA on appropriate development plans for botanical drugs and these differ from nonbotanical drugs and synthetic mimics and forms of botanical drugs. The USFDA also published a draft document "Cannabis and cannabis-derived compounds. Quality considerations for clinical research - Guidance for industry" (USFDA 2020).

New Dietary Ingredient Notification (NDIN)

USFDA requires that a NDIN must be submitted for a dietary ingredient which was not previously marketed in the USA before October 15, 1994, as defined in the Dietary Supplement Health & Education Act or DSHEA (USFDA 2021). A database of submitted 75-day Premarket Notifications (https://www.fda.gov/food/new-dietary-ingredients-ndi-notification-process/submitted-75-day-premarket-notifications-new-dietary-ingredients) are available on FDA's website and CBD and full spectrum hemp extracts can be found on this list; however, at this time, all manufacturers of CBD-containing extracts have received letters from FDA stating that their products cannot be used in dietary supplements.

European Regulations

In December of 2020, the European Monitoring Centre for Drugs and Drug Addiction published "Low-THC cannabis products in Europe" in which the regulation of CBD products is described (EMCDDA 2020). They outline the very complex regulatory environment in Europe which often varies by country. The European Commission has stated that cannabinoids derived from the hemp plant (*Cannabis sativa L.*) are considered novel foods. The Novel Food Regulation (EU) No. 2015/2283 entered into force on January 1, 2018, and an ingredient is considered a novel food if it had not already been sold as an ingredient before May 15, 1997.

Toxicologic Evaluation

Regulatory toxicology is focused on protecting the health of humans and other animals. The objectives of preclinical in vitro and in vivo testing of hemp phytochemicals for toxicological effects are to establish their safety in humans and domestic animals. These studies do not establish beneficial health effects. Preclinical studies generally are a series of studies that start with in vitro studies to establish their safety in cell culture and bacterial systems and then progress to animal studies.

Research Standards

Toxicology studies, in particular those used to evaluate safety, should comply with the applicable government-regulated research standards and these requirements vary between countries. Compliance with guidelines such as OECD ensure that the studies are well designed and conducting the studies in compliance with GLPs ensures that they are well conducted and repeatable. Examples of some applicable standards are given in Table 1.

In Vitro Toxicology

Testing for Genotoxicity and Mutagenicity

Genotoxicity studies are conducted to evaluate the potential for substances to induce genetic alterations in somatic cells, germ cells, or both, by a variety of mechanisms. The OECD Guidance Document No. 238 notes that genetic alterations manifest long after the exposure and those genetic alterations may lead to cancer or degenerative diseases (OECD 2016). A battery of tests is generally recommended when evaluating

Table 1 Government-defined research standards

Research standard	References
OECD Guidelines for Testing of Chemicals [Section 4 (Test No. 408): Health Effects, Repeated Dose 90-Day Oral Toxicity Study in Rodents (1998)]	OECD (2018)
OECD (1999). OECD Series on Principles of Good Laboratory Practice (GLP) and Compliance Monitoring	OECD (1998)
US Food and Drug Administration (FDA) (2007). US FDA Toxicological Principles for the Safety Assessment of Food Ingredients (Redbook 2000, Revised 2007 IV.C. 4. a. Subchronic Toxicity Studies with Rodents [2003])	USFDA (2007)
US Food and Drug Administration (USFDA) (2018). US FDA Good Laboratory Practices	USFDA (2018)
Guide for the Care and Use of Laboratory Animals (8th ed.). Washington, DC: National Academy Press.	NRC (2011)

a substance for the potential to cause damage to DNA (EFSA 2017; OECD 2016; Kirkland et al. 2011). Genetic toxicology studies are conducted to detect two types of DNA damage; the direct and irreversible damage that can be transmitted to the next generation of cells, often called mutagenicity and the early, often reversible DNA damage (OECD 2016). The use of a battery of genotoxicity tests rather than a single test has been widely accepted due to the range of mechanisms that can be involved in causing damage to DNA (Hayes and Kruger 2014; OECD 2016; EFSA 2017; EMA 2012). There are both in vitro and in vivo tests for genotoxicity and as discussed earlier, a combination of tests is usually recommended. Hundreds of tests have been developed that can be used to identify the potential of a substance to cause DNA damage but only a small number of these are now recommended for routine use (Hayes and Kruger 2014). A summary of a few of these studies based on the OECD guidelines can be found in Table 2.

In Vivo Toxicology

Testing in Animals

Animal toxicity studies are designed to identify and characterize toxic effects of the test substance that would occur during use by the target species (Monticello et al. 2017). The purpose of toxicity testing CBD preparations in animal is to determine the dose response curve for toxicity, identify specific toxicity for the CBD preparation, and estimate a safe intake level (Marx et al. 2018). Important decisions in study design are appropriate government-specified standards, selection of the species, strain, sex, and age the of test animals as well as the parameters that are used to assess toxicity (Table 3). Specific information on drug metabolism and other uniqueness when selecting the species and strain of the animals must be considered (Monticello et al. 2017). Animal testing must include the route of exposure (oral, dermal, and inhalation) as the intended route of administration for the marketed product. All studies in animals should comply with regulatory requirements for animal studies in the countries where the product is intended to be marketed.

Table 2 Summary of genotoxicity studies

Tests for gene mutations	
Bacterial reverse mutation assay	This is often referred to as the "Ames test" and is used to identify base-pair substitutions and frameshift mutations which result from insertions or deletions (OECD 2016). The study is conducted in multiple strains of *Salmonella typhimurium* and often *Escherichia coli* as well
In vitro mammalian cell gene mutation tests (with the *Hprt* or *xprt* genes)	This test is used to evaluate if the test material can induce gene mutations at the hypoxanthine-guanine phosphoribosyl transferase (*Hprt*) or xanthine-guanine phosphoribosyl transferase (*xprt*) reporter gene and can be performed using a number of well-established cell lines or mammalian peripheral lymphocytes (OECD 2016). As per the OECD (2016) Guideline, the most common cell lines used are the CHO, CHL, and V79 Chinese Hamster cell lines, the L5178 mouse lymphoma cells as well as the TK6 human lymphoblastoid cells
In vitro mammalian cell gene mutation tests (with the thymidine kinase gene)	This test is used to evaluate if the test material can induce gene mutations at the thymidine kinase (*TK*) reporter gene (OECD 2016). Specific TK heterozygous cell lines are used for this test
Tests for Chromosomal Abnormalities The OECD (2016) Guideline states that there are two endpoints that can be used to determine if a test material causes chromosomal damage and/or aneuploidy, these being chromosomal aberrations and micronuclei.	
In vitro mammalian chromosomal aberration test	This test is used to determine if the test material can induce structural chromosomal aberrations in established cell lines or primary cell cultures
In vitro mammalian cell micronucleus test	The induction of chromosomal breaks and aneuploidy by the test material in primary human or other mammalian peripheral blood lymphocytes or established cell lines by the test material is identified with this test
In vivo mammalian erythrocyte micronucleus test	This study is usually conducted in laboratory rodents and is used to identify if a test material can induce micronuclei in bone marrow erythroblasts or peripheral blood
In vivo mammalian bone marrow chromosomal aberration test	This study is also usually conducted in laboratory rodents. It is used to determine if the test material can induce structural chromosomal aberrations in the cells of the bone marrow
Tests for primary DNA damage	
In vivo mammalian alkaline comet assay	This assay evaluates the potential for a test material to induce primary DNA damage and can detect single- and double-strand breaks

Acute Dose Range Finding Studies (DFRs)

DFRs generally are the first stage in assessing the acute toxicity in female and male laboratory animals. The objectives of DRFs are to identify organ toxicity, clinical signs of intoxication, and minimally invasive parameters that can be used to identify intoxication in subsequent studies. The parameters in DFRs generally include feed consumption, body weights, clinical assessment, clinical chemistry, hematology, and anatomical pathology. The DRFs can be a single escalating dose study or a multiple dose study with daily dosing for a specified time. The stairstep design is an

Table 3 In vivo animal studies parameters

Study/Parameter	Description
Regulations	Government-regulated study design standards
Test article	Chemical description, identification of contaminations, preparation for dosing, and route of administration
Selection of test animal	Recognized commonly used species, strain, sex, and age
Clinical assessment and neurobehavior	Physical examination, behavior, locomotion, coordination, motor activity, and functional observation battery in an open field
Ophthalmology	Detection of anatomical changes in the eyes (veterinary ophthalmologist)
Food consumption	Effect on appetite
Body weight	Effect of test substance on body weight and weight gains
Endocrinology	Minimally should include thyroid function parameters, serum glucose levels used as an indirect test for pancreatic islet cell function
Reproduction	Follows regulated protocols for developmental toxicity, reproductive function, and multigenerational studies
Hematology	Effect on red and white blood cells and rapidly multiplying cells in the erythroid and myeloid and lymphocyte series and production of platelets
Clinical chemistry	Blood clotting and damage to organ systems and homeostasis
Macroscopic pathology and organ weights	Visual and texture examination of all organs. Organ weights should be normalized to body weight or brain weight
Histopathology	Microscopic observations at the tissue, cellular, and subcellular levels, special staining interpretation (veterinary pathologist)
Urinalysis	Kidney function and pathology
Skin irritation studies	Products for topical application
Unscheduled deaths	Are deaths test substance related, require complete pathology

increasing dose level sequence administering a single dose at each escalating step with a 48-h observational interval between each dose. Fourteen-day dosing regimens are used in DFRs for CBD preparations.

Subchronic and Chronic Studies

The purpose of subchronic and chronic studies is to identify the longer-term toxicity in an animal model using specified parameters (Table 2). These studies should include a 28-day recovery period and an example of these studies have been published by Marx et al. (2018) and Dziwenka et al. (2020). The 28-day recovery period provides key information on the reversibility of toxic effects observed in the subchronic and chronic studies. Data from the subchronic and chronic studies can be used to calculate the no observed adverse effect level (NOAEL) (Dziwenka et al. 2020). Dose regimens for subchronic and chronic studies are selected from the range finding studies.

Pharmacological and Pharmacokinetic Studies

Biochemical studies in laboratory animals and cell cultures identify the upregulation, downregulation, and inhibition of drug metabolizing enzymes. Output from these studies can be used to predict unwanted and adverse interactions with synthetic and phytomedications and supplements. The biotransformation pathways of CBD and metabolites of CBD can also be identified. Biochemical studies can also be used to identify specific receptors and provide insight for desirable effects, e.g., changes in the inflammatory index. Biochemical studies also show the effects of CBD on important enzymes in biotransformation pathways of both prescription and nonprescription drugs (Abu-Sawwa et al. 2020). The best predictors of potential adverse effects must receive consideration (Monticello et al. 2017).

Developmental Studies

Developmental studies are used to determine teratology and effects on embryonic survival and live births. Example of the fetal effects observed include early embryonic mortalities, cleft palate, exencephalies, limb and tail malformations, and the numbers of dead and live pups delivered (Parasuraman 2011). Developmental studies provide information on the safety of products used during pregnancy.

Multigenerational Studies

Multigenerational studies are used to assess the toxic effects of the test substance on fertility, stillborn, and parameters that evaluate the health of F1 generation.

Available Forms of CBD

CBD is available to both the general public and medical professionals in many products and in many forms. The expected route of exposure for the product in humans must be taken into consideration when designing a preclinical safety study. While products which are taken topically or via inhalation are available, the focus of this chapter will be on orally consumed products.

There are a variety of orally consumed CBD-containing products which need to be differentiated when evaluating safety and designing preclinical studies. One highly purified form of CBD, Epidiolex®, has been approved as a drug. Other oral products available on the market which have been the subject of much discussion are the CBD-containing extracts prepared from *Cannabis sativa* L. containing less than 0.3% THC by dry weight, also referred to as industrial hemp. Marinotti and Sarill (2020) discuss the differentiation of full-spectrum hemp extracts from CBD isolates and the differences with respect to safety. They stated that the differences between hemp extracts, distillates, and purified or isolates are informally defined as shown in Table 4.

CBD is the most abundant nonpsychotropic cannabinoid found in CBD-rich extracts; however, it is not the only phytochemical present. It is important to consider the product being evaluated for safety – is it purified CBD or is it a CBD-containing hemp extract? As noted by Andre et al. (2016) and may others, hundreds of phytochemicals have been described in hemp products and studies continue on their bioactivity. This variety of phytochemicals can impact the assessment of safety if the test material used in the studies is not well characterized. Given natural

Table 4 Differences in CBD content of various products produced from industrial hemp (modified from Marinotti and Sarill 2020)

Product	CBD content (%)
Hemp extract	10–25
Distillate	25–80
Purified or isolate	>95

[a]Modified from Marinotti and Sarill (2020)

variation in botanical extracts, it is important to ensure that specifications are set for the product and that the manufacturing process ensures consistency between production lots. This assurance of consistency allows for the conclusions of the safety studies to be applied to all production lots of the products.

Recently, there has been a significant increase in the public's interest in products containing CBD and a corresponding increase in studies that can be found in the published literature regarding the safety of CBD in both humans and companion animals as well as laboratory species. The preclinical studies used to gain this information must be well designed and take differences in metabolism of CBD between the animal species selected and humans into consideration.

Standards for Enabling Applications to Humans

The translational value of data from animal studies to humans has been questioned and work has been done to improve the reproducibility (Percie du Sert et al. 2018, 2020). The Animal Research: Reporting of In Vivo Experiments (ARRIVE) guidelines, as stated on the website, provide a checklist of recommendations when reporting animal-based research with the intention of maximizing the quality and reliability of published research by ensuring the publications have enough detail to add to the scientific knowledge base. These guidelines were developed in 2010 and since then others, such as (Freedman et al. 2015), discuss the economical impacts of low reproducibility rates in research. Leenaars et al. (2019) conducted a review to answer the following question: "What is the observed range of the animal-to-human translation success (and failure) rates within the currently available empirical evidence?". They found that the translational success varied widely and concluded that translational success may be unpredictable, meaning that it may not be clear initially if the results of an animal study will contribute to the body of translational knowledge. Percie du Sert et al. (2020) note that adherence to the ARRIVE guidelines has been inconsistent and that the expected improvements in the quality of animal research publications have not been realized. The guidelines were recently updated to assist in the usability in research. Not only is the design of the studies and careful selection of the animal models used important, the clear and transparent reporting of the research method and findings are essential to reproducibility as noted by Percie du Sert et al. (2018, 2020). Clear disclosure of the CBD product being tested needs to be included in the study being reported.

Although these challenges exist, conducting studies in animals are still required. As noted by Brubaker and Lauffenburger (2020), "the experiments required to understand disease biology to the degree required for ascertaining effective treatments cannot be performed in human subjects, translation from animals to humans is necessary." While this statement is not specifically addressing safety evaluations, it none the less applies.

The biotransformation pathways of CBD and metabolites of CBD can also be identified using studies conducted in laboratory animals. In addition, biochemical studies can also be used to identify specific receptors and provide insight for desirable effects, e.g., changes in the inflammatory index. When designing and evaluating any preclinical study, the differences between species with respect to differences in metabolism must be understood and considered.

Cerne (2020) conducted a review to assess what information is available on the acute and chronic toxicological effects of CBD. Much of the information reviewed is from studies with Epidiolex®. Epidiolex® is a highly purified form of CBD approved by the US Food and Drug Administration (USFDA) and the European Medicines Agency (EMA) as a treatment for seizures associated with Lennox-Gastaut and Dravet syndrome, in patients 2 years of age or older (Cerne 2020). The authors, and others, conclude that although multiple studies have been conducted, there are significant gaps in the data which require additional preclinical and clinical studies to be conducted inclusive of the mechanism of action (Abu-Sawwa et al. 2020).

The increasing interest in the use of CBD and CBD-containing products in companion animals has led to an increase in information available on the pharmacokinetics and safety of CBD in animal species other than the laboratory rat or mouse. There are a number of recent pharmacokinetic studies conducted with CBD-containing products in laboratory beagles by Bartner et al. (2018), Chicoine et al. (2020), Deabold et al. (2019), Gamble et al. (2018), and Vaughn et al. (2020, 2021). Gamble et al. (2018) and Verrico et al. (2020) conducted safety and/or efficacy studies of CBD-containing materials in dogs with osteoarthritis and Kulpa et al. (2021) conducted a study to evaluate the safety of escalating doses of three cannabinoid oils in healthy cats. Vaughn et al. 2020 conducted a study to evaluate the safety of escalating cannabinoid doses in dogs and Ryan et al. (2021) has reported on the pharmacokinetics and tolerance of horses to CBD.

It is important to review all of these publications, as well as the other available preclinical safety publications available regarding CBD and CBD-containing products, with a clear picture of the test material used in each one. As stated by Cogan (2020), the concept of an entourage effect with cannabis was first expressed in 1998. The definition of an entourage effect is still not clearly outlined, and Cogan (2020) discusses that the proposed interactions of THC and CBD are one of the most common entourage effects discussed in the literature. Regardless of the possibility of interactions between phytochemicals, including CBD, in the test material occurring or not, thorough characterization of the test material is important in order to fully interpret the results of any preclinical studies.

Potential Future Direction with Preclinical Studies

Information on CBD and CBD-containing extracts is currently changing at a phenomenal rate. New studies and reviews are continuously being published, however there is still a knowledge gap regarding the safety of CBD. Cerne (2020) summarizes a list of recommended studies that are needed to complete the safety profile of CBD which include suggested preclinical studies to evaluate the toxicity of the CBD metabolite 7-COOH-cannabidiol. Included in the list of recommended studies for both 7-COOH-cannabidiol and CBD are reproductive and developmental studies, studies in juvenile animals, and longer-term carcinogenicity studies. Concerns have also been raised regarding the potential for CBD consumption to have an adverse effect on the liver and male reproductive tract (Abu-Sawwa et al. 2020; Carvalho et al. 2020; Dziwenka et al. 2020). Concerns have been raised regarding the possibility of liver toxicity following the ingestion of CBD and the potential for CBD-drug interactions (Watkins et al. 2021; Ewing et al. 2019). Additional preclinical studies in these areas will provide valuable safety information.

As discussed earlier, and also recommended by Cerne (2020), research evaluating the potential for CBD-drug interactions is an important area for future preclinical study. Vazquez et al. (2020) state that a drug-drug interaction is where one drug/compound alters the clinical effect of another but that the interactions are not necessarily adverse. The authors discuss the effects of cannabinoids on CYP450 isoenzymes, glucuronosyltransferases (UGT's) as well as efflux transporters and conclude that information on interactions between cannabinoids and other medications is limited. Much of the information in the literature is regarding potential interactions between CBD and antiseizure medications (Abu-Sawwa et al. 2020; Dos Santos et al. 2021; Gottschling et al. 2020; Patsalos et al. 2020; Schaiquevich et al. 2020; VanLandingham et al. 2020). Others, such as Devinsky et al. (2014) and Stout and Cimino (2014), have reviewed the effect of CBD on CYP450 isoforms. Preclinical studies utilized to gather additional information on the potential effects of CBD on the metabolism of other compounds need to consider differences in metabolism between animal species and humans.

The design, selection of the animal model, detailed characterization of the CBD-containing test material, conduct, and transparency in the reporting of the findings of any preclinical studies are all critical aspects to ensure that good quality information is available on the metabolism and safety of CBD.

Applications to Other Areas of Addiction

There is increasing evidence, especially in controlled laboratory animal studies, that CBD is beneficial as an adjunct therapeutic and as a primary therapeutic in the treatment of substance abuse disorders. In narcotic substance use disorder, there is evidence in laboratory animals that CBD has inhibitory effects on opioid reward–

associated learning and memories, cue-induced heroin-seeking, and opioid withdrawal. CBD protects the liver from cocaine and ethyl alcohol induced liver hepatotoxicity (Galaj et al. 2019; Galaj and Xi 2020). CBD has been shown to reduce self-administration of ethyl alcohol in rats (Maccioni et al. 2021). Studies in laboratory animals show CBD is beneficial to prevent liver injury in alcohol addiction (Jiang et al. 2021). In nicotine-dependent rats, treatment with CBD alleviated exacerbated signs of somatic withdrawal and increased sensitivity to pain (Smith et al. 2021). Daldegan-Bueno et al. (2021) found preclinical evidence that CBD is beneficial in treating amphetamine addiction disorders. For CBD to have a claim for substance use disorders, it will require approval as a drug by the regulatory agencies in the majority of countries.

Key Points

- Cannabidiol (CBD) is extracted from hemp (*Cannabis sativa*).
- CBD does not have psychotropic effects in humans and animals.
- Growing consumption of CBD-rich extracts for its potential health benefits in both humans and companion animals.
- CBD is regulated for consumer protection by the USFDA and European Union.
- When health claims are made for CBD, the regulatory agencies regulate CBD as a drug and the health claim has to be scientifically proven.

Dictionary of Terms

Acute toxicity study – is a toxicology study to observe substances administered in single or multiple doses for short term, generally 24–72 h.

Biotransformation – is the chemical changes to CBD by enzymes and other bodily chemical process.

Cannabidiol – is one of 85 cannabinoids identified within the Cannabis plant that has a molecular weight of 314.5.

Crude hemp extracts – are the crude product after extraction with a solvent before refinement. Different solvents can be used that enhance the content of CBD in the crude extract.

CYP450 enzymes – a group of enzymes that generally catalyze chemical metabolism of drugs and toxic substances. These enzymes can genetically be up- and downregulated by increasing or decreasing their formation from protein precursors. These enzymes can also be inhibited by drugs and toxic substances.

Delta9-tetrahydrocannabinol – is the primary psychotropic chemical in hemp.

Dietary ingredient – is a substance that increases the dietary intake and can be a concentrated form of a substance.

Genotoxicity – is the study of toxic substances on the fidelity of a genome.

In vitro – in glass.

In vivo – in life.

Nonpsychotropic – does not affect behavior, mood, perception, or thoughts.

Pharmacokinetic study – determines the absorption, distribution, and elimination of the test substance.

Pharmacological study – is a study or series of studies to determine the actions of a substance and its interactions with biochemical and physiological processes.

Subchronic study – is a toxicology study using a daily dosing schedule for a period of 28 days. These studies can include a recovery period during which the test substance is not administered.

Teratology – is the study to determine the effects of chemical and physical agents on prenatal development.

Toxicology – is the study of the adverse biological effects of a chemical or physical agent.

Summary Points

- US Congress passed legislation legalizing hemp that contain <0.3% THC exempting hem products from the Controlled Substance Act.
- The USFDA has responsibility of ensuring that CBD is not harmful and there is scientific data to support health claims made for CDB.
- CBD is a phytochemical extracted from hemp and is a licensed drug (Epidiolex®) for Lennox- Gastaut and Dravet syndromes.
- CBD products are new dietary ingredients that cannot be used in formulating dietary supplements.
- The European Commission considers the cannabinoids as novel foods.
- Hemp extracts containing <0.3% THC must be safe for ingestion and generally require toxicity testing.
- Toxicology studies to determine the safety of non-THC hemp extracts should follow the OECD and/or USFDA Guidelines.

References

Abu-Sawwa R, Scutt B, Park Y (2020) Emerging use of Epidiolex (cannabidiol) in epilepsy. J Pediatr Pharmacol Ther 25(6):485–499. https://doi.org/10.5863/1551-6776-25.6.485

Andre CM, Hausman JF, Guerriero G (2016) *Cannabis sativa:* the plant of the thousand and one molecules. Front Plant Sci 7:19. https://doi.org/10.3389/fpls.2016.00019

Bartner LR, McGrath S, Rao S, Hyatt LK, Wittenburg LA (2018) Pharmacokinetics of cannabidiol administered by 3 delivery methods at 2 different dosages to healthy dogs. Can J Vet Res 82(3): 178–183

Britch SC, Babalonis S, Walsh SL (2021) Cannabidiol: pharmacology and therapeutic targets. Psychopharmacology 238(1):9–28. https://doi.org/10.1007/s00213-020-05712-8

Brubaker DK, Lauffenburger DA (2020) Translating preclinical models to humans. Science 367 (6479):742–743. https://doi.org/10.1126/science.aay8086

Carvalho RK, Andersen ML, Mazaro-Costa R (2020) The effects of cannabidiol on male reproductive system: a literature review. J Appl Toxicol 40(1):132–150. https://doi.org/10.1002/jat.3831

Cerne K (2020) Toxicological properties of delta9-tetrahydrocannabinol and cannabidiol. Arh Hig Rada Toksikol 71(1):1–11. https://doi.org/10.2478/aiht-2020-71-3301

Chicoine A, Illing K, Vuong S, Pinto KR, Alcorn J, Cosford K (2020) Pharmacokinetic and safety evaluation of various oral doses of a novel 1:20 TH:CBD cannabis herbal extract in dogs. Front Vet Sci 7:583404. https://doi.org/10.3389/fvets.2020.583404

Cogan PS (2020) The 'entourage effect' or 'Hodge-podge hashish': the questionable rebranding, marketing, and expectations of cannabis polypharmacy. Expert Rev Clin Pharmacol 13(8):835–845. https://doi.org/10.1080/17512433.2020.1721281

Daldegan-Bueno D, Maia LO, Glass M, Jutras-Aswad D, Fischer B (2021) Coexposure of cannabinoids with amphetamines and biological, behavioural and health outcomes: A scoping review of animal and human studies. Psychopharmacology (Berl). https://doi.org/10.1007/s00213-021-05960-2

Deabold KA, Schwark WS, Wolf L, Wakshlag JJ (2019) Single-dose pharmacokinetics and preliminary safety assessment with use of CBD-rich hemp nutraceutical in healthy dogs and cats. Animals (Basel) 9(10). https://doi.org/10.3390/ani9100832

Devinsky O, Cilio MR, Cross H, Fernandez-Ruiz J, French J, Hill C, . . . Friedman D (2014) Cannabidiol: pharmacology and potential therapeutic role in epilepsy and other neuropsychiatric disorders. Epilepsia 55(6):791–802. https://doi.org/10.1111/epi.12631

Dos Santos RG, Hallak JEC, Crippa JAS (2021) Neuropharmacological effects of the main phytocannabinoids: a narrative review. Adv Exp Med Biol 1264:29–45. https://doi.org/10.1007/978-3-030-57369-0_3

Dziwenka M, Coppock RW, McCorkle A, Palumbo E, Ranmirez C (2020) Safety assessment of a hemp extract using genotoxicity and oral repeat-dose toxicity studies in Sprague-Dawley rats. Toxicol Rep 7:376–385

EFSA Scientific Committee (2017) Clarification of some aspects related to genotoxicity assessment. EFSA J 15(12):e05113. https://doi.org/10.2903/j.efsa.2017.5113

EMA (2012) ICH guideline S2 (R1) on genotoxicity testing and data interpretation for pharmaceuticals intended for human use. Step 5. (EMA/CHMP/ICH/126642/2008). European Medicines Agency, London. https://www.ema.europa.eu/en/ich-s2-r1-genotoxicity-testing-data-interpretation-pharmaceuticals-intended-human-use. Accessed 23 Sept 2021

EMCDDA (2020) Low-THC cannabis products in Europe. European Monitoring Centre for Drugs and Drug Addiction, Lisbon. Retrieved from https://www.emcdda.europa.eu/publications/ad-hoc-publication/low-thc-cannabis-products-europe_en

Ewing LE, McGill MR, Yee EU, Quick CM, Skinner CM, Kennon-McGill S,. . . Koturbash I (2019) Paradoxical patterns of sinusoidal obstruction syndrome-like liver injury in aged female CD-1 mice triggered by cannabidiol-rich cannabis extract and acetaminophen co-administration. Molecules 24(12). https://doi.org/10.3390/molecules24122256

Freedman LP, Cockburn IM, Simcoe TS (2015) The economics of reproducibility in preclinical research. PLoS Biol 13(6):e1002165. https://doi.org/10.1371/journal.pbio.1002165

Galaj E, Xi ZX (2020) Possible receptor mechanisms underlying cannabidiol effects on addictive-like behaviors in experimental animals. Int J Mol Sci 22(1). https://doi.org/10.3390/ijms22010134

Galaj E, Bi GH, Yang HJ, Xi ZX (2019) Cannabidiol attenuates the rewarding effects of cocaine in rats by cb2, 5-th1a and trpv1 receptor mechanisms. Neuropharmacology:107740. https://doi.org/10.1016/j.neuropharm.2019.107740

Gamble LJ, Boesch JM, Frye CW, Schwark WS, Mann S, Wolfe L,. . . Wakshlag JJ (2018) Pharmacokinetics, safety, and clinical efficacy of cannabidiol treatment in osteoarthritic dog. Front Vet Sci 5:165

Gottschling S, Ayonrinde O, Bhaskar A, Blockman M, D'Agnone O, Schecter D, . . . Cyr C (2020) Safety considerations in cannabinoid-based medicine. Int J Gen Med 13:1317–1333. https://doi.org/10.2147/IJGM.S275049

Hayes AW, Kruger CL (eds) (2014) Hayes' principles and methods of toxicology, vol 1, 6th edn. CRC Press, Boca Raton

Jiang X, Gu Y, Huang Y, Zhou Y, Pang N, Luo J,. . . Yang L (2021) CBD alleviates liver injuries in alcoholics with high-fat high-cholesterol diet through regulating NLRP3 inflammasome-pyroptosis pathway. Front Pharmacol 12:724747. https://doi.org/10.3389/fphar.2021.724747

Kirkland D, Reeve L, Gatehouse D, Vanparys P (2011) A core in vitro genotoxicity battery comprising the Ames test plus the in vitro micronucleus test is sufficient to detect rodent carcinogens and in vivo genotoxins. Mutat Res 721(1):27–73. https://doi.org/10.1016/j.mrgentox.2010.12.015

Kulpa JE, Paulionis LJ, Eglit GM, Vaughn DM (2021) Safety and tolerability of escalating cannabinoid doses in healthy cats. J Feline Med Surg:1098612X211004215. https://doi.org/10.1177/1098612X211004215

Leenaars CHC, Kouwenaar C, Stafleu FR, Bleich A, Ritskes-Hoitinga M, De Vries RBM, Meijboom FLB (2019) Animal to human translation: a systematic scoping review of reported concordance rates. J Transl Med 17(1):223. https://doi.org/10.1186/s12967-019-1976-2

Maccioni P, Bratzu J, Carai MAM, Colombo G, Gessa GL (2021) Reducing effect of cannabidiol on alcohol self-administration in Sardinian alcohol-preferring rats. Cannabis Cannabinoid Res. https://doi.org/10.1089/can.2020.0132

Marinotti O, Sarill M (2020) Differentiating full-spectrum hemp extracts from CBD isolates: implications for policy, safety and science. J Diet Suppl 17(5):517–526. https://doi.org/10.1080/19390211.2020.1776806

Martin LJ, Banister SD, Bowen MT (2021) Understanding the complex pharmacology of cannabidiol: mounting evidence suggests a common binding site with cholesterol. Pharmacol Res 166:105508. https://doi.org/10.1016/j.phrs.2021.105508

Marx TK, Reddeman R, Clewell AE, Endres JR, Beres E, Vertesi A,. . . Szakonyine IP (2018). An assessment of the genotoxicity and subchronic toxicity of a supercritical fluid extract of the aerial parts of hemp. J Toxicol 2018:8143582. https://doi.org/10.1155/2018/8143582

Monticello TM, Jones TW, Dambach DM, Potter DM, Bolt MW, Liu M, . . . Kadambi VJ (2017) Current nonclinical testing paradigm enables safe entry to first-in-human clinical trials: the IQ consortium nonclinical to clinical translational database. Toxicol Appl Pharmacol 334:100–109. https://doi.org/10.1016/j.taap.2017.09.006

NRC (2011) Guide for the care and use of laboratory animals, 8th edn. National Academy Press, Washington, DC. www.nap.edu/catalog/18952/guide-for-the-care-and-use-of-laboratory-animals-eighth

Nuapia Y, Tutu H, Chimuka L, Cukrowska E (2020) Selective extraction of cannabinoid compounds from cannabis seed using pressurized hot water extraction. Molecules 25(6). https://doi.org/10.3390/molecules25061335

OECD (1998) OECD series on principles of good laboratory practice and compliance monitoring number 1. OECD principles on good laboratory practice (as revised in 1997). OECD, Paris. Retrieved from Https://www.oecd.org/chemicalsafety/testing/oecdseriesonprinciplesofgoodlaboratorypracticeglpandcompliancemonitoring.htm

OECD (2016) Overview of the set of OECD genetic toxicology test guidelines and updates performed in 2014–2015: series on testing and assessment No. 238. OECD, Paris. Retrieved from https://www.oecd.org/publications/overview-on-genetic-toxicology-tgs-9789264274761-en.htm

OECD (2018) Test no. 408: repeated dose 90-day Oral toxicity study in rodents, OECD guidelines for the testing of chemicals, section 4. OECD Publishing, Paris. https://doi.org/10.1787/9789264070707-en

Parasuraman S (2011) Toxicological screening. J Pharmacol Pharmacother 2(2):74–79. https://doi.org/10.4103/0976-500X.81895

Patsalos PN, Szaflarski JP, Gidal B, VanLandingham K, Critchley D, Morrison G (2020) Clinical implications of trials investigating drug-drug interactions between cannabidiol and enzyme inducers or inhibitors or common antiseizure drugs. Epilepsia 61(9):1854–1868. https://doi.org/10.1111/epi.16674

Pellati F, Borgonetti V, Brighenti V, Biagi M, Benvenuti S, Corsi L (2018) *Cannabis sativa* L. and nonpsychoactive cannabinoids: their chemistry and role against oxidative stress, inflammation, and cancer. Biomed Res Int 2018:1691428. https://doi.org/10.1155/2018/1691428

Percie du Sert NP, Hurst V, Ahluwalia A, Alam S, Altman DG, Avey MT, ... Holgate ST (2018) Revision of the ARRIVE guidelines: rationale and scope. BMJ Open Sci 2(1):e000002. https://doi.org/10.1136/bmjos-2018-000002

Percie du Sert N, Hurst V, Ahluwalia A, Alam S, Avey MT, Baker M, ... Wurbel H (2020) The ARRIVE guidelines 2.0: updated guidelines for reporting animal research. PLoS Biol 18(7): e3000410. https://doi.org/10.1371/journal.pbio.3000410

Ryan D, McKemie DS, Kass PH et al (2021) Pharmacokinetics and effects on arachidonic acid metabolism of low doses of cannabidiol following oral administration to horses. Drug Test Anal 13:1305–1317. https://doi.org/10.1002/dta.3028

Schaiquevich P, Riva N, Maldonado C, Vazquez M, Caceres-Guido P (2020) Clinical pharmacology of cannabidiol in refractory epilepsy. Farm Hosp 44(5):222–229. https://doi.org/10.7399/fh.11390

Smith LC, Tieu L, Suhandynata RT, Boomhower B, Hoffman M, Sepulveda Y,... George O (2021) Cannabidiol reduces withdrawal symptoms in nicotine-dependent rats. Psychopharmacology 238(8):2201–2211. https://doi.org/10.1007/s00213-021-05845-4

Stout SM, Cimino NM (2014) Exogenous cannabinoids as substrates, inhibitors, and inducers of human drug metabolizing enzymes: a systematic review. Drug Metab Rev 46(1):86–95. https://doi.org/10.3109/03602532.2013.849268

US Food and Drug Administration (FDA) (2007) US FDA toxicological principles for the safety assessment of food ingredients [Redbook 2000, Revised 2007 IV.C. 4. a. Subchronic toxicity studies with rodents (2003)]. https://www.fda.gov/media/79074/download

US Government (2018) Hemp farming act (2018). Accessed via. https://www.congress.gov/bill/115th-congress/senate-bill/2667/text. Accessed 15 May 2021

USFDA (2016) Botanical drug development guidance for industry. USFDA, Washington, DC. Retrieved from https://www.fda.gov/regulatory-information/search-fda-guidance-documents/botanical-drug-development-guidance-industry

USFDA (2018) US FDA good laboratory practices. https://www.accessdata.fda.gov/scripts/cdrh/cfdocs/cfcfr/CFRSearch.cfm?CFRPart=58

USFDA (2020) Cannabis and cannabis-derived compounds: quality considerations for clinical research – guidance for industry (draft guidance). Available via USFDA. https://www.fda.gov/regulatory-information/search-fda-guidance-documents/cannabis-and-cannabis-derived-compounds-quality-considerations-clinical-research-guidance-industry. Accessed 15 Aug 2021

USFDA (2021) New dietary ingredients (NDI) notification process. Retrieved from https://www.fda.gov/food/dietary-supplements/new-dietary-ingredients-ndi-notification-process

VanLandingham KE, Crockett J, Taylor L, Morrison G (2020) A phase 2, double-blind, placebo-controlled trial to investigate potential drug-drug interactions between cannabidiol and clobazam. J Clin Pharmacol 60(10):1304–1313. https://doi.org/10.1002/jcph.1634

Vaughn D, Kulpa J, Paulionis L (2020) Preliminary investigation of the safety of escalating cannabinoid doses in healthy dogs. Front Vet Sci 7:51. https://doi.org/10.3389/fvets.2020.00051

Vaughn DM, Paulionis LJ, Kulpa JE (2021) Randomized, placebo-controlled, 28-day safety and pharmacokinetics evaluation of repeated oral cannabidiol administration in healthy dogs. Am J Vet Res 82(5):405–416. https://doi.org/10.2460/ajvr.82.5.405

Vazquez M, Guevara N, Maldonado C, Guido PC, Schaiquevich P (2020) Potential pharmacokinetic drug-drug interactions between cannabinoids and drugs used for chronic pain. Biomed Res Int 2020:3902740. https://doi.org/10.1155/2020/3902740

Verrico CD, Wesson S, Konduri V, Hofferek CJ, Vazquez-Perez J, Blair E, ... Halpert MM (2020) A randomized, double-blind, placebo-controlled study of daily cannabidiol for the treatment of canine osteoarthritis pain. Pain 161(9):2191–2202. https://doi.org/10.1097/j.pain.0000000000001896

Watkins PB, Church RJ, Li J, Knappertz V (2021) Cannabidiol and abnormal liver chemistries in healthy adults: results of a phase I clinical trial. Clin Pharmacol Ther 109(5):1224–1231. https://doi.org/10.1002/cpt.2071

Cannabis Use and Sleep

64

Renée Martin-Willett, Ashley Master, L. Cinnamon Bidwell, and Sharon R. Sznitman

Contents

Sleep and Health 1371
Sleep Disorders 1372
Existing Treatments for Sleep Disorders 1375
Cannabis and Sleep 1376
Effects of Cannabis on Sleep Disorders 1377
Comorbid Sleep Disturbance with Other Diagnoses 1379
Routes of Administration for Cannabinoids 1382
Inhaled Versus Edible Cannabinoids 1382
Synthetic Versus Plant-Derived Cannabinoids 1383
Differential Effects of Cannabinoids and Other Compounds 1384
Long-Term Use of Cannabis and Cannabis Use Disorder (CUD) 1386
Applications to Other Areas of Substance Use Disorders 1386
Implications and Future Directions 1387
Comparison of Plant-Based and Synthetic Cannabinoids in Relation to Sleep 1387
The Effects of Mode of Administration, Dosages, and Potencies 1388
Data Needed to Capture Pre-Onset of Use, Short-Term Use, and Long-Term Use 1388
Comparison of Cannabis Use Exclusively as a Sleep Aid Versus the Effects of Cannabis Use for Comorbid Conditions on Sleep Outcomes 1388
Comparison of Sleep Outcomes Between Recreational and Medical Cannabis Users 1389

R. Martin-Willett · A. Master
Department of Psychology and Neuroscience, University of Colorado Boulder, Boulder, CO, USA
e-mail: rema8106@colorado.edu; asso6774@colorado.edu

L. C. Bidwell
Department of Psychology and Neuroscience, University of Colorado Boulder, Boulder, CO, USA

Institute of Cognitive Science, University of Colorado Boulder, Boulder, CO, USA
e-mail: lcb@colorado.edu

S. R. Sznitman (✉)
School of Public Health, University of Haifa, Faculty of Social Welfare and Health Sciences, Haifa, Israel
e-mail: sznitman@research.haifa.ac.il

V. B. Patel, V. R. Preedy (eds.), *Handbook of Substance Misuse and Addictions*,
https://doi.org/10.1007/978-3-030-92392-1_70

Conclusion 1389
Mini Dictionary 1389
Summary Points 1390
References 1391

Abstract

Cannabis has long been associated with sleep disturbance, but the precise nature of this relationship remains unclear. The limited effectiveness and tolerability of existing sleep aids indicates a critical need for viable alternatives. Cannabis may prove such an alternative, as a growing proportion of cannabis users report a beneficial effect of cannabis on a range of sleep disturbances. Further, emerging clinical evidence supports the use of cannabis and cannabis-derived compounds in the treatment of sleep disorders, as well as disordered sleep secondary to other diagnoses such as chronic pain, post-traumatic stress disorder (PTSD), and depression. However, these results are often inconsistent across studies, likely due to a combination of varying user characteristics – such as duration and frequency of use – and different formulations and potencies employed by different research designs. Additionally, extensive research supports a bidirectional relationship between sleep and cannabis use, such that sleep disturbance increases cannabis use and risk of misuse, while long-term cannabis use increases risk of sleep disturbance. To explicate the complex relationship between cannabis and sleep, we propose the following directions for future research: 1) comparison of plant-based and synthetic cannabinoids in relation to sleep; 2) comparison of different modes of administration, dosages, and potencies; 3) comparison of different durations of cannabis use (i.e., pre-onset of use, short-term use, and long-term use); 4) comparison of cannabis use exclusively as a sleep aid versus effects of cannabis on sleep outcomes comorbid with other conditions; and 5) comparison of sleep outcomes between recreational and medical cannabis users.

Keywords

Sleep · Cannabis · Alcohol · Sleep disturbance · Insomnia

Sleep disturbance is commonly associated with cannabis use. Extensive research supports a bidirectional relationship between sleep and cannabis use, such that sleep disturbance increases cannabis use and risk of misuse, while long-term cannabis use increases risk of sleep disturbance (Breslau et al. 1996; Haario et al. 2013). In addition to this known risk, there is mounting evidence that cannabis can also be of benefit to sleep disturbances in certain circumstances, though there is a need for continued research in the area. Unfortunately, while cannabis use is increasingly legal in US states and internationally, the current legal environment highly restricts researchers' ability to study cannabis use on the legal market (see Fig. 1) (Hutchison et al. 2019; MacCallum and Russo 2018), including in relation to sleep. This chapter will provide an overview of common sleep disorders as well as a review of the

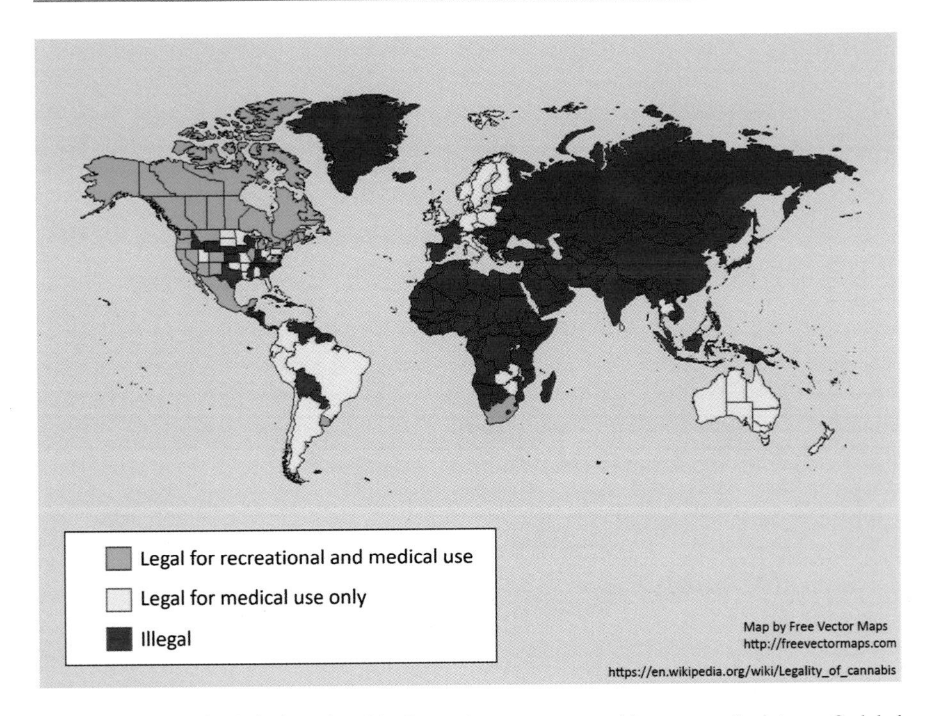

Fig. 1 Global Cannabis legality. This figure is meant to provide a general picture of global cannabis legality and purposefully employs broad category definitions. For our purposes, "legal" refers to policies in which adult use is not penalized; "medical use" refers to policies in which THC may only be used as a treatment for a qualifying medical condition(s); "recreational use" refers to adult use of THC without a need for medical qualification

current data on bidirectional associations and effects between sleep and cannabis. An overview of cannabis pharmacology in relation to sleep and current limitations of the research will then be discussed. Finally, implications of the research findings concerning cannabis and sleep and future directions to guide research and public health and policy will be discussed.

Sleep and Health

Sleep behaviors are governed by *circadian rhythms*, which are physiological and behavioral changes that occur on a 24-hour cycle (Hasler et al. 2012). The *sleep/wake system* is a circadian rhythm that maintains homeostasis by balancing our need for sleep (i.e., "sleep drive") with our need to be awake. The sleep drive builds with continued wakefulness, ultimately causing us to feel tired and fall asleep; once asleep, homeostasis is achieved, and the sleep drive is replaced by a growing need for alertness that increases with continued sleep and eventually prompts awakening (Fuller et al. 2006). The most model of the regulation of sleep is Borbély's two-process model, which proposes that sleep relies on two processes working seamlessly together. *Process S* is the accumulation of sleep-inducing substances in the brain – the longer someone is awake, the stronger their desire will be for sleep. *Process C* controls the timing of the body's internal biological processes as well as alertness levels. Put simply, the first process causes a pressure to fall asleep, while the second dictates the daily rhythm or timing of sleep (Borbély et al. 2016).

Human sleep is characterized by alternations between two distinct phases: *non-rapid eye movement sleep* (about 80% of sleep) and *rapid eye movement (REM) sleep* (about 20% of sleep). Non-REM sleep is comprised of three stages (N1, N2, and N3), with each successive stage associated with increased depth and restfulness of sleep. REM sleep, where most dreaming occurs, is characterized by physical paralysis and increased brain activity relative to non-REM sleep. Although the exact purpose of REM sleep is currently unknown, preliminary evidence suggests a role in memory consolidation and other cognitive and physiological processes (Fraigne et al. 2014; Peever and Fuller 2017).

Key fact: Sleep disturbance is linked to obesity, diabetes, and cardiovascular disease as well as emotional processing, stress management, and resilience.

Sleep disturbance is linked to a wide range of adverse physical and mental health outcomes. Poor sleep is associated with increased risk of cardiometabolic diseases such as obesity (Knutson 2012), diabetes (Shan et al. 2015), and hypertension, as well as cardiovascular diseases such as hypercholesterolemia, and atherosclerosis (Cappuccio et al. 2011). Sleep deprivation causes neurocognitive impairment, specifically in regard to working memory, executive functioning, and processing speed (Goel et al. 2009; Killgore 2010). Sleep is also related to many aspects of mental health, including emotional processing (Tempesta et al. 2018), stress management (Almojali et al. 2017), and resilience in the face of hardship (Wang et al. 2020). Further, sleep disturbance is associated with general mortality, such that short sleep duration predicts a 10–12% increased risk of death, while long sleep duration predicts a 30–38% increased risk of death (Cappuccio et al. 2010; Gallicchio and Kalesan 2009). An overview of the most common sleep disorders and their treatments are provided in the following section.

Sleep Disorders

Many people experience sleep disturbance at some point in their lives (Grandner 2017). For example, poor sleep is common in college students (Lund et al. 2010) and perinatal women (Tomfohr et al. 2015) and is also associated with high levels of poverty (Grandner et al. 2015). Fortunately, most cases of sleep disturbance are transient and eventually resolve on their own, but severe cases may constitute *sleep disorders* – persistent, debilitating sleep disturbances that are not attributable to other causes (K. Pavlova and Latreille 2019). This section describes cardinal symptoms and prevalence of six main categories of sleep disorders (see Table 1).

Key fact: The incidence rates of sleep disorders has been increasing globally over the past 30 years, with higher prevalence in lower- and middle-income countries (Sexton-Radek et al. 2020).

Table 1 Sleep disorder categories and status in cannabis research

Sleep disorder category	Notable examples	Preliminary evidence for cannabis as treatment?
Insomnia disorder Chronically insufficient quantity and quality of sleep	Sleep-onset insomnia Sleep-maintenance insomnia Late insomnia	Yes
Hypersomnia disorders Excessive sleepiness and unintended lapses into sleep during daytime	Hypersomnolence disorders Narcolepsy	No
Circadian rhythm disorders Misalignment between internal sleep/wake rhythms and external patterns of light and darkness	Delayed sleep phase syndrome Advanced sleep phase syndrome	Yes
Breathing-related sleep disorders Pauses in breathing during sleep that cause awakenings during the night	Obstructive sleep apneaCentral sleep apneaComplex sleep apnea	Yes
Parasomnias Abnormal behaviors that occur during non-REM or REM stages of sleep	Somnambulance Night terrors Nightmare disorder REM sleep behavior disorder	Yes (REM sleep behavior disorder)
Restless legs syndrome Overwhelming urge to move the legs during evening and nighttime hours	N/A	Yes

This table briefly describes cardinal symptoms of six main categories of sleep disorders, notable examples of each, and whether empirical evidence from cannabis research supports cannabis as a viable treatment

Insomnia disorder is characterized by difficulty initiating and/or maintaining sleep, associated with significant daytime consequences, impairment, or distress and present despite adequate opportunity for sleep (Vargas et al. 2020). There are three main types of insomnia: *sleep-onset insomnia* involves trouble falling asleep at bedtime; *sleep-maintenance insomnia* involves numerous or prolonged awakenings during the night; *late insomnia* involves early-morning awakening with difficulty falling back asleep (American Psychiatric Association 2013). Global estimates indicate that up to 30% of adults report at least one symptom of insomnia, while 6–10% meet criteria for insomnia disorder (Roth 2007). Insomnia is most prevalent among women and older adults and often comorbid with other medical and psychiatric conditions (American Psychiatric Association 2013).

Hypersomnia disorders are characterized by prolonged primary sleep periods, frequent naps, or difficulty awakening after abrupt awakenings accompanied with distress or impairment (Bollu et al. 2018). *Hypersomnolence disorder* is characterized by abnormally long sleep duration (> 9 h/day) and difficulty staying alert after awakening. *Narcolepsy* is a disorder of acute onset rapid eye movement sleep characterized by excessive daytime sleepiness and accompanied by frequent, unpredictable, and uncontrollable sleep episodes (termed "sleep attacks"). Narcolepsy can be divided into type 1, in which sleep attacks are accompanied with *cataplexy*, a sudden loss of muscle tone that is often precipitated by strong emotions, or type 2 (without cataplexy) (Slowik et al. 2021). Narcolepsy is rare, only affecting 0.02–0.04% of adults. Hypersomnolence affects 1% of the US and European populations. Both are equally prevalent in men and women (American Psychiatric Association 2013).

Circadian rhythm disorders (CRD) are caused by misalignment of internal sleep/wake rhythms with external patterns of light and darkness. Examples of CRD include *delayed sleep phase syndrome* (sleep onset occurs later than desired) and *advanced sleep phase syndrome* (sleep onset occurs earlier than desired). CRD can be caused by external factors such as jet lag and shift work (e.g., nighttime shift work or shift work rotating between day and night). It is important to note that affected individuals report normal quality and quantity of sleep when allowed to set their own schedule – problems arise when endogenous rhythms do not conform to environmental expectations. Prevalence ranges between 0.17% and 1% in adults (American Psychiatric Association 2013).

Sleep-disordered breathing or *sleep-related breathing disorders* are characterized by pauses in breathing during sleep that result in frequent awakenings throughout the night. There are three main types of breathing-related sleep disorders: *obstructive sleep apnea (OSA)* is a cessation of airflow caused by collapse of the upper airway during sleep; *central sleep apnea* is a cessation of airflow due to inconsistent respiratory effort; *complex sleep apnea* is a combination of obstructive and central sleep apneas (Pavlova and Latreille 2019). OSA is the most common breathing-related sleep disorder, affecting 1–2% of children, 2–15% of middle-age adults, and over 20% of older adults (American Psychiatric Association 2013).

Key fact: Obstructive sleep apnea is the most common sleep-related breathing disorder and can occur at any age.

Parasomnias are abnormal behaviors that occur during specific stages of sleep (Fleetham and Fleming 2014). Parasomnias associated with non-REM sleep include *somnambulism* (sleepwalking) and *night terrors* (recurrent episodes of abrupt awakening accompanied by intense fear and associated autonomic arousal). Parasomnias that occur during REM sleep include *REM sleep behavior disorder* (characterized by loss of the usual muscle atonia that occurs during REM sleep, resulting in abnormal movements during REM sleep that may cause injury to the sleeper or bed partner) and *nightmare disorder* (frequent distressing and threatening dreams). Prevalence varies considerably between different parasomnias. For example, somnambulism is fairly common, as 29.2% of adults experience at least one episode of sleepwalking during their lives (although only 1–5% meet criteria for sleepwalking disorder). Conversely, REM sleep behavior disorder is relatively rare, affecting only 0.38–0.5% of adults (American Psychiatric Association 2013).

Restless legs syndrome (RLS) is a parasomnia that is characterized by an overwhelming urge to move the legs that worsens during evening and nighttime hours. RLS is associated with significant sleep latency and fragmented sleep. The urge to move the legs is often relieved by physical activity, which causes affected individuals to remain awake and active during the night (American Psychiatric Association 2013). RLS is fairly common, with an average prevalence of 15% across studies (although estimates are as low as 2–7% when strict diagnostic criteria are employed) (American Psychiatric Association 2013; Innes et al. 2011). RLS is most common in women and older adults (Innes et al. 2011).

Overall, shared commonalities across sleep disorders are a disruption of daily functioning, diminished quality of life, and increased risk of adverse health outcomes. Additionally, varying clinical presentations and diffuse or unknown etiology render the symptoms of disordered sleep challenging to alleviate.

Existing Treatments for Sleep Disorders

Current pharmacological treatments for sleep disorders are numerous and diverse. Insomnia is typically treated using non-benzodiazepine hypnotics, also known as "z-drugs," such as zolpidem (Ambien), eszopiclone (Lunesta), and zaleplon (Sonata). Medications approved for narcolepsy and daytime sleepiness are stimulants (Dexedrine, Ritalin), non-stimulant wake-promoting medications such as modafinil/armodafinil, and other medications such as sodium oxybate. Parasomnias and RLS can be managed using dopamine agonists such as carbidopa/levodopa (Sinemet) and pramipexole (Mirapex) (Ramar and Olson 2013). As a group, prescription sleep aids are generally effective at mitigating sleep disturbances, but such benefits are often accompanied by a diverse range of adverse side effects (e.g., headaches, dizziness, compulsive behaviors, and even additional sleep disturbances such as daytime sleepiness and somnambulance) and potential for abuse, tolerance, and dependence (Ramar and Olson 2013). Over-the-counter antihistamine or antihistamine/analgesic-type drugs (OTC "sleep aids") as well as herbal and nutritional substances (e.g., valerian and melatonin) are not recommended in the treatment of chronic insomnia due to the relative lack of efficacy and safety data, despite widespread use (Riemann et al. 2015; Schutte-Rodin et al. 2008).

Side effects and addictive potential of pharmacological sleep aids can be avoided through the use of non-pharmacological interventions. *Bright light therapy* (i.e., exposure to light as a means of "resetting" abnormal sleep/wake patterns) is a noninvasive, cost effective treatment for circadian rhythm disorders that is associated with minimal side effects (Gooley 2008; Ramar and Olson 2013). The American Academy of Sleep Medicine recommends *cognitive behavioral therapy* for insomnia (CBT-I; Cognitive Behavioral Therapy is an Effective Treatment for Chronic Insomnia 2009). However, there are barriers and challenges to implementing CBT-I, including a lack of access to adequately trained clinicians as well as the time-consuming nature of treatment (Morin 2017; Riemann et al. 2017). OSA and other breathing-related sleep disorders are typically treated using a *continuous positive airway pressure (CPAP) machine*, a mechanical device that facilitates breathing by keeping the airway clear during sleep. CPAP machines are highly effective, but many patients find the equipment cumbersome and uncomfortable, which ultimately leads to poor treatment adherence (Weaver et al. 2014).

Key fact: Current pharmacological treatments for disordered sleep are usually hypnotics or dopamine agonists, while non-pharmacological treatments such as bright light therapy or CBT are also in use.

In sum, standard pharmacological sleep aids are generally effective at managing their respective treatment targets, but improvements may be compromised by adverse side effects and high potential for abuse or dependence. Furthermore, the long-term safety/efficacy of pharmacological sleep aids is also in question due to risk of falls, daytime sleepiness, and increased dementia risk. Although non-pharmaceutical treatments elicit few physical side effects, they may be difficult to access (e.g., CBT – due to high costs and substantial time commitment) and can lead to unacceptable reductions in quality of life (e.g., restrictive and uncomfortable CPAP machines). These deficiencies indicate a critical need for alternative treatments that are effective, accessible, and well-tolerated. While cannabis has achieved wide accessibility and is increasingly used as a sleep aid, data are needed to determine its efficacy and viability as an alternative to conventional treatments.

Cannabis and Sleep

For much of the past century, substances such as alcohol, opium, barbiturates, and benzodiazepines were standard treatments for most sleep disturbances (Tringale and Jensen 2011). These substances facilitate sleep in the short term, but repeated use may lead to dependence or addiction, which ultimately exacerbates existing sleep disturbances or precipitates new sleep problems (Ek et al. 2021). Acute effects of substance use on sleep largely depend upon the substance in question. For example, stimulants such as cocaine and amphetamines cause light, restless, and disrupted sleep, whereas depressants (e.g., benzodiazepines, alcohol) and opiates (e.g., heroin) initially act as sedatives but cause sleep disruptions later in the night (e.g., increased night awakenings) due to acute withdrawal effects (Angarita et al. 2016). In contrast, cannabis use may have benefits as a sleep aid without the many side effects associated with other substances, as evidenced by a recent review of clinical trials suggesting positive effects from cannabinoid administration (Kuhathasan et al. 2019). This section will discuss how cannabis is currently being used as a sleep aid by the public and the current state of the research on cannabinoids on sleep disorders and disrupted sleep comorbid with other conditions.

Across the United States and internationally, policies governing the use of cannabis generally make a distinction between recreational and medical use, with separate regulations and laws for different type of users. However, the reality of legalized cannabis use and the motivations driving use among the public likely do not fall into discreet “medical” and “recreational” categories. For example, in a recent community study of over 700 Canadian users, 80% of participants who reported medically motivated use also reported concurrent recreational use (Turna et al. 2020). Within medical use, the most common conditions cited include chronic pain, anxiety and depression, and disordered sleep concurrently with other conditions, as well as on its own (Kosiba et al. 2019; Kvamme et al. 2021;

Lintzeris et al. 2018). Although no regulatory body has recommended cannabis for sleep disturbances, users report that the use of cannabis improves sleep (Bonn-Miller et al. 2014; Hazekamp et al. 2013; Walsh et al. 2013), with cannabis use for sleep occurring across age groups but most commonly among middle and older adult groups (Haug et al. 2017; Lin et al. 2016).

While there are no nationally representative data to indicate how many people use cannabis specifically to alleviate disordered sleep symptoms, there are studies that suggest that use for this purpose is widespread, has been occurring for many years, and is increasing. Even 20 years ago, over half of the sample in a small study of medical cannabis use reported improvement in sleep from cannabis (Ogbome et al. 2000). Recent cannabis dispensary data also strongly suggest that cannabis is increasingly being used on the recreational market as a sleep aid. In one survey study, 74% of dispensary customers endorsed cannabis use for sleep improvement (Bachhuber et al. 2019), and aggregate level data suggests that OTC sleep aids are being substituted with the use of cannabis (Piper et al. 2017). This substitution appears to extend to both older adults (Abuhasira et al. 2019; Baumbusch and Sloan Yip 2021) and adolescents (Blevins et al. 2016). Finally, a strong negative relationship was observed at the county level in the US state of Colorado between OTC sleep aid sales and dispensary operations. In other words, once a dispensary began operating in a given county, OTC sleep aid sales declined over 240% on average over the course of the 1-year study (Doremus et al. 2019). Importantly, cannabis comes in many formulations with varying levels of Δ9-tetrahydrocannabinol (THC; the cannabinoid more strongly associated with drug reward properties) and cannabidiol (CBD; a nonintoxicating cannabinoid), the two primary cannabinoids which both have different pharmacologies and effects. Given these data, the research on the effects of cannabis and cannabinoids on sleep is highly relevant to public health. The following section will provide key results in this area, for both sleep disorders and disrupted sleep comorbid with other conditions.

Effects of Cannabis on Sleep Disorders

Insomnia. Cannabis is assumed to be an effective short-term treatment for insomnia and other sleep disturbances (Winiger et al. 2021), as medical cannabis users often report using cannabis to alleviate sleep latency and other symptoms of insomnia (Tringale and Jensen 2011). However, there is less consensus in clinical research on cannabis and insomnia.

Several studies suggest a beneficial effect of cannabis on insomnia. Tringale and Jensen (2011) found that medicinal cannabis users – both with and without reported sleep problems – experienced significantly reduced sleep latency after cannabis use, although effect sizes were larger in users who reported sleep disturbance. Another study on medical users suggested that effects of cannabis on sleep disturbance may depend on cannabinoid content, as individuals with insomnia and greater sleep latency reported using cannabis with higher CBD concentrations, and sleep

Table 2 Pharmaceutical cannabinoids commonly used in sleep research

Generic name	Brand name(s)	Formulation	Mode of administration	Indications supported by empirical evidence	
				Sleep disorders	Comorbidities
Dronabinol	Marinol Syndros	Synthetic THC	Oral	Insomnia Obstructive sleep apnea	Chronic pain[a]
Nabilone	Cesamet	Synthetic THC	Oral	N/A	Post-traumatic stress disorder Chronic pain[a] Fibromyalgia[a]
Naboximols	Sativex	THC-CBD 1:1	Oromucosal spray	N/A	Chronic pain[a] Muscle spasms[a] Multiple sclerosis[a] Fibromyalgia[a]

This table provides basic information on pharmaceutical cannabinoids commonly used in clinical research on sleep disorders and/or sleep disturbance comorbid with other conditions
[a]Regulatory approval for respective Indication in one or more nations

medication use was associated with the use of lower THC concentrations (Belendiuk et al. 2015).

Other studies found that natural and synthetic THC (specifically dronabinol) are associated with decreased sleep latency in healthy populations, although effects may vary according to the frequency of cannabis use (Gorelick et al. 2013) and cannabinoid content (Nicholson et al. 2004; see Table 2 for an overview of commonly used synthetic cannabinoids). Specifically, Gorelick et al. (2013) found that beneficial effects of cannabis decreased over time, suggesting a potential effect of tolerance. Nicholson et al. (2004) used a blinded, placebo-controlled design (three conditions: 15 mg THC, 5 mg THC/5 mg CBD, and 15/mg THC/15 mg CBD) to determine differential effects of cannabinoids and dose on sleep and related behaviors in young adults. They found that THC alone produced sedative effects, but such effects were not present following equal doses of THC and CBD. Rather, the THC–CBD condition was associated with less restful sleep, as evidenced by decreased stage N3 sleep (i.e., slow-wave sleep) relative to the other conditions.

In contrast, a study using a sample of self-identified alcohol and/or cannabis users found that cannabis and alcohol are both associated with poor sleep quality, with greater severity in users of both alcohol and cannabis (Ogeil et al. 2015). Overall, these preliminary findings suggest that the effects of cannabis on insomnia are impacted by cannabis product characteristics such as dose and cannabinoid content, as well as user characteristics such as the frequency of cannabis use, comorbid sleep disturbance, and co-occurring use of other substances.

Obstructive sleep apnea. Reduced quality of life and poor treatment adherence caused by CPAP machines – the standard treatment for OSA – have prompted investigation of cannabinoids as potential alternative treatments. Preliminary research was conducted using animal models. In a pioneering study, Carley et al. (2002) used Sprague-Dawley rats to examine the role of cannabinoids in regulating breathing during sleep. Results showed that THC – along with the endocannabinoid *oleamide* – reduced the frequency of apneic events, suggesting that cannabinoids can potentially suppress serotonin-mediated symptoms of OSA. In a subsequent study by Calik et al. (2014), researchers injected dronabinol (synthetic THC) directly into the nodose ganglia of Sprague-Dawley rats with the aim of reducing serotonin-induced apneas. Results showed that dronabinol reduced serotonin-induced apneas, possibly by regulating upper airway muscles that facilitate breathing during sleep. Taken together, these results from animal models show promising therapeutic potential that justifies continued research on dronabinol in humans.

A proof-of-concept study by Prasad et al. (2013) investigated the safety, tolerability, and efficacy of dronabinol in decreasing the frequency and severity of OSA symptoms in adult humans. Results showed that dronabinol was well tolerated and effective in reducing apneic events. A subsequent study by the same research team examined the effects of dronabinol on sleep as measured by EEG. The authors found that dronabinol was associated with changes in delta and theta frequencies and increased ultradian rhythms, both of which correlated with improvement in apneas and a reduced feeling of sleepiness (Farabi et al. 2014). Initial research conducted in animal models and preliminary work in humans suggest that synthetic THC may have therapeutic potential in treatment of OSA.

Parasomnias. Although few studies have investigated cannabis as treatment for parasomnias, early evidence indicates a promising effect of cannabis on restless legs syndrome (RLS) and REM behavior disorder (RBD). A pioneering study of six patients with treatment-resistant RLS found that all six patients reported total relief of RLS symptoms – as well as increased sleep quality – following self-administration of cannabis (Megelin and Ghorayeb 2017). This effect was replicated in a follow-up study, wherein 11 of 12 patients reported significant improvement of RLS symptoms after using cannabis (Ghorayeb 2020).

To date, only one study has investigated the effects of cannabis in treating RBD. Chagas et al. (2014) used an open-label case study design to assess the efficacy of CBD in reducing RBD symptoms in four adults with Parkinson's disease. Results showed that CBD was well tolerated and significantly reduced behaviors associated with RBD. Specifically, of the four participants, three reported zero episodes of RBD following treatment (compared to baseline frequency of 2–7 RBS episodes per week), and one reported a single episode of RBD following treatment. These promising preliminary findings justify further examination of the effects of cannabis on parasomnias, ideally using larger samples and randomized placebo-controlled research designs.

Comorbid Sleep Disturbance with Other Diagnoses

Sleep disturbance frequently co-occurs with mental disorders, including depression, anxiety, and suicidality (Breslau et al. 1996), and other conditions such as chronic pain and cancer, all of which have detrimental effects on sleep. Many such conditions – including chronic pain, post-traumatic stress disorder, and cancer – are common indications for medical cannabis (Boehnke et al. 2019), but evidence is limited as to specific effects of cannabis on sleep for these patients. Nevertheless, despite limited scientific evidence, therapeutic use of cannabis is steadily increasing as more jurisdictions legalize cannabis (Boehnke et al. 2019). This section outlines research on the use of cannabis to improve sleep disturbance comorbid with other conditions.

Depression and anxiety. Sleep disturbance and cannabis use often coincide with negative emotions, most notably depression and anxiety, but it is presently unclear if cannabis relieves or exacerbates these symptoms. A nascent body of research shows a beneficial effect of cannabinoids on affective symptoms (Sarris et al. 2020). CBD appears to be particularly effective at ameliorating sleep complaints in individuals experiencing anxiety (Sarris et al. 2020; Shannon et al. 2019a). Conversely, other findings indicate a negative correlation between cannabis use and both mood and sleep quality. For example, Hser et al. (2017) conducted a secondary analysis on data from a cannabis use disorder medication trial and found that both quality of sleep and symptoms of depression and anxiety improved following cessation of cannabis use in adults aged 18–50.

Key fact: Depression and anxiety are ranked by the World Health Organization (WHO) as the first and sixth leading causes of disability, respectively, worldwide (Depression and other common mental disorders: Global health estimates 2017).

Clinical research has worked to elucidate details of this putative bidirectional relationship by examining cannabis as treatment for sleep disturbance in populations with clinically significant affective disorders. Major depressive disorder (MDD) is a psychiatric condition characterized by continuous low mood and loss of interest or pleasure in enjoyable activities and is highly comorbid with both sleep disturbance and cannabis use (American Psychiatric Association 2013). Individuals with MDD endorse using cannabis for sleep-initiating effects and managing and coping with symptoms of depression (Babson et al. 2013). This aligns with findings that cannabis use increases according to severity of sleep disturbance and depression symptoms (Feingold et al. 2017; Feingold and Weinstein 2021). Alas, perceived benefits of cannabis are undermined by observational and epidemiological studies showing no evidence of beneficial long-term effects of cannabis on depression-related outcomes (Feingold and Weinstein 2021).

Babson et al. (2013) examined the relationship between MDD, cannabis use, and perceived sleep quality in a sample of medical cannabis users. Consistent with previous research on both clinical and subthreshold populations, greater severity of depression was significantly associated with greater frequency of cannabis use. The authors found an unexpected moderating effect of perceived sleep quality on the relationship between MDD and cannabis use, such that participants with the most severe depression symptoms and good perceived sleep quality reported the most problematic cannabis use. This pattern suggests that medical cannabis users with heightened levels of depression symptoms may use cannabis, at least in part, to improve sleep quality. Future research should clarify this relationship and seek to replicate findings using both synthetic and plant-derived cannabinoids.

Post-traumatic stress disorder. Post-traumatic stress disorder (PTSD) is often accompanied by sleep disturbance in the form of insomnia and frequent nightmares. Emerging research suggests THC and related synthetics may alleviate PTSD-related sleep disturbances. Fraser (2009) examined the effect of nabilone (synthetic THC) in managing treatment-resistant nightmares associated with PTSD. Results showed nabilone increased sleep duration and reduced frequency and intensity of nightmares. Subsequent research produced similar results, suggesting nabilone may be a promising alternative treatment for PTSD-related sleep disturbance (Jetly et al. 2015). Further research should determine if this beneficial effect of nabilone can be achieved using commercially available THC products derived from whole-plant cannabis.

Chronic pain. Chronic pain significantly diminishes the potential for restful sleep. Much research on this topic was conducted using nabiximols (Sativex), a THC–CBD oromucosal spray, as treatment for sleep disturbance co-occurring with chronic pain. A review of seven early placebo-controlled clinical trials (phase II–phase 3) showed nabiximols was associated with significantly greater self-reported sleep quality in chronic pain patients in all seven studies. Interestingly, effects of tolerance were minimal, as extension studies found up to 40% of patients reported "very good" sleep quality despite relatively long drug exposure and no escalation of dose (Russo et al. 2007). In contrast, other studies found no significant effect of nabiximols on sleep duration, although subjective improvements in sleep quality were noted (Ware and Ferguson 2015). Ware et al. (2010) investigated the effectiveness of nabilone as compared to amitriptyline, an antidepressant commonly used to treat nerve pain, in improving sleep among patients with fibromyalgia. Patients in both conditions showed improvements in sleep, although treatment with nabilone was associated with greater improvements in sleep compared to amitriptyline.

Key fact: Chronic pain patients are among the most highly studied for cannabis and sleep and consistently report improved sleep quality across studies.

Other comorbid sleep conditions. Cannabis has been shown to relieve other common sleep-disrupting symptoms such as muscle spasms. Moderate evidence indicates that cannabinoids, primarily nabiximols, are an effective treatment to improve short term sleep outcomes in individuals with obstructive sleep apnea syndrome, fibromyalgia (Ware et al. 2010), chronic pain, and multiple sclerosis (Zettl et al. 2016). Findings are similar with respect to fatigue, as studies among patients with irritable bowel disease, Crohn's disease, Parkinson's disease, and multiple sclerosis, for whom fatigue is a serious issue, found that cannabis users reported less fatigue than nonusers. Taken together, results suggest that cannabis may indirectly improve sleep by ameliorating physical discomfort that prevents adequate sleep.

Effects of cannabis on cancer-related sleep disturbance represent a promising, yet understudied, direction for further research. Sleep disturbance is extremely common in cancer patients, with a prevalence as high as 80%. Further, cancer-related fatigue – a common and debilitating side effect of cancer and its treatment – is often comorbid with sleep disorders (Palesh et al. 2010). However, despite robust associations between cancer and sleep disturbance, no studies have specifically investigated cannabis as a treatment for cancer-related sleep disorders or fatigue. Future research should examine the viability of cannabis as a sleep aid in cancer patients.

To summarize, the research to date gives promising early evidence for the use of cannabis or cannabis-derived compounds both in the treatment of some sleep disorders as well as symptoms of disordered sleep secondary to other diagnoses, such as chronic pain, PTSD, or depression. However, most data suggest that duration and frequency of use are both central to the efficacy of cannabis to relieve symptoms and that the use of cannabis for sleep is not without risks. Furthermore, the fact that the public is administering highly diverse forms of cannabis on the legal market further complicates our understanding of how cannabis use may be related to sleep outcomes as well as highlights our need to understand the different pharmacokinetic (PK) effects of inhaled, edible, topical, plant-derived, and synthetic cannabis.

Routes of Administration for Cannabinoids

Cannabinoids can be administered in a number of different ways, especially in regions where cannabis is legally and commercially available. Many legal jurisdictions boast an increasing array of options that includes cannabis flower, concentrates, edibles, topical products such as lotions or transdermal patches (Borodovsky et al. 2016), and synthetic derivations. Widespread legalization, commercialization, and decades of selective breeding have resulted in significant increases in cannabis potency on the legal market (i.e., cannabinoid concentration in a given product, expressed as percent of total weight) compared to that of previous decades (ElSohly et al. 2016). Given that synthetic derivations of cannabis are the most frequent form employed in clinical trials, it is increasingly critical to understand the different pharmacokinetic effects of the most common forms of cannabis in relation to medically motivated use and sleep in particular. A comparison of these different forms and their properties is thus provided below.

Inhaled Versus Edible Cannabinoids

Emerging research suggests that inhaled and orally consumed ("edible") forms of cannabis have different PK effects. Inhalation swiftly delivers cannabinoids from the lungs to the brain via the bloodstream, producing near-immediate effects that last 2–4 h (Huestis et al. 1992). Conversely, edibles are broken down and absorbed in the digestive system, resulting in effects that are delayed (30–60 min after dosing) yet longer-lasting (up to 6 h) (Poyatos et al. 2020). Studies comparing blood cannabinoid concentration following inhaled and oral administration found that maximum blood concentration (C_{max}) of orally consumed cannabinoids is consistently lower than C_{max} after inhaling a similar dose. Cannabinoid absorption (measured by the correlation between dose and C_{max}) was higher for oral formulations compared to inhaled forms (Poyatos et al. 2020).

Key fact: Inhalation of cannabis produces near-immediate effects that last 2–4 h, while effects of edibles are delayed by 30–60 min but can last up to 6 h.

Despite significant PK differences, oral and inhaled forms are similar in terms of subjective effects such as mood changes, feelings of intoxication, cognitive impairment, food intake, feelings of being "high" or "stoned," and psychomotor performance (Chait and Zacny 1992; Hart et al. 2002). However, one study found that orally consumed cannabis was associated with lower ratings of positive subjective effects and higher ratings of negative subjective effects (Ewusi Boisvert et al. 2020). Other evidence indicates subjective effects of edible cannabis are more susceptible to tolerance and therefore closely related to the frequency of use (Hart et al. 2002; Newmeyer et al. 2017).

PK differences between inhaled and oral cannabinoids, specifically in terms of onset and duration of acute intoxication, may yield distinct effects on sleep and sleep disturbance, although no studies have directly examined this possibility. The rapid intoxication that follows inhalation suggests inhaled forms may facilitate faster sleep onset (i.e., decreased sleep latency). However, acute effects will likely subside a few hours after dosing and fail to prevent early awakening during the night. Conversely, effects of edibles will be delayed by 30–60 min after dosing, but once asleep, the longer-lasting effects may allow fewer awakenings during the night. Taken together, inhalation may be better suited for improving difficulties with sleep onset, while edibles are more effective in reducing problems associated with sleep maintenance. It should be noted, however, that delayed intoxication following oral administration could be mitigated by dosing 30–60 min before bedtime. These presumed differential effects of inhaled and oral cannabinoids are clinically promising (e.g., patients will be able to make more informed treatment decisions) and present a compelling opportunity for further clinical research.

Synthetic Versus Plant-Derived Cannabinoids

Because of regulatory barriers with the use of many forms of cannabis in clinical research, controlled trials of cannabis are often conducted using *synthetic cannabinoids*, which are created in a laboratory rather than extracted from the cannabis plant. Synthetic cannabinoids are similar to their naturally occurring counterparts (most often THC) in most respects – they interact with the same cannabinoid receptors (CB_1 and CB_2) and elicit similar physiological and subjective effects (Castaneto et al. 2014). However, some evidence suggests synthetic cannabinoids are associated with increased frequency and severity of adverse drug reactions compared to plant-derived cannabinoids (Castaneto et al. 2014; Papaseit et al. 2018; Winstock et al. 2015).

Synthetic cannabinoids are chemically pure and therefore often used in rigorously controlled clinical trials that prioritize internal validity (in fact, synthetic cannabinoids were originally created for research purposes (Papaseit et al. 2018)).

Unfortunately, clinical trial procedures seldom align with the way cannabis is used naturalistically and have not kept up with rapid and drastic legal market changes (e.g., expansion of edibles, increasing THC potency). Real-world users are free to choose their preferred cannabis product and route of administration and self-titrate their dose until they achieve the desired state of intoxication or other desired effect (e.g., pain relief, sleep). Further, most cannabis users consume commercially available products made from whole plant cannabis, which contains numerous chemical compounds that vary considerably from synthetic formulations but also between individual plants. At present, few studies have directly compared synthetic and plant-derived cannabinoids with THC, so further research is needed to confirm these findings and evaluate possible mechanisms. Any differences between synthetic and plant-derived cannabinoids may have profound implications for research on cannabis and sleep.

Differential Effects of Cannabinoids and Other Compounds

One substantial difference between synthetic and plant-based formulations is the presence of multiple cannabinoids and other compounds in the latter form. The effects of cannabinoids such as THC and CBD are increasingly believed to have differential effects on sleep through mechanisms of the endocannabinoid system. The cannabinoid type 1 receptor (CB_1) within the endocannabinoid system (ECS) is involved in the modulation of light-induced phase shifts, with CB_1 receptors active in brain regions central to circadian rhythms, including the thalamus and the dorsal and median raphe nuclei (Pacher et al. 2006; Sanford et al. 2008). Some current pharmacological treatments for disordered sleep involve the direct administration of endocannabinoid neurotransmitters, such as anandamide (AEA) or 2-arachidonoylglycerol (2-AG), or the modulation of related compounds, such as the enzyme fatty acid amide hydrolase (FAAH), wherein the increased tone of AEA and 2-AG (or the decreased tone of FAAH) has been associated with improved sleep (Kesner and Lovinger 2020; see Fig. 2).

Key fact: Some treatments for disordered sleep involve modifying the tone of endocannabinoids with the goal of modulating circadian rhythms.

Both THC and CBD bind to CB_1, wherein THC is a partial agonist for CB_1, CBD acts as a weak CB_1 agonist (Thomas et al. 2007), and both exogenous cannabinoids have effects on AEA and FAAH. Some work suggests that THC diminishes circadian rhythms in humans (Nicholson et al. 2004; Perron et al. 2001) and reduces sleep onset latency (SOL) and REM sleep, while increasing slow-wave sleep (SWS) in the short term and decreasing SWS in the long term (Kaul et al. 2021). Though understudied, CBD is nonintoxicating and dose dependent (Shannon et al. 2019b) and may have positive effects on sleep outcomes. Specifically, high doses of CBD have a sedative effect, while low doses have a stimulating effect (Carlini and Cunha 1981; Conroy and Arnedt 2014; Nicholson et al. 2004; Russo et al. 2007), though long-term effects have not been studied (Kaul et al. 2021). Research is mixed as to whether CBD may also have a synergistic relationship to THC, such that

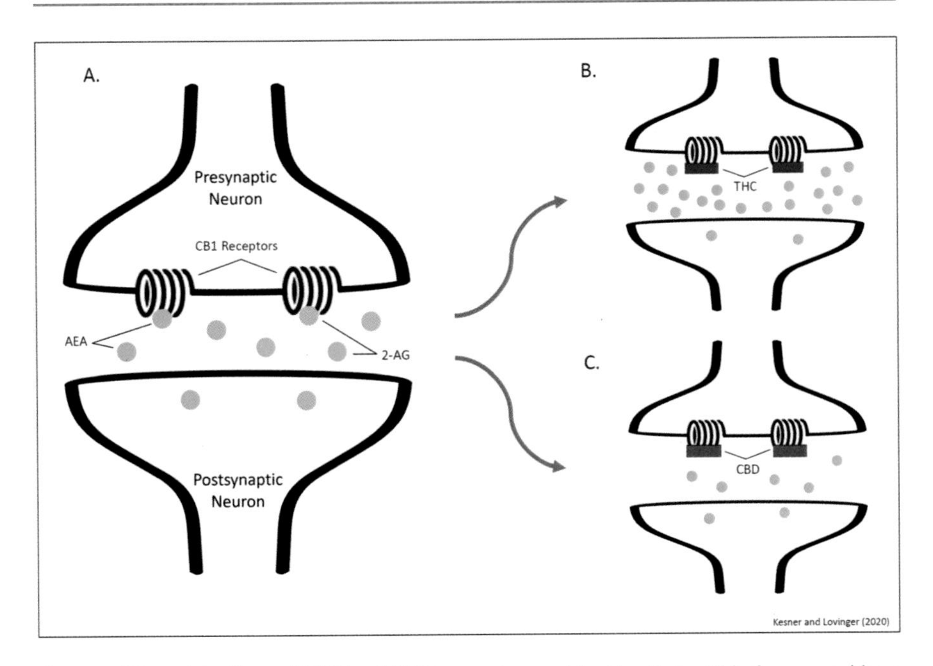

Fig. 2 Differential effects of THC and CBD on endocannabinoid activity. This figure provides a simplified depiction of the differential effects of THC and CBD on endocannabinoid activity. (**a**) ECS neurotransmitters anandamide (AEA) and 2-arachidonoylglycerol (2-AG) are released from postsynaptic neurons to bind to CB1 receptors on presynaptic neurons. (**b**) THC partially binds to CB1 receptors, which increases endocannabinoid activity while possibly disrupting circadian rhythms. (**c**) CBD binds weakly to CB1 receptors, eliciting a dose-dependent effect on both ECS activity and sleep outcomes. High doses appear to have a sedative effect while low doses appear to have a stimulating effect

coadministration of CBD may mitigate intoxication, impaired cognition, and subjective affective effects of THC (Bhattacharyya et al. 2010; Demirakca et al. 2011). Whether the synergistic relationship between these two cannabinoids has any effect on sleep processes is yet to be studied in depth. One study using EEG monitoring reported that CBD at higher doses countered the sedative effects of THC, as well as increased "awake" activity during sleep in a sample of young adults (Nicholson et al. 2004).

Even less attention has been paid in the literature to the relationship between sleep and other constituent compounds of the cannabis plant, such as other cannabinoids or terpenes. There are 100 s of compounds within the cannabis plant that fall into these two categories but remain greatly understudied. It is hypothesized that they have varying synergistic relationships with THC and CBD (Russo 2011), otherwise known as "entourage effects" (Ben-Shabat et al. 1998), but there is no research date on the relationship between these effects and sleep. Simultaneously, preclinical research on terpenes – unsaturated hydrocarbons found in the oils of the plant – such as linalool (Xu et al. 2021), limonene (Park et al. 2011), citral and myrcene (Do Vale et al. 2002), and phytoncide (Woo and Lee 2020) may have effects on sleep processes.

Key fact: The "entourage effect" hypothesis suggests that the constituent components of cannabis such as cannabinoids and terpenes have varying synergistic relationships with each other, modifying the effects of compounds on their own.

Taken together, while the data on THC and CBD suggest potential benefit for sleep from both compounds separately and together, the effects of these compounds vary greatly depending on the mode of administration, whether the product is synthetic or plant-based, and the THC potency of the product. It will be important for future research to account for these critical factors, as their relationship to both positive and negative effects of cannabis on sleep.

Long-Term Use of Cannabis and Cannabis Use Disorder (CUD)

It is possible that long-term regular cannabis use, and especially the use of high THC products, leads to tolerance to sleep-inducing effects (Babson et al. 2017; Freeman and Winstock 2015), yet no studies have examined this (Colizzi and Bhattacharyya 2018). Potential development of tolerance to sleep-inducing effects might in turn be associated with escalation of dose and frequency of use, in order to achieve the sought out benefits of cannabis, which might be associated with cannabis use disorder (CUD) (Fergusson et al. 2003). In other words, chronic use of cannabis may cause habituation to the sleep-inducing and slow-wave sleep-enhancing properties of cannabis, leading to CUD. Regular users may find themselves in a vicious cycle of using cannabis to manage sleep, habituating to the effects, and using more cannabis in order to obtain the desired impact, resulting in problematic patterns of use. While sleep disruption has been demonstrated to be a consistently primary factor in cannabis withdrawal and relapse (Kesner and Lovinger 2020), no research to date has examined transition to CUD or tolerance to sleep-inducing effects in medical users, and among recreational users, there are no studies that have examined tolerance to sleep-inducing effects.

Chronic use of cannabis is associated with a large array of sleep deficits including sleep quality problems, sleep disturbances, prolonged latency to sleep onset, lower sleep duration, and insomnia. Conroy et al. (2016) found that daily cannabis users reported more insomnia symptoms and decreased sleep quality compared to both non-daily users and nonusers. Interestingly, sleep scores were similar between non-daily users and nonusers, which suggests occasional users might not experience the same magnitude of cannabis-related sleep disturbance as reported by daily users. Sleep disturbances are the hallmark of cannabis withdrawal and may serve to maintain use and predict relapse. Studies have demonstrated a link between quit success and rates of lapse/relapse to cannabis use. For example, Budney et al. (2008) found that 65% of cannabis users reported poor sleep as a primary reason for lapse/relapse to cannabis.

Applications to Other Areas of Substance Use Disorders

In addition to CUD, there are other well-documented connections between substance use and disrupted sleep. Alcohol has long been documented to disrupt sleep quality and be related to daytime impairment (Park et al. 2015; Vitiello 1997) and greater risk for OSA (Burgos-Sanchez et al. 2020), and yet it is often used to self-medicate sleep disruptions due to its acute sedative effects (Park et al. 2015; Vitiello 1997). Similarly, smoking also has been consistently associated with sleep disturbance and sleep-related disordered breathing (Amiri and Behnezhad 2020) and, like alcohol, a cyclical pattern of poor sleep, precipitating greater cravings and withdrawal (Purani et al. 2019). In fact, not only is disrupted sleep a risk factor for relapse in alcohol use but also it is likely a universal risk factor for relapse across many classes of substances (Brower and Perron 2010). In the case of illicit drug use, there is increasing evidence that while sleep and drug addiction share many neurobiological processes, different substance have negative effects on the different aspects of sleep or sleep stages and that these negative effects can persist long after substance use is discontinued (Gordon 2019). Many people perceive OTC sleep aids and herbal remedies for disrupted sleep to be safe and effective compared to self-medication with other substances such as alcohol. However, even these substances can be associated with undesirable side effects, tolerance and decreased efficacy, or dependence (Randall et al. 2008). Given the challenges associated with the use of any pharmacological sleep intervention, it will be important to continue to understand what the safest and most efficacious treatments for disrupted sleep are.

Implications and Future Directions

While there is some evidence for a relationship between cannabis use and sleep disturbance, there is also increasing evidence that cannabis can be of benefit to sleep disturbances in certain circumstances. Medical cannabis laws and policies are rapidly changing as more people increasingly use cannabis for therapeutic benefits such as aiding sleep. Data suggests that OTC sleep aids are being increasingly substituted with the use of cannabis to improve sleep disturbance with or without comorbidity with other conditions such as depression, PTSD, and chronic pain. There is no reason to believe that this trend will reverse; thus, there is a burgeoning need for research to better inform public policy and personal choice when it comes to cannabis use for sleep. Future directions for the field should work to quickly disseminate findings in the following areas.

Comparison of Plant-Based and Synthetic Cannabinoids in Relation to Sleep

Synthetic cannabinoids are used both as legal pharmacological agents, in clinical research settings, as well as illegal drugs. Unlike plant-based cannabinoids, synthetics are full agonists and have higher affinity for CB_1 receptors (Le Boisselier et al. 2017). While legal synthetics such as nabilone have been investigated for use to support sleep (such as in the case of PTSD (Sholler et al. 2020), there are risks associated with illicit cannabinoids such as prolonged effects and a higher abuse liability that may also impact sleep outcomes (Alves et al. 2020; Mills et al. 2015). Importantly, there are no studies to date comparing the effects of synthetic and plant-based cannabis on sleep. Future research is needed to understand whether important factors such as PK differences or entourage effects modify the effects of cannabis on sleep.

The Effects of Mode of Administration, Dosages, and Potencies

The cannabinoid content of cannabis used in most existing studies to date is either unknown (observational studies) or limited in terms of dose and potencies (Suraev et al. 2020). Randomized control trials (RCTs) tend to measure the effect of only one or two cannabinoids that are administrated according to a pre-set research protocol, and these conditions bear little resemblance to real-world use, which include long-term use (Cohen et al. 2016; Sznitman et al. 2020), ad libitum administration, administration by inhalation (MacCallum and Russo 2018), and whole plant product use (Clark et al. 2004; Ware et al. 2003). While RCTs with emphasis on internal validity play an important role in the scientific literature, there is a growing need to test the relationship between cannabis use and sleep using long-term follow-up data with high external validity to validate related experimental and laboratory findings.

Data Needed to Capture Pre-Onset of Use, Short-Term Use, and Long-Term Use

As noted above, most real-world cannabis use to treat symptoms such as sleep disturbances is long term (Cohen et al. 2016; Sznitman et al. 2020), and naturalistic research often does not capture pre-onset of use symptom levels. Furthermore, little to no research has been conducted on sleep outcomes that specifically compares short-term and long-term use of cannabis. Given that the data current available suggests that the benefits of cannabis for sleep decrease with long-term use (Babson et al. 2017), more research is needed over longer time frames to understand this relationship over months or years.

Comparison of Cannabis Use Exclusively as a Sleep Aid Versus the Effects of Cannabis Use for Comorbid Conditions on Sleep Outcomes

To reach a better understanding of how cannabis influences sleep, research should examine whether cannabis use infers direct or indirect beneficial effects on sleep. For example, research that examined cannabis and sleep in the realm of chronic pain has reported on sleep outcomes (Russo et al. 2007; Ware et al. 2010; Ware and Ferguson 2015). Yet, these studies have not tested whether the effects on sleep are direct or if they achieve their sleep effects through a reduction in pain symptoms. A better understanding of direct and indirect effects will help elucidate the mechanisms underlying sleep effects of cannabis. Furthermore, examining the effects of cannabis on sleep in the realm of pain reduction may open up a rare window into examining how sleep expectations influence cannabis use effects on sleep. Indeed, it is possible that positive sleep expectations are low in chronic pain patients (or patients who use for other non-sleep symptoms), and thus, comparing sleep effects in these populations to patients who are explicitly using cannabis as sleep aid may aid in further understanding of the mechanisms by which cannabis relates to sleep.

Comparison of Sleep Outcomes Between Recreational and Medical Cannabis Users

Sleep problems may be particularly prevalent in medical cannabis patients, as the conditions that are typically providing access to medical cannabis licenses (e.g. pain, PTSD, cancer) are associated with sleep disturbances (Breslau et al. 1996). Recreational users may have fewer sleep problems than medical users, but long-term regular use of cannabis produces tolerance and dependence which in turn lead to sleep problems (Babson et al. 2017; Freeman and Winstock 2015). As such, frequent and high potency THC recreational users may also be suffering from sleep disturbances at high rates. Disentangling causes of sleep problems (cannabis dependence vs. primary health problems being treated with cannabis) is important to better understand both the benefits and potential risks of cannabis in relation to sleep disturbances. This could be achieved by following and comparing cannabis users who use cannabis recreationally, who use cannabis primarily as a sleep aid, and who use cannabis primarily to treat a sleep-comorbid condition.

Conclusion

Sleep disturbance is linked to a wide range of adverse physical and mental health outcomes, including mortality. Current pharmacological treatments for sleep disorders are numerous and diverse, and there is increasing evidence from preclinical research and RCTs that cannabis may be a promising treatment for primary sleep disorders or comorbid sleep disturbances. Cannabis use is associated with sleep disturbance; however, there is increasing evidence that cannabis can be of benefit to sleep disturbances in certain circumstances, such as comorbidity with insomnia, OSA, depression, PTSD, among others. More research is needed to understand the risks and benefits of cannabis, and its component cannabinoids, in relation to sleep for different types of users.

Mini Dictionary

- *Δ9-tetrahydrocannabinol (THC)* – A lipid phytocannabinoid constituent of the cannabis plant that is responsible for the psychoactive properties of cannabis.

- *Cannabidiol (CBD)* – A lipid phytocannabinoid constituent of the cannabis plant that, along with THC, most commonly accounts for the extracted contents of the cannabis plant. CBD is non-intoxicated and is believed to have potential synergistic effects with THC as well as anti-inflammatory properties.
- *Cannabis use disorder (CUD)* – A substance use disorder characterized by the Diagnostic and Statistical Manual (DSM) as continued, chronic use of cannabis despite functional and behavior impairment that is clinically significant.
- *Circadian rhythms* – Physiological and behavioral changes that occur on a 24-hour cycle.
- *Endogenous cannabinoids* – Endogenous lipid neurotransmitters expressed throughout the nervous system.
- *Exogenous cannabinoids* – Exogenous lipid-based compounds such as phytocannabinoids that interact with the same cannabinoid receptor sites as endogenous cannabinoids.
- *Late insomnia* – A form of insomnia that involves early-morning awakening with difficulty falling back asleep.
- *Nabiximols (Sativex)* – A pharmaceutical extract of THC and CBD administered as an oral mucosal drug approved to treat symptoms of pain and spasticity.
- *Parasomnias* – Abnormal behaviors that occur during specific stages of sleep.
- *REM sleep – A sleep stage* characterized by physical paralysis and increased brain activity relative to non-REM sleep.
- *Sleep disorders* – Persistent, debilitating sleep disturbances that are not attributable to other causes.
- *Sleep/wake system* – A circadian rhythm that maintains homeostasis by balancing our need for sleep with our need to stay awake and alert during the day.
- *Sleep-maintenance insomnia* – A sleep disorder that involves numerous or prolonged awakenings during the night.
- *Sleep-onset insomnia* – A sleep disorder that involves trouble falling asleep at bedtime.

Summary Points

1. The limited effectiveness and tolerability of existing sleep aids indicates a critical need for viable alternatives.
2. Findings on cannabis and sleep are often inconsistent across studies, likely due to a combination of varying user characteristics – such as duration and frequency of use – and different formulations and potencies employed by different research designs.
3. Some research supports a bidirectional relationship between sleep and cannabis use, such that sleep disturbance increases cannabis use and risk of misuse, while long-term cannabis use increases risk of sleep disturbance.
4. Other emerging research supports cannabis and cannabis-derived compounds in the treatment of sleep disorders, as well as sleep disturbance secondary to other diagnoses such as chronic pain, post-traumatic stress disorder (PTSD), and depression.

5. Future research directions on cannabis and sleep should include 1) comparison of plant-based and synthetic cannabinoids in relation to sleep; 2) comparison of different modes of administration, dosages, and potencies; 3) comparison of different durations of cannabis use (i.e., pre-onset of use, short-term use, and long-term use); 4) comparison of cannabis use exclusively as a sleep aid versus effects of cannabis on sleep outcomes comorbid with other conditions; and 5) comparison of sleep outcomes between recreational and medical cannabis users.

References

Abuhasira R, Ron A, Sikorin I et al (2019) Medical cannabis for older patients – treatment protocol and initial results. J Clin Med 8(11):1819. https://doi.org/10.3390/jcm8111819. MDPI AG

Almojali AI, Almalki SA, Alothman AS et al (2017) The prevalence and association of stress with sleep quality among medical students. J Epidemiol Glob Health 7(3):169–174. https://doi.org/10.1016/j.jegh.2017.04.005. Elsevier Ltd

Alves VL, Gonçalves JL, Aguiar J et al (2020) The synthetic cannabinoids phenomenon: from structure to toxicological properties. A review. Crit Rev Toxicol. https://doi.org/10.1080/10408444.2020.1762539. Taylor and Francis Ltd

American Psychiatric Association (2013) Diagnostic and statistical manual of mental disorders, 5th edn. American Psychiatric Association, Arlington. https://doi.org/10.1176/appi.books.9780890425596

Amiri S, Behnezhad S (2020) Smoking and risk of sleep-related issues: a systematic review and meta-analysis of prospective studies. Can J Public Health 111(5):775–786. https://doi.org/10.17269/S41997-020-00308-3. Springer

Angarita GA, Emadi N, Hodges S et al (2016) Sleep abnormalities associated with alcohol, cannabis, cocaine, and opiate use: a comprehensive review. Addict Sci Clin Pract. https://doi.org/10.1186/s13722-016-0056-7. BioMed Central Ltd

Babson KA, Boden MT, Bonn-Miller MO (2013) Sleep quality moderates the relation between depression symptoms and problematic cannabis use among medical cannabis users. Am J Drug Alcohol Abuse 39(3):211–216. https://doi.org/10.3109/00952990.2013.788183

Babson KA, Sottile J, Morabito D (2017) Cannabis, cannabinoids, and sleep: a review of the literature. Curr Psychiatry Rep 19(23):1–12. https://doi.org/10.1007/s11920-017-0775-9

Bachhuber M, Arnsten JH, Wurm G (2019) Use of cannabis to relieve pain and promote sleep by customers at an adult use dispensary. J Psychoactive Drugs 51(5):400–404. https://doi.org/10.1080/02791072.2019.1626953. Routledge

Baumbusch J, Sloan Yip I (2021) Exploring new use of cannabis among older adults. Clin Gerontol 44(1):25–31. https://doi.org/10.1080/07317115.2020.1746720. Routledge

Belendiuk KA, Babson KA, Vandrey R et al (2015) Cannabis species and cannabinoid concentration preference among sleep-disturbed medicinal cannabis users. Addict Behav 50:178–181. https://doi.org/10.1016/j.addbeh.2015.06.032. Elsevier Ltd

Ben-Shabat S, Fride E, Sheskin T et al (1998) An entourage effect: inactive endogenous fatty acid glycerol esters enhance 2-arachidonoyl-glycerol cannabinoid activity. Eur J Pharmacol 353(1): 23–31. https://doi.org/10.1016/S0014-2999(98)00392-6

Bhattacharyya S, Morrison PD, Fusar-Poli P et al (2010) Opposite effects of Δ-9-tetrahydrocannabinol and cannabidiol on human brain function and psychopathology. Neuropsychopharmacology 35(3):764–774. https://doi.org/10.1038/npp.2009.184. Nature Publishing Group

Blevins CE, Banes KE, Stephens RS et al (2016) Change in motives among frequent cannabis-using adolescents: predicting treatment outcomes. Drug Alcohol Depend 167:175–181. https://doi.org/10.1016/j.drugalcdep.2016.08.018. Elsevier Ireland Ltd

Boehnke KF, Gangopadhyay S, Clauw DJ et al (2019) Qualifying conditions of medical cannabis license holders in the United States. Health Aff 38(2):295–302. https://doi.org/10.1377/hlthaff.2018.05266. Project HOPE

Bollu PC, Manjamalai S, Thakkar M et al (2018) Hypersomnia. Mo Med 115(1):85. Missouri State Medical Association

Bonn-Miller MO, Babson KA, Vandrey R (2014) Using cannabis to help you sleep: heightened frequency of medical cannabis use among those with PTSD. Drug Alcohol Depend 136(1):162–165. https://doi.org/10.1016/j.drugalcdep.2013.12.008

Borbély AA, Daan S, Wirz-Justice A et al (2016) The two-process model of sleep regulation: a reappraisal. J Sleep Res 25(2):131–143. https://doi.org/10.1111/JSR.12371

Borodovsky JT, Crosier BS, Lee DC et al (2016) Smoking, vaping, eating: is legalization impacting the way people use cannabis? Int J Drug Policy 36:141–147. https://doi.org/10.1016/j.drugpo.2016.02.022. Elsevier B.V

Breslau N, Roth T, Rosenthal L et al (1996) Sleep disturbance and psychiatric disorders: a longitudinal epidemiological study of young adults. Biol Psychiatry 39(6):411–418. https://doi.org/10.1016/0006-3223(95)00188-3. Elsevier USA

Brower KJ, Perron BE (2010) Sleep disturbance as a universal risk factor for relapse in addictions to psychoactive substances. Med Hypotheses 74(5):928–933. https://doi.org/10.1016/J.MEHY.2009.10.020. Churchill Livingstone

Budney AJ, Vandrey RG, Hughes JR et al (2008) Comparison of cannabis and tobacco withdrawal: severity and contribution to relapse. J Subst Abus Treat 35(4):362–368. https://doi.org/10.1016/J.JSAT.2008.01.002. Pergamon

Burgos-Sanchez C, Jones NN, Avillion M et al (2020) Impact of alcohol consumption on snoring and sleep apnea: a systematic review and meta-analysis. Otolaryngol–Head Neck Surg 163(6): 1078–1086. https://doi.org/10.1177/0194599820931087. SAGE Publications, Los Angeles

Calik MW, Radulovacki M, Carley DW (2014) Intranodose ganglion injections of dronabinol attenuate serotonin-induced apnea in Sprague-Dawley rat. Respir Physiol Neurobiol 190(1): 20–24. https://doi.org/10.1016/j.resp.2013.10.001

Cappuccio FP, D'Elia L, Strazzullo P et al (2010) Sleep duration and all-cause mortality: a systematic review and meta-analysis of prospective studies. Sleep 33(5):585–592. https://doi.org/10.1093/sleep/33.5.585. American Academy of Sleep Medicine

Cappuccio FP, Cooper D, Delia L et al (2011) Sleep duration predicts cardiovascular outcomes: a systematic review and meta-analysis of prospective studies. Eur Heart J. https://doi.org/10.1093/eurheartj/ehr007

Carlini EA, Cunha JM (1981) Hypnotic and antiepileptic effects of Cannabidiol. J Clin Pharmacol 21(S1):417S–427S. https://doi.org/10.1002/j.1552-4604.1981.tb02622.x. John Wiley & Sons, Ltd

Carley DW, Paviovic S, Janelidze M, Radulovacki M. (2002) Functional role for cannabinoids in respiratory stability during sleep. Sleep. 15;25(4):391–8

Castaneto MS, Gorelick DA, Desrosiers NA et al (2014) Synthetic cannabinoids: epidemiology, pharmacodynamics, and clinical implications. Drug Alcohol Depend 144:12–41. https://doi.org/10.1016/j.drugalcdep.2014.08.005. Elsevier Ireland Ltd

Chagas MHN, Eckeli AL, Zuardi AW et al (2014) Cannabidiol can improve complex sleep-related behaviours associated with rapid eye movement sleep behaviour disorder in Parkinson's disease patients: a case series. J Clin Pharm Ther 39(5):564–566. https://doi.org/10.1111/jcpt.12179. Blackwell Publishing Ltd

Chait LD, Zacny JP (1992) Reinforcing and subjective effects of oral Δ9-THC and smoked marijuana in humans. Psychopharmacology 107(2–3):255–262. https://doi.org/10.1007/BF02245145. Springer-Verlag

Clark AJ, Ware MA, Yazer E et al (2004) Patterns of cannabis use among patients with multiple sclerosis. Neurology 62(11):2098–2100. https://doi.org/10.1212/01.WNL.0000127707.07621.72. Lippincott Williams and Wilkins

Cognitive Behavioral Therapy is an Effective Treatment for Chronic Insomnia (2009). https://aasm.org/cognitive-behavioral-therapy-is-an-effective-treatment-for-chronic-insomnia/. Accessed 30 July 2021

Cohen NL, Heinz AJ, Ilgen M et al (2016) Pain, cannabis species, and cannabis use disorders. J Stud Alcohol Drugs 77(3):515–520. https://doi.org/10.15288/jsad.2016.77.515. Alcohol Research Documentation Inc

Colizzi M, Bhattacharyya S (2018) Cannabis use and the development of tolerance: a systematic review of human evidence. Neurosci Biobehav Rev 93:1–25. https://doi.org/10.1016/j.neubiorev.2018.07.014. Elsevier Ltd

Conroy DA, Arnedt JT (2014) Sleep and substance use disorders: an update. Curr Psychiatry Rep. https://doi.org/10.1007/s11920-014-0487-3. Current Medicine Group LLC 1

Conroy, DA, Kurth, ME, Strong, DR, Brower, KJ, & Stein, MD (2016) Marijuana use patterns and sleep among community-based young adults. J Addict Dis 35(2):135–143. https://doi.org/10.1080/10550887.2015.1132986

Demirakca T, Sartorius A, Ende G et al (2011) Diminished gray matter in the hippocampus of cannabis users: possible protective effects of cannabidiol. Drug Alcohol Depend 114(2–3):242–245. https://doi.org/10.1016/j.drugalcdep.2010.09.020. Elsevier Ireland Ltd

World Health Organization (2017) Depression and other common mental disorders: global health estimates. Geneva

Do Vale TG, Furtado EC, Santos JG et al (2002) Central effects of citral, myrcene and limonene, constituents of essential oil chemotypes from Lippia alba (mill.) N.E. Brown. Phytomedicine 9(8):709–714. https://doi.org/10.1078/094471102321621304. Urban & Fischer

Doremus JM, Stith SS, Vigil JM (2019) Using recreational cannabis to treat insomnia: evidence from over-the-counter sleep aid sales in Colorado. Complement Ther Med 47:102207. https://doi.org/10.1016/j.ctim.2019.102207. Churchill Livingstone

Ek J, Jacobs W, Kaylor B et al (2021) Addiction and sleep disorders. In: Advances in experimental medicine and biology. Springer, pp 163–171. https://doi.org/10.1007/978-3-030-61663-2_12

ElSohly MA, Mehmedic Z, Foster S et al (2016) Changes in cannabis potency over the last 2 decades (1995–2014): analysis of current data in the United States. Biol Psychiatry 79(7): 613–619. https://doi.org/10.1016/j.biopsych.2016.01.004. Elsevier

Ewusi Boisvert E, Bae D, Pang RD et al (2020) Subjective effects of combustible, vaporized, and edible cannabis: results from a survey of adolescent cannabis users. Drug Alcohol Depend 206. https://doi.org/10.1016/j.drugalcdep.2019.107716. Elsevier Ireland Ltd

Farabi SS, Prasad B, Quinn L et al (2014) Impact of dronabinol on quantitative electroencephalogram (qEEG) measures of sleep in obstructive sleep apnea syndrome. J Clin Sleep Med 10(01): 49–56. https://doi.org/10.5664/jcsm.3358. American Academy of Sleep Medicine

Feingold D, Weinstein A (2021) Cannabis and depression. In: Advances in experimental medicine and biology. Springer, pp 67–80. https://doi.org/10.1007/978-3-030-57369-0_5

Feingold D, Rehm J, Lev-Ran S (2017) Cannabis use and the course and outcome of major depressive disorder: a population based longitudinal study. Psychiatry Res 251:225–234. https://doi.org/10.1016/J.PSYCHRES.2017.02.027. Elsevier

Fergusson DM, Horwood LJ, Lynskey MT et al (2003) Early reactions to cannabis predict later dependence. Arch Gen Psychiatry 60(10):1033–1039. https://doi.org/10.1001/archpsyc.60.10.1033. American Medical Association

Fleetham JA, Fleming JAE (2014) Parasomnias. CMAJ 186(8):E273–E280. https://doi.org/10.1503/cmaj.120808. Canadian Medical Association

Fraigne JJ, Grace KP, Horner RL et al (2014) Mechanisms of REM sleep in health and disease. Curr Opin Pulm Med 20(6):527–532. https://doi.org/10.1097/MCP.0000000000000103

Fraser GA (2009) The use of a synthetic cannabinoid in the management of treatment-resistant nightmares in Posttraumatic Stress Disorder (PTSD). CNS Neurosci Ther 15(1):84–88. https://doi.org/10.1111/j.1755-5949.2008.00071.x. John Wiley & Sons, Ltd (10.1111)

Freeman TP, Winstock AR (2015) Examining the profile of high-potency cannabis and its association with severity of cannabis dependence. Psychol Med 45(15):3181–3189. https://doi.org/10.1017/S0033291715001178. Cambridge University Press

Fuller PM, Gooley JJ, Saper CB (2006) Neurobiology of the sleep-wake cycle: sleep architecture, circadian regulation, and regulatory feedback. J Biol Rhythms 21(6):482–493. https://doi.org/10.1177/0748730406294627. Sage Publications, Thousand Oaks

Gallicchio L, Kalesan B (2009) Sleep duration and mortality: a systematic review and meta-analysis. J Sleep Res 18(2):148–158. https://doi.org/10.1111/j.1365-2869.2008.00732.x. John Wiley & Sons, Ltd

Ghorayeb I (2020) More evidence of cannabis efficacy in restless legs syndrome. Sleep Breath 24(1):277–279. https://doi.org/10.1007/S11325-019-01978-1

Goel N, Rao H, Durmer JS et al (2009) Neurocognitive consequences of sleep deprivation. Semin Neurol 29(4):320–339. https://doi.org/10.1055/s-0029-1237117

Gooley JJ (2008) Treatment of circadian rhythm sleep disorders with light. Ann Acad Med Singap 37(8):669

Gordon HW (2019) Differential effects of addictive drugs on sleep and sleep stages. J Addict Res (OPAST Group) 3(2). https://doi.org/10.33140/JAR.03.02.01. NIH Public Access

Gorelick DA, Goodwin RS, Schwilke E et al (2013) Tolerance to effects of high-dose oral Δ9-tetrahydrocannabinol and plasma cannabinoid concentrations in male daily cannabis smokers. J Anal Toxicol 37(1):11–16. https://doi.org/10.1093/jat/bks081

Grandner MA (2017) Sleep, health, and society. Sleep Med Clin 12(1):1–22. https://doi.org/10.1016/j.jsmc.2016.10.012. W.B. Saunders

Grandner MA, Jackson NJ, Izci-Balserak B et al (2015) Social and behavioral determinants of perceived insufficient sleep: analysis of the behavioral risk factor surveillance system. Front Neurol 6. https://doi.org/10.3389/fneur.2015.00112. Frontiers Media S.A

Haario P, Rahkonen O, Laaksonen M et al (2013) Bidirectional associations between insomnia symptoms and unhealthy behaviours. J Sleep Res 22(1):89–95. https://doi.org/10.1111/j.1365-2869.2012.01043.x

Hart CL, Ward AS, Haney M et al (2002) Comparison of smoked marijuana and oral D 9-tetrahydrocannabinol in humans. Psychopharmacology 164:407–415. https://doi.org/10.1007/s00213-002-1231-y

Hasler BP, Smith LJ, Cousins JC et al (2012) Circadian rhythms, sleep, and substance abuse. Sleep Med Rev 16(1):67–81. https://doi.org/10.1016/j.smrv.2011.03.004

Haug NA, Padula CB, Sottile JE et al (2017) Cannabis use patterns and motives: a comparison of younger, middle-aged, and older medical cannabis dispensary patients. Addict Behav 72:14–20. https://doi.org/10.1016/j.addbeh.2017.03.006. NIH Public Access

Hazekamp A, Ware MA, Muller-Vahl KR et al (2013) The medicinal use of cannabis and cannabinoids – an international cross-sectional survey on administration forms. J Psychoactive Drugs 45(3):199–210. https://doi.org/10.1080/02791072.2013.805976. Routledge

Hser YI, Mooney LJ, Huang D et al (2017) Reductions in cannabis use are associated with improvements in anxiety, depression, and sleep quality, but not quality of life. J Subst Abus Treat 81:53–58. https://doi.org/10.1016/j.jsat.2017.07.012. Elsevier Inc

Huestis MA, Sampson AH, Holicky BJ et al (1992) Characterization of the absorption phase of marijuana smoking. Clin Pharmacol Ther 52(1):31–41. https://doi.org/10.1038/clpt.1992.100

Hutchison KE, Bidwell LC, Ellingson JM et al (2019) Medical cannabis research: rapid progress requires innovative research designs. Value Health 22(11):1289–1294

Innes KE, Selfe TK, Agarwal P (2011) Prevalence of restless legs syndrome in north American and Western European populations: a systematic review. Sleep Med 12(7):623–634. https://doi.org/10.1016/j.sleep.2010.12.018. Elsevier

Jetly R, Heber A, Fraser G et al (2015) The efficacy of nabilone, a synthetic cannabinoid, in the treatment of PTSD-associated nightmares: a preliminary randomized, double-blind, placebo-controlled cross-over design study. Psychoneuroendocrinology 51:585–588. https://doi.org/10.1016/j.psyneuen.2014.11.002. Elsevier Ltd

Kaul M, Zee PC, Sahni AS (2021) Effects of cannabinoids on sleep and their therapeutic potential for sleep disorders. Neurotherapeutics. https://doi.org/10.1007/s13311-021-01013-w. Springer Science and Business Media Deutschland GmbH

Kesner AJ, Lovinger DM (2020) Cannabinoids, endocannabinoids and sleep. Front Mol Neurosci. https://doi.org/10.3389/fnmol.2020.00125. Frontiers Media S.A
Killgore WDS (2010) Effects of sleep deprivation on cognition. Prog Brain Res 185:105–129. https://doi.org/10.1016/B978-0-444-53702-7.00007-5. Elsevier B.V
Knutson KL (2012) Does inadequate sleep play a role in vulnerability to obesity? Am J Hum Biol 24(3):361–371. https://doi.org/10.1002/ajhb.22219
Kosiba JD, Maisto SA, Ditre JW (2019) Patient-reported use of medical cannabis for pain, anxiety, and depression symptoms: systematic review and meta-analysis. Soc Sci Med 233:181–192. https://doi.org/10.1016/J.SOCSCIMED.2019.06.005. Pergamon
Kuhathasan N, Dufort A, MacKillop J et al (2019) The use of cannabinoids for sleep: a critical review on clinical trials. Exp Clin Psychopharmacol. https://doi.org/10.1037/pha0000285. American Psychological Association Inc
Kvamme SL, Pedersen MM, Alagem-Iversen S et al (2021) Beyond the high: mapping patterns of use and motives for use of cannabis as medicine. NAD Nordic Stud Alcohol Drugs 38(3):270–292. https://doi.org/10.1177/1455072520985967. SAGE Publications Ltd
Le Boisselier R, Alexandre J, Lelong-Boulouard V et al (2017) Focus on cannabinoids and synthetic cannabinoids. Clin Pharmacol Ther 101(2):220–229. https://doi.org/10.1002/cpt.563. Nature Publishing Group
Lin LA, Ilgen MA, Jannausch M et al (2016) Comparing adults who use cannabis medically with those who use recreationally: results from a national sample. Addict Behav 61:99–103. https://doi.org/10.1016/J.ADDBEH.2016.05.015. Pergamon
Lintzeris N, Driels J, Elias N et al (2018) Medicinal cannabis in Australia, 2016: the Cannabis as Medicine Survey (CAMS-16). Med J Aust 209(5):211–216. https://doi.org/10.5694/MJA17.01247. John Wiley & Sons, Ltd
Lund HG, Reider BD, Whiting AB et al (2010) Sleep patterns and predictors of disturbed sleep in a large population of college students. J Adolesc Health 46(2):124–132. https://doi.org/10.1016/j.jadohealth.2009.06.016
MacCallum CA, Russo EB (2018) Practical considerations in medical cannabis administration and dosing. Eur J Intern Med. https://doi.org/10.1016/j.ejim.2018.01.004. Elsevier B.V
Megelin T, Ghorayeb I (2017) Cannabis for restless legs syndrome: a report of six patients. Sleep Med 36:182–183. https://doi.org/10.1016/J.SLEEP.2017.04.019
Mills B, Yepes A, Nugent K (2015) Synthetic cannabinoids. Am J Med Sci. https://doi.org/10.1097/MAJ.0000000000000466. Lippincott Williams and Wilkins
Morin CM (2017) Issues and challenges in implementing clinical practice guideline for the management of chronic insomnia. J Sleep Res 26(6):673–674. https://doi.org/10.1111/JSR.12639. John Wiley & Sons, Ltd
Newmeyer MN, Swortwood MJ, Abulseoud OA et al (2017) Subjective and physiological effects, and expired carbon monoxide concentrations in frequent and occasional cannabis smokers following smoked, vaporized, and oral cannabis administration. Drug Alcohol Depend 175:67–76. https://doi.org/10.1016/j.drugalcdep.2017.02.003. Elsevier Ireland Ltd
Nicholson AN, Turner C, Stone BM et al (2004) Effect of Δ9-tetrahydrocannabinol and cannabidiol on nocturnal sleep and early-morning behavior in young adults. J Clin Psychopharmacol 24(3):305–313. https://doi.org/10.1097/01.jcp.0000125688.05091.8f
Ogbome AC, Smart RG, Weber T et al (2000) Who is using cannabis as a medicine and why: an exploratory study. J Psychoactive Drugs 32(4):435–443. https://doi.org/10.1080/02791072.2000.10400245. Taylor & Francis Group
Ogeil RP, Phillips JG, Rajaratnam SMW et al (2015) Risky drug use and effects on sleep quality and daytime sleepiness. Hum Psychopharmacol. https://doi.org/10.1002/hup.2483
Pacher P, Bátkai S, Kunos G (2006) The endocannabinoid system as an emerging target of pharmacotherapy. Pharmacol Rev. https://doi.org/10.1124/pr.58.3.2. NIH Public Access
Palesh OG, Roscoe JA, Mustian KM et al (2010) Prevalence, demographics, and psychological associations of sleep disruption in patients with cancer: University of Rochester Cancer Center-

community clinical oncology program. J Clin Oncol 28(2):292–298. https://doi.org/10.1200/JCO.2009.22.5011

Papaseit E, Pérez-Mañá C, Pérez-Acevedo AP et al (2018) Cannabinoids: from pot to lab. Int J Med Sci 15(12):1286–1295. https://doi.org/10.7150/ijms.27087. Ivyspring International Publisher

Park HM, Lee JH, Yaoyao J et al (2011) Limonene, a natural cyclic terpene, is an agonistic ligand for adenosine A2A receptors. Biochem Biophys Res Commun 404(1):345–348. https://doi.org/10.1016/j.bbrc.2010.11.121. Academic Press

Park S-Y, Oh M-K, Lee B-S et al (2015) The effects of alcohol on quality of sleep. Kor J Fam Med 36(6):294. https://doi.org/10.4082/KJFM.2015.36.6.294. Korean Academy of Family Medicine

Pavlova MK, Latreille V (2019) Sleep disorders. Am J Med 132(3):292–299. https://doi.org/10.1016/j.amjmed.2018.09.021

Peever J, Fuller PM (2017) The biology of REM sleep. Curr Biol 27(22):R1237–R1248. https://doi.org/10.1016/j.cub.2017.10.026. Cell Press

Perron RR, Tyson RL, Sutherland GR (2001) Δ9-tetrahydrocannabinol increases brain temperature and inverts circadian rhythms. Neuroreport 12(17):3791–3794. https://doi.org/10.1097/00001756-200112040-00038

Piper BJ, DeKeuster RM, Beals ML et al (2017) Substitution of medical cannabis for pharmaceutical agents for pain, anxiety, and sleep. J Psychopharmacol 31(5):569–575. https://doi.org/10.1177/0269881117699616

Poyatos L, Pérez-Acevedo AP, Papaseit E et al (2020) Oral administration of cannabis and Δ-9-tetrahydrocannabinol (Thc) preparations: a systematic review. Medicina (Lithuania) 56(6):1–28. https://doi.org/10.3390/medicina56060309

Prasad B, Radulovacki MG, Carley DW (2013) Proof of concept trial of dronabinol in obstructive sleep apnea. Front Psych 4. https://doi.org/10.3389/fpsyt.2013.00001

Purani H, Friedrichsen S, Allen AM (2019) Sleep quality in cigarette smokers: associations with smoking-related outcomes and exercise. Addict Behav 90:71–76. https://doi.org/10.1016/J.ADDBEH.2018.10.023. Pergamon

Ramar K, Olson EJ (2013) Management of common sleep disorders. Am Fam Physician 88(4):231–238

Randall S, Roehrs TA, Roth T (2008) Over-the-counter sleep aid medications and insomnia. Primary Psychiatry 15(5):52–58. https://www.researchgate.net/publication/228358857. Accessed 16 Aug 2021

Riemann D, Nissen C, Palagini L et al (2015) The neurobiology, investigation, and treatment of chronic insomnia. Lancet Neurol. https://doi.org/10.1016/S1474-4422(15)00021-6. Lancet Publishing Group

Riemann D, Baglioni C, Bassetti C et al (2017) European guideline for the diagnosis and treatment of insomnia. J Sleep Res 26(6):675–700. https://doi.org/10.1111/jsr.12594. Blackwell Publishing Ltd

Roth T (2007) Insomnia: definition, prevalence, etiology, and consequences. J Clin Sleep Med 3(5):S7–S8. https://doi.org/10.5664/jcsm.26929. American Academy of Sleep Medicine

Russo EB (2011) Taming THC: potential cannabis synergy and phytocannabinoid-terpenoid entourage effects. Br J Pharmacol 163(7):1344–1364. https://doi.org/10.1111/j.1476-5381.2011.01238.x. Blackwell Publishing Ltd

Russo EB, Guy GW, Robson PJ (2007) Cannabis, pain, and sleep: lessons from therapeutic clinical trials of sativexρ, a cannabis-based medicine. Chem Biodivers. https://doi.org/10.1002/cbdv.200790150

Sanford AE, Castillo E, Gannon RL (2008) Cannabinoids and hamster circadian activity rhythms. Brain Res 1222:141–148. https://doi.org/10.1016/j.brainres.2008.05.048. Elsevier

Sarris J, Sinclair J, Karamacoska D et al (2020) Medicinal cannabis for psychiatric disorders: a clinically-focused systematic review. BMC Psychiatry 20(1). https://doi.org/10.1186/s12888-019-2409-8. BioMed Central

Schutte-Rodin S, Broch L, Buysse D et al (2008) Clinical guideline for the evaluation and management of chronic insomnia in adults. J Clin Sleep Med 4(5):487–504. https://doi.org/10.5664/JCSM.27286. American Academy of Sleep Medicine

Sexton-Radek K, Burkes B, Levitt T et al (2020) Global sleep health in a COVID-19 virus-infected world. Int Med 2(2):99–101. https://doi.org/10.5455/im.102662
Shan Z, Ma H, Xie M et al (2015) Sleep duration and risk of type 2 diabetes: a meta-analysis of prospective studies. Diabetes Care 38(3):529–537. https://doi.org/10.2337/dc14-2073. American Diabetes Association Inc
Shannon S, Lewis N, Lee H et al (2019a) Cannabidiol in anxiety and sleep: a large case series. Perm J 23:18–041. https://doi.org/10.7812/TPP/18-041. NLM (Medline)
Shannon S, Lewis N, Lee H et al (2019b) Cannabidiol in anxiety and sleep: a large case series. Perm J 23. https://doi.org/10.7812/TPP/18-041. Kaiser Permanente
Sholler DJ, Huestis MA, Amendolara B et al (2020) Therapeutic potential and safety considerations for the clinical use of synthetic cannabinoids. Pharmacol Biochem Behav. https://doi.org/10.1016/j.pbb.2020.173059. Elsevier Inc
Slowik JM, Collen JF, Yow AG (2021) Narcolepsy. StatPearls Publishing. https://www.ncbi.nlm.nih.gov/books/NBK459236/. Accessed 30 July 2021
Suraev AS, Marshall NS, Vandrey R et al (2020) Cannabinoid therapies in the management of sleep disorders: a systematic review of preclinical and clinical studies. Sleep Med Rev 53:101339. https://doi.org/10.1016/j.smrv.2020.101339. Elsevier BV
Sznitman SR, Vulfsons S, Meiri D et al (2020) Medical cannabis and insomnia in older adults with chronic pain: a cross-sectional study. BMJ Support Palliat Care 10:415. https://doi.org/10.1136/bmjspcare-2019-001938
Tempesta D, Socci V, De Gennaro L et al (2018) Sleep and emotional processing. Sleep Med Rev 40:183–195. https://doi.org/10.1016/j.smrv.2017.12.005. W.B. Saunders Ltd
Thomas A, Baillie GL, Phillips AM et al (2007) Cannabidiol displays unexpectedly high potency as an antagonist of CB 1 and CB 2 receptor agonists in vitro. Br J Pharmacol 150(5):613–623. https://doi.org/10.1038/sj.bjp.0707133. John Wiley & Sons, Ltd
Tomfohr LM, Buliga E, Letourneau NL et al (2015) Trajectories of sleep quality and associations with mood during the perinatal period. Sleep 38(8):1237–1245. https://doi.org/10.5665/sleep.4900. Associated Professional Sleep Societies, LLC
Tringale R, Jensen C (2011) Cannabis and insomnia. Depression 4:0–68
Turna J, Balodis I, Munn C et al (2020) Overlapping patterns of recreational and medical cannabis use in a large community sample of cannabis users. Compr Psychiatry 102:152188. https://doi.org/10.1016/J.COMPPSYCH.2020.152188. W.B. Saunders
Vargas I, Nguyen AM, Muench A et al (2020) Acute and chronic insomnia: what has time and/or hyperarousal got to do with it? Brain Sci 10(2). https://doi.org/10.3390/BRAINSCI10020071. Multidisciplinary Digital Publishing Institute (MDPI)
Vitiello MV (1997) Sleep, alcohol and alcohol abuse. Addict Biol 2(2):151–158. https://doi.org/10.1080/13556219772697
Walsh Z, Callaway R, Belle-Isle L et al (2013) Cannabis for therapeutic purposes: patient characteristics, access, and reasons for use. Int J Drug Policy 24(6):511–516. https://doi.org/10.1016/j.drugpo.2013.08.010. Elsevier
Wang J, Zhang X, Simons SR et al (2020) Exploring the bi-directional relationship between sleep and resilience in adolescence. Sleep Med 73:63–69. https://doi.org/10.1016/j.sleep.2020.04.018. Elsevier B.V
Ware MA, Ferguson G (2015) Review article: sleep, pain and cannabis. J Sleep Disord Ther 04(02). https://doi.org/10.4172/2167-0277.1000191
Ware MA, Doyle CR, Woods R et al (2003) Cannabis use for chronic non-cancer pain: results of a prospective survey. Pain 102(1–2):211–216. https://doi.org/10.1016/s0304-3959(02)00400-1. Elsevier
Ware MA, Fitzcharles MA, Joseph L et al (2010) The effects of nabilone on sleep in fibromyalgia: results of a randomized controlled trial. Anesth Analg 110(2):604–610. https://doi.org/10.1213/ANE.0b013e3181c76f70
Weaver TE, Calik MW, Farabi SS et al (2014) Innovative treatments for adults with obstructive sleep apnea. Nat Sci Sleep. https://doi.org/10.2147/NSS.S46818. Dove Medical Press Ltd

Winiger EA, Hitchcock LN, Bryan AD et al (2021) Cannabis use and sleep: expectations, outcomes, and the role of age. Addict Behav 112. https://doi.org/10.1016/j.addbeh.2020.106642. Elsevier Ltd

Winstock A, Lynskey M, Borschmann R et al (2015) Risk of emergency medical treatment following consumption of cannabis or synthetic cannabinoids in a large global sample. J Psychopharmacol 29(6):698–703. https://doi.org/10.1177/0269881115574493. Sage

Woo J, Lee CJ (2020) Sleep-enhancing effects of phytoncide via behavioral, electrophysiological, and molecular modeling approaches. Exp Neurobiol. https://doi.org/10.5607/en20013. Korean Society for Neurodegenerative Disease

Xu L, Li X, Zhang Y et al (2021) The effects of linalool acupoint application therapy on sleep regulation. RSC Adv 11(11):5896–5902. https://doi.org/10.1039/d0ra09751a. Royal Society of Chemistry

Zettl UK, Rommer P, Hipp P et al (2016) Evidence for the efficacy and effectiveness of THC-CBD oromucosal spray in symptom management of patients with spasticity due to multiple sclerosis. Ther Adv Neurol Disord. https://doi.org/10.1177/1756285615612659

Sleep and Cannabis Online Resources

https://med.stanford.edu/insomnia.html
https://sleepeducation.org
https://www.cdc.gov/sleep/resources.html
https://www.nhlbi.nih.gov/health-topics/education-and-awareness/sleep-health
https://www.sleepassociation.org
https://www.sleepfoundation.org

65 The Reward System: What It Is and How It Is Altered in Cannabis Users

Natasha L. Mason, Peter van Ruitenbeek, and Johannes G. Ramaekers

Contents

Introduction 1400
The Reward System 1401
Acute Effects of Cannabis on the Reward System 1402
Acute Effect of THC on Resting State Functional Connectivity in Occasional Users 1403
Acute Effect of THC on Neurotransmission in Occasional Users 1407
Acute Effect of THC on Task-Related Brain Activity in Occasional Users 1410
Acute Effect of THC on Resting State Functional Connectivity and Neurotransmission in Chronic Users 1411
Acute Effect of THC on Task-Related Brain Activity in Chronic Users 1412
Persisting Effects of Cannabis on the Reward System 1412
Chronic Cannabis Use and Resting State Functional Connectivity 1412
Chronic Cannabis Use and Neurotransmission 1412
Chronic Cannabis Use and Task-Related Brain Activity 1423
Conclusion 1425
Application to Addiction 1428
Dorsal Striatal Dominance 1429
Increased Incentive Salience 1430
Decrease Response to Natural Reward 1430
Application to Public Health 1431
Summary Statements (5–15) 1431
Key Facts (5 Single Sentences) 1432
Mini-Dictionary of Terms 1432
References 1433

Abstract

Cannabis is the most commonly used illicit drug, most often reported to be used for its euphoric and relaxing effects. It is suggested that cannabis' interaction with the brain's reward system in particular may be of specific relevance to both the

N. L. Mason (✉) · P. van Ruitenbeek · J. G. Ramaekers
Department of Neuropsychology and Psychopharmacology, Faculty of Psychology and Neuroscience, Maastricht University, Maastricht, Netherlands
e-mail: natasha.mason@maastrichtuniversity.nl

V. B. Patel, V. R. Preedy (eds.), *Handbook of Substance Misuse and Addictions*, https://doi.org/10.1007/978-3-030-92392-1_71

euphoric and motivational effects of the drug and subsequently to the development of patterns of frequent, chronic use. Thus by understanding where and how cannabis acts on the system, insight may be obtained into whether and the extent to which cannabis has abuse liability from a biological perspective. Overall, research suggests that cannabis perturbs the brain's reward system via its action on dopaminergic and glutamatergic functioning. In occasional cannabis users, THC acutely increases dopamine and glutamate throughout the system, which disrupts fronto-striatal functional connectivity at rest, and blunts the neural response to rewarding stimuli. However, the effects of cannabis on the reward system are dynamic and change over time, according to frequency of use. Chronic cannabis users display opposite changes in dopaminergic and glutamatergic neurotransmission, suggesting the development of neuroadaptations following repeated cannabis use. Studies also suggest that cannabis has abuse liability, with chronic cannabis users displaying hyperresponsive reward circuitry following cannabis-related cues and reduced neural markers of cognitive control over habitual behavior, and some mixed evidence exists for hyporesponsiveness of the reward system towards natural rewards. In light of the growing therapeutic and recreational use of cannabis, it is suggested that governmental bodies should implicate public policy to mitigate the possibility that individual cannabis use develops into addiction.

Keywords

Cannabis · THC · Addiction · Dopamine · Glutamate · Reward · Neuroimaging · Nucleus accumbens · fMRI · Magnetic resonance spectroscopy · Functional connectivity

Abbreviations

BOLD	Blood-oxygen-level-dependent
CB1	cannabinoid receptor type 1
fMRI	functional magnetic resonance imaging
GABA	gamma-aminobutyric acid
MRS	magnetic resonance spectroscopy
Nac	nucleus accumbens
PET	positron emission tomography
THC	tetrahydrocannabinol
VTA	ventral tegmental area

Introduction

Cannabis is the most commonly used illicit drug, with an estimated 4% of the global population reportedly using the substance (UNODC 2020). Given the changing legal landscape and increased interest in therapeutic use, the prevalence of (long-term) cannabis use is expected to increase (Hall and Lynskey 2016). Thus, as cannabis use increases, and the perception of risk of use decreases (Johnston et al. 2018), a pertinent question is how cannabis use affects the brain and whether there are long-term (neurobiological) consequences (Zehra et al. 2018). Furthermore, as 10% of those who recreationally consume cannabis develop daily use patterns (World Health Organization 2016), it is of particular importance to understand the effect on neuro-circuitry which may underlie this increase and persistence of use. The most cited reason to sustain recreational cannabis use is due to cannabis' ability to induce acute feelings of euphoria and relaxation (Kettner et al. 2019), a common shared property of other drugs of abuse (Wise and Bozarth 1985). Second, daily use may signal the presence of addiction-associated brain mechanisms increasing motivational drive to consume cannabis. It is suggested that cannabis' interaction with the brain's reward system in particular may be of specific relevance to both the euphoric and motivational effects of the drug (Robinson and Berridge 1993, 2008; Kringelbach and Berridge 2012) and subsequently to the development of patterns of frequent, chronic use.

The Reward System

Reward is defined as any event that increases the probability of a response with a positive hedonic element (Koob and Volkow 2016). This definition encompasses a range of potential hedonic events with diverse rewarding outcomes, such as eating appetizing food, listening to music, and using (addictive) drugs (Kringelbach and Berridge 2012). That said, regardless of the type of rewarding event, reward processes appear to be similarly mediated in the brain via well-developed meso-corticolimbic circuitry, referred to collectively as the reward system (Kringelbach and Berridge 2012). The reward system consists of both subcortical and cortical brain regions, which are connected via various neurotransmitter projections, and can be divided into different pathways according to structure and function. Examples of such important subdivisions include the mesolimbic and the mesocortical dopaminergic pathways. Namely, upon presentation of a stimulus or cue that indicates a reward, dopaminergic neurons in the ventral tegmental area (VTA) respond, increasing transmission of dopamine throughout the brain. In the mesolimbic pathway, this includes projections to the nucleus accumbens (NAc), a brain region broadly implicated in acquiring behaviors in response to and eliciting behaviors in anticipation of rewarding stimuli. In the mesocortical pathway, this includes projections to prefrontal cortical regions such as the orbitofrontal cortex, medial frontal cortex, and the anterior cingulate, brain regions implicated in executive and inhibitory control, as well as motivation and salience attribution (Pierce and Kumaresan 2006; Volkow et al. 2011).

As well as via dopaminergic pathways, the reward system also receives major sources of innervation from glutamatergic projections. For example, the NAc receives further input from glutamatergic neurons of the hippocampus and amygdala, which are implicated in learning, conditioning, and memory. Additionally, glutamatergic afferents from the prefrontal cortex feedback to the VTA and to the

NAc, where they further modulate dopaminergic neurons. These projections form synapses with excitatory and inhibitory (GABAergic) pathways in the NAc, which relay back to the cortex and through the thalamus (Bonelli and Cummings 2007). Taken together, the glutamatergic pathways interacting with the reward system suggest a role in both acquiring stimulus-response associations and executive control.

In sum, the reward system consists of mesocorticolimbic circuitry which connects via dopaminergic, glutamatergic, and GABAergic neurotransmission. Of the brain regions implicated in this circuitry, the VTA and the NAc play central roles in the processing of rewarding events in order to predict future reward which provides motivation to perform behavior directed at obtaining that reward, such as the use of recreational drugs (Lupica et al. 2004). Thus by understanding where and how cannabis acts on the system, insight may be obtained into whether and the extent to which cannabis has abuse liability from a biological perspective.

Acute Effects of Cannabis on the Reward System

Once ingested, the main psychoactive component of cannabis (delta-9-tetrahydro-cannabinol; THC) binds to G-protein-coupled cannabinoid (CB1) receptors in the brain (Hashimotodani et al. 2007; Mackie 2008), which are abundantly located at presynaptic terminals or axons on glutamatergic and GABAergic neurons (Freund et al. 2003). The expression of CB1 receptors varies according to brain area and neuronal cell types. Namely, CB1 receptors exhibit higher expression on GABAergic neurons and are predominantly found in the basal ganglia, including the NAc, and at lower levels throughout the cortex, including frontal cortical areas, the hippocampus, and amygdala (Van Waes et al. 2012). Activation of CB1 receptors subsequently results in a suppression of glutamate and GABA release from presynaptic terminals, and CB1 receptor signaling results in inhibition of both glutamatergic and GABAergic synaptic transmission (Freund et al. 2003; Hashimotodani et al. 2007; Ramaekers et al. 2020). Due to the predominantly presynaptic location of CB1 receptors, and the powerful inhibitory effects on both glutamatergic and GABAergic transmission in the basal ganglia and beyond, CB1 receptor activation and signaling can modulate a wide range of neurotransmitter circuits, including the reward system.

Multiple human neuroimaging studies have been conducted in order to assess acute cannabis-induced alterations in brain activity (reviewed in Bloomfield et al. 2019, Gunasekera et al. 2020). Studies of metabolic brain activity, utilizing methodologies such as functional magnetic resonance imaging (fMRI), xenon-enhanced computed tomography, positron emission tomography (PET), and arterial spin labeling, have generally found acute increments in cerebral blood flow and metabolism in reward-related frontal and subcortical regions (Mathew et al. 1989, 1992a, b; Van Hell et al. 2011). These studies have demonstrated that the brain regions modulated by THC broadly overlap with regions implicated in the reward system. That said, as these regions also contain the highest concentrations of CB1 receptors, these metabolic changes may be due to direct endocannabinoid effects, rather than reflecting processes mediated via reward circuitry (Bloomfield et al. 2016). Thus in order to establish more direct effects of cannabis (and subsequently THC) on reward-related function, studies have utilized fMRI, PET, and magnetic resonance spectroscopy (MRS) to assess functional connectivity (FC) between areas of the reward system, neurometabolite concentrations such as dopamine, glutamate, and GABA in reward system brain areas, and have employed tasks on which performance is modulated by the reward system. Importantly, as there is evidence of differential effects of occasional versus repeated cannabis exposure on the reward system, studies conducted in these different populations have demonstrated that the effects of THC on reward-related circuitry are dynamic, and change over time, which may signal abuse potential.

Acute Effect of THC on Resting State Functional Connectivity in Occasional Users

Utilizing fMRI to assess functional connectivity changes at rest, studies have mainly found acute THC-induced reductions in functional connectivity in occasional users between areas of the reward system (Tables 1 and 3). Across these studies, occasional users have been broadly defined as those who have used cannabis between <10 times in their life, up to those who use <3 times a week. The most common focus of these studies has been investigating functional connectivity between striatal areas, including the putamen, caudate, and NAc, and the rest of the brain (Mason et al. 2019; Crane and Phan 2021; Ramaekers et al. 2016; Grimm et al. 2018). Three out of the five studies found THC acutely decreased synchronicity between the NAc and other areas of the reward system, including the ventral pallidum (involved in reward; hedonic experience (Kringelbach and Berridge 2012)), the prefrontal cortex and midcingulate areas (involved in executive and inhibitory control), and the anterior insula and thalamus (both involved in the salience network, which detects salient stimuli and subsequently generates a relevant behavioral response) (Mason et al. 2019; Ramaekers et al. 2016). Conversely, one study did not find any changes in functional connectivity between the dorsal striatum (putamen and caudate) and the rest of the brain (Grimm et al. 2018), whereas another study found an *increase* in functional connectivity between the right nucleus accumbens and right medial and dorsomedial prefrontal cortex (Crane and Phan 2021) after oral ingestion of THC. That said, these studies found either insufficient blood THC concentration levels during times of scanning (Grimm et al. 2018) or did not collect pharmacokinetic data at the time of scanning (Crane and Phan 2021). This is important to note, as the pharmacokinetic profile of oral formulations of THC are slower and less intense than inhaled THC; thus it could be suggested that the discrepancy between the vaporized (Mason et al. 2019; Mason et al. 2021; Ramaekers et al. 2016) and orally ingested cannabis (Grimm et al. 2018; Crane and Phan 2021)) could be due to the window of maximal THC effects happening outside of the scanner in the latter studies. In accordance with this suggestion, previous studies have found that THC-induced

Table 1 Acute and chronic effects of THC on functional connectivity between brain regions of the reward system

Reference	A/C	Population	Paradigm	Measurement	Seed	SN	VTA	St	Nac	VP	Amy	Hip	mPF	ACC	OFC	Ins	TPJ	Tha
Klumpers, 2012	A	OU	Rest	BOLD	Salience network													
Grim, 2018	A	OU	Rest	BOLD	Putamen													
	A				Caudate													
Mason, 2018	A	OU	Rest	BOLD	NAc													
Bossong, 2019	A	OU	Rest	BOLD	Insula													
	A	OU	Rest	BOLD	Medial superior frontal cortex													
	A	OU	Rest	BOLD	Middle orbital frontal gyrus													
Wall, 2019	A	OU	Rest	BOLD	Insula													
Crane, 2021	A	OU	Rest	BOLD	NAc													
	A				Putamen													
	A				Caudate													
Mason, 2019	A	OU	Rest	BOLD	ROI													
	A	CU	Rest	BOLD	ROI													
Ramaekers, 2016	A	FR	Rest	BOLD	Nac													
van Hell, 2012	A	OU	Task - reward processing	BOLD	ROI													
Jansma, 2013	A	OU	Task - reward processing	BOLD	ROI													
Freeman, 2018	A	OU	Task - reward processing	BOLD	ROI													
de Sousa Fernandes, 2016	A	FR	Task - reward processing	BOLD	ROI													
Borgwardt, 2008	A	OU	Task - impulsivity	BOLD	Whole brain													
Atakan, 2012	A	OU	Task - impulsivity	BOLD	Whole brain													
Bhattacharyya, 2015	A	OU	Task - impulsivity	BOLD	Whole brain													
Jager, 2006	C	CU vs NU	Task - executive function/attention	BOLD	ROI													

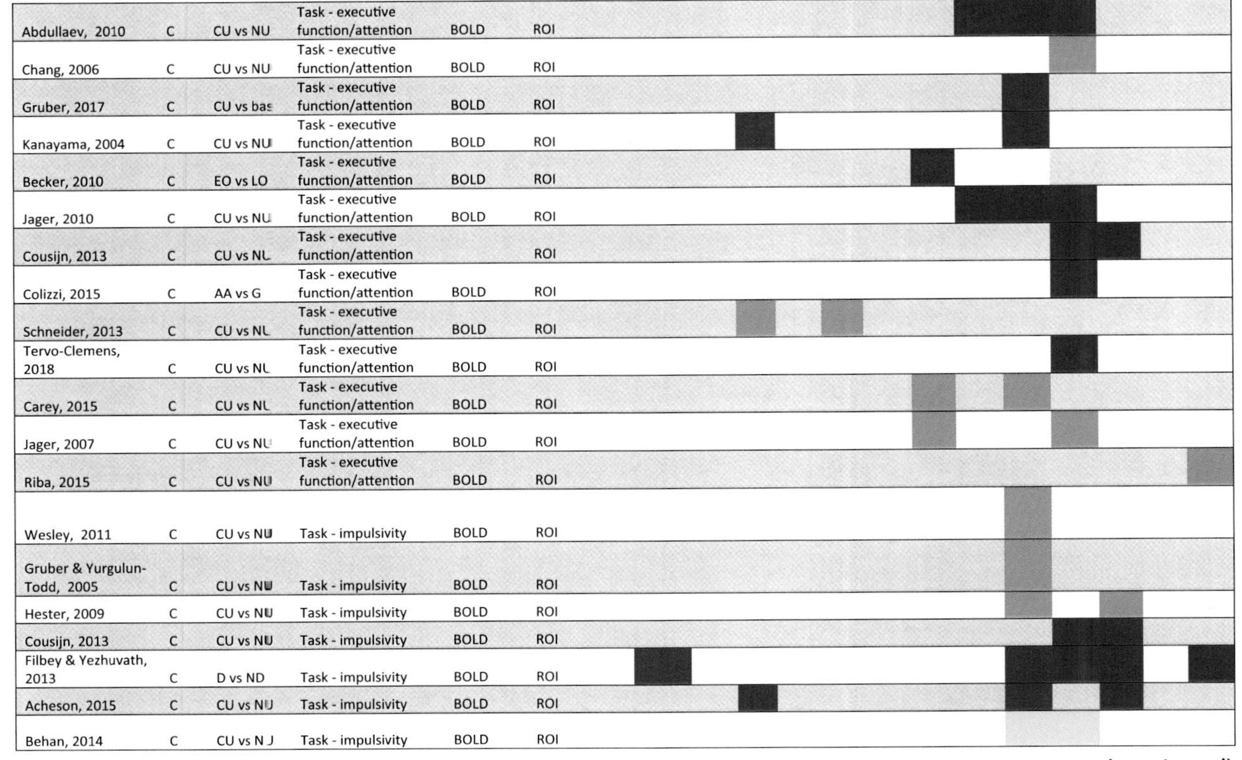

Abdullaev, 2010	C	CU vs NU	Task - executive function/attention	BOLD	ROI
Chang, 2006	C	CU vs NU	Task - executive function/attention	BOLD	ROI
Gruber, 2017	C	CU vs bas	Task - executive function/attention	BOLD	ROI
Kanayama, 2004	C	CU vs NU	Task - executive function/attention	BOLD	ROI
Becker, 2010	C	EO vs LO	Task - executive function/attention	BOLD	ROI
Jager, 2010	C	CU vs NU	Task - executive function/attention	BOLD	ROI
Cousijn, 2013	C	CU vs NU	Task - executive function/attention		ROI
Colizzi, 2015	C	AA vs G	Task - executive function/attention	BOLD	ROI
Schneider, 2013	C	CU vs NU	Task - executive function/attention	BOLD	ROI
Tervo-Clemens, 2018	C	CU vs NU	Task - executive function/attention	BOLD	ROI
Carey, 2015	C	CU vs NU	Task - executive function/attention	BOLD	ROI
Jager, 2007	C	CU vs NU	Task - executive function/attention	BOLD	ROI
Riba, 2015	C	CU vs NU	Task - executive function/attention	BOLD	ROI
Wesley, 2011	C	CU vs NU	Task - impulsivity	BOLD	ROI
Gruber & Yurgulun-Todd, 2005	C	CU vs NU	Task - impulsivity	BOLD	ROI
Hester, 2009	C	CU vs NU	Task - impulsivity	BOLD	ROI
Cousijn, 2013	C	CU vs NU	Task - impulsivity	BOLD	ROI
Filbey & Yezhuvath, 2013	C	D vs ND	Task - impulsivity	BOLD	ROI
Acheson, 2015	C	CU vs NU	Task - impulsivity	BOLD	ROI
Behan, 2014	C	CU vs N J	Task - impulsivity	BOLD	ROI

(continued)

Table 1 (continued)

Nestor, 2010	C	CU vs NU	Task - reward processing	BOLD	ROI
Jager, 2013	C	CU vs NU	Task - reward processing	BOLD	ROI
Enzi, 2015	C	CU vs NU	Task - reward processing	BOLD	ROI
van Hell, 2010	C	CU vs NU	Task - reward processing	BOLD	ROI
Ford, 2014	C	CU vs NU	Task - reward processing	BOLD	ROI
Yip, 2014	C	CU vs NU	Task - reward processing	BOLD	ROI
Vingerhoets, 2016	C	CU vs Bas	Task - reward processing	BOLD	ROI
Zhou, 2019	C	CU vs NU	Task - reward processing	BOLD	ROI
de Sousa Fernandes Perna, 2016	C	CU vs NU vs AL	Task - reward processing	BOLD	ROI
Filbey & Dunlop, 2014	C	DU vs NDU	Task - reward processing	BOLD	ROI
Lichtenstein, 2017	C	ES vs SH,SL	Task - reward processing	BOLD	Nucleus accumbens
Cheng , 2014	C	CU vs NU	Rest	BOLD	ROI
Lopez-Larson, 2015	C	CU vs NU	Rest	BOLD	Orbitofrontal cortex
Pujol, 2014	C	CU vs NU	Rest	BOLD	Anterior insula
Manza, 2018	C	CU vs NU	Rest	BOLD	FC subcortical circuits
Newman, 2020	C	CU vs NU	Rest	BOLD	dACC
Mason, 2021	C	CU vs OU	Rest	BOLD	ROI
	C				Nucleus accumbens
Blanco-Hinojo, 2017	C	CU vs NU	Rest	BOLD	Dorsal caudate
	C				Dorsal putamen
	C				Nucleus accumbens
	C				Ventral putamen
Zhou, 2018	C	CU vs NU	Rest	BOLD	Ventral striatum
	C				Dorsal striatum

Key: blue = decrease, red = increase = no change*

changes in the reward system (Mason et al. 2019), and reward system-dependent behaviors (Ramaekers et al. 2009), are dose-dependent and only take place after a certain minimum threshold of THC is reached in blood.

Acute Effect of THC on Neurotransmission in Occasional Users

It has been suggested that a reduction of functional connectivity between the striatum and regions of the reward system such as the thalamus and frontal cortex reflect increases in dopaminergic neurotransmission throughout the mesocorticolimbic circuit (Ramaekers et al. 2016; Mason et al. 2019; Ramaekers et al. 2020; Ramaekers et al. 2021). Namely, the VTA is proposed to be under inhibitory control of GABAergic and glutamatergic interneurons, on which presynaptic CB1 receptors are located (Bloomfield et al. 2016). When THC binds to these CB1 receptors, it inhibits their suppression of the VTA, which results in stimulation of dopamine release from the VTA to the striatum and other parts of the circuit. Although most evidence of the effect of cannabinoid agonists on dopaminergic stimulation in the striatum stems from preclinical models (Gardner 2005), a few PET studies have been performed in humans (Bossong et al. 2009; Stokes et al. 2009, 2010; Bossong and Kahn 2016) (Tables 2 and 4). Together these studies have shown that acute administration of THC in occasional cannabis users results in reduced [11C]-raclopride binding (consistent with increased dopamine levels) in certain subdivisions of the striatum. Namely, compared to placebo, THC-induced elevations in dopamine were seen in the ventral striatum (consisting of the NAc), but not in the pre- or post-commisural putamen or dorsal caudate (Bossong and Kahn 2016), demonstrating regionally selective effects of THC on dopaminergic functioning, contained to the ventral striatum. As the main output neurons from the NAc are GABAergic medium spiny neurons, the functional consequence of such an increase of dopamine in this area would be a decrement of functional connectivity to the basal ganglia, ventral pallidum, and other areas of the reward circuitry (Salgado and Kaplitt 2015), as demonstrated in previous studies with cannabis and other dopaminergic drugs (Ramaekers et al. 2013; Mason et al. 2019; Ramaekers et al. 2016).

Table 1 (continued) *A* acute, *C* chronic, *SN* substantia nigra, *VTA* ventral tegmental area, *St* striatum, *Nac* nucleus accumbens, *VP* ventral pallidum, *Amy* amygdala, *hip* hippocampus, *mPF* medial prefrontal cortex, *Acc* anterior cingulate cortex, *OFC* orbitofrontal cortex, *ins* anterior insula, *TPJ* temporal parietal junction, *Tha* thalamus, *bas* baseline, *CD* cannabis disorder, *CU* chronic user, *D* dependent user, *DSM* diagnostic and statistical manual of mental disorders, *EO* early onset user, *ES* escalating use, *FR* frequent user, *INH* inhalation, *LO* late onset users, *ND* non-dependent user, *NU* non-user, *NU* non-user, *OU* occasional user, *ROI* region of interest, *SH* stable high use, *SL* stable low use

**no-change was marked if the analysis focused on this area (ROI, or specific voxel placement). If the area did not show a statistical difference in a whole-brain seed-to-voxel analysis, this was not marked, as a lack of change could also be attributable to an issue with multiple comparisons*

Table 2 Acute and chronic effects of THC on neurotransmitters in brain regions of the reward system

Reference	A/C	Population	Paradigm	Measurement	SN	VTA	St	Nac	VP	Amy	Hip	mPF	ACC	OFC	Ins	TPJ	Tha
Bossong 2009	A	OU	Rest	Dopamine release													
Stokes, 2009 & 2010	A	OU	Rest	Dopamine release													
Bossong, 2016	A	OU	Rest	Dopamine release													
Colizzi 2018	A	OU	Rest	Glutamate													
Mason, 2018 & 2019	A	OU	Rest	Glutamate													
Mason, 2018 & 2019	A	OU	Rest	GABA													
Mason, 2019	A	CU	Rest	Glutamate													
Mason, 2019	A	CU	Rest	GABA													
Chang, 2006	C	CU vs NU	MRS	Glutamate													
Prescot 2011	C	CU vs NU	MRS	Glutamate													
Prescot, 2013	C	CU vs NU	MRS	Glutamate													
Muetzel, 2013	C	CU vs NU	MRS	Glutamate													
Sung, 2013	C	CU vs NU	MRS	Glutamate													
Rigucci, 2018	C	CU vs NU	MRS	Glutamate													
Newman, 2019	C	CU vs NU	MRS	Glutamate													
Watts, 2020	C	CU vs NU	MRS	Glutamate													
Mason, 2021	C	CU vs OU	MRS	Glutamate													
Prescot, 2013	C	CU vs NU	MRS	GABA													
Mason, 2021	C	CV vs OU	MRS	GABA													
Urban, 2012	C	AU vs NU	PET	Response to dopamine challenge													
Wiers, 2016	C	CU vs NU	PET	Response to dopamine challenge													

Volkow, 2014	C	CU vs NU	PET	Response to dopamine challenge
Mizrahi, 2013	C	CU	PET	Dopamine release
Mizrahi, 2014	C	CU vs NO	PET	Dopamine release
van de Giessen, 2017	C	CU vs NU	PET	Dopamine release
Leroy et, 2014	C	CU vs HC	PET	Dopamine transporter
Bloomfield, 2014	C	CU	PET	Dopamine synthesis
Bloomfield, 2014	C	CU vs NU	PET	Dopamine synthesis
Albrecht, 2013	C	CU vs NU	PET	D2 receptor availability
Urban, 2012	C	AU vs NU	PET	D2/D3 receptor availability
Volkow, 2014	C	AU vs NU	PET	D2/D3 receptor availability
Sevy, 2008	C	AU vs NU	PET	D2/D3 receptor availability
Tomasi, 2015	C	CU vs NU	PET/fMRI	D2/D3 receptor modulation
Kamp, 2019	C	Meta-analysis	PET	D2/D3 receptor availability

Key: blue = decrease, red = increase, yellow = no change*

Key: blue = decrease, red = increase, yellow = no change*
A acute, *C* chronic, *SN* substantia nigra, *VTA* ventral tegmental area, *St* striatum, *Nac* nucleus accumbens, *VP* ventral pallidum, *Amy* amygdala, *hip* hippocampus, *mPF* medial prefrontal cortex, *Acc* anterior cingulate cortex, *OFC* orbitofrontal cortex, *ins* anterior insula, *TPJ* temporal parietal junction, *Tha* thalamus, *bas* baseline, *CD* cannabis disorder, *CU* chronic user, *D* dependent user, *DSM* diagnostic and statistical manual of mental disorders, *EO* early onset user, *ES* escalating use, *FR* frequent user, *INH* inhalation, *LO* late onset users, *ND* non-dependent user, *NU* non-user, *NU* non-user, *OU* occasional user, *ROI* region of interest, *SH* stable high use, *SL* stable low use
**no change was marked if the analysis focused on this area (ROI, or specific voxel placement). If the area did not show a statistical difference in a whole-brain seed-to-voxel analysis, this was not marked, as a lack of change could also be attributable to an issue with multiple comparisons*

An additional neurochemical consequence of dopaminergic stimulation in the NAc, and subsequent reduction in functional connectivity from the NAc to the ventral pallidum, is a decrease of GABAergic inhibitory tone to the thalamus, resulting in an increase of glutamatergic signaling to the prefrontal cortex, the VTA, and the NAc (Ramaekers et al. 2016). In accordance with this proposed circuitry, acute pharmacological challenge studies with THC have found that THC increases glutamate concentration levels in the striatum, in occasional cannabis users (Colizzi et al. 2020; Mason et al. 2019, 2021) (Tables 2 and 4). Additionally, Mason et al. (2019) found that the THC-induced increments in striatal glutamate were strongly correlated with THC-induced changes of functional connectivity between the NAc and other areas of the reward system, which has led to the proposition that increased stimulatory glutamatergic input from the prefrontal cortex to the NAc synergizes with cannabis-induced increases in dopaminergic input from the VTA to the NAc, which leads to further perturbation of the reward system (Ramaekers et al. 2020).

Acute Effect of THC on Task-Related Brain Activity in Occasional Users

Only a few fMRI studies have examined the acute effect of THC on brain activity, while participants engaged in cognitive tasks that require the recruitment of the reward circuitry (Tables 1 and 5). These cognitive tasks include assessments of reward processing and response inhibition. In general, fMRI studies that have either presented rewarding stimuli or employed monetary incentive or impulsivity tasks have found attenuation in areas of the reward system compared to placebo, albeit activation seems to be brain-region and task-dependent.

Two studies assessed the effect of THC on brain activity while individuals were exposed to stimuli that have been shown to stimulate dopamine release, namely, listening to music (Freeman et al. 2018), and drug associated marketing cues (De Sousa Fernandes Perna et al. 2017). Both studies found that ingestion of THC attenuated striatal activation in response to these rewarding stimuli, providing further support that THC increases (tonic) dopamine levels in the striatum. Specifically, rewarding stimuli have been shown previously to increase phasic dopamine release in the striatum (Schultz 2007), which makes the striatal response to reward (response sensitivity) vary with the availability of tonic dopamine; reward sensitivity is found to be high, when tonic dopamine is low and vice versa (Cools and D'Esposito 2011). Thus a phasic response to rewarding stimuli would decrease in the presence of THC-induced elevations in tonic dopamine, leading to an attenuation of the striatal response as seen in these studies (De Sousa Fernandes Perna et al. 2017).

Utilizing an established reward paradigm, which provides a measure of sensitivity to anticipation of reward as well as sensitivity to notification that the reward has been won, two studies have assessed THC-induced changes in the neural response to a monetary incentive delay task, with mixed results (Van Hell et al. 2012; Jansma et al. 2013). In both studies, participants showed similar behavioral responses to reward after receiving THC or placebo, with faster responses if a reward could be won, but no drug-specific effect. In regard to THC-induced brain changes, Jansma et al. (2013) found that THC attenuated nucleus accumbens activity, but not caudate putamen activity, during monetary reward anticipation, with no effect on neural activity during reward feedback. On the other hand, van Hell et al. (2012) found THC administration attenuated inferior parietal cortex, inferior temporal gyrus, and posterior cingulate activity during reward feedback compared to placebo, but not during reward anticipation. Although inconsistent in regard to the stage (anticipation vs feedback) THC-induced changes took place, both studies were consistent in that they did not find any drug-induced changes in trials in which there was no possibility to win a reward. Additionally, they are consistent with previous studies using this paradigm, which have found that anticipation of a reward activates ventral striatal regions, whereas reward feedback activates more frontal regions (Knutson et al. 2001a, b). Thus, just as during exposure to rewarding stimuli, it would be hypothesized that since THC exposure already increases dopamine in the reward system, this would result in a blunting effect on reward anticipation and feedback while intoxicated and subsequent attenuation of neural responses in areas that make up the reward system.

As reviewed in Gunasekera et al. (2021), studies which have assessed impulsivity have consistently found THC *increased* hippocampal, as well as striatal, and particularly caudate, activation, compared to placebo (Borgwardt et al. 2008). Simultaneously, attenuation of activation in the prefrontal cortex and anterior cingulate area (Atakan et al. 2013; Bhattacharyya et al. 2015; Borgwardt et al. 2008) was found during the task, whereas effects on anterior insula activity have been mixed (Atakan et al. 2013; Bhattacharyya et al. 2015). Importantly, such studies found activation differences with no significant difference in task performance (mean inhibition errors), suggesting that this region-dependent hyper- and hypoactivation may represent compensatory effort needed when individuals are under the influence of THC, to operate optimally in response-inhibition/impulsivity tasks.

Acute Effect of THC on Resting State Functional Connectivity and Neurotransmission in Chronic Users

To the best of our knowledge, only one study has examined the acute effect of THC on resting state functional connectivity and neurotransmission in chronic cannabis users. Mason et al. (2019) found that compared to placebo, THC did not alter synchronicity between the NAc and other areas of the reward system, suggesting a blunted dopaminergic response after THC. This is in contrast to occasional users, in which decreased synchronicity was found, as has been discussed previously. Additionally in the same study, THC did not acutely alter glutamate concentrations in the striatum and the anterior cingulate cortex. Taken together, results suggest repeated and frequent cannabis use results in a blunted response to THC in the reward system. Due to the association between THC-induced changes in the reward system and the impairing and rewarding effects of the drug (reviewed in Ramaekers et al. (2021)), it has been suggested that this blunted reward system response may underlie the acute tolerance to these effects, witnessed in frequent and chronic cannabis users (reviewed in Ramaekers et al. (2020)).

Acute Effect of THC on Task-Related Brain Activity in Chronic Users

To the best of our knowledge, no studies have examined the acute effect of THC on brain activity in chronic cannabis users, while participants engaged in cognitive tasks that require the recruitment of reward circuitry, representing a research gap in the literature.

Persisting Effects of Cannabis on the Reward System

Chronic Cannabis Use and Resting State Functional Connectivity

Chronic cannabis use has been primarily associated with increased functional connectivity within the ventral striatum (Filbey and Dunlop 2014; Manza et al. 2018), amygdala and hippocampus (Filbey and Dunlop 2014; Newman et al. 2020), and prefrontal areas (Filbey and Dunlop 2014; Cheng et al. 2014; Lopez-Larson et al. 2015; Pujol et al. 2014)(Tables 1 and 3). Increments in functional connectivity have also been associated with age of onset of drug use (Filbey and Dunlop 2014) and cannabis use frequency (Lopez-Larson et al. 2015). One study revealed no change in functional connectivity of chronic cannabis users as compared to occasional cannabis users (Mason et al. 2021), whereas another study (Lichenstein et al. 2017) showed that chronic cannabis users that followed an escalating trajectory of cannabis use frequency showed a distinct pattern of negative functional connectivity between the NAc and medial prefrontal cortex, relative to chronic cannabis users whose pattern of use remained stable (high or low). In the escalating trajectory group, a negative NAc-medial prefrontal cortex connectivity was linked to higher levels of depressive symptoms, anhedonia, and lower educational attainment.

Chronic Cannabis Use and Neurotransmission

A range of studies have employed MRS and PET imaging to assess dopaminergic function in chronic cannabis users (Tables 2 and 4). These studies have consistently shown that the capacity of chronic cannabis users to synthesize striatal dopamine is significantly reduced (Bloomfield et al. 2014a) and associated to levels of apathy, a prominent symptom of cannabis use disorder (Bloomfield et al. 2014b). Chronic cannabis users also displayed a blunted response to dopaminergic challenges with d-amphetamine (Urban et al. 2012; Van De Giessen et al. 2017) and methylphenidate (Volkow et al. 2014; Wiers et al. 2016), as evidenced by lower levels of dopamine release in the striatum as compared to controls. Striatal dopamine levels were lower

Table 3 Neuroimaging studies of the acute and chronic effects of THC on reward-related circuitry at rest

Reference	A/C	Population	Population definition	Drug and dose	Route	Modality	Paradigm	Comparison	Sample Size	Analysis	Behavioral correlate	Task performance
Klumpers et al. 2012	A	OU	<1x/week	THC; 2 mg or 6 mg	INH	fMRI	Rest	THC vs placebo	12	ROI		
Grimm et al. 2018	A	OU	Not specified	THC; 10 mg	PO	fMRI	Rest	THC vs placebo	16	Seed to voxel		
Mason et al. 2019	A	OU	<3x/week	THC; 300 ug/kg	INH	fMRI & MRS	Rest & (1)H-MRS	THC vs placebo	10	Seed to voxel; glutamate concentrations	Subjective high	Sustained attention
Bossong et al. 2019	A	OU	<1x/week	THC; 6 mg + 1 mg repeated doses	INH	fMRI	Rest	THC vs placebo	39	Seed to voxel	Subjective high	
Wall et al. 2019	A	OU	<3x/week	THC; 8 mg	INH	fMRI	Rest	THC vs placebo	17	Seed to voxel		
Crane and Phan 2021	A	OU	<10x/lifetime	THC; 7.5 mg	PO	fMRI	Rest	THC vs placebo	24 vs 22	Seed to voxel	Euphoria	
Mason et al. 2019	A	OU & CU	OU = <3x/week; CU >4x/week	THC; 300 ug/kg	INH	fMRI & MRS	Rest & (1)H-MRS	THC vs placebo; OU vs CU	12 vs 12	Seed to voxel; ROI to ROI; glutamate/GABA		
Ramaekers et al. 2016	A	FR	15x/month	THC; 450 ug/kg	INH	fMRI	Rest	THC vs placebo	122	Seed to voxel		Cognitive impulsivity
Cheng et al. 2014	C	CU	12.8/w			fMRI	Rest	CU vs NU	12 vs 13	FC	–	–
Lopez-Larson et al. 2015	C	CU	14.8/w			fMRI	Rest	CU vs NU	43 vs 31	Seed to voxel	Impulsivity	–

(continued)

Table 3 (continued)

Reference	A/C	Population	Population definition	Drug and dose	Route	Modality	Paradigm	Comparison	Sample Size	Analysis	Behavioral correlate	Task performance
Pujol et al. 2014	C	CU	899/y			fMRI	Rest	CU vs NU	28 vs 29	Seed to voxel	–	–
Manza et al. 2018	C	CU	Human connectome			fMRI	Rest	CU vs NU	30 vs 30	FC	–	–
Newman et al. 2020	C	CU	30.2x/mo			fMRI	Rest	CU vs NU	23 vs 23	ROI		
Mason et al. 2019	C	CU	> 5 days/ week			fMRI	Rest	CU vs OU	12 vs 12	Seed to voxel; ROI to ROI; glutamate concentrations		No change
Blanco-Hinojo et al. 2017	C	CU	Onset<16y, >14/week for 2y			fMRI	Rest	CU vs NU	28 vs 29	Seed to voxel	Motor control/ verbal fluence/ emotional picture viewing	CU: < arousal judgement
Zhou et al. 2018	C	CU	DSM-IV diagnosis, 28 d/month, 78 months			fMRI	Rest	CD vs NU	24 vs 22	FC	–	–

A acute, *C* chronic, *AU* abstinent user, *bas* baseline, *CD* cannabis disorder, *CU* chronic user, *D* dependent user, *DSM* diagnostic and statistical manual of mental disorders, *EO* early onset user, *ES* escalating use, *FR* frequent user, *INH* inhalation, *LO* late onset users, *ND* non-dependent user, *NU* non-user, *NU* non-user, *OU* occasional user, *ROI* region of interest, *SH* stable high use, *SL* stable low use

Table 4 Neuroimaging studies of the acute and chronic effects of THC on neurotransmission in reward-related circuitry

Reference	A/C	Population	Population definition	Drug and dose	Route	Modality	Paradigm	Comparison	Sample size	Analysis	Behavioral correlate	Task performance
Bossong et al. 2009	A	OU	>4x/year; <1x/week	THC; 8 mg	INH	PET	[11C]-raclopride binding	THC vs placebo	7	Dopamine release		
Mason et al. 2019	A	OU	<3x/week	THC; 300 ug/kg	INH	fMRI & MRS	Rest & (1) H-MRS	THC vs placebo	10	Seed to voxel; glutamate concentrations	Subjective high	Sustained attention
Stokes et al. 2009, 2010	A	OU	20x/lifetime	THC; 10 mg	PO	PET	[11C]-raclopride binding		13	Dopamine release		
Bossong et al. 2015	A	OU	Between 20x/lifetime and < 1x/week	THC; 10 mg and 8 mg	PO and INH	PET	[11C]-raclopride binding	THC vs placebo	20	Dopamine release		
Colizzi et al. 2020	A	OU	Abstinent 6 months	THC; 1.19 mg/2 ml	IV	MRS	(1)H-MRS	THC vs placebo	16	Glutamate	Psychomimetic symptoms	
Mason et al. 2019	A	OU	OU = <3x/week; CU >4x/week	THC; 300 ug/kg	INH	fMRI & MRS	Rest & (1) H-MRS	THC vs placebo	12	Seed to voxel; ROI to ROI; glutamate; GABA		Sustained attention
Chang et al. 2006a	C	CU	230/lifetime			MRS	(1)H-MRS	CU vs NU	51 vs 30	Glutamate	Executive function; memory	CU: Increased RT and errors
Prescot et al. 2011	C	CU	1367/lifetime			MRS	(1)H-MRS	CU vs NU	17 vs 17	Glutamate		
Prescot et al. 2013	C	CU	1124/lifetime			MRS	(1)H-MRS	CU vs NU	13 vs 16	Glutamate/GABA		
Muetzel et al. 2013	C	CU	25x/m			MRS	(1)H-MRS	CU vs NU	27 vs 26	Glutamate		

(continued)

Table 4 (continued)

Reference	A/C	Population	Population definition	Drug and dose	Route	Modality	Paradigm	Comparison	Sample size	Analysis	Behavioral correlate	Task performance
Sung et al. 2013	C	CU	1099/lifetime			MRS	(1)H-MRS	CU vs NU	8 vs 10	Glutamate/N-acetylaspartate		
Rigucci et al. 2018	C	CU/OC	CU > 3x/week			MRS	(1)H-MRS	CU/OC vs NU	18 vs 33	Glutamate	Executive function	CU/OU: Decrease in memory, attention, motor speed
Newman et al. 2019	C	CU	33x/mo			MRS	(1)H-MRS	CU vs NU	26 vs 24	Glutamate		
Watts et al. 2020	C	CU	1.39 gr/day			MRS	(1)H-MRS	CU vs NU	26 vs 47	Glutamate		
Mason et al. 2019	C	CU	>5d/week			MRS	(1)H-MRS	Placebo	12	Glutamate/GABA	Executive function; attention	No change
Urban et al. 2012	C	AU	517 puffs/mo			PET	[11C] raclopride	AU vs NU	16 vs 16	Dopamine release,D2/3R		
Wiers et al. 2016	C	CU	6.8 days/w			PET	[18F]-FDG	CU vs NU	24 vs 24	Dopamine release		
Volkow et al. 2014	C	CU	4.9 days/w			PET	[11C] raclopride	CU vs NU	24 vs 24	Dopamine release		
Mizrahi et al. 2013	C	CU	15.5x/w			PET	[11C]-(+)-PHNO	CU vs NU	13 vs 12	Dopamine release		
Mizrahi et al. 2014	C	CU	4892/lifetime			PET	[11C]-(+)-PHNO	CU vs NU	12 vs 12	Dopamine release		
Van De Giessen et al. 2017	C	CU	79.2 gr/m			PET	[11C]-(+)-PHNO	CU vs NU	11 vs 12	Dopamine release	Executive function; memory	No change
	C	CU	4.8x/day			PET	[11C]PE2I	CU vs HC				

Leroy et al. 2012									13 vs 11	Dopamine transporter		
Bloomfield et al. 2014b	C	CU	28.1 gr/mo			PET	[18F]-DOPA	CU	14	Dopamine synthesis		
Bloomfield et al. 2014a	C	CU	26.3 gr/mo			PET	[18F]-DOPA	CU vs NU	19 vs 19	Dopamine synthesis		
Albrecht et al. 2013	C	CU	46.6x/mo			PET	[11C] raclopride	CU vs NU	10 vs 8	D2 receptor availability		
Volkow et al. 2014	C	AU	4.8 /day			PET	[11C] raclopride	AU vs NU	24 vs 24	D2/D3 receptor availability		
Sevy et al. 2008	C	AU	16gr/d			PET	[18F]-FDG	AU vs NU	6 vs 6	D2/D3 receptor availability		
Tomasi et al. 2015	C	CU	5x/d			PET/ fMRI	[11C] raclopride	CU vs NU	18 vs 14	D2/D3 receptor modulation		
Hermann et al. 2007	C	CU	–			MRS	(1)H-MRS	CU vs NU	13 vs 13	N-acetylaspartate	Impulsivity	CU: Decreased performance

A acute, *C* chronic, *AU* abstinent user, *bas* baseline, *CD* cannabis disorder, *CU* chronic user, *D* dependent user, *DSM* diagnostic and statistical manual of mental disorders, *EO* early onset user, *ES* escalating use, *FR* frequent user, *INH* inhalation, *LO* late onset users, *ND* non-dependent user, *NU* non-user, *NU* non-user, *OU* occasional user, *ROI* region of interest, *SH* stable high use, *SL* stable low use

Table 5 Neuroimaging studies of the acute and chronic effects of THC during reward-related tasks

Reference	A/C	Population	Population definition	Drug and dose	Route	Modality	Paradigm	Comparison	Sample size	Analysis	Behavioral correlate	Task performance
Borgwardt et al. 2008	A	OU	<15x/ lifetime	THC; 10 mg	PO	fMRI	Task based	THC vs placebo	10	Whole brain	Impulsivity	No change
Atakan et al. 2013	A	OU	<15x/ lifetime	THC; 10 mg	PO	fMRI	Task based	THC vs placebo	21	Whole brain	Impulsivity	No change
Bhattacharyya et al. 2015	A	OU	<25x/ lifetime	THC; 10 mg	PO	fMRI	Task based	THC vs placebo	36	Whole brain	Impulsivity	No change
Van Hell et al. 2012	A	OU	>/= 4x/year; <1x/week	THC; 8 mg	INH	fMRI	Task based	THC vs placebo	11	ROI	Reward processing	No change
Jansma et al. 2013	A	OU	>/= 4x/year; <1x/week	THC; 6 mg	INH	fMRI	Task based	THC vs placebo vs NU	11 vs 10	ROI	Reward processing	No change
Freeman et al. 2018	A	OU	≥4x/year; ≤3 times/wk	THC; 8 mg	INH	fMRI	Task based	THC vs placebo	16	ROI	Reward processing	Increased ratings of wanting to listen to music
de Sousa Fernandes et al. 2017	A	FR	≥3x/week; <19 times/ wk	THC; 300 ug/kg	INH	fMRI	Task based	THC vs placebo vs NU	21 vs 20	ROI	Reward processing	FR: Increased positive association with marketing cues
Jager et al. 2006	C	CU	350x/y			fMRI	Task based	CU vs NU	10 vs 10	ROI	Executive function/ attention	No change

Abdullaev et al. 2010	C	CU	71–196 days/y			fMRI	Task based	CU vs NU	14 vs 14	ROI	Executive function/ attention	CU: Increase RT and errors
Chang et al. 2006b	C	CU	> 5 days / week			fMRI	Task based	CU vs NU	12 vs 19	ROI	Executive function/ attention	No change
Gruber et al. 2017	C	CU	5.3x/w			fMRI	Task based	CU vs bas	45	ROI	Exexutive function/ attention	Decrease RT and errors, increase accuracy
Kanayama et al. 2004	C	CU	19.200/ lifetime			fMRI	Task based	CU vs NU	12 vs 10	ROI	Executive function/ memory	No change
Becker et al. 2010	C	CU (EO and LO)	17.2x/m vs 9.9x/m			fMRI	Task based	EO vs LO	26 vs 17	ROI	Executive function/ memory	EO: Increase RT
Jager et al. 2010	C	CU	741x/y			fMRI	Task based	CU vs NU	21 vs 24	ROI	Executive function/ memory	No change
Cousijn et al. 2013a	C	CU	4.9x/w			fMRI	Task based	CU vs NU	31 vs 41	ROI	Executive function/ memory	No change
Colizzi et al. 2015	C	CU	–			fMRI	Task based	AA genotype vs G genotype	81 vs 117	ROI	Executive function/ memory	G carrier: Decrease accuracy
Sneider et al. 2013	C	CU	> 5 days / week			fMRI	Task based	CU vs NU	11 vs 7	ROI	Executive function/ memory	CU: Decreased performance
Tervo-Clemens et al. 2018	C	CU	1.45x/day			fMRI	Task based	CU vs NU	46 vs 15	ROI	Executive function/ memory	CU: Increased performance

(continued)

Table 5 (continued)

Reference	A/C	Population	Population definition	Drug and dose	Route	Modality	Paradigm	Comparison	Sample size	Analysis	Behavioral correlate	Task performance
Carey et al. 2015	C	CU	72,5x/m			fMRI	Task based	CU vs NU	15 vs 15	ROI	Executive function/ memory	CU: Decreased error-rate correction performance
Jager et al. 2007	C	CU	1900x lifetime			fMRI	Task based	CU vs NU	20 vs 20	ROI	Executive function/ memory	No change
Riba et al. 2015	C	CU	5x/day			fMRI	Task based	CU vs NU	16 vs 16	ROI	Executive function/ memory	CU: Increased sensitivity to false memory
Wesley et al. 2011	C	CU	29.4x/m			fMRI	Task based	CU vs NU	16 vs 16	ROI	Impulsivity	CU: More errors
Gruber and Yurgelun-Todd 2005	C	CU	39.4x/week			fMRI	Task based	CU vs NU	9 vs 9	ROI	Impulsivity	CU: Increase commission errors
Hester et al. 2009	C	CU	76.3x/m			fMRI	Task based	CU vs NU	16 vs 16	ROI	Impulsivity	CU: Decrease error awareness
Cousijn et al. 2013b	C	CU	4.9x/w			fMRI	Task based	CU vs NU	32 vs 41	ROI	Impulsivity	No change
	C	CU (D and ND)	3.4 vs 4x / day			fMRI	Task based	D vs ND	44 vs 30	ROI	Impulsivity	No change

Filbey and Yezhuvath 2013												
Acheson et al. 2015	C	CU	>5/week			fMRI	Task based	CU vs NU	14 vs 14	ROI	Impulsivity	Not reported
Behan et al. 2014	C	CU	178.4x/m			fMRI	Task based	CU vs NU	17 vs 18	ROI	Impulsivity	CU:Decrease accuracy
Nestor et al. 2010	C	CU	7258/lifetime			fMRI	Task based	CU vs NU	14 vs 14	ROI	Reward processing	No change
Jager et al. 2013	C	CU	4006/lifetime			fMRI	Task based	CU vs NU	21 VS 24	ROI	Reward processing	No change
Enzi et al. 2015	C	CU	13.3/w			fMRI	Task based	CU vs NU	15 vs 15	ROI	Reward processing	No change
Van Hell et al. 2010	C	CU	3841/lifetime			fMRI	Task based	CU vs NU	14 VS 13	ROI	Reward processing	No change
Ford et al. 2014	C	CU	22/m			fMRI	Task based	CU vs NU	15 vs 17	ROI	Reward processing	No change
Yip et al. 2014	C	CU (abstinent)	–			fMRI	Task based	CU vs NU	20 vs 20	ROI	Reward processing	No change
Vingerhoets et al. 2016	C	CU	2.6–3.1gr/w			fMRI	Task based	CU vs bas	23	ROI	Reward processing	CU: Increase drug cue reactivity
Zhou et al. 2019	C	CU	984–1583/ lifetime			fMRI	Task based	CU vs NU	38 vs 44	ROI	Reward processing	CU: Increase drug cue reactivity
Lichenstein et al. 2017	C	CU (ES, SH, SL)	9,5/m			fMRI	Task based	ES vs SH, SL		FC	Reward processing	No change

(continued)

Table 5 (continued)

Reference	A/C	Population	Population definition	Drug and dose	Route	Modality	Paradigm	Comparison	Sample size	Analysis	Behavioral correlate	Task performance
									26 vs 11 vs 111			
Filbey and Dunlop 2014	C	CU	80.8/3mo			fMRI	Task based	CU vs NU	31 vs 24	FC	Reward processing	–

A acute, *C* chronic, *AU* abstinent user, *bas* baseline, *CD* cannabis disorder, *CU* chronic user, *D* dependent user, *DSM* diagnostic and statistical manual of mental disorders, *EO* early onset user, *ES* escalating use, *FR* frequent user, *INH* inhalation, *LO* late onset users, *ND* non-dependent user, *NU* non-user, *NU* non-user, *OU* occasional user, *ROI* region of interest, *SH* stable high use, *SL* stable low use

in chronic cannabis users as compared to non-using controls as suggested by a higher binding affinity of a D2/D3 receptors ligand (Mizrahi et al. 2013), although dopamine release to stress did not differ between groups. In cannabis users with psychotic proneness, the striatal dopamine response to stress was higher as compared to a group of individuals with clinical high risk for schizophrenia and with no history of cannabis use (Mizrahi et al. 2014). PET studies assessing dopamine transporter availability in cannabis users reported reduced availability in the striatum, thalamus, and middle cingulate (Leroy et al. 2012) as compared to non-cannabis using controls. PET studies assessing D2/D3 receptor density have generally not reported any difference between cannabis users and controls (Urban et al. 2012; Van De Giessen et al. 2017; Volkow et al. 2014), although negative correlations between D2 receptor availability and current history of cannabis use (Albrecht et al. 2013) and age of first use (Urban et al. 2012) have been found. A recent meta-analysis of D2/D3 receptor binding studies in cannabis users also concluded that no significant difference in receptor availability compared to controls exists (Kamp et al. 2019). Interestingly, modulation of D2/D3 receptors in the ventral striatum and dorsal caudate was disrupted in cannabis users as compared to controls. Overall, these findings suggest that chronic cannabis users display a disruption in striatal dopamine function and in D2/D3 receptor signaling.

A limited number of imaging studies has investigated glutamate-related metabolites in chronic cannabis users as compared to non-cannabis using controls. A range of studies has shown reductions in glutamate in (frontal white matter of) the anterior cingulate (Chang et al. 2006a; Prescot et al. 2011, 2013), although no change in glutamate has also been reported (Watts et al. 2020; Newman et al. 2019). Reduction of glutamate levels in the basal ganglia has been reported as well (Chang et al. 2006a; Muetzel et al. 2013). In one of the latter studies, the striatal glutamate reduction was only reported in female cannabis users (Muetzel et al. 2013). A MRS study in concomitant cannabis and methamphetamine users reported no difference in frontal glutamate levels as compared to controls, but that study may have suffered from a small sample size and polydrug use of the target population (Sung et al. 2013). Finally, a recent study revealed no difference in striatal and anterior cingulate cortex levels of glutamate in chronic cannabis users as compared to occasional users of cannabis; however chronic users did show a blunted glutamatergic response to an acute cannabis challenge (Mason et al. 2021).

Only two studies have assessed GABA concentrations in chronic cannabis users. One research team reported a 15% reduction in GABA concentrations in the anterior cingulate as compared to non-cannabis using controls (Prescot et al. 2013). Another research project did not find any differences in striatal and anterior cingulate cortex GABA frontal glutamate levels in chronic and occasional cannabis users (Mason et al. 2021).

Chronic Cannabis Use and Task-Related Brain Activity

A range of fMRI studies have examined brain activity in chronic users while engaged in cognitive task performance that requires the recruitment of the reward circuitry (Tables 1 and 5). These cognitive tasks include assessments of executive control and attention, memory and learning, impulse control, and reward processing.

fMRI studies assessing the impact of chronic cannabis use on executive function as compared to non-using controls have repeatedly reported hyperactivation in the prefrontal cortex when engaged in tasks requiring working memory and decision-making (Becker et al. 2010; Kanayama et al. 2004; Jager et al. 2010; Cousijn et al. 2013b; Colizzi et al. 2015) and attention (Abdullaev et al. 2010; Chang et al. 2006b; Gruber et al. 2017). In about 50% of these studies, task performance in chronic users however did not significantly differ from that of the control group (Kanayama et al. 2004; Jager et al. 2010; Cousijn et al. 2013a, b; Chang et al. 2006b; Tervo-Clemmens et al. 2018) or even showed performance improvement (Tervo-Clemmens et al. 2018), whereas the remaining studies reported increased response time or decreased accuracy (Becker et al. 2010; Colizzi et al. 2015; Abdullaev et al. 2010; Gruber et al. 2017). In contrast to most studies, some studies have reported decrements in prefrontal activation (Chang et al. 2006b) or the absence of differential activation in the prefrontal cortex when comparing chronic users to controls (Jager et al. 2006). Overall these findings suggest that prefrontal hyperactivation reflects increased compensatory efforts needed to optimize performance during tasks requiring executive function and that depending on the success of the compensatory effort, task performance might be worse, similar, or better as compared to controls.

In fMRI studies focusing on BOLD activation during tasks requiring learning and memory, a consistent pattern of hypoactivation of prefrontal and striatal areas seems to emerge. Reductions in brain activity have been demonstrated in the striatum (Sneider et al. 2013; Riba et al. 2015), the hippocampus (Carey et al. 2015; Jager et al. 2007), and prefrontal areas (Carey et al. 2015; Jager et al. 2007; Riba et al. 2015). The majority of these studies also reported performance deficits in parallel to the pattern of hypoactivation in these memory-related network areas, such as impaired error-related learning (Carey et al. 2015), deficits in retrieval (Sneider et al. 2013), and increased sensitivity to false memory formation (Riba et al. 2015). These findings are in support of a wide range of clinical studies showing that chronic cannabis use is associated with deficits in memory and learning (Bossong et al. 2014; Broyd et al. 2016).

Studies focusing on brain activation during impulsivity tasks in chronic users as compared to non-users have provided mixed findings. A number of them have reported hypoactivation in prefrontal brain areas of chronic cannabis users (Wesley et al. 2011; Gruber and Yurgelun-Todd 2005; Hester et al. 2009), whereas others reported hyperactivation in striatal and prefrontal areas (Filbey and Yezhuvath 2013; Acheson et al. 2015; Cousijn et al. 2013b) or the absence of differences in prefrontal activity when compared to controls (Behan et al. 2014). It seems of interest that those studies that reported deficits in impulse control (i.e., increased error rate, impaired inhibition, impaired error awareness) in chronic cannabis users (Wesley et al. 2011; Gruber and Yurgelun-Todd 2005; Hester et al. 2009; Behan et al. 2014) also reported a concurrent hypoactivity or no change in brain activation in prefrontal brain areas. In studies that reported hyperactivity in striatal and prefrontal areas in chronic cannabis users, no change in impulsive control was observed compared to non-using controls (Filbey and Yezhuvath 2013, Acheson et al. 2015, Cousijn et al. 2013b). In line with results from studies assessing executive functioning, these results also suggest that hyperactive brain activation represents compensatory effort needed to operate optimally in impulsivity tasks, whereas hypoactivation might arise when compensation fails and loss of impulse control occurs.

Cross-sectional studies employing monetary incentive tasks or cue reactivity tasks to assess reward processing in chronic cannabis users and controls have provided mixed results as well. There is evidence of striatal activation (Nestor et al. 2010; Jager et al. 2013) and deactivation in anticipation of reward (Van Hell et al. 2010) in chronic cannabis users. Absence of striatal activation in anticipation of reward (Ford et al. 2014) and striatal activation in neutral trials when no reward was to be expected (Jager et al. 2013) have also been reported. Reward feedback has been associated with increased activity in striatal and prefrontal areas (Van Hell et al. 2010; Enzi et al. 2015; Yip et al. 2014) in chronic cannabis users, while some studies reported no change in response to reward feedback (Jager et al. 2013; Ford et al. 2014). In all of these studies, actual performance of chronic cannabis users and controls did not significantly differ from each other. Performance differences were only observed in two studies that employed a cue reactivity task to measure reward processing (Vingerhoets et al. 2016; Zhou et al. 2019). In one of these studies, increased drug cue reactivity was not associated with any change in striatal activity as compared to controls, although cue-induced striatal activation in chronic cannabis users did predict the severity of their cannabis use disorder (Vingerhoets et al. 2016). The other study (Zhou et al. 2019) reported increased ventral striatal reactivity and striatal frontal coupling in response to drug cues. An exploratory analysis revealed that ventral striatal reactivity in dependent cannabis users was strongly associated with craving. In addition, dependent cannabis users also selectively exhibited dorsal striatal reactivity, whereas non-dependent cannabis users did not. Overall these studies suggest a change in brain processing of reward in chronic cannabis users that in turn however does not automatically produce a noticeable change in associated behavioral responses as assessed with neuropsychological tests.

Conclusion

Taken together, evidence suggests that the effects of THC on reward-related circuitry are dynamic and change over time. Namely, in occasional cannabis users, THC acutely increases dopamine throughout the reward system, as evident from studies assessing THC-induced changes in functional connectivity within the circuit (Ramaekers et al. 2016; Mason et al. 2019) and those assessing brain activity while participants engaged in cognitive tasks which require recruitment of reward circuitry (Bhattacharyya et al. 2015; Borgwardt et al. 2008; De Sousa Fernandes Perna et al. 2017). Additionally, alterations in functional connectivity, dopaminergic transmission, and glutamatergic transmission within the reward system have been found to be significantly associated with both the impairing (Mason et al. 2019; Ramaekers et al. 2016) and the rewarding (Mason et al. 2019, Ramaekers et al. 2016)

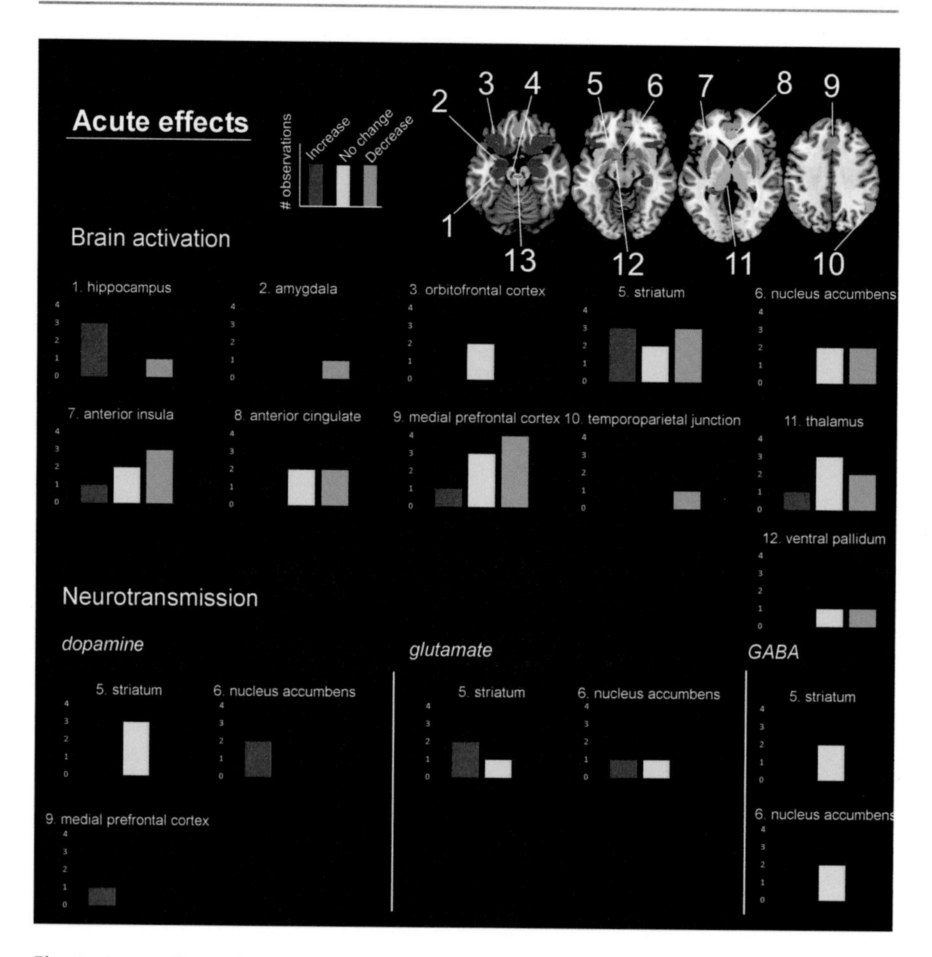

Fig. 1 **Acute effects of cannabis on brain activation and measures of neurotransmission.** *Top right* Brain areas that make up the reward system. 1 = hippocampus, 2 = amygdala, 3 = orbitofrontal cortex, 4 = substantia nigra, 5 = striatum, 6 = nucleus accumbens, 7 = insula, 8 = anterior cingulate, 9 = medial prefrontal cortex, 10 = temporoparietal junction, 11 = thalamus, 12 = ventral pallidum, 13 = ventral tegmental area. Bar graphs represent the number of observations that indicated increased (red), no change (yellow), or decreased (blue) brain activation or measures of dopamine, glutamate, or GABA signaling following acute administration of cannabis

effects of cannabis in occasional users, suggesting that the impact on neural activity within this system underlies many of the behavioral changes that take place after ingestion of THC (Ramaekers et al. 2021).

Conversely, in those who use the drug frequently, a blunted dopaminergic and glutamatergic response in the reward system is found, in response to a THC challenge (Mason et al. 2021). Whereas in the long-term, compared to the acute brain changes, chronic cannabis use seems to induce opposite neural effects (Figs. 1 and 2). For example, acutely THC has been found to increase glutamate and dopamine in the striatum and NAc, whereas sober chronic cannabis users

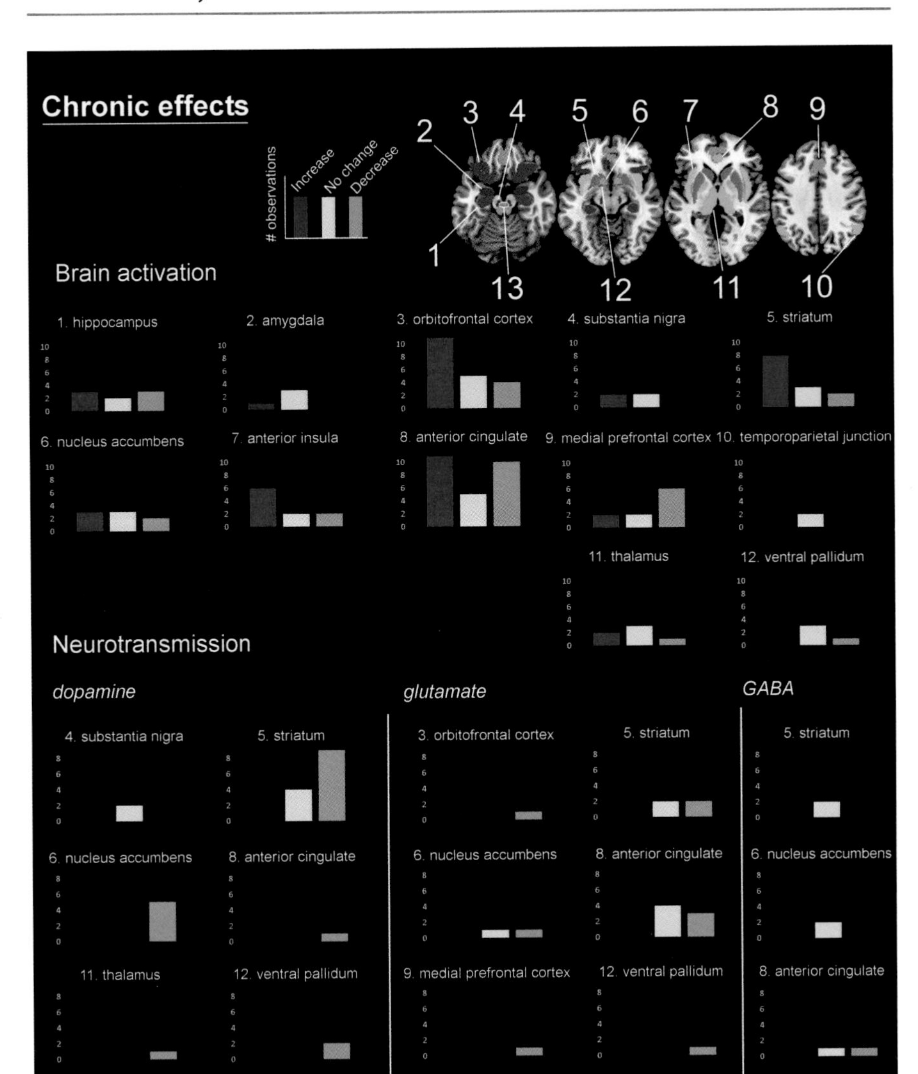

Fig. 2 Effects of chronic cannabis use on brain activation and measures of neurotransmission. *Top right* Brain areas that make up the reward system. 1 = hippocampus, 2 = amygdala, 3 = orbitofrontal cortex, 4 = substantia nigra, 5 = striatum, 6 = nucleus accumbens, 7 = insula, 8 = anterior cingulate, 9 = medial prefrontal cortex, 10 = temporoparietal junction, 11 = thalamus, 12 = ventral pallidum, 13 = ventral tegmental area. Bar graphs represent the number of observations that indicated increased (red), no change (yellow), or decreased (blue) brain activation or measures of dopamine, glutamate, or GABA signaling in chronic cannabis users

demonstrate a decrease of glutamate and glutamate-related metabolites and lower levels of dopamine release and dopamine transporter availability (Figs. 1 and 2, Table 2).

As reviewed in Ramaekers et al. (2020), these functional and neurochemical changes in the brain induced by repeated use of cannabis and THC are suggested to result from CB1 receptor downregulation, namely, a reduction in the number and signaling efficacy of CB1 receptors, as a homeostatic response (Hirvonen et al. 2012). It is noteworthy that downregulation of CB1 receptors appears to be region-specific, occurring to a larger extent, and more rapidly, in areas that make up the reward system (Hirvonen et al. 2012; Ramaekers et al. 2020). However such changes have been found to be reversible, with normalization of CB1 receptor availability taking place rapidly upon termination of cannabis use (Hirvonen et al. 2012). Thus, taken together, evidence suggests that acutely cannabis perturbs the brain's reward system via its action on dopaminergic and glutamatergic functioning, whereas repeated use of cannabis induces neuroadaptations in the brain's reward system, potentially via CB1 receptor downregulation as a homeostatic response. That said, future studies assessing the acute effects of thc on CB1 receptor availability in chronic cannabis users are necessary to confirm the latter hypothesis.

Application to Addiction

Substance use disorder has been characterized by a number of behavioral changes for which biological correlates have been identified (for review see Koob and Volkow (2016)). Within the context of the reward system, substance use disorder patients display habitual behavior which is dominant over goal-directed behavior (Everitt and Robbins 2005, 2016). Where initially drug taking is aimed at achieving the effects that a particular drug has, in substance use disorder patients, a stimulus associated with the drug has become sufficient to elicit drug-seeking and drug-taking behavior (Everitt and Robbins 2005, 2016). This habitual behavior is associated with dorsal striatal activation dominance (dorsolateral striatum, i.e., putamen in humans) (e.g., (Vollstadt-Klein et al. 2010; Sjoerds et al. 2013; Zhukovsky et al. 2019)). Second, substance use disorder patients show increased responsiveness to addiction-related cues (incentive salience/sensitization: (Robinson and Berridge 1993, 2001; Berridge and Robinson 2016)). Neural correlates of the increased incentive salience of addiction-related cues are represented by higher/more activation of the ventral striatum (i.e., NAc) compared with non-substance use disorder patients. In addition, addiction-related cue-induced craving is associated with increased activation of brain areas governing behavioral control and goal determination (e.g., anterior cingulate, dorsolateral prefrontal cortex, orbitofrontal cortex), suggesting behavior to be aimed at obtaining the substance of addiction (Kober et al. 2016; Lee et al. 2005; Risinger et al. 2005; Volkow et al. 2005; Jasinska et al. 2014). Finally, lower responsiveness of the same system to natural rewards represents the lack of interest in every day rewards and the anhedonic state often displayed by substance use disorder patients (Koob and Volkow 2016).

The neural characterizations of the reward system responsiveness observed in substance use disorder can be used as markers for addiction-like processes in long-term cannabis users and can help determine whether they show addiction-related brain changes. Evidence for these changes can take various forms, but mostly consist of human neuroimaging data. Within this approach, task-based and resting state functional connectivity, structural differences in gray and white matter, task-related activation, and differences in neurotransmitter synthesis and receptor binding in relevant brain areas may signal addiction relevant changes.

Dorsal Striatal Dominance

A potential prominent role of the dorsal striatum in cannabis-dependent subject's behavior is supported by structural brain changes. THC increased dendritic spine density in the posterior dorsomedial striatum in mice (Fernandez-Cabrera et al. 2018), and long-term cannabis users show more gray matter volume in the putamen and pallidum compared with non-users (Moreno-Alcazar et al. 2018). In addition, cannabis users (with psychotic-like symptoms) show a decrease in dopamine synthesis capacity in the putamen (Bloomfield et al. 2014b), and greater striatal activation and putamen volumes have been associated with poor treatment outcomes (Yip et al. 2014). Finally, increased cue reactivity of the putamen in cannabis users has been associated with dependence and problem severity in cannabis users at 3-year follow-up (Vingerhoets et al. 2016).

It may be expected that functional connectivity between dorsal striatum and frontal cortex decreases, marking reduced cognitive control over dorsal striatal elicited habitual behavior, a notion that is supported by differences between long-term and short-users in the acute effects of cannabis on anterior cingulate connectivity (Mason et al. 2021). In further support, decreased resting state functional connectivity between the dorsal striatum and anterior cingulate and dorsal medial prefrontal cortex has been observed in long-term cannabis users in two studies (Blanco-Hinojo et al. 2017; Zhou et al. 2018). However, in one of these studies (Blanco-Hinojo et al. 2017), a decrease in ventral striatal-anterior cingulate functional connectivity was observed, while in the other study increased connectivity was observed between ventral striatum and medial prefrontal cortex/anterior cingulate cortex (Zhou et al. 2018). In support of the latter finding, larger local functional connectivity in the ventral striatum has been found in cannabis-dependent users compared with non-users (Manza et al. 2018).

The potential changes in ventral striatal-frontal cortex functional connectivity may be associated with changes in glutamate levels. Dorsal anterior cingulate-NAc functional connectivity linearly decreases as a function of monthly cannabis use and dorsal anterior cingulate glutamate levels (Newman et al. 2020). Reductions in glutamate levels in the anterior cingulate of long-term users further support changes in goal-directed behavior (Chang et al. 2006a; Prescot et al. 2011, 2013), but see Watts et al. (2020).

Taken together, these functional and structural changes in structures governing goal-directed and habitual behavior are in line with reduced cognitive control over dorsal striatal-associated habitual behavior; however the changes in ventral striatal functional connectivity are equivocal. As direct assessments of goal-directed versus habitual behavior and associated neural activation in long-term cannabis users are still lacking, strong conclusions cannot be drawn at this point.

Increased Incentive Salience

Addiction-related cues-induced increased signaling of incentive value and the neural correlates have also been observed in cannabis users. For example, dependent and nondependent cannabis users have shown increased responsiveness of the ventral striatum in response to cannabis-related cues (Zhou et al. 2019) and marketing videos (De Sousa Fernandes Perna et al. 2017). Heavy users with high-problem severity have shown an increased mesolimbic (ventral tegmental area, orbitofrontal cortex, anterior cingulate, striatum) response to cannabis-related cues (Cousijn et al. 2013a). Moreover, increased activation of ventral tegmental area, thalamus, anterior cingulate, insula, amygdala, orbitofrontal cortex, and nucleus accumbens in response to cannabis-associated tactile stimuli has been observed in 72 h abstinent users, with fronto-striatal activation being associated with problem severity (Filbey et al. 2009, 2016; Filbey and Dunlop 2014). The above described hyperresponsive networks in response to cannabis-related cues suggest increased signaling of potential reward which may motivate cannabis-seeking behavior.

Decrease Response to Natural Reward

The often observed phenomenon of decreased neural response to rewards other than addiction-related has also been observed in cannabis users, but findings are mixed. Reduced activation in lateral orbitofrontal cortex during performance on an Iowa gambling task has been observed in 25-day abstinent users, particularly in heavy users (Bolla et al. 2005). Long-term cannabis users have shown a smaller response of the NAc during reward anticipation compared with non-users (Van Hell et al. 2010). In addition, lower functional connectivity between NAc and medial prefrontal cortex in response to receiving monetary reward has been shown in a group with escalating dose of cannabis use over time compared with stable high/low dose (Lichenstein et al. 2017). In contrast, no difference (Enzi et al. 2015) or larger responses of the rewards system in long-term users to monetary incentives have also been observed, for example, during a task comprising both anticipation and reception of monetary rewards (Acheson et al. 2015). Moreover, in a well-designed study separating monetary incentive anticipation from reception, long-term frequent cannabis users displayed increased NAc activation during anticipation of a "win" outcome, which was correlated with lifetime cannabis use (Nestor et al. 2010).

To conclude, there is evidence for long-term cannabis users to display brain changes that suggest dominance of dorsal striatal structures potentially contributing to drug-taking behavior. However, the evidence for a clear shift from ventral striatal to dorsal striatal activation is equivocal due to mixed findings concerning ventral striatal changes. The suggested hyperresponsiveness of the ventral striatum to addiction-related cues appears more consistent, such that long-term cannabis users show increased responsiveness. In contrast, long-term cannabis users appear not to show a clear reduction in responsiveness to anticipation and reception of rewards other than addiction-related. In support, (Bossong et al. 2015) only found a modest increase in striatal dopamine release compared with other drugs of abuse, potentially signaling limited abuse liability of cannabis.

Application to Public Health

As discussed above, there is evidence to suggest that cannabis has abuse liability from a biological perspective, namely, action on the brain's reward system. This conclusion is particularly important in light of the changing legalization status of cannabis, and the growing therapeutic interest for a range of different disorders, and suggests that special attention should be paid when navigating this landscape. Importantly, steps can be taken to try to mitigate the possibility that individual's cannabis use does not develop into a use disorder (addiction). In regard to therapeutic cannabis, governmental granting bodies can incentivize research to investigate the potential of low, therapeutic doses, or cannabis products with low THC concentrations, which provide symptomatic relief but do not perturb the brain's reward system, thus potentially reducing abuse liability. In regard to recreational use, governments can control the cost of cannabis products via taxation, which has been shown to be a successful public health policy for other legal drugs like alcohol and nicotine (Budney et al. 2019). Finally, it is suggested that governments should regulate the use of marketing and advertising strategies aimed to normalize and initiate cannabis product use (Budney et al. 2019). This is a particularly important aspect of public policy, as cannabis users have been shown to be hyperresponsive to cannabis-related cues and display reduced cognitive control over habitual behaviors, and in regard to sensitivity to marketing tactics, it has been found that especially younger individuals are vulnerable targets.

Summary Statements (5–15)

- In occasional cannabis users, THC acutely increases dopamine throughout the reward system, as evident from studies assessing THC-induced functional connectivity within the circuit, those assessing brain activity while participants engaged in reward-related tasks, and PET imaging studies.
- Those who use cannabis frequently display an acute blunted dopaminergic and glutamatergic response in the reward system, which may explain their tolerance to some of the impairing and rewarding effects of cannabis.
- THC acutely blunts the neural response in the striatum/nucleus accumbens to rewarding stimuli, including music, drug-associated cues, and monetary incentive.
- fMRI studies comparing brain activation in the reward circuit of chronic cannabis users and controls often report changes in brain processing in the absence of any change in behavioral responses as assessed with neuropsychological tests.

- Hyperactive brain activation in the reward circuit of chronic cannabis users might represent compensatory effort needed to operate optimally in neurocognitive tasks, whereas hypoactivation might arise when compensation fails and loss of neurocognitive control occurs.
- Chronic cannabis users display reduced levels of dopamine, glutamate, and GABA in the reward circuit.
- Chronic cannabis users display hyperresponsive reward circuitry following cannabis-related cues.
- Chronic cannabis are hypothesized to display reduced cognitive control over dorsal striatal (i.e., habitual) behavior.
- Evidence for a typical hyporesponsive reward system in long-term cannabis users to non-addiction-related stimuli is mixed.
- Government granting bodies can incentivize research to investigate the potential of low, therapeutic doses, or cannabis products with low THC concentrations, which provide symptomatic relief but do not perturb the brain's reward system, thus potentially reducing abuse liability.
- Governments should regulate marketing and advertisement of cannabis products, as cannabis users have been found to be hyperresponsive to cannabis-related cues and display reduced cognitive control over habitual behaviors.

Key Facts (5 Single Sentences)

1) Cannabis perturbs the brain's reward system via its action on dopaminergic and glutamatergic functioning.
2) The effects of cannabis on the reward system are dynamic and change over time, according to frequency of use.
3) Acute and chronic cannabis use produce opposite change in dopaminergic, glutamatergic, and GABAergic neurotransmission in the reward system, suggesting the development of neuradaptions following repeated cannabis exposure.
4) There is evidence to suggest that cannabis has abuse liability from a biological perspective, namely, enhanced responding toward cannabis predicting cues, and markers of reduced cognitive control over basal ganglia structures governing habitual responding.
5) Controlled studies on the brain's response to acute cannabis exposure in chronic users are scarce, but needed.

Mini-Dictionary of Terms

Cannabinoids: Compounds found in cannabis or that are synthetically produced to mimic naturally occurring cannabinoids.

Chronic cannabis users: In the reviewed studies, defined broadly as those who use cannabis at least one time a day.

Functional connectivity: A measure of similarity or correlation between brain signals arising from anatomically separated brain regions that indicates that the regions are functionally connected.

Functional magnetic resonance imaging (fMRI): A noninvasive technique for measuring and mapping brain activity based on changes in blood oxygen level-dependent signals that indicate underlying neural activity.

Occasional cannabis users: In the reviewed studies, defined broadly as those who have used cannabis between <10 times in their life, up to those who use <3 times a week.

Positron emission tomography (PET): A magnetic resonance imaging technique that uses radioactive substances known as radiotracers to visualize and measure changes in metabolic processes and in other physiological activities such as receptor occupancy.

Proton magnetic resonance spectroscopy (MRS): A noninvasive imaging technique that allows measurement of chemicals that are present in relatively high concentrations in the brain (in the millimolar range) such as glutamate, GABA, and other markers of metabolic activity.

Striatum: A small group of subcortical brain structures, including the caudate and putamen (dorsal striatum) and the nucleus accumbens (ventral striatum). The dorsal striatum is often studied more in the context of movement, whereas the ventral striatum and nucleus accumbens have been extensively studied for its role in reward-related processes.

Tetrahydrocannabinol (THC): The cannabis plant's primary component for causing psychoactive effects, including both the rewarding and impairing effects of the drug. It is one of over 100 cannabinoids that have been identified in the cannabis plant. In experimental research studies, it is often given in an isolated form.

References

Abdullaev Y, Posner MI, Nunnally R, Dishion TJ (2010) Functional MRI evidence for inefficient attentional control in adolescent chronic cannabis abuse. Behav Brain Res 215:45–57

Acheson A, Ray KL, Hines CS, Li K, Dawes MA, Mathias CW, Dougherty DM, Laird AR (2015) Functional activation and effective connectivity differences in adolescent marijuana users performing a simulated gambling task. J Addict 2015:783106

Albrecht DS, Skosnik PD, Vollmer JM, Brumbaugh MS, Perry KM, Mock BH, Zheng QH, Federici LA, Patton EA, Herring CM, Yoder KK (2013) Striatal D(2)/D(3) receptor availability is inversely correlated with cannabis consumption in chronic marijuana users. Drug Alcohol Depend 128:52–57

Atakan Z, Bhattacharyya S, Allen P, Martin-Santos R, Crippa JA, Borgwardt SJ, Fusar-Poli P, Seal M, Sallis H, Stahl D, Zuardi AW, Rubia K, Mcguire P (2013) Cannabis affects people differently: inter-subject variation in the psychotogenic effects of Delta9-tetrahydrocannabinol: a functional magnetic resonance imaging study with healthy volunteers. Psychol Med 43: 1255–1267

Becker B, Wagner D, Gouzoulis-Mayfrank E, Spuentrup E, Daumann J (2010) The impact of early-onset cannabis use on functional brain correlates of working memory. Prog Neuro-Psychopharmacol Biol Psychiatry 34:837–845

Behan B, Connolly CG, Datwani S, Doucet M, Ivanovic J, Morioka R, Stone A, Watts R, Smyth B, Garavan H (2014) Response inhibition and elevated parietal-cerebellar correlations in chronic adolescent cannabis users. Neuropharmacology 84:131–137

Berridge KC, Robinson TE (2016) Liking, wanting, and the incentive-sensitization theory of addiction. Am Psychol 71:670–679

Bhattacharyya S, Atakan Z, Martin-Santos R, Crippa J, Kambeitz J, Malhi S, Giampietro V, Williams S, Brammer M, Rubia K (2015) Impairment of inhibitory control processing related to acute psychotomimetic effects of cannabis. Eur Neuropsychopharmacol 25:26–37

Blanco-Hinojo L, Pujol J, Harrison BJ, Macia D, Batalla A, Nogue S, Torrens M, Farre M, Deus J, Martin-Santos R (2017) Attenuated frontal and sensory inputs to the basal ganglia in cannabis users. Addict Biol 22:1036–1047

Bloomfield MA, Morgan CJ, Egerton A, Kapur S, Curran HV, Howes OD (2014a) Dopaminergic function in cannabis users and its relationship to cannabis-induced psychotic symptoms. Biol Psychiatry 75:470–478

Bloomfield MA, Morgan CJ, Kapur S, Curran HV, Howes OD (2014b) The link between dopamine function and apathy in cannabis users: an [18F]-DOPA PET imaging study. Psychopharmacology 231:2251–2259

Bloomfield MA, Ashok AH, Volkow ND, Howes OD (2016) The effects of Delta(9)-tetrahydrocannabinol on the dopamine system. Nature 539:369–377

Bloomfield MAP, Hindocha C, Green SF, Wall MB, Lees R, Petrilli K, Costello H, Ogunbiyi MO, Bossong MG, Freeman TP (2019) The neuropsychopharmacology of cannabis: a review of human imaging studies. Pharmacol Ther 195:132–161

Bolla KI, Eldreth DA, Matochik JA, Cadet JL (2005) Neural substrates of faulty decision-making in abstinent marijuana users. NeuroImage 26:480–492

Bonelli RM, Cummings JL (2007) Frontal-subcortical circuitry and behavior. Dialogues Clin Neurosci 9:141

Borgwardt SJ, Allen P, Bhattacharyya S, Fusar-Poli P, Crippa JA, Seal ML, Fraccaro V, Atakan Z, Martin-Santos R, O'carroll C, Rubia K, Mcguire PK (2008) Neural basis of Delta-9-tetrahydrocannabinol and cannabidiol: effects during response inhibition. Biol Psychiatry 64:966–973

Bossong MG, Kahn RS (2016) The salience of reward. *JAMA*. Psychiatry 73:777–778

Bossong MG, Van Berckel BN, Boellaard R, Zuurman L, Schuit RC, Windhorst AD, Van Gerven JM, Ramsey NF, Lammertsma AA, Kahn RS (2009) Delta 9-tetrahydrocannabinol induces dopamine release in the human striatum. Neuropsychopharmacology 34:759–766

Bossong MG, Jager G, Bhattacharyya S, Allen P (2014) Acute and non-acute effects of cannabis on human memory function: a critical review of neuroimaging studies. Curr Pharm Des 20: 2114–2125

Bossong MG, Mehta MA, Van Berckel BN, Howes OD, Kahn RS, Stokes PR (2015) Further human evidence for striatal dopamine release induced by administration of 9-tetrahydrocannabinol (THC): selectivity to limbic striatum. Psychopharmacology 232:2723–2729

Bossong MG, van Hell HH, Schubart CD, van Saane W, Iseger TA, Jager G, van Osch MJP, Jansma JM, Kahn RS, Boks MP, Ramsey NF (2019) Acute effects of Δ9-tetrahydrocannabinol (THC) on resting state brain function and their modulation by COMT genotype. Eur Neuropsychopharm 29(6):766–776. https://doi.org/10.1016/j.euroneuro.2019.03.010

Broyd SJ, Van Hell HH, Beale C, Yucel M, Solowij N (2016) Acute and chronic effects of cannabinoids on human cognition-a systematic review. Biol Psychiatry 79:557–567

Budney AJ, Sofis MJ, Borodovsky JT (2019) An update on cannabis use disorder with comment on the impact of policy related to therapeutic and recreational cannabis use. Eur Arch Psychiatry Clin Neurosci 269:73–86

Carey SE, Nestor L, Jones J, Garavan H, Hester R (2015) Impaired learning from errors in cannabis users: dorsal anterior cingulate cortex and hippocampus hypoactivity. Drug Alcohol Depend 155:175–182

Chang L, Cloak C, Yakupov R, Ernst T (2006a) Combined and independent effects of chronic marijuana use and HIV on brain metabolites. J Neuroimmune Pharmacol 1:65–76

Chang L, Yakupov R, Cloak C, Ernst T (2006b) Marijuana use is associated with a reorganized visual-attention network and cerebellar hypoactivation. Brain 129:1096–1112

Cheng H, Skosnik PD, Pruce BJ, Brumbaugh MS, Vollmer JM, Fridberg DJ, O'donnell BF, Hetrick WP, Newman SD (2014) Resting state functional magnetic resonance imaging reveals distinct brain activity in heavy cannabis users - a multi-voxel pattern analysis. J Psychopharmacol 28: 1030–1040

Colizzi M, Fazio L, Ferranti L, Porcelli A, Masellis R, Marvulli D, Bonvino A, Ursini G, Blasi G, Bertolino A (2015) Functional genetic variation of the cannabinoid receptor 1 and cannabis use interact on prefrontal connectivity and related working memory behavior. Neuropsychopharmacology 40:640–649

Colizzi M, Weltens N, Mcguire P, Lythgoe D, Williams S, Van Oudenhove L, Bhattacharyya S (2020) Delta-9-tetrahydrocannabinol increases striatal glutamate levels in healthy individuals: implications for psychosis. Mol Psychiatry 25:3231–3240

Cools R, D'Esposito M (2011) Inverted-U-shaped dopamine actions on human working memory and cognitive control. Biol Psychiatry 69:e113–e125

Cousijn J, Goudriaan AE, Ridderinkhof KR, Van Den Brink W, Veltman DJ, Wiers RW (2013a) Neural responses associated with cue-reactivity in frequent cannabis users. Addict Biol 18: 570–580

Cousijn J, Wiers RW, Ridderinkhof KR, Van Den Brink W, Veltman DJ, Porrino LJ, Goudriaan AE (2013b) Individual differences in decision making and reward processing predict changes in cannabis use: a prospective functional magnetic resonance imaging study. Addict Biol 18: 1013–1023

Crane NA, Phan KL (2021) Effect of Delta9-tetrahydrocannabinol on frontostriatal resting state functional connectivity and subjective euphoric response in healthy young adults. Drug Alcohol Depend 221:108565

De Sousa Fernandes Perna EB, Theunissen EL, Kuypers KP, Evers EA, Stiers P, Toennes SW, Witteman J, Van Dalen W, Ramaekers JG (2017) Brain reactivity to alcohol and cannabis marketing during sobriety and intoxication. Addict Biol 22:823–832

Enzi B, Lissek S, Edel MA, Tegenthoff M, Nicolas V, Scherbaum N, Juckel G, Roser P (2015) Alterations of monetary reward and punishment processing in chronic cannabis users: an FMRI study. PLoS One 10:e0119150

Everitt BJ, Robbins TW (2005) Neural systems of reinforcement for drug addiction: from actions to habits to compulsion. Nat Neurosci 8:1481–1489

Everitt BJ, Robbins TW (2016) Drug addiction: updating actions to habits to compulsions ten years on. Annu Rev Psychol 67:23–50

Fernandez-Cabrera MR, Higuera-Matas A, Fernaud-Espinosa I, Defelipe J, Ambrosio E, Miguens M (2018) Selective effects of Delta9-tetrahydrocannabinol on medium spiny neurons in the striatum. PLoS One 13:e0200950

Filbey FM, Dunlop J (2014) Differential reward network functional connectivity in cannabis dependent and non-dependent users. Drug Alcohol Depend 140:101–111

Filbey F, Yezhuvath U (2013) Functional connectivity in inhibitory control networks and severity of cannabis use disorder. Am J Drug Alcohol Abuse 39:382–391

Filbey FM, Schacht JP, Myers US, Chavez RS, Hutchison KE (2009) Marijuana craving in the brain. Proc Natl Acad Sci U S A 106:13016–13021

Filbey FM, Dunlop J, Ketcherside A, Baine J, Rhinehardt T, Kuhn B, Dewitt S, Alvi T (2016) fMRI study of neural sensitization to hedonic stimuli in long-term, daily cannabis users. Hum Brain Mapp 37:3431–3443

Ford KA, Wammes M, Neufeld RW, Mitchell D, Theberge J, Williamson P, Osuch EA (2014) Unique functional abnormalities in youth with combined marijuana use and depression: an FMRI study. Front Psych 5:130

Freeman TP, Pope RA, Wall MB, Bisby JA, Luijten M, Hindocha C, Mokrysz C, Lawn W, Moss A, Bloomfield MAP, Morgan CJA, Nutt DJ, Curran HV (2018) Cannabis dampens the effects of music in brain regions sensitive to reward and emotion. Int J Neuropsychopharmacol 21:21–32

Freund TF, Katona I, Piomelli D (2003) Role of endogenous cannabinoids in synaptic signaling. Physiol Rev 83:1017–1066

Gardner EL (2005) Endocannabinoid signaling system and brain reward: emphasis on dopamine. Pharmacol Biochem Behav 81:263–284

Grimm O, Loffler M, Kamping S, Hartmann A, Rohleder C, Leweke M, Flor H (2018) Probing the endocannabinoid system in healthy volunteers: Cannabidiol alters fronto-striatal resting-state connectivity. Eur Neuropsychopharmacol 28:841–849

Gruber SA, Yurgelun-Todd DA (2005) Neuroimaging of marijuana smokers during inhibitory processing: a pilot investigation. Brain Res Cogn Brain Res 23:107–118

Gruber SA, Sagar KA, Dahlgren MK, Gonenc A, Smith RT, Lambros AM, Cabrera KB, Lukas SE (2017) The grass might be greener: medical marijuana patients exhibit altered brain activity and improved executive function after 3 months of treatment. Front Pharmacol 8:983

Gunasekera B, Davies C, Martin-Santos R, Bhatthacharyya S (2020) The yin and Yang of cannabis-a systematic review of human neuroimaging evidence of the differential effects of delta-9-tetrahydrocannabinol and cannabidiol. Biological Psychiatry: Cognitive Neuroscience and Neuroimaging 6:636–645

Gunasekera B, Diederen K, Bhattacharyya S (2021) Cannabinoids, reward processing, and psychosis. Psychopharmacology (Berl)

Hall W, Lynskey M (2016) Evaluating the public health impacts of legalizing recreational cannabis use in the United States. Addiction 111:1764–1773

Hashimotodani Y, Ohno-Shosaku T, Kano M (2007) Endocannabinoids and synaptic function in the CNS. Neuroscientist 13:127–137

Hermann D, Sartorius A, Welzel H, Walter S, Skopp G, Ende G, Mann K (2007) Dorsolateral Prefrontal Cortex N-Acetylaspartate/Total Creatine (NAA/tCr) Loss in Male Recreational Cannabis Users. Biological Psychiatry 61(11):1281–1289. https://doi.org/10.1016/j.biopsych.2006.08.027

Hester R, Nestor L, Garavan H (2009) Impaired error awareness and anterior cingulate cortex hypoactivity in chronic cannabis users. Neuropsychopharmacology 34:2450–2458

Hirvonen J, Goodwin R, Li C-T, Terry G, Zoghbi S, Morse C, Pike V, Volkow N, Huestis M, Innis R (2012) Reversible and regionally selective downregulation of brain cannabinoid CB 1 receptors in chronic daily cannabis smokers. Mol Psychiatry 17:642–649

Jager G, Kahn RS, Van Den Brink W, Van Ree JM, Ramsey NF (2006) Long-term effects of frequent cannabis use on working memory and attention: an fMRI study. Psychopharmacology 185:358–368

Jager G, Van Hell HH, De Win MM, Kahn RS, Van Den Brink W, Van Ree JM, Ramsey NF (2007) Effects of frequent cannabis use on hippocampal activity during an associative memory task. Eur Neuropsychopharmacol 17:289–297

Jager G, Block RI, Luijten M, Ramsey NF (2010) Cannabis use and memory brain function in adolescent boys: a cross-sectional multicenter functional magnetic resonance imaging study. J Am Acad Child Adolesc Psychiatry 49:561–572, 572 e1-3

Jager G, Block RI, Luijten M, Ramsey NF (2013) Tentative evidence for striatal hyperactivity in adolescent cannabis-using boys: a cross-sectional multicenter fMRI study. J Psychoactive Drugs 45:156–167

Jansma JM, Van Hell HH, Vanderschuren LJ, Bossong MG, Jager G, Kahn RS, Ramsey NF (2013) THC reduces the anticipatory nucleus accumbens response to reward in subjects with a nicotine addiction. Transl Psychiatry 3:e234

Jasinska AJ, Stein EA, Kaiser J, Naumer MJ, Yalachkov Y (2014) Factors modulating neural reactivity to drug cues in addiction: a survey of human neuroimaging studies. Neurosci Biobehav Rev 38:1–16

Johnston, L. D., Miech, R. A., O'malley, P. M., Bachman, J. G., Schulenberg, J. E. & Patrick, M. E. 2018. Monitoring the future national survey results on drug use, 1975–2017: overview, key findings on adolescent drug use

Kamp F, Proebstl L, Penzel N, Adorjan K, Ilankovic A, Pogarell O, Koller G, Soyka M, Falkai P, Koutsouleris N, Kambeitz J (2019) Effects of sedative drug use on the dopamine system: a systematic review and meta-analysis of in vivo neuroimaging studies. Neuropsychopharmacology 44:660–667

Kanayama G, Rogowska J, Pope HG, Gruber SA, Yurgelun-Todd DA (2004) Spatial working memory in heavy cannabis users: a functional magnetic resonance imaging study. Psychopharmacology 176:239–247

Kettner H, Mason NL, Kuypers KP (2019) Motives for classical and novel psychoactive substances use in psychedelic polydrug users. Contemp Drug Probl 46:304–320

Klumpers LE, Cole DM, Khalili-Mahani N, Soeter RP, te Beek ET, Rombouts SARB, van Gerven JMA (2012) Manipulating brain connectivity with δ9-tetrahydrocannabinol: A pharmacological resting state FMRI study. NeuroImage 63(3):1701–1711. https://doi.org/10.1016/j.neuroimage.2012.07.051

Knutson B, Adams CM, Fong GW, Hommer D (2001a) Anticipation of increasing monetary reward selectively recruits nucleus accumbens. J Neurosci 21:RC159-RC159

Knutson B, Fong GW, Adams CM, Varner JL, Hommer D (2001b) Dissociation of reward anticipation and outcome with event-related fMRI. Neuroreport 12:3683–3687

Kober H, Lacadie CM, Wexler BE, Malison RT, Sinha R, Potenza MN (2016) Brain activity during cocaine craving and gambling urges: an fMRI study. Neuropsychopharmacology 41:628–637

Koob GF, Volkow ND (2016) Neurobiology of addiction: a neurocircuitry analysis. Lancet Psychiatry 3:760–773

Kringelbach ML, Berridge KC (2012) The joyful mind. Sci Am 307:40–45

Lee JH, Lim Y, Wiederhold BK, Graham SJ (2005) A functional magnetic resonance imaging (FMRI) study of cue-induced smoking craving in virtual environments. Appl Psychophysiol Biofeedback 30:195–204

Leroy C, Karila L, Martinot JL, Lukasiewicz M, Duchesnay E, Comtat C, Dolle F, Benyamina A, Artiges E, Ribeiro MJ, Reynaud M, Trichard C (2012) Striatal and extrastriatal dopamine transporter in cannabis and tobacco addiction: a high-resolution PET study. Addict Biol 17: 981–990

Lichenstein SD, Musselman S, Shaw DS, Sitnick S, Forbes EE (2017) Nucleus accumbens functional connectivity at age 20 is associated with trajectory of adolescent cannabis use and predicts psychosocial functioning in young adulthood. Addiction 112:1961–1970

Lopez-Larson MP, Rogowska J, Yurgelun-Todd D (2015) Aberrant orbitofrontal connectivity in marijuana smoking adolescents. Dev Cogn Neurosci 16:54–62

Lupica CR, Riegel AC, Hoffman AF (2004) Marijuana and cannabinoid regulation of brain reward circuits. Br J Pharmacol 143:227–234

Mackie K (2008) Cannabinoid receptors: where they are and what they do. J Neuroendocrinol 20: 10–14

Manza P, Tomasi D, Volkow ND (2018) Subcortical local functional Hyperconnectivity in cannabis dependence. Biol Psychiatry Cogn Neurosci Neuroimaging 3:285–293

Mason NL, Theunissen EL, Hutten N, Tse DHY, Toennes SW, Stiers P, Ramaekers JG (2019) Cannabis induced increase in striatal glutamate associated with loss of functional corticostriatal connectivity. Eur Neuropsychopharmacol 29:247–256

Mason NL, Theunissen EL, Hutten N, Tse DHY, Toennes SW, Jansen JFA, Stiers P, Ramaekers JG (2021) Reduced responsiveness of the reward system is associated with tolerance to cannabis impairment in chronic users. Addict Biol 26:e12870

Mathew RJ, Wilson W, Tant S (1989) Acute changes in cerebral blood flow associated with marijuana smoking. Acta Psychiatr Scand 79:118–128

Mathew RJ, Wilson WH, Humphreys DF, Lowe JV, Wiethe KE (1992a) Changes in middle cerebral artery velocity after marijuana. Biol Psychiatry 32:164–169

Mathew RJ, Wilson WH, Humphreys DF, Lowe JV, Wiethe KE (1992b) Regional cerebral blood flow after marijuana smoking. J Cereb Blood Flow Metab 12:750–758

Mizrahi R, Suridjan I, Kenk M, George TP, Wilson A, Houle S, Rusjan P (2013) Dopamine response to psychosocial stress in chronic cannabis users: a PET study with [11C]−+-PHNO. Neuropsychopharmacology 38:673–682

Mizrahi R, Kenk M, Suridjan I, Boileau I, George TP, Mckenzie K, Wilson AA, Houle S, Rusjan P (2014) Stress-induced dopamine response in subjects at clinical high risk for schizophrenia with and without concurrent cannabis use. Neuropsychopharmacology 39:1479–1489

Moreno-Alcazar A, Gonzalvo B, Canales-Rodriguez EJ, Blanco L, Bachiller D, Romaguera A, Monte-Rubio GC, Roncero C, Mckenna PJ, Pomarol-Clotet E (2018) Larger gray matter volume in the basal ganglia of heavy cannabis users detected by voxel-based morphometry and subcortical volumetric analysis. Front Psych 9:175

Muetzel RL, Marjanska M, Collins PF, Becker MP, Valabregue R, Auerbach EJ, Lim KO, Luciana M (2013) In vivo (1)H magnetic resonance spectroscopy in young-adult daily marijuana users. Neuroimage Clin 2:581–589

Nestor L, Hester R, Garavan H (2010) Increased ventral striatal BOLD activity during non-drug reward anticipation in cannabis users. NeuroImage 49:1133–1143

Newman SD, Cheng H, Schnakenberg Martin A, Dydak U, Dharmadhikari S, Hetrick W, O'Donnell B (2019) An investigation of neurochemical changes in chronic cannabis users. Front Hum Neurosci 13:318

Newman SD, Cheng H, Kim DJ, Schnakenberg-Martin A, Dydak U, Dharmadhikari S, Hetrick W, O'Donnell B (2020) An investigation of the relationship between glutamate and resting state connectivity in chronic cannabis users. Brain Imaging Behav 14:2062–2071

Organization WH (2016) Health and social effects of nonmedical cannabis use (the). World Health Organization

Pierce RC, Kumaresan V (2006) The mesolimbic dopamine system: the final common pathway for the reinforcing effect of drugs of abuse? Neurosci Biobehav Rev 30:215–238

Prescot AP, Locatelli AE, Renshaw PF, Yurgelun-Todd DA (2011) Neurochemical alterations in adolescent chronic marijuana smokers: a proton MRS study. NeuroImage 57:69–75

Prescot AP, Renshaw PF, Yurgelun-Todd DA (2013) Gamma-amino butyric acid and glutamate abnormalities in adolescent chronic marijuana smokers. Drug Alcohol Depend 129:232–239

Pujol J, Blanco-Hinojo L, Batalla A, Lopez-Sola M, Harrison BJ, Soriano-Mas C, Crippa JA, Fagundo AB, Deus J, De La Torre R, Nogue S, Farre M, Torrens M, Martin-Santos R (2014) Functional connectivity alterations in brain networks relevant to self-awareness in chronic cannabis users. J Psychiatr Res 51:68–78

Ramaekers JG, Kauert G, Theunissen E, Toennes SW, Moeller M (2009) Neurocognitive performance during acute THC intoxication in heavy and occasional cannabis users. J Psychopharmacol 23:266–277

Ramaekers J, Evers E, Theunissen E, Kuypers K, Goulas A, Stiers P (2013) Methylphenidate reduces functional connectivity of nucleus accumbens in brain reward circuit. Psychopharmacology 229:219–226

Ramaekers J, Van Wel J, Spronk D, Franke B, Kenis G, Toennes S, Kuypers K, Theunissen E, Stiers P, Verkes R (2016) Cannabis and cocaine decrease cognitive impulse control and functional corticostriatal connectivity in drug users with low activity DBH genotypes. Brain Imaging Behav 10:1254–1263

Ramaekers JG, Mason NL, Theunissen EL (2020) Blunted highs: Pharmacodynamic and behavioral models of cannabis tolerance. Eur Neuropsychopharmacol 36:191–205

Ramaekers JG, Mason NL, Kloft L, Theunissen EL (2021) The why behind the high: determinants of neurocognition during acute cannabis exposure. Nat Rev Neurosci 22:439–454

Riba J, Valle M, Sampedro F, Rodriguez-Pujadas A, Martinez-Horta S, Kulisevsky J, Rodriguez-Fornells A (2015) Telling true from false: cannabis users show increased susceptibility to false memories. Mol Psychiatry 20:772–777

Rigucci S, Xin L, Klauser P, Baumann PS, Alameda L, Cleusix M, Jenni R, Ferrari C,Pompili M, Gruetter R, Do KQ, Conus P (2018) Cannabis use in early psychosis is associated with reduced glutamate levels in the prefrontal cortex. Psychopharmacology 235(1):13–22. https://doi.org/10.1007/s00213-017-4745-z

Risinger RC, Salmeron BJ, Ross TJ, Amen SL, Sanfilipo M, Hoffmann RG, Bloom AS, Garavan H, Stein EA (2005) Neural correlates of high and craving during cocaine self-administration using BOLD fMRI. NeuroImage 26:1097–1108

Robinson TE, Berridge KC (1993) The neural basis of drug craving: an incentive-sensitization theory of addiction. Brain Res Brain Res Rev 18:247–291

Robinson TE, Berridge KC (2001) Incentive-sensitization and addiction. Addiction 96:103–114

Robinson TE, Berridge KC (2008) Review. The incentive sensitization theory of addiction: some current issues. Philos Trans R Soc Lond Ser B Biol Sci 363:3137–3146

Salgado S, Kaplitt MG (2015) The nucleus accumbens: a comprehensive review. Stereotact Funct Neurosurg 93:75–93

Schultz W (2007) Multiple dopamine functions at different time courses. Annu Rev Neurosci 30: 259–288

Sevy S, Smith GS, Ma Y, Dhawan V, Chaly T, Kingsley PB, Kumra S, Abdelmessih S, Eidelberg D (2008) Cerebral glucose metabolism and D2/D3 receptor availability in young adults with cannabis dependence measured with positron emission tomography. Psychopharmacology 197(4):549–556. https://doi.org/10.1007/s00213-008-1075-1

Sjoerds Z, De Wit S, Van Den Brink W, Robbins TW, Beekman AT, Penninx BW, Veltman DJ (2013) Behavioral and neuroimaging evidence for overreliance on habit learning in alcohol-dependent patients. Transl Psychiatry 3:e337

Sneider JT, Gruber SA, Rogowska J, Silveri MM, Yurgelun-Todd DA (2013) A preliminary study of functional brain activation among marijuana users during performance of a virtual water maze task. J Addict 2013:461029

Stokes PR, Mehta MA, Curran HV, Breen G, Grasby PM (2009) Can recreational doses of THC produce significant dopamine release in the human striatum? NeuroImage 48: 186–190

Stokes PR, Egerton A, Watson B, Reid A, Breen G, Lingford-Hughes A, Nutt DJ, Mehta MA (2010) Significant decreases in frontal and temporal [11C]-raclopride binding after THC challenge. NeuroImage 52:1521–1527

Sung YH, Carey PD, Stein DJ, Ferrett HL, Spottiswoode BS, Renshaw PF, Yurgelun-Todd DA (2013) Decreased frontal N-acetylaspartate levels in adolescents concurrently using both methamphetamine and marijuana. Behav Brain Res 246:154–161

Tervo-Clemmens B, Simmonds D, Calabro FJ, Day NL, Richardson GA, Luna B (2018) Adolescent cannabis use and brain systems supporting adult working memory encoding, maintenance, and retrieval. NeuroImage 169:496–509

Tomasi D, Wang G-J, Volkow ND (2015) Human Brain Mapping 36(8):3154–3166. https://doi.org/10.1002/hbm.22834

UNODC (2020) World drug report 2020. Available https://wdr.unodc.org/wdr2020/index.html

Urban NB, Slifstein M, Thompson JL, Xu X, Girgis RR, Raheja S, Haney M, Abi-Dargham A (2012) Dopamine release in chronic cannabis users: a [11c]raclopride positron emission tomography study. Biol Psychiatry 71:677–683

Van De Giessen E, Weinstein JJ, Cassidy CM, Haney M, Dong Z, Ghazzaoui R, Ojeil N, Kegeles LS, Xu X, Vadhan NP, Volkow ND, Slifstein M, Abi-Dargham A (2017) Deficits in striatal dopamine release in cannabis dependence. Mol Psychiatry 22:68–75

Van Hell HH, Vink M, Ossewaarde L, Jager G, Kahn RS, Ramsey NF (2010) Chronic effects of cannabis use on the human reward system: an fMRI study. Eur Neuropsychopharmacol 20: 153–163

Van Hell HH, Bossong MG, Jager G, Kristo G, Van Osch MJ, Zelaya F, Kahn RS, Ramsey NF (2011) Evidence for involvement of the insula in the psychotropic effects of THC in humans: a double-blind, randomized pharmacological MRI study. Int J Neuropsychopharmacol 14: 1377–1388

Van Hell HH, Jager G, Bossong MG, Brouwer A, Jansma JM, Zuurman L, Van Gerven J, Kahn RS, Ramsey NF (2012) Involvement of the endocannabinoid system in reward processing in the human brain. Psychopharmacology 219:981–990

Van Waes V, Beverley JA, Siman H, Tseng KY, Steiner H (2012) CB1 cannabinoid receptor expression in the striatum: association with Corticostriatal circuits and developmental regulation. Front Pharmacol 3:21

Vingerhoets WA, Koenders L, Van Den Brink W, Wiers RW, Goudriaan AE, Van Amelsvoort T, De Haan L, Cousijn J (2016) Cue-induced striatal activity in frequent cannabis users independently predicts cannabis problem severity three years later. J Psychopharmacol 30:152–158

Volkow ND, Wang GJ, Ma Y, Fowler JS, Wong C, Ding YS, Hitzemann R, Swanson JM, Kalivas P (2005) Activation of orbital and medial prefrontal cortex by methylphenidate in cocaine-addicted subjects but not in controls: relevance to addiction. J Neurosci 25:3932–3939

Volkow ND, Wang G-J, Fowler JS, Tomasi D, Telang F (2011) Addiction: beyond dopamine reward circuitry. Proc Natl Acad Sci 108:15037–15042

Volkow ND, Wang GJ, Telang F, Fowler JS, Alexoff D, Logan J, Jayne M, Wong C, Tomasi D (2014) Decreased dopamine brain reactivity in marijuana abusers is associated with negative emotionality and addiction severity. Proc Natl Acad Sci U S A 111:E3149–E3156

Vollstadt-Klein S, Wichert S, Rabinstein J, Buhler M, Klein O, Ende G, Hermann D, Mann K (2010) Initial, habitual and compulsive alcohol use is characterized by a shift of cue processing from ventral to dorsal striatum. Addiction 105:1741–1749

Wall MB, Pope R, Freeman TP, Kowalczyk OS, Demetriou L, Mokrysz C, Hindocha C, Lawn W, Bloomfield MAP, Freeman AM, Feilding A, Nutt D Curran HV (2019) Dissociable effects of cannabis with and without cannabidiol on the human brain's resting-state functional connectivity. J Neuropsychopharm 33(7):822–830. https://doi.org/10.1177/0269881119841568

Watts JJ, Garani R, Da Silva T, Lalang N, Chavez S, Mizrahi R (2020) Evidence that cannabis exposure, abuse, and dependence are related to glutamate metabolism and glial function in the anterior cingulate cortex: a (1)H-magnetic resonance spectroscopy study. Front Psych 11:764

Wesley MJ, Hanlon CA, Porrino LJ (2011) Poor decision-making by chronic marijuana users is associated with decreased functional responsiveness to negative consequences. Psychiatry Res 191:51–59

Wiers CE, Shokri-Kojori E, Wong CT, Abi-Dargham A, Demiral SB, Tomasi D, Wang GJ, Volkow ND (2016) Cannabis abusers show Hypofrontality and blunted brain responses to a stimulant challenge in females but not in males. Neuropsychopharmacology 41:2596–2605

Wise R, Bozarth M (1985) Brain mechanisms of drug reward and euphoria. Psychiatr Med 3: 445–460

Yip SW, Devito EE, Kober H, Worhunsky PD, Carroll KM, Potenza MN (2014) Pretreatment measures of brain structure and reward-processing brain function in cannabis dependence: an exploratory study of relationships with abstinence during behavioral treatment. Drug Alcohol Depend 140:33–41

Zehra A, Burns J, Liu CK, Manza P, Wiers CE, Volkow ND, Wang G-J (2018) Cannabis addiction and the brain: a review. J Neuroimmune Pharmacol 13:438–452

Zhou F, Zimmermann K, Xin F, Scheele D, Dau W, Banger M, Weber B, Hurlemann R, Kendrick KM, Becker B (2018) Shifted balance of dorsal versus ventral striatal communication with frontal reward and regulatory regions in cannabis-dependent males. Hum Brain Mapp 39: 5062–5073

Zhou X, Zimmermann K, Xin F, Zhao W, Derckx RT, Sassmannshausen A, Scheele D, Hurlemann R, Weber B, Kendrick KM, Becker B (2019) Cue reactivity in the ventral striatum characterizes heavy cannabis use, whereas reactivity in the dorsal striatum mediates dependent use. Biol Psychiatry Cogn Neurosci Neuroimaging 4:751–762

Zhukovsky P, Puaud M, Jupp B, Sala-Bayo J, Alsio J, Xia J, Searle L, Morris Z, Sabir A, Giuliano C, Everitt BJ, Belin D, Robbins TW, Dalley JW (2019) Withdrawal from escalated cocaine self-administration impairs reversal learning by disrupting the effects of negative feedback on reward exploitation: a behavioral and computational analysis. Neuropsychopharmacology 44:2163–2173

Attitudes and Cannabis Legalization 66

Jennifer D. Ellis and Stella M. Resko

Contents

Introduction 1442
Attitudes Towards Cannabis Use and Changes over Time in the United States 1442
Attitudes Towards Cannabis Use and Changes over Time Outside of the United States 1444
Reasons for Positive and Negative Attitudes Towards Cannabis Legalization 1446
Correlates of Favoring and Opposing Legalization 1448
Applications to Other Areas of Addiction 1450
Applications to Areas of Public Health 1450
Mini-Dictionary of Terms 1451
Key Facts 1451
Summary Points 1452
References 1452

Abstract

Cannabis policy has drastically evolved in recent years in the United States and elsewhere. As policy has changed, attitudes and perceptions of risk have also changed. The purpose of the present chapter was to (1) review how policy and attitudes related to cannabis legalization have changed over time, (2) explore common reasons for having positive and negative attitudes towards cannabis legalization, and (3) explore correlates of favoring and opposing legalization. Attitudes towards cannabis and legalization have become increasingly favorable over time, although youth cannabis use and road safety remain prominent concerns. Men, younger individuals, individuals who are politically liberal, and individuals with past exposure to cannabis are generally more likely to support

J. D. Ellis (✉)
Department of Psychiatry, Johns Hopkins University, Baltimore, MD, USA
e-mail: jellis36@jhmi.edu

S. M. Resko
School of Social Work, Wayne State University, Detroit, MI, USA
e-mail: stella@wayne.edu

V. B. Patel, V. R. Preedy (eds.), *Handbook of Substance Misuse and Addictions*,
https://doi.org/10.1007/978-3-030-92392-1_72

legalization, although more work is needed to explore whether these correlates have changed over time and to examine differences across cultures.

Keywords

Cannabis · Marijuana · THC · Legalization · Decriminalization · Recreational use · Drug policy · Correlates · Attitudes · Public perceptions

Introduction

As shown in Fig. 1, recreational and medical cannabis policy has drastically evolved in recent years. In 1996, California became the first US state to legalize medical cannabis, and in 2012 Colorado became the first state to legalize recreational cannabis. As of August of 2021 (Fig. 2), 18 states have legalized cannabis for recreational use. Cannabis policy has evolved in some countries outside of the United States as well. Uruguay was the first country to legalize recreational cannabis in 2013, and legal sales of cannabis in their pharmacies began in 2017. Canada passed legislation allowing for recreational use in 2018. Although cannabis remains illegal in much of Australia, the Capital Territory, which includes Canberra, legalized cannabis for personal use, though no recreational market exists. Public perceptions have evolved along with these policies and influenced attitudes towards cannabis.

Attitudes Towards Cannabis Use and Changes over Time in the United States

In the United States, public opinion polls demonstrate how attitudes towards recreational cannabis legalization have become increasingly more favorable over time. In 1969, results from the Gallup Organization poll indicated that only 12% of

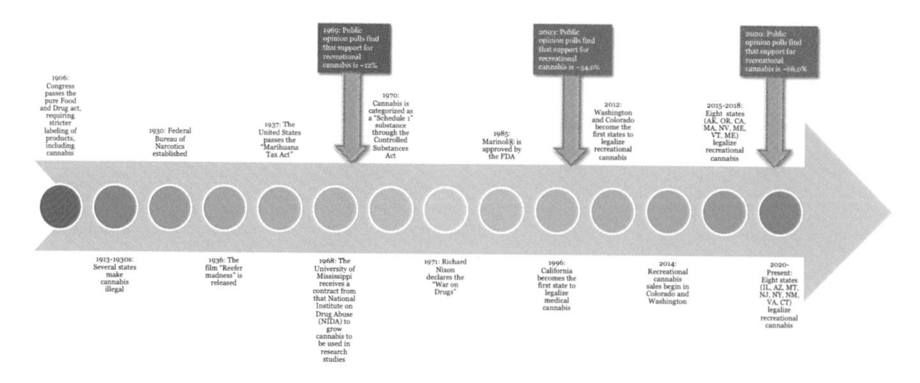

Fig. 1 History of cannabis policy and attitudes in the United States. Cannabis policy has drastically evolved in the United States over the past century, and changes in policy have often been reflected in public attitudes and perceptions towards cannabis use

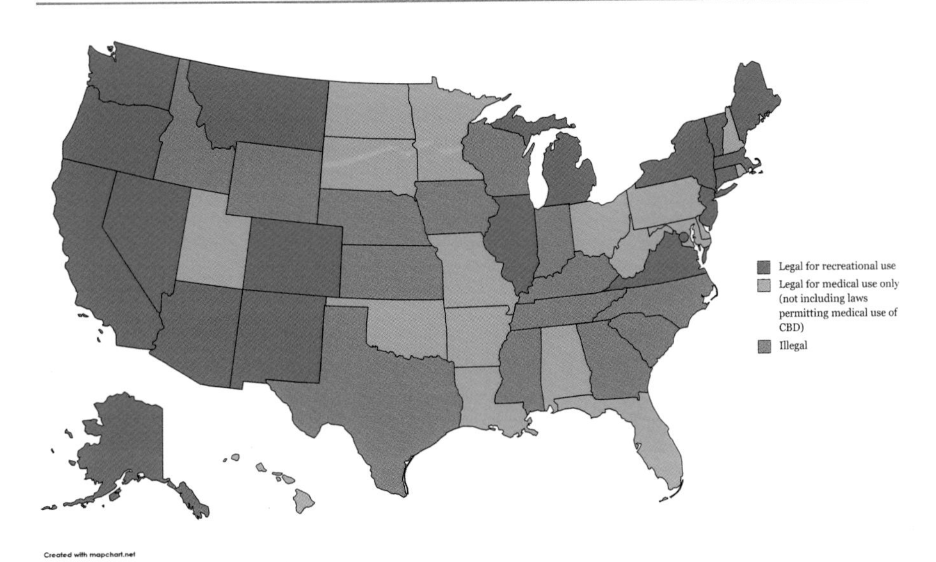

Fig. 2 Legality of psychoactive cannabis by state. The figure shows cannabis policy in the United States. Of note, cannabis policy is complicated, and many cannabinoids (including delta-9-THC) remain illegal at the federal level. Some states where psychoactive cannabis is illegal for recreational and medical use have policies which permit use of cannabidiol products containing limited or no THC for medical use

Americans thought cannabis should be legal for recreational purposes, whereas that number had increased to 34% in 2003 (Millhorn et al. 2009). Results from the General Social Survey (GSS) suggested that support for cannabis legalization increased from 17.7% in 1988 to 57.4% in 2014 (Schnabel and Sevell 2017). In November of 2020, results from Gallup suggested that support for legalization reached a record 68% (Brenan 2020).

Increases in support for legalization have generally coincided with decreases in perceived risk in the United States. For example, a study of parents in Washington State found that support for adult use increased and perceived harm of regular cannabis use decreased between 1985 and 2014 (Kosterman et al. 2016). Results from the National Survey on Drug Use and Health suggested that perceptions that regular cannabis posed great risk decreased between 2002 and 2012, while perceptions that it posed no risk increased (Okaneku et al. 2015). Monitoring the future data also suggests that perceived risk has declined among adolescents over the past 20 years (Danseco et al. 1999; Miech et al. 2017; Terry-McElrath et al. 2017; Johnston et al. 2021). Coverage in the news, social media, and advertisements also became more favorable between 2003 and 2018 (Park and Holody 2018). However, changes in perceived risk also appeared to vary by type of cannabis; perceptions that edibles posed no harm increased between 2016 and 2018, while perceptions of no harm from smoking declined during that same time period (Reboussin et al. 2019). This finding suggests that although individuals may be increasingly aware of risks associated with smoking, this may be less true for other forms of cannabis that have recently gained popularity.

It is unclear whether changes in policy are driven by changes in perception or if public perceptions change following legalization. Some researchers suggest that legalization has little to no impact on attitudes towards cannabis generally. For example, a study of adolescents living in states where legalization for recreational use occurred found that legalization was not associated with lower perceived harm (Bailey et al. 2020). Further, perceptions in risk, norms, or attitudes related to cannabis did not significantly change following recreational legalization in Washington among adolescents enrolled in a Seattle-based clinical trial for cannabis use (Blevins et al. 2018). Similar evidence was found among college students living in Washington, a legal use state, relative to Wisconsin, a non-legalization state. Legalization status was not associated with more liberal changes in attitudes (Barker and Moreno 2021). Finally, a phone survey of adolescents in Washington and Wisconsin found that participants reported that legalization did not influence most of their self-reported attitudes about cannabis or intentions to use it. However, legalization did influence attitudes regarding safety (e.g., lack of potential health risks) (Moreno et al. 2016).

In contrast, other work has suggested changes in perceived risk following legalization. Results from the National Survey on Drug Use and Health compared Colorado to nonmedical states on perceived risk; in Colorado, perceiving great risk in using cannabis one to two times per week decreased between 2007–2008 and 2010–2011 (i.e., before and after the recreational market had been established; Schuermeyer et al. 2014). Additionally, a study of undergraduates surveyed before and after passage of Initiative 71 in the District of Columbia found that positive attitudes towards cannabis, perceptions that cannabis use is normative, and willingness to use increased following legalization. However, increases in positive attitudes and willingness to use cannabis were only observed among abstinent or experimental users. Intentions to use cannabis increased in abstinent, experimental, or light users, and normative beliefs increased among moderate and heavy users only (Clarke et al. 2018). Thus, relationships between perceptions of cannabis use and legalization are likely bidirectional and influenced by individual use characteristics (see Fig. 3).

Attitudes Towards Cannabis Use and Changes over Time Outside of the United States

Similar shifts in attitudes have also been observed outside of the United States. An early study of students and teachers at a Canadian university found 62.5% of students surveyed and 43.4% of teachers favored legalization (Paul 1977). A more recent survey conducted in 2014 in Canada suggested that most adults in Ontario supported decriminalizing or legalizing cannabis (Fischer et al. 2016). Interestingly, in contrast to the United States, a general population survey in Canada found ratings

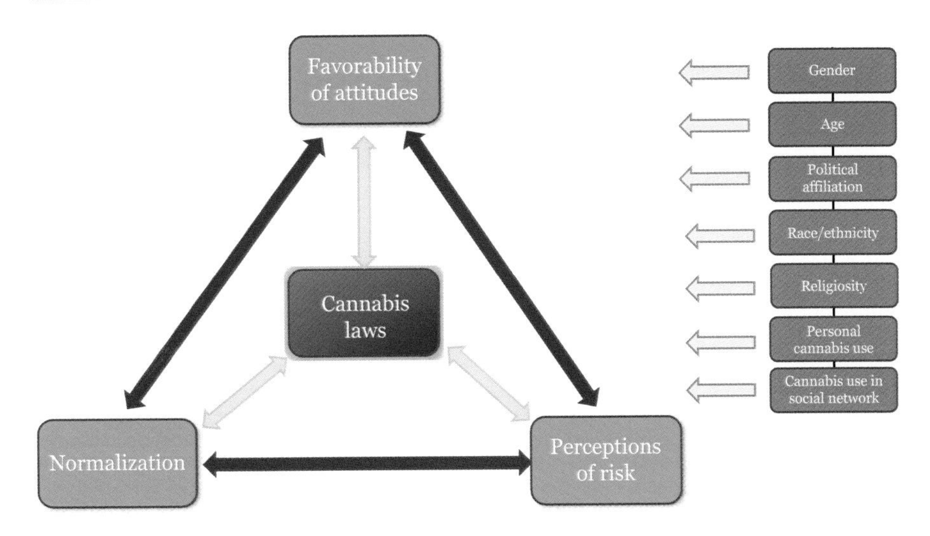

Fig. 3 Conceptual model depicting interactions between cannabis policy, attitudes, and individual characteristics. Work suggests that favorability of attitudes, perceptions or risk, and normalization of cannabis evolve along with cannabis laws. Personal characteristics also influence individual attitudes towards cannabis and support for legalization

of the seriousness of cannabis use increased between 2008 and 2018 while staying the same for alcohol and tobacco (Cunningham and Koski-Jännes 2019).

Further, a 2014 study in Australia suggested that participants showed a strong preference for legalization or over civil penalties over both criminalization and cannabis cautioning (i.e., in which law enforcement confiscates small amounts of cannabis and provides psychoeducation) (Shanahan et al. 2014). Similarly, findings from the Australian National Drug Strategy Household Survey suggested that support for criminalization decreased over time and support for legalization increased (Kaur et al. 2020). In Iran, where cannabis remains illegal, qualitative evidence suggests religious authorities were open to regulation of cannabis by the government (Ghiabi et al. 2018).

Other work suggests considerable support for medical cannabis in many countries. A 2015 survey, for example, found 78% of adults in Israel and 51% of adults in Norway support medical cannabis legalization (Sznitman and Bretteville-Jensen 2015). However, in some other countries, support for medical cannabis is high, whereas support for recreational cannabis is low. For example, a 2017 study in Serbia suggested overwhelming support for medical cannabis and low levels of support towards recreational cannabis use (Gazibara et al. 2017). In addition, a survey of general practitioners in Ireland in 2017 found that although 58.6% were opposed to the decriminalization of cannabis, 58.6% supported cannabis for medical uses (Crowley et al. 2017). Thus, more work is needed to understand better the nuances of these views and how perspectives towards cannabis have changed.

Reasons for Positive and Negative Attitudes Towards Cannabis Legalization

Changes in cannabis policy have led to intense public debate. A number of papers have explored the reasons that people support and oppose legalization, as well as correlates of endorsing particular opinions. A summary of these opinions is shown in Table 1. For example, reasons for favoring legalization include increased safety with regulation of products (Alon et al. 2021; Resko et al. 2019), perceptions that cannabis is less addictive and more socially acceptable, and a lower health risk than other substances, including legal substances, such as tobacco and alcohol (Asbridge et al. 2016; Chen-Sankey et al. 2020; Månsson and Ekendahl 2013; Resko et al. 2019), as well as the potential for legalization to increase tax revenue (McGinty et al. 2016, 2017; Resko et al. 2019; Osborne and Fogel 2017).

Effects of criminalization of cannabis use on minority communities, the criminal justice system, and the illegal drug trade have been a common argument in favor of legalization. In fact, an online panel survey cited prison overcrowding as one of the most commonly endorsed reasons in favor of legalization (McGinty et al. 2017), and the increasing burden on the criminal justice system generally was the second most commonly endorsed reason for supporting legalization among adults in Michigan (Resko et al. 2019). Discussion of legalization as a way to minimize criminal justice system involvement has centered around three central themes: (1) reducing costs associated with policing and incarcerating individuals for cannabis use, (2) reducing crime associated with black market sales and opposing drug cartels, and (3) reducing injustice associated with cannabis criminalization (McGinty et al. 2016, McGinty et al. 2017; Osborne and Fogel 2017; Resko et al. 2019). These findings from self-report data are also consistent with a media content analysis, which suggested that reduction in criminal justice involvement and costs was the most common pro-legalization argument between 2010 and 2014 (McGinty et al. 2016). Of note,

Table 1 Some of the common reasons for supporting and opposing legalization of cannabis for recreational use identified across studies

Reasons for supporting legalization	Reasons for opposing legalization
Beliefs that cannabis is beneficial, especially with regard to health	Concerns about cannabis-impaired driving
Beliefs that legalization will reduce black market sales	Concerns about use will increase, especially among youth, parents, and pregnant women
Increase ability to conduct research	Gateway drug hypothesis
Reduce burden on criminal justice system/reduce incarceration costs	Increasing potency of cannabis products
Reduce effects of criminalization on marginalized communities	Not enough research
Low perceptions of risk, especially relative to other substances	Perception that cannabis is harmful
Perception that legalization will increase safety (regulation of products)	Potential normalization
Tax revenue	

the criminal justice system and criminalization of drug use disproportionately impacts marginalized communities, including communities of color (Koch, Lee, and Lee 2016; Cole et al. 2018; Fritz 2021), and some proponents of this argument view legalization of cannabis as one strategy to reduce mass incarceration. These findings from self-report data are also consistent with a media content analysis, which suggested that reduction in criminal justice involvement and costs was the most common pro-legalization argument between 2010 and 2014 (McGinty et al. 2016).

On the flip side, concerns about the potential for increases in cannabis use among adolescents have become one of the most common reasons given for opposing legalization. Online surveys have repeatedly found that concerns about youth health were commonly endorsed as reasons opposing legalization (McGinty et al. 2017; Resko et al. 2019). Similarly, a content analysis from news stories found that discussion that cannabis may harm youth was one of the most common anti-legalization arguments made between 2010 and 2014 (McGinty et al. 2016). A qualitative study of adolescent substance use treatment providers in Denver found that providers believed that legalization contributed to normalization and increases in access, often undermining substance use treatment efforts (Sobesky and Gorgens 2016).

Use by parents and pregnant women is also a concern. An anonymous survey of pregnant women in Maryland suggested that 10% of the sample stated that if cannabis were legalized, they would use more during pregnancy (Mark et al. 2017). Most parents in Washington State were opposed to adolescent use and cannabis use around children but also incorrectly believed the legal age of use to be 18 in Washington. In this sample, increases in use and cannabis use disorder were observed over time among parents who used cannabis, both before and after cannabis was made legal and retail stores opened (Kosterman et al. 2016). Other findings suggest that, among adults with children living in the home, the effects of medical cannabis laws on use have been particularly pronounced among older and highly educated age groups (Goodwin et al. 2021).

However, despite these concerns, evidence that legalization of cannabis increases cannabis use among youth has been mixed. Results from the National Youth Tobacco Survey, a national survey of adolescents in 6–12 grade, found that youth in states with legal cannabis (medical and/or recreational) had greater likelihood of having used cannabis in e-cigarettes at least once (Nicksic et al. 2020). Results from the National Survey on Drug Use and Health suggested that cannabis use disorders were more prevalent in adolescents aged 12–17 and young adults aged 18–25 in Colorado relative to states without medical cannabis legalization (Schuermeyer et al. 2014). Although data from the Treatment Episode Dataset – Admissions (TEDS-A) suggested that treatment admissions for cannabis use among adolescents declined between 2008 and 2017 and these declines were greater in states with legal cannabis (Mennis and Stahler 2020), these declines may indicate potential declines in perceived harm or lower stigma of cannabis, rather than declining cannabis problems. Finally, a qualitative study of adolescents in San Francisco suggested that participants who had used cannabis at least once generally perceived cannabis as safe to use. Respondents cited both legalization and use by people in their lives as reasons for considering that cannabis is safe (Friese 2017).

In contrast, data from the Youth Risk Behavioral Surveillance Survey suggested no differences in adolescent cannabis use between states that did and did not enact medical cannabis policy (Choo et al. 2014). Data from Monitoring the Future suggests that adolescent cannabis use has not increased from 1991 to 2016 across levels of perceived risk (Terry-McElrath et al. 2017). Further, evidence from a clinical trial for adolescents using cannabis before and after legalization in Seattle found that there were no differences in substance use, but cannabis-related problems (measured by the Marijuana Problems Index) and cannabis use disorder symptoms did increase (Blevins et al. 2018). A study comparing two cohorts of adolescents in Washington recruited before and after legalization for nonmedical use (vs. medical only) found that past 30-day cannabis use was slightly, but not significantly, higher in the second cohort (Mason et al. 2016).

Another common concern regarding legalization is road safety. An online panel survey found that concerns about motor vehicle crashes were one of the most common arguments against legalization (McGinty et al. 2017), and one study found that over half of respondents believed that legalizing cannabis would negatively impact road safety (Resko et al. 2020). Further, a media content analysis found that cannabis-impaired driving was a common anti-legalization argument raised in news stories between 2010 and 2014 (McGinty et al. 2016). These concerns are not unfounded, as some work suggests that driving after cannabis use is more common in states with legal recreational cannabis, despite greater knowledge of risks associated with driving after use in these states (Lensch et al. 2020). An interesting direction for future work may be examining how support for legalization changes following the development of new roadside technologies. For example, a survey of adults in the United States suggested that support for legalization would be higher if a reliable roadside sobriety test could be administered (Looby et al. 2007).

Correlates of Favoring and Opposing Legalization

Several studies have explored correlates of attitudes towards legalization. Correlates of supporting legalization are depicted in Fig. 4. Early work done in the 1970s suggested that political ideology (Baer 1973), geographic region (Fisher et al. 1974), and past cannabis experience (Baer 1973; Fisher et al. 1974) were associated with perspectives on cannabis and legalization. In more present studies, younger age (Fischer et al. 2016; Ellis et al. 2019), liberal political affiliation (Looby et al. 2007; Palamar 2014; Collingwood et al. 2018; Ellis et al. 2019), and male gender (Palamar 2014; Fischer et al. 2016; Ellis et al. 2019) have been associated with favoring legalization of cannabis. Religiosity (Palamar 2014; Collingwood et al. 2018) and race/ethnicity (Looby et al. 2007; Palamar 2014) have also been associated with favoring legalization, although these findings have been observed in fewer studies.

Gender differences in attitudes towards legalization are somewhat counterintuitive, as women tend to be more liberal than men about other political issues but tend to be more conservative with regard to cannabis legalization. Gender differences in

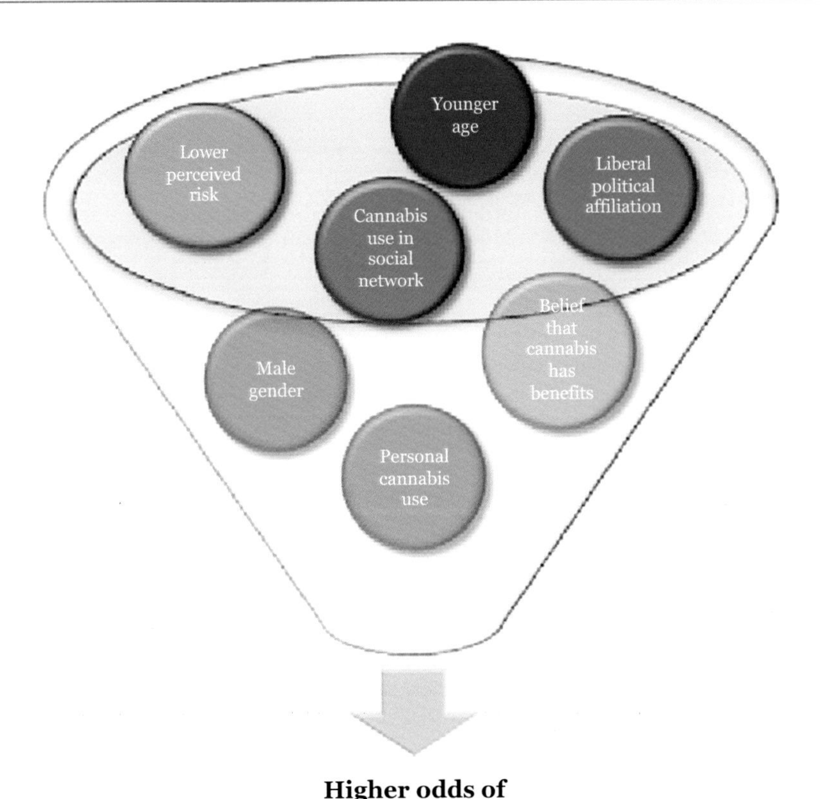

Fig. 4 Correlates of supporting legalization of cannabis for recreational use. Previous work suggests that support for legalization of cannabis is associated with a number of individual factors, including those depicted above

perceptions of cannabis legalization may be due to greater religiosity among women and findings that men are more likely to encounter and use cannabis (Elder and Greene 2019). Gender differences may also be related to greater concern about the present lack of regulation among women. For example, one study found that gender differences in the likelihood of supporting legalization dissipated if a reliable roadside test could be administered (Looby et al. 2007).

Familiarity with cannabis may be associated with lower perceived risk and greater likelihood of supporting legalization. Past or present use of cannabis and other substances is a robust correlate of favoring legalization (Palamar 2014; Cohn et al. 2017; Gazibara et al. 2017; Pearson et al. 2017; Ellis et al. 2019). Having a family member or friend requiring medical cannabis (Gazibara et al. 2017) is also a robust correlate of favoring legalization for medical use. Among adolescents, having friends that don't approve of cannabis use is associated with a lower likelihood of support for legalization (Palamar 2014). Similarly, a study of college students at two universities found that individuals who had more favorable perceptions of cannabis were more likely to have more friends who used cannabis (Berg et al. 2015). Lower perceived risk is also a correlate of favoring legalization, and individuals who supported legalization were less likely to be concerned about potency, road safety, employee safety, or emergency department visits (Resko et al. 2020).

With regard to medical cannabis, beliefs that cannabis has medical benefits and exposure to patient testimonials have been linked to favoring legalization of cannabis for medical use. One study found that beliefs that cannabis has medical benefits were related to support for medical use (Sznitman and Bretteville-Jensen 2015). Further, in an experimental study, participants were randomly assigned to different video conditions about medical cannabis. Participants shown a video that included patient testimonials were more likely to show increased positive attitudes, beliefs, and intentions about medical cannabis (Sznitman and Lewis 2018).

However, more research is needed, as some work suggests that there may be cross-cultural differences in correlates of favoring legalization and that correlates many vary in different countries. For example, a study of correlates of favoring legalization in Uruguay, the United States, and El Salvador suggested that individuals with children were less likely to support legalization in the United States and El Salvador but not Uruguay. Religiosity was negatively related, and years of education were positively related to supporting legalization in Uruguay and El Salvador but not the United States. Liberal political ideology was associated with favoring legalization in Uruguay and the United States but not El Salvador. However, in all three countries, having tried cannabis was associated with supporting legalization (Cruz et al. 2016). Thus, more work is needed to explore whether correlates of favoring or opposing legalization of cannabis generalize in different countries.

Applications to Other Areas of Addiction

Changes in cannabis policy have provoked further discussion about federal drug policy generally in the United States. Just as criminalization of cannabis has been described as disproportionately harming marginalized communities, criminalization of other substances has been similarly criticized (Miron and Partin 2021). Additionally, a push for a regulated market for other substances has gained popularity. For example, in November 2020, Oregon passed Measure 109, which legalized regulation of psilocybin, which has already been decriminalized in a number of jurisdictions. Thus, understanding how perceptions related to other substances, as well as other addictive behaviors such as gambling, remains an important area for future work as it is possible that attitudes towards other substances will also evolve over time.

Applications to Areas of Public Health

Rapidly changing attitudes towards cannabis have important implications for public health, as access to legal cannabis is rapidly expanding for individuals 21 and older in the United States and in other countries. Moving forward, continuing to monitor of how public perceptions of cannabis and attitudes towards cannabis legalization change will be needed as public policy continues to shift and cannabis regulation is advanced. Examining whether correlates of favoring legalization change will also be important to track. Research on global differences in attitudes towards cannabis and perception of risk for different cannabis products will also be relevant directions for future work. Finally, a useful direction for future work may be examining support for different regulatory strategies (i.e., legalization with no regulated market, limitations on potency of products), and examining attitudes towards technologies that may assist with cannabis regulation (i.e., roadside testing) will be beneficial as an increasing number of countries legalize cannabis.

Mini-Dictionary of Terms

- Cannabidiol/CBD: A cannabinoid that is generally viewed as nonintoxicating and has been approved for treating certain medical conditions (e.g., EPIDIOLEX ® for epilepsy). CBD is also commercially available in many states.
- Cannabis roadside sobriety test: A test that can be administered if impaired driving is suspected to examine whether an individual is currently impaired by cannabis. Unlike alcohol, there is not currently a widely used breathalyzer test for cannabis, meaning that police often rely on field sobriety tests.
- Decriminalization: The removal of criminal penalties for cannabis use. Actual decriminalization policies vary widely but often require payment of a fine.
- Legalization (medical): Legally allowing the use of cannabis to treat or alleviate symptoms resulting from a medical condition. Some jurisdictions permit medical use of psychoactive cannabis, whereas others allow cannabidiol (CBD) products containing little or no THC for medical use.
- Legalization (recreational): The removal of penalties for nonmedical cannabis use. Often involves establishment of a recreational cannabis market.
- Medical cannabis/medical use: Use of cannabis to treat or alleviate symptoms resulting from a medical condition.
- Psychoactive cannabis: Cannabis from marijuana plants (rather than hemp cannabis plants) that contains nontrivial amounts of THC and produces subjective changes in mood, bodily sensations, thoughts, etc.
- Recreational cannabis market: State regulation of cannabis cultivation, transportation, and sales for recreational use.
- Recreational cannabis/recreational use: Use of cannabis by adults for nonmedical purposes.

Key Facts

Key facts of changing cannabis legalization attitudes:

- A number of countries have passed recreational or medical cannabis laws in recent years.

- 18 states have legalized cannabis for recreational use in the United States, despite the fact that cannabis remains illegal at the federal level.
- Perceived risk of cannabis has declined in the United States.
- Despite declines in perceived risk, concerns remain, including concerns about motor vehicle safety and youth use.
- Perceptions of risk appear to be moderated by individual characteristics, including demographics and past experiences of use.

Summary Points

- Attitudes towards cannabis and cannabis legalization have greatly changed in recent years.
- Arguments in favor of legalization include the potential for criminal justice reform, reducing impacts on marginalized communities, tax revenue, and perceptions that cannabis poses less risk than other substances.
- Arguments opposing legalization include concerns about youth use, use by parents, and road safety.
- Some individuals may be more or less likely to support legalization. For example, younger age, more liberal political ideology, male gender, lower perceived risk, and experiences with cannabis are associated with greater likelihood of supporting legalization.
- Some cross-cultural differences have been observed in attitudes towards cannabis legalization and correlates of favoring legalization, although more research is needed.

References

Alon L, Bruce D, Blocker O et al (2021) Perceptions of quality and safety in cannabis acquisition amongst young gay and bisexual men living with HIV/AIDS who use cannabis: impact of legalisation and dispensaries. Int J Drug Policy 88:103035

Asbridge M, Valleriani J, Kwok J et al (2016) Normalization and denormalization in different legal contexts: comparing cannabis and tobacco. Drugs Educ Prev Pol 23(3):212–223

Baer DJ (1973) Attitudes about marijuana and political views. Psychol Rep 32(3):1051–1054

Bailey JA, Epstein M, Roscoe JN, Oesterle S, Kosterman R, Hill KG (2020) Marijuana legalization and youth marijuana, alcohol, and cigarette use and norms. American journal of preventive medicine 59(3):309–316

Barker AK, Moreno MA (2021) Effects of recreational marijuana legalization on college students: a longitudinal study of attitudes, intentions, and use behaviors. J Adolesc Health 68(1):110–115

Berg CJ, Stratton E, Schauer GL et al (2015) Perceived harm, addictiveness, and social acceptability of tobacco products and marijuana among young adults: marijuana, hookah, and electronic cigarettes win. Subst Use Misuse 50(1):79–89

Blevins CE, Marsh E, Banes KE et al (2018) The implications of cannabis policy changes in Washington on adolescent perception of risk, norms, attitudes, and substance use. Subst Abuse 12:1178221818815491

Brenan M (2020) Support for legal marijuana inches up to new high of 68%. Gallup, November, 6, 2020

Chen-Sankey JC, Jewett BJ, Orozco L et al (2020) "Hey, I got to smoke some weed": favorable perceptions of marijuana use among non-college-educated young adult cigarette smokers. Subst Use Misuse 55(1):48–55
Choo EK, Benz M, Zaller N et al (2014) The impact of state medical marijuana legislation on adolescent marijuana use. J Adolesc Health 55(2):160–166
Clarke P, Dodge T, Stock ML (2018) The impact of recreational marijuana legislation in Washington, DC on marijuana use cognitions. Subst Use Misuse 53(13):2165–2173
Cohn AM, Johnson AL, Rose SW et al (2017) Support for marijuana legalization and predictors of intentions to use marijuana more often in response to legalization among US young adults. Subst Use Misuse 52(2):203–213
Cole DM, Thomas DM, Field K et al (2018) The 21st century cures act implications for the reduction of racial health disparities in the US criminal justice system: a public health approach. J Racial Ethn Health Disparities 5(4):885–893
Collingwood L, O'Brien BG, Dreier S (2018) Evaluating ballot initiative support for legalised marijuana: the case of Washington. Int J Drug Policy 56:6–20
Crowley D, Collins C, Delargy I et al (2017) Irish general practitioner attitudes toward decriminalisation and medical use of cannabis: results from a national survey. Harm Reduct J 14(1):1–8
Cruz JM, Queirolo R, Boidi MF (2016) Determinants of public support for marijuana legalization in Uruguay, the United States, and El Salvador. J Drug Issues 46(4):308–325
Cunningham JA, Koski-Jännes A (2019) The last 10 years: any changes in perceptions of the seriousness of alcohol, cannabis, and substance use in Canada? Subst Abuse Treat Prev Policy 14(1):1–6
Danseco ER, Kingery PM, Coggeshall MB (1999) Perceived risk of harm from marijuana use among youth in the USA. Sch Psychol Int 20(1):39–56
Elder L, Greene S (2019) Gender and the politics of marijuana. Soc Sci Q 100(1):109–122
Ellis JD, Resko SM, Szechy K et al (2019) Characteristics associated with attitudes toward marijuana legalization in Michigan. J Psychoactive Drugs 51(4):335–342
Fischer B, Ialomiteanu AR, Russell C et al (2016) Public opinion towards cannabis control in Ontario: strong but diversified support for reforming control of both use and supply. Can J Criminol Crim Justice 58(3):443–459
Fisher G, Steckler A, Strantz I et al (1974) The legalization of marihuana: views of several American populations of users and non-users. J Psychedelic Drugs 6(3):333–349
Friese B (2017) "Is marijuana even a drug?" A qualitative study of how teens view marijuana use and why they use it. J Psychoactive Drugs 49(3):209–216
Fritz KG (2021) The importance of rights to the argument for the decriminalization of drugs. Am J Bioeth 21(4):46–48
Gazibara T, Prpic M, Maric G et al (2017) Medical cannabis in Serbia: the survey of knowledge and attitudes in an urban adult population. J Psychoactive Drugs 49(3):217–224
Ghiabi M, Maarefvand M, Bahari H et al (2018) Islam and cannabis: legalisation and religious debate in Iran. Int J Drug Policy 56:121–127
Goodwin RD, Kim JH, Cheslack-Postava K et al (2021) Trends in cannabis use among adults with children in the home in the United States, 2004–2017: impact of state-level legalization for recreational and medical use. Addiction 116:2770
Johnston LD, Miech RA, O'Malley PM et al (2021) Monitoring the future national survey results on drug use 1975–2020: overview, key findings on adolescent drug use. Institute for Social Research, University of Michigan, Ann Arbor
Kaur N, Keyes KM, Hamilton AD et al (2020) Trends in cannabis use and attitudes toward legalization and use among Australians from 2001–2016: an age-period-cohort analysis. Addiction 116:1152
Koch DW, Lee J, Lee K (2016) Coloring the war on drugs: Arrest disparities in black, brown, and white. Race and Social Problems 8(4):313–325. https://doi.org/10.1007/s12552-016-9185-6
Kosterman R, Bailey JA, Guttmannova K et al (2016) Marijuana legalization and parents' attitudes, use, and parenting in Washington State. J Adolesc Health 59(4):450–456

Lensch T, Sloan K, Ausmus J et al (2020) Cannabis use and driving under the influence: behaviors and attitudes by state-level legal sale of recreational cannabis. Prev Med 141:106320

Looby A, Earleywine M, Gieringer D (2007) Roadside sobriety tests and attitudes toward a regulated cannabis market. Harm Reduct J 4(1):1–6

Månsson J, Ekendahl M (2013) Legitimacy through scaremongering: the discursive role of alcohol in online discussions of cannabis use and policy. Addict Res Theory 21(6):469–478

Mark K, Gryczynski J, Axenfeld E et al (2017) Pregnant women's current and intended cannabis use in relation to their views toward legalization and knowledge of potential harm. J Addict Med 11(3):211–216

Mason WA, Fleming CB, Ringle JL et al (2016) Prevalence of marijuana and other substance use before and after Washington State's change from legal medical marijuana to legal medical and nonmedical marijuana: cohort comparisons in a sample of adolescents. Subst Abuse 37(2):330–335

McGinty EE, Samples H, Bandara SN et al (2016) The emerging public discourse on state legalization of marijuana for recreational use in the US: analysis of news media coverage, 2010–2014. Prev Med 90:114–120

McGinty EE, Niederdeppe J, Heley K et al (2017) Public perceptions of arguments supporting and opposing recreational marijuana legalization. Prev Med 99:80–86

Mennis J, Stahler GJ (2020) Adolescent treatment admissions for marijuana following recreational legalization in Colorado and Washington. Drug Alcohol Depend 210:107960

Miech R, Johnston L, O'Malley PM (2017) Prevalence and attitudes regarding marijuana use among adolescents over the past decade. Pediatrics 140(6):e20170982

Millhorn M, Monaghan M, Montero D et al (2009) North Americans' attitudes toward illegal drugs. J Hum Behav Soc Environ 19(2):125–141

Miron J, Partin E (2021) Ending the war on drugs is an essential step toward racial justice. Am J Bioeth 21(4):1–3

Moreno MA, Whitehill JM, Quach V et al (2016) Marijuana experiences, voting behaviors, and early perspectives regarding marijuana legalization among college students from 2 states. J Am Coll Heal 64(1):9–18

Nicksic NE, Do EK, Barnes AJ (2020) Cannabis legalization, tobacco prevention policies, and cannabis use in E-cigarettes among youth. Drug Alcohol Depend 206:107730

Okaneku J, Vearrier D, McKeever RG et al (2015) Change in perceived risk associated with marijuana use in the United States from 2002 to 2012. Clin Toxicol 53(3):151–155

Osborne GB, Fogel C (2017) Perspectives on cannabis legalization among Canadian recreational users. Contemp Drug Probl 44(1):12–31

Palamar JJ (2014) An examination of opinions toward marijuana policies among high school seniors in the United States. J Psychoactive Drugs 46(5):351–361

Park SY, Holody KJ (2018) Content, exposure, and effects of public discourses about marijuana: a systematic review. J Health Commun 23(12):1036–1043

Paul MK (1977) Comparative attitudes of university students and school teachers on the use and legalization of marijuana. J Drug Educ 7(4):323–335

Pearson MR, Liese BS, Dvorak RD et al (2017) College student marijuana involvement: perceptions, use, and consequences across 11 college campuses. Addict Behav 66:83–89

Reboussin BA, Wagoner KG, Sutfin EL et al (2019) Trends in marijuana edible consumption and perceptions of harm in a cohort of young adults. Drug Alcohol Depend 205:107660

Resko S, Ellis J, Early TJ et al (2019) Understanding public attitudes toward cannabis legalization: qualitative findings from a statewide survey. Subst Use Misuse 54(8):1247–1259

Resko SM, Szechy KA, Early TJ et al (2020) Perceptions of public health consequences of marijuana legalization. Addict Res Theory 29:255–262

Schnabel L, Sevell E (2017) Should Mary and Jane be legal? Americans' attitudes toward marijuana and same-sex marriage legalization, 1988–2014. Public Opin Q 81(1):157–172

Schuermeyer J, Salomonsen-Sautel S, Price RK et al (2014) Temporal trends in marijuana attitudes, availability and use in Colorado compared to non-medical marijuana states: 2003–11. Drug Alcohol Depend 140:145–155

Shanahan M, Gerard K, Ritter A (2014) Preferences for policy options for cannabis in an Australian general population: a discrete choice experiment. Int J Drug Policy 25(4):682–690

Sobesky M, Gorgens K (2016) Cannabis and adolescents: exploring the substance misuse treatment provider experience in a climate of legalization. Int J Drug Policy 33:66–74

Sznitman SR, Bretteville-Jensen AL (2015) Public opinion and medical cannabis policies: examining the role of underlying beliefs and national medical cannabis policies. Harm Reduct J 12(1): 1–10

Sznitman SR, Lewis N (2018) Examining effects of medical cannabis narratives on beliefs, attitudes, and intentions related to recreational cannabis: a web-based randomized experiment. Drug Alcohol Depend 185:219–225

Terry-McElrath YM, O'Malley PM, Patrick ME et al (2017) Risk is still relevant: time-varying associations between perceived risk and marijuana use among US 12th grade students from 1991 to 2016. Addict Behav 74:13–19

67 Impact of Parental Cannabis

Implications for Public Health

Nicolas Berthelot, Maude Morneau, and Carl Lacharité

Contents

Introduction 1458
State of Knowledge Regarding Cannabis Use by Parents 1458
  Portrait of Parents Using Cannabis 1458
  Impact of Cannabis Use on the Ability to Respond to Children's Needs 1459
  Risk of Abuse or Neglect When Using Cannabis 1461
  Impact of Cannabis Use on Domains of Functioning Related to Parenting 1461
  Impact of Parental Cannabis Use on Offspring Development 1462
What Is the Perception of Parents Regarding Their Use of Cannabis? 1463
New Directions for Scientific Research on Parental Cannabis Use 1464
Policies, Procedures, and Public Health Measures Regarding Parental Cannabis Use 1464
Applications to Other Areas of Addiction 1465
Key Facts on Parents Who Use Cannabis and on the Development of the Child 1466
Summary Points 1467
References 1467

Abstract

This chapter aims to review the current knowledge about the effects of parental cannabis use on parenting behaviors and offspring development and to discuss the covering of the issue of parental cannabis use by mass media and public health organizations. Existing research has generally concluded that parental cannabis use is a significant risk factor for parenting and child development. However, there is still a paucity of empirical studies on this topic, and existing research presents important limitations, restraining our ability to conclude about the

N. Berthelot (✉)
Department of Nursing Sciences, Université du Québec à Trois-Rivières, Trois-Rivières, QC, Canada
e-mail: nicolas.berthelot@uqtr.ca

M. Morneau · C. Lacharité
Department of Psychology, Université du Québec à Trois-Rivières, Trois-Rivières, QC, Canada
e-mail: maude.morneau@uqtr.ca; carl.lacharite@uqtr.ca

V. B. Patel, V. R. Preedy (eds.), *Handbook of Substance Misuse and Addictions*,
https://doi.org/10.1007/978-3-030-92392-1_73

dangers of using cannabis when caring for a child. At this point, very little is known about the circumstances under which the use of cannabis is a risk factor for parenting and about the mechanisms through which parental cannabis use influences offspring development. The lack of hard facts addressing these issues allows for mass media to promote opinion-based publications that praise the parental use of cannabis.

Keywords

Cannabis · Marijuana · Drugs · Parents · Mother · Parenting · Offspring · Child development · Maltreatment · Policies · Review

Introduction

Generally, public health organizations recommend that the use of cannabis by parents should be avoided, considering the possible brain damage a direct exposure to the substance may have in developing children and adolescents (Berthelot et al. 2020). Such recommendations are mainly based on studies of pregnant women who used cannabis during pregnancy and of the use of cannabis during adolescence (Rey et al. 2004), a phenomenon that would be between 1.7 and 7.1 times more frequent in offspring of users (O'Loughlin et al. 2019). However, these recommendations are counterbalanced by a massive popular literature promoting the benefits of using cannabis as a parent (Berthelot et al. 2020). In an attempt to clarify this issue, the present chapter will (1) review the current knowledge on the effects of parental cannabis use on parenting and offspring development, (2) discuss how the topic of parental cannabis use is covered in and by mass media, and (3) present some examples of policies and public health measures that address parental cannabis use.

State of Knowledge Regarding Cannabis Use by Parents

Portrait of Parents Using Cannabis

Little data on the prevalence of parental cannabis use is currently available. A recent survey with 3300 respondents performed by the *Quebec National Institute of Public Health* during the COVID-19 pandemic in the province of Quebec, Canada – where cannabis use has been legal since 2018 – showed that 16% of adults living with at least one child below 18 years old reported having used cannabis during the last month, the majority (79%) for recreational purpose (Institut National de Santé Publique du Québec 2021). Among the users, 36% used it at least once a week and 41% at least once a day. As regards American samples, Goodwin et al. (2021) used the data from the 2017 National Survey on Drug Use and Health to evaluate the association between cannabis legalization and cannabis use among 22 308 adults with children in the home. Overall, around 11% of adults reported having used cannabis during the last month, and around 4% reported daily cannabis use. Prevalence rates of past-month cannabis use were higher in states with recreational cannabis laws (12%), followed by states with medical cannabis laws (9%) and without legal cannabis use (6%). While the participants from the previous surveys reported living in a household with children, they were not necessarily one of the primary caregivers, and existing studies involving parents of a young child would suggest lower prevalence rates. For instance, Freisthler et al. (2015) questioned 3023 parents or legal tutors of children below 13 years old from California in 2009 – before the legalization of cannabis for recreational use – on their use of cannabis. Five percent of the sample ($n = 129$) reported having used cannabis at least once during the last year. Overall, we remain poorly informed about the prevalence of parental cannabis use, but existing data suggests that the phenomenon is relatively frequent and that millions of parents in Western populations do or would use cannabis.

Even less is known about the characteristics of the parents who use cannabis and about the context in which they take the substance (e.g., in presence of the child or not). It seems that, in adults living in a household that includes children, cannabis use would be more frequent in younger adults, in males, and in people with very low income. However, this phenomenon reaches all subgroups of the population, including adults with college education and sufficient income, particularly in states where recreational use is legal (Goodwin et al. 2021).

Impact of Cannabis Use on the Ability to Respond to Children's Needs

As shown in Fig. 1, parental cannabis use may impact offspring development in two ways. First, the use of cannabis by parents may increase the risk of directly exposing children to the substance through in utero exposure, secondhand smoke, family values promoting cannabis use, and an increased accessibility to the substance. Second, parental cannabis use may also affect children indirectly via a negative effect of cannabis on the parents' capacity to deliver adequate care as well as on their mental health, cognitive functioning, attachment behaviors, and their capacities to efficiently recognize, reflect on, and respond to their children's mental states.

There is, however, a paucity of studies directly assessing the impact of cannabis use on parenting behaviors and on the ability of parents to respond to their children's needs. First, a study by Brook et al. (2006) with 258 African-American and young Puerto Rican parents, 34% of which reported having used cannabis at least once during the last year, found a negative association between cannabis use and self-report affection toward their children. They further observed that the positive effect of some protective personality factors in parents on child-rearing behaviors was offset by the effect of marijuana use. Second, using a different sample of 248 young

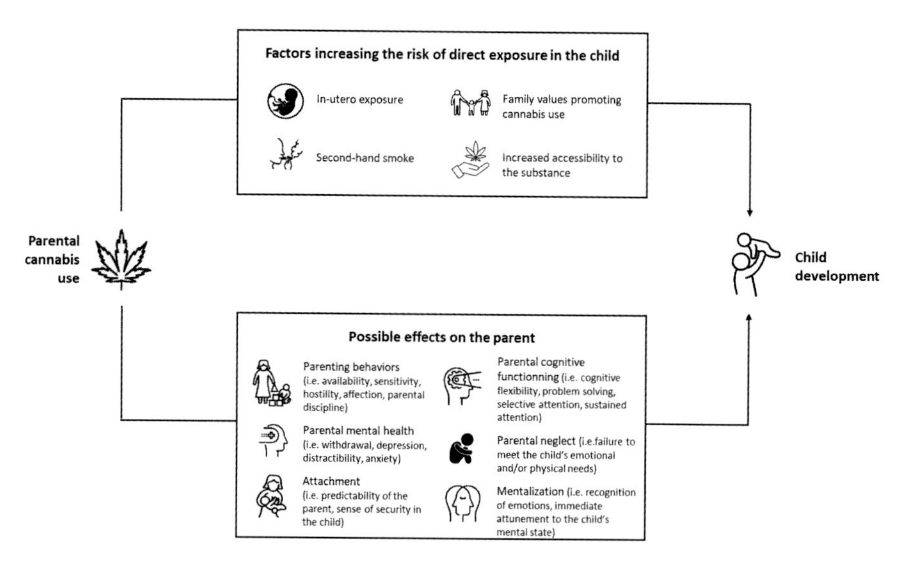

Fig. 1 Potential mediators of the effect of parental cannabis use on child development. (Reprinted from the Journal of the American Academy of Child and Adolescent Psychiatry, 59(3), Berthelot, N., Garon-Bissonnette, J., Drouin-Maziade, C., Duguay, G., Milot, T., Lemieux, R., Lacharité, C., St-Laurent, D., Dubois-Comtois, K., Parental cannabis use: Contradictory discourses in the media, governmental publications and the scientific literature, 333-335, Copyright (2020), with permission from Elsevier)

parents (60% mothers), Brook et al. (2000) observed that parents who did not use cannabis or used the substance occasionally reported greater affection (OR = 2.02) and more time spent with the child (OR = 2.33) than parents frequently using cannabis. This potentially negative impact of a frequent use of marijuana was, however, offset by the protective personality variable of maternal sensitivity (e.g., perceiving oneself as being gentle or compassionate). These findings also find support in the dissertation of Maalouf (2010) who used data from a two-generation cohort involving 1700 mothers and their children ($n = 4489$) to assess the mediating role of parenting skills in the transmission of marijuana use. He found that 10–14-year-old children of mothers using cannabis reported less respectful relationships and less effective discipline with their mother than offspring of mothers not using cannabis. Children of mothers using cannabis were especially more likely to report their wishes to have their mothers spend more time with them. A recent study, however, suggests that the impact of cannabis use on child-rearing behaviors may be moderated by the severity of cannabis use. Indeed, in their multigenerational longitudinal study of 363 children and adolescents, Hill et al. (2018) observed that parental cannabis use did not impair parenting, as evaluated by the children, when the parents did not meet the criteria of a cannabis use disorder. In contrast, offspring of parents who met the criteria of a cannabis use disorder reported lower levels of positive parenting.

Risk of Abuse or Neglect When Using Cannabis

It is well-documented that parents with problematic substance use are at increased risk of maltreating their children (Wells 2009). However, the specific association between parental cannabis use and parental maltreatment remains ambiguous. According to Moore and Stuart (2005), the use of cannabis would increase the risk of violence and aggression through an alteration of the substance with cognitive functions involved in the treatment of complex and conflictual information and with behavioral inhibition. A meta-analysis on the association between cannabis use and aggressive behaviors (Ostrowsky 2011) however revealed highly contradictory findings: some studies observed no associations between cannabis use and aggression (Barrett et al. 2011; Green et al. 2010; Marie et al. 2008; Pedersen and Skardhamar 2010), others found that using cannabis increased the risk of aggression (Feingold et al. 2008; Huas et al. 2008; Moore et al. 2008; Swartout and White 2010), and others found a negative association between cannabis use and aggression (Kaplan et al. 2001; White and Hansell 1998). As regards the association between parental cannabis use and parental maltreatment, more specifically, Freisthler and Gruenewald (2014) observed that parents who had used cannabis in the past year reported engaging in physical abuse three times more frequently than those who had not. However, current cannabis use was not related to self-reported supervisory neglect and was inversely related to physical neglect. This suggests that cannabis use may be associated with some types of maltreatment and not others. More research is definitely needed to clarify this important issue.

Impact of Cannabis Use on Domains of Functioning Related to Parenting

The use of cannabis may lead to impairments in cognitive functions involved in the regulation of emotions and of parenting behaviors, such as learning, attention, working memory, episodic memory, processing speed, and executive functions (Fernandez-Serrano et al. 2011; Lovell et al. 2020; Petker et al. 2019; Volkow et al. 2016; Zimmermann et al. 2017). These neuropsychological impairments can in turn interfere with parents' judgment during parent-child interactions and increase the risk of inconsistent care or inadequate responses to the needs of the child (Child Welfare Information Gateway 2009; Conley et al. 2004; Deater-Deckard et al. 2012). However, the indirect association between parental cannabis use and inadequate parental behaviors via cognitive impairments remains to be confirmed using an experimental design.

The use of cannabis may also indirectly affect parenting by triggering psychiatric symptoms. Indeed, on the one hand, psychiatric symptoms have been shown to impede the availability of parents to respond to their children's needs (Licata et al. 2016) and to negatively affect offspring development (Goodman et al. 2011). On the other hand, higher prevalence of anxiety disorders (Kedzior and Laeber 2014;

Xue et al. 2021), depressive disorders (Lev-Ran et al. 2014), psychotic disorders (Marconi et al. 2016), and manic symptoms (Gibbs et al. 2015) has been reported in adults using cannabis. However, causal pathways have not been confirmed yet, and the direction of the association remains to be clarified.

Impact of Parental Cannabis Use on Offspring Development

Most studies on the impact of parental cannabis use on offspring development mainly focused on offspring of women who used cannabis during pregnancy. These studies suggest that prenatal exposure to cannabis would increase the risk of cognitive deficits and of mental health problems during childhood (El Marroun et al. 2009; Goldschmidt et al. 2000, 2004, 2008; Noland et al. 2005). The studies on the effect of postnatal parental cannabis use mainly focused on risky behaviors during adolescence. They showed, for instance, that offspring of users would be more inclined to use cannabis than offspring of nonusers (Bailey et al. 2016; Johnson et al. 1984; O'Loughlin et al. 2019) and would use the substance for the first time earlier in their development (Sokol et al. 2018). In addition, daughters of fathers with a lifetime cannabis use disorder (Cho 2018) and children of mothers with chronic cannabis use (De Genna et al. 2015) reported having been initiated to sexuality at a considerably younger age than offspring of parents who did not use cannabis or did not meet the criteria of a cannabis use disorder. Finally, Marmorstein and colleagues (Marmorstein 2009) showed that parental cannabis dependence increased the risk for alcohol (OR = 1.95) and drug dependence (OR = 1.38) in their adolescents but did not elevate the risk for ADHD, oppositional defiant disorder, conduct disorder, antisocial behavior, and nicotine dependence. The authors concluded that parental cannabis dependence would be more weakly associated with offspring externalizing problems than dependence on other drugs.

Studies involving younger children are scarce. In their longitudinal study of 332 pregnant adolescents followed up until 16 years postpartum, De Genna and colleagues (De Genna et al. 2015) observed that offspring of mothers who used marijuana over a decade were more likely to have internalizing problems at ages 10 and 14 and externalizing problems at age 10 than offspring of non-using mothers and of mothers who eventually quit using cannabis. In their study of 247 young, unmarried, low-income, minority mothers and their children followed from pregnancy to 3 years postpartum, Eiden et al. (2018) observed that higher cannabis use across the infant toddler period predicted higher behavior problems at 2 years, even when controlling for prenatal cannabis use. They further reported that the frequency of cannabis use between 2 and 16 months was positively correlated with the severity of child emotional reactivity, somatic complaints, anxiety/depression, attentional problems, and aggressive behavior at 3 years.

In conclusion, empirical studies on the effect of cannabis use on parenting and child development are scarce. Previous research generally concluded that parental cannabis use is a significant risk factor for parenting and child development, but most studies presented important limitations. For instance, they mainly relied on self-report measures and rarely considered potentially confounding variables, whereas parental cannabis use typically coexists with other risk factors known to affect parenting and to have intergenerational repercussions (Garon-Bissonnette et al. 2019). Furthermore, we still do not know under which circumstances the use of cannabis is a risk factor for parenting. For instance, the study of Hill et al. (2018) showed that the use of cannabis would not be a significant risk factor for parenting difficulties when the criteria of a substance use disorder are not met. Such a finding is intriguing and calls for further research on the specific effect of cannabis on parenting, knowing that cannabis use disorders are strongly associated with other psychiatric issues (such as other drug use, psychosis, mood disorders, anxiety disorders, and personality disorders; Hasin and Walsh 2021). Finally, the mechanisms through which parental cannabis use could influence offspring development remain unknown and need to be investigated using rigorous experimental designs.

What Is the Perception of Parents Regarding Their Use of Cannabis?

A review of publications in online media, print news, and print media on parental cannabis use showed that these publications generally promoted the use of cannabis by parents (Berthelot et al. 2020). Indeed, these publications commonly cited users who considered that cannabis contributed to making them better parents, increased their appreciation of their children, and strengthened their bond. Such a positive portrayal of parental cannabis use was observed not only in media devoted to the promotion of cannabis (e.g., Leafly; Enochs 2018) but also in popular media, such as The New York Times (Wolfe 2012), New York Daily News (Loreto 2017), Today's Parent (Goldberg 2018), The Guardian (Halperin 2018), or Cosmopolitan (Grover 2015). Numerous groups on social media in different countries also promote cannabis use by parents. For instance, the Facebook group "The Cannavist Mom" has approximately 40 000 members. Books, such as *Weed Mom* (Brand 2020), are also dedicated to promoting a "cannabis-friendly family life."

In spite of this abundance of articles, publications, and blogs publicizing the use of cannabis by parents, the majority of parents would not share this opinion. Indeed, in their longitudinal study involving 395 parents (56% mothers) from the state of Washington, where cannabis has been legal since 2012, Kosterman et al. (2016) observed that 52% of parents approved the use of cannabis in adults but that 89% disapproved the use of cannabis when caring for children. Similarly, 93% condemned the use of cannabis in situations where children can see the caregiver using cannabis or know what he/she is doing. These results, which remain to be reproduced and extended, suggest that sanctioning cannabis use in the presence of children remains a marginal phenomenon.

At this point, we know very little about parents' motivations for using cannabis. Some argue that using cannabis would increase their productivity and permit them to accomplish household chores more efficiently (Loreto 2017; Sabourin 2019; Stump 2017). Others claim that using cannabis would contribute to making them more patient and peaceful during interactions with their children (Goldberg 2018; Loreto 2017; Sabourin 2019; Schulte 2015; Thurstone et al. 2013) and would increase their interest in communicating and playing with their children (Goldberg 2018; Halperin 2018; Sabourin 2019). Yet some parents would use cannabis mainly as a treatment to alleviate physical pain or psychological problems (Sabourin 2019; Schulte 2015). This, however, remains anecdotic, and qualitative and quantitative research is required to get a better understanding of the motivation behind parental use of cannabis when caring for their children.

New Directions for Scientific Research on Parental Cannabis Use

There is a paucity of studies addressing the issue of parental cannabis use. We argue that scientific research on parental cannabis use is urgently needed to inform parents and professionals and to counterbalance the striking number of opinion-based publications on this topic. First, more rigorous studies are definitely required to advance our understanding of the association between cannabis use and parenting practices. In this regard, the recent legalization of cannabis in different countries and multiple states across America provides a unique opportunity for implementing experimental research protocols that may contribute to clarifying whether or not there are causal pathways between the use of cannabis and parenting impairments. Second, we still know very little about (1) the prevalence of parental cannabis use, (2) the motivations of parents for using cannabis when caring for children, (3) the perception parents have of the impact of cannabis use on their behaviors and on their children, as well as (4) the circumstances under which they use the substance. Population surveys and qualitative studies are urgently needed to address these questions. Finally, further studies will be needed to evaluate the success of public health measures to inform about the risk of using cannabis when caring for a child and to evaluate the usefulness and value of clinical guidelines that also consider parental cannabis use in child welfare decision-making.

Policies, Procedures, and Public Health Measures Regarding Parental Cannabis Use

Governmental and paragovernmental publications covering the topic of parental cannabis use are generally at the complete opposite of mass media publications: they mostly argue that using cannabis when caring for children is unsafe and may have damaging consequences (Berthelot et al. 2020). For instance, in Canada, where cannabis has been legal since 2018, the government argues that using cannabis may

(1) reduce a person's ability to pay attention, make decisions, or react to emergencies, (2) affect how parents respond to the needs of their children and how to keep them safe, and (3) negatively affect parent-child interactions and attachment (Health Canada 2018). To our knowledge, there are still very little policies and public health measures specifically addressing the issue of parental cannabis use. Interestingly, in 2016, the Colorado School of Public Health, in collaboration with the Kempe Center for the Prevention and Treatment of Child Abuse and Neglect and the Children's Hospital Colorado, conducted a health impact assessment to inform new state policies about how the use of cannabis by caregivers should be considered in child welfare decision-making (Ng and Tung 2016). That report led to a certain number of recommendations related to mandatory reporting practices and child welfare screening decisions. It was namely recommended that a child protection report be recorded (1) when the use of cannabis by an adult who cares for a child threatens or possibly harms the health or welfare of the child, (2) when a newborn tests positive for THC at birth, (3) when there is reasonable suspicion of purposeful or negligent pediatric exposure to or ingestion of marijuana, and (4) when the manufacture, distribution, production, or cultivation practices of marijuana are suspected of creating an environment that is injurious to the child (Ng and Tung 2016, p. 7).

Applications to Other Areas of Addiction

The issue of cannabis use by parents is unique, and there is a definite risk of considering substance use by parents as a homogeneous phenomenon. On the one hand, comparing cannabis to more severe substances would be prejudicial. Indeed, some substances, such as narcotics, stimulants, and hallucinogens, may have a more definite impact on parenting than cannabis and probably deserve to be treated differently in clinical, public health, and child welfare practices. On the other hand, many publications that advocate the right and option of parents to use cannabis make a simplistic comparison between cannabis use and alcohol use. They argue that most societies do not condemn the use of alcohol by parents and that, consequently, using cannabis when caring for children should be socially accepted. Interestingly, no one contends that using alcohol increases the ability to care for children, whereas a number of publications on cannabis promote the use of cannabis by parents (Berthelot et al. 2020). Accordingly, public health practice should consider both substances differently.

In conclusion, the recent legalization of cannabis in different countries and states across America calls for new policies, procedures, and public health measures regarding the use of cannabis by parents. Such courses of action could guide the different networks of services concerned by the health and well-being of children and parents. Public health organizations, however, have access to very limited data to inform their recommendations, given the poor quality of scientific evidence regarding the impact of cannabis use on parenting and child development (Ng and Tung 2016). This lack of hard facts addressing these issues allows for mass media to

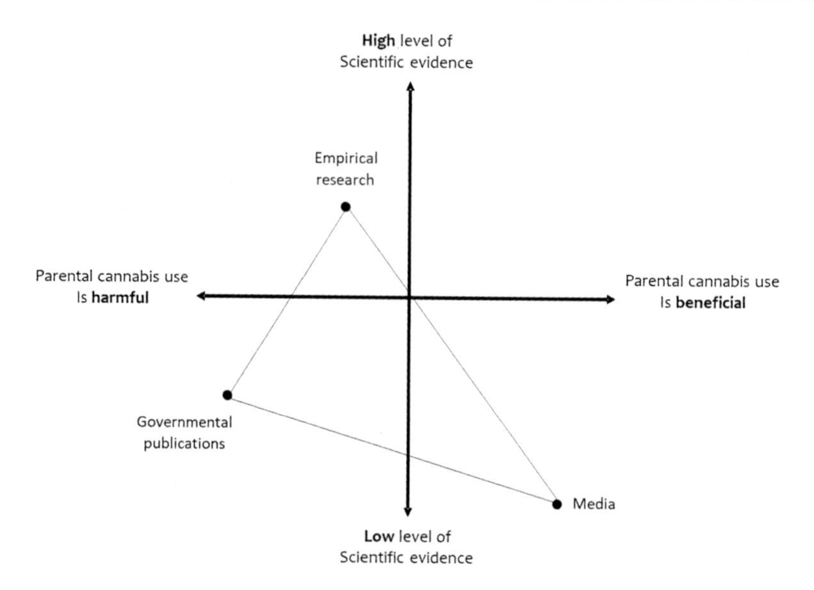

Fig. 2 Different positions concerning the effects of parental cannabis use on parenting according to the level of scientific evidence. (Reprinted from the Journal of the American Academy of Child and Adolescent Psychiatry, 59(3), Berthelot, N., Garon-Bissonnette, J., Drouin-Maziade, C., Duguay, G., Milot, T., Lemieux, R., Lacharité, C., St-Laurent, D., Dubois-Comtois, K., Parental cannabis use: Contradictory discourses in the media, governmental publications and the scientific literature, 333-335, Copyright (2020), with permission from Elsevier)

promote opinion-based publications that praise the parental use of cannabis (see Fig. 2). Scientific research on parental cannabis use should be considered, therefore, an urgent priority.

Key Facts on Parents Who Use Cannabis and on the Development of the Child

- The recreational use of cannabis is legal in Canada, Georgia, Mexico, South Africa, Uruguay, and in multiple states in the United States.
- Many adults with children in the home report using cannabis. However, the prevalence of cannabis use by parents and the circumstances under which they use the substance remains largely unknown.
- There is a paucity of rigorous empirical research on the effect of using cannabis on parenting behaviors.
- Existing evidence suggests negative associations between the use of cannabis by parents and attachment behaviors, as well as their offspring development.
- Publications on parental cannabis use in mass media generally promote the use of cannabis by parents.

Summary Points

- The use of cannabis by parents is relatively frequent and would concern at least 5% of parents.
- Negative associations were reported between cannabis use and some parental behaviors, such as in the demonstration of affection by parents.
- The mechanisms through which parental cannabis use influences offspring development remain unknown. Preliminary evidence suggests that parental cannabis use may affect children via a negative effect of cannabis on the capacity of parents to deliver adequate care as well as on their mental health, cognitive functioning, and attachment behaviors.
- It is not clear whether the use of cannabis by parents increases the risk of child maltreatment.
- Offspring of users would be more inclined to have internalized and externalized problems.
- We still do not know under which circumstances the use of cannabis is a risk factor for parenting, and available data suggest that the negative effect of cannabis may be limited to parents with a cannabis use disorder.
- A massive popular literature promotes the benefits of using cannabis as a parent, but the use of cannabis in the presence of children remains condemned by the majority of adults.
- There are still very few policies and public health measures addressing the issue of parental cannabis use.

References

Bailey JA, Hill KG, Guttmannova K et al (2016) Associations between parental and grandparental marijuana use and child substance use norms in a prospective, three-generation study. J Adolesc Health 59(3):262–268

Barrett EL, Mills KL, Teesson M (2011) Hurt people who hurt people: violence amongst individuals with comorbid substance use disorder and post traumatic stress disorder. Addict Behav 36(7): 721–728

Berthelot N, Garon-Bissonnette J, Drouin-Maziade C et al (2020) Parental cannabis use: contradictory discourses in the media, government publications, and the scientific literature. J Am Acad Child Adolesc Psychiatry 59(3):333–335

Brand DS (Ulysses Press) (2020) Weed Mom: The canna-curious woman's guide to healthier relaxation, happier parenting, and chilling TF out. Berkeley, Canada

Brook JS, Richter L, Whiteman M (2000) Effects of parent personality, upbringing, and marijuana use on the parent-child attachment relationship. J Am Acad Child Adolesc Psychiatry 39(2): 240–248

Brook JS, Balka EB, Fei K et al (2006) The effects of parental tobacco and marijuana use and personality attributes on child rearing in African-American and Puerto Rican young adults. J Child Fam Stud 15(2):153–164

Child Welfare Information Gateway (2009) Protecting children in families affected by substance use disorders. In: Child abuse and neglect user manual series. US Department of Health and Human Services. https://www.childwelfare.gov/pubs/usermanuals/substanceuse/

Cho BY (2018) Associations of father's lifetime cannabis use disorder with child's initiation of cannabis use, alcohol use, and sexual intercourse by child gender. Subst Use Misuse 53(14): 2330–2338

Conley CS, Caldwell MS, Flynn M et al (2004) Parenting and mental health. Handb Paren Theory Res Prac 276–295

De Genna NM, Goldschmidt L, Cornelius MD (2015) Maternal patterns of marijuana use and early sexual behavior in offspring of teenage mothers. Matern Child Health J 19(3):626–634

Deater-Deckard K, Wang Z, Chen N et al (2012) Maternal executive function, harsh parenting, and child conduct problems. J Child Psychol Psychiatry 53(10):1084–1091

Eiden RD, Zhao J, Casey M et al (2018) Pre-and postnatal tobacco and cannabis exposure and child behavior problems: bidirectional associations, joint effects, and sex differences. Drug Alcohol Depend 185:82–92

El Marroun H, Tiemeier H, Steegers EA et al (2009) Intrauterine cannabis exposure affects fetal growth trajectories: the Generation R Study. J Am Acad Child Adolesc Psychiatry 48 (12):1173–1181

Enochs E (2018) We need to destigmatize parents who use cannabis. https://www.leafly.ca/news/lifestyle/destigmatizing-parents-who-smoke-marijuana. Accessed 20 Sept 2021

Feingold A, Kerr DC, Capaldi DM (2008) Associations of substance use problems with intimate partner violence for at-risk men in long-term relationships. J Fam Psychol 22(3):429

Fernandez-Serrano MJ, Pérez-García M, Verdejo-García A (2011) What are the specific vs. generalized effects of drugs of abuse on neuropsychological performance? Neurosci Biobehav Rev 35(3):377–406

Freisthler B, Gruenewald PJ (2014) Examining the relationship between the physical availability of medical marijuana and marijuana use across fifty California cities. Drug Alcohol Depend 143: 244–250

Freisthler B, Gruenewald PJ, Wolf JP (2015) Examining the relationship between marijuana use, medical marijuana dispensaries, and abusive and neglectful parenting. Child Abuse Negl 48: 170–178

Garon-Bissonnette J, Morneau M, Duguay G et al (2019) Cannabis use during pregnancy does not occur in the absence of other risk factors affecting child neurodevelopment. Poster accepted for presentation at 66th annual meeting for American Academy of Child and Adolescent Psychiatry, Chicago, USA, 14–19 October 2019

Gibbs M, Winsper C, Marwaha S et al (2015) Cannabis use and mania symptoms: a systematic review and meta-analysis. J Affect Disord 171:39–47

Goldberg J (2018) Parents who smoke pot. https://www.todaysparent.com/family/parenting/parents-who-smoke-pot/. Accessed 10 Aug 2021

Goldschmidt L, Day NL, Richardson GA (2000) Effects of prenatal marijuana exposure on child behavior problems at age 10. Neurotoxicol Teratol 22(3):325–336

Goldschmidt L, Richardson GA, Cornelius MD et al (2004) Prenatal marijuana and alcohol exposure and academic achievement at age 10. Neurotoxicol Teratol 26(4):521–532

Goldschmidt L, Richardson GA, Willford J et al (2008) Prenatal marijuana exposure and intelligence test performance at age 6. J Am Acad Child Adolesc Psychiatry 47(3): 254–263

Goodman SH, Rouse MH, Connell AM et al (2011) Maternal depression and child psychopathology: a meta-analytic review. Clin Child Fam Psychol Rev 14(1):1–27

Goodwin RD, Kim JH, Cheslack-Postava K et al (2021) Trends in cannabis use among adults with children in the home in the United States, 2004–2017: impact of state-level legalization for recreational and medical use. Addiction

Green KM, Doherty EE, Stuart EA et al (2010) Does heavy adolescent marijuana use lead to criminal involvement in adulthood? Evidence from a multiwave longitudinal study of urban African Americans. Drug Alcohol Depend 112(1-2):117–125

Grover L (2015) Marijuana makes me a better mom. https://www.cosmopolitan.com/lifestyle/a43211/marijuana-mom/. Accessed 20 Sept 2021

Halperin A (2018) Cannabis strengthened our bond: can pot make you a better parent? https://www.theguardian.com/society/2018/apr/16/cannabis-marijuana-parenting-children-drugs. Accessed 10 Aug 2021

Hasin D, Walsh C (2021) Cannabis use, cannabis use disorder, and comorbid psychiatric illness: a narrative review. J Clin Med 10(1):15

Health Canada (2018) Thinking about using cannabis while parenting? In: Cannabis use, effects and risks. Government of Canada. https://www.canada.ca/en/health-canada/services/drugs-medication/cannabis/health-effects/parents.html. Accessed 30 Sep 2021

Hill M, Sternberg A, Suk HW et al (2018) The intergenerational transmission of cannabis use: Associations between parental history of cannabis use and cannabis use disorder, low positive parenting, and offspring cannabis use. Psychol Addict Behav 32(1):93

Huas C, Hassler C, Choquet M (2008) Has occasional cannabis use among adolescents also to be considered as a risk marker? Eur J Pub Health 18(6):626–629

Institut National de Santé Publique du Québec (2021) Pandémie et consommation de cannabis, de tabac et d'alcool. In: COVID-19: Sondage sur les attitudes et comportements des adultes québécois. Quebec National Institute of Public Health. https://www.inspq.qc.ca/covid-19/sondages-attitudes-comportements-quebecois/consommation-mai-2021. Accessed 10 June 2021

Johnson GM, Shontz FC, Locke TP (1984) Relationships between adolescent drug use and parental drug behaviors. Adolescence 19(74):295–299

Kaplan HB, Tolle GC Jr, Yoshida T (2001) Substance use-induced diminution of violence: a countervailing effect in longitudinal perspective. Criminology 39(1):205–224

Kedzior KK, Laeber LT (2014) A positive association between anxiety disorders and cannabis use or cannabis use disorders in the general population-a meta-analysis of 31 studies. BMC Psychiatry 14(1):1–22

Kosterman R, Bailey JA, Guttmannova K et al (2016) Marijuana legalization and parents' attitudes, use, and parenting in Washington State. J Adolesc Health 59(4):450–456

Lev-Ran S, Roerecke M, Le Foll B et al (2014) The association between cannabis use and depression: a systematic review and meta-analysis of longitudinal studies. Psychol Med 44(4): 797–810

Licata M, Zietlow AL, Träuble B et al (2016) Maternal emotional availability and its association with maternal psychopathology, attachment style insecurity and theory of mind. Psychopathology 49(5):334–340

Loreto M (2017) 5 ways smoking marijuana can make you a better parent. https://www.nydailynews.com/life-style/5-ways-smoking-marijuana-better-parent-article-1.3394051. Accessed 10 Aug 2021

Lovell ME, Akhurst J, Padgett C et al (2020) Cognitive outcomes associated with long-term, regular, recreational cannabis use in adults: a meta-analysis. Exp Clin Psychopharmacol 28 (4):471–494

Maalouf WE (2010) The role of parenting skills in the intergenerational transmission of marijuana use behavior. Thesis, Johns Hopkins University

Marconi A, Di Forti M, Lewis CM et al (2016) Meta-analysis of the association between the level of cannabis use and risk of psychosis. Schizophr Bull 42(5):1262–1269

Marie D, Fergusson DM, Boden JM (2008) Links between ethnic identification, cannabis use and dependence, and life outcomes in a New Zealand birth cohort. Aust Nz J Psychiat 42(9):780–788

Marmorstein NR (2009) Longitudinal associations between alcohol problems and depressive symptoms: early adolescence through early adulthood. Alcohol Clin Exp Res 33(1):49–59

Moore TM, Stuart GL (2005) A review of the literature on marijuana and interpersonal violence. Aggress Violent Behav 10(2):171–192

Moore TM, Stuart GL, Meehan JC et al (2008) Drug abuse and aggression between intimate partners: a meta-analytic review. Clin Psychol Rev 28:247–274

Ng V, Tung G (2016) Marijuana and child abuse and neglect: a health impact assessment. Colorado School of Public Health. https://coloradosph.cuanschutz.edu/docs/librariesprovider151/default-document-library/mj-cw-hia-final-report-11-3-2016.pdf?sfvrsn=ed49ffb9_0. Accessed 22 Aug 2021

Noland JS, Singer LT, Short EJ et al (2005) Prenatal drug exposure and selective attention in preschoolers. Neurotoxicol Teratol 27(3):429–438

O'Loughlin JL, Dugas EN, O'Loughlin EK et al (2019) Parental cannabis use is associated with cannabis initiation and use in offspring. J Pediatr 206:142–147

Ostrowsky MK (2011) Does marijuana use lead to aggression and violent behavior? J Drug Educ 41 (4):369–389

Pedersen W, Skardhamar T (2010) Cannabis and crime: findings from a longitudinal study. Addiction 105(1):109–118

Petker T, Owens MM, Amlung MT et al (2019) Cannabis involvement and neuropsychological performance: findings from the Human Connectome Project. J Psychiatry Neurosci 44(6):414

Rey JM, Martin A, Krabman P (2004) Is the party over? Cannabis and juvenile psychiatric disorder: the past 10 years. J Am Acad Child Adolesc Psychiatry 43(10):1194–1205

Sabourin C (2019) « Meilleure mère » grâce au cannabis. https://www.lesoleil.com/actualite/insolite/meilleure-mere-grace-au-cannabis-265573cd2971a799ea4b98b6990fd15c. Accessed 12 Aug 2021

Schulte B (2015) Even where it's legal for parents to smoke pot: what about the kids? https://www.washingtonpost.com/local/even-where-its-legal-for-parents-to-smoke-pot-what-about-the-kids/2015/06/06/dd4549c8-f977-11e4-9030-b4732caefe81_story.html. Accessed 10 Aug 2021

Sokol NA, Okechukwu CA, Chen JT et al (2018) Maternal cannabis use during a child's lifetime associated with earlier initiation. Am J Prev Med 55(5):592–602

Stump S (2017) « Marijuana moms » say smoking pot makes them better parents. https://www.today.com/parents/marijuana-moms-say-smoking-pot-makes-them-better-parents-t114510. Accessed 12 Aug 2021

Swartout KM, White JW (2010) The relationship between drug use and sexual aggression in men across time. J Interpers Violence 25(9):1716–1735

Thurstone C, Binswanger I, Corsi K et al (2013) Medical marijuana use and parenting: a qualitative study. Adolesc Psychiatry 3(2):190–194

Volkow ND, Swanson JM, Evins AE et al (2016) Effects of cannabis use on human behavior, including cognition, motivation, and psychosis: a review. JAMA Psychiatry 73(3):292–297

Wells K (2009) Substance abuse and child maltreatment. Pediatr Clin N Am 56(2):345–362

White HR, Hansell S (1998) Acute and long-term effects of drug use on aggression from adolescence into adulthood. J Drug Issues 28(4):837–858

Wolfe M (2012) Pot for parents. https://www.nytimes.com/2012/09/08/opinion/how-pot-helps-parenting.html. Accessed 30 Sept 2021

Xue S, Husain MI, Zhao H et al (2021) Cannabis use and prospective long-term association with anxiety: a systematic review and meta-analysis of longitudinal studies: Usage du cannabis et association prospective à long terme avec l'anxiété: une revue systématique et une méta-analyse d'études longitudinales. Can J Psychiatr 66(2):126–138

Zimmermann K, Walz C, Derckx RT et al (2017) Emotion regulation deficits in regular marijuana users. Hum Brain Mapp 38(8):4270–4279

Public Health Issues of Legalizing Cannabis

Considerations for Future Studies

Steven R. Boomhower

Contents

Introduction 1472
Biological Aspects 1473
Public Health Aspects 1476
Evaluating the Health Effects of Cannabis 1480
Applications to Other Areas of Addiction 1484
Applications to Public Health 1485
Mini-dictionary of Terms 1485
Key Facts of Cannabis and Public Health 1485
Summary Points 1486
References 1486

Abstract

Cannabis has been used by humans for centuries and contains a number of cannabinoid and non-cannabinoid compounds. In the United States, cannabis has a history of and continues to follow a complicated legislative path, with many states legalizing the recreational or medicinal use of cannabis or decriminalizing its use. There have been a number of studies of the therapeutic potential of cannabis and cannabinoids over the past several decades, and there now exists several cannabinoid-based medications for the treatment of various medical conditions. There has also been emerging evidence of adverse health effects linked to cannabis use. Due to legislative changes in cannabis use and possession, individuals have increasingly looked to studies of cannabis health effects to inform decisions related to cannabis and public health. Thus, it is particularly important that future observational studies of cannabis and health effects strive to produce accurate and reliable study results. Study design considerations related to

S. R. Boomhower (✉)
Gradient, Boston, MA, USA

Harvard Division of Continuing Education, Harvard University, Cambridge, MA, USA
e-mail: sboomhower@fas.harvard.edu; sboomhower@gradientcorp.com

V. B. Patel, V. R. Preedy (eds.), *Handbook of Substance Misuse and Addictions*,
https://doi.org/10.1007/978-3-030-92392-1_74

chemical constituents, exposure measurement, health outcome assessment, study design, confounding variables, and the dose-response relationship should be considered in designing future studies and when drawing conclusions related to cannabis-health outcomes in populations.

Keywords

Chemical constituents · Cannabis · Confounding variables · Dose-response relationship · Health outcome assessment · Exposure measurement · Legalization · Medical marijuana · Pharmacokinetics · Study design

Abbreviations

AIDS	acquired immunodeficiency syndrome
CB1	cannabinoid-1 receptor
CB2	cannabinoid-2 receptor
CBD	cannabidiol
CBN	cannabinol
CDC	Centers for Disease Control and Prevention
EVALI	e-cigarette or vaping associated lung injury
FDA	United States Food and Drug Administration
NASEM	National Academies of Sciences, Engineering, and Medicine
THC	Δ9-tetrahydrocannabinol
US	United States

Introduction

Cannabis is the genus of flowering plants belonging to the Cannabaceae family, which was first named by the German physician and botanist, Leonhart Fuchs, in 1542 (Hancock and McKim 2017). However, the earliest mention of cannabis is thought to be in Ancient Egyptian religious passages carved into stone walls of pyramids around 2350 BCE (Hancock and McKim 2017). Since then, a number of species of cannabis have been discovered, which include *Cannabis sativa*, *Cannabis indica*, and *Cannabis ruderalis*. Cannabis comprises many chemicals, including cannabinoids (e.g., Δ9-tetrahydrocannabinol [THC] and cannabidiol [CBD]) and non-cannabinoid chemicals (e.g., terpenoids or flavonoids). In the United States, cannabis has a history of and continues to follow a complicated legislative path, with many states legalizing the recreational use of cannabis. With access to cannabis becoming easier due in part to the loosening of cannabis regulatory laws, there is growing importance for understanding the health effects of cannabis use. Although there now exist a few cannabinoid-based, FDA-approved medications, the science of cannabis health effects remains in its infancy. Future studies of cannabis use and health outcomes – particularly as they relate to public health – must consider a number of factors related to study design in order to ensure robust and reliable scientific findings. This chapter discusses the pharmacokinetic and neurobiological factors of cannabis, the use of cannabinoids in medicine, a brief review of the history of cannabis legislation in the United States, current rates and prevalence of cannabis use, and study design considerations (i.e., chemical constituents, exposure measurement, health outcome assessment, study design, confounding variables, and the dose-response relationship). Scientific and medical professionals should consider these factors in designing future studies and when drawing conclusions related to cannabis-health outcomes in populations.

Biological Aspects

Pharmacokinetics of cannabinoids. There are two primary routes of administration for cannabis – inhalation via smoking or vaping and oral ingestion. Once cannabis is administered, its chemical constituents (e.g., THC and CBD) are absorbed into the body. Absorption describes the process by which chemicals move into the body and/or bloodstream. Cannabinoids from smoked cannabis are readily and rapidly absorbed into the circulatory system from the respiratory tract. Blood THC concentrations typically peak within the first 30 min after smoking, though the amount of absorbed THC will depend on the depth of inhalation (i.e., puff volume) as well as puff frequency (National Academies of Sciences, Engineering, and Medicine [NASEM] 2017; Hancock and McKim 2017). In general, the bioavailability of THC following smoking or vaping is similar – ranging from approximately 10–50% (Hancock and McKim 2017). In contrast to cannabis inhalation, ingestion of cannabis results in peak blood THC concentrations following 1–4 h after administration (NASEM 2017; Spindle et al. 2020). Further, because of the high lipid solubility and low water solubility of cannabinoids, oral administration of cannabis typically results in lower THC and CBD bioavailability than inhalation. In general, the bioavailability of THC following oral administration ranges from approximately 5–20% (Spindle et al. 2020; Hancock and McKim 2017).

Following the absorption of cannabinoids into the circulatory system, they are distributed throughout the body. Distribution describes the process by which an absorbed chemical travels throughout the body to various target organs or tissues. With respect to cannabis' psychoactive effects (mediated primarily by THC), cannabinoids readily pass the blood-brain barrier and interact with the endogenous cannabinoid neurocircuitry (i.e., the endocannabinoid neurotransmitter system). The endocannabinoid neurotransmitter system comprises both endogenous cannabinoids (i.e., anandamide and 2-arachidonoylglycerol) and cannabinoid receptors (NASEM 2017; Hancock and McKim 2017). The two known cannabinoid receptors in the body are cannabinoid-1 (CB1) and cannabinoid-2 (CB2) receptors, whose crystal structures have only recently been described (Hua et al. 2016; Li et al. 2019). CB1 receptors are primarily expressed in the central nervous system and mediate much of the cognitive and behavioral effects of cannabinoid compounds (Fig. 1). CB2 receptors are primarily expressed in the peripheral nervous system and immune system and mediate some of the non-psychoactive effects (e.g., anti-inflammatory, anti-nausea, or analgesic effects) of cannabinoids (NASEM 2017). Cannabinoids

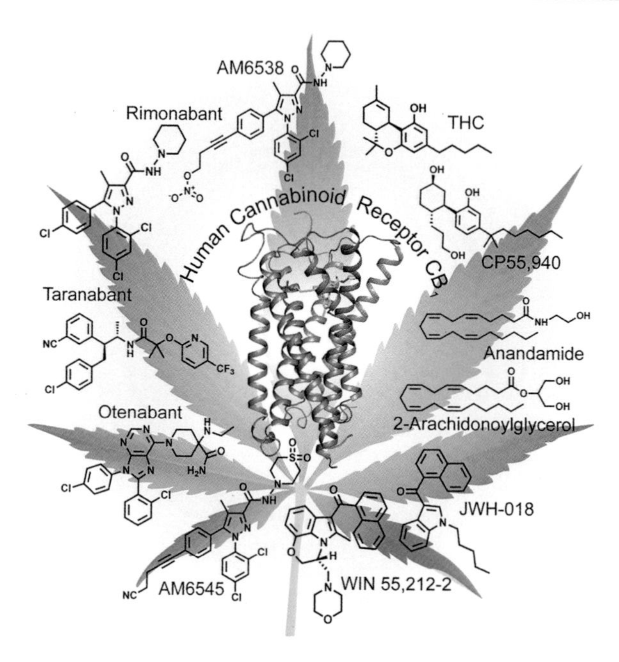

Fig. 1 The human cannabinoid-1 (CB1) receptor and various cannabinoid compounds. The CB1 receptor is primarily expressed in the central nervous system and is activated by endogenous cannabinoids (i.e., endocannabinoids), such as anandamide or 2-arachidonoylglycerol, or other cannabinoid agonists, such as Δ9-tetrahydrocannabinol (THC), CP55,940, JWH-018, or WIN55,212-2. The CB1 receptor is blocked by cannabinoid antangonists, such as AM6538, AM6545, rimonbant, tranabant, or otenabant. (Reprinted from Cell, Volume 167, Issue 3, Hua et al., Crystal Structure of the Human Cannabinoid Receptor CB1, 750–762, 2016, with permission from Elsevier)

tend to accumulate in body fat due to their high lipid solubility, and body fat acts as a long-term storage site in which cannabinoid molecules are released back into the circulation over days, weeks, or months with repeated cannabis use (Hancock and McKim 2017).

Cannabinoids begin to be metabolized and excreted from the body very shortly after they are absorbed (Huestis et al. 1992; Spindle et al. 2020). Metabolism refers to the process by which chemicals are transformed by bodily processes, and excretion refers to the process by which chemicals (or their byproducts) are eliminated from the body. Cannabinoids undergo a large degree of first-pass metabolism, which refers to the enzymatic breakdown of chemicals within the blood stream (Hancock and McKim 2017). In the liver, THC is metabolized into 11-OH-THC, which is then metabolized into THC-COOH, THC-COOH glucuronide, and other metabolites (Hancock and McKim 2017; Spindle et al. 2020). 11-OH-THC is considered to be equipotent to THC in terms of its psychoactive effects, and THC-COOH and THC-COOH glucuronide are inactive metabolites (NASEM 2017; Hancock and McKim 2017). THC and its metabolites are mostly excreted in feces (approximately

65%) and urine (approximately 20%) (Hancock and McKim 2017). The half-life of cannabinoids and their metabolites varies considerably within and between individuals due to a number of factors such as dose, frequency of use, and lipid deposition (i.e., the slow release of THC from fat stores). The half-life of THC ranges from approximately 30 h to 4 days (Hancock and McKim 2017). It should be noted that some evidence suggests that other chemical constituents of cannabis, such as CBD and cannabinol (CBN), can also affect the rate of metabolism and excretion of THC (Hancock and McKim 2017). Knowledge of the pharmacokinetics of THC metabolism and excretion can also be used to determine when recent use may have occurred. For example, some investigators have developed models of the time-course of THC metabolite concentrations to predict the time elapsed since cannabis use (e.g., Huestis et al. 1992).

Cannabinoids in medicine. Perhaps one of the most compelling reasons for the legalization of cannabis has been the recognition of therapeutic effects of THC and CBD. Although cannabis has been used to treat various ailments throughout history (Hancock and McKim 2017), the majority of rigorous scientific studies (e.g., randomized clinical trials) of the therapeutic potential of cannabis have been conducted only in the last few decades. Indeed, many studies have provided evidence of the therapeutic potential of cannabinoids in humans and nonhumans, including its effects on pain management (i.e., as an antinociceptive or analgesic) and appetite (Leung 2011). Synthetic cannabinoids (i.e., pharmaceutical-grade compounds) designed to mimic the actions of compounds found in cannabis first began appearing in the 1980s. Since then, only a few cannabinoid drugs have been approved for medical use across the world.

Presently, the US Food and Drug Administration (FDA) has approved four medications that contain cannabinoids for the treatment of health conditions. Table 1 lists these compounds and their approved indications. Interestingly, some of these drugs (e.g., Marinol and Syndros) contain THC, which is also a Schedule I drug under the Controlled Substances Act and considered to have high abuse potential and no medical use. However, upon its FDA approval in 1985, Marinol was designated a Schedule II drug (i.e., medically useful but high abuse potential) and then rescheduled as a Schedule III drug (i.e., medically useful and moderate/low abuse potential) in 1999 (64 Fed. Reg. 35928 (July 2, 1999); 21 CFR Section 1308.13(g)(1)). Although not yet

Table 1 Cannabinoid-based drugs approved for clinical use in the United States

Brand name	Generic name	Clinical uses
Epidiolex	Cannabidiol	Seizures associated with Lennox-Gastaut syndrome, Dravet syndrome, or tuberous sclerosis complex
Marinol	Dronabinol/ THC	Chemotherapy-associated nausea and vomiting; AIDS-associated loss of appetite and weight loss
Syndros	Dronabinol/ THC	Chemotherapy-associated nausea and vomiting; AIDS-associated loss of appetite and weight loss
Cesamet	Nabilone	Chemotherapy-associated nausea and vomiting

AIDS Acquired immunodeficiency syndrome, THC Δ9-tetrahydrocannabinol

approved for use in the United States, it is also worth mentioning that nabiximols (Sativex), an oromucosal spray containing a 1:1 ratio of THC and CBD (along with other minor cannabinoids), has been approved for the treatment of spasticity (i.e., muscle stiffness and spasm) due to multiple sclerosis in the United Kingdom and European Union. Nabiximols are currently being evaluated in a number of clinical trials in the United States for the treatment of spasticity due to multiple sclerosis.

Although some of the cannabinoids found in the drugs listed in Table 1 occur naturally in cannabis (e.g., THC and CBD), the FDA has not approved cannabis for medical use in any condition to date. There are a number of reasons for this, including that (1) there is an insufficient amount of information regarding cannabis' benefits versus risks from randomized clinical trials, and (2) the chemical constituents in cannabis lack consistency in terms of their concentrations to allow for accurate dosing, which makes evaluating cannabis as a whole-plant medicine difficult (Freeman et al. 2021; Vandrey et al. 2015). That is not to say, however, that individuals cannot take cannabis as "medical marijuana." Indeed, many states have legalized the use of cannabis to treat various ailments so long as one obtains approval from a medical doctor (see Table 2). Medical-marijuana patients report using cannabis to treat many symptoms, including sleep problems, pain, and anxiety (Walsh et al. 2013). Historical milestones related to the legalization of medical marijuana are discussed in more detail in the following section.

Unfortunately, not all cannabinoid drugs have encountered success as pharmacotherapeutics despite promising data regarding efficacy. For example, rimonabant (Accomplia), a CB1 antagonist and inverse agonist was first developed by Sanofi-Aventis in 2006 and was marketed in Europe as an appetite suppressant and anti-obesity drug. Indeed, rimonabant showed promising results, with participants experiencing dramatic weight loss and improved cardiovascular outcomes (Christensen et al. 2007), and was eventually approved for use in 56 countries (though not in the United States) under the trade name Zimulti. However, upon a review of post-marketing data in 2008, rimonabant was removed from the market due to evidence of an increased risk of psychiatric disorders, including suicidality, depression, and anxiety, compared to placebo (Christensen et al. 2007; Hancock and McKim 2017). Although not used as a medical treatment today, rimonabant continues to be used as a tool in preclinical studies to assess the involvement of the endocannabinoid neurotransmitter system in eating (Boomhower and Rasmussen 2014; Boomhower et al. 2013; Rasmussen et al. 2012), perhaps in hopes that improved cannabinoid drugs may be developed for use in metabolic disorders or obesity.

Public Health Aspects

Historical milestones in legalization. The legalization of cannabis in the United States has a rich history. The practice of smoking cannabis and use of the word "marijuana" are believed to have been introduced in the United States in the early

Table 2 Legal status[a] of recreational and medicinal cannabis use and decriminalization status in the United States

State	Recreational use	Medicinal	Decriminalized
Alabama	Mixed	Legal	No
Alaska	Legal	Legal	Yes
Arizona	Legal	Legal	Yes
Arkansas	Mixed	Legal	No
California	Legal	Legal	Yes
Colorado	Legal	Legal	Yes
Connecticut	Legal	Legal	Yes
Delaware	Mixed	Legal	Yes
District of Columbia	Legal	Legal	Yes
Florida	Mixed	Legal	No
Georgia	Mixed	Illegal	No
Hawaii	Mixed	Legal	Yes
Idaho	Illegal	Illegal	No
Illinois	Legal	Legal	Yes
Indiana	Mixed	Illegal	No
Iowa	Mixed	Illegal	No
Kansas	Illegal	Illegal	No
Kentucky	Mixed	Illegal	No
Louisiana	Mixed	Legal	No
Maine	Legal	Legal	Yes
Maryland	Mixed	Legal	Yes
Massachusetts	Legal	Legal	Yes
Michigan	Legal	Legal	Yes
Minnesota	Mixed	Legal	Yes
Mississippi	Mixed	Legal	Yes
Missouri	Mixed	Legal	Yes
Montana	Legal	Legal	Yes
Nebraska	Mixed	Illegal	Yes
Nevada	Legal	Legal	Yes
New Hampshire	Mixed	Legal	Yes
New Jersey	Legal	Legal	Yes
New Mexico	Legal	Legal	Yes
New York	Legal	Legal	Yes
North Carolina	Mixed	Illegal	Yes
North Dakota	Mixed	Legal	Yes
Ohio	Mixed	Legal	Yes
Oklahoma	Mixed	Legal	No
Oregon	Legal	Legal	Yes
Pennsylvania	Mixed	Legal	No
Rhode Island	Mixed	Legal	Yes
South Carolina	Illegal	Illegal	No
South Dakota	Legal	Legal	Yes

(continued)

Table 2 (continued)

State	Recreational use	Medicinal	Decriminalized
Tennessee	Illegal	Illegal	No
Texas	Mixed	Illegal	No
Utah	Mixed	Legal	No
Vermont	Legal	Legal	Yes
Virginia	Legal	Legal	Yes
Washington	Legal	Legal	Yes
West Virginia	Mixed	Legal	No
Wisconsin	Mixed	Illegal	No
Wyoming	Illegal	Illegal	No

[a]Data reflect state marijuana laws as of July 2021. Changes in cannabis legislation may have occurred since these data were published

1900s, and upon an increase in use of marijuana in California, cannabis was promptly outlawed in the state in 1913 (Mead 2019; Hancock and McKim 2017). There are a number of theories for why cannabis began to be banned throughout many US states in the early 1900s (Mead 2019), but the most likely reason is thought to be due to its perceived association with illegal activity and violence with a lack of reliable scientific data to the contrary at the time. By 1936, 48 states had laws regulating the possession, use, or sale of cannabis, which co-occurred with the infamous anti-cannabis film *Reefer Madness* that was released that same year. The United States was not alone in enacting legislation to limit cannabis use at the time – other countries such as Canada and the United Kingdom began imposing restrictions on cannabis possession in the 1920s, with some of the first international controls on cannabis occurring in 1928 (Hancock and McKim 2017). In 1970, the US federal government passed the Controlled Substances Act, which determined that marijuana had no potential medical use and a high potential for abuse as a Schedule I drug. As a Schedule I drug, the use, possession, sale, growth, and distribution of cannabis (as well as cannabis mimetics, or drugs that share mechanisms of action with cannabis) remain illegal under US federal law.

Following changing attitudes toward cannabis that were, in part, driven by recognition of its potential medical uses, US states began permitting the cultivation, possession, and use of cannabis for certain medical purposes (Mead 2019). In 1996, as part of the Compassionate Use Act in response to the acquired immunodeficiency syndrome (AIDS) crisis, California became the first state to approve cannabis cultivation and possession (Mead 2019; Hancock and McKim 2017). Although medical use was generally limited in the following years in California (as well as other states that began permitting medical marijuana, such as Oregon and Washington), an increasing number of physicians willing to provide permission to qualifying patients as well as increased availability of dispensaries contributed to medical marijuana growth (Mead 2019). Finally, in 2012, Colorado became the first state to approve the recreational use of cannabis by adults. Since then, a number of states have approved recreational and medical use of cannabis and/or decriminalized its use (Table 2).

Prevalence of cannabis use. With decriminalization and legalization of cannabis use in the United States, it is assumed that both a greater proportion of individuals may administer cannabis and/or administer cannabis at higher rates. One of the most robust datasets for information related to cannabis use in the United States comes from the Monitoring the Future survey (Johnston et al. 2021). The Monitoring the Future survey has been conducted for over 40 years and includes several ongoing, longitudinal surveys of nationally representative samples of high school students, college students, young adults, and adults. Survey takers are asked to self-report their use of cannabis ("marijuana" on the survey) during a period of time. For example, survey takers are asked to report on whether they have ever used marijuana ("Lifetime"), and whether they have used marijuana at least once in the previous year ("Past Year"), once in the previous month ("Past Month"), or nearly every day (i.e., 21 of 30 days) in the last month ("Daily"). Table 3 shows lifetime, past year, past month, and daily prevalence of marijuana use in students living in the United States. These data include marijuana use in the form of smoking, vaping, and edibles. According to these results, nearly 40–50% of students have tried marijuana in their lifetime by the 12th grade. Further, the number of students using marijuana "daily" has increased from 2017 to 2020, such that approximately 5.8–6.9% of 12th graders report using marijuana nearly every day.

Although cannabis use reached its highest prevalence in the late 1970s, cannabis is the most frequently used illicit drug among students and adults to date (Johnston et al. 2021). Rates of cannabis use are influenced by a number of factors, including availability, social acceptability, and perceived risk of harm (Hancock and McKim 2017; Johnston et al. 2021). In 2014, the percentage of students who believed that

Table 3 Prevalence of marijuana use in United States 8th graders, 10th graders, and 12th graders from 2017 to 2020

		Year of survey			
Age group	Prevalence	2017	2018	2019	2020[a]
8th graders	Lifetime	13.5%	13.9%	15.2%	14.8%
	Past year	10.1%	10.5%	11.8%	11.4%
	Past month	5.5%	5.6%	6.6%	6.5%
	Daily	0.8%	0.7%	1.3%	1.1%
10th graders	Lifetime	30.7%	32.6%	34%	33.3%
	Past year	25.5%	27.5%	28.8%	28%
	Past month	15.7%	16.7%	18.4%	16.6%
	Daily	2.9%	3.4%	4.8%	4.4%
12th graders	Lifetime	45%	43.6%	43.7%	43.7%
	Past year	37.1%	35.9%	35.7%	35.2%
	Past month	22.9%	22.2%	22.3%	21.1%
	Daily	5.9%	5.8%	6.4%	6.9%

Source: Johnston et al. (2021)

[a]Data collection for 2020 stopped prematurely due to the COVID-19 pandemic. According to the National Institutes of Drug Abuse (NIDA), survey completion rates in 2020 were approximately 25% of the previous years' completion rates, gathered from a broad geographic range, and statistically weighted to be nationally representative

regular cannabis smoking posed a risk of harm reached all-time lows and remains generally low – this is particularly important in that, historically, low levels of perceived risk tend to track and sometimes predict increases in use (Hancock and McKim 2017). Data from the Monitoring the Future Survey will continue to be an important tool as changes to the legal status of recreational cannabis use occur across the United States.

Evaluating the Health Effects of Cannabis

That cannabinoids may have potential therapeutic benefit for individuals is an exciting prospect. Indeed, the legalization of cannabis and cannabis derivatives in many US states has arguably allowed for more scientific study of the health effects of cannabis, particularly in observational studies of the general population. However, there is growing evidence that suggests there are risks associated with cannabis use, particularly repeated use (NASEM 2017). Some states have even begun mandating that cannabis-containing products have warnings regarding cannabis use. For example, the California Office of Environmental Health Hazard Assessment lists cannabis smoke as a carcinogen and cannabis and THC as a developmental toxicant under Proposition 65 (Tomar et al. 2009; Campbell et al. 2019). As scientific knowledge of cannabis health effects grows, a number of factors must be considered in designing studies to ensure reliable results and conclusions are made (Temple et al. 2010) – particularly as those in science, medicine, regulation, and litigation begin (and continue) to rely on cannabis health studies to assess the potential risks of cannabis use. The following points are limitations or sources of uncertainty related to the conduct and interpretation of cannabis health studies that should be controlled for (or minimized) in designing future studies, particularly when drawing conclusions related to cannabis-health outcomes in populations. These points are summarized in Fig. 2.

Chemical constituents. As cannabis is a whole-plant, it not only contains a number of chemicals in addition to cannabinoids but also may be exposed to contaminants as part of the cultivation or storage process. For example, biological contaminants (e.g., fungus and bacteria), heavy metals, pesticides, and other chemicals may be present in cannabis preparations (Leung 2011; NASEM 2017). Additionally, cannabis may also be mixed with other drugs (e.g., tobacco or stimulants) to enhance its psychoactive effects or to alleviate its side effects (NASEM 2017). Pesticide and solvent contamination can also result from various extraction and inhalation methods for some dosing formulations (Thomas and Pollard 2016).

With respect to studies of cannabis health effects, considering the extent of contamination present in cannabis products is particularly important. A good illustration of this comes from a series of cases of e-cigarette or vaping associated lung injury (EVALI) in the United States in 2019 (Centers for Disease Control and Prevention [CDC] 2020; Krishnasamy et al. 2020). In the majority of cases, individuals reported using THC vaping products before the onset of EVALI symptoms;

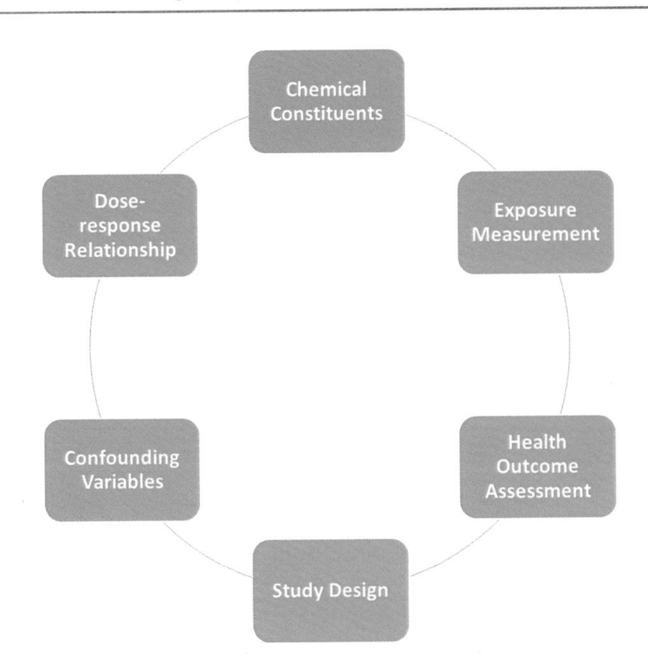

Fig. 2 Study aspects that inform evaluations of the health effects of cannabis. A number of study aspects are useful for determining whether cannabis use is associated with health effects. Though not a comprehensive list, scientific and medical professionals must consider chemical constituents (i.e., the extent to which cannabis may contain other, non-cannabinoid compounds), exposure measurement (i.e., reliable estimates of cannabis intake), health outcome assessment (i.e., reliable and objective assessments of health endpoints of interest), study design (i.e., the extent to which a study's design permits causal inferences), confounding variables (i.e., the extent to which variables associated with cannabis use and health outcomes of interest are controlled), and the dose-response relationship (i.e., whether there is a dose-dependent change in the health outcome of interest) when drawing conclusions related to cannabis-health outcomes in populations

however, upon examination of bronchoalveolar lavage fluid samples, elevated concentrations of vitamin E acetate were detected (CDC 2020; Krishnasamy et al. 2020). Indeed, many of the THC-containing vaping products linked to EVALI cases had used vitamin E acetate as a diluent, which was likely combusted during the vaping process, produced ketene gas, and resulted in severe lung injury (CDC 2020). Thus, it was not the case that vaped THC produced EVALI; rather, that chemicals in the diluent (i.e., vitamin E acetate) produced EVALI.

Exposure measurement. Obtaining a detailed exposure history to cannabis is essential to population studies of cannabis health effects. This is particularly difficult though, in that the preparation of cannabis for use among individuals is highly variable. For example, the amount of cannabis in smokable joints has been shown to vary substantially, ranging from approximately 0.07 to 0.88 g of cannabis per joint (van der Pol et al. 2013; NASEM 2017). Estimation of dose is further complicated by evidence of variability in THC potency among cannabis joints and edibles, particularly across the last few decades. For example, cannabis joints were shown to range from 1.1 to 24.7% in THC concentration (van der Pol et al. 2013), and the amount of THC in cannabis edibles has been shown to range from 1 to 1,236 mg (Vandrey et al. 2015). With respect to the evolution of THC potency across time, herbal- and resin-based cannabis THC concentrations have increased by approximately 0.29% and 0.57% per year (respectively) since 1970 (Freeman et al. 2021).

In addition to variability in the concentration of THC and other cannabinoids in cannabis, self-report also presents a source of uncertainty in exposure assessment. Indeed, many observational studies of cannabis health effects quantify cannabis exposure via self-report measures (e.g., surveys or questionnaires) (NASEM 2017). Self-report measures of cannabis use can be inaccurate, incomplete, or imprecise for a number of reasons, including poor memory, social norms related to illicit drug use, or limited knowledge of cannabis administration (NASEM 2017). Indeed, self-reports of the amount of cannabis smoked (measured as grams of cannabis per joint) as well as cannabis potency (measured on a visual analogue scale) were generally poor predictors of objective measures of cannabis amount and potency in individuals (van der Pol et al. 2013). Similarly, reliance on self-reported frequency of cannabis use also is a limitation of cannabis health studies, particularly when arbitrary classification systems are employed that do not readily distinguish between frequency of use (e.g., "regular users," "heavy users," or "non-users") (Temple et al. 2010). Future observational studies of cannabis users should consider implementing reliable, objective, and accurate measures of cannabis use.

Health outcome assessment. Accurate and objective characterization of the health effect(s) of interest in studies is also important for establishing reliable cannabis health effect associations. A number of observational studies rely on self-reported health effects or symptoms (e.g., Walsh et al. 2013; NASEM 2017). Similar to the issues discussed above, participant self-reports of health outcomes can be limited; however, when self-report measures must be used, investigators should ensure the survey's or questionnaire's reliability and validity. When feasible, objective and reliable health assessments performed by a medical professional or investigator should be used in observational studies of cannabis health effects. Further, providing information on health outcomes at various intervals throughout studies (e.g., in longitudinal studies that follow participants over many years) would also help improve precision of study findings (NASEM 2017). Related to the reporting of health outcomes, it is also important for investigators to report effect sizes (rather than mere statistical significance) and consider reported effect sizes in the context of clinical significance (Temple et al., 2010). Stated differently, a statistically significant difference between cannabis users and non-users in a study may not necessarily be clinically significant. For example, a relatively small deficit in spatial memory following cannabis use observed in a laboratory setting may have no impact on an individual's performance in navigating real-world settings (e.g., work, home, or community).

Study design. There are a number of study designs that investigators can implement in observational studies of cannabis use – each with its own strengths and limitations. The primary study designs in observational studies are ecological, cross-sectional, case-control, cohort, and randomized clinical trials. *Ecological studies* assess whether the occurrence of a health effect in a population (usually defined by geographic region, workplace, or duration of time) correlates with the occurrence of drug exposure (Webster 2007). Because ecological studies do not collect individual data, it is not possible to determine whether a study participant was exposed to a drug or whether a participant displayed a health effect. Thus, ecological studies do not provide evidence of a causal relationship between cannabis exposure and a health effect (Bonita et al. 2006). *Cross-sectional studies* provide information about individuals' exposures and health effects at one point in time (Rothman and Greenland 2008). Typically, the overall prevalence of the health outcome of interest is compared among groups of individuals (e.g., cannabis users and non-users); however, it is not possible to ascertain whether cannabis use preceded the health outcome of interest in cross-sectional studies because both exposure history and health outcome assessments are conducted at similar time points. Similar to ecological studies, cross-sectional studies do not provide evidence of a causal relationship between cannabis exposure and a health effect (Bonita et al. 2006). *Case-control studies* identify groups of individuals with (case) or without (control) a health outcome of interest, and then compare or estimate the exposure history between each group (Paneth et al. 2002). Case-control studies are useful for health outcomes that are rare (e.g., schizophrenia); however, it can be difficult to retroactively estimate an individual's cannabis use history, particularly if it occurred many years prior. Care must also be taken to ensure appropriate controls are selected. *Cohort studies* follow a group of individuals across time, during which each participant's relevant exposures and health effects are assessed (Rothman and Greenland 2008). Importantly, prospective cohort studies document a group of participants' exposures and then follow them for a number of years. When conducted appropriately, cohort studies can provide information regarding a causal relationship between cannabis exposure and a health effect. However, attrition (dropping out) of participants can also impact the results of cohort studies. Finally, *randomized clinical trials* take advantage of experimental control in that participants are randomly assigned to various treatment groups and then health outcomes are observed over one or multiple sessions. For example, participants may be assigned to smoked cannabis treatment, ingested cannabis treatment, or a control condition, and then complete health assessments in the future. When conducted appropriately, randomized clinical trials provide the greatest certainty with respect to causal relationships between cannabis use and a health effect. However, randomized clinical trials also must consider appropriate blinding conditions – that is, study investigators and participants should not know the treatments that are being administered to minimize placebo or expectation effects. Further, randomized clinical trials are typically not implemented to study adverse health effects in individuals because it would not be ethical to knowingly assign individuals to a treatment group that would cause harm.

Confounding variables. The assessment and control of confounding variables is particularly important in cannabis health studies (NASEM 2017; Temple et al. 2010). Confounding variables are factors that are associated with both cannabis use and the health outcome(s) of interest; thus, controlling for them in analyses has the potential to attenuate or even eliminate statistically significant associations between cannabis use and a given health effect. Depending on the health outcome of interest, a number of confounding variables must be considered. For example, in studies of cannabis use and intelligence (or other measures of cognition), variables such as the quality of the home environment, parental intelligence, socioeconomic status, and history of mental health disorders (among other relevant factors) should be measured and analyzed (NASEM 2017). Related to the issue of confounding, cannabis users may be overrepresented in a particular population that has the health effect of interest. For example, cannabis (and other drug) use tends to be comorbid with other psychological disorders, including psychotic disorders (Temple et al. 2010; NASEM 2017). Thus, it becomes unclear whether deficits in cognitive functioning among individuals with psychotic orders (e.g., schizophrenia) are related to a comorbid diagnosis, cannabis use alone, or both. This is particularly relevant in studies of cannabis use and psychological outcomes, such as affective disorders or drug use, in which common risk factors like childhood adversity are implicated in both (Temple et al. 2010; Rabiee et al. 2020).

Dose-response relationship. A central tenant of toxicology is the concept that "the dose makes the poison," attributed to Paracelsus. This tenant describes the dose-response curve, or the relationship between the dose of a drug and a response (e.g., a measure of a health effect) and that the effects of a chemical are usually proportional to the concentration of the chemical in the body (Hancock and McKim 2017). Dose-response relationships (or dose-response curves) can provide information as to whether data collected in a study provide evidence that cannabis use is associated with a particular health effect. For example, that increased doses of cannabis are associated with increasingly reduced chronic neuropathic pain provides evidence of a cannabis-health association (Andreae et al. 2015); however, the absence of a dose-response relationship would provide evidence against a chemical-health association (e.g., Zuardi et al. 2017). Observational studies of cannabis health effects should ensure that data are collected in such a way as to assess whether dose-response relationships are present, including collecting health observations at a range of cannabis doses as well as a control (or unexposed) condition.

Applications to Other Areas of Addiction

Study design considerations related to chemical constituents, exposure measurement, health outcome assessment, study design, confounding variables, and the dose-response relationship are highly relevant to addiction, both as it relates to cannabis and addiction to other drugs. For example, along with cannabis, scientists are gaining an appreciation for the potential therapeutic effects of hallucinogens, such as psilocybin (Johnson and Griffiths 2017). Psilocybin is a psychedelic compound that is found in many species of fungi (i.e., mushrooms). In many respects, psilocybin and cannabis are similar with respect to their legislative history in the United States as well as their scientific "rediscovery" in terms of their potential therapeutic effects. However, many hallucinogens (like cannabis) remain as Schedule I drugs (i.e., considered to have not medical benefit and be highly addictive). Although the potential therapeutic effects of hallucinogens are compelling (Johnson and Griffiths 2017), ensuring that evidence regarding their potential adverse effects is accurate and reliable is also important, particularly with respect to the study design considerations in Fig. 2. Hallucinogens are taken at much lower rates in the United States compared to cannabis, and the legalization of hallucinogens in the United States has yet to take as firm a hold as cannabis legalization. Thus, long-term observational studies of hallucinogen users are likely many years away.

Applications to Public Health

A careful balance must be struck with respect to the legalization of recreational cannabis use and minimizing the risks of cannabis use. For example, emerging evidence suggests that cannabis use can impair driving ability and may increase the risk of motor vehicle collisions (Rogeberg and Elvik 2016). Further, unintentional cannabis ingestion by children also represents a public health concern (Richards et al. 2017). Thus, it will be important for public health officials and legislators to consider how best to educate the public with respect to the risks of cannabis use. To date, there are observational studies that provide strong evidence that cannabis use is associated with some adverse effects (e.g., psychotic symptoms), but there are many health outcomes that have not been conclusively linked to cannabis use (NASEM 2017). The topics discussed in this chapter, particularly those presented in Fig. 2, are important for establishing accurate and reliable evidence of the potential risks of cannabis use.

Mini-dictionary of Terms

- *Absorption* is the process by which chemicals move into the body and/or bloodstream,
- *Bioavailability* is the proportion of drug that is contained in the circulation (blood stream) and is available to affect physiology.
- *Cannabis Mimetics* are drugs that share mechanisms of action with cannabis.
- *Distribution* describes the process by which an absorbed chemical travels throughout the body to various target organs or tissues.
- *Excretion* refers to the process by which chemicals (or their by-products) are eliminated from the body.
- *First-pass Metabolism* refers to the enzymatic breakdown of chemicals within the blood stream.
- *Half-life* refers to the amount of time required for 50% of the concentration of an absorbed chemical to be excreted from the body.
- *Metabolism* refers to the process by which chemicals are transformed by bodily processes.

Key Facts of Cannabis and Public Health

- Cannabis contains many chemicals, including cannabinoids and non-cannabinoids.
- Cannabis is the most frequently used illicit drug in the United States.

- Some cannabinoids have been approved for the treatment of various medical conditions.
- Although recreational cannabis use is legal in many US states, researchers are still studying whether cannabis use is associated with adverse effects.
- Robust studies of cannabis use and health outcomes will consider a number of study design considerations, such as those shown in Fig. 2.

Summary Points

- Cannabis use in humans has occurred over centuries, dating back to the Ancient Egyptians.
- The primary manner in which people administer cannabis is by smoking or ingesting it.
- Cannabis contains a number of cannabinoids that interact with the endocannabinoid neurotransmitter system, which comprises two endogenous cannabinoids (anandamide and 2-arachidonoylglycerol) and two cannabinoid receptor subtypes (CB1 and CB2).
- THC is metabolized into both active and inactive metabolites, which are then excreted from the body in feces and urine.
- To date, there are four FDA-approved medications that contain cannabinoids that are used to treat medical conditions.
- The legal pathway of cannabis has been complicated throughout United States history; however, many US states now have legalized the recreational or medicinal use of cannabis and/or have decriminalized cannabis use.
- Cannabis is one of the most highly used illicit drugs in the United States, with approximately 40–50% of students reporting that they have used cannabis in their lifetime by the 12th grade and approximately 5.8–6.9% of 12th graders reporting that they have used cannabis nearly every day.
- California has begun mandating that cannabis-containing products have warnings regarding cannabis use and have determined that cannabis smoke is a carcinogen and cannabis and THC are developmental toxicants.
- Study design considerations related to chemical constituents, exposure measurement, health outcome assessment, study design, confounding variables, and the dose-response relationship should be considered in designing future studies and when drawing conclusions related to cannabis-health outcomes in populations.

References

Andreae MH, Carter GM, Shaparin N, Suslov K, Ellis RJ, Ware MA, Abrams DI, Prasad H, Wilsey B, Indyk D, Johnson M (2015) Inhaled cannabis for chronic neuropathic pain: a meta-analysis of individual patient data. J Pain 16(12):1221–1232

Bonita R, Beaglehole R, Kjellstrom T (2006) Basic epidemiology. World Health Organization, Geneva, Switzerland

Boomhower SR, Rasmussen EB (2014) Haloperidol and rimonabant increase delay discounting in rats fed high-fat and standard-chow diets. Behav Pharmacol 25(8):705

Boomhower SR, Rasmussen EB, Doherty TS (2013) Impulsive-choice patterns for food in genetically lean and obese Zucker rats. Behav Brain Res 241:214–221

Campbell M et al (2019) Evidence on the developmental toxicity of cannabis (marijuana) smoke and delta-9-THC. California EPA: Reproductive and cancer hazard assessment branch of the office of environmental health hazard assessment, California, USA

Centers for Disease Control and Prevention (2020) Outbreak of lung injury associated with the use of e-cigarette, or vaping, products. Accessed at: https://www.cdc.gov/tobacco/basic_information/e-cigarettes/severe-lung-disease.html

Christensen R, Kristensen PK, Bartels EM, Bliddal H, Astrup A (2007) Efficacy and safety of the weight-loss drug rimonabant: a meta-analysis of randomised trials. Lancet 370(9600):1706–1713

Freeman TP, Craft S, Wilson J, Stylianou S, ElSohly M, Di Forti M, Lynskey MT (2021) Changes in delta-9-tetrahydrocannabinol (THC) and cannabidiol (CBD) concentrations in cannabis over time: systematic review and meta-analysis. Addiction 116(5):1000–1010

Hancock S, McKim W (2017) Drugs and behavior: an introduction to behavioral pharmacology. Pearson, USA

Hua T, Vemuri K, Pu M, Qu L, Han GW, Wu Y, Zhao S, Shui W, Li S, Korde A, Laprairie RB (2016) Crystal structure of the human cannabinoid receptor CB1. Cell 167(3):750–762

Huestis MA, Henningfield JE, Cone EJ (1992) Blood cannabinoids. I. Absorption of THC and formation of 11-OH-THC and THCCOOH during and after smoking marijuana. J Anal Toxicol 16(5):276–282

Johnson MW, Griffiths RR (2017) Potential therapeutic effects of psilocybin. Neurotherapeutics 14 (3):734–740

Johnston LD, Miech RA, O'Malley PM, Bachman JG, Schulenberg JE, Patrick ME (2021) Monitoring the future national survey results on drug use 1975–2020: overview, key findings on adolescent drug use. Institute for Social Research, University of Michigan, Ann Arbor

Krishnasamy VP, Hallowell BD, Ko JY, Board A, Hartnett KP, Salvatore PP, Danielson M, Kite-Powell A, Twentyman E, Kim L, Cyrus A (2020) Update: characteristics of a nationwide outbreak of e-cigarette, or vaping, product use–associated lung injury—United States, August 2019–January 2020. Morb Mortal Wkly Rep 69(3):90

Leung L (2011) Cannabis and its derivatives: review of medical use. J Am Board Family Med 24 (4):452–462

Li X, Hua T, Vemuri K, Ho JH, Wu Y, Wu L, Popov P, Benchama O, Zvonok N, Qu L, Han GW (2019) Crystal structure of the human cannabinoid receptor CB2. Cell 176(3):459–467

Mead A (2019) Legal and regulatory issues governing cannabis and cannabis-derived products in the United States. Front Plant Sci 10:697

National Academies of Sciences, Engineering, and Medicine (2017) The health effects of cannabis and cannabinoids: the current state of evidence and recommendations for research

Paneth N, Susser E, Susser M (2002) Origins and early development of the case-control study: Part 1, Early evolution. Sozial-und Präventivmedizin 47(5):282–288

Rabiee R, Lundin A, Agardh E, Forsell Y, Allebeck P, Danielsson AK (2020) Cannabis use, subsequent other illicit drug use and drug use disorders: a 16-year follow-up study among Swedish adults. Addict Behav 106:106390

Rasmussen EB, Reilly W, Buckley J, Boomhower SR (2012) Rimonabant reduces the essential value of food in the genetically obese Zucker rat: an exponential demand analysis. Physiol Behav 105(3):734–741

Richards JR, Smith NE, Moulin AK (2017) Unintentional cannabis ingestion in children: a systematic review. J Pediatr 190:142–152

Rogeberg O, Elvik R (2016) The effects of cannabis intoxication on motor vehicle collision revisited and revised. Addiction 111(8):1348–1359

Rothman KJ, Greenland S (2008) Modern epidemiology. Lippincott Williams & Wilkins

Spindle TR, Cone EJ, Herrmann ES, Mitchell JM, Flegel R, LoDico C, Bigelow GE, Vandrey R (2020) Pharmacokinetics of cannabis brownies: a controlled examination of Δ9-tetrahydrocannabinol and metabolites in blood and oral fluid of healthy adult males and females. J Anal Toxicol 44(7):661–671

Temple EC, Brown RF, Hine DW (2010) The 'grass ceiling': limitations in the literature hinder our understanding of cannabis use and its consequences. Addiction 106(2):238–244

Thomas BF, Pollard GT (2016) Preparation and distribution of cannabis and cannabis-derived dosage formulations for investigational and therapeutic use in the United States. Front Pharmacol 7:285

Tomar RS, Beaumont J, Hsieh JCY (2009) Evidence on the carcinogenicity of marijuana smoke. California EPA: Reproductive and Cancer Hazard Assessment Branch of the Office of Environmental Health Hazard Assessment, California, USA

van der Pol P, Liebregts N, de Graaf R, Korf DJ, van den Brink W, van Laar M (2013) Validation of self-reported cannabis dose and potency: an ecological study. Addiction 108(10):1801–1808

Vandrey R, Raber JC, Raber ME, Douglass B, Miller C, Bonn-Miller MO (2015) Cannabinoid dose and label accuracy in edible medical cannabis products. JAMA 313(24):2491–2493

Walsh Z, Callaway R, Belle-Isle L, Capler R, Kay R, Lucas P, Holtzman S (2013) Cannabis for therapeutic purposes: patient characteristics, access, and reasons for use. Int J Drug Policy 24(6): 511–516

Webster TF (2007) Bias magnification in ecologic studies: a methodological investigation. Environ Health 6(1):1–17

Zuardi AW, Rodrigues NP, Silva AL, Bernardo SA, Hallak JE, Guimarães FS, Crippa JA (2017) Inverted U-shaped dose-response curve of the anxiolytic effect of cannabidiol during public speaking in real life. Front Pharmacol 8:259

Over-the-Counter Cannabidiol (CBD) 69

Leticia Shea

Contents

OTC Medications 1490
Dietary Supplements 1491
How Is CBD Regulated? 1492
What Differences Exist Between Prescription CBD and "OTC" CBD? 1493
CBD Drug (And Supplement!) Interactions 1494
CBD Pharmacogenomics 1498
What Is Cannabidiol and How Does It Work? 1506
Topical CBD 1507
CBD Adverse Effects 1508
Applications to Public Health 1512
Key Facts 1512
Mini Dictionary 1512
Key Summary Points 1513
References 1514

Abstract

Cannabidiol (CBD) is commonly referred to as the "non-psychoactive" cannabinoid found in *Cannabis*. Although CBD does not equate to getting "high," additional studies are needed to evaluate both safety and efficacy. Unfortunately, the step to determine safety and efficacy prior to being readily available to the public was skipped for this compound. Over-the-counter (OTC) CBD is readily available, and the side effects and precautions that have been determined in clinical trials are not provided to consumers on the labeling information. OTC CBD creates a conundrum to truly determining if and what benefit(s) may exist

L. Shea (✉)
Department of Pharmacy Practice, School of Pharmacy, Regis University, Denver, CO, USA
e-mail: Lshea@regis.edu

V. B. Patel, V. R. Preedy (eds.), *Handbook of Substance Misuse and Addictions*,
https://doi.org/10.1007/978-3-030-92392-1_75

with this compound due to the extreme variability in products and concentrations. This chapter aims to outline what is currently known regarding CBD, illegally available OTC.

Keywords

Cannabidiol · CBD · Cannabinoids · Over-the-counter · OTC · Dietary supplements · THC · Tetrahydrocannabinol · Full spectrum · Pharmacogenomics · Drug interactions · Drug safety

Abbreviations

AHRQ	The Agency for Healthcare Research and Quality
AUC	Area under the curve
CB1	Cannabinoid 1 receptor
CBC	Cannabichromene
CBD	Cannabidiol
CBDA	Cannabidiolic acid
CBDV	Cannabidivarin
CBG	Cannabigerol
CBN	Cannabinol
CYP	Cytochrome
DSHEA	The Dietary Supplement Health and Education Act of 1994
GABA	Gamma-aminobutyric acid; main inhibitory neurotransmitter
NSAIDs	Nonsteroidal anti-inflammatory drugs
OTC	Over-the-counter
THC	Δ^9-Tetrahydrocannabinol
TTO	Tea tree oil

Cannabidiol (CBD), the "non-psychoactive" cannabinoid, is one of many non-psychoactive **cannabinoids** found in *Cannabis*; however, the lack of psychoactive activity hardly defines the compound. CBD has become exceedingly accessible to individuals, with claims found on the over-the-counter (OTC) labeling far outreaching what science has determined to be safe or efficacious. Generally, when medication or supplements are available to the public, they fall under the delineation of **OTC medications** or **dietary supplements**. There is a clear distinction between these two types of products.

OTC Medications

Companies hoping to bring their product to the OTC market must submit an application to the Division of Nonprescription Drug Products in the Office of Drug Evaluation (FDA, OTC 2020). Some of the products are drugs that have been available only as prescription, while others are new drug products. Although there is a difference in the processes for prescription to OTC versus new product to OTC, both incorporate expert review for safety and efficacy. This is done through several avenues such as postmarketing safety data, review of efficacy and safety data related to ***controlled clinical trials***, review of clinical pharmacology, statistical analysis, and chemistry (FDA, OTC 2020). Once the product has been determined to be both safe and efficacious for consumer use, generally for a specific set of time, it may then be approved for OTC status. It is important to note that OTC medications contain very specific dosing and approved length of use limitations. For example, omeprazole was approved as an OTC medication (from prescription) but only in the setting in which it is used for 2 weeks (Prilosec 2018). If an individual determines that they require the use of this medication for longer than 2 weeks, then it is recommended to seek additional medical attention so that a provider may evaluate and monitor their condition and response to the medication (Prilosec 2018). When a medication is approved as OTC, it does not suggest that they are safe for everyone, nor should these medications be utilized for chronic (long-term) use. Ibuprofen, a common nonsteroidal anti-inflammatory drug (NSAID), is approved for short-term OTC use at doses at or below 400 mg (Motrin 2007). The ibuprofen tablets/capsules available as OTC are 200 mg, and the approved OTC dosing for adults is 200–400 mg orally every 4 to 6 h as needed for pain (Motrin 2007). If an individual is to take this drug daily, they should be monitored by their primary care provider and/or other providers. NSAIDs can increase cardiovascular risk, initiate or perpetuate harm to the kidneys and the gastrointestinal tract (Motrin 2007). These risks associated with NSAIDs must be included on package labeling as well as inside the package insert. All OTC medications are required to share their safety profile, adverse events, and warning information in their package inserts.

Dietary Supplements

Dietary supplements do not have safety or efficacy requirements as seen with products sold as OTC medications. Dietary supplements are assumed safe until proven otherwise. Furthermore, dietary supplements are not required to report adverse events that have occurred in clinical trials. For example, if vitamin E was regulated as a medication, all vitamin E packaging would be required to include that vitamin E has been associated with an increased risk of mortality in certain populations, and exhibited an increased risk for heart failure and hospitalization associated with heart failure (Hayden et al. 2007; Lonn et al. 2005). Specifically, Hayden et al. determined an increase in mortality was seen in vitamin E users with a history of stroke, coronary bypass graft surgery, or myocardial infarction (Hayden et al. 2007). Another trial exhibited patients taking Vitamin E, in comparison to placebo, had a higher risk of heart failure as well as hospitalization *for* heart failure (Lonn et al. 2005). Unfortunately for consumers, none of this information is included in vitamin E packaging.

The Dietary Supplement Health and Education Act of 1994 (DSHEA) mandates that it is the *manufacturers'* jurisdiction to ensure safety and validation for all claims stated on their product (FDA, Dietary Supplements 2019). This is a sharp contrast from medications, where safety data is analyzed by an unaffiliated party prior to marketing and consumer access. If a new dietary ingredient is brought to market, it is the manufacturer's responsibility to notify the FDA of its use and demonstrate why it is believed to be safe (FDA, Dietary Supplements 2019; Eichner et al. 2016). Since the enactment of DSHEA, well over 51,000 supplements have been brought to market, but less than 1% have provided notifications (Eichner et al. 2016). Relying on manufacturers to self-report ingredients is inhibitory toward public safety, as studies have clearly shown that many dietary supplements contain pharmaceuticals, banned or discouraged use ingredients (Eichner et al. 2016; Cohen et al. 2021). The lack of reporting has facilitated the availability of supplements with questionable safety.

How Is CBD Regulated?

So, the question is as follows: Where does CBD belong? Is it regulated as an OTC medication or a dietary supplement? The answer is: neither. CBD is only approved as a prescription drug under the brand name, Epidiolex® for very rare seizure disorders (Abernethy 2019; Epidiolex 2018; FDA, Drug Trials Snapshots 2018). The confusion perhaps begins with the Agriculture Improvement Act of 2018 (Farm Bill, PL 115-334), in which hemp was removed from the definition of marijuana (Abernethy 2019). The "Farm Bill" removes *Cannabis sativa L.* with low concentrations of delta-9-tetrahydrocannabinol (THC) (specifically less than 0.3% THC dry weight) from being considered a controlled substance. *Cannabis sativa L.* has many cannabinoids present, but how it is grown and removed from the ground impacts the concentrations of these constituents and thus the regulatory status in which the plant belongs. Hemp seeds do not contain CBD or THC and are permitted to be used legally in US food (Abernethy 2019). This is not the case for parts of the hemp plant that contain cannabinoids such as CBD and THC. It remains illegal to market CBD as a dietary supplement or to be added to food items (Abernethy 2019). Regardless, "OTC" CBD remains widely accessible (Shea et al. 2020a).

CBD was approved for prescription use following 4 clinical trials of patients with severe forms of epilepsy known as Lennox-Gastaut syndrome and Dravet syndrome (Epidiolex 2018; FDA, Drug Trials Snapshots 2018). These double-blinded clinical trials were performed to evaluate the safety and efficacy of CBD *in addition to* other epilepsy medications in patients with severely uncontrolled (refractory) epilepsy. It is important to recognize several factors when considering the onslaught of CBD available for consumers without a prescription. CBD was studied in a very select population that does not properly represent the general population in the United States. For example, when considering all 4 clinical trials that resulted in the approval of Epidiolex®, 77% of the patients were less than 18 years of age, 86% of the patients were white, and 100% of the patients suffered from a severe seizure disorder and were on additional epilepsy medication(s) (Epidiolex 2018; FDA, Drug Trials Snapshots 2018). Individuals with these disorders exhibit excessive excitation in the brain (Wallace et al. 2016). There are several pathophysiological mechanisms proposed for Dravet syndrome, predominately resulting from genetic mutations of the SCN1A gene (Wallace et al. 2016). Inhibition of GABAergic inhibitory neurons (inhibition of the inter-neurons that inhibit excitation) and increased sodium density resulting in glutamatergic excitatory neurons hyperexcitability are some of the models with evidence (Wallace et al. 2016). Lennox-Gastaut syndrome most often occurs in result to brain injury, but there is also evidence of cortical hyperexcitability during brain development (Asadi-Pooya 2018; Camfield 2011). There remains variability, but the underlying consistency is excessive neuronal excitation that is not exhibited in individuals without epilepsy, i.e., the majority of individuals in the United States.

What Differences Exist Between Prescription CBD and "OTC" CBD?

Many OTC CBD products are labeled as "full spectrum" (Shea et al. 2020a). Full spectrum implies the existence of additional active compounds (cannabinoids, terpenes, and other biological compounds) in the CBD extract (Shea et al. 2020a; Pavlovic et al. 2018). Discrepancies occur depending on the plant strain and extraction method utilized (Shea et al. 2020a; Pavlovic et al. 2018). Standardization of how "full spectrum" extracts are performed does not exist, so consumers should remain aware that actual active compounds will differ, regardless that the product label only states "CBD" (Shea et al. 2020a; Pavlovic et al. 2018; Shea et al. 2020a, b).

Numerous studies investigating the quality and quantity of active cannabinoids present in OTC CBD products have revealed copious "full spectrum" CBD products to contain more THC than the permitted threshold of less than 0.3% THC (Shea et al. 2020a, b; Pavlovic et al. 2018; Hazekamp 2018; Bonn-Miller et al. 2017; US Food and Drug Administration 2020).

Concerns are warranted for unregulated CBD as adverse events/poor outcomes can be compounded (pun intended) by several factors:

- Drug interactions
- Disease interactions
- Pharmacogenomic differences

Table 1 provides a simplified comparison of what consumers can expect when comparing OTC CBD to prescription CBD.

Table 1 Prescription CBD versus OTC CBD products

Prescription CBD	OTC CBD
Highly purified	Variability in content and purity (i.e., "full spectrum")
Only contains CBD	May contain additional cannabinoids (and other active compounds)
Available as oral solution	Available in numerous formulations (oral, sublingual, edible, inhalant, topical, transdermal, etc.) that have not been studied in humans for efficacy or safety
Available as 100 mg/mL	Available in variable doses and concentrations

CBD Drug (And Supplement!) Interactions

CBD requires extensive cytochrome P450 (CYP) metabolism. The CYP enzymes are located throughout the body, but CBD and the majority of all drugs are metabolized via this system in the liver. Obtaining a foundational understanding of this process is important to understand the context in which CBD may impact individuals on other medications (or supplements). The most predominant isoform responsible for drug metabolism (accounting for the metabolism of approximately 30% of the currently available medications on the market) is CYP3A4 (Doohan et al. 2021). CBD has been found to be a partial inhibitor of this enzyme (Doohan et al. 2021; Yamaori 2011). CYP2D6 and CYP2C9 are also extremely important for drug metabolism, required for 20% and 13%, respectively, of all drugs currently on the market (Doohan et al. 2021). There is contrasting data as to whether CBD or other cannabinoids have clinically significant activity at CYP2D6, but the data is strong regarding several cannabinoids having potent inhibitory action at CYP2C9 (Doohan et al. 2021). CYP2C19 is required for the metabolism of 7% of all drugs currently on the market, which may seem mediocre in comparison to the other CYP enzymes mentioned, but when you consider the thousands of medications currently marketed, it is a number that should not be taken lightly. Additionally, these percentages are based on the total number of drugs, not the prevalence of their use. Thus, drugs that are highly prevalent (such as clopidogrel, metabolized by CYP2C19) are going to be seen often, and CBD taken concomitantly may lead to grave interactions and side effects. CBD has exhibited potent inhibition at CYP2C19, suggesting that CBD should be taken very cautiously for anyone on any medications or supplements metabolized by CYP3A4, CYP2C9, and CYP2C19 (Doohan et al. 2021; Jiang et al. 2013; Yamaori 2011, 2013; Yamaori et al. 2011a, b; Rong et al. 2018).

CBD is both a **substrate** and an **inhibitor** for certain CYP450 enzymes (Ujváry and Hanuš 2016). Substrate indicates that CBD is a chemical entity that is acted upon by an enzyme (CYP2C19, for example) in which a new compound is created in the reaction – generally a compound that may be excreted from the body. At times, these compounds may also have pharmacological activity. It is suspected that CBD does have some active metabolites, but currently no human studies have been performed to confirm the biological activity of CBD metabolites (Ujváry and Hanuš 2016).

It can be daunting to understand what "an inhibitor" equates to, since the outcome is also dependent on the type of drugs being administered. Figures 1 and 2 provide a simplified depiction of the roles CYP enzymes play dependent on whether a drug is an "active" drug or a "pro" drug. CBD is considered an "active" drug, in which it exerts its effect prior to being metabolized (i.e., acted upon by CYP enzymes). However, as mentioned already, it is also believed that CBD may have active metabolites. The most prevalent metabolites of CBD are hydroxylated 7-carboxyl derivatives of CBD (Ujváry and Hanuš 2016). Human studies are needed to evaluate the activity of this and other CBD metabolites.

As discussed already, OTC CBD products generally contain more than just CBD (Pavlovic et al. 2018; Shea et al. 2020a, b; Hazekamp 2018; Bonn-Miller et al. 2017;

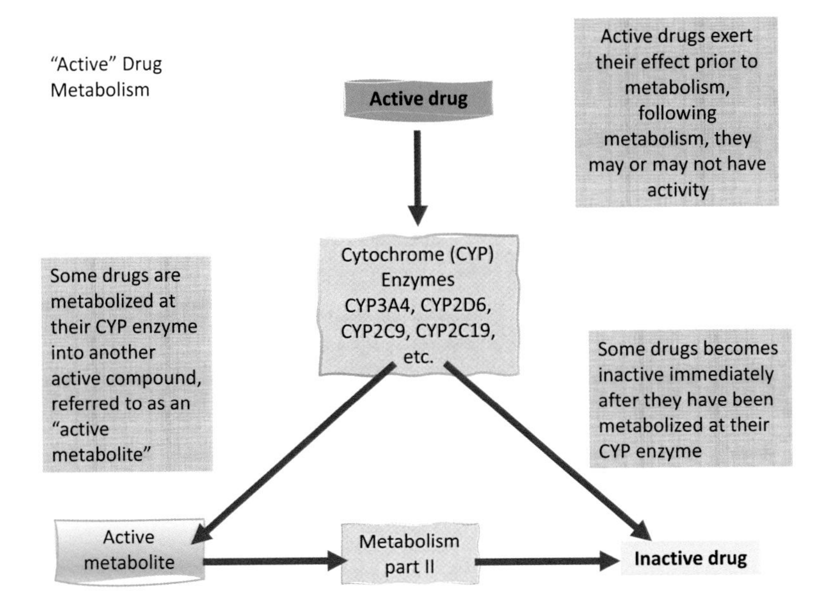

Fig. 1 Active drug metabolism depiction

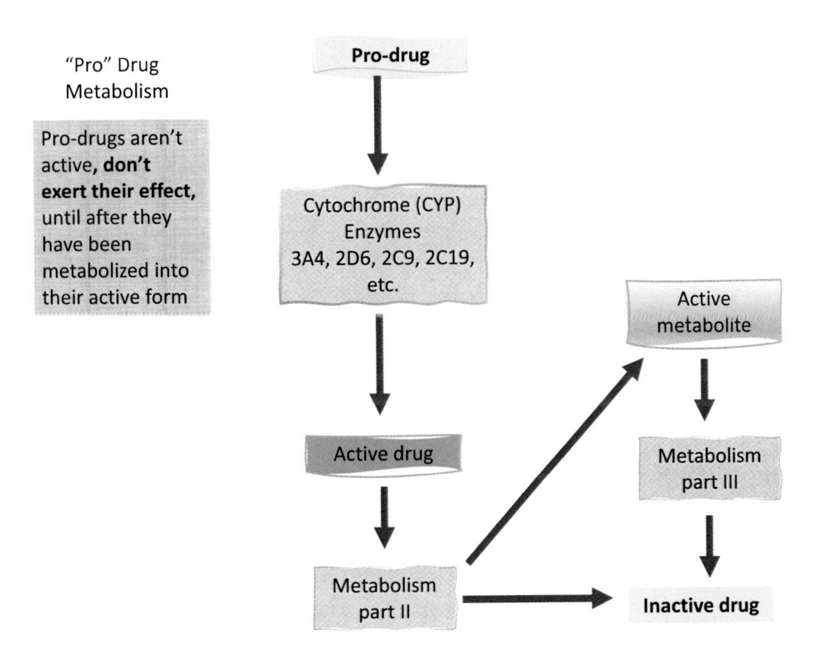

Fig. 2 "Pro-drug" metabolism depiction

Table 2 Oral CBD products ("Full Spectrum") = more drug interactions?

	Cytochrome P450 enzymes						
Cannabinoid	2A6	2B6	2C9	2C19	2D6	3A4	1A2
CBN	W	**W**		W	W	W	**I**
CBD	W	**I**	I	**I**	W	**I**	
CBG		W	I	W			W
THC	W	**I**	W[a]		W	W	

Cannabis products containing THC
W, Weak inhibition; I, Inhibition
[a]THC exhibits weak inhibition, but THC acid exhibits stronger inhibition which may result in clinically significant inhibition when consuming

US Food and Drug Administration 2020). This variability provides a conundrum as to what to expect from the product as well as how it will interact with the body (and other medications/supplements consumed).

Table 2 provides some of the cannabinoids that may be present at variable concentrations in OTC CBD products. In a study analyzing OTC CBD products sold in retail pharmacies, the majority of the products were listed as "full spectrum" (Shea et al. 2020a). It may be prudent to consider drug interactions beyond those of simply CBD, as other cannabinoids also have metabolism through CYP enzymes. Table 2 outlines the common CYPP450 enzymes and indicates what role each cannabinoid may have at these sites (Doohan et al. 2021; Jiang et al. 2013; Yamaori 2011, 2013; Yamaori et al. 2011; Rong et al. 2018). Additionally, some patients may exhibit stronger reactions to the medications based on genetic variations of their CYP activity. This will be discussed further under the pharmacogenomic considerations for CBD section.

CBD has the potential to have significant drug-drug or drug-supplement interactions considering the extensive CYP activity; however, the majority of the data currently available for CBD and drug interactions are based on interactions specific to medications taken for epilepsy.

A trial that evaluated the drug interaction of CBD with clobazam (an antiepileptic medication metabolized through CYP3A4 and CYP2C19) resulted in both an increase of exposure to clobazam and clobazam's active metabolite, norclobazam (Geffrey et al. 2015).

What is needed for public safety is to evaluate CBD (and other cannabinoid constituents) in the context of the most common health conditions exhibited in the United States and corresponding medications (i.e., heart disease and medications to manage or prevent heart conditions). The Agency for Healthcare Research and Quality (AHRQ) evaluates medical expenditures and provides a list of the medications most commonly prescribed each year (Medical Expenditures Panel Survey 2018). When reviewing this list, it is important to consider how many interactions may be possible if individuals are choosing to use oral OTC CBD while taking any of these commonly prescribed medications. Figure 3 provides some of the most common medications prescribed that share sites of metabolism with CBD. The concern for sharing sites of metabolism with CBD is that there is a high likelihood

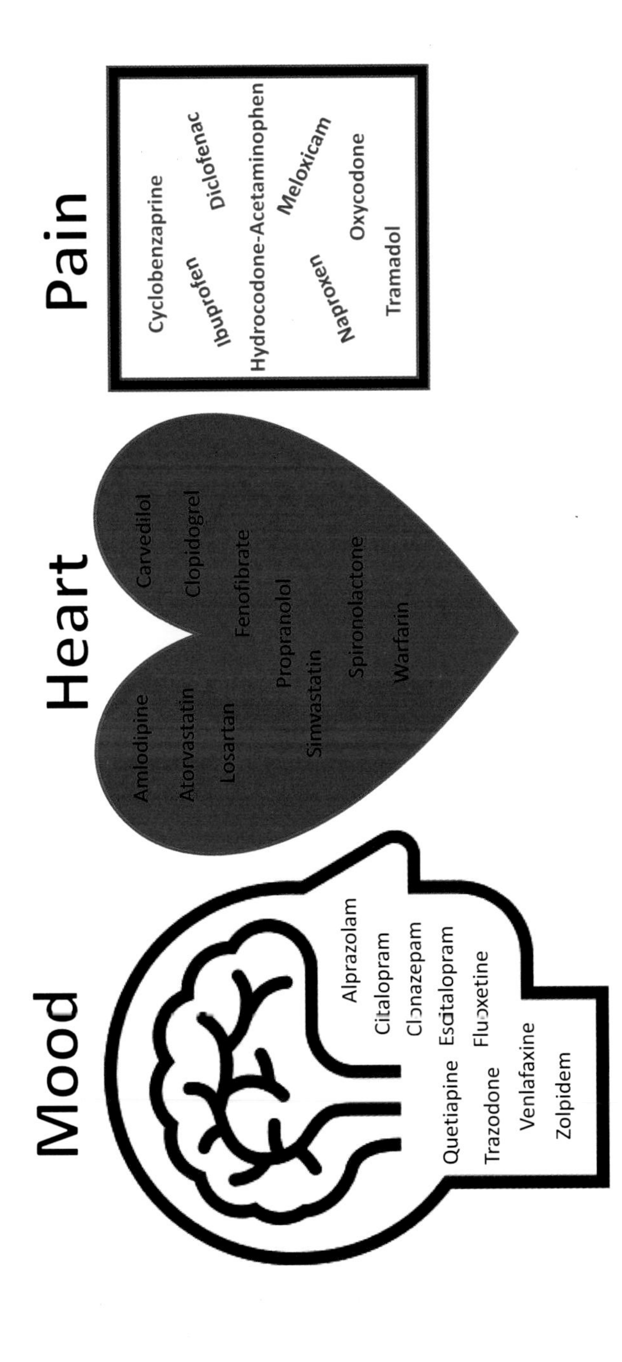

Fig. 3 Commonly prescribed medications that share sites of metabolism with CBD

this will lead to increased exposure to either CBD and/or the other drug(s) sharing the site of metabolism. More drug exposure = more side effects/poor health outcomes. Simvastatin, rated as #10 out of the top 200 drugs currently prescribed in the United States, not only has CYP metabolism predominately through CYP3A4, but also possesses minor CYP2D6 activity. Since CBD has CYP3A4 and minor CYP2D6 inhibition, it is reasonable to consider this may lead to a clinically significant drug interaction. Signs and symptoms of a clinically significant drug interaction between CBD and simvastatin would be myopathy (muscle pain, muscle cramps), with an increased risk for rhabdomyolysis as well (Williams and Feely 2002). Most likely, the significance of this interaction would result due to CYP3A4 inhibition, but CYP2D6 activity should not be ignored as mutated CYP2D6 alleles have been shown to be responsible for certain individuals having an intolerance to simvastatin. Thus, although minor inhibition of CYP2D6 seems irrelevant, it is not in the setting in patients with alleles that result in them being “CYP2D6 poor metabolizers” (Mulder et al. 2001).

CBD Pharmacogenomics

Clinically significant drug-gene interactions have been established for several medications; however, CBD is not one of them. Many genes have been suggested to interact with CBD as well as other cannabinoids (Hryhorowicz et al. 2018). Individuals with **genotypes** that are associated with CYP3A4, 2C19, and 2C9 poor metabolism may see an accumulation or increased exposure to CBD. Increased exposure to CBD puts an individual at higher risk of experiencing the side effects exhibited in CBD clinical trials (See Table 3).

This section provides hypothetical considerations since CBD pharmacogenomics, especially the CBD available over the counter, has not been evaluated in clinical pharmacogenomic studies. This section is created utilizing what is known about CBD (significant to activity at CYP3A4, CYP2C19, and CYP2C9) and how this may impact individuals that have genetic variations at one or more of the genes that code for these enzymes. First and foremost, an individual that exhibits poor metabolism at any of the CYP enzymes that play a role in CBD metabolism is likely to have increased exposure to CBD and thus increased risk for side effects. Additionally, they are more likely to have significant drug interactions with other drugs or supplements metabolized through these pathways, augmenting their risk for side effects (either from increased exposure of CBD or increased exposure to other medications/supplements). Conversely, CBD may also *decrease* the efficacy of drugs if they are prodrugs (See Fig. 2 for prodrug depiction). CYP2C19 functionality has been associated with a profound impact on the prodrug clopidogrel, in which **phenotype** variations can impact clopidogrel safety and efficacy (Plavix 2020). An individual with decreased or increased CYP2C19 expression may present with subtherapeutic or supratherapeutic clopidogrel levels, respectively (Plavix 2020). As previously mentioned, CYP2C19 is one of the primary enzymes involved in the metabolism of CBD. If an individual is taking clopidogrel and CBD, a valid

Table 3 CBD studies for indications outside of seizure-activity

Year published	Disease state studied	CBD dosing	Clinical trial description	*n*
2006	Sublingual cannabinoids on intraocular pressure (Tomida et al. 2006)	5 mg THC 20 mg CBD 40 mg CBD Sublingual	Randomized double-blinded placebo-controlled Intraocular pressure was decreased when given THC ($p = 0.026$) and increased when given 40 mg CBD ($p = 0.028$) No effect with 20 mg CBD	6
2011	Anxiolytic effects of CBD in generalized social anxiety disorder (Crippa et al. 2011)	400 mg CBD	Randomized double-blinded, placebo-controlled trial Treatment-naïve participants with social anxiety disorder Oral CBD associated with decreased subjective anxiety ($p < 0.001$), and reduced ECD uptake in the left parahippocampal gyrus, hippocampus, and inferior temporal gyrus ($p < 0.001$) was exhibited – areas in which are thought to play a role in anxiety Side effects not reported	10
2011	CBD as anxiolytic for simulated public speaking in treatment-naïve social phobia patients (Bergamaschi et al. 2011)	600 mg CBD single dose	Randomized double-blinded, placebo-controlled trial CBD significantly reduced anxiety, cognitive impairment, discomfort in speech performance, and anticipation Side effects not reported	24
2012	Evaluation of CBD, anandamide signaling, and psychotic symptoms in schizophrenia (Leweke et al. 2012)	800 mg/day divided in four doses (titrated up from 200 mg/day)	Double-blinded, randomized, parallel-group, controlled trial (CBD versus amisulpride) Differences were not significant (CI = −12.6,14.6; $p = 0.884$) between CBD and amisulpride CBD group exhibited fewer extrapyramidal symptoms ($p = 0.006$), less weight gain ($p = 0.010$), lower prolactin increase, and indicator of sexual dysfunction ($P < 0.001$) Suggestive that CBD may be a modality where further research is needed to evaluate its role as an antipsychotic	42

(continued)

Table 3 (continued)

Year published	Disease state studied	CBD dosing	Clinical trial description	n
2013	CBD and cigarette consumption in tobacco smokers (Morgan et al. 2013)	CBD metered dose inhaler providing 400 μg CBD dissolved in absolute ethanol ≈ 5%	Randomized double-blinded, placebo-controlled trial Smokers randomized to receive an CBD inhaler ($n = 12$) or placebo ($n = 12$) for 1 week No differences in number of cigarettes smoked were seen in placebo group. CBD group exhibited ~40% decrease in cigarettes smoked No changes in cravings exhibited in either group Side effects not reported	24
2014	CBD in the treatment of patients with Parkinson's disease (Chagas et al. 2014)	75 mg/day or 300 mg/day of CBD	Randomized clinical trial No significant differences in motor and general symptoms scores, nor were neuroprotective effects evident Well-being and quality of life scores for 300 mg CBD PDQ-39, ($p = 0.05$)	23
2015	CBD for the prevention of graft-versus-host-disease after hematopoietic cell transplantation (Yeshurun et al. 2015)	300 mg/day CBD oral	Observational study All patients also on standard therapy: cyclosporine, methotrexate, and filgrastim CBD noncompliance primarily associated with mucositis and nausea Improvement in graft-versus-host disease symptoms seen on day 100, but no difference at 12 months	48
2016	Oral CBD doses and effects of smoked cannabis (Haney et al. 2016)	200, 400, or 800 mg CBD 90 min prior to cannabis administration	Randomized double-blinded, placebo-controlled trial Oral CBD did not alter the effects of THC from smoked cannabis	31
2017	Oral CBD and abuse liability in marijuana smokers (Babalonis et al. 2017)	200, 400, and 800 mg CBD taken in addition to smoking marijuana	Randomized double-blinded, placebo-controlled trial evaluating abuse liability of oral CBD in addition to marijuana CBD did not display abuse risk ($p > 0.5$; no difference from placebo) Marijuana increased abuse rating ($p < 0.05$)	31
2017	Low-dose CBD for Crohn's disease. (Naftali et al. 2017)	10 mg CBD twice daily	Randomized double-blinded, placebo-controlled trial of oral CBD for Crohn's disease No significant difference from placebo	20

2018	CBD as adjunctive therapy in schizophrenia (McGuire et al. 2018)	1000 mg/day (10 ml of 100 mg/mL oral solution in two divided doses)	Double-blind parallel-group trial Psychotic symptoms were reduced compared to placebo (95% CI −2.5,−0.2; $p = 0.019$) Negative symptoms difference did not attain significance No difference in level of functioning Side effects: Gastrointestinal events (18.6%), diarrhea (9.3%), and nausea (7.0%)	90
2018	Effect of CBD on medial temporal, midbrain, and striatal dysfunction in people at high risk of psychosis (Bhattacharyya et al. 2018)	Single oral dose of 600 mg CBD	Randomized, placebo-controlled trial MRI exhibited CBD group had increased activation in the right caudate during encoding and increase activation in the parahippocampal gyrus and midbrain during recall compared to placebo, but lower activation compared to control group 33 clinical high-risk, antipsychotic medication naïve participants; 19 healthy patients as control	52
2018	Pharmacokinetics of highly purified CBD in healthy subjects (Taylor et al. 2018)	Single ascending dose: 1500, 3000, 4500, or 6000 mg CBD Multiple dose: 750 or 1500 mg CBD twice daily Food effect: 1500 mg CBD single dose	Randomized double-blinded, placebo-controlled trial Time to maximum plasma concentration was ~4–5 h High fat meal increased CBD plasma exposure but did not impact half-life and Tmax Side effects: diarrhea, headache	68
2018	The effects of CBD on cognition and symptoms in patients with schizophrenia (Boggs et al. 2018)	600 mg/day (300 mg BID) × 6 weeks	Randomized double-blinded, placebo-controlled trial Placebo-treated subjects improved over time ($P = 0.03$) CBD not associated with improvement Sedation more prevalent in CBD group compared to placebo	36
2018	Abuse potential assessment of CBD in recreational polydrug users (Schoedel et al. 2018)	Single dose of Epidiolex; 750 mg, 1500 mg, or 4500 mg Compared to alprazolam and dronabinol	Randomized double-blinded, placebo-controlled trial "Drug-liking" was significantly different from placebo for higher CBD doses (1500 mg and 4500 mg, $p = 0.04$ and 0.002, respectively) but not for 750 mg dose ($p = 0.51$) Alprazolam and dronabinol had significantly higher Drug-Liking, Overall-Liking, and Take Drug Again VAS Emax values compared with all doses	43

(continued)

Table 3 (continued)

Year published	Disease state studied	CBD dosing	Clinical trial description	n
			of CBD ($P \leq 0.004$) CBD group participants discontinuation due to elevated liver enzymes ($n = 1$), QT-prolongation ($n = 1$), and hypersensitivity ($n = 1$) Most common side effects reported in CBD group: somnolence, diarrhea, and upset stomach	
2018	Chronic pain treatment with CBD in kidney transplant (Cuñetti et al. 2018)	Increased from 50 to 150 mg twice daily for 3 weeks	Observational study Seven patients assessed: Two achieved optimal pain control; four had partial response; and one achieved no change in pain control Side effects reported include the following: nausea, dry mouth, dizziness, and intermittent episodes of heat	7
2018	Endocannabinoid system in healthy volunteers: CBD and fronto-striatal resting-state connectivity (Tomida et al. 2018)	10 mg THC or 600 mg CBD single dose oral capsule	Randomized double-blinded, placebo-controlled trial CBD yielded higher brain connectivity compared to placebo and THC In schizophrenia, altered fronto-striatal connectivity has been designated as an intermediate phenotype Suggestive for possible role regarding antipsychotic effect	16
	CBD on persecutory ideation and anxiety in a high trait paranoid group (Hundal et al. 2018)	600 mg CBD single dose	Randomized double-blinded, placebo-controlled trial CBD scores not statistically significant ($P = 0.15$) CBD exhibited no significant difference in any parameters analyzed in comparison to placebo Side effects reported in CBD group: sedation ($n = 5$), dizziness ($n = 2$), and nausea ($n = 2$)	32
2019	CBD in subjects at high risk for psychosis (Wilson et al. 2019)	600 mg CBD	Randomized double-blinded, placebo-controlled trial Reaction time was significantly slower overall in high-risk CBD group ($p < 0.001$) compared to high-risk placebo group No differences in activation in the hippocampus-midbrain-striatum between any of the groups Total 33 antipsychotic-naïve subjects at high risk for psychosis compared with 19 healthy controls	52

2019	Effects of CBD on brain excitation in adults with and without autism spectrum disorder (Pretzsch et al. 2019)	Single oral dose of 600 mg CBD	Randomized double-blinded, placebo-controlled trial CBD increased glutamate in the basal ganglia; it decreased glutamate in the dorsomedial prefrontal cortex (DMPFC) while also increasing GABA in the DMPFC Decrease in glutamate and increase in GABA support other studies suggestive of sedative qualities associated with CBD	34
2019	Palmitoylethanolamide and CBD and inflammation-induced hyperpermeability of the human gut (Couch et al. 2019)	600 mg CBD or PEA administered with 600 mg of aspirin	Randomized double-blinded, placebo-controlled trial Aspirin-induced inflammation caused an increase in urinary concentration of mannitol and lactulose over the 6-h study period ($P < 0.0001$ and $P < 0.001$, respectively CBD group exhibited decrease in mannitol and lactulose concentrations ($P < 0.0001$) Suggestive CBD may have some preventive effect on inflammation-induced hyperpermeability of the gut, but additional studies warranted as individuals were all healthy and do not exhibit a truly inflamed gut	30
2019	CBD and cravings and anxiety in drug-abstinent individuals with heroin use disorder (Hurd et al. 2019)	400 mg or 800 mg, once daily for 3 consecutive days	Randomized double-blinded, placebo-controlled trial Cravings in placebo group were significantly higher after drug cues in comparison to either CBD group $p = 0.0047$ Anxiety higher in the placebo group compared to either CBD group $p = 0.0079$ Diarrhea most commonly reported side effect in CBD groups	42
2019	Vaporized THC and CBD alone and in combination in frequent and infrequent cannabis users (Solowij et al. 2019)	CBD 400 mg CBD/THC 400 mg/4 mg THC 8 mg	Randomized, controlled trial Examined measures of intoxication following administration of vaporized THC and CBD, alone and in combination, to frequent and infrequent cannabis users At 55 minutes following inhalation administration of CBD, scores were statistically different from placebo Both groups studied reported feeling intoxicated by high-dose CBD administered alone ($p = 0.005$)	36

(continued)

Table 3 (continued)

Year published	Disease state studied	CBD dosing	Clinical trial description	n
2020	Topical CBD for peripheral neuropathy of lower extremities (Xu et al. 2020)	250 mg/3 fl. Oz (topical)	Randomized double-blinded, placebo-controlled trial Topically delivered CBD oil demonstrated significant reduction in the following [in comparison to placebo oil]: intense pain ($p = 0.00901$), sharp pain ($p = 0.00000255$), cold ($p = 0.0434$), and itchy sensations ($p = 0.00108$)	29
2020	Pharmacokinetics of synthetic CBD in healthy volunteers (Izgelov et al. 2020)	90 mg CBD	Single oral administration of CBD in sesame oil and SNEDSS (formulation to increase bioavailability) resulted in significant increased AUC and Cmax values compared to the administration of CBD as powder at the same dose A ~7-fold increase in AUC and ~22-fold increase in Cmax for CBD-SNEDDS compared to powder An ~8-fold increase in AUC and ~17-fold increase in Cmax for CBD-sesame oil compared to powder Formulations impact bioavailability of CBD Side effects reported were as follows: somnolence, abdominal pain, and flatulence	12
2020	Abrupt withdrawal of CBD (Taylor et al. 2020)	Part 1: 750 mg CBD (Epidiolex®) twice daily Part 2: 750 mg CBD (Epidiolex®) daily or placebo	Randomized, double-blinded trial Healthy male and female participants aged 18–45 years No significant signs of withdrawal experienced **Most common adverse events** reported in CBD group: Diarrhea 63.3% Headache 50% Abdominal pain 46.7% Nausea 43.3% Fatigue 33.3% Dizziness 23.3% Somnolence 23.3% **Discontinuation/withdrawal AEs** Skin and subcutaneous tissue disorders 23.3%	45

			Generalized skin rash 20% Drug-induced liver injury 6.7% Eosinophilia* 6.7% Hepatobiliary disorders * one patient experienced both eosinophilia and drug-induced liver injury	
2021	CBD and liver chemistries in healthy adults (Watkins et al. 2021)	Day 1: 200 mg caffeine + CBD-matched placebo Day 3: 250 mg CBD Days 4,5: 250 mg BID Days 6,7: 500 mg morning and 250 mg evening Days 8,9: 500 mg BID Days 10,11: 750 mg q am, 500 mg q pm Days 12–27: 750 mg BID	Open-label, fixed single sequence drug-trial Healthy adults evaluated for CBD safety respective to liver activity Peak serum alanine aminotransferase (ALT) values greater than the upper limit of normal (ULN) were seen in 44% of the participants. The value exceeded 5 × ULN in 31% of the participants. Thus, 31% met the international consensus criteria for drug-induced liver injury All ALT elevations above the ULN began within 2–4 weeks of initial exposure to CBD Most common adverse events reported were diarrhea (50%) and abdominal pain (31%)	16

interaction would exist, regardless of whether the patient was a CYP2C19 poor or normal metabolizer. The validity of concern is that the interaction would be more severe for a patient. A patient that is a CYP2C19 poor metabolizer means that clopidogrel would be even less effective as the effectiveness of clopidogrel to provide its antiplatelet activity is dependent on the conversion (metabolism via CYP2C19) into the active metabolite (See Fig. 2 for prodrug depiction). Clopidogrel is prescribed to reduce the rate of heart attacks and strokes in individuals at risk for these cardiovascular events. Based on CBD and its known inhibition of CYP2C19, this would be detrimental toward the efficacy of clopidogrel. The overarching principle is that CBD is yet to be studied and evaluated in individuals that exhibit poor metabolism at these CYP sites of metabolism. Additional studies are warranted to determine what doses may be safe for individuals with poor metabolism as well as what benefit, if any, it may have for the numerous claims found on OTC CBD labeling in this population.

What Is Cannabidiol and How Does It Work?

CBD is but one of many cannabinoids present in the *Cannabis* plant. It remains difficult to confirm the direct mechanism(s) of CBD as much of what is known clinically is based on highly purified pharmaceutical-grade CBD in the setting of rare seizure disorders, ***and*** in combination with other medications. Additionally, many studies performed that include CBD also contain THC, which dilutes scientific knowledge of what one can expect from CBD, alone. The claims of benefit for CBD are growing, but much of the science is lost in the grandeur of the claims. A prospective cohort study evaluating cannabinoids in the setting of chronic pain and the impact on opioid use provided hopeful results on a strategy to diminish the use of opioids in those suffering from chronic pain (Capano et al. 2020). The authors describe the product as "hemp-derived soft gels." Furthermore, the name of the study is: *Evaluation of the effects of* CBD hemp *extract on opioid use and quality of life indicators in chronic pain patients*. What is important to highlight is that the soft gels contained more than CBD. Each soft gel contained 15.7 mg CBD (a very small dose), 0.5 mg THC (the definition of hemp requires less than 0.3% THC), 0.3 mg **CBDV**, 0.9 mg **CBDA**, and 0.8 mg **CBC**. This product contains active ingredients with numerous pharmacologic targets beyond CBD, alone. Another study with promising results for improvement in ulcerative colitis published their results under the following title: *A randomized, double-blind, placebo-controlled, parallel-group, pilot study of cannabidiol-rich botanical extract in the symptomatic treatment of ulcerative colitis* (Irving et al. 2018). Although the product did contain CBD, it also contained THC, which limits how the results can be extrapolated in regard to CBD. The title is embracing the CBD component, but it fails to give credit where credit is due. The cannabinoid with the most evidence in pain relief remains to be pharmaceutical grade THC or THC-like compounds, although evidence remains conflicting (Stockings et al. 2018).

Fortunately, more studies are now being performed truly evaluating CBD (and CBD-only) outside the setting of epilepsy. Considering the mass availability of CBD to the public, taking a look at these studies is warranted. Table 3 provides a targeted review of studies evaluating CBD for indications other than epilepsy. These studies were selected because they evaluate the response from CBD formulations that do not contain other cannabinoids. Some studies have a comparator group taking a formulation containing THC, but there is a group with CBD only, which provides insight as to what can be gleaned from this compound, alone. Pharmacokinetic studies are included.

The CBD products readily available to the public contain other cannabinoids with variability in the amount of CBD as well as additional cannabinoids (Shea et al. 2020a). CBD may act as a negative allosteric modulator at the cannabinoid 1 receptor (CB1); however, activity is dependent on the concentration of CBD present (Straiker et al. 2018). CBD may lead to suppression of excitation, which is consistent to what has been seen in clinical trials evaluating CBD for augmented treatment in refractory forms of epilepsy; however, anticonvulsive effects have been studied in multiple models of seizure and were not mediated by CB1 receptor activity (Iannotti et al. 2014). This is strongly suggestive that CBD has activity beyond cannabinoid receptors (Iannotti et al. 2014; De Petrocellis et al. 2011).

Studies evaluating CBD in patient populations outside of severe epilepsy are supportive of CBD having a CNS-depressant effect, although the parameters measured are different, from subjective questionnaires to magnetic resonance spectroscopy.

The mechanism of action for CBD must be considered within the context of the following variables:

- **Concentration of CBD**: Higher levels of CBD are more likely to have allosteric modulation at CB1 receptor.
- **Concentration of other cannabinoids**: Other cannabinoids have different mechanisms and receptor activity which may impact the overall effect of CBD.
- **Coadministration with other drugs**: CBD is highly metabolized in the liver by enzymes necessary to metabolize many other medications; as such, this can lead to variability of drug exposure dependent on the coadministered medications and/or supplements and their sites of metabolism.
- **Route of administration**: CBD has poor oral bioavailability, so inhaled administration is going to provide a different effect than oral and topical administration. All different routes will provide a different effect from CBD (+/− other cannabinoids).

Topical CBD

Clinical trials utilizing topical CBD (only) are scarce, but one published study indicated that topical CBD application may provide benefit in the setting of neuropathic pain (Xu et al. 2020). Additional studies are needed to evaluate the safety and efficacy of topical CBD formulations. In a study evaluating OTC CBD products, the majority of topical CBD products contained additional active ingredients (Shea et al. 2020a). Table 4 provides an overview of these additional active ingredients commonly found in topical OTC CBD products (Shea et al. 2020a).

CBD Adverse Effects

Epidiolex® studies have demonstrated side effects from oral CBD to include behavioral changes, sleep disturbances, liver injury (and/or elevated liver enzymes), rashes, and gastrointestinal upset (Epidiolex, 2018). A review performed evaluating adverse effects of CBD from randomized controlled trials supported these findings and reported some of the most common side effects associated with oral CBD to be elevated transaminases (liver enzymes), sedation, and lethargy (Dos Santos et al. 2020). The most common side effects reported in the studies evaluating CBD provided in Table 4 include diarrhea, dizziness, gastrointestinal events, nausea, and sedation (McGuire et al. 2018; Taylor et al. 2018; Boggs et al. 2018; Schoedel et al. 2018; Cuñetti et al. 2018). Taylor et al. provided frequencies of adverse events in their study: diarrhea (63.3%), headache (50%), abdominal pain (46.7%), nausea (43.3%), fatigue (33.3%), dizziness (23.3%), and somnolence (23.3%) (Taylor et al. 2020). Additionally important to note were the side effects that led to the withdrawal from the study. Although not attaining the same prevalence as the most common side effects, they are of concern when considering the massive availability of oral CBD to patients not being monitored or followed. Side effects that resulted in withdrawal from the study included the following: skin and subcutaneous tissue disorders (23.3%), generalized skin rash (20%), drug-induced liver injury (6.7%), eosinophilia (6.7%), and hepatobiliary disorders (6.7%) (Taylor et al. 2020). Drug-induced liver injury is of growing concern with CBD. It was exhibited in Epidiolex® studies, but it has been seen in other CBD clinical trials as well. A study specifically evaluating CBD safety in regard to liver activity exhibited drug-induced liver injury in 31% of their patients (Watkins et al. 2021). Overall, the most common side effects associated with oral CBD include somnolence, dizziness, nausea, abdominal pain, and diarrhea, but elevated liver enzymes might also need to be added to that list.

Factors that increase patient exposure are more likely to result in adverse effects. These factors include the following:

- Genetic polymorphisms resulting in poor metabolism of CBD
- Taking oral CBD with other drugs/supplements metabolized by the same CYP enzymes

It is important to consider that the adverse events or side effects most commonly associated with CBD are from studies evaluating oral formulations, not topical. There are currently no human studies evaluating or reporting side effects of topical CBD.

Table 4 Additional active ingredients commonly found in *topical* CBD products

Active ingredient	Mechanism of action	Comment
Arnica	**Active compound**: sesquiterpene lactone helenalin, 11alpha,13-dihydrohelenalin, and its ester (Lyss et al. 1997) **Mechanism of action**: inhibition of NFkappaB-mediated inflammation (Lyss et al. 1997; Widrig et al. 2007)	**Efficacy**: In a study comparing topical arnica ($n = 100$) to topical ibuprofen ($n = 98$), arnica was found to be noninferior to topical NSAID therapy (Lyss et al. 1997) **Side effects/adverse events**: The following side effects have been reported with the use of arnica: skin irritation/itching, reddening, and allergic eczema (Lyss et al. 1997) **Caution**: In order to determine skin sensitivity/response to topical therapy, a small patch of skin should be tested prior to applying to a larger surface area. This is especially important in patients with a history of having sensitive skin, allergies, or eczema
Camphor bark	**Active compound**: Both stereoisomers (+)-camphor and (−)-camphor activate TRP channels (Xu et al. 2005) **Mechanism of action**: desensitization of TRPV1 and blocking of TRPA1 may provide the analgesic effects of camphor (Xu et al. 2005)	**Efficacy**: One study found pain relief from knee osteoarthritis from a camphor containing cream. The camphor was determined to be the cause of immediate pain relief due to sensory effects of temperature changes at the site (Cohen et al. 2003) **Side effects/adverse events**: Topical application of camphor products is not likely to cause toxicity in adults; however, the ingestion of 3.5 g of camphor can cause death, and 2.0 g has been shown to lead to toxicity; the immediate collapse of an infant has been reported after the *application* of a small dose to the nostrils, so it is paramount that camphor-containing products are not applied to infants (Chen et al. 2013) A study on dermal patches of camphor provided insight on how minimally camphor is absorbed in adults, even at high doses for extended periods of time. From the low systemic absorption and short half-life, the authors concluded that topical camphor is unlikely to accumulate even with twice daily application of 8-h exposures (Martin et al. 2004) **Caution**: Camphor has been shown to cause toxicity when ingested or when applied inside the nostrils. The ingestion or use of camphor containing products in any other way but topically is not recommended. When used topically, camphor is minimally absorbed through the skin even at high doses for extended periods of time; therefore, topical use on intact skin should be safe for adults.
Capsicum	**Active compounds**: Capsaicin (Kozukue et al. 2005) **Mechanism of action**: Activates TRPV1 leading to sensory	**Efficacy**: Low-concentration topical capsaicin has been found to be modestly effective for osteoarthritis. Capsaicin patches have also been found to reduce back pain (Anand and Bley 2011) **Side effects/adverse reactions**: Local, transient, application site reactions, mainly pain and

(continued)

Table 4 (continued)

Active ingredient	Mechanism of action	Comment
	neuronal depolarization. (Anand and Bley 2011) Topical application initially results in feelings of heat and burning; however, repeated applications cause a persistent local effect on cutaneous nociceptors decreasing the sensation of heat and burning but maintaining pain relief at the site of application (Anand and Bley 2011)	erythema, are most commonly seen with topical application (Anand and Bley 2011) At high concentrations, more adverse events have been reported, such as more pain, pruritus, swelling, and transient variable elevations in blood pressure (Barkin 2013) **Caution**: Burning sensation upon initial application should be expected. This sensation should diminish over time, while still providing pain relief. The concentration of capsicum in CBD product is not listed, so precaution should be considered. Reports of burns have been submitted through the FDA adverse event reporting system from the use of OTC products containing active ingredients of menthol, methyl salicylate, or *capsaicin* (U.S. Food and Drug Administration 2016). Due to this, products should be used with caution that contain capsaicin/capsicum and applied to a small area to monitor for adverse events before larger area use
Menthol peppermint	**Active compound**: The majority of analgesic properties are thought to be from the(−)-menthol isomer; however, additional isomers present in this plant may attribute to activity (Pergolizzi Jr et al. 2018) **Mechanism of action**: Topically, it acts on activity-dependent voltage-gated neuron channels causing a localized anesthetic effect (Pergolizzi Jr et al. 2018). It causes a cooling sensation, cutaneous vasodilation (Pergolizzi Jr et al. 2018)	**Efficacy**: Menthol has been found to significantly reduce pain compared to ice ($p = 0.02$) (Pergolizzi Jr et al. 2018) **Side effects/adverse reactions**: Menthol when applied topically is minimally systemically absorbed and has a short half-life. Some adverse effects of localized burning have been reported (Martin et al. 2004; Barkin 2013) **Caution**: Reports of burns have been submitted through the FDA adverse event-reporting system from the use of OTC products containing active ingredients of **menthol**, methyl salicylate, or capsaicin (U.S. Food and Drug Administration 2016; Arif 2015; Grimes 1999). Due to this, products should be used with caution that contain menthol and applied to a small area to monitor for adverse events before a larger surface area is considered
White willow bark	**Active compound**: Topically, it is known that salicylic acid has activity (Shara and Stohs 2015) Other salicylate present in white	**Efficacy**: Current literature is lacking in what topical application of white willow bark may provide. The majority of the literature evaluating white willow bark is oral ingestion or activity respective to salicylic acid. As such, it is difficult to determine the efficacy when the concentration of salicylic acid is not determined in topical white willow bark formulations

	willow bark may or may not have topical activity via this form of administration **Mechanism of action**: Salicylate acid provides anti-inflammatory mechanisms; however, it is only one of the several salicylate compounds present in white willow bark. The mechanisms of each of these entities via topical application is not known.	**Side effects/adverse events**: Side effects associated with topical salicylic acid are dryness, exfoliation, crusting, and burning, and hypopigmentation has occurred in patients with darker skin tones (Arif 2015; Grimes 1999). Side effects increase proportionally to the concentration of salicylic acid applied. **Caution**: Avoid use in patients with salicylate allergies
Tea tree oil (TTO)	**Active compound**: terpinen-4-ol **Mechanism of action**: inhibits cytokine production by human monocytes and reduces production of interleukin-8 by human keratinocyte cells (Hammer 2015)	**Efficacy**: When used topically for acne, it has been shown to reduce inflammatory lesions better than placebo and better than baseline (before treatment with TTO) (Hammer 2015) **Side effects/adverse events**: Minor pruritus, burning, stinging, scaling, itching, redness, and dryness have been reported as adverse events from application of TTO (Hammer 2015) **Caution**: With products that contain TTO, minor pruritus, burning, stinging, scaling, itch, redness, and dryness may occur. These events have been reported after topical application, and systemic effects should not be expected because TTO has shown to have poor topical absorption (Hammer 2015)
Trolamine salicylate	**Active compound**: trolamine salicylate **Mechanism of action**: topical NSAID (nonsteroidal anti-inflammatory) (Mason et al. 2004)	**Efficacy**: Topical trolamine salicylate was found to reduce pain in comparison to placebo in hand osteoarthritis, but other studies indicated no difference between trolamine salicylate and placebo in knee osteoarthritis pain (Rothacker et al. 1998; Algozzine et al. 1982) **Side effects**: When trolamine salicylate is applied topically, salicylic acid is not detected systemically (Morra et al. 1996). Thus, side effects should not be expected **Caution**: Avoid use in patients with salicylate allergies. Data on the product is lacking, use with caution

Applications to Public Health

In this chapter, we have reviewed the extensive variability regarding OTC CBD and how much remains to be determined regarding the safety and efficacy of CBD, especially the CBD readily available OTC or online. In particular, many individuals may also be consuming THC, an illegal entity, under the illusion they are only taking CBD. Clinical trials have suggested efficacy for some conditions, but the variability in product ingredients and quality leaves OTC CBD to be more of a health gamble than a modality for treatment. If it is to become a treatment modality, more studies are needed to evaluate for whom it will provide benefit, *and* the appropriate dosing recommendations to do so. Additional attention is also warranted in regard to other cannabinoids: Do they diminish or augment the desired pharmacological effect? Much pharmacological knowledge remains to be determined.

Key Facts

- CBD available OTC is not regulated.
- Many OTC CBD products also contain other cannabinoids.
- Some OTC CBD products labeled as CBD-only have been found to contain THC.
- Oral CBD has the potential to have many drug-drug or drug-supplement interactions.
- Side effects commonly associated with CBD include diarrhea, headache, abdominal pain, nausea, fatigue, dizziness, and somnolence.
- Serious adverse effects associated with CBD include subcutaneous tissue disorders, generalized skin rash, and drug-induced liver injury.

Mini Dictionary

- **AUC**: area under the curve; total amount of drug exposure.
- **Cannabichromene (CBC)**: cannabinoid present in *Cannabis sativa L*; nonpsychoactive.
- **Cannabidiolic acid (CBDA)**: predominant cannabinoid found in *Cannabis sativa L*; precursor to CBD; and nonpsychoactive.
- **Cannabidivarin (CBDV)**: cannabinoid found in *Cannabis sativa L*; nonpsychoactive.
- **Cannabinoids**: compounds found in *Cannabis*, sometimes referred to as phytocannabinoids. Hundreds of cannabinoids have been isolated, but the most common remain to be THC followed by CBD. Some occur more often in their acid form or may occur in acid form based on the processing of the plant.
- **Controlled clinical trials**: trials to evaluate safety and efficacy with a comparison group which may include a placebo or a different treatment. “Blinded” means either the participants or evaluators (clinicians) are blind to the drug being administered. Double-blinded refers to both parties being unaware of the drug

being administered. Double-blinded controlled clinical trials exhibit the most strength in evidence. How an individual perceives a drug can impact its efficacy and safety. Additionally, how a clinician feels a drug may work can also impact their behavior. Double-blinded results are most likely to indicate a drug's true efficacy and safety results.

- **Dietary supplements**: Any products that are taken by mouth that contain a "dietary ingredient," including vitamins, minerals, amino acids, herbs (or "botanicals"), and substances used to "supplement" the diet. In the United States, supplements are governed by those that make them, meaning it is the responsibility of the manufacturer's responsibility to ensure safety, as pre-marketing safety is not required. Dietary supplements are not required to be proven safe prior to being available on the market.
- **Full spectrum**: CBD extract that contains additional active cannabinoids, often stated to include the other cannabinoids and compounds present in the hemp plant under the claim that this provides additional benefit. The additional benefit is not founded by any scientific evidence.
- **Gamma-aminobutyric acid (GABA)**: main inhibitory neurotransmitter, meaning this neurotransmitter causes the neurons it interacts with less likely to fire an action potential, often leading to sedative effects as seen with alcohol.
- **Genotype**: the genetic instructions of an organism; the instructions inherited from each parent. Example: A patient has genotype that is determined via one allele from each parent.
- **Over-the-counter (OTC) medications**: medications that have been studied in clinical trials and have been reviewed and approved for OTC status by the Division of Nonprescription Drug Products in the Office of Drug Evaluation.
- **Phenotype**: the traits exhibited by an organism which are influenced by the genotype, but also environmental influences will determine the expression of the genes which may alter characteristics and traits exhibited.
- **Δ^9-Tetrahydrocannabinol (THC)**: prevalent compound found in *Cannabis sativa L*; psychoactive.

Key Summary Points

- CBD available OTC is not a regulated product, so product variability should be expected.
- Many CBD products available contain other cannabinoids that may alter the response a patient has from CBD.
- The majority of topical CBD products contain additional active compounds.
- Some CBD products labeled as CBD-only have been found to contain THC.
- OTC CBD has not been studied in clinical trials to ensure safety or efficacy. Product formulations and the amount of CBD within differ greatly from the products studied in clinical trials.
- Oral CBD has a high potential to have many drug-drug or drug-supplement interactions.

- CBD metabolism may be impacted by genetic variations in how individuals metabolize drugs.
- OTC CBD labeling does not inform consumers of side effects that have occurred in clinical trials. Side effects commonly associated with CBD include diarrhea, headache, abdominal pain, nausea, fatigue, dizziness, and somnolence.
- Serious adverse effects associated with CBD include subcutaneous tissue disorders, generalized skin rash, and drug-induced liver injury.

References

Abernethy A (2019) Hemp production & 2018 farm bill. https://www.fda.gov/news-events/congressional-testimony/hemp-production-and-2018-farm-bill-07252019. Accessed 22 July 2021

Algozzine GJ, Stein GH, Doering PL et al (1982) Trolamine salicylate cream in osteoarthritis of the knee. JAMA 247(9):1311–1313

Anand P, Bley K (2011) Topical capsaicin for pain management: therapeutic potential and mechanisms of action of the new high-concentration capsaicin 8% patch. Br J Anaesth 107(4):490–502

Arif T (2015) Salicylic acid as a peeling agent: a comprehensive review. Clin Cosmet Investig Dermatol 8:455–461

Asadi-Pooya AA (2018) Lennox-Gastaut syndrome: a comprehensive review. Neurol Sci 39(3):403–414

Babalonis S, Haney M, Malcolm RJ, Lofwall MR et al (2017) Oral cannabidiol does not produce a signal for abuse liability in frequent marijuana smokers. Drug Alcohol Depend 172:9–13

Barkin RL (2013) The pharmacology of topical analgesics. Postgrad Med 125(4 Suppl 1):7–18

Bergamaschi MM, Queiroz RH, Chagas MH, de Oliveira DC et al (2011) Cannabidiol reduces the anxiety induced by simulated public speaking in treatment-naïve social phobia patients. Neuropsychopharmacology 36(6):1219–1226

Bhattacharyya S, Wilson R, Appiah-Kusi E, O'Neill A et al (2018) Effect of cannabidiol on medial temporal, midbrain, and striatal dysfunction in people at clinical high risk of psychosis: a randomized clinical trial. JAMA Psychiat 75(11):1107–1117

Boggs DL, Surti T, Gupta A, Gupta S et al (2018) The effects of cannabidiol (CBD) on cognition and symptoms in outpatients with chronic schizophrenia a randomized placebo controlled trial. Psychopharmacology 235(7):1923–1932

Bonn-Miller MO, Loflin MJE, Thomas BF et al (2017) Labeling accuracy of cannabidiol extracts sold online. JAMA 318(17):1708–1709

Camfield PR (2011) Definition and natural history of Lennox-Gastaut syndrome. Epilepsia 52 (Suppl 5):3–9

Capano A, Weaver R, Burkman E (2020) Evaluation of the effects of CBD hemp extract on opioid use and quality of life indicators in chronic pain patients: a prospective cohort study. Postgrad Med 132(1):56–61

Chagas MH, Zuardi AW, Tumas V, Pena-Pereira MA et al (2014) Effects of cannabidiol in the treatment of patients with Parkinson's disease: an exploratory double-blind trial. J Psychopharmacol 28(11):1088–1098

Chen W, Vermaak I, Viljoen A (2013) Camphor – a fumigant during the Black Death and a coveted fragrant wood in ancient Egypt and Babylon – a review. Molecules 18(5):5434–5454

Cohen M, Wolfe R, Mai T et al (2003) A randomized, double blind, placebo controlled trial of a topical cream containing glucosamine sulfate, chondroitin sulfate, and camphor for osteoarthritis of the knee [published correction appears in J Rheumatol. 2003 Nov;30(11):2512]. J Rheumatol 30(3):523–528

Cohen PA, Travis JC, Vanhee C, Deuster P et al (2021) Nine prohibited stimulants found in sports and weight loss supplements: deterenol, phenpromethamine (Vonedrine), oxilofrine, octodrine, beta-methylphenylethylamine (BMPEA), 1,3-dimethylamylamine (1,3-DMAA),

1,4-dimethylamylamine (1,4-DMAA), 1,3-dimethylbutylamine (1,3-DMBA) and higenamine. Clin Toxicol (Phila) 23:1–7

Couch DG, Cook H, Ortori C, Barrett D et al (2019) Palmitoylethanolamide and cannabidiol prevent inflammation-induced hyperpermeability of the human gut in vitro and in vivo-a randomized, placebo-controlled, double-blind controlled trial. Inflamm Bowel Dis 25(6): 1006–1018

Crippa JA, Derenusson GN, Ferrari TB, Wichert-Ana L et al (2011) Neural basis of anxiolytic effects of cannabidiol (CBD) in generalized social anxiety disorder: a preliminary report. J Psychopharmacol 25(1):121–130

Cuñetti L, Manzo L, Peyraube R, Arnaiz J et al (2018) Chronic pain treatment with cannabidiol in kidney transplant patients in Uruguay. Transplant Proc 50(2):461–464

De Petrocellis L, Ligresti A, Moriello AS et al (2011) Effects of cannabinoids and cannabinoid-enriched Cannabis extracts on TRP channels and endocannabinoid metabolic enzymes. Br J Pharmacol 163(7):1479–1494

Doohan PT, Oldfield LD, Arnold JC, Anderson LL (2021) Cannabinoid interactions with cytochrome P450 drug metabolism: a full-spectrum characterization. AAPS J 23(4):91

Dos Santos RG, Guimarães FS, Crippa JAS, Hallak JEC et al (2020) Serious adverse effects of cannabidiol (CBD): a review of randomized controlled trials. Expert Opin Drug Metab Toxicol 16(6):517–526

Eichner S, Maguire M, Shea LA, Fete MG (2016) Banned and discouraged-use ingredients found in weight loss supplements. J Am Pharm Assoc 56(5):538–543

Epidiolex®(cannabidiol) package insert (2018). https://www.accessdata.fda.gov/drugsatfda_docs/label/2018/210365lbl.pdf. Accessed 27 July 2021

Geffrey AL, Pollack SF, Bruno PL, Thiele EA (2015) Drug-drug interaction between clobazam and cannabidiol in children with refractory epilepsy. Epilepsia 56(8):1246–1251

Grimes PE (1999) The safety and efficacy of salicylic acid chemical peels in darker racial-ethnic groups. Dermatol Surg 25(1):18–22

Hammer KA (2015) Treatment of acne with tea tree oil (melaleuca) products: a review of efficacy, tolerability and potential modes of action. Int J Antimicrob Agents 45(2):106–110

Haney M, Malcolm RJ, Babalonis S, Nuzzo PA et al (2016) Oral cannabidiol does not alter the subjective, reinforcing or cardiovascular effects of smoked cannabis. Neuropsychopharmacology 41(8):1974–1982

Hayden KM, Welsh-Bohmer KA, Wengreen HJ, Zandi PP et al (2007) Risk of mortality with vitamin E supplements: the Cache County study. Am J Med 120(2):180–184

Hazekamp A (2018) The trouble with CBD oil. Med Cannabis Cannabinoids 1:65–72

Hryhorowicz S, Walczak M, Zakerska-Banaszak O, Słomski R, Skrzypczak-Zielińska M (2018) Pharmacogenetics of Cannabinoids. Eur J Drug Metab Pharmacokinet 43(1):1–12. https://doi.org/10.1007/s13318-017-0416-z

Hundal H, Lister R, Evans N, Antley A et al (2018) The effects of cannabidiol on persecutory ideation and anxiety in a high trait paranoid group. J Psychopharmacol 32(3):276–282

Hurd YL, Spriggs S, Alishayev J, Winkel G et al (2019) Cannabidiol for the reduction of cue-induced craving and anxiety in drug-abstinent individuals with heroin use disorder: a double-blind randomized placebo-controlled trial. Am J Psychiatry 176(11):911–922

Iannotti FA, Hill CL, Leo A et al (2014) Nonpsychotropic plant cannabinoids, cannabidivarin (CBDV) and cannabidiol (CBD), activate and desensitize transient receptor potential vanilloid 1 (TRPV1) channels in vitro: potential for the treatment of neuronal hyperexcitability. ACS Chem Neurosci 5(11):1131–1141

Irving PM, Iqbal T, Nwokolo C, Subramanian S et al (2018) A randomized, double-blind, placebo-controlled, parallel-group, pilot study of cannabidiol-rich botanical extract in the symptomatic treatment of ulcerative colitis. Inflamm Bowel Dis 24(4):714–724

Izgelov D, Davidson E, Barasch D, Regev A et al (2020) Pharmacokinetic investigation of synthetic cannabidiol oral formulations in healthy volunteers. Eur J Pharm Biopharm 154:108–115. https://doi.org/10.1016/j.ejpb.2020.06.021

Jiang R, Yamaori S, Okamoto Y et al (2013) Cannabidiol is a potent inhibitor of the catalytic activity of cytochrome P450 2C19. Drug Metab Pharmacokinet 28(4):332–338

Kozukue N, Han JS, Kozukue E et al (2005) Analysis of eight capsaicinoids in peppers and pepper-containing foods by high-performance liquid chromatography and liquid chromatography-mass spectrometry. J Agric Food Chem 53(23):9172–9181

Leweke FM, Piomelli D, Pahlisch F, Muhl D et al (2012) Cannabidiol enhances anandamide signaling andalleviates psychotic symptoms of schizophrenia. Transl Psychiatry 2(3):e94

Lonn E, Bosch J, Yusuf S, Sheridan P et al (2005) Effects of long-term vitamin E supplementation on cardiovascular events and cancer: a randomized controlled trial. JAMA 293(11):1338–1347

Lyss G, Schmidt TJ, Merfort I et al (1997) Helenalin, an anti-inflammatory sesquiterpene lactone from arnica, selectively inhibits transcription factor NF-kappaB. Biol Chem 378(9):951–961

Martin D, Valdez J, Boren J et al (2004) Dermal absorption of camphor, menthol, and methyl salicylate in humans. J Clin Pharmacol 44(10):1151–1157

Mason L, Moore RA, Edwards JE et al (2004) Systematic review of efficacy of topical rubefacients containing salicylates for the treatment of acute and chronic pain. BMJ 328(7446):995

McGuire P, Robson P, Cubala WJ, Vasile D, Morrison PD, Barron R, Taylor A, Wright S (2018) Cannabidiol (CBD) as an adjunctive therapy in schizophrenia: a multicenter randomized controlled trial. Am J Psychiatry 175(3):225–231

Medical Expenditure Panel Survey (MEPS) (2007–2017) (2018) Agency for Healthcare Research and Quality (AHRQ), Rockville, MD. ClinCalc DrugStats Database version 20.0. https://clincalc.com/DrugStats/Top200Drugs.aspx. Accessed 17 July 2020

Morgan CJ, Das RK, Joye A, Curran HV et al (2013) Cannabidiol reduces cigarette consumption in tobacco smokers: preliminary findings. Addict Behav 38(9):2433–2436

Morra P, Bartle WR, Walker SE et al (1996) Serum concentrations of salicylic acid following topically applied salicylate derivatives. Ann Pharmacother 30(9):935–940

Motrin®Ibuprofen package insert (2007). https://www.accessdata.fda.gov/drugsatfda_docs/label/2007/017463s105lbl.pdf

Mulder AB, van Lijf HJ, Bon MA et al (2001) Association of polymorphism in the cytochrome CYP2D6 and the efficacy and tolerability of simvastatin. Clin Pharmacol Ther 70(6):546–551

Naftali T, Mechulam R, Marii A, Gabay G et al (2017) Low-dose cannabidiol is safe but not effective in the treatment for Crohn's disease, a randomized controlled trial. Dig Dis Sci 62(6):1615–1620

Pavlovic R, Nenna G, Calvi L et al (2018) Quality traits of "cannabidiol oils": cannabinoids content, terpene fingerprint and oxidation stability of European commercially available preparations. Molecules 23(5):1230

Pergolizzi JV Jr, Taylor R Jr, LeQuang JA et al (2018) The role and mechanism of action of menthol in topical analgesic products. J Clin Pharm Ther 43(3):313–319

Plavix (clopidogrel) [prescribing information] (2020) Bridgewater, NJ: Bristol-Myers Squibb/Sanofi Pharmaceuticals Partnership

Pretzsch CM, Freyberg J, Voinescu B, Lythgoe D et al (2019) Effects of cannabidiol on brain excitation and inhibition systems; a randomised placebo controlled single dose trial during magnetic resonance spectroscopy in adults with and without autism spectrum disorder. Neuropsychopharmacology 44(8):1398–1405

Prilosec®omeprazole package insert (2018). https://www.prilosecpackets.com/_resources/Prilosec-PI-2018.pdf. Accessed 1 Sept 2021

Rong C, Carmona NE, Lee YL et al (2018) Drug-drug interactions as a result of co-administering THC and CBD with other psychotropic agents. Expert Opin Drug Saf 17(1):51–54

Rothacker DQ, Lee I, Littlejohn TW 3rd (1998) Effectiveness of a single topical application of 10% trolamine salicylate cream in the symptomatic treatment of osteoarthritis. J Clin Rheumatol 4(1):6–12

Schoedel KA, Szeto I, Setnik B, Sellers EM et al (2018) Abuse potential assessment of cannabidiol (CBD) in recreational polydrug users: a randomized, double-blind, controlled trial. Epilepsy Behav 88:162–171

Shara M, Stohs SJ (2015) Efficacy and safety of white willow bark (Salix alba) extracts. Phytother Res 29:1112–1116

Shea LA, Leeds M, Bui D, Mujica M et al (2020a) "Over-the-counter" cannabidiol (CBD) sold in the community pharmacy setting in Colorado. Drugs Therapy Perspect 36:573–582

Shea LA, Goldwire MA, Hymel D, Bui D (2020b) Colorado community pharmacists' survey and their perspectives regarding marijuana. SAGE Open Med 8:2050312120938215. https://doi.org/10.1177/2050312120938215. PMID: 32821385; PMCID: PMC7412924

Solowij N, Broyd S, Greenwood LM, van Hell H et al (2019) A randomised controlled trial of vaporised Δ9-tetrahydrocannabinol and cannabidiol alone and in combination in frequent and infrequent cannabis users: acute intoxication effects. Eur Arch Psychiatry Clin Neurosci 269(1): 17–35

Stockings E, Campbell G, Hall W, Nielsen S et al (2018) Cannabis and cannabinoids for the treatment of people with chronic noncancer pain conditions: a systematic review and meta-analysis of controlled and observational studies. Pain 159(10):1932–1954

Straiker A, Dvorakova M, Zimmowitch A, Mackie K (2018) Cannabidiol inhibits endocannabinoid signaling in autaptic hippocampal neurons. Mol Pharmacol 94(1):743–748

Taylor L, Gidal B, Blakey G, Tayo B et al (2018) A phase I, randomized, double-blind, placebo-controlled, single ascending dose, multiple dose, and food effect trial of the safety, tolerability and pharmacokinetics of highly purified cannabidiol in healthy subjects. CNS Drugs 32(11): 1053–1067

Taylor L, Crockett J, Tayo B, Checketts D et al (2020) Abrupt withdrawal of cannabidiol (CBD): a randomized trial. Epilepsy Behav 104(Pt A):106938

Tomida I, Azuara-Blanco A, House H, Flint M et al (2006) Effect of sublingual application of cannabinoids on intraocular pressure: a pilot study. J Glaucoma 15(5):349–353

Tomida O, Löffler M, Kamping S, Hartmann A et al (2018) Probing the endocannabinoid system in healthy volunteers: Cannabidiol alters fronto-striatal resting-state connectivity. Eur Neuropsychopharmacol 28(7):841–849

U.S. Food and Drug Administration (2016) FDA Drug Safety Communication: rare cases of serious burns with the use of over-the-counter topical muscle and joint pain relievers. http://www.fda.gov/Drugs/DrugSafety/ucm318858.htm. Accessed 6 Apr 2017

U.S. Food and Drug Administration (FDA) (2018) Drug trials snapshots: epidiolex. https://www.fda.gov/drugs/drug-approvals-and-databases/drug-trials-snapshots-epidiolex. Accessed 8 July 2021

U.S. Food and Drug Administration (FDA) (2019) Dietary supplements. https://www.fda.gov/food/dietary-supplements. Accessed 8 July 2021

U.S. Food and Drug Administration (FDA) (2020) Over-the-Counter (OTC) nonprescription drugs. https://www.fda.gov/drugs/how-drugs-are-developed-and-approved/over-counter-otc-nonprescription-drugs. Accessed 8 July 2021

Ujváry I, Hanuš L (2016) Human metabolites of cannabidiol: a review on their formation, biological activity, and relevance in therapy. Cannabis Cannabinoid Res 1(1):90–101

Wallace A, Wirrell E, Kenney-Jung DL (2016) Pharmacotherapy for Dravet syndrome. Paediatr Drugs 18(3):197–208

Watkins PB, Church RJ, Li J, Knappertz V (2021) Cannabidiol and abnormal liver chemistries in healthy adults: results of a phase I clinical trial. Clin Pharmacol Ther 109(5):1224–1231

Widrig R, Suter A, Saller R et al (2007) Choosing between NSAID and arnica for topical treatment of hand osteoarthritis in a randomised, double-blind study. Rheumatol Int 27:585–591

Williams D, Feely J (2002) Pharmacokinetic-pharmacodynamic drug interactions with HMG-CoA reductase inhibitors. Clin Pharmacokinet 41(5):343–370

Wilson R, Bossong MG, Appiah-Kusi E, Petros N et al (2019) Cannabidiol attenuates insular dysfunction during motivational salience processing in subjects at clinical high risk for psychosis. Transl Psychiatry 9(1):203

Xu H, Blair NT, Clapham DE (2005) Camphor activates and strongly desensitizes the transient receptor potential vanilloid subtype 1 channel in a vanilloid-independent mechanism. J Neurosci 25(39):8924–8937

Xu DH, Cullen BD, Tang M, Fang Y (2020) The effectiveness of topical cannabidiol oil in symptomatic relief of peripheral neuropathy of the lower extremities. Curr Pharm Biotechnol 21(5):390–402

Yamaori S, Ebisawa J, Okushima Y et al (2011a) Potent inhibition of human cytochrome P450 3A isoforms by cannabidiol: role of phenolic hydroxyl groups in the resorcinol moiety. Life Sci 88: 730–736

Yamaori S, Okamoto Y, Yamamoto I et al (2011b) Cannabidiol, a major phytocannabinoid, as a potent atypical inhibitor for CYP2D6. Drug Metab Dispos 39(11):2049–2056

Yeshurun M, Shpilberg O, Herscovici C, Shargian L et al (2015) Cannabidiol for the prevention of graft-versus-host-disease after allogeneic hematopoietic cell transplantation: results of a phase II study. Biol Blood Marrow Transplant 21(10):1770–1775

Linking Cannabis and Homicide: Comparison with Alcohol

70

Oybek Nazarov and Guohua Li

Contents

Introduction 1520
Drugs and Violence 1521
Cannabis and Homicide 1522
Pharmacological Disinhibition 1523
Economic Compulsiveness 1523
Risky Situation 1524
Homicide and Suicide Comparison 1524
Alcohol and Homicide 1525
Alcohol Consumption Pattern 1525
Concurrent Use of Cannabis and Alcohol and Homicide 1526
Interaction Between Cannabis and Alcohol 1526
Summary and Suggestions 1527
Applications to Other Substance Use Disorders 1528
Other Drugs and Violence 1528
Applications to Other Areas of Public Health 1529
Implications Beyond Violence 1529
Mini-Dictionary 1529
Key Facts 1529
Summary Points 1530
References 1530

O. Nazarov
The University of Queensland, School of Medicine, Mayne Medical Reception, Herston, QLD, Australia
e-mail: o.nazarov@uqconnect.edu.au

G. Li (✉)
Department of Anesthesiology, Vagelos College of Physicians and Surgeons, Columbia University, New York, NY, USA
e-mail: gl2240@cumc.columbia.edu

V. B. Patel, V. R. Preedy (eds.), *Handbook of Substance Misuse and Addictions*,
https://doi.org/10.1007/978-3-030-92392-1_77

Abstract

The use of cannabis, alcohol, and other drugs is a major risk factor for assaultive injuries and violent deaths. Cannabis is one of the most frequently detected drugs among homicide victims as well as perpetrators. It is evident that as more countries move toward legalizing cannabis, this drug is playing an increasingly important role in homicide victimization and perpetration.

Keywords

Alcohol · Cannabis · Drugs · Homicide · Injury · Violence

Abbreviations

CDC	Centers for Disease Control and Prevention
NVDRS	National Violent Death Reporting System
OR	Odds ratio
Δ-9-THC	Delta-9-tetrahydrocannabinol
BAC	Blood alcohol concentration

Introduction

Homicide is the third leading cause of death among young people aged 15 to 34 in the United States, according to the Centers for Disease Control and Prevention (CDC) (CDC 2018). The US homicide rate is over seven times the rate in other industrialized countries (Grinshteyn and Hemenway 2016). Research indicates a significant link between the use of alcohol and cannabis and homicide (Darke et al. 2009; Nazarov and Li 2020). In a recent study, Nazarov and Li (2020) analyzed toxicological data from the 2004–2016 National Violent Death Reporting System (NVDRS) and found that 37.5% of homicide victims tested positive for alcohol, 31.0% for cannabis, and 11.4% for both (Fig. 1). They also noted that the prevalence of cannabis detected in homicide victims increased from 22.3% to 42.1% over this time period in both sexes and across all age and racial groups (Fig. 2), whereas alcohol involvement showed a slight decrease. Given the high prevalence of cannabis and alcohol detected in homicide victims, it is important to understand the causal role of these substances in homicide incidents. With more states legalizing cannabis for medical and recreational use, assessing and mitigating the risk of injury associated with cannabis has become a thorny public policy issue.

In this chapter, we review epidemiologic studies examining the role of cannabis and alcohol use in violence perpetration and victimization, identify research gaps, and outline future directions.

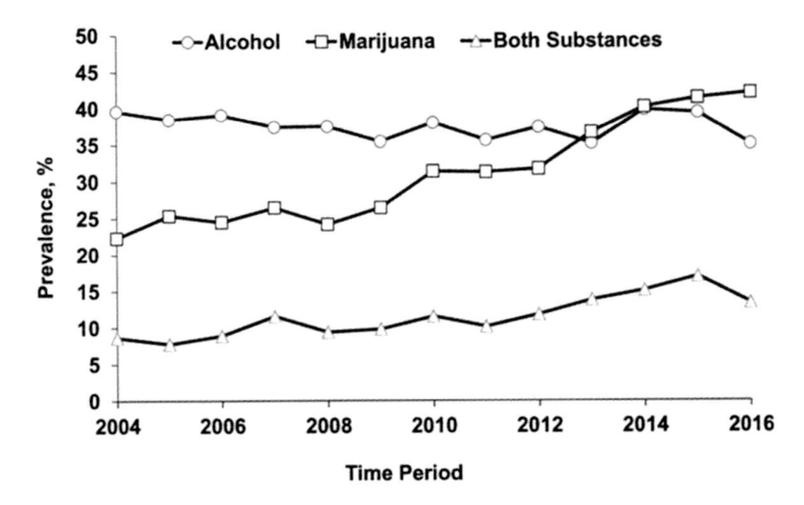

Fig. 1 Prevalence of alcohol, cannabis, and both substances in the United States between 2004 and 2016. Adapted from (Nazarov and Li 2020)

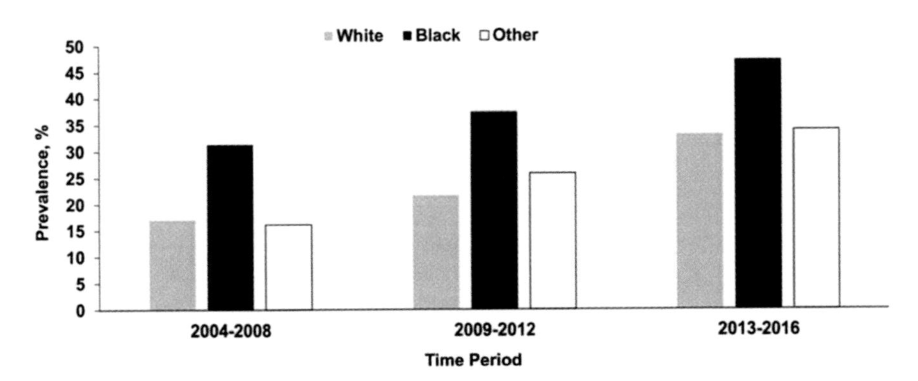

Fig. 2 Cannabis consumption in the United States over time among different groups of the population. Adapted from (Nazarov and Li 2020)

Drugs and Violence

The World Health Organization (WHO) classified drug use as "harmful drug use" and "drug dependence" (WHO 2018). Using drugs for nonmedical purposes appears to be increasing in many parts of the world. Its criminality makes it difficult to quantify drug users precisely; reported data are often scarce and unrepresentative (Darke et al. 2012).

Substance abuse is a major public health issue, and people with substance use disorder already have significantly higher mortality rates than their peers

(Wilcox et al. 2004). For example, alcohol use disorder is linked to a twofold increase in all-cause mortality (Darke et al. 2009). The major causes of death associated with substance use disorder are usually a disease or a medical condition (e.g., human immunodeficiency virus (HIV), hepatic cirrhosis, and overdose). However, a significant proportion of substance user deaths are the result of violence, either perpetrated by others against the person (homicide) or self-inflicted (suicide) (Darke et al. 2012). The causes of such high rates of violent death vary. Homicide rates may also be higher due to the proximal effects of the drug in question (e.g., disinhibition from alcohol intoxication, paranoia from psychostimulant use), which can lead to violent situations. Illicit drug use raises the distal risk of violence because high levels of crime are committed to support such use or to protect drug dealing networks (European Monitoring Centre for Drugs and Drug Addiction 2018; WHO 2018).

Cannabis and Homicide

Cannabis is one of the most frequently detected drugs among homicide victims as well as perpetrators. Goldstein (1985) developed the tripartite conceptual framework for understanding the relationships between the drug-homicide nexus. This framework applies to both perpetrators and victims of violence and to cannabis, alcohol, and other drugs. Under this framework, cannabis and alcohol are causally linked to violence (in particular homicide) through three pathways (Fig. 3) (Goldstein 1985).

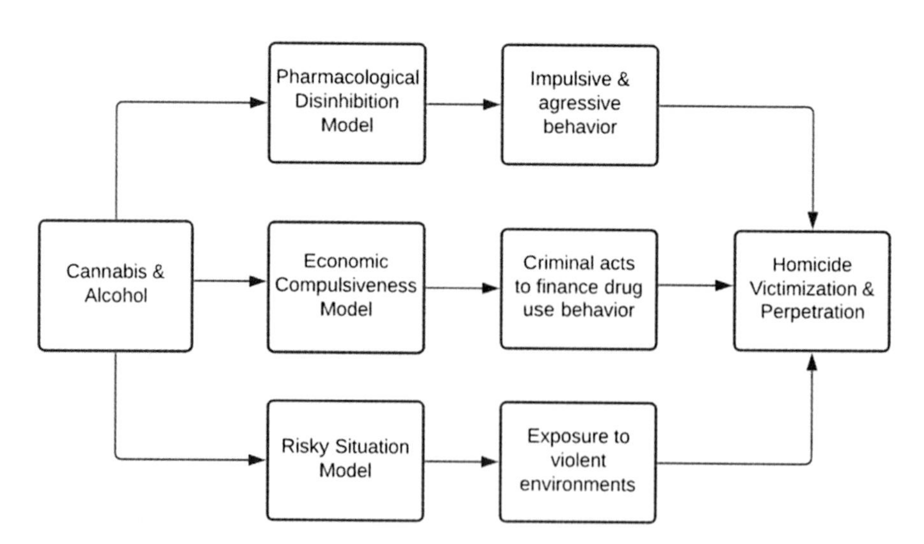

Fig. 3 The tripartite conceptual framework depicting the connection of cannabis and alcohol on homicide

Pharmacological Disinhibition

First, the psychopharmacological effects of cannabis and alcohol, including acute and chronic effects as well as withdrawal symptoms, may increase the user's propensity of excitability, irrationality, impulsiveness, and aggressiveness. The psychopharmacological effects of alcohol and other drugs have been studied extensively. For instance, the pharmacological disinhibition model posits that alcohol impacts the prefrontal cortex area of the brain responsible for impulse control, judgment, and interpretation of social cues, resulting in impulsive or aggressive behaviors (Exum 2006). Similarly, it is evident that cannabis use impairs cognitive functions, inhibits impulse control, and increases aggressive behaviors (Yanowitch and Coccaro 2011). Reingle et al. (2012) analyzed data for 9,421 adolescents participating in the National Longitudinal Study of Adolescent Health and found that cannabis use during adolescence is associated with a twofold increased risk of perpetration of and victimization by intimate partner violence in early adulthood. Moreover, withdrawal from chronic cannabis use may instigate irritability and heighten the risk of conflict and aggression (Bonnet and Preuss 2017). Among chronic cannabis users, the major pathway linking cannabis to violence appears to be through increased paranoia and other psychotic episodes, wherein the delusional perpetrators believed they were in danger from the victims (Darke et al. 2012).

A review article by Miller et al. (2020) suggested that chronic consumption of cannabis increases violence rates. They examined 14 incidents of violence among chronic cannabis users and found that the main causes of the homicide cases were paranoia, psychosis, aggressiveness, personality change, and hallucinations (Miller et al. 2020). It is also evident that in chronic cannabis users, panic attacks, confusion, hallucinations, suspiciousness, and paranoia are common, influencing users' cognition in ways that enhance violent responses to perceived provocations (Meier et al. 2012).

Some cannabis compounds act on central endocannabinoid receptors, which regulate many behavioral functions, including aggression. While cannabis consumption can induce mild euphoria and relaxation in some users, adverse acute psychopharmacological effects are prevalent. Meier et al. (2012) reported that even a single dose of cannabis could trigger impairments in behavioral regulation underpinning the control of impulsivity and aggression by modifying the normal functioning of its underlying natural substrate, the ventrolateral prefrontal cortex.

Economic Compulsiveness

Second, economic compulsiveness may pose cannabis and other drug users to a heightened risk of committing economically oriented crimes, such as robbery, to finance their compulsive substance use behaviors. The economic compulsiveness pathway is not primarily driven by impulsiveness but by the motivation to obtain money to pay for drugs, and the related violence usually results from situational and contextual factors when the economic crime is perpetrated, such as the offender's nervousness, firearm use, the victim's reaction, and the intervention of a third party.

Risky Situation

Finally, the systemic mechanism refers to violence resulting from the inherently aggressive nature of the illicit drug distribution system, such as territorial disputes between rival dealers and retaliatory killings. Numerous studies have examined the relationship between cannabis use and homicide; many of them have relied on toxicological testing data for victims and perpetrators (Darke and Duflou 2008; Darke et al. 2009, 2012; Darke 2010; Auckloo and Davies 2019; Nazarov and Li 2020). These studies indicate that about 6–42% of homicide victims and 5–11% of perpetrators had consumed cannabis and that cannabis was much more frequently detected in homicide victims than in suicide victims (Darke et al. 2009; Kuhns and Maguire 2012; Sheehan et al. 2013). This tripartite conceptual framework can be further extended to other psychoactive drugs in order to coherently classify the interrelationship between other drugs and violence.

Homicide and Suicide Comparison

The association of cannabis consumption with homicide and suicide was studied in a cross-sectional study conducted in Australia (Darke et al. 2009). Psychoactive substances were found in more than half of the cases through autopsy. Cannabis was more frequently detected in homicide victims than in suicides (odds ratio (OR) 2.39). Furthermore, homicide victims were significantly more likely to test positive for delta-9-tetrahydrocannabinol (Δ-9-THC) in blood samples, implying that the victims might be under the influence of cannabis at the time of death.

Darke et al. (2009) also estimated the ORs for different substances among homicide victims compared to suicide deaths. Cannabis was detected in 22.1% of the homicide victims, more than twice as likely as in suicides. Compared with the prevalence of daily use of cannabis in the Australian general population (about 2%), cannabis use was associated with an 11-fold increase in homicide victimization. Similarly, Nazarov and Li (2020) found that cannabis was detected in homicide victims about three times as common as expected based on the prevalence of cannabis use in the US general population. Furthermore, the prevalence of cannabis found in homicide victims varied by age and ethnicity and was exceptionally high in adolescent and black victims (Nazarov and Li 2020). Similar findings were reported by Sheehan et al. (2013). Cannabis was more likely to be involved in homicides, whereas antidepressants and opiates were more likely to be involved in suicides. There existed marked differences in drug use patterns between sexes: drugs associated with homicide were more prevalent in males, whereas drugs associated with suicide were more prevalent in females. Considering these differences in drug use patterns is necessary for developing tailored interventions to reduce substance abuse and violence.

Alcohol and Homicide

Experimental studies have found a dose-response relationship between blood alcohol concentration (BAC) and aggression, with the effects becoming significant at the level of 0.05 g/dL and rising with higher BAC levels (Duke et al. 2011). Approximately 40% of homicide victims had consumed alcohol prior to the fatal injury (Nazarov and Li 2020). Excessive drinking can result in more severe forms of violence, which can quickly escalate into extremely dangerous situations. The short- and long-term effects of alcohol distort a person's mental abilities, contributing to an increased risk of committing violent crimes (WHO 2018).

Although the link between alcohol and homicide is well documented, only a few recent studies explored the role of alcohol in homicide victimization in the United States. Naimi et al. (2016) examined how common alcohol was involved in homicide victimization, as well as the sociodemographic and other factors that were linked to alcohol involvement in homicide victimization. They analyzed BAC data recorded in the NVDRS from 17 states. The results indicated that almost 40% of all homicide victims had a positive BAC and males were twice more likely to have BAC higher than 0.08% than females. The study also identified the independent predictors for victims to have a BAC higher than 0.08%: being a male, Hispanic, American Indian, having a history of partner violence, and non-firearm homicide (Naimi et al. 2016).

Alcohol Consumption Pattern

Alcohol use by either the perpetrator, the victim, or both is frequently a contributing factor in homicide. The link between alcohol use and homicide is most pronounced in societies where drinking is frequently heavy enough to induce intoxication such as nations in Northern and Eastern Europe (Rossow 2001; Pridemore and Chamlin 2006). According to meta-analyses of studies conducted in societies where drinking to intoxication is common, 48% of both victims and perpetrators had been drinking at the time of the homicide incidents, and 37% of offenders and 33–35% of victims had consumed enough alcohol to be intoxicated (Kuhns et al. 2009, 2011).

Several studies have indicated that the association between alcohol and homicide is stronger in countries with an intoxication-oriented drinking pattern than in countries with a more moderate drinking pattern (Rossow 2001; Pridemore and Chamlin 2006). Norström (2011) examined the alcohol-homicide link in "dry," "moderate," and "wet" states of the United States based on alcohol sales data and found no conclusive evidence that homicide rates were positively associated with alcohol consumption levels.

Concurrent Use of Cannabis and Alcohol and Homicide

Present evidence suggests that the prevalence of concurrent use of cannabis and alcohol has increased by 53.9% between 2004 and 2016 (Nazarov and Li 2020). Toxicological testing data from random roadside surveys also found that drivers using cannabis were 50–66% more likely to use alcohol, compared with those not using cannabis (with an adjusted OR of 1.5) (Li and Chihuri 2020).

Concurrent use of cannabis and alcohol is the most common polydrug combination (Earleywine and Newcomb 1997; Martin et al. 1996; Nazarov and Li 2020; Li and Chihuri 2020). The use of both alcohol and cannabis at the same time (i.e., simultaneous use) could be more harmful than using both substances separately or even concurrently. Due to the widespread use of cannabis and alcohol and the high prevalence of concurrent use, conditions specific to simultaneous use can have significant consequences for polydrug users. Studies have linked simultaneous cannabis and alcohol use to more detrimental consequences involving psychological distress, psychopathology, and drug dependency (Margolese et al. 2004; Barnwell and Earleywine 2006).

A study based on the toxicology results obtained from 1,780 homicide victims found that 40–65% of the victims were positive for both alcohol and other drugs (Kuhns et al. 2012). Rivara and colleagues (1997) used a case-control design to assess the association between chronic substance use and violent death. They analyzed 388 homicide cases and an equal number of controls identified through medical examiner reports and found that subjects who reportedly used both alcohol and illicit drugs were at markedly increased risk of homicide relative to those who used neither substance (OR 12.0). These findings suggest that while alcohol and cannabis can each contribute to increased homicide victimization, using them together increased the risk to a level that is higher than the sum of the effects of the two substances when used separately.

Interaction Between Cannabis and Alcohol

Concurrent use of cannabis and alcohol poses a serious concern because these two drugs could interact with each other. Psychoactive substances can be complementary in various modes of use, with the use of one being positively associated with the use of another. They can, on the other hand, substitute for one another; if one becomes too expensive, unavailable, or dangerous, another can be used in its place. If the supply of the usual substance is cut off, finding a supply of a cross-dependent substance as a substitute becomes a matter of urgency for users with substance use disorder (Kiepek et al. 2018; WHO 2018). Alcohol has shown to be a complementary substance for other psychoactive drugs (e.g., nicotine) and risk-taking behaviors (e.g., driving at excessive speed and running red lights and speeding while driving) (Cameron and Williams 2001; Pierani and Tiezzi 2009; Tauchmann et al. 2013).

Studies of substitution or complementarity between cannabis and alcohol were conducted primarily in adolescents and college students, and the results have been inconsistent. Although decriminalization of cannabis use in some Australian states coincided with higher alcohol use, analysis of Australian population surveys found "some evidence to suggest that cannabis and alcohol are substitutes" (Cameron and Williams 2001). A study of adolescents in the United States found evidence of substitution in the youngest cohort (around 13 years old) – binge drinking decreased after medical cannabis became available – but no significant change in those aged 15 and 17 years old (Cerdá et al. 2018).

Williams et al. (2004), on the other hand, reported evidence that alcohol and cannabis were complementary among college students in the United States. Similarly, Pape et al. (2009) found complementarity among European teenagers: 80% of Norwegians aged 14–20 years who used cannabis also drank alcohol, and the majority of 15–16-year-olds who used cannabis also drank alcohol in 35 European countries. In a study based on national drug survey data in Australia, Zhao and Harris (2004) found no significant effects in terms of complementarity versus substitution for any use of cannabis on alcohol consumption (Zhao and Harris 2004).

As more US states move toward legalizing cannabis as a harm reduction strategy (e.g., for controlling the opioid epidemic), there is an urgent need to better understand the relationships between cannabis use and opioid use and between cannabis use and alcohol use and the individual and joint effects of these substances on violence, overdose, and other injuries.

Summary and Suggestions

Several characteristics of alcohol and cannabis are worth noting. With the ratification of the 21st Amendment to the US Constitution, the prohibition of alcohol in the United States ended in 1933 (Smentkowski 2020). On the other hand, to facilitate the war on drugs, cannabis was classified as a schedule 1 drug through the Controlled Substance Act of 1970 (Gabay 2013). One of the few similarities between alcohol and cannabis is that they both metabolize through the liver (Rao and Topiwala 2020). The active components of the two substances are different (ethanol in alcohol and Δ-9-THC in cannabis). So are the biological mechanism and pharmacokinetics through which they are metabolized in the body and eliminated from the body (Huestis 2007; Rao and Topiwala 2020). Due to these characteristics, alcohol is removed much faster from the body due to its hydrophilic property than lipophilic cannabis (Huestis 2007; Rao and Topiwala 2020). In addition, while alcohol acts on the central nervous system as a depressant, cannabis may serve as a stimulant, a hallucinogenic, and a depressant (Rao and Topiwala 2020; Cravanas Jr and Frei 2020), which makes it more difficult to predict the effect of cannabis in different individuals than the effect of alcohol.

Existing research indicates that cannabis use and alcohol use are commonly involved in homicide victimization and perpetration and are each associated with a substantially increased risk of homicide victimization and perpetration (Table 1). However, limitations in the relevant epidemiologic literature leave many questions unanswered. A review of drug-related homicide in Europe uncovered three key

Table 1 Summary of epidemiologic evidence for cannabis use and homicide in comparison with alcohol use

	Victims		Perpetrators	
Substance	Prevalence	Estimated Odds Ratio	Prevalence	Estimated Odds Ratio
Cannabis	31.0%[1]	OR=2.4[2]	5.0–31.0%[3]	OR=2.90[4]
Alcohol	37.5%[1]	OR=2.1[3]	40.0–50.0%[3]	OR=3.64[5]

Ref:1-Nazarov and Li 2020; 2-Darke et al. 2009; 3-Darke 2010; 4-Emma et al. 2016, 5-Hedlund et al. 2018

obstacles that hindered monitoring of drug-related homicide (European Monitoring Centre for Drugs and Drug Addiction 2018): missing and incomplete data, lack of comparability in testing and recording, and inadequate data quality. These data issues need to be addressed in order to evaluate and monitor the risk of violence associated with cannabis and alcohol consumption.

Applications to Other Substance Use Disorders

Other Drugs and Violence

The association of psychoactive illicit drugs, such as cannabis, opioids, and psychostimulants, with homicide and suicide was studied in a cross-sectional study conducted in Australia (Darke et al. 2009). Psychoactive substances were found in more than half of the cases through autopsy. Cannabis was one of the most present illicit drugs followed by opioids in homicide victims compared to suicide. Additionally, they found that homicide cases were also significantly more likely to have Δ-9-THC present, meaning that individuals were under an active influence of the drug at the time of death.

A study by Sheehan et al. (2013) found that certain drugs are associated with homicide more often than suicide. Marijuana, cocaine, and amphetamines were significantly more likely to be present among homicide decedents. On the contrary, antidepressants and opiates were more often associated with suicide. Differences were also detected within the gender: drugs associated with homicide were more prevalent among males, while drugs associated with suicide were more likely to be used in females. Considering these differences may be extremely useful for tailored interventions, as one suits all approach is never successful (especially in such complicated matters as substance abuse).

Delaveris et al. (2014) analyzed autopsy reports of nonnatural death (accidents, suicide, and homicide) decedents to document the prevalence of polydrug use. The study population was 20–59-year-old individuals, who died by nonnatural cause of which 15% were due to suicide and 3% homicide, and toxicological tests identified any illicit drug in the body. The research showed that more than 75% of eligible autopsy cases were accidental intoxications with polydrug found in all manner of death. The study also indicated intoxication suicides had the highest number of substances with the total substance profile similar to accidental intoxications. The authors concluded that polydrug findings are common in adults who die from an unnatural cause while using illicit drugs.

Applications to Other Areas of Public Health

Implications Beyond Violence

Another study comparing individual and joint effects of cannabis and alcohol use was a case-control study by Chihuri et al. (2017) that demonstrated the effects of both cannabis and alcohol beyond implications of violence. They analyzed 1,944 fatal crash accidents against 7,719 controls, who were drivers who participated in the 2007 National Roadside Survey of Alcohol and Drug Use by Drivers. The results indicated that fatal cases were significantly more likely to test positive for cannabis, alcohol, and both substances. The adjusted ORs were 16.3, 1.5, and 25.1 for those testing positive for alcohol and negative for cannabis, positive for cannabis and negative for alcohol, and positive for both substances, respectively. These findings reaffirm that while alcohol and cannabis are each responsible for higher fatality rates, using them together increases the risks significantly higher than just the sum of their separate effects.

Mini-Dictionary

Endocannabinoid receptors: A protein molecule to which cannabis binds and exerts its effect

Delta-9-tetrahydrocannabinol (Δ-9-THC): The main psychoactive ingredient of cannabis

Depressant: A substance that acts to reduce the activity in the central nervous system

Hallucinogenic: A substance that causes hallucinations

Lipophilic: A substance that has a tendency to combine or dissolve in fats

Pharmacokinetics: Describes the movement of a substance into, through, and out of the body

Polydrug: A combination of more than one drug/substance

Key Facts

- Psychoactive effects of both alcohol and cannabis may predispose a person to become a homicide victim or perpetrator.
- The risk of violence is much higher when cannabis and alcohol are consumed simultaneously or concurrently than when they are consumed separately.
- Cannabis is more frequently detected among homicide victims than among suicide victims.

- About 37% of homicide victims tested positive for alcohol, 31.0% for cannabis, and 11.4% for both.
- The prevalence of cannabis detected in homicide victims almost doubled from 2004 to 2016 in both sexes and across all age and racial groups in the United States.

Summary Points

The prevalence of cannabis detected among homicide victims is increasing, while alcohol remains relatively stable.

Pathways linking cannabis use to violence include pharmacological disinhibition, economic compulsiveness, and risky situation.

The prevalence of cannabis detected among homicide victims is much higher than in suicide victims.

Alcohol is the most commonly detected substance among homicide victims, particularly in societies where drinking to intoxication is common.

The concurrent use of cannabis and alcohol is the most common polydrug combination.

References

Auckloo MBKM, Davies BB (2019) Post-mortem toxicology in violent fatalities in Cape Town, South Africa: a preliminary investigation. J Forensic Legal Med 63:18–25. https://doi.org/10.1016/j.jflm.2019.02.005

Barnwell SS, Earleywine M (2006) Simultaneous alcohol and cannabis expectancies predict simultaneous use. Subst Abuse Treat Prev Policy 1:29. https://doi.org/10.1186/1747-597X-1-29

Bonnet U, Preuss U (2017) The cannabis withdrawal syndrome: current insights. Subst Abus Rehabil 8. https://doi.org/10.2147/sar.s109576

Cameron L, Williams J (2001) Cannabis, alcohol and cigarettes: substitutes or complements? Econ Rec 77(236):19–34. https://doi.org/10.1111/1475-4932.00002

Centers for Disease Control and Prevention (2018) 10 leading causes of death by age group, United States. https://www.cdc.gov/injury/images/lc-charts/leading_causes_of_death_by_age_group_2018_1100w850h.jpg. Accessed March 25, 2022.

Cerdá M, Sarvet A, Wall M, Feng T, Keyes K, Galea S, Hasin D (2018) Medical marijuana laws and adolescent use of marijuana and other substances: alcohol, cigarettes, prescription drugs, and other illicit drugs. Drug Alcohol Depend 183:62–68. https://doi.org/10.1016/j.drugalcdep.2017.10.021

Chihuri S, Li G, Chen Q (2017) Interaction of marijuana and alcohol on fatal motor vehicle crash risk: a case-control study. Inj Epidemiol 4(1):8. https://doi.org/10.1186/s40621-017-0105-z

Cravanas B Jr, Frei K (2020) The effects of Cannabis on hallucinations in Parkinson's disease patients. J Neurol Sci 15(419):117206. https://doi.org/10.1016/j.jns.2020.117206. Epub 2020 Oct 22

Darke S (2010) The toxicology of homicide offenders and victims: a review. Drug Alcohol Rev 29 (2):202–215. https://doi.org/10.1111/j.1465-3362.2009.00099.x

Darke S, Degenhardt L, Mattick R (2012) Mortality amongst illicit drug users epidemiology, causes and intervention. Cambridge University Press, New York

Darke S, Duflou J (2008) Toxicology and circumstances of death of homicide victims in New South Wales, Australia 1996–2005. J Forensic Sci 53(2):447–451. https://doi.org/10.1111/j.1556-4029.2008.00679.x

Darke S, Duflou J, Torok M (2009) Drugs and violent death: comparative toxicology of homicide and non-substance toxicity suicide victims. Addiction 104(6):1000–1005. https://doi.org/10.1111/j.1360-0443.2009.02565.x

Delaveris GJM, Teige B, Rogde S (2014) Non-natural manners of death among users of illicit drugs: substance findings. Forensic Sci Int 238:16–21. https://doi.org/10.1016/j.forsciint.2014.02.009

Earleywine M, Newcomb MD (1997) Concurrent versus simultaneous polydrug use: prevalence, correlates, discriminant validity, and prospective effects on health outcomes. Exp Clin Psychopharmacol 5:353–364. https://doi.org/10.1037/1064-1297.5.4.353

Emma E, McGinty S, Choksy G, Wintemute J (2016) The relationship between controlled substances and violence. Epidemiol Rev 38(1):5–31. https://doi.org/10.1093/epirev/mxv008

European Monitoring Centre for Drugs and Drug Addiction (2018) Drug-related homicide in Europe: a first review of the data and literature. EMCDDA Papers

Exum ML (2006) Alcohol and aggression: an integration of findings from experimental studies. J Crim Just 34(2):131–145. https://doi.org/10.1016/j.jcrimjus.2006.01.008

Gabay M (2013) The federal controlled substances act: schedules and pharmacy registration. Hosp Pharm 48(6):473–474. https://doi.org/10.1310/hpj4806-473

Goldstein PJ (1985) The drugs/violence nexus: a tripartite conceptual framework. J Drug Issues 15 (4):493–506. https://doi.org/10.1177/002204268501500406

Grinshteyn E, Hemenway D (2016) Violent death rates: the US compared with other high-income OECD countries, 2010. Am J Med 129(3):266–273. https://doi.org/10.1016/j.amjmed.2015.10.025

Hedlund J, Forsman J, Sturup J, Masterman T (2018) Pre-offense alcohol intake in homicide offenders and victims: a forensic-toxicological case-control study. J Forensic Legal Med 56: 55–58. https://doi.org/10.1016/j.jflm.2018.03.004. Epub 2018 Mar 6

Huestis MA (2007) Human cannabinoid pharmacokinetics. Chem Biodivers 4(8):1770–1804. https://doi.org/10.1002/cbdv.200790152

Kiepek N, Beagan B, Harris J (2018) A pilot study to explore the effects of substances on cognition, mood, performance, and experience of daily activities. Perform Enhanc Health 6(1):3–11. https://doi.org/10.1016/j.peh.2018.02.003

Kuhns J, Maguire E (2012) Drug and alcohol use by homicide victims in Trinidad and Tobago, 2001–2007. Forensic Sci Med Pathol **8**:243–251. https://doi.org/10.1007/s12024-011-9305-y

Kuhns J, Wilson D, Clodfelter T, Maguire E, Ainsworth S (2011) A meta-analysis of alcohol toxicology study findings among homicide victims. Addiction 106(1):62–72. https://doi.org/10.1111/j.1360-0443.2010.03153.x

Kuhns J, Wilson D, Maguire E, Ainsworth S, Clodfelter T (2009) A meta-analysis of marijuana, cocaine and opiate toxicology study findings among homicide victims. Addiction 104(7):1122–1131. https://doi.org/10.1111/j.1360-0443.2009.02583.x

Li G, Chihuri S (2020) Is marijuana use associated with decreased use of prescription opioids? Toxicological findings from two US national samples of drivers. Subst Abuse Treat Prev Policy 15:12. https://doi.org/10.1186/s13011-020-00257-7

Margolese HC, Malchy L, Negrete JC, Tempier R, Gill K (2004) Drug and alcohol use among patients with schizophrenia and related psychoses: levels and consequences. Schizophr Res 67: 157–166. https://doi.org/10.1016/S0920-9964(02)00523-6

Martin CS, Kaczynski NA, Maisto SA, Tarter RE (1996) Polydrug use in adolescent drinkers with and without DSM-IV alcohol abuse and dependence. Alcohol Clin Exp Res 20:1099–1108. https://doi.org/10.1111/j.1530-0277.1996.tb01953.x

Meier MH, Caspi A, Ambler A, Harrington H, Houts R, Keefe RS, McDonald K, Ward A, Poulton R, Moffitt TE (2012) Persistent cannabis users show neuropsychological decline from childhood to midlife. Proc Natl Acad Sci U S A 109(40):15980. https://doi.org/10.1073/pnas.1206820109

Miller NS, Ipeku R, Oberbarnscheidt T (2020) A review of cases of marijuana and violence. Int J Environ Res Public Health 17(5):1–14. https://doi.org/10.3390/ijerph17051578

Naimi T, Xuan Z, Cooper S, Coleman S, Hadland S, Swahn M, Heeren T (2016) Alcohol involvement in homicide victimization in the United States. Alcohol Clin Exp Res 40(12): 2614–2621. https://doi.org/10.1111/acer.13230

Nazarov O, Li G (2020) Trends in alcohol and marijuana detected in homicide victims in 9 US states: 2004–2016. Injury Epidemiol 7(1):2. https://doi.org/10.1186/s40621-019-0229-4

Norström T (2011) Alcohol and homicide in the United States: is the link dependent on wetness? Drug Alcohol Rev 30(5). https://doi.org/10.1111/j.1465-3362.2011.00295.x

Pape H, Rossow I, Storvoll EE (2009) Under double influence: assessment of simultaneous alcohol and cannabis use in the general youth populations. Drug Alcohol Depend 101(1–2):69–73. https://doi.org/10.1016/j.drugalcdep.2008.11.002

Pierani P, Tiezzi S (2009) Addiction and interaction between alcohol and tobacco consumption. Empir Econ 37(1):1–23. https://doi.org/10.1007/s00181-008-0220-3

Pridemore WA, Chamlin MB (2006) A time-series analysis of the impact of heavy drinking on homicide and suicide mortality in Russia, 1956–2002. Addiction 101(12):1719–1729. https://doi.org/10.1111/j.1360-0443.2006.01631.x

Rao R, Topiwala A (2020) Alcohol use disorders and the brain. Addiction 115(8):1580–1589. https://doi.org/10.1111/add.15023. Wiley Online Library

Reingle JM, Jennings WG, Maldonado-Molina MM (2012) Risk and protective factors for trajectories of violent delinquency among a nationally representative sample of early adolescents. Youth Violence Juvenile Justice 10(3):261–277. https://doi.org/10.1177/1541204011431589

Rossow I (2001) Alcohol and homicide: a cross-cultural comparison of the relationship in 14 European countries. Addiction 96(SUPPL1):77–92. https://doi.org/10.1080/09652140020021198

Sheehan C, Roger R, Williams G IV, Boardman J (2013) Gender differences in the presence of drugs in violent deaths. Addiction 108(3):547–555. https://doi.org/10.1111/j.1360-0443.2012.04098.x

Smentkowski Brian P (2020) "Twenty-first amendment". Encyclopedia Britannica, https://www.britannica.com/topic/Twenty-first-Amendment. Accessed 9 May 2021

Tauchmann H, Lenz S, Requate T, Schmidt C (2013) Tobacco and alcohol: complements or substitutes? Empir Econ 45(1). https://doi.org/10.1007/s00181-012-0611-3

WHO (2018) Global status report on alcohol and health 2018, Global status report on alcohol. Available at: http://www.who.int/substance_abuse/publications/global_alcohol_report/msbgsruprofiles.pdf%0Ahttp://www.ncbi.nlm.nih.gov/pubmed/29355346

Wilcox HC, Conner KR, Caine ED (2004 Dec) Association of alcohol and drug use disorders and completed suicide: an empirical review of cohort studies. Drug Alcohol Depend 7(76 Suppl): S11–S19. https://doi.org/10.1016/j.drugalcdep.2004.08.003

Williams J, Pacula R, Chaloupka F, Wechsler H (2004) Alcohol and marijuana use among college students: economic complements or substitutes? Health Econ 13(9):825–843. https://doi.org/10.1002/hec.859

Yanowitch R, Coccaro EF (2011) The neurochemistry of human aggression. Adv Genet 75:151–170. https://doi.org/10.1016/B978-0-12-380858-5.00005-8

Zhao X, Harris MN (2004) Demand for marijuana, alcohol and tobacco: participation, levels of consumption and cross-equation correlations. Econ Rec 80(251):394–410. https://doi.org/10.1111/j.1475-4932.2004.00197.x

Part VII

Caffeine

Caffeine Consumption over Time

71

Gabrielle Rabelo Quadra, Emília Marques Brovini,
Joyce Andreia dos Santos, and José R. Paranaíba

Contents

Introduction 1536
Patterns and Trends of Caffeine Consumption 1538
Global and Regional Coffee Consumption Over Time 1538
Continental Patterns of Coffee Consumption 1540
Caffeine Consumption According to Age 1543
Public Health Perspectives 1544
Is Caffeine Addictive? 1544
Effects on Mental and Physical Health 1544
Current Strategies and Prevention 1545
Environmental Issue: Another Point to Be Explored 1546
Applications to Other Areas of Addiction 1546
Applications to Public Health 1547
Mini-Dictionary of Terms 1548
Key Facts of Caffeine Consumption Over Time 1548
Summary Points 1549
References 1549

Abstract

Caffeine is one of the most consumed substances worldwide, and although it is present in many food products in different concentrations, coffee is likely the most significant product in terms of caffeine concentration and consumption.

G. R. Quadra (✉) · J. A. dos Santos · J. R. Paranaíba
Departamento de Biologia, Laboratório de Ecologia Aquática, Programa de Pós-Graduação em Biodiversidade e Conservação da Natureza, Universidade Federal de Juiz de Fora, Juiz de Fora, Brazil
e-mail: gabrielle.quadra@ecologia.ufjf.br; santos.joyce@ecologia.ufjf.br; jose.paranaiba@ecologia.ufjf.br

E. M. Brovini
Laboratório de Química Tecnológica e Ambiental (LQTA), Programa de Pós-Graduação em Engenharia Ambiental, Universidade Federal de Ouro Preto, Ouro Preto, Brazil
e-mail: emilia.brovini@engenharia.ufjf.br

V. B. Patel, V. R. Preedy (eds.), *Handbook of Substance Misuse and Addictions*,
https://doi.org/10.1007/978-3-030-92392-1_78

Despite being known and used by humankind for hundreds of years, the patterns of consumption and environmental risks are not fully understood. Therefore, global spatial and temporal caffeine consumption was investigated over the last 20 years, and health perspectives were discussed. An increase of 37% in per capita coffee consumption was observed in the last two decades worldwide, mainly in the Middle East and North Africa (84.2%) and upper middle-income countries (86.1%). Although there is still controversy on whether it is an addictive substance, it is worth noting that risks associated with its high consumption exist, mainly by more sensitive people and when mixing it with other substances, such as alcohol.

Keywords

Coffee · Alcohol · Anxiety · Soft drinks · Environment · Europe · Energy drinks · Per capita consumption · Health risks · Tea · Tobacco

Abbreviations

B.C	Before Christ
EAP	East Asia and Pacific
ECA	Europe and Central Asia
EFSA	European Food Safety Authority
FDA	U.S. Food and Drug Administration
g	Gram or grams
GDP	Gross domestic product
GNI	Gross national income
HDI	Human development index
LAC	Latin America and Caribbean
MENA	Middle East and North Africa
mg	Milligram or milligrams
mg/kg/day	Milligram per kilogram per day
mg/kg	Milligram per kilogram
mg/L	Milligram per liter
NA	North America
ng/L	Nanogram per liter
SA	South Asia
SSA	Sub-Saharan Africa
Tg	Teragram
WHO	World Health Organization

Introduction

The caffeine history starts in 1819 when Friedlieb Ferdinand Runge (Germany) isolated the compound and named it. However, some speculations mention that caffeine-based plants were discovered in Paleolithic times, about 700,000 B.C, and were used for pharmacological purposes (Weinberg and Bealer 2019). Nowadays, coffee, tea, and cola are the most popular drinks globally, making caffeine possibly the most consumed psychoactive substance (Diogo et al. 2013; Weinberg and Bealer 2019). Not only drinks contain caffeine but also other food products (e.g., chocolates), medicines (e.g., analgesics, appetite suppressants, and stimulants) and personal care products (Buerge et al. 2003; Diogo et al. 2013).

In addition to a cup of coffee, energy drink has increasingly gained popularity over the years, mainly by students (Olsen 2013). Energy drink companies have been aggressively marketing toward college students since at least 40% drink a cup of coffee a day (Olsen 2013). But this is not just an American reality. Europeans consume much denser coffee than Americans, indicating more caffeine consumption per ingested dose (Qi Li 2013). In Asia, caffeine intake is mainly through coffee and tea, which are traditional beverages in the continent, where Chinese and Indians ingest it to keep alert and prevent sleepiness (Gera et al. 2016; Chei et al. 2018). Soft drinks are the primary sources of caffeine for children, representing 50–64% of the total caffeine consumption by this group, as well as chocolates that, despite having lower caffeine concentrations, are consumed in several products (Frary et al. 2005). Caffeine-based drugs are mainly consumed by adults and the elderly, sometimes intermittently, and self-medication leads to overconsumption and potential health issues (Carrillo Benitez 2000). Although caffeine is found in many products in different concentrations, coffee represents one of the highest caffeine concentrations among them (Mitchell et al. 2014) (Fig. 1).

Caffeine acts by blocking adenosine receptors and is classified as a methylxanthine, a group of central nervous system stimulants (Carrillo Benitez 2000; Diogo et al. 2013). Approximately 95% of the ingested caffeine is metabolized in the human body (Tang-Liu et al. 1983), and its removal rates in wastewater treatment

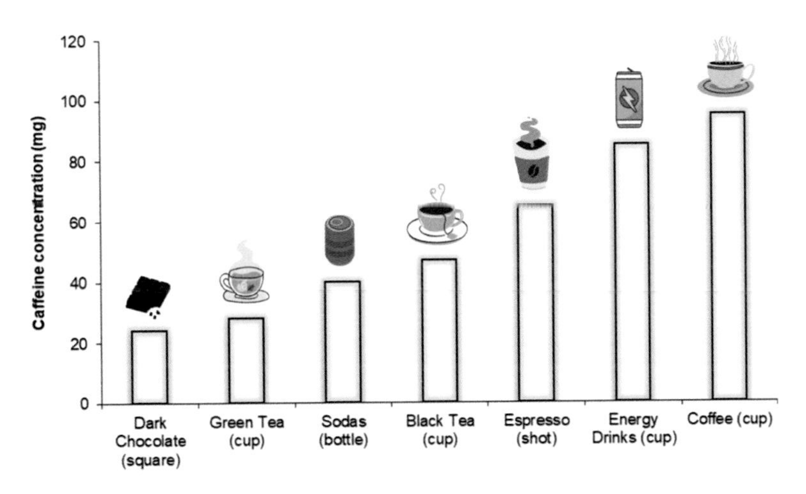

Fig. 1 Concentration of caffeine (mg) in different products. Data source: Harvard, EFSA (European Food Safety Authority) and My Food Data. The graph was created in Excel and the figure with icons in Canva

plants are relatively high (Bruton et al. 2010; Camacho-Muñoz et al. 2012). However, as the consumption is increasing and sewage treatment coverage is not sufficient worldwide, caffeine has been used as a tracer for domestic sewage in the environment, with caffeine being found in different matrices, including drinking water (Strauch et al. 2008; Bruton et al. 2010; Quadra et al. 2020).

Although caffeine is known as a safe compound and provides some benefits, high consumption may be toxic to humans (Price and Fligner 1990). Moreover, once in the environment, caffeine may pose a risk to aquatic and terrestrial organisms (Bruton et al. 2010). In this context, understand the global patterns of caffeine consumption may be helpful to support public health actions. In this chapter, the global spatial (i.e., countries) and temporal (i.e., from 2000 to 2019) caffeine consumption patterns were investigated, spotlighting possible impacts on global public health. All data used here were collected from the World Bank (total population) and International Coffee Organization (domestic consumption and non-member import). Coffee was used as a proxy for caffeine consumption since it contains a higher amount of caffeine and it is consumed worldwide.

Patterns and Trends of Caffeine Consumption

Global and Regional Coffee Consumption Over Time

Caffeine consumption increased globally from 2000 to 2019 and it is strongly related to global population growth (Fig. 2). A previous study has shown the global increase in caffeine consumption until 2013 (Quadra et al. 2020). Coupled with that, the per capita coffee consumption is also increasing (Fig. 2). Between 2000 and 2009, the global per capita coffee consumption increased about 15%, and between 2009 and 2019, the rise was even higher, reaching about 19%. In total, over the previous two decades (2000–2019), per coffee capita consumption increased about 37%.

Although the global per capita coffee consumption is increasing, this is not a trend for all investigated countries (190 counties out of 195 – considering the Holy See and the State of Palestine), indicating distinct regional patterns of coffee consumption. Quadra and colleagues also showed a high positive relationship between per capita caffeine consumption and time for most of the countries (from 2000 to 2013; Quadra et al. 2020). Considering the seven global regions classification, based on the World Bank, it was possible to observe that Europe and Central Asia and North America had the highest per capita coffee consumption in 2000 (Fig. 3). The Middle East and North Africa had the highest percentage of increase in the last two decades (84.2%), followed by East Asia and Pacific (71.4%), Europe and Central Asia (67.5%), South Asia (23%), North America (15.8%), and sub-Saharan Africa (14.1%). In contrast, in the Latin America and the Caribbean, there was almost no increase (0.04%).

Those observed trends may be related to gross national income (GNI). High-income countries had the highest per capita coffee consumption in 2000, which does not mean they had the highest increase in the last decades (Fig. 4). Indeed, the GNI

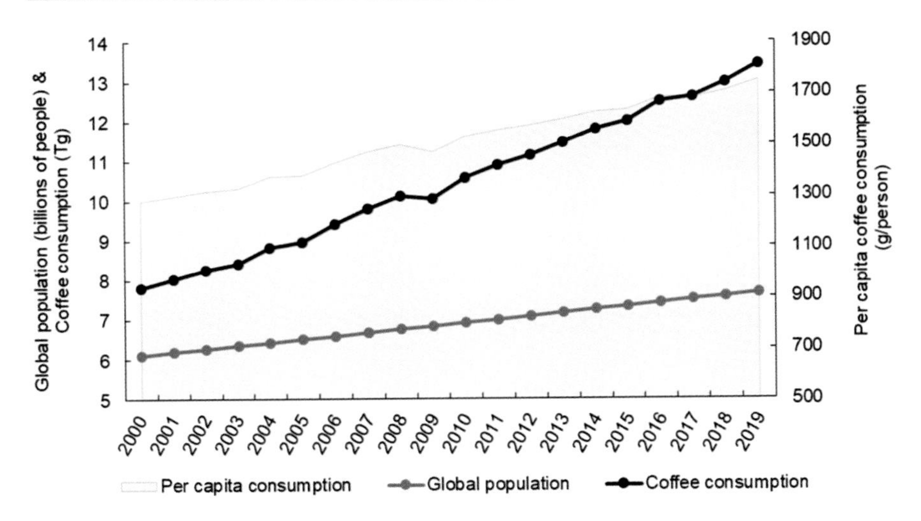

Fig. 2 The primary y-axis represents the global population in billions of people and global coffee consumption in teragrams (Tg). The secondary y-axis represents the per capita coffee consumption in grams per person. Data source: World Bank and International Coffee Organization. The graph was created in Excel

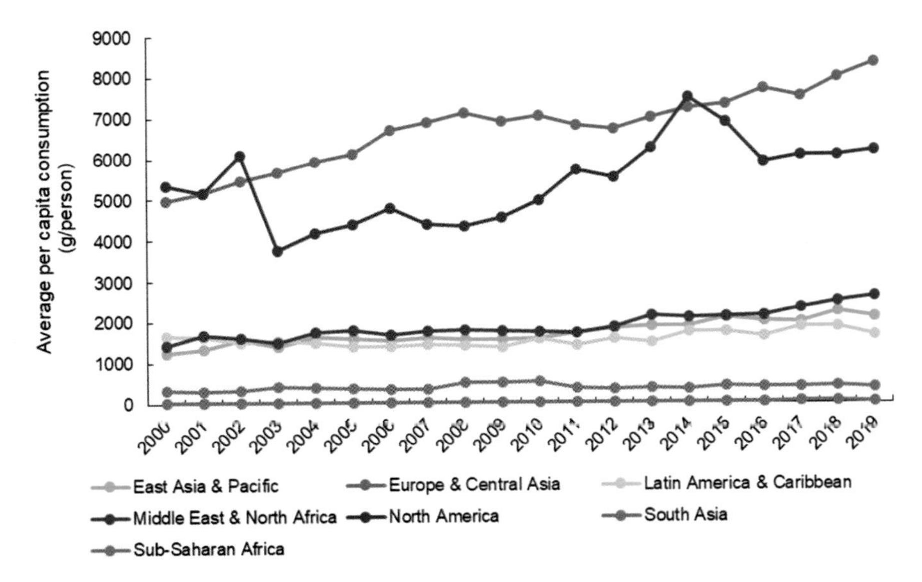

Fig. 3 The y-axis represents the average per capita coffee consumption in grams per person. Different colors represent each global region. Data source: World Bank and International Coffee Organization. The graph was created in Excel

class with the higher percentage of increase of per capita coffee consumption in the previous two decades was upper middle-income countries (86.1%), followed by high-income countries (49%), lower middle-income countries (45.7%), and low-income

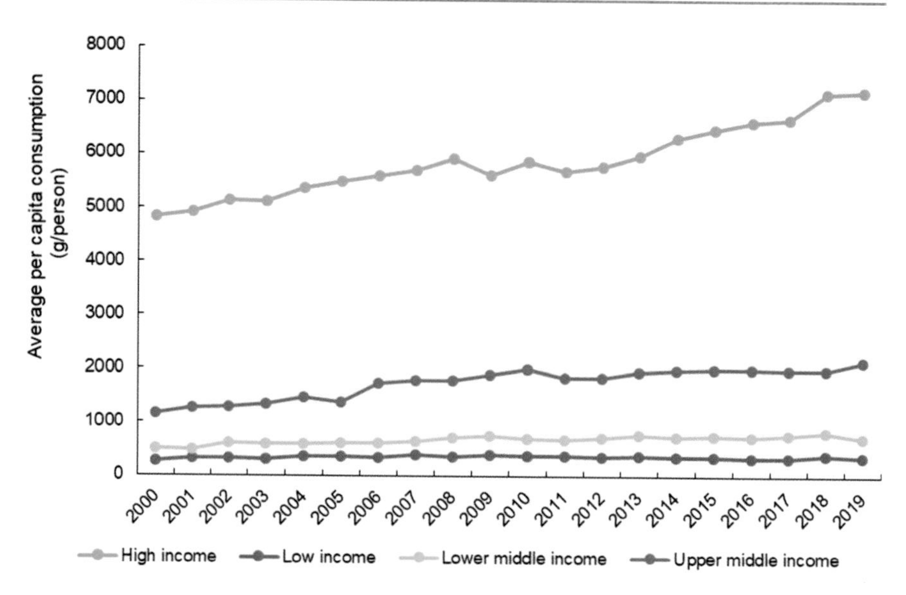

Fig. 4 The y-axis represents the average per capita coffee consumption in grams per person. The different colors represent each gross national income (GNI) class. Data source: World Bank and International Coffee Organization. The graph was created in Excel

countries (38.8%). Correlation between per capita coffee consumption and human development index (HDI) and gross domestic product (GDP) was previously shown, in which countries with high HDI and GDP showed higher coffee consumption, with the opposite also being confirmed (Quadra et al. 2020).

Despite not showing the most remarkable growth, it is essential to note the highest overall per capita coffee consumption for high-income countries (Fig. 5). The relationship between personal income and coffee consumption by the population is clear. Furthermore, the wide variation between coffee consumption data from Europe and Central Asia and sub-Saharan Africa was also remarkable (Fig. 5). These patterns of between-countries consumption will be further explored in the next topic.

Continental Patterns of Coffee Consumption

Different patterns of coffee consumption were observed between continents. For example, since 2000, Europe has shown the highest per capita coffee consumption, especially in Scandinavian countries (Fig. 6). In 2010, Canada also showed a higher per capita coffee consumption, together with other European countries. In 2019, in general, Europe showed a higher per capita coffee consumption compared to other continents (Fig. 6). In Africa, only a few countries stand out with higher per capita coffee consumption across the years (2000, 2010, and 2019). This higher consumption pattern in European countries and lower consumption in African countries was also shown by Quadra et al. (2020), but here a more refined spatial and temporal

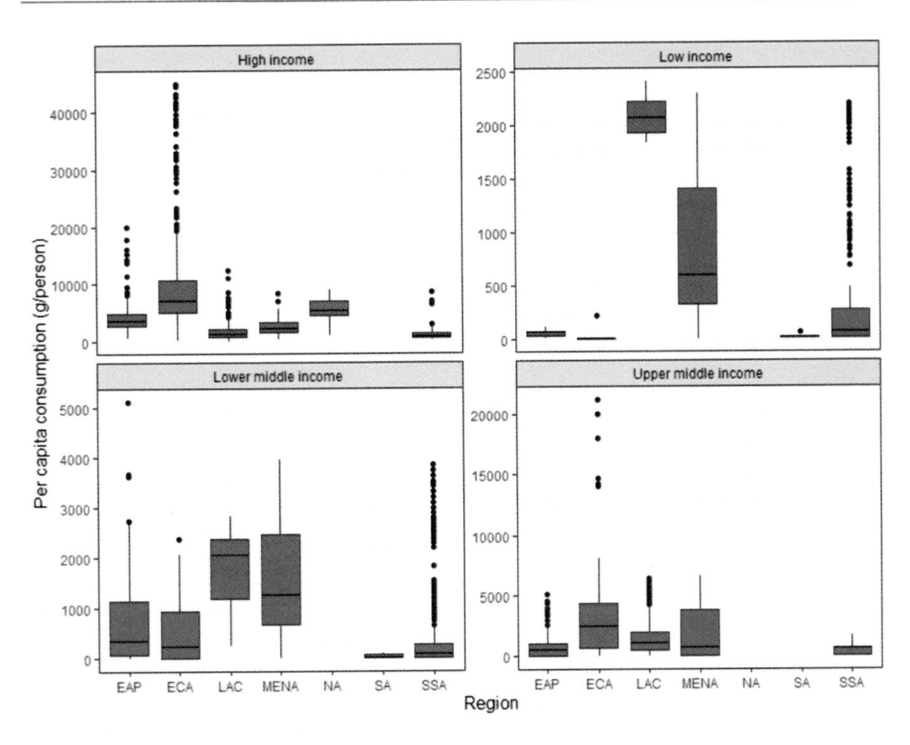

Fig. 5 The lines within the boxes indicate the median, the boxes delimit the 25th and 75th percentiles, and the whiskers delimit the fifth and 95th percentiles. The dots represent outliers. Note the different scales between graphs. EAP, East Asia and Pacific; ECA, Europe and Central Asia; LAC, Latin America and Caribbean; MENA, Middle East and North Africa; NA, North America; SA, South Asia; SSA, sub-Saharan Africa. Data source: World Bank and International Coffee Organization. The graph was created in R software

assessment was provided. It is also noteworthy that most countries in Africa and Latin America are known as coffee exporters, while countries in the northern hemisphere, in general, are importers. Another study also showed the role of European countries in the global patterns of caffeine consumption, highlighting these countries as the most significant coffee consumers, mainly for fresh-brewed type (Reyes and Cornelis 2018). Caffeine ingestion through tea is more evident in Africa and Asia and the Pacific. Latin America and the Caribbean showed the highest percentage of caffeine intake by carbonated drinks (soda and energy drinks), although coffee consumption is also high for some countries. In North America, Canada showed increased consumption of fresh-brewed coffee and herbal/fruit tea, while the USA showed a high caffeine intake by noncola carbonates besides fresh-brewed coffee (Reyes and Cornelis 2018).

Considering the 179 countries investigated (11 countries were excluded from this analysis since they had zero values as coffee consumption in the database in the last two decades), 121 showed an enhanced per capita coffee consumption over the last two decades, ranging from 2% to 1,211,643%. The five countries with the highest

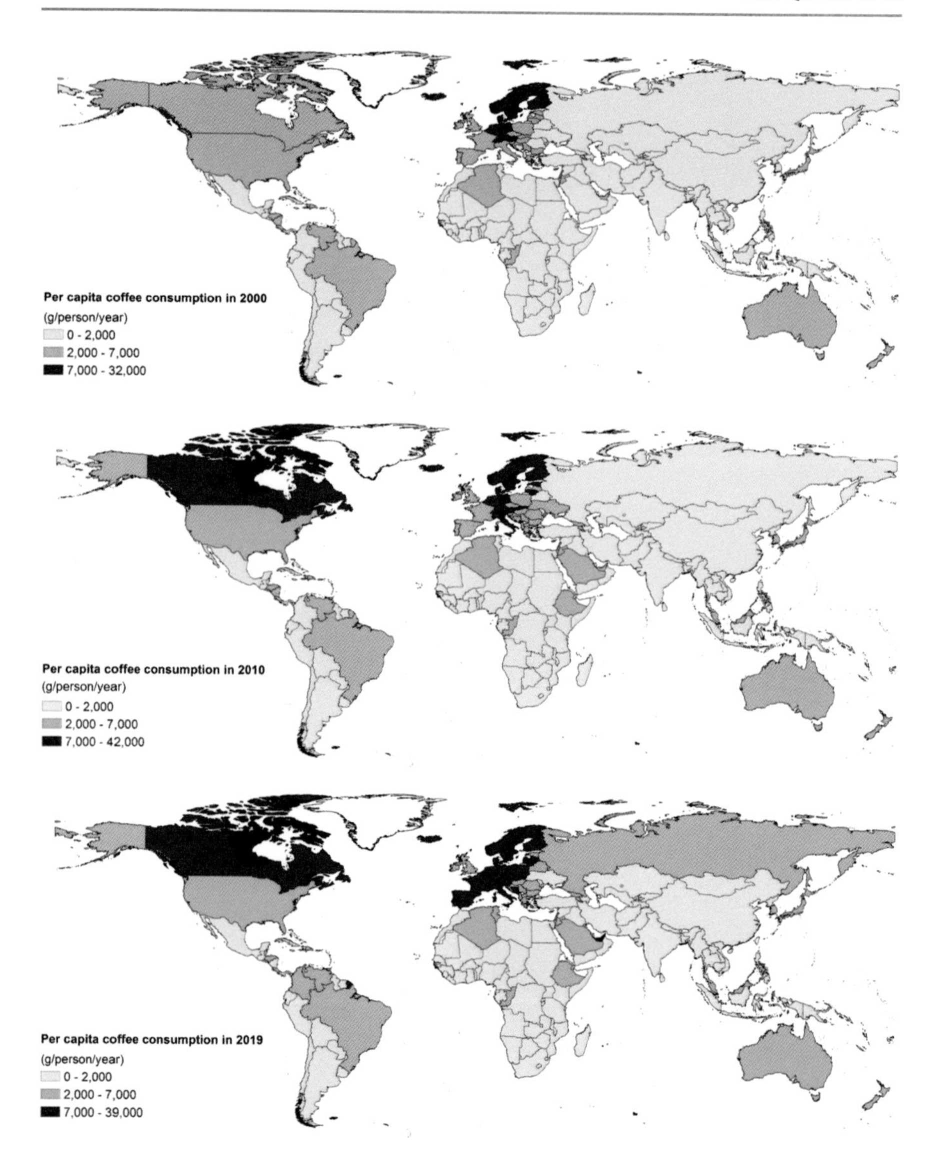

Fig. 6 Coffee consumption is presented as grams per person per year. Hollow countries mean that data was not available. Note that darker colors represent higher coffee consumption. Data source: World Bank and International Coffee Organization. The map was created in ArcGis (ESRI, v. 10.3.1)

increase were Myanmar, Kyrgyz Republic, Iran, Djibouti, and Mauritania. Sri Lanka, Norway, and Cuba showed very similar values of coffee consumption over time, with percentages over the last two decades of 0.5, −0.3, and – 0.4%, respectively. A total of 55 countries showed a negative trend over time, meaning that the per capita coffee consumption in these countries decreased in the last decades,

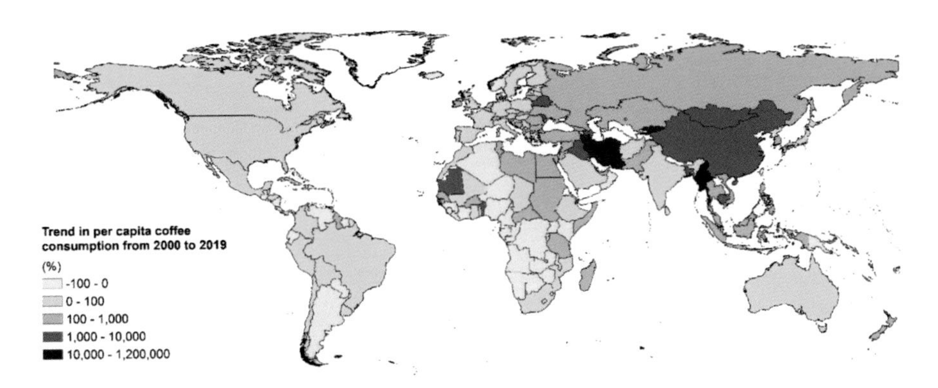

Fig. 7 The percentage of increase was evaluated considering the per capita coffee consumption in 2019 in relation to 2000. Hollow countries mean that data was not available. Note that darker colors represent higher consumption. Data source: World Bank and International Coffee Organization. The map was created in ArcGis (ESRI, v. 10.3.1)

ranging from −3% to −100%. The five countries with the highest decreasing trend over time were Zambia, Saint Kitts and Nevis, Togo, British Virgin Islands, and Tonga (Fig. 7).

Caffeine Consumption According to Age

The pattern of caffeine consumption varies significantly among age groups. For example, teenagers drink more energy drinks than adults, in which caffeine intake may be mainly through coffee or tea, depending on the region (Olsen 2013; Qi Li 2013; Mitchell et al. 2014; Gera et al. 2016; Chei et al. 2018). On the other hand, caffeine ingestion by children is especially via chocolate and soft drinks (Frary et al. 2005). Although children and teenagers do not consume much caffeine through coffee – a product that has the highest caffeine concentrations – the consumption of other caffeine-based products is higher, which may increase daily caffeine consumption. For example, a study performed in the USA showed that people from 2–5 years had a 90th percentile caffeine intake equal to 3.7 mg/kg/day, while, from 6–12 years, caffeine intake was 2.7 mg/kg/day, and from 13–17 years caffeine intake was 2.9 mg/kg/day (Mitchell et al. 2014). College students, on the other hand, are one of the largest segments of caffeine consumption (90th percentile caffeine intakes of 3.9–4.2 mg/kg/day in the USA; Mitchell et al. 2014). This consumption is closely related to college activities, such as exams and homework (Olsen 2013). Due to these factors, major brands of coffee and energy drinks carry out effective marketing at universities, attracting students' attention and increasing the consumption of caffeinated beverages (Olsen 2013).

However, the biggest consumers of caffeine are the adult and the elderly. For example, the caffeine intake by these groups is up to 5.9 mg/kg/day in the USA (90th percentile; Mitchell et al. 2014). The elderly generally drink beverages with a higher concentration of caffeine than other age groups (Mitchell et al. 2014). This trend can partially be explained by the consumption of medicines as well as by using caffeine as a way to relieve symptoms such as tiredness and headaches (Ágoston et al. 2018).

Public Health Perspectives

Is Caffeine Addictive?

There is an enormous controversy and debate about whether caffeine is addictive.

Studies pointed out that caffeine influences the nervous system and, thus, is considered a psychoactive substance that may lead to addiction (Gupta and Gupta 1999; Budney et al. 2013). According to Gupta and Gupta (1999), caffeine can cause dependence and abstinence, but the degree of addiction is lower than other drugs such as tobacco, alcohol, and cocaine. Favrod-Coune and Broers (2021) pointed out that caffeine-withdrawal syndrome can be confused or underestimated, which may occur after a rapid withdrawal of the regularly consumed substance, even on intakes of 100 mg/day (Juliano and Griffiths 2004). Another study also concluded that caffeine consumption is more related to a dedicated habit than a compulsive addiction (Satel 2006).

On the other hand, some studies show positive effects of caffeine consumption. Although studies that assess the risks and benefits of coffee consumption are very complex since several factors affect how a substance will act in the human body, George et al. (2008) and Pourshahidi et al. (2016) demonstrated through a literature review that caffeine consumption might improve metabolic health, physical performance, and antioxidant system. The authors mention that, in fact, the caffeine consumption risks are more associated with populations more sensitive to stimulants, as well as other lifestyle habits, such as smoking, alcohol ingestion, and others. The WHO (World Health Organization) does not indicate any risk of caffeine addiction, although there are indications of daily consumption limits and more susceptible populations to adverse effects (WHO 2021).

Therefore, caffeine meets some criteria to be considered a drug with the potential for addiction, but controlled consumption is safe and may bring benefits. It is necessary to know the withdrawal symptoms better in order to prevent possible adverse effects. Hence, despite being a well-known substance used by humans for hundreds of years, conclusive studies with more reliable data are needed.

Effects on Mental and Physical Health

In the human body, caffeine acts by changing intracellular calcium, antagonizing the adenosine and benzodiazepine receptors, and inhibiting phosphodiesterases (Gupta and Gupta 1999). These mechanisms cause the enhance of neurotransmitters and potentiate the response of cells to neurotransmitter activation (Gupta and Gupta 1999). Consequently, caffeine can cause changes in the cardiac, gastrointestinal, nervous, and renal systems, as well as changes in mood and sleep patterns (Leonard et al. 1987). However, only at toxic plasma levels of caffeine these reactions may occur, and, even at high concentrations, some bodies also may develop tolerance to acute and chronic effects of caffeine (Leonard et al. 1987; Gupta and Gupta 1999).

Evidence shows that excessive coffee intake can also cause psychiatric disorders. Caffeine is related to increased anxiety and sleep disorders, exacerbating psychosis (Winston et al. 2005). In patients who already have mental disorders, caffeine can cause hostility and increase psychotic symptoms (Winston et al. 2005). These symptoms may vary depending on age and sex (Jee et al. 2020). For example, caffeine increases anxiety disorders and insomnia in teenagers. The probability of developing depression decreases in adult women, while, in adolescence, women are at a higher risk of depression than men (Jee et al. 2020).

Moderate daily caffeine intake by adults (up to 400 mg/day) is not associated with negative effects, such as cardiovascular diseases, increased incidence of cancer, calcium balance, and effects on male fertility (Nawrot et al. 2003). However, reproductive-aged women and children may require control over daily caffeine intake once they may be in risk subgroups (Ennis 2014). The WHO warns of preterm birth or stillbirth risks, reduced birth weight, and growth changes (WHO 2021). However, Browne and colleagues did not show evidence of caffeine consumption and malformation of the fetus (Browne et al. 2007). Other studies also did not show an association between moderate caffeine intake and body disorders (Winkelmayer et al. 2005; Barger-Lux et al. 1990). Therefore, adverse effects caused by caffeine consumption may vary mainly due to daily-ingested dose and, consequently, the type of ingested product, age group, and personal emotional stability.

Current Strategies and Prevention

Currently, there are no formal regulations for caffeine consumption but only recommendations by different agencies. The FDA (U.S. Food and Drug Administration) and EFSA, for example, cite 400 mg/day, which is about four to five cups of coffee, as an amount unlikely to raise concerns for healthy adults (FDA 2018; Coffee & Health 2021). Toxic effects, such as seizures, may occur with rapid caffeine consumption of ~1200 mg (FDA 2018). However, caffeine presents a wide-range sensibility, depending on the metabolism of each person (FDA 2018). Therefore, caution is always necessary, especially for children or even teenagers and young adults, with excessive intake, mixing with alcohol and other drugs (FDA 2018; Mayo Clinic 2020). Attention is also necessary for pregnant or breastfeeding or even for those trying to become pregnant, in which the recommendation is to consume less than 200 mg/day of caffeine (WHO 2016; Mayo Clinic 2020). People that drink more than four cups of coffee a day need to be alert for the side effects, such as headache, upset stomach, insomnia, nervousness, irritability, or fast heartbeat, and should limit the consumption if one or more of those side effects appear (FDA 2018; Mayo Clinic 2020). Attention is also necessary with those taking medicines, such as ephedrine, theophylline, or echinacea, since caffeine may interact and cause adverse effects (Mayo Clinic 2020). Some tips for those who want to reduce the caffeine consumption are as follows: observe the ingested amount, cut it gradually, consume decaffeinated beverages, short the brew time or drink herbal teas, and check the labels of the products since caffeine is present in many of them (Mayo Clinic 2020).

Therefore, despite being considered a safe substance and present in daily life, it is a substance liable to cause addiction, being necessary precautions, especially for more sensitive populations.

Environmental Issue: Another Point to Be Explored

Although higher concentrations are needed to cause toxic effects in humans, caffeine may cause damage in minor concentrations once in the environment. As previously mentioned, caffeine is highly metabolized in the human body; its removal in sewage treatment plants and degradation in the environment are also relatively high compared to other organic compounds, but as consumption is part of the everyday life of many people, caffeine is continuously load into the environment (Tang-Liu et al. 1983; Thomas and Foster 2005; Bruton et al. 2010; Camacho-Muñoz et al. 2012). The literature regarding the ecotoxicological effects of caffeine is diverse, and adverse effects were observed from ng/L to mg/L. To name a few examples, oxidative stress and cellular damage in mollusks (Del Rey et al. 2011; Aguirre-Martínez et al. 2015; Cruz et al. 2016) affect negatively microbial activity, respiration, and biomass (Bunch and Bernot 2011; Rosi-Marshall et al. 2013) and behavior and neuromuscular effects in fish (Chen et al. 2008, Steele et al. 2018). Moreover, when caffeine was mixed with other pharmaceuticals, a synergetic effect was found affecting aquatic communities' composition (Lawrence et al. 2012), and then mixture effects should be taken into account. Some studies performed a risk assessment of caffeine and found risks mainly related to chronic effects in aquatic ecosystems (Rodríguez-Gil et al. 2018; Dafouz et al. 2018; Di Lorenzo et al. 2019; Quadra et al. 2020).

Although not directly linked to public health, effects on aquatic ecosystems can affect humans for several reasons. When affecting primary or secondary producers, there is a tendency to imbalance the food chain, affecting edible organisms and directly affecting fish and mollusks, as previously mentioned. Caffeine may also lead to the loss of ecosystem services such as depuration or even affecting biogeochemical cycles, which are fundamental to biological processes. Therefore, despite the benefits to humans, higher concentrations in the environment bring risks that will undoubtedly affect human life. Thus, caffeine regulation goes beyond direct public health issues.

Applications to Other Areas of Addiction

Another critical point of discussion is whether caffeine consumption may increase the consumption of other addictive substances and vice versa. For example, a review study concluded that the relationship between caffeine and tobacco consumption is strong (Swanson et al. 1994). However, another review also found the same relationship, although it was more related to coffee consumption than caffeine itself, as the authors found no association between tobacco and tea consumption (Istvan and Matarazzo 1984). Phillips and Ogeil (2015) also reported the relationship between tobacco and caffeine consumption, but it was stronger in people with a propensity for depression, low self-esteem, or psychological distress. Another study performed in the Netherlands and the United Kingdom also showed a link between tobacco and caffeine consumption, concluding that each cigarette smoked per day represented an increase in 3.7 mg of caffeine consumption in the Netherlands and 8.4 mg in the United Kingdom (Treur et al. 2016). The behavioral or pharmacological effect may explain the relationship between caffeine and tobacco consumption: coffee-drinking is more common between inter-cigarette intervals, and smoking is more common immediately after coffee consumption (Emurian et al. 1982). However, it is unclear whether this stimulus to consumption is actually caused by the behavioral or pharmacological effect (Swanson et al. 1994).

Other authors proposed that the increase in stress and alcohol consumption is associated with a corresponding increase in both coffee and cigarette consumption (Conway et al. 1981). However, the relationship between caffeine and alcohol consumption is unclear. According to Klatsky et al. (1977), there was a decrease in caffeine consumption among people who frequently consume alcoholic beverages. On the other hand, Dawber et al. (1974) noted a positive relationship between coffee consumption (> six cups of coffee/day) and alcohol consumption by men. The result of the positive relationship was corroborated by Cameron and Boehmer (1982). Caffeine consumption, mainly through energy drinks, can increase alcohol consumption since energy drinks cause agitation and lead to higher alcohol consumption (Kuhns et al. 2010). Moreover, commonly consumed drinks are based on mixing some alcoholic beverages and energy drinks. There is a widespread belief that caffeine outweighs the adverse effects of alcohol and, therefore, they are consumed together (López-Cruz et al. 2013). However, caffeine and alcohol together may facilitate aggressive and violent actions (Kuhns et al. 2010). Thus, some factors favor the possibility of intoxication by alcohol and caffeine mixture, such as nightlife, acceptance of drunkenness, and legal and illegal drugs, especially in young people. However, to target and educate young people, more in-depth research must be done about the adverse effects of caffeine combined with other widely used substances.

Applications to Public Health

Although it is considered a safe substance and its consumption brings daily benefits to humankind, some precautions need to be taken with caffeine consumption. As already mentioned, high caffeine consumption may alter the function of cardiac, gastrointestinal, nervous, and renal systems (Leonard et al. 1987). Moreover, excessive caffeine intake may also cause psychiatric disorders, such as anxiety and sleep disorders (Winston et al. 2005). More than four cups of coffee a day can have adverse effects (FDA 2018; Mayo Clinic 2020). However, some populations are at a higher risk, such as reproductive-aged women and children (Ennis 2014; WHO 2021). For children and teenagers, some researchers believe that because brain and body development is still taking place, the risks of addiction, heightened agitation, and increased obesity in the future, mainly due to soft drink consumption, are real (Temple 2009). Moreover, caffeine has the potential to increase sleep and anxiety disorders in teenagers (Jee et al. 2020). However, it is difficult to generalize the results of the studies, which may even bring misinterpretations because the physical and mental condition dramatically influences how the substance interferes in the body (Rockett 2002). Thus, as caffeine can be considered a substance with the potential to cause addiction, the high consumption, the mixture with other addictive substances, and coupled consumption with medicines need to be taken into account for all consumers.

Mini-Dictionary of Terms

- **Addictive:** Dependence on something, usually a substance, which means it is difficult to stop doing or ingesting once started.
- **Carbonated drinks:** Beverages that contain dissolved carbon dioxide.
- **Fresh-brewed:** Something that is newly made. It is a type of coffee that is made using gravity where hot water dissolves the powder and then is filtered.
- **Methylxanthine:** A group of central nervous system stimulants.
- **Patterns:** A repeated arrangement.
- **Sensitive population:** People who are more vulnerable due to different factors and/or conditions, such as age, disease, pregnancy, among others.
- **Trends:** A direction of change or development, tendency to follow a certain way.

Key Facts of Caffeine Consumption Over Time

- The caffeine history starts in 1819 when a scientist isolated and named it. However, there are rumors that caffeine-based plants were discovered about 700,000 B.C and were used for pharmacological purposes.
- Caffeine is one of the most consumed psychoactive substances worldwide.
- Caffeine is present in several products not only in coffee, soft drinks, tea, and chocolates but also in medicines and personal care products.
- Caffeine consumption varies among age groups, in which adults and the elderly are the biggest consumers.
- Caffeine consumption also varies among regions, where ingestion through tea is more common in Africa, Asia, and the Pacific, through soda and energy drinks in Latin America and the Caribbean, and fresh-brewed coffee in North America.
- Caffeine meets some criteria to be considered a substance with the potential for addiction. Indeed, some studies pointed out caffeine dependence and abstinence, but the degree is lower than other drugs such as tobacco, alcohol, and cocaine.

- Moderate caffeine intake by adults (up to 400 mg/day) is not associated with negative effects.
- Some studies showed that caffeine consumption might have benefits, such as improving metabolic health, physical performance, and antioxidant system.
- Excessive coffee intake may cause psychiatric disorders, such as anxiety and sleep disorders, and cause side effects, such as headache, upset stomach, irritability, and fast heartbeat.
- Some studies found a positive correlation between caffeine consumption and tobacco and alcohol consumption.
- Assessing the risks and benefits of caffeine consumption is complex because several factors affect how the substance will act in the human body.

Summary Points

- Between 2000 and 2019, the global per capita coffee consumption increased about 37%.
- The Middle East and North Africa had the highest percentage of per capita coffee consumption increase in the last two decades.
- The upper middle-income countries had the highest percentage of per capita coffee consumption increase in the last two decades.
- Since 2000, Europe has shown the highest per capita coffee consumption, especially in Scandinavian countries.
- In 2010, Canada also showed a higher per capita coffee consumption.
- In 2019, in general, Europe showed a higher per capita coffee consumption compared to other continents.
- In Africa, only a few countries stand out with high per capita coffee consumption across the evaluated years (2000, 2010, and 2019).
- Caffeine can be considered a substance with the potential to cause addiction, and high consumption, the mixture with other addictive substances, and coupled consumption with medicines need precautions.
- More in-depth research is necessary about the adverse effects of caffeine, mainly considering the consumption coupled with other substances.

References

Ágoston C, Urbán R, Király O et al (2018) Why do you drink caffeine? The development of the motives for caffeine consumption questionnaire (MCCQ) and its relationship with gender, age and the types of caffeinated beverages. Int J Ment Heal Addict 16:981–999

Aguirre-Martínez GV, DelValls AT, Martín-Díaz ML (2015) Yes, caffeine, ibuprofen, carbamazepine, novobiocin and tamoxifen have an effect on *Corbicula fluminea* (Müller, 1774). Ecotoxicol Environ Saf 120:142–154

Barger-Lux MJ, Heaney RP, Stegman MR (1990) Effects of moderate caffeine intake on the calcium economy of premenopausal women. Am J Clin Nutr 52:722–725

Browne ML, Bell EM, Druschel CM et al (2007) Maternal caffeine consumption and risk of cardiovascular malformations. Birth Defects Res A Clin Mol Teratol 79:533–543

Bruton T, Alboloushi A, de la Garza B et al (2010) Fate of caffeine in the environment and Ecotoxicological considerations. In: Contaminants of emerging concern in the environment: ecological and human health considerations. American Chemical Society, Washington, DC, pp 257–273

Budney AJ, Brow PC, Griffiths RR et al (2013) Caffeine withdrawal and dependence: a convenience survey among addiction professionals. J Caffeine Res 3(2):67–71

Buerge II, Poiger T, Müller MD et al (2003) Caffeine, an anthropogenic marker for wastewater contamination of surface waters. Environ Sci Technol 37:691–700

Bunch AR, Bernot MJ (2011) Distribution of nonprescription pharmaceuticals in Central Indiana streams and effects on sediment microbial activity. Ecotoxicology 20:97–109

Camacho-Muñoz D, Martín J, Santos J et al (2012) Effectiveness of conventional and low-cost wastewater treatments in the removal of pharmaceutically active compounds. Water Air Soil Pollut 223:2611–2621

Cameron R, Boehmer J (1982) And coffee too. Int J Addict 17:569–574

Carrillo JA, Benitez J (2000) Clinically significant pharmacokinetic interactions between dietary caffeine and medications. Clin Pharmacokinet 39:127–153

Chei C, Loh JK, Soh A et al (2018) Coffee, tea, caffeine, and risk of hypertension: the Singapore Chinese health study. Eur J Nutr 57:1333–1342

Chen YH, Huang YH, Wen CC et al (2008) Movement disorder and neuromuscular change in zebrafish embryos after exposure to caffeine. Neurotoxicol Teratol 30:440–447

Coffee & Health. Guidelines on caffeine intake. https://www.coffeeandhealth.org/topic-overview/guidelines-on-caffeine-intake/. Accessed May 2021

Conway TL, Vickers RR Jr, Ward HW et al (1981) Occupational stress and variation in cigarette, coffee, and alcohol consumption. J Health Soc Behav 22:155–165

Cruz D, Almeida Â, Calisto V et al (2016) Caffeine impacts in the clam *Ruditapes philippinarum*: alterations on energy reserves, metabolic activity and oxidative stress biomarkers. Chemosphere 160:95–103

Dafouz R, Cáceres N, Rodríguez-Gil JL et al (2018) Does the presence of caffeine in the marine environment represent an environmental risk? A regional and global study. Sci Total Environ 615:632–642

Dawber TR, Kannel WB, Gordon T (1974) Coffee and cardiovascular disease: observations from the Framingham study. N Engl J Med 291:871–874

Del Rey ZR, Granek EF, Buckley BA (2011) Expression of HSP70 in *Mytilus californianus* following exposure to caffeine. Ecotoxicology 20:855

Di Lorenzo T, Castaño-Sánchez A, Di Marzio WD et al (2019) The role of freshwater copepods in the environmental risk assessment of caffeine and propranolol mixtures in the surface water bodies of Spain. Chemosphere 220:227–236

Diogo JS, Silva LS, Pena A et al (2013) Risk assessment of additives through soft drinks and nectars consumption on Portuguese population: a 2010 survey. Food Chem Toxicol 62:548–553

EFSA – European Food Safety Authority. Caffeine. https://www.efsa.europa.eu/sites/default/files/corporate_publications/files/efsaexplainscaffeine150527.pdf. Accessed May 2021

Emurian HH, Nellis MJ, Brady JV et al (1982) Event time-series relationship between cigarette smoking and coffee drinking. Addict Behav 7:441–444

Ennis D (2014) The effects of caffeine on health: the benefits outweigh the risks. Perspectives 6:2

Favrod-Coune T, Broers B (2021) Addiction to caffeine and other xanthines. In: El-Guebaly N, Carrà G, Galanter M et al (eds) Textbook of addiction treatment. Springer, Cham

FDA – U.S. Food & Drug Administration (2018) How much caffeine is too much? https://www.fda.gov/consumers/consumer-updates/spilling-beans-how-much-caffeine-too-much. Accessed May 2021

Frary CD, Johnson RK, Wang MQ (2005) Food sources and intakes of caffeine in the diets of persons in the United States. J Am Diet Assoc 105:110–113

George SE, Ramalakshmi K, Mohan Rao LJ (2008) A perception on health benefits of coffee. Crit Rev Food Sci Nutr 48:464–486

Gera M, Kalra S, Gupta P (2016) Caffeine intake among adolescents in Delhi. Ind J Commun Med 41:151–153

Gupta BS, Gupta U (1999) Caffeine and behavior: current views and research trends. CRC Press. Boca Raton, Florida, USA

Harvard T.H. Chan. School of Public Health. Caffeine. https://www.hsph.harvard.edu/nutritionsource/caffeine/. Accessed May 2021

International Coffee Organization. https://www.ico.org/new_historical.asp?section=Statistics. Accessed May 2021

Istvan J, Matarazzo J (1984) Tobacco, alcohol, and caffeine use: a review of their interrelationships. Psychol Bull 95:301–326

Jee HJ, Lee SG, Bormate KJ et al (2020) Effect of caffeine consumption on the risk for neurological and psychiatric disorders: sex differences in human. Nutrients 12:3080

Juliano LM, Griffiths RR (2004) A critical review of caffeine withdrawal: empirical validation of symptoms and signs, incidence, severity, and associated features. Psychopharmacology 176:1

Klatsky AL, Friedman GD, Siegelaub AB et al (1977) Alcohol consumption among white, black, or oriental men and women: Kaiser-Permanente multiphasic health examination data. Am J Epidemiol 105:311–323

Kuhns JB, Clodfelter TA, Bersot HY (2010) Examining and understanding the joint role of caffeine and alcohol in facilitating violent offending and victimization. Contemp Drug Probl 37:267–287

Lawrence JR, Zhu B, Swerhone GD et al (2012) Molecular and microscopic assessment of the effects of caffeine, acetaminophen, diclofenac, and their mixtures on river biofilm communities. Environ Toxicol Chem 31:508–517

Leonard TK, Watson RR, Mohs ME (1987) The effects of caffeine on various body systems: a review. J Am Diet Assoc 87:1048–1053

López-Cruz L, Salamone JD, Correa M (2013) The impact of caffeine on the behavioral effects of ethanol related to abuse and addiction: a review of animal studies. J Caffeine Res 3:9–21

Mayo Clinic (2020) Caffeine. https://www.mayoclinic.org/healthy-lifestyle/nutrition-and-healthy-eating/in-depth/caffeine/art-20045678. Accessed May 2021

Mitchell DC, Knight CA, Hockenberry J et al (2014) Beverage caffeine intakes in the US. Food Chem Toxicol 63:136–142

My Food Data. Top 10 food and drinks high in caffeine. https://www.myfooddata.com/articles/high-caffeine-foods-and-drinks.php#:~:text=High%20caffeine%20foods%20and%20drinkscaffeine%20is%20as%20an%20average. Accessed May 2021

Nawrot P, Jordan S, Eastwood J et al (2003) Effects of caffeine on human health. Food Addit Contam 20:1–30

Olsen NL (2013) Caffeine consumption habits and perceptions among University of new Hampshire students. Honors Theses Capstones 103:1–68

Phillips JG, Ogeil R (2015) Decision-making style, nicotine and caffeine use and dependence. Hum Psychopharmacol Clin Exp 30:442–450

Pourshahidi LK, Navarini L, Petracco M et al (2016) A comprehensive overview of the risks and benefits of coffee consumption. Compr Rev Food Sci Food Saf 15:671–684

Price KR, Fligner DJ (1990) Treatment of caffeine toxicity with esmolol. Ann Emerg Med 19: 44–46

Qi H, Li S (2013) Dose-response meta-analysis on coffee, tea and caffeine consumption with risk of Parkinson's disease. Geriatr Gerontol Int 14:430–439

Quadra GR, Paranaíba JR, Vilas-Boas J et al (2020) A global trend of caffeine consumption over time and related-environmental impacts. Environ Pollut 256:113343

Reyes CM, Cornelis MC (2018) Caffeine in the diet: country-level consumption and guidelines. Nutrients 10:1772

Rockett I (2002) Caffeine "addiction" in high school youth: evidence of an adverse health relationship. Addict Res Theory 10:31–42

Rodríguez-Gil JL, Cáceres N, Dafouz R et al (2018) Caffeine and paraxanthine in aquatic systems: global exposure distributions and probabilistic risk assessment. Sci Total Environ 612: 1058–1071
Rosi-Marshall EJ, Kincaid DW, Bechtold HA et al (2013) Pharmaceuticals suppress algal growth and microbial respiration and alter bacterial communities in stream biofilms. Ecol Appl 23:583–593
RStudio Team. RStudio: Integrated Development for R (2020) RStudio. PBC, Boston. http://www.rstudio.com/
Satel S (2006) Is caffeine addictive? A review of the literature. Am J Drug Alcohol Abuse 32: 493–502
Steele WB, Mole RA, Brooks BW (2018) Experimental protocol for examining behavioral response profiles in larval fish: application to the neuro-stimulant caffeine. J Vis Exp 137:57938
Strauch G, Möder M, Wennrich R et al (2008) Indicators for assessing anthropogenic impact on urban surface and groundwater. J Soils Sediments 8:23–33
Swanson JA, Lee JW, Hopp JW (1994) Caffeine and nicotine: a review of their joint use and possible interactive effects in tobacco withdrawal. Addict Behav 19:229–256
Tang-Liu D, Williams R, Riegelman S (1983) Disposition of caffeine and its metabolites in man. J Pharmacol Exp Ther 224:180–185
Temple JL (2009) Caffeine use in children: what we know, what we have left to learn, and why we should worry. Neurosci Biobehav Rev 33:793–806
Thomas PM, Foster GD (2005) Tracking acidic pharmaceuticals, caffeine, and triclosan through the wastewater treatment process. Environ Toxicol Chem Int J 24:25–30
Treur JL, Taylor AE, Ware JJ et al (2016) Associations between smoking and caffeine consumption in two European cohorts. Addiction 111:1059–1068
Weinberg BA, Bealer BK (2019) The world of caffeine: the science and culture of the world's most popular drug. Routledge, New York and London
WHO. World Health Organization (2016) WHO recommendations on antenatal care for a positive pregnancy experience. World Health Organization
WHO. World Health Organization. Restricting caffeine intake during pregnancy. https://www.who.int/elena/titles/caffeine-pregnancy/en/. Accessed May 2021
Winkelmayer WC, Stampfer MJ, Willett WC et al (2005) Habitual caffeine intake and the risk of hypertension in women. JAMA 294:2330–2335
Winston AP, Hardwick E, Jaberi N (2005) Neuropsychiatric effects of caffeine. Adv Psychiatr Treat 11:432–439
World Bank. https://data.worldbank.org/. Accessed May 2021

List of Useful Website

Canva: https://www.canva.com/
Coffee & Health: https://www.coffeeandhealth.org/
European Food Safety Authority: https://www.efsa.europa.eu/
Harvard T.H. Chan. School of Public Health: https://www.hsph.harvard.edu/
International Coffee Organization: https://www.ico.org/
Mayo Clinic: https://www.mayoclinic.org/
My Food Data: https://www.myfooddata.com/
R Team: http://www.rstudio.com/
Simple maps: https://simplemaps.com/data/world-cities
U.S. Food & Drug Administration: https://www.fda.gov/
World Bank: https://www.worldbank.org/en/home
World Health Organization: https://www.who.int/

Caffeine and Alcohol

72

Beyond Commonplaces Suggested by the Presence of Caffeine in Energy Drinks

Laura Dazzi, Alessandra T. Peana, Rossana Migheli, Riccardo Maccioni, Romina Vargiu, Biancamaria Baroli, Elio Acquas, and Valentina Bassareo

Contents

Introduction 1554
Alcohol's Pharmacological and Toxicological Profile 1555
Caffeine's Pharmacological and Toxicological Profile 1556
Preclinical Studies 1556
Energy Drinks 1557
AMED and Its Consequences 1560
Applications to Other Areas of Addiction 1562

L. Dazzi · R. Maccioni · B. Baroli
Department of Life and Environmental Sciences, University of Cagliari, Cagliari, Italy
e-mail: laura.dazzi@unica.it; bbaroli@unica.it

A. T. Peana
Department of Chemistry and Pharmacy, University of Sassari, Sassari, Italy
e-mail: apeana@uniss.it

R. Migheli
Department of Experimental Medical and Surgical Sciences, University of Sassari, Sassari, Italy
e-mail: rmigheli@uniss.it

R. Vargiu
Department of Biomedical Sciences, University of Cagliari, Cagliari, Italy
e-mail: rvargiu@unica.it

E. Acquas (✉)
Department of Life and Environmental Sciences, Center of Excellence for the Study of Neurobiology of Addiction, University of Cagliari, Cagliari, Italy
e-mail: acquas@unica.it

V. Bassareo
Department of Biomedical Sciences and Center of Excellence for the Study of Neurobiology of Addiction, University of Cagliari, Cagliari, Italy
e-mail: bassareo@unica.it

V. B. Patel, V. R. Preedy (eds.), *Handbook of Substance Misuse and Addictions*,
https://doi.org/10.1007/978-3-030-92392-1_79

Applications to Other Areas of Public Health 1566
Mini-Dictionary of Terms 1566
Summary Points 1567
References 1568

Abstract

The mixed consumption of caffeinated and alcoholic beverages, both characterized by high concentrations of their psychopharmacologically active constituents, has recently seen, in particular in adolescents and young adults, an impressive boost characterized by a binge-like drinking behavior aimed at obtaining higher levels of alcohol intoxication. This rise of dysregulated consumption, grounded on the fallacious belief that caffeine might reduce the sedative and locomotor impairing effects of high alcohol intake, overall increases the intrinsic potential of alcohol to induce addiction and promote other negative consequences on health directly related to such excessive intake. Moreover, both caffeine and alcohol are endowed with known biphasic effects, and the consequences of their interactions may strictly depend on several factors including doses and modalities of consumption. Although several preclinical studies confirmed the ability of caffeinated and alcoholic drinks to influence each other's effects, their results remain highly inconclusive. In fact, these studies have been mainly focused on characterizing the effects of the interaction between alcohol and the main ingredient of energy drinks, caffeine, and did not take into consideration that energy drinks are extremely variable in their caffeine's content and also include other psychopharmacologically active ingredients. The present chapter takes the challenge to synthetically present a critical perspective on the lights and shadows of preclinical evidence on this critical topic that is related to potentially serious implications on public health.

Keywords

Adenosine receptors · Alcohol · Alcoholic beverages · Alcohol mixed energy drinks (AMED) · Binge-like drinking · Caffeine · Energy drinks · Gateway effect

Introduction

Caffeine and alcohol, two chemicals that share ancient roots and a significant presence in the development of human civilization, somehow compete for the reputation of being the most consumed psychopharmacologically active substance in the world (Morgan et al. 2013). Caffeine and alcohol also share the property of being endowed with complex, not univocal, pharmacological profiles. These, at least in part, are characterized by the property of being grounded on different mechanisms of action depending on the dose, the molecular target, and the biological site (Lê et al. 2001; Nehlig et al. 1992). The present chapter is devoted to characterizing, in the perspective of the potential drawbacks on individuals' and public health, the consequences of caffeine's and alcohol's interaction following combined or mixed consumption. In this regard, it appears critical to point out that both substances are freely available, cheap, and unanimously overall well tolerated and represent, at least in Western and civilized countries, a substantial part of eating habits. This apparently trivial, but also obvious and common to both substances', property urges clinicians, as well as neurobiologists, to pay increasingly higher attention to the modalities and consequences associated with their combined use. Last but not least, it is worth mentioning that the above twinning between caffeine and alcohol finds its issue of divergence in the literature on their addictive potential: while, in fact, there is a general consensus on the addictive potential of alcohol (Witkiewitz et al. 2019), this does not apply to caffeine that, despite some attempts, still lacks of being included in the list of addictive substances (Heinz et al. 2020). Alcohol's abnormal/heavy consumption itself has been related, besides addiction (alcohol use disorder, AUD), to several serious issues, and indeed it may act as the Trojan horse responsible for many other serious negative consequences that impact mainly on the liver and the cardiovascular system (Axley et al. 2019; Rehm et al. 2017). On the other hand, as it will be discussed below, an uncontrolled heavy intake of caffeine, relatively common in energy drink consumers, may cause serious cardiovascular problems (Whayne 2015). Thus, alcohol, due to its addictive profile, may trigger its abnormal/heavy consumption and therefore be responsible for serious individual and public health problems (Abrahao et al. 2017); on the other hand, caffeine, although being devoid of addictive properties, may self-promote its excessive consumption because of its mood and attention enhancer profile (Nehlig et al. 1992). Their mixed consumption may be promoted by the fallacious belief that at high volumes energy drinks may reduce the sedative and locomotor impairing effects of high alcohol intake, hence being responsible for many undesired effects (Ferreira et al. 2006). The present chapter is intended to go beyond the short pharmacological and toxicological characterization of both substances described in the following paragraphs, in order to focus on their interaction with a perspective free of the bias that presently envisions the consumption of high amounts of caffeinated beverages (energy drinks) as a costless strategy to increase the intake of alcoholic drinks.

Alcohol's Pharmacological and Toxicological Profile

Alcohol's molecule, due to its small size and amphiphilicity, easily crosses any biological membranes reaching every district in the body exerting both peripheral and central effects. Alcohol's effects are dose-dependent and range from behavioral stimulation and euphory to deep sedation (up to coma) with a wide range of intermediate conditions involving the motivational (Gilpin and Koob 2008), motor (Harrison et al. 2017), cognitive (Spear 2016), mnemonic (Spear 2016), and vital functions' (Vonghia et al. 2008) domains, whose detailed description is outside the scope of the present chapter. The acute and chronic assumption of alcohol also induces several peripheral effects including hypothermia (Vonghia et al. 2008), diuresis (due to inhibition of vasopressin secretion), gastric and salivary secretion, arrhythmias (extension of QT interval), liver (cirrhosis and fibrosis), and pancreatic damages (Mihic et al. 2017). Moreover, alcohol is classified as a type 1 carcinogenic compound and represents a direct causal factor of liver cancer and a risk factor for mouth, throat, larynx esophageal, and gut cancer (Mihic et al. 2017).

Caffeine's Pharmacological and Toxicological Profile

Caffeine is mostly known as a central and peripheral stimulant. Its pharmacological actions are attributable to its ability to antagonize adenosine's A1 and A2A receptors and to inhibit phosphodiesterases, thus activating intracellular calcium mobilization (Nehlig et al. 1992). Peripheral caffeine's pharmacological actions extend from the stimulation of fat degradation during lipolysis to the increase in aortic pressure and respiratory frequency (Nehlig et al. 1992). Caffeine's central stimulating effects include increased arousal, alertness, and attention and facilitation of the wake state and of cognitive function (Nehlig et al. 1992).

Preclinical Studies

In the last years, a growing number of publications have focused on evaluating the effect of the coadministration of caffeine and alcohol, in the attempt to demonstrate the ability of caffeine to antagonize some of alcohol's pharmacological actions (for review, see Lopez-Cruz et al. 2013). However, the studies, rather than clarifying the interaction between the two drugs, yielded conflicting results. Accordingly, while some data suggested that caffeine is able to (i) potentiate the increase in locomotor activity induced by low doses of alcohol (Waldeck 1974; Sudakov et al. 2003; Hilbert et al. 2013; Lopez-Cruz et al. 2013), (ii) abolish the stimulant effect of higher doses (Lopez-Cruz et al. 2013), (iii) attenuate the motor impairment induced by alcohol (Connole et al. 2004), (iv) increase alertness and reduce the sedative effect of alcohol (El Yacoubi et al. 2003), and (v) reduce the alcohol-induced memory impairments (Spinetta et al. 2008) and its anxiolytic effect (Gulick and Gould 2009; Prediger et al. 2004), others showed either no effects or a potentiating action of caffeine on alcohol-induced effects (Dar et al. 1987). The data appear even more confusing when it comes to evaluating the ability of caffeine to modulate alcohol intake (Lopez-Cruz et al. 2013; Fernandes et al. 2020). While some studies have shown that caffeine increases the intake of an alcoholic solution at low doses but fails to elicit the same effect at higher doses (Kunin et al. 2000), others suggested that high doses of caffeine can reduce alcohol intake (Rezvani et al. 2013). Moreover, some of them failed to show any modulatory action of caffeine on alcohol intake (Fernandes et al. 2020; Carvalho et al. 2012).

These conflicting results arise from the profound differences in the protocols used (forced vs. voluntary alcohol or caffeine intake), in the doses of caffeine administered (low, moderate or high), in the type of administration (acute vs. chronic) of both alcohol and caffeine, and finally in the gender and strain of rats or mice used in the experiments.

Moreover, many of these most recent studies were inspired by the clinical observation of the increasing habit, mostly by adolescents and young adults, of consuming high doses of caffeine through the ingestion of high volumes of energy drinks. Notably, as it will be pointed out elsewhere in this chapter, energy drinks do not contain just caffeine, and, unfortunately, these studies did not take into account that caffeine is not the only psychoactive ingredient of energy drinks. In fact, other substances such as taurine and guaranà extracts, among others, are able to modify alcohol-induced effects per se (de Sanctis et al. 2017; Tarragon et al. 2021).

Energy Drinks

Energy drinks are caffeinated beverages that, in the last decade, have become very popular among adolescents and young adults (Degirmenci et al. 2018; Mansour et al. 2019) for their stimulant effects and performance-enhancing properties, which are claimed to be beneficial for high school and university students, athletes, and people who need to have the maximum efficiency for as long as needed (up to many hours) (Fig. 1).

The stimulant effects of energy drinks depend on their high concentration of caffeine and sucrose and on the presence of taurine and various B vitamins, such as nicotinamide, pyridoxine, and riboflavin, as well as ginseng and guaranà seed extracts (Aranda and Morlock 2006; Iyadurai and Chung 2007). The composition of these beverages and the ease of obtaining them promote their use and abuse and,

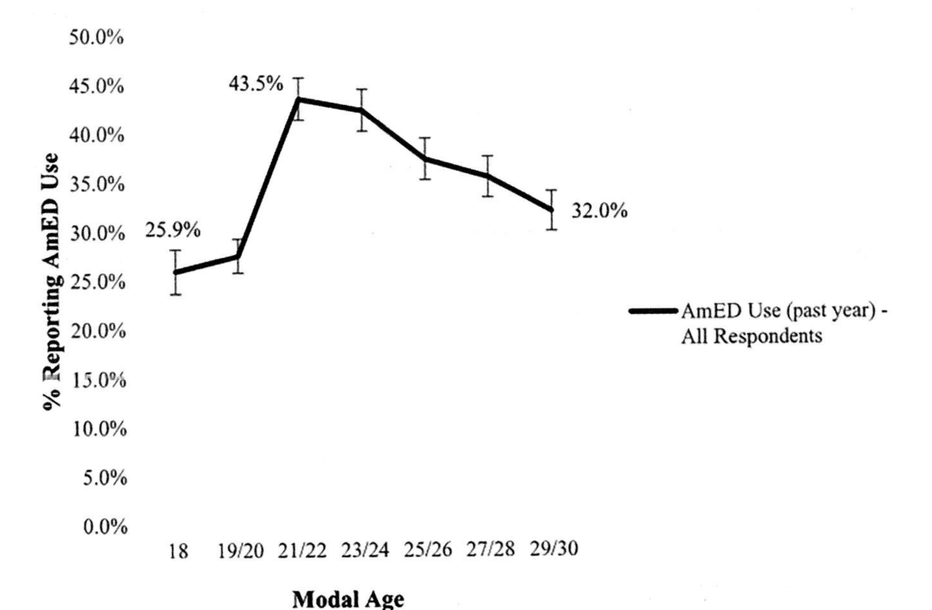

Fig. 1 Overall prevalence of past 12-month AMED use from modal ages 18 to 29/30. Note: N (unwtd) = 2222. Percentages were calculated using attrition weights. 95% confidence intervals are based on standard errors obtained using Taylor linearization. (Reproduced under permission (Elsevier license number: 5126420261718) from Patrick et al. (2018))

due to the high concentrations of caffeine and taurine, increase the diffusion of their negative effects on the central nervous system (CNS) and cardiovascular system. A robust literature of epidemiological studies and case reports demonstrate that energy drink consumption induces cerebral vasculopathy (Worrall et al. 2005), acute mania (Machado-Vieira et al. 2001; Quadri et al. 2018), epileptic seizures (Iyadurai and Chung 2007; Calabrò et al. 2012), coronary artery vasospasm (Wilson et al. 2012), and severe cardiac arrest or myocardial ischemia (Berger and Alford 2009; Lippi et al. 2016). On the other hand, very few preclinical studies on animals have been reported on this topic. Recently, Vargiu et al. (2021) published an original study on the effect of the chronic consumption, during adolescence, of Red Bull, a known energy drink, on mesocortical and mesolimbic dopamine transmission (Fig. 2) and cardiovascular system (Fig. 3) in adult rats. Authors of this study found that chronic

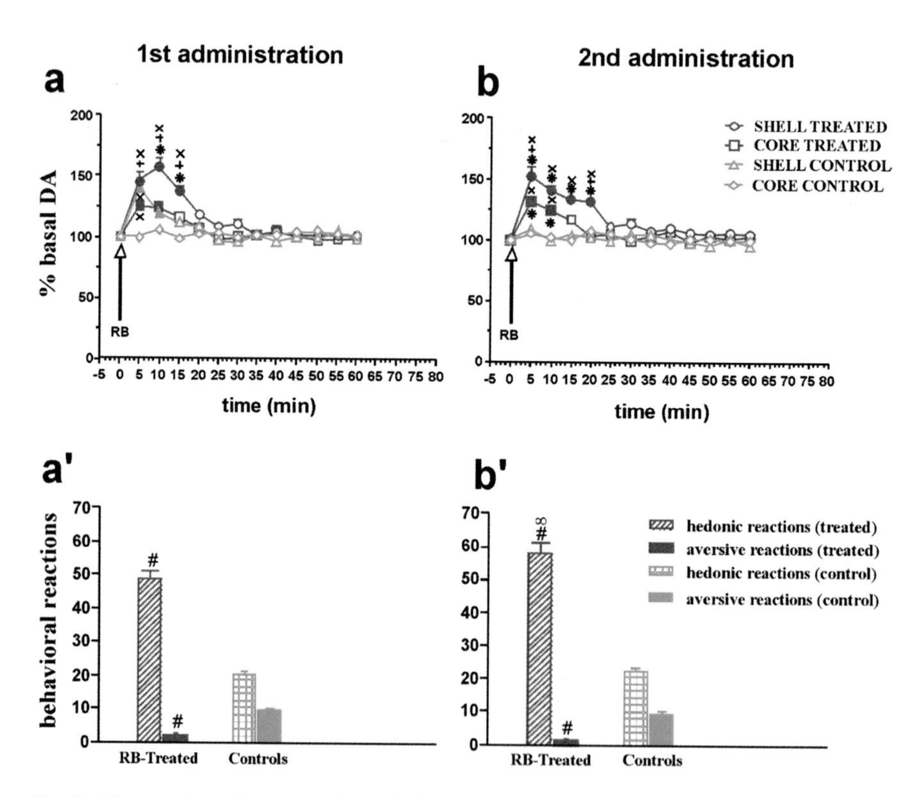

Fig. 2 Changes in nucleus accumbens shell and core dialysate dopamine after two subsequent intraoral administrations of Red Bull (RB) (2 mL) in Red Bull-treated and control rats. The figure also shows the score of hedonic and aversive taste reactions during intraoral Red Bull infusion. (**a** and **b**): Dopamine transmission. Filled symbols indicate $p < 0.001$ vs. basal values; $^{*}p < 0.05$ vs. dopamine responsiveness in the shell of control rats; $^{+}p < 0.05$ vs. dopamine responsiveness in the core of Red Bull-treated rats; $p < 0.05$ vs. DA responsiveness in the core of control rats. Statistical analysis: four-way ANOVA. (**a**′ and **b**′): Taste reactions: $^{\#}p < 0.001$ vs. control rats; $^{\infty}p < 0.001$ vs. first administration. Statistical analysis: two-way ANOVA. (Reproduced under a Creative Commons CC BY 4.0 license from Vargiu et al. (2021))

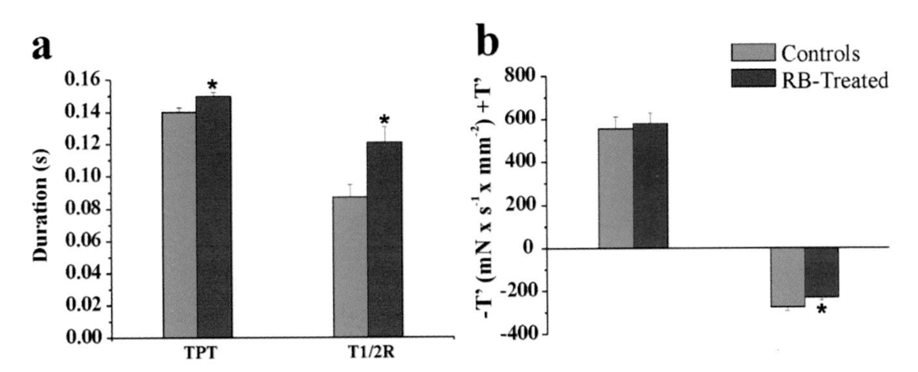

Fig. 3 Isometric contractility indices in controls and Red Bull (RB)-treated LVPMs (left ventricular papillary muscle). (**a**) TPT, time to peak tension, and $T_{1/2}$ R, half-time of relaxation. (**b**) +T′, peak rate of tension rise, and -T′, peak rate of tension fall. Values are expressed as the mean ± SEM; $^{*}p < 0.05$. Statistical analysis: Student's t-test. (Reproduced under a Creative Commons CC BY 4.0 license from Vargiu et al. (2021))

voluntary intake of elevated amounts of Red Bull from adolescence to adulthood increases dopamine release in the nucleus accumbens shell, an important cerebral area involved in the rewarding mechanisms and in the responsiveness to drugs of abuse (Di Chiara et al. 2004). Notably, after such Red Bull repeated administration, dopamine transmission in the nucleus accumbens shell was affected with a non-adaptive increase, a mechanism similar to that observed after repeated administration of drugs of abuse (Bassareo et al. 2003; Lecca et al. 2006a, b, 2007a, b; Bassareo et al. 2017). These results may explain the capability of energy drinks, such as Red Bull, to induce, mostly in adolescents, their compulsive intake. Furthermore, Vargiu et al. (2021) reported that chronic Red Bull consumption in rats maintained at rest had no effect on heart rate and increased systolic and diastolic blood pressure and the double product (systolic blood pressure multiplied by the pulse rate), indicating an overall increased cardiac workload. In addition, long-term Red Bull treatment induced early and hidden papillary contractility impairment. In conclusion, the authors of this study suggest that the pressor effects of chronic Red Bull treatment appear to be due to vascular effects rather than to increased cardiac contractility.

Moreover, the side effects of energy drinks on the CNS and cardiovascular system are increasing as a result of the trend to mix them with alcohol (spirits) and fruit juice to obtain palatable cocktails. In fact, this mix may potentiate the adverse effects observed in the nervous, cardiovascular, and gastrointestinal systems (Munteanu et al. 2018). These authors studied the long-term effects of Red Bull intake, alone or in combination with alcohol, on the ventricular myocardium of rats and reported that the morphological and ultrastructural alterations induced by the energy drinks in the cardiac muscle, such as enlarged intermyofibrillar spaces and disrupted cristae of mitochondria, were very similar to those produced by alcohol consumption and by the mix of energy drinks and alcohol in Wistar rats. Moreover, several studies investigated the effect of the consumption of energy drinks in combination with alcohol and showed that energy drinks significantly reduce the immediate effects of alcoholic intoxication, which may lead to an increased consumption of alcoholic drinks (Arria et al. 2011). In this regard, Ferreira et al. (2006) reported that, when combined with alcohol, Red Bull attenuates the perception of alcoholic intoxication.

The intake of energy drinks and alcoholic beverages (alcohol mixed energy drinks, AMED), above all in adolescents and young adults, may promote a binge-like modality of assumption in the attempt to drink alcohol for longer and achieve higher levels of intoxication.

Repeated exposure to alcohol during adolescence also increases motivation for its consumption (Spear 2018; Volkow et al. 2010). Finally, a further point of concern is that adolescents who frequently consume energy drinks are exposed to a higher risk of alcohol abuse and use of illegal drugs (Arria et al. 2010, 2017; Terry-McElrath et al. 2014; Woolsey et al. 2014) as well as to a lower perception of the risk of using them (Jackson and Leal 2018). These studies strengthen the argument in support of the inclusion of energy drinks in the gateway hypothesis (Figs. 6 and 7) (Galimov et al. 2020).

AMED and Its Consequences

Epidemiological studies from different countries reported that the habit to mix energy drinks with alcohol is becoming widespread especially among adolescents, often underage (Curran and Marczinski 2017) (Fig. 1). This habit is four times more frequent among college students, with 30–40% of them reporting using AMED at least once a month (Mallett et al. 2015; Patrick et al. 2018). This rise in AMED consumption is accompanied by an increase in alcohol-related problems, and in the admissions to the emergency department of individuals with a high level of intoxication after AMED consumption (Substance Abuse and Mental Health Service Administration, Center for Behavioral Health Statistics and Quality 2013), and in the AMED-related calls to poison control centers. Therefore, in 2010, the Food and Drug Administration prohibited the sale of the premixed combination of energy drinks and alcohol in the USA. However, the availability of energy drinks and alcohol allows the consumers to prepare their own mix. As a consequence, the percentage of people consuming AMED continues to increase (Curran and Marczinski 2017).

Several studies reported the higher association of AMED with risky behaviors such as driving while drunk, getting involved in bars' fights, or engaging in unprotected sex (Mallett et al. 2014, 2015; Miller 2012; Thombs et al. 2010). Snipes and Benotsch (2013) also reported higher consumption of illicit drugs in AMED users than in alcohol-only consumers. Survey studies indicate that AMED consumers are more likely to be young adults (between 15 and 23 years old), male, and higher alcohol and illicit drug consumers with respect to AMED nonusers (Marczinski and Fillmore 2014) (Fig. 4). The difficulty in finding a positive statistical correlation between AMED consumption and engagement in risky behavior, however, has led some authors to suggest that the association might be due to a more impulsive attitude of AMED consumers that makes them, with respect to the general

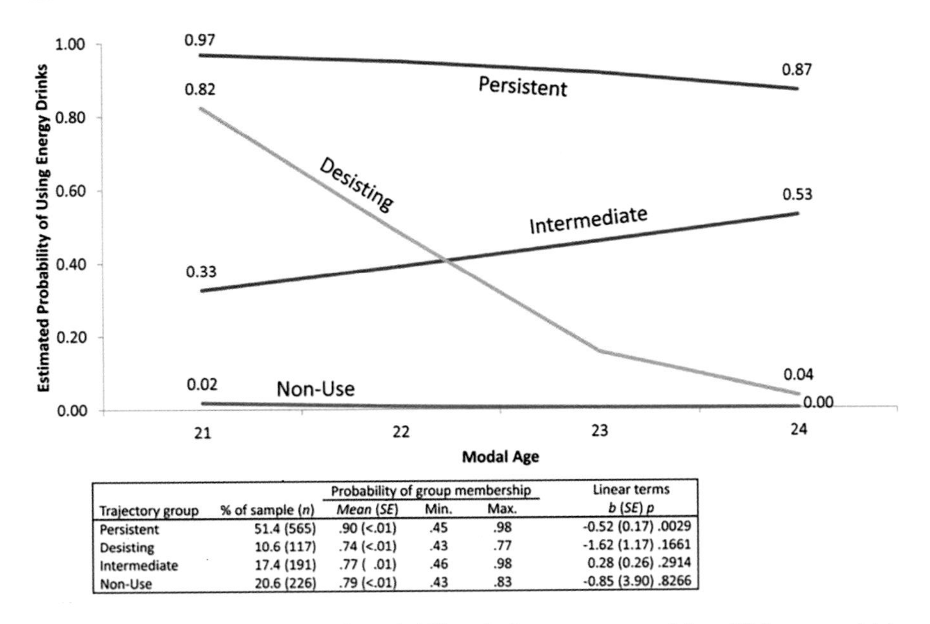

Trajectory group	% of sample (n)	Probability of group membership Mean (SE)	Min.	Max.	Linear terms b (SE) p
Persistent	51.4 (565)	.90 (<.01)	.45	.98	-0.52 (0.17) .0029
Desisting	10.6 (117)	.74 (<.01)	.43	.77	-1.62 (1.17) .1661
Intermediate	17.4 (191)	.77 (.01)	.46	.98	0.28 (0.26) .2914
Non-Use	20.6 (226)	.79 (<.01)	.43	.83	-0.85 (3.90) .8266

Fig. 4 Estimated marginal means for probability of substance use at modal age 25, by energy drink trajectory group membership ($n = 863$). Note: Results adjusted for the effects of gender, race, parents' education, sensation-seeking, other caffeine consumption, and the corresponding substance use measure at modal age 21. Matching pairs of superscripted letters denote statistically significant differences in probability of a given substance use outcome ($p < 0.05$). A significant difference in NPA is reported between the Desisting and Intermediate groups, but the overall $\chi 2$ for the trajectory group variable did not attain statistical significance in that model ($p = 0.051$). AUD, alcohol use disorder; NPS, nonmedical use of prescription stimulants; NPA, nonmedical use of prescription analgesics. (Reproduced under permission (Elsevier license number: 5126960494376) from Arria et al. (2017))

population, more likely to engage in risky behaviors (Verster et al. 2018). Arria and coworkers (Arria et al. 2011) conducted a longitudinal study in a cohort of college students in the USA, concluding that heavier energy drink consumers were at significantly greater risk for alcohol-related problems and to develop alcohol dependence confirming previous findings by other authors (Miller 2008a, b).

The vast majority of survey data indicate that young people mix energy drinks with alcohol to mask some of the sedative effects of alcohol (Marczinski and Fillmore 2014), reduce the feeling of drunkenness, and consume higher doses of alcohol, thus accelerating and prolonging the drinking episode (Arria et al. 2011). Energy drinks may thus increase alcohol assimilation, reduce the time to reach drunkenness, and at the same time reduce alcohol-induced sedation (Thombs et al. 2011). However, even though AMED consumers might perceive themselves as less intoxicated, the association between energy drinks and alcohol does not reduce the breath alcohol concentration (BRAC) nor the alteration in motor coordination induced by alcohol intake (Ferreira et al. 2006; Marczinski and Fillmore 2006). An example of this aberrant perception is the condition, known as "wide-awake drunkenness," thought to be responsible for most of the risky behavior in which AMED consumers engage, in the wrong belief to be able to function normally.

Results derived from the surveys on the effect of AMED might lack accuracy when it comes to ascertaining the exact amount of substances taken, whether the consumption of energy drinks and alcohol was contemporaneous or not, and the objective measure of motor coordination after AMED intake. To overcome the possible confounding data, surveys and field work have been reproduced in the lab, where these variables can be more easily controlled. Laboratory studies in humans allowed to randomly assign participants to different experimental groups and, more importantly, to conduct a within-subject design testing where each subject was evaluated for every condition (Marczinski and Fillmore 2014). The results confirmed the findings from survey studies and indicated that AMED reduced the sedative effect of alcohol but did not modify the objective alteration in motor coordination (Marczinski et al. 2011). They also showed that energy drinks augment the priming effect of a low dose of alcohol, increasing the desire for more alcohol (Marczinski et al. 2011).

As described in previous paragraphs, animal studies have been more focused on the effect of the mixed administration of alcohol with caffeine (for review, see Lopez-Cruz et al. 2013), showing that caffeine is able to potentiate the increase in locomotor activity induced by low doses of alcohol and to abolish the stimulant effect of higher doses (Waldeck 1974; Sudakov et al. 2003; Hilbert et al. 2013; Lopez-Cruz et al. 2013); attenuates the motor impairment induced by alcohol (Connole et al. 2004); increases alertness and reduces the sedative effect of alcohol (El Yacoubi et al. 2003); reduces the alcohol-induced memory impairments (Spinetta et al. 2008); and has anxiolytic effects (Gulick and Gould 2009; Prediger et al. 2004). More recently (Porru et al. 2020), caffeine has been shown to antagonize the ability of alcohol to induce conditioned place preference and place aversion.

However, while being the main component of energy drinks, caffeine is not the only one (de Sanctis et al. 2017). Most of the other components – taurine, ginseng, guarana, and sugar – have the ability to interfere with the rewarding and stimulating effects of alcohol alone (de Sanctis et al. 2017; Tarragon et al. 2021), and the effect of their combination should be taken into consideration.

Applications to Other Areas of Addiction

In this chapter, we reviewed the literature to shed light on the different influences of energy drinks and caffeine intake on alcohol pharmacological effects.

Laboratory studies in humans report that AMED augments the priming effect of a low dose of alcohol, increasing the desire for more alcohol and reducing its sedative effect but failing to modify alcohol's induced objective alteration of motor coordination. This fact makes AMED consumers prone to engage in risky behaviors, such as driving while drunk. The association between energy drinks and alcohol seems to promote alcohol intake facilitating the onset of its addiction as well as of dependence on other licit and illicit behaviors and compounds such as

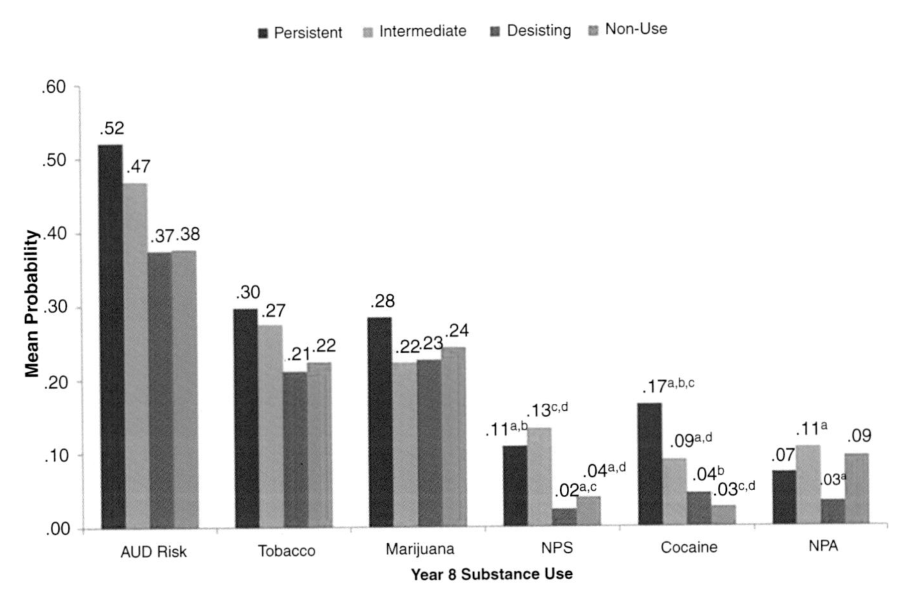

Fig. 5 Estimated marginal means for probability of substance use at modal age 25, by energy drink trajectory group membership (n = 863). Note: Results adjusted for the effects of gender, race, parents' education, sensation-seeking, other caffeine consumption, and the corresponding substance use measure at modal age 21. Matching pairs of superscripted letters denote statistically significant differences in probability of a given substance use outcome ($p < 0.05$). A significant difference in NPA is reported between the Desisting and Intermediate groups, but the overall chi-square for the trajectory group variable did not attain statistical significance in that model ($p = 0.051$). AUD, alcohol use disorder; NPS, nonmedical use of prescription stimulants; NPA, nonmedical use of prescription analgesics. (Reproduced under permission (Elsevier license number: 5126960494376) from Arria et al. (2017))

cigarette smoking and the use of tranquilizers, sleeping pills, and painkillers (Benkert and Abel 2020) (Fig. 5). Moreover, energy drinks are caffeinated beverages containing not only high concentrations of caffeine but also other psychoactive ingredients such as taurine and guaranà extract. Thus, it should be constantly kept in mind that data from studies on the interaction between caffeine and alcohol cannot be used to make inferences on the consequences of the interactions between energy drink and alcoholic beverage consumption and, of course, also the other way round. Thus, it appears that this topic needs to be addressed with clear experimental designs and a rigorous approach to allow collecting meaningful and translationally valuable data. As an example, of the return from such an approach, by analyzing the studies on the combined administration of caffeine with alcohol, we recently observed that caffeine, at low, pharmacologically meaningful doses, prevents alcohol-elicited associative learning and/or alcohol's reinforcing properties by antagonizing the ability of alcohol to induce place conditioning, a validated preclinical model to assess the reinforcing properties of drugs and predict their ability to transfer their motivational value to unconditioned

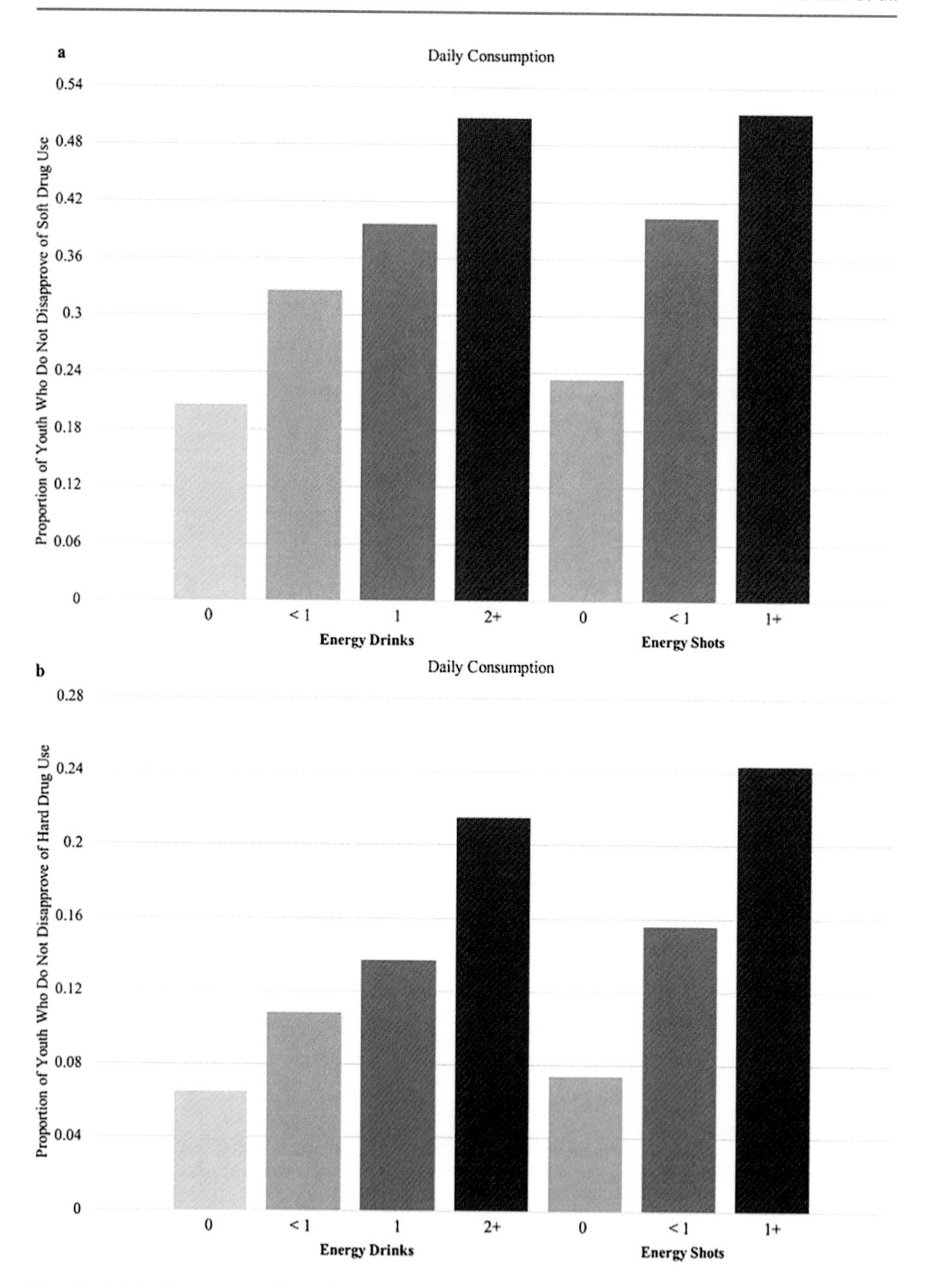

Fig. 6 (**a**) Daily consumption of energy drinks/shots and the proportion of youth who do not disapprove of soft drug use. (**b**) Daily consumption of energy drinks/shots and the proportion of youth who do not disapprove of hard drug use. (Reproduced under permission (Elsevier license number: 5126971336393) from Jackson and Leal (2018))

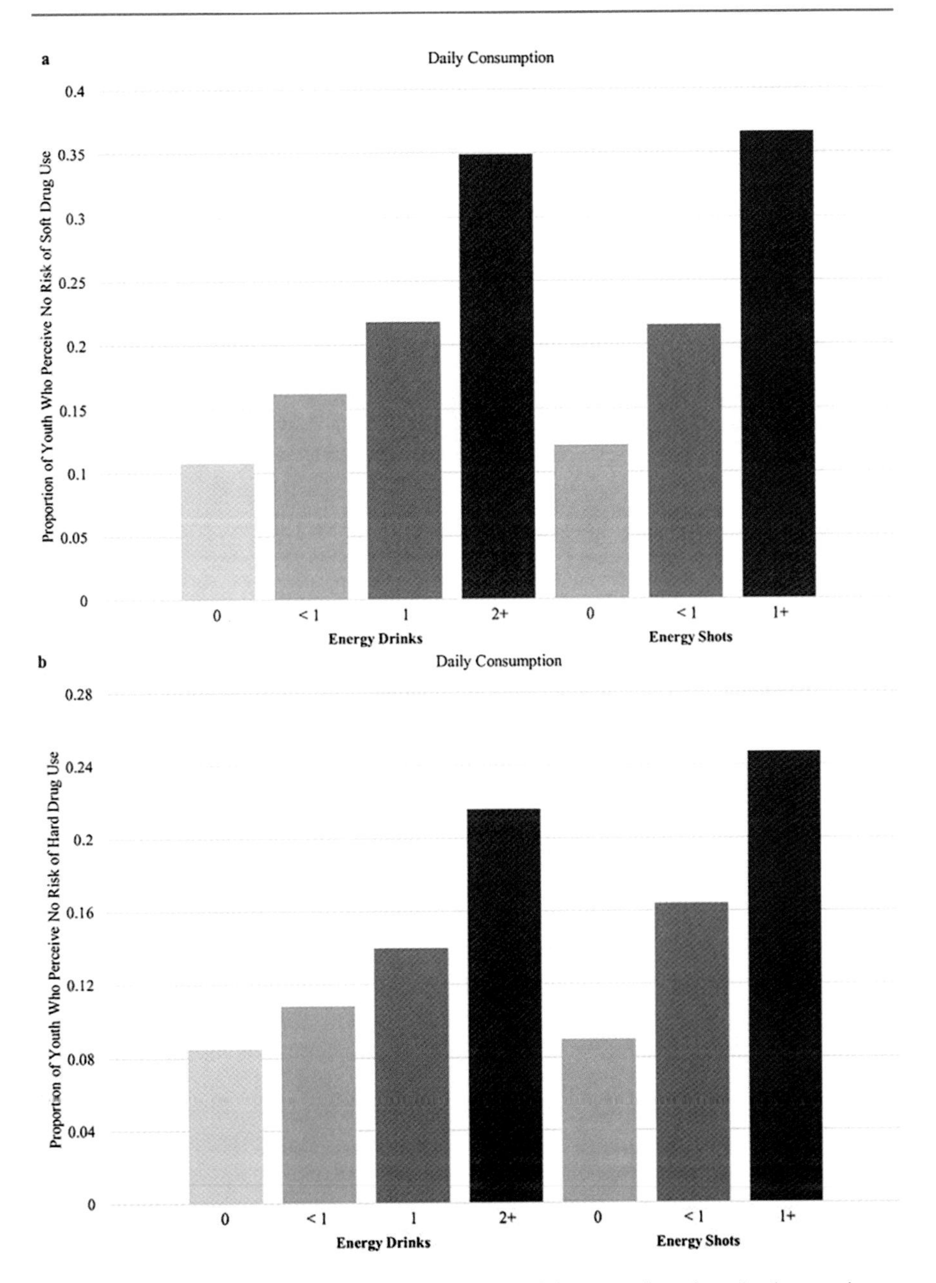

Fig. 7 (**a**) Daily consumption of energy drinks/shots and the proportion of youth who perceive no risk of *soft* drug use. (**b**) Daily consumption of energy drinks/shots and the proportion of youth who perceive no risk of *hard* drug use. (Reproduced under permission (Elsevier license number: 5126971336393) from Jackson and Leal (2018))

environmental stimuli (Porru et al. 2020). In other words, experimental evidence suggests that caffeine, given alone, is able to interfere with some alcohol's actions that may play an important role in the development of alcohol dependence. Thus, although further studies, strictly controlled in terms of all critical variables (doses, timing, modalities of the administrations) involved, are necessary to deepen some aspects of caffeine properties on alcohol effects, we are encouraged to conclude that caffeine could prove to be a valuable tool in the fight against some phases (acquisition, development) of alcohol addiction (Figs. 6 and 7).

Applications to Other Areas of Public Health

In keeping with the aim of reviewing the consequences of the interaction between caffeine and alcohol to their impact on public health, though applying the distinction to take into account the role of energy drinks, the present chapter dealt with addiction-related issues, mostly referred to alcohol and alcoholic beverages. However, as also pointed out in two short sections of the chapter, excessive consumption of alcoholic and caffeinated beverages brings about a significant number of serious reasons of concern in terms of individual's and public health. However, in the context to succinctly extend this analysis to other areas of public health, it appears relevant adding to the above concerns, the evidence related to the consequences of the consumption of sugar-sweetened beverages (energy drinks) in terms of increasing the risk of developing obesity and metabolic syndrome.

Mini-Dictionary of Terms

Alcoholic beverages: In the broadest sense, this expression indicates any kind of drink with a significant presence of alcohol (ethyl alcohol). In alcoholic beverages, alcohol's concentration is expressed as volume (ml) of pure alcohol per 100 ml of volume of the beverage. Another way to indicate such beverages is "alcoholic drinks" although this might be confusing because the word "drink" also indicates a unit of measure, often used to indicate the degree of dependence on alcohol; a "drink" is meant either a 330 ml can of beer or a 150 ml glass of wine or a 40 ml shot of spirits.

AMED: This acronym stands for alcohol mixed energy drinks, a commonly used term to indicate a variety of combinations of energy drinks and alcoholic beverages whose consumption takes place under a binge drinking modality, for example, vodka energy (34 ml of vodka and 64 ml of energy drink).

Binge-like drinking: Intense, compulsive modality of consumption of a beverage; originally referred to alcoholic drinks (binge drinking), this expression is presently adopted to indicate the modality of compulsively drinking whatever beverage.

Biphasic effect: The property of some compounds to elicit opposite effects depending on the dose. Both alcohol and caffeine have biphasic effects, respectively, on mood and locomotor activity.

Energy drinks: A type of drink that contains licit psychostimulant compounds, mainly caffeine, but also, e.g., guaranà extracts and taurine. These drinks differ substantially from classical coffees or teas because of the high content of caffeine per serve, which is not always explicit in the ingredient list. Energy drinks have been and still are the object of very intense advertising campaigns that place a great emphasis on their potential effects on improving cognitive performance, increasing attention and reaction speed, and also increasing endurance and muscle strength.

Gateway effect: Based on longitudinal studies (i.e., studies grounded on looking at the relationship between variables over an extended period of time), this is an expression that indicates the statistical probability of a given event. Gateway effect is commonly used to signify that the consumption of a substance or a mix of substances, e.g., energy drinks, may result in an increased probability of consuming other substances.

Risk factor: A substance or in general a condition (variable) that upon acute or repeated presentation may increase the probability of happening a given consequence.

Summary Points

- Caffeine and alcohol, two chemicals that share ancient roots and a significant presence in the development of human civilization, also compete for the reputation of being the most consumed psychopharmacologically active substance in the world.
- As both substances are freely available, cheap, and well tolerated, their consumption is widely spread. In particular among adolescents, alcohol is consumed by way of alcoholic drinks, whereas caffeine is taken mainly by way of energy drinks. This represents a threat to individuals' and public health and a growing concern for clinicians and neurobiologists.
- The intake of energy drinks and alcoholic beverages (AMED), which has risen, above all in adolescents and young adults, is still presently boosted by the fallacious belief that at high doses energy drinks may reduce the sedative and locomotor impairing effects of high alcohol intake.
- AMED consumption may promote a binge-like modality of assumption in the attempt to drink alcohol for longer and achieve higher levels of intoxication.
- A growing number of publications have focused on evaluating the effect of the coadministration of caffeine (the main ingredient of energy drinks) and alcohol, in the attempt to demonstrate the ability of caffeine to antagonize some of the pharmacological undesired actions of alcohol.
- Animal studies have been focused on the effect of the mixed administration of alcohol with caffeine, showing that caffeine is able (i) to potentiate the increase in locomotor activity induced by low doses of alcohol and abolish the inhibitory effects of higher doses, (ii) to attenuate the motor impairment induced by alcohol, (iii) to increase alertness and reduce the sedative effect of alcohol, and (iv) to reduce the alcohol-induced memory impairments and anxiolytic effects. Such preclinical studies rather than clarifying the interaction between the two drugs yielded conflicting results.

- Although being the main component of energy drinks, caffeine is not the only one, and most of the other components – taurine, ginseng, guarana, and sugar – have the ability to interfere with the rewarding and stimulating effects of alcohol alone; therefore, the effect of their combination should be taken into consideration.

References

Abrahao KP, Salinas AG, Lovinger DM (2017) Alcohol and the brain: neuronal molecular targets, synapses, and circuits. Neuron 96(6):1223–1238. https://doi.org/10.1016/j.neuron.2017.10.032

Aranda M, Morlock G (2006) Simultaneous determination of riboflavin, pyridoxine, nicotinamide, caffeine and taurine in energy drinks by planar chromatography-multiple detection with confirmation by electrospray ionization mass spectrometry. J Chromatogr 1131(1–2):253–260. https://doi.org/10.1016/j.chroma.2006.07.018

Arria AM, Caldeira KM, Kasperski SJ et al (2010) Increased alcohol consumption, nonmedical prescription drug use, and illicit drug use are associated with energy drink consumption among college students. J Addict Med 4(2):74–80. https://doi.org/10.1097/adm.0b013e3181aa8dd4

Arria AM, Caldeira KM, Kasperski SJ et al (2011) Energy drink consumption and increased risk for alcohol dependence. Alcohol Clin Exp Res 35(2):365–375. https://doi.org/10.1111/j.1530-0277.2010.01352.x

Arria AM, Caldeira KM, Bugbee BA et al (2017) Trajectories of energy drink consumption and subsequent drug use during young adulthood. Drug Alcohol Depend 179:424–432. https://doi.org/10.1016/j.drugalcdep.2017.06.008

Axley PD, Richardson CT, Singal AK (2019) Epidemiology of alcohol consumption and societal burden of alcoholism and alcoholic liver disease. Clin Liver Dis 23(1):39–50. https://doi.org/10.1016/j.cld.2018.09.011

Bassareo V, De Luca MA, Aresu M et al (2003) Differential adaptive properties of accumbens shell dopamine responses to ethanol as a drug and as a motivational stimulus. Eur J Neurosci 17(7):1465–1472. https://doi.org/10.1046/j.1460-9568.2003.02556.x

Bassareo V, Cucca F, Frau R et al (2017) Changes in dopamine transmission in the nucleus accumbens shell and core during ethanol and sucrose self-administration. Front Behav Neurosci 11:71. https://doi.org/10.3389/fnbeh.2017.00071

Benkert R, Abel T (2020) Heavy energy drink consumption is associated with risky substance use in young Swiss men. Swiss Med Wkly 150:w20243. https://doi.org/10.4414/smw.2020.20243

Berger AJ, Alford K (2009) Cardiac arrest in a young man following excess consumption of caffeinated "energy drinks". Med J Aust 190(1):41–43. https://doi.org/10.5694/j.1326-5377.2009.tb02263.x

Calabrò RS, Italiano D, Gervasi G et al (2012) Single tonic-clonic seizure after energy drink abuse. Epilepsy Behav 23(3):384–385. https://doi.org/10.1016/j.yebeh.2011.12.010

Carvalho C, Silveira da Cruz J, Takahashi R (2012) Prolonged exposure to caffeinated alcoholic solutions prevents the alcohol deprivation effect in rats. J Caffeine Res 2(2):83–89. https://doi.org/10.1089/jcr.2012.0013

Connole L, Harkin A, Maginn M (2004) Adenosine A1 receptor blockade mimics caffeine's attenuation of ethanol-induced motor incoordination. Basic Clin Pharmacol Toxicol 95(6):299–304. https://doi.org/10.1111/j.1742-7843.2004.pto950509.x

Curran CP, Marczinski CA (2017) Taurine, caffeine and energy drinks: reviewing the risks to the adolescent brain. Birth Defect Res 109(20):1640–1648. https://doi.org/10.1002/bdr2.1177

Dar MS, Jones M, Close G et al (1987) Behavioral interactions of ethanol and methylxanthines. Psychopharmacology 91(1):1–4. https://doi.org/10.1007/bf00690916

De Sanctis V, Soliman N, Soliman ST et al (2017) Caffeinated energy drinks consumption among adolescents and potential health consequences associated with their use: a significant public health hazard. Acta Biomed 88(2):222–231. https://doi.org/10.23750/abm.v88i2.6664

Degirmenci N, Fossum IN, Strand TA et al (2018) Consumption of energy drinks among adolescents in Norway: a cross-sectional study. BMC Public Health 18(1):1391. https://doi.org/10.1186/s12889-018-6236-5

Di Chiara G, Bassareo V, Fenu S, Se Luca MA, Spina L, Cadoni C, Acquas E, Carboni E, Valentini V, Ledda D (2004) Dopamine and drug addiction: the nucleus accumbens shell connection. Neuropharmacology 47 Suppl 1:227–241. https://doi.org/10.1016/j.neuropharm.2004.06.032

El Yacoubi M, Ledent C, Parmentier M et al (2003) Caffeine reduces hypnotic effects of alcohol through adenosine A2A receptor blockade. Neuropharmacology 45(7):977–985. https://doi.org/10.1016/s0028-3908(03)00254-5

Ferreira SE, de Mello MT, Pompeia S et al (2006) Effects of energy drink ingestion on alcohol intoxication. Alcohol Clin Exp Res 30(4):598–605. https://doi.org/10.1111/j.1530-0277.2006.00070.x

Fernandes PR, Almeida FB, da Cunha MMMV, Feddern CF, Freese L, Barros HMT (2020) The effects of caffeine on alcohol oral self-administration behavior in rats. Physiol Behav 223:112966. https://doi.org/10.1016/j.physbeh.2020.112966

Galimov A, Hanewinkel R, Hansen J et al (2020) Association of energy drink consumption with substance-use initiation among adolescents: a 12-month longitudinal study. J Psychopharmacol 34(2):221–228. https://doi.org/10.1177/0269881119895545

Gilpin NW, Koob GF (2008) Neurobiology of alcohol dependence: focus on motivational mechanisms. Alcohol Res Health 31(3):185–195

Gulick D, Gould TJ (2009) Effects of ethanol and caffeine on behavior in C57BL/6 mice in the plus-maze discriminative avoidance task. Behav Neurosci 123(6):1271–1278. https://doi.org/10.1037/a0017610

Harrison NL, Skelly MJ, Grosserode EK et al (2017) Effects of acute alcohol on excitability in the CNS. Neuropharmacology 122:36–45. https://doi.org/10.1016/j.neuropharm.2017.04.007

Heinz A, Daedelow LS, Wackerhagen C et al (2020) Addiction theory matters – why there is no dependence on caffeine or antidepressant medication. Addict Biol 25(2):e12735. https://doi.org/10.1111/adb.12735

Hilbert ML, May CE, Griffin WC (2013) Conditioned reinforcement and locomotor activating effects of caffeine and ethanol combinations in mice. Pharmacol Biochem Behav 110:168–173. https://doi.org/10.1016/j.pbb.2013.07.008

Iyadurai SJ, Chung SS (2007) New-onset seizures in adults: possible association with consumption of popular energy drinks. Epilepsy Behav 10(3):504–508. https://doi.org/10.1016/j.yebeh.2007.01.009

Jackson DB, Leal WE (2018) Energy drink consumption and the perceived risk and disapproval of drugs: monitoring the future, 2010–2016. Drug Alcohol Depend 188:24–31. https://doi.org/10.1016/j.drugalcdep.2018.03.022

Kunin D, Gaskin S, Rogan F et al (2000) Caffeine promotes ethanol drinking in rats. Examination using a limited-access free choice paradigm. Alcohol 21(3):271–277. https://doi.org/10.1016/s0741-8329(00)00101-4

Lê AD, Kiianmaa K, Cunningham CL et al (2001) Neurobiological processes in alcohol addiction. Alcohol Clin Exp Res 25(5 Suppl ISBRA):144S–151S. https://doi.org/10.1111/j.1530-0277.2001.tb02389.x

Lecca D, Cacciapaglia F, Valentini V et al (2006a) Monitoring extracellular dopamine in the rat nucleus accumbens shell and core during acquisition and maintenance of intravenous WIN 55,212-2 self-administration. Psychopharmacology 188(1):63–74. https://doi.org/10.1007/s00213-006-0475-3

Lecca D, Cacciapaglia F, Valentini V et al (2006b) Preferential increase of extracellular dopamine in the rat nucleus accumbens shell as compared to that in the core during acquisition and maintenance of intravenous nicotine self-administration. Psychopharmacology 184(3–4):435–446. https://doi.org/10.1007/s00213-005-0280-4

Lecca D, Cacciapaglia F, Valentini V et al (2007a) Differential neurochemical and behavioral adaptation to cocaine after response contingent and noncontingent exposure in the rat. Psychopharmacology 191(3):653–667. https://doi.org/10.1007/s00213-006-0496-y

Lecca D, Valentini V, Cacciapaglia F et al (2007b) Reciprocal effects of response contingent and noncontingent intravenous heroin on in vivo nucleus accumbens shell versus core dopamine in the rat: a repeated sampling microdialysis study. Psychopharmacology 194(1):103–116. https://doi.org/10.1007/s00213-007-0815-y

Lippi G, Cervellin G, Sanchis-Gomar F (2016) Energy drinks and myocardial ischemia: a review of case reports. Cardiovasc Toxicol 16(3):207–212. https://doi.org/10.1007/s12012-015-9339-6

López-Cruz L, Salamone JD, Correa M (2013) The impact of caffeine on the Behavioral effects of ethanol related to abuse and addiction: a review of animal studies. J Caffeine Res 3(1):9–21. https://doi.org/10.1089/jcr.2013.0003

Machado-Vieira R, Viale CI, Kapczinski F (2001) Mania associated with an energy drink: the possible role of caffeine, taurine, and inositol. Can J Psychiatr 46(5):454–455. https://doi.org/10.1177/070674370104600524

Mallett KA, Marzell M, Scaglione N (2014) Are all alcohol and energy drink users the same? Examining individual variation in relation to alcohol mixed with energy drink use, risky drinking, and consequences. Psychol Addict Behav 28(1):97–104. https://doi.org/10.1037/a0032203

Mallett KA, Scaglione N, Reavy R et al (2015) Longitudinal patterns of alcohol mixed with energy drink use among college students and their associations with risky drinking and problems. J Stud Alcohol Drugs 76(3):389–396. https://doi.org/10.15288/jsad.2015.76.389

Mansour B, Amarah W, Nasralla E (2019) Energy drinks in children and adolescents: demographic data and immediate effects. Eur J Pediatr 178(5):649–656. https://doi.org/10.1007/s00431-019-03342-7

Marczinski CA, Fillmore MT (2006) Clubgoers and their trendy cocktails: implications of mixing caffeine into alcohol on information processing and subjective reports of intoxication. Neuropsychopharmacol 14(4):450–458. https://doi.org/10.1037/1064-1297.14.4.450

Marczinski CA, Fillmore MT, Bardgett ME, Howard MA (2011) Effects of energy drinks mixed with alcohol on behavioral control: risks for college students consuming trendy cocktails. Alcohol Clin Exp Res 35(7):1282–1292. https://doi.org/10.1111/j.1530-0277.2011.01464.x

Marczinski CA, Fillmore MT (2014) Energy drinks mixed with alcohol: what are the risks? Nutr Rev 72(Suppl 1):98–107. https://doi.org/10.1111/nure.12127

Mihic SJ, Koob GF, Mayfield J et al (2017) Ethanol, Chapter 23. In: Brunton LL, Hilal-Dandan R, Knollmann BC (eds) Goodman & Gilman's: the pharmacological basis of therapeutics, 13th edn. McGraw-Hill Education, New York

Miller KE (2008a) Energy drinks, race, and problem behaviors among college students. J Adolesc Health 43(5):490–497. https://doi.org/10.1016/j.jadohealth.2008.03.003

Miller KE (2008b) Wired: energy drinks, jock identity, masculine norms, and risk taking. J Am Coll Heal 56(5):481–490. https://doi.org/10.3200/jach.56.5.481-490

Miller KE (2012) Alcohol mixed with energy drink use and sexual risk-taking: casual, intoxicated, and unprotected sex. J Caffeine Res 2(2):62–69. https://doi.org/10.1089/jcr.2012.0015

Morgan CJ, Noronha LA, Muetzelfeldt M et al (2013) Harms and benefits associated with psychoactive drugs: findings of an international survey of active drug users. J Psychopharmacol 27(6):497–506. https://doi.org/10.1177/0269881113477744

Munteanu C, Rosioru C, Tarba C, Lang C (2018) Long-term consumption of energy drinks induces biochemical and ultrastructural alterations in the heart muscle. Anatol J Cardiol 19(5):326–323. https://doi.org/10.14744/AnatolJCardiol.2018.90094

Nehlig A, Daval JL, Debry G (1992) Caffeine and the central nervous system: mechanisms of action, biochemical, metabolic and psychostimulant effects. Brain Res Brain Res Rev 17(2): 139–170. https://doi.org/10.1016/0165-0173(92)90012-b

Patrick ME, Veliz P, Linden-Carmichael A et al (2018) Alcohol mixed with energy drink use during young adulthood. Addict Behav 84:224–230. https://doi.org/10.1016/j.addbeh.2018.03.022

Porru S, Maccioni R, Bassareo V et al (2020) Effects of caffeine on ethanol-elicited place preference, place aversion and ERK phosphorylation in CD-1 mice. J Psychopharmacol 34(12):1357–1370. https://doi.org/10.1177/0269881120965892

Prediger RD, Batista LC, Takahashi RN (2004) Adenosine A1 receptors modulate the anxiolytic-like effect of ethanol in the elevated plus-maze in mice. Eur J Pharmacol 499(1–2):147–154. https://doi.org/10.1016/j.ejphar.2004.07.106

Quadri S, Harding L, Lillig M (2018) An energy drink-induced manic episode in an adolescent. Prim Care Companion CNS Disord 20(6):18102318. https://doi.org/10.4088/pcc.18l02318

Rehm J, Gmel GE Sr, Gmel G et al (2017) The relationship between different dimensions of alcohol use and the burden of disease-an update. Addiction 112(6):968–1001. https://doi.org/10.1111/add.13757

Rezvani AH, Sexton HG, Johnson J et al (2013) Effects of caffeine on alcohol consumption and nicotine self-administration in rats. Alcohol Clin Exp Res 37(9):1609–1617. https://doi.org/10.1111/acer.12127

Snipes DJ, Benotsch EG (2013) High-risk cocktails and high-risk sex: examining the relation between alcohol mixed with energy drink consumption, sexual behavior, and drug use in college students. Addict Behav 38(1):1418–1423. https://doi.org/10.1016/j.addbeh.2012.07.011

Spear LP (2016) Consequences of adolescent use of alcohol and other drugs: studies using rodent models. Neurosci Biobehav Rev 70:228–243. https://doi.org/10.1016/j.neubiorev.2016.07.026

Spear LP (2018) Effects of adolescent alcohol consumption on the brain and behaviour. Nat Rev Neurosci 19(4):197–214. https://doi.org/10.1038/nrn.2018.10

Spinetta MJ, Woodlee MT, Feinberg LM et al (2008) Alcohol-induced retrograde memory impairment in rats: prevention by caffeine. Psychopharmacology 201(3):361–371. https://doi.org/10.1007/s00213-008-1294-5

Substance Abuse and Mental Health Service Administration, Center for Behavioral Health Statistics and Quality (2013) The DAWN Report: Update on emergency department visits involving energy drinks: A continuing public health concern. Rockville, MD

Sudakov SK, Rusakova IV, Medvedeva OF (2003) Effect of chronic caffeine consumption on changes in locomotor activity of WAG/G and Fischer-344 rats induced by nicotine, ethanol, and morphine. Bull Exp Biol Med 136(6):563–565. https://doi.org/10.1023/b:bebm.0000020204.54037.be

Tarragon E, Calleja-Conde J, Giné E (2021) Alcohol mixed with energy drinks: what about taurine? Psychopharmacology 238(1):1–8. https://doi.org/10.1007/s00213-020-05705-7

Terry-McElrath YM, O'Malley PM, Johnston LD (2014) Energy drinks, soft drinks, and substance use among United States secondary school students. J Addict Med 8(1):6–13. https://doi.org/10.1097/01.adm.0000435322.07020.53

Thombs DL, O'Mara RJ, Tsukamoto M et al (2010) Event-level analyses of energy drink consumption and alcohol intoxication in bar patrons. Addict Behav 35(4):325–330. https://doi.org/10.1016/j.addbeh.2009.11.004

Thombs D, Rossheim M, Barnett TE et al (2011) Is there a misplaced focus on AMED? Associations between caffeine mixers and bar patron intoxication. Drug Alcohol Depend 116(1–3):31–36. https://doi.org/10.1016/j.drugalcdep.2010.11.014

Vargiu R, Broccia F, Lobina C et al (2021) Chronic red bull consumption during adolescence: effect on mesocortical and mesolimbic dopamine transmission and cardiovascular system in adult rats. Pharmaceuticals (Basel) 14(7):609. https://doi.org/10.3390/ph14070609

Verster JC, Benson S, Johnson SJ et al (2018) Alcohol mixed with energy drink (AMED): a critical review and meta-analysis. Hum Psychopharmacol 33(2):e2650. https://doi.org/10.1002/hup.2650

Volkow ND, Wang GJ, Fowler JS et al (2010) Addiction: decreased reward sensitivity and increased expectation sensitivity conspire to overwhelm the brain's control circuit. BioEssays 32(9):748–755. https://doi.org/10.1002/bies.201000042

Vonghia L, Leggio L, Ferrulli A et al (2008) Acute alcohol intoxication. Eur J Intern Med 19(8):561–567. https://doi.org/10.1016/j.ejim.2007.06.033

Waldeck B (1974) Ethanol and caffeine: a complex interaction with respect to locomotor activity and central catecholamines. Psychopharmacologia 36(3):209–220. https://doi.org/10.1007/bf00421803

Whayne TF Jr (2015) Coffee: a selected overview of beneficial or harmful effects on the cardiovascular system? Curr Vasc Pharmacol 13(5):637–648

Wilson RE, Kado HS, Samson R et al (2012) A case of caffeine-induced coronary artery vasospasm of a 17-year-old male. Cardiovasc Toxicol 12(2):175–179. https://doi.org/10.1007/s12012-011-9152-9

Witkiewitz K, Litten RZ, Leggio L (2019) Advances in the science and treatment of alcohol use disorder. Sci Adv 5(9):eaax4043. https://doi.org/10.1126/sciadv.aax4043

Woolsey CL, Barnes LB, Jacobson BH et al (2014) Frequency of energy drink use predicts illicit prescription stimulant use. Subst Abus 35(1):96–103. https://doi.org/10.1080/08897077.2013.810561

Worrall BB, Phillips CD, Henderson KK (2005) Herbal energy drinks, phenylpropanoid compounds, and cerebral vasculopathy. Neurology 65(7):1137–1138. https://doi.org/10.1212/01.wnl.0000178985.35765.e0

Caffeine and Anxiety-Like Behavior

73

Anderson Ribeiro-Carvalho, Ana C. Dutra-Tavares,
Cláudio C. Filgueiras, Alex C. Manhães, and Yael Abreu-Villaça

Contents

Introduction: Caffeine Exposure at Adulthood 1574
Developmental Exposure to Caffeine 1576
Mechanisms Related to Anxiety Induced by Caffeine 1579
Susceptibility to Anxiety Effects of Caffeine 1582
Applications to Other Areas of Addiction 1583
Application to Public Health 1584
Mini-Dictionary of Terms 1585
Key Facts Regarding Susceptibility to Anxiety Effects of Caffeine 1585
Summary Points 1585
References 1585

Abstract

Caffeine is the most frequently consumed psychoactive substance in the world. Despite its safety, caffeine consumption has been linked to negative consequences on mood. Here, we describe the effects of caffeine consumption on anxiety-related behaviors. These effects are dependent of several factors such as tolerance, genetic polymorphism, mental health status, sex, and age. Special attention will be paid to the effects of caffeine during pregnancy and adolescence. This chapter also addresses mechanisms associated with the effects of caffeine on anxiety, which are, at least in part, mediated by adenosine receptors. Polymorphisms in genes controlling the expression of these receptors have been implicated in susceptibility to anxiety caused by caffeine consumption. Caffeine use

A. Ribeiro-Carvalho (✉)
Departamento de Ciências, Faculdade de Formação de Professores, Universidade do Estado do Rio de Janeiro, São Gonçalo, Brazil
e-mail: anderson.carvalho@uerj.br

A. C. Dutra-Tavares · C. C. Filgueiras · A. C. Manhães · Y. Abreu-Villaça
Departamento de Ciências Fisiológicas, Instituto de Biologia Roberto Alcantara Gomes, Universidade do Estado do Rio de Janeiro, Rio de Janeiro, Brazil

V. B. Patel, V. R. Preedy (eds.), *Handbook of Substance Misuse and Addictions*,
https://doi.org/10.1007/978-3-030-92392-1_80

and anxiety in patients with mental disorders will also be addressed. The issues that have already been identified regarding caffeine effects on anxiety recommends moderation in its consumption and should guide policy formulation by drug/food regulatory agencies.

Keywords

Caffeine · Anxiety · Developmental exposure · Substance abuse · Adenosine receptors · Mental disorders · Energy drinks · Gene polymorphisms · Panic disorder · Dose response · Drug addiction · Withdrawal symptoms

List of Abbreviations

A1R	Adenosine receptor A1
A2R	Adenosine receptor A2
BDNF	Brain-derived neurotrophic factor
BNST	Bed nucleus of stria terminalis
CPA	N6-Cyclopentyladenosine
CREB	cAMP-response element-binding protein
DASS-21	Self-reported Depression Anxiety Stress Scale
ED	Energy drinks
fMRI	Functional magnetic resonance imaging
GABA	γ-aminobutyric acid
GAD-7	Generalized Anxiety Disorder-7 scale
GFP	Green fluorescent protein
HPA	Hypothalamic–pituitary–adrenal
MC4	Melanocortin-4
MEG	Source-localized magnetoencephalography
NPSR	Neuropeptide S receptor
PET	Positron emission tomography
POMS	Profile of Mood States questionnaire
PVN	Paraventricular hypothalamic nucleus
α-MSH	Alpha-melanocyte stimulating hormone

Introduction: Caffeine Exposure at Adulthood

A consensus exists regarding the safety of caffeine consumption in moderate amounts by adult humans, a fact that is particularly important since it is the most frequently consumed psychoactive substance in the world, being present in relevant amounts in products such as coffee, tea, sodas, energy drinks, and chocolate bars (IOM 2014; EFSA 2015). Interestingly, there is extensive evidence of the beneficial health effects associated with the consumption of this methylxanthine in amounts corresponding to less than 400 mg of caffeine (approximately 6 cups of espresso) per day or less for adults (Guest et al. 2021; Laatar et al. 2021). However, excessive doses, of over 1200 mg/day, have been linked to negative outcomes (Turnbull et al.

2016). Although unsafe, effectively toxic, intake levels require the individual to consume 2000 mg/day or more, potentially lethal doses requiring more than 5000 mg/day (Willson 2018), a range of undesirable, albeit generally short-lasting and readily reversible, neurophysiological effects have already been described with far lower doses (Willson 2018).

Increased anxiety, defined here as an emotion characterized by feelings of uneasiness and apprehensive thoughts, has been identified as a possible outcome of caffeine consumption (van Calker et al. 2019). It must be pointed out that susceptibility to the anxiogenic effects of caffeine consumption in adults not only depends on the dose that is being ingested but also varies depending on factors such as: 1) development of tolerance in habitual consumers (Turnbull et al. 2016); 2) mental health status (Naftalovich et al. 2020); 3) sex (Jee et al. 2020); 4) differences in the metabolism of caffeine (Fulton et al. 2018). In general, high doses of caffeine, of more than 700 mg/day, are needed to make the identification of increased anxiety more consistent (Turnbull et al. 2016). Below this level of consumption, results vary considerably, with different studies showing outcomes ranging from mild anxiolytic effects to anxiogenic ones (Fiani et al. 2021). Some studies have observed significant associations between caffeine intake and perceived levels of anxiety. For example, a study by Bertasi and collaborators (2021) showed a positive correlation between the Generalized Anxiety Disorder-7 (GAD-7) scale scores and the weekly caffeine intake in young US college students. Scores were above 5 for most of the students that drank more than 10 cups per week. In fact, ingestion of six cups of coffee a day has been linked with higher risk of developing anxiety and panic disorders (Kendler et al. 2006). Consumption of caffeine-containing energy drinks (ED), particularly prevalent in young adults, has also been associated with increased anxiety. Kaur and collaborators (2020), using a cohort from a prospective population-based study in Australia (Raine Study), indicated that young men (20 to 22 years old) that changed from non-ED consumers to ED consumers across a two-year follow-up showed increased anxiety scores in the self-reported Depression Anxiety Stress Scale (DASS-21). Contrastingly, it has also been reported that consumption of 500 mL of ED (containing 120 mg of caffeine) results in a reduction of anxiety, as indicated by the Profile of Mood States (POMS) questionnaire (Chtourou et al. 2019).

In trying to assess how caffeine consumption affects the human brain in terms of metabolism, function, and connectivity, a number of studies used positron emission tomography (PET), functional magnetic resonance imaging (fMRI), and source-localized magnetoencephalography (MEG). For example, a reduction in cerebral blood flow in the entire brain was observed 30 min after the consumption of 200 mg of caffeine (Chang et al. 2018). Furthermore, a reduction in metabolic activity, also 30 min after caffeine ingestion, was observed in the putamen, caudate, nucleus pallidum, and insula (Park et al. 2014), regions that have been associated with the modulation of anxiety levels (Tremblay et al. 2015). Acute caffeine consumption was also shown to reduce functional connectivity in the brain, as indicated by both fMRI and MEG (Wong et al. 2012; Tal et al. 2013), a finding that has been associated with increased anxiety (Tung et al. 2021). The effects of caffeine on the brain are not limited to a short period following consumption since long-term exposure to this drug has also been shown to affect brain connectivity. A study by Magalhães and collaborators (2021) has shown that habitual coffee drinkers have a brain functional connectivity that differs from that of non-coffee drinkers. Using resting-state fMRI, this group showed that habitual drinkers had a dose-dependent reduction in functional connectivity in the right precuneus (somatosensory network) and in the right insula (limbic network). By offering coffee to the non-coffee drinkers, these authors further evidenced that the patterns of functional connectivity in the limbic network of these subjects became indistinguishable from that of habitual drinkers 30 min after caffeine consumption. Interestingly, although stress levels were increased in habitual drinkers of both sexes, only men showed a positive association between caffeine dose and anxiety levels (Magalhães et al. 2021). This last result is in line with previous studies that indicated that: 1) adult men, but not women, show a dose-dependent increase in anxiety levels after consumption of coffee having different concentrations of caffeine (Botella and Parra 2003); 2) young adult men, but not women, that consumed more than 250 mL/day of energy drink experienced increased anxiety symptoms (Trapp et al. 2014); 3) in children (secondary school, England), high doses of caffeine, particularly above 1000 mg per week, were associated with increased risk of high anxiety in boys but not in girls (Richards and Smith 2015). Sex, therefore, constitutes a relevant factor in assessing the impact of caffeine consumption on anxiety levels (Jee et al. 2020). However, assessing the mechanisms that might explain these sex differences in susceptibility is a complicated endeavor, particularly when the fact that women show higher risk for anxiety disorders than men is considered (Altemus et al. 2014).

Although consumption of caffeine in moderate amounts is generally safe for adult humans, developmental exposure to this drug may have negative impacts. As it will be shown below, both short- and long-term detrimental effects of caffeine exposure during gestation, infancy, and adolescence on the brain have already been identified.

Developmental Exposure to Caffeine

Studies have shown that chronic consumption of high doses of caffeine during gestation downregulates the A1 receptor (A1R) and the Gi protein coupled to this receptor in the fetal brain (León et al. 2002) as well as the A1R and A2R in the neonatal brain (Lorenzo et al. 2010). Given the fact that adenosine controls the release of several neurotransmitters, perinatal caffeine exposure promotes a number of changes in neurotransmitter and receptor systems that play important roles during brain development, such as the serotoninergic, glutamatergic, GABAergic, and cholinergic ones (León et al. 2005; Silva et al. 2008; Tchekalarova et al. 2014). In addition, chronic caffeine exposure affects the levels of BDNF, CREB, and other proteins that are important for synaptogenesis (Mioranzza et al. 2014; Alhowail and Aldubayan 2020). Taken together, these actions during development may alter neurobiological processes essential for brain growth and wiring, resulting in the wide range of long-lasting neurobehavioral impairments observed in individuals developmentally exposed to caffeine. It is important to notice that the behavioral outcomes may depend on genetic background, dose of caffeine, and period of exposure.

During pregnancy, caffeine metabolism is reduced and its averaged half-life can increase from 3 h in nonpregnant women to 10 h during the last 4 weeks of pregnancy (Knutti et al. 1982). Caffeine crosses the placenta as well as the fetal blood–brain barrier, and given the immaturity of the caffeine-degrading enzyme systems, its half-life can range from 50 to 95 h in fetuses (Rorabaugh 2021). Thus, the regular consumption of caffeine during gestation may lead to its accumulation in the fetus. Several studies have investigated possible associations between maternal caffeine consumption and childhood neurobehavioral outcomes, although this issue still remains a matter of debate. Regarding anxiety, few studies are available, and the results are inconclusive. Tea consumption of more than 8 cups/day at 15 weeks of gestation was associated with an increased risk of anxiety-depressive disorder in 11-year-old offspring (Hvolgaard Mikkelsen et al. 2017). However, in the same study, coffee consumption of more than 8 cups/day (which contains twice as much caffeine by volume than tea) was not associated with anxiety-depressive disorders (Hvolgaard Mikkelsen et al. 2017). Prenatal maternal dietary caffeine intake from coffee, tea, and cola (assessed by questionnaire at 14–18 week of gestation) was not associated with a higher risk for emotional symptoms in 5-year-old offspring (Loomans et al. 2012). Similarly, total maternal caffeine intake and caffeine intake from different sources (coffee, tea, and caffeinated soft drinks) were not associated with a higher risk of anxiety in the offspring at 8 years of age (Berglundh et al. 2021). Some preclinical studies show that developmental exposure to caffeine affects anxiety-like behavior later in life, but results are also not consistent. Adult Swiss mice exposed to caffeine via drinking water (0.3 g/L) during the entire gestation and lactation periods show an increase in anxiety-related behaviors, such as greater number of fecal pellets in the open field test, higher number of attempts in light-dark box, and decreased percentage of entries in open arms in elevated plus maze test (Laureano-Melo et al. 2016). In contrast, adult GIN [green fluorescent protein (GFP)–expressing inhibitory neurons] mice exposed to caffeine via drinking water (0.3 g/L) from 15 days before mating up to postnatal day 15 do not display alterations in anxiety-like behaviors in the elevated plus maze (Silva et al. 2013). Adolescent rats administered with higher doses of caffeine (15–20 mg/Kg) through gavage over postnatal days 2–6 showed less anxiety than controls in the elevated plus maze and dark–light transition (Pan and Chen 2007).

As the child grows and transitions into adolescence, he or she becomes gradually more independent regarding the intake of caffeinated products, self-regulation becoming increasingly more important. Two relevant issues associated with this transition are that the adolescent brain is still undergoing significant ontogenetic changes, rendering it particularly susceptible to the effects of psychostimulants, and that adolescents are usually not sufficiently mature to correctly assess the possible consequences of their actions, which help explain their increased propensity for displaying risk-taking behavior when compared to adults. As if to underscore the risks involved in the aforementioned transition, the consumption of energy drinks by teenagers has markedly increased in the last decades, a fact that is being closely followed by marked increases in the number of reported adverse effects of energy drinks consumption in this age group (Harris and Munsell 2015). Furthermore, an increase in the number of emergency hospitalizations associated with excessive energy drink intake in adolescents has been reported (Pennington et al. 2010). Although these beverages are composed of many components, caffeine is the main ingredient in the majority of energy drinks and its content ranges from 50 to over 280 mg per can or bottle (McLellan and Lieberman 2012), which is much more than what is usually present in a cup of coffee (50 to 100 mg) or a can of cola (40 to 60 mg) (Gray et al. 2012). These products are often strategically marketed toward the young consumer, so much so that 30–50% of adolescents and young adults consume energy drinks (Seifert et al. 2011). Nowak and Jasionowski (2016) showed that energy drinks were consumed by 69% of young athletes and 17% drank every day or 1–3 times a week (Nowak and Jasionowski 2016). Caffeinated beverages are often consumed by adolescents and young adults with the aim of boosting performance and endurance, enhancing alertness, physical ability and cognitive performance, or as a coping strategy in the management of stressful academic situations (Babu et al. 2008).

Although consumption of a few caffeinated beverages daily may not seem to be a matter of concern, the fact is that young individuals may be ingesting proportionally more caffeine than adults when parameters such as body mass are considered (Luebbe and Bell 2009). Yet, despite their widespread, frequently excessive, use and negative health consequences, little is known about the potential mental health effects of caffeine consumption among young people, particularly on anxiety. Although some studies have observed that anxiety was unrelated to caffeine use among adolescents and young adults (Temple et al. 2009; Temple and Ziegler 2011), other reports described an association between caffeine and anxiety or stress, particularly when large amounts of caffeine were involved. Bernstein et al. (2002) found that caffeine-dependent adolescents (mean caffeine consumption: 244.4 ± 173.0 mg/day) scored significantly higher on an anxiety inventory than non-dependent ones (Bernstein et al. 2002). Marmorstein (2016) also described a positive correlation between coffee consumption with panic and anxiety symptoms among early adolescents, replicating observations made in adults, although the effects appeared to occur at lower doses, which most likely reflects the lower body mass of adolescents (Marmorstein 2016).

Larger effects of caffeine seem to occur in sensitive individuals, such as psychiatric patients (Richards and Smith 2015). Individuals who experience somatic symptoms of anxiety may find that higher quantities of caffeine increase the intensity of their symptoms. Furthermore, to some youths who are more sensitive to bodily sensations related to an anxiety state, the stimulating effects of caffeine or its withdrawal are perceived more intensely. Thus, anxiety sensitivity affects caffeine consumption, leading to either avoidance or greater consumption (Luebbe 2011). For instance, Marmorstein (2016), in a 16-month longitudinal study, described that social anxiety was protective against increases in energy drink consumption, suggesting that youth who avoid certain social settings may be relatively protected against the use of energy drinks (Marmorstein 2016). In contrast, Whalen et al.

(2007) found that youth with depression and comorbid anxiety disorders consumed greater amounts of caffeine per day than those without these disorders (Whalen et al. 2007). The aforementioned data mostly indicates that symptoms of anxiety are a consequence of increased caffeine consumption. Interestingly, the self-medication hypothesis has been proposed to link substance use disorders to a variety of mental disorders (Turner et al. 2018). In this scenario, youth with mental illnesses might use caffeine to relieve apathy and lethargy, or to improve attention and physical performance (Chelben et al. 2008; Richards and Smith 2015). Although not specifically related to anxiety, but consistent with this idea, caffeine use decreased across an 8-week treatment protocol for youth with major depressive disorder (Whalen et al. 2007). It is worth mentioning that despite the beneficial effects of caffeine, youths generally submit themselves to a cycle of high levels of caffeine intake followed by cessation, a pattern that might lead to anxiety-related symptoms or worsen those that are already present (Whalen et al. 2007).

Studies that investigated sex differences in caffeine-induced anxiety during adolescence are far and few in between. Nevertheless, two studies observed sex differences in caffeine-induced anxiety in young individuals (Trapp et al. 2014; Richards and Smith 2015): total caffeine intake was associated with increased anxiety only in young males. Both studies also showed that young males consumed more caffeine than similarly aged females. Thus, although it appears that young males are more vulnerable to the harmful effects of caffeine than females, this increased vulnerability could be the consequence of greater consumption of caffeine by males, an issue that needs further clarification. In this regard, it has already been shown that caffeine produces greater arousal effects in young males when compared to females, and that adolescent males are more likely to have caffeine-reinforcing effects than females (Adan et al. 2008; Temple et al. 2009). Besides that, as mentioned above, energy drinks are often marketed toward young males, which might contribute to greater consumption by this demographic segment (Trapp et al. 2014).

As previously shown, increased consumption of caffeinated beverages by youths is related to their desire to improve some abilities in dealing with academic routines or to self-medicate impairments associated with neuropsychiatric disorders. Considering that this use pattern is potentially dangerous, young people should be aware of the potentially harmful effects associated with caffeinated beverages consumption. Young individuals should be oriented to adequately self-regulate the consumption of caffeine-containing products and to engage in alternative and healthier ways to increase energy levels such as getting an adequate diet and sleep.

Mechanisms Related to Anxiety Induced by Caffeine

There is some evidence pointing to a dual effect of caffeine on anxiety, with low doses promoting anxiolytic-like behavior responses (Hughes et al. 2014) while, at high doses, anxiogenic effects prevail (Jain et al. 1995). However, while the anxiolytic effects are not always identified (Sweeney et al. 2016), the increase in anxiety levels as caffeine intake increases is consistently demonstrated, so much so that, in animal models, most studies that investigate candidate therapeutic drugs for anxiety disorders use caffeine to induce an anxiogenic state (Hale et al. 2010; Khurana and Bansal 2019).

Caffeine acutely activates neurons in brain regions involved with anxiety responses, such as the hippocampus, the bed nucleus of stria terminalis (BNST), the lateral septum, the amygdala, the paraventricular hypothalamic nucleus (PVN), the locus coeruleus, and the lateral parabrachial nucleus, as demonstrated by the increased expression of the immediate early gene c-fos (Fig. 1a; Savchenko and Boughter 2011). The classic mechanism of action of caffeine is the reduction of adenosinergic transmission in the brain by its action on G-coupled A1 and A2A receptors (A1R and A2AR, respectively). Therefore, the modulation of anxiety by caffeine is, at least in part, mediated by its nonselective antagonism of ARs. However, whether there is an AR subtype that mediates its anxiogenic effects is still a matter of debate (van Calker et al. 2019). In this regard, the involvement of each AR subtype in the caffeine-mediated modulation of affective state can be inferred by the impact of AR knockout mice and selective AR agonists and antagonists on anxiety levels. Mice lacking A1R (Johansson et al. 2001; Giménez-Llort et al. 2002) display enhanced anxiety, which is consistent with evidence that selective activation of A1R by administration of N6-Cyclopentyladenosine (CPA) induces anxiolytic-like behavior (Jain et al. 1995; Florio et al. 1998). Interestingly, while A2AR knockout mice are also more anxious than wild-type ones (Deckert 1998), this effect is not mimicked by selective A2AR antagonists (El Yacoubi et al.

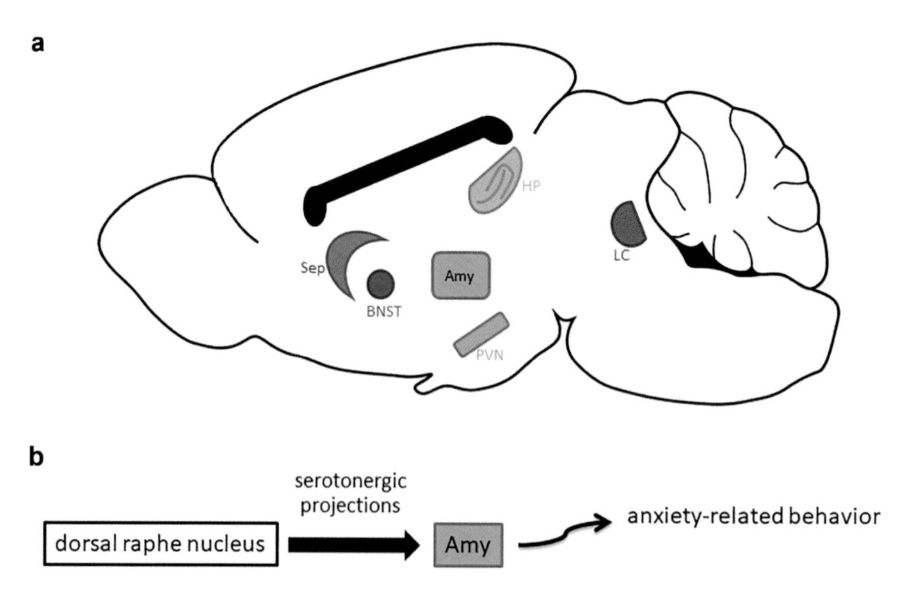

Fig. 1 Caffeine activates neurons in brain regions involved with anxiety responses. (**a**) Brain regions that possibly mediate caffeine anxiogenic effects in rodents; (**b**) some studies suggest that caffeine-evoked serotonergic activation of the dorsal raphe nucleus to basolateral amygdala (Amy) pathway is relevant for the modulation of anxiety-related behavior

2000). These data suggest that both A1 and A2A receptors subtypes play a role in anxiety.

In addition to caffeine's direct effect on ARs, several studies have demonstrated interactions of the adenosinergic system with other neurotransmitter systems involved in the pathogenesis of anxiety, including the serotonergic one. Acute caffeine has a widespread stimulatory effect on serotonergic neurons in the dorsal raphe nucleus, together with decreased expression of genes that control serotonergic signaling, tph2 and slc22a3, genes that encode tryptophan hydroxylase, the rate-limiting enzyme in the biosynthesis of brain serotonin, and Slc22a3, a sodium independent, low affinity, high capacity serotonin transporter expressed in serotonergic neurons (Arnold et al. 2019). It should be noted, however, that other studies show a more restricted pattern of caffeine-evoked activation on specific subpopulations of serotonergic neurons of the raphe nuclei that project to the basolateral amygdaloid nucleus (Fig. 1b), a region important for emotional appraisal and modulation of anxiety-related responses (Abrams et al. 2005). In terminal regions such as the hippocampus, caffeine increases the release of serotonin, an effect mediated by its blockade of A1Rs at presynaptic terminals (Okada et al. 1999).

Studies in zebrafish (de Carvalho et al. 2019) and rodent models (Khurana and Bansal 2019) suggest that brain oxidative stress represents a biochemical mechanism involved in anxiety-like behavior evoked by caffeine. Agents that minimize oxidative stress prevent caffeine-induced anxiogenic behavior as well as caffeine-induced increase in oxidative stress markers and decrease in enzymes of antioxidant defense in hippocampus, amygdala, and the prefrontal cortex of rats (Patki et al. 2015). Caffeine prooxidant effects may be related to its ability to antagonize the uptake of Ca2+ in intracellular stores and to evoke Ca2+ outflux from the endoplasmic reticulum. The consequent increase in cytoplasmic Ca2+ has been associated with increased biogenesis of free radicals and reduced cellular antioxidant levels (Peng and Jou 2010). The blockage of L-type Ca2+-channel reverses caffeine-induced anxiety and brings the associated brain oxido-nitrosative stress biomarkers back to control levels (Khurana and Bansal 2019).

The anxiogenic nature of caffeine has led to the investigation of the association between the dysregulation of hypothalamic–pituitary–adrenal (HPA) axis and the enhanced anxiety behavior mediated by caffeine. Even though a causal role has not been established, in rodents, anxiogenic caffeine doses elevate plasma adrenocorticotropin hormone and corticosterone levels (Nicholson 1989; Patz et al. 2006). Adolescence may be a period of greater sensitivity, as evidence of dysfunctional HPA axis due to adolescent exposure persists into adulthood in the absence of continued caffeine consumption (O'Neill et al. 2016). There is also evidence that alpha-melanocyte stimulating hormone (α-MSH), acting via its MC4 receptor in the amygdala, a crucial locus for processing anxiety-related behavior, may mediate anxiogenic effects of caffeine. In this regard, pre-exposure to α-MSH, or to an MC4 receptor agonist, RO27-3225, in the amygdala, potentiates caffeine-induced anxiogenic behavior. The combined administration of α-MSH or RO27-3225 with chronic caffeine delays the development of tolerance and prevents withdrawal-induced anxiety-like behavior (Bhorkar et al. 2014).

While it is established that caffeine affects anxiety levels both in humans and in animal models, and that ARs-mediated reduction of adenosinergic transmission takes part in caffeine's modulatory actions, other mechanisms are either directly or indirectly involved. Future studies are needed to expand our knowledge on caffeine biological targets and mechanisms of action, as well as to define their relative relevance on mediating anxiety.

Susceptibility to Anxiety Effects of Caffeine

During the last decade, accumulating evidence has demonstrated that caffeine effects on mood may be affected by several factors. There are great interindividual variations in the effects of acute caffeine exposure. Preclinical and human studies indicate that both genetic and environmental factors impact caffeine-induced anxiety alterations. Some psychological disorders also increase susceptibility to the anxiogenic effects of caffeine. On the other hand, caffeine use predisposes anxiety alterations generated by other conditions such as drug dependence.

Genetic variations influence physiological responses to caffeine consumption. It is well established that some gene polymorphisms are relevant for caffeine anxiogenic effect. While a polymorphism in the gene that encodes for the CYP1A2 isoform, an enzyme responsible for caffeine metabolism, may be relevant for some interindividual differences (Nehlig 2018), the genetic variation of the AR gene seems to be crucial to caffeine-induced anxiety effects. Alsene and colleagues (2003) demonstrated that the adenosine receptor A2A gene is associated with the anxiogenic action of caffeine in healthy individuals (Alsene et al. 2003). The 1976T/T and the 2592Tins/Tins genotypes generated greater increases in subjective experience of anxiety after 150 mg oral dose of caffeine freebase administration than other genotypic groups. Gajewska et al. (2013), using a prepulse inhibition model, indicated that women with A2A 1976TT genotype are more susceptible to experiencing anxiety following caffeine exposure. In this study, prepulse inhibition was impaired by caffeine in women with this risk genotype (A2A 1976TT) when compared to male with the same genotype, while no significant effects were observed in the non-risk genotype or placebo group (Gajewska et al. 2013). Despite these findings, moderate and high caffeine consumers seem to have tolerance to anxiogenic effects of caffeine regardless of genetic predisposition (Rogers et al. 2010). Associations between A2A and dopamine D2 receptor gene polymorphisms also seem to be relevant in explaining interindividual variance in susceptibility to caffeine-induced anxiety (Childs et al. 2008). Polymorphisms in the neuropeptide S system are also candidates to explain the interindividual differences in anxiety induced by caffeine. The neuropeptide S receptor (NPSR) is expressed in the amygdaloid complex and the paraventricular hypothalamic nucleus (Xu et al. 2007) and its activation elicits anxiolytic effects (Leonard et al. 2008). Domschke et al. (2012) demonstrated that, in carriers of the more active NPSR TT genotype, caffeine exposure resulted in an increased magnitude of the acoustic startle reflex in the neutral emotional condition and decreased startle magnitude in response to unpleasant stimuli (Domschke et al. 2012).

Several environmental factors may affect caffeine effects on brain function. Since the effects of caffeine on anxiety are dose-dependent, alterations on caffeine metabolism could change anxiety levels. Factors that slow metabolism and, consequently, increase serum caffeine could enhance susceptibility to its anxiogenic effects. A number of such factors have already been described: Pregnancy, liver disorders, and co-exposure to several other drugs (Carrillo and Benitez 2000; Grosso and Bracken 2005). Even a physical fatigue state seems to be relevant to the anxiety effects of caffeine. Individuals with low trait physical fatigue report an increase in feelings of anxiety, while caffeine reduces anxiety in individuals with high trait physical fatigue (Fuller et al. 2021). Future studies are needed to investigate the brain mechanisms that underlie caffeine interactions related to anxiety-induced behaviors.

Studies have shown that some mental disorders increase susceptibility to caffeine anxiogenic effects. Even though an universal association pattern between psychiatric disorders and caffeine phenotypes has not been identified, caffeine-induced anxiogenic effects have been described in panic disorder, social anxiety, and major depression concurrent with panic attacks (Nardi et al. 2007, 2009; Masdrakis et al. 2008). While 480 mg of caffeine does not elicit panic attacks in healthy individuals, these are triggered in about 60% of panic disorder and 50% of performance social anxiety disorder individuals. Two possibilities may explain this association: firstly, susceptibility to caffeine anxiogenic effects and these mental disorders could be caused by the same underlying genetic and/or environmental factors. On the other hand, this association could represent a causal relationship, so that mental disorders increase the risk of caffeine-induced anxiogenic effects and vice versa (Fig. 2). Interestingly, there is evidence in support of both possibilities. Adenosine receptor A2A polymorphisms are reported to increased susceptibility to panic disorder and other anxiety-related phenotypes (Hohoff et al. 2010). Caffeine may also interact with other substances in altering anxiety levels, a possibility that could have relevant implications regarding other substance use disorders.

Applications to Other Areas of Addiction

Caffeine use can predispose anxiety alterations generated by other substance use. A history of caffeine use has been associated with higher anxiety scores in young adult cigarette smokers (Dosh et al. 2010). Preclinical studies also demonstrated that caffeine or caffeine beverages (energy drinks) could induce anxiety-like behaviors in association with ethanol exposure (Hughes 2011; Krahe et al. 2017). The mixture of caffeine and sucrose also seems to evoke anxiety-like behavior under certain conditions (Xu and Reichelt 2018). Since increased anxiety during drug withdrawal has been considered one of the most important factors in relapse, anxiety effects induced by caffeine during drug withdrawal are relevant to addiction treatment. Interestingly, preclinical studies suggest that history of caffeine use could increase

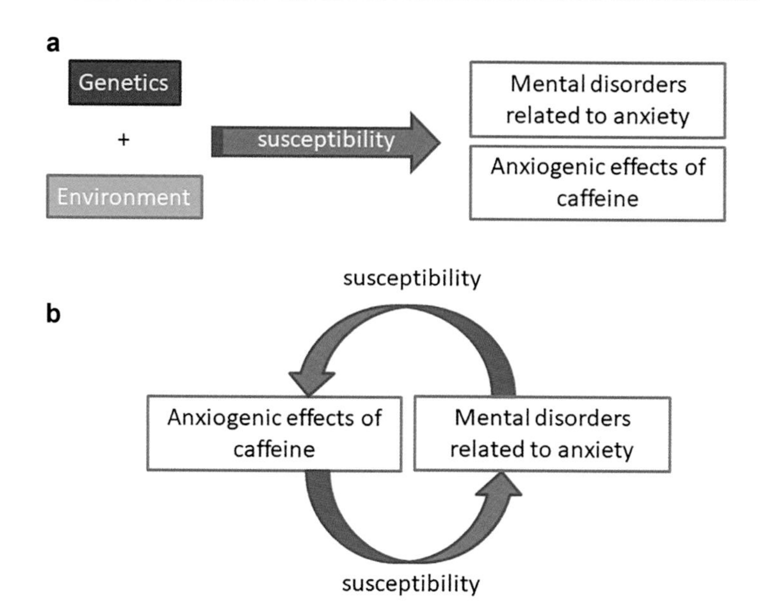

Fig. 2 Association between mental disorders (see main text) and susceptibility to anxiogenic effects of caffeine. (**a**) Environmental and genetic factors may underlie both conditions; (**b**) possibility of a bidirectional causal relationship

anxiety disorder susceptibility precipitated by withdrawal to other drugs. Exposure to caffeine increases anxiogenic-like effects associated with nicotine and alcohol withdrawal in rodents (Matovu and Alele 2018; da Silva Gonçalves et al. 2019). If a similar effect occurs in humans, caffeine-induced anxiogenic effects could facilitate relapse to drug use during a period of abstinence. In this sense, drug addicted persons who attempt to quit may benefit from reducing caffeine intake.

Application to Public Health

The association between caffeine consumption and anxiety-related behaviors is complex, depending not only on the ingested dose but also on the age of exposure, genetic profile, sex, exposure to other drugs, and other factors. Despite being considered a safe substance to consume, the associations among caffeine use, anxiety, and some mental disorders such as panic and substance use disorder are a matter of great concern. The recent public health problems generated by high consumption of caffeinated drinks by adolescents, especially in co-exposure with alcoholic drinks, reinforce the idea that a prudent approach should be considered when assessing the safety of caffeine during brain development. The observed effects of caffeine on anxiety advises limiting consumption of this substance to moderate doses and should inform drug/food regulatory agencies in establishing public policies regarding caffeine consumption, particularly during development and by individuals who have mental health comorbidities.

Mini-Dictionary of Terms

- **BDNF** – brain-derived neurotrophic factor is a protein recognized by its regulatory role in brain development.
- **c-fos** – c-fos is a protein used as an indirect marker of neuronal activity.
- **CREB** – cAMP-response element-binding protein is a cellular transcription factor and has a well-documented role in neuronal plasticity.
- **Gene polymorphism** – polymorphism involves one of two or more variants of a specific DNA sequence. In general, each allele must also occur in the population at a rate of at least 1%.
- **Receptor downregulation** – term used when there is a reduction in the cell expression of the receptor or its affinity.

Key Facts Regarding Susceptibility to Anxiety Effects of Caffeine

- There are great interindividual variations in levels of caffeine-induced anxiety.
- Factors that slow caffeine metabolism and, consequently, increase serum caffeine also increase susceptibility to its anxiogenic effects.
- Developmental exposure to caffeine may cause long-lasting alterations on anxiety levels.
- Polymorphisms in the adenosine receptor gene affect susceptibility to caffeine-induced anxiety.
- Some psychiatric disorders increase susceptibility to caffeine anxiogenic effect.

Summary Points

- High caffeine consumption increases anxiety levels.
- This effect is dependent of several factors such as tolerance, genetic profile, mental health status, sex, and age.
- At low to moderate concentrations, caffeine effects are mediated by adenosine receptor antagonism.
- Caffeine-evoked serotonergic activation of the dorsal raphe nucleus to basolateral amygdala pathway is relevant for the modulation of anxiety-related behavior.
- Both genetic and environmental factors impact caffeine-induced anxiety levels.

References

Abrams JK et al (2005) Serotonergic systems associated with arousal and vigilance behaviors following administration of anxiogenic drugs. Neuroscience 133(4):983–997. https://doi.org/10.1016/j.neuroscience.2005.03.025

Adan A et al (2008) Early effects of caffeinated and decaffeinated coffee on subjective state and gender differences. Prog Neuro-Psychopharmacol Biol Psychiatry 32(7):1698–1703. https://doi.org/10.1016/j.pnpbp.2008.07.005

Alhowail A, Aldubayan M (2020) Mechanisms underlying cognitive impairment induced by prenatal caffeine exposure. Eur Rev Med Pharmacol Sci 24(22):11909–11913. https://doi.org/10.26355/eurrev_202011_23849

Alsene K et al (2003) Association between A2a receptor gene polymorphisms and caffeine-induced anxiety. Neuropsychopharmacology 28(9):1694–1702. https://doi.org/10.1038/sj.npp.1300232

Altemus M, Sarvaiya N, Neill Epperson C (2014) Sex differences in anxiety and depression clinical perspectives. Front Neuroendocrinol 35(3):320–330. https://doi.org/10.1016/j.yfrne.2014.05.004

Arnold MR et al (2019) Effects of chronic caffeine exposure during adolescence and subsequent acute caffeine challenge during adulthood on rat brain serotonergic systems. Neuropharmacology 148:257–271. https://doi.org/10.1016/j.neuropharm.2018.12.019

Babu KM, Church RJ, Lewander W (2008) Energy drinks: the new eye-opener for adolescents. Clin Pediatr Emerg Med 9(1):35–42. https://doi.org/10.1016/j.cpem.2007.12.002

Berglundh S et al (2021) Maternal caffeine intake during pregnancy and child neurodevelopment up to eight years of age – results from the Norwegian mother, father and child cohort study. Eur J Nutr 60(2):791–805. https://doi.org/10.1007/s00394-020-02280-7

Bernstein GA et al (2002) Caffeine dependence in teenagers. Drug Alcohol Depend 66(1):1–6. https://doi.org/10.1016/S0376-8716(01)00181-8

Bertasi RAO et al (2021) Caffeine intake and mental health in college students. Cureus 13(4): e14313. https://doi.org/10.7759/cureus.14313

Bhorkar AA et al (2014) Involvement of the central melanocortin system in the effects of caffeine on anxiety-like behavior in mice. Life Sci 95(2):72–80. https://doi.org/10.1016/j.lfs.2013.12.014

Botella P, Parra A (2003) Coffee increases state anxiety in males but not in females. Hum Psychopharmacol 18(2):141–143. https://doi.org/10.1002/hup.444

Carrillo JA, Benitez J (2000) Clinically significant pharmacokinetic interactions between dietary caffeine and medications. Clin Pharmacokinet 39(2):127–153. https://doi.org/10.2165/00003088-200039020-00004

Chang D et al (2018) Caffeine caused a widespread increase of resting brain entropy. Sci Rep 8(1): 2700. https://doi.org/10.1038/s41598-018-21008-6

Chelben J et al (2008) Effects of amino acid energy drinks leading to hospitalization in individuals with mental illness. Gen Hosp Psychiatry 30(2):187–189. https://doi.org/10.1016/j.genhosppsych.2007.10.002

Childs E et al (2008) Association between ADORA2A and DRD2 polymorphisms and caffeine-induced anxiety. Neuropsychopharmacology 33(12):2791–2800. https://doi.org/10.1038/npp.2008.17

Chtourou H et al (2019) Acute effects of an "energy drink" on short-term maximal performance, reaction times, psychological and physiological parameters: insights from a randomized double-blind, placebo-controlled, counterbalanced crossover trial. Nutrients 11(5). https://doi.org/10.3390/nu11050992

da Silva Gonçalves B et al (2019) Lifelong exposure to caffeine increases anxiety-like behavior in adult mice exposed to tobacco smoke during adolescence. Neurosci Lett 696:146. https://doi.org/10.1016/j.neulet.2018.12.026

de Carvalho TS et al (2019) Oxidative stress mediates anxiety-like behavior induced by high caffeine intake in zebrafish: protective effect of alpha-tocopherol. Oxidative Med Cell Longev 2019:1–9. https://doi.org/10.1155/2019/8419810

Deckert J (1998) The adenosine A2A receptor knockout mouse: a model for anxiety? Int J Neuropsychopharmacol 1(2):S1461145798001217. https://doi.org/10.1017/S1461145798001217

Domschke K et al (2012) Modification of caffeine effects on the affect-modulated startle by neuropeptide S receptor gene variation. Psychopharmacology 222(3):533–541. https://doi.org/10.1007/s00213-012-2678-0

Dosh T et al (2010) A comparison of the associations of caffeine and cigarette use with depressive and ADHD symptoms in a sample of young adult smokers. J Addict Med 4(1):52–54. https://doi.org/10.1097/ADM.0b013e3181b508ec

El Yacoubi M et al (2000) The anxiogenic-like effect of caffeine in two experimental procedures measuring anxiety in the mouse is not shared by selective A 2A adenosine receptor antagonists. Psychopharmacology 148(2):153–163. https://doi.org/10.1007/s002130050037
European Food Safety Authority (EFSA) (2015) Scientific opinion on the safety of caffeine. EFSA panel on dietetic products, nutrition and allergies (NDA). EFSA J 13(5):4102
Fiani B et al (2021) The neurophysiology of caffeine as a central nervous system stimulant and the resultant effects on cognitive function. Cureus 13(5):e15032. https://doi.org/10.7759/cureus.15032
Florio C et al (1998) Adenosine A 1 receptors modulate anxiety in CD1 mice. Psychopharmacology 136(4):311–319. https://doi.org/10.1007/s002130050572
Fuller DT, Smith ML, Boolani A (2021) Trait energy and fatigue modify the effects of caffeine on mood, cognitive and fine-motor task performance: a post-hoc study. Nutrients 13(2):412. https://doi.org/10.3390/nu13020412
Fulton JL et al (2018) Impact of genetic variability on physiological responses to caffeine in humans: a systematic review. Nutrients 10(10). https://doi.org/10.3390/nu10101373
Gajewska A et al (2013) Effects of ADORA2A gene variation and caffeine on prepulse inhibition: a multi-level risk model of anxiety. Prog Neuro-Psychopharmacol Biol Psychiatry 40:115–121. https://doi.org/10.1016/j.pnpbp.2012.08.008
Giménez-Llort L et al (2002) Mice lacking the adenosine A 1 receptor are anxious and aggressive, but are normal learners with reduced muscle strength and survival rate. Eur J Neurosci 16(3): 547–550. https://doi.org/10.1046/j.1460-9568.2002.02122.x
Gray B, Das K, J. and Semsarian, C. (2012) Consumption of energy drinks: a new provocation test for primary arrhythmogenic diseases? Int J Cardiol 159(1):77–78. https://doi.org/10.1016/j.ijcard.2012.05.121
Grosso LM, Bracken MB (2005) Caffeine metabolism, genetics, and perinatal outcomes: a review of exposure assessment considerations during pregnancy. Ann Epidemiol 15(6):460–466. https://doi.org/10.1016/j.annepidem.2004.12.011
Guest NS et al (2021) International society of sports nutrition position stand: caffeine and exercise performance. J Int Soc Sports Nutr 18(1):1. https://doi.org/10.1186/s12970-020-00383-4
Hale MW et al (2010) Multiple anxiogenic drugs recruit a parvalbumin-containing subpopulation of GABAergic interneurons in the basolateral amygdala. Prog Neuro-Psychopharmacol Biol Psychiatry 34(7):1285–1293. https://doi.org/10.1016/j.pnpbp.2010.07.012
Harris JL, Munsell CR (2015) Energy drinks and adolescents: what's the harm? Nutr Rev 73(4): 247–257. https://doi.org/10.1093/nutrit/nuu061
Hohoff C et al (2010) Adenosine A2A receptor gene: evidence for association of risk variants with panic disorder and anxious personality. J Psychiatr Res 44(14):930–937. https://doi.org/10.1016/j.jpsychires.2010.02.006
Hughes RN (2011) Adult anxiety-related behavior of rats following consumption during late adolescence of alcohol alone and in combination with caffeine. Alcohol 45(4):365–372. https://doi.org/10.1016/j.alcohol.2010.10.006
Hughes RN et al (2014) Evidence for anxiolytic effects of acute caffeine on anxiety-related behavior in male and female rats tested with and without bright light. Behav Brain Res 271:7–15. https://doi.org/10.1016/j.bbr.2014.05.038
Hvolgaard Mikkelsen S et al (2017) Maternal caffeine consumption during pregnancy and behavioral disorders in 11-year-old offspring: a Danish National Birth Cohort Study. J Pediatr 189: 120–127.e1. https://doi.org/10.1016/j.jpeds.2017.06.051
Institute of Medicine (IOM) (2014) Caffeine in food and dietary supplements: examining safety: workshop summary. National Academies Press. www.nap.edu
Jain N et al (1995) Anxiolytic activity of adenosine receptor activation in mice. Br J Pharmacol 116 (3):2127–2133. https://doi.org/10.1111/j.1476-5381.1995.tb16421.x
Jee HJ et al (2020) Effect of caffeine consumption on the risk for neurological and psychiatric disorders: sex differences in human. Nutrients 12(10). https://doi.org/10.3390/nu12103080
Johansson B et al (2001) Hyperalgesia, anxiety, and decreased hypoxic neuroprotection in mice lacking the adenosine A1 receptor. Proc Natl Acad Sci 98(16):9407–9412. https://doi.org/10.1073/pnas.161292398

Kaur S et al (2020) Consumption of energy drinks is associated with depression, anxiety, and stress in young adult males: evidence from a longitudinal cohort study. Depress Anxiety 37(11):1089–1098. https://doi.org/10.1002/da.23090

Kendler KS, Myers J, Gardner CO (2006) Caffeine intake, toxicity and dependence and lifetime risk for psychiatric and substance use disorders: an epidemiologic and co-twin control analysis. Psychol Med 36(12):1717–1725. https://doi.org/10.1017/S0033291706008622

Khurana K, Bansal N (2019) Lacidipine attenuates caffeine-induced anxiety-like symptoms in mice: role of calcium-induced oxido-nitrosative stress. Pharmacol Rep 71(6):1264–1272. https://doi.org/10.1016/j.pharep.2019.07.008

Knutti R, Rothweiler H, Schlatter C (1982) The effect of pregnancy on the pharmacokinetics of caffeine. 187–192. https://doi.org/10.1007/978-3-642-68511-8_33

Krahe TE et al (2017) Energy drink enhances the behavioral effects of alcohol in adolescent mice. Neurosci Lett 651. https://doi.org/10.1016/j.neulet.2017.04.050

Laatar R et al (2021) Caffeine consumption improves motor and cognitive performances during dual tasking in middle-aged women. Behav Brain Res 412:113437. https://doi.org/10.1016/j.bbr.2021.113437

Laureano-Melo R et al (2016) Behavioral profile assessment in offspring of Swiss mice treated during pregnancy and lactation with caffeine. Metab Brain Dis 31(5):1071–1080. https://doi.org/10.1007/s11011-016-9847-5

León D et al (2002) Adenosine A1 receptor down-regulation in mothers and fetal brain after caffeine and theophylline treatments to pregnant rats. J Neurochem 82(3):625–634. https://doi.org/10.1046/j.1471-4159.2002.01008.x

León D et al (2005) Effect of chronic gestational treatment with caffeine or theophylline on Group I metabotropic glutamate receptors in maternal and fetal brain. J Neurochem 94(2):440–451. https://doi.org/10.1111/j.1471-4159.2005.03211.x

Leonard SK et al (2008) Pharmacology of neuropeptide S in mice: therapeutic relevance to anxiety disorders. Psychopharmacology 197(4):601–611. https://doi.org/10.1007/s00213-008-1080-4

Loomans EM et al (2012) Caffeine intake during pregnancy and risk of problem behavior in 5-to 6-year-old children. Pediatrics 130(2):e305–e313. https://doi.org/10.1542/peds.2011-3361

Lorenzo AM et al (2010) Maternal caffeine intake during gestation and lactation down-regulates adenosine A 1 receptor in rat brain from mothers and neonates. J Neurosci Res 88(6):1252–1261. https://doi.org/10.1002/jnr.22287

Luebbe AM (2011) Child and adolescent anxiety sensitivity, perceived subjective effects of caffeine and caffeine consumption. J Caffeine Res 1(4):213–218. https://doi.org/10.1089/jcr.2011.0020

Luebbe AM, Bell DJ (2009) Mountain dew ® or mountain don't?: a pilot investigation of caffeine use parameters and relations to depression and anxiety symptoms in 5th- and 10th-grade students. J Sch Health 79(8):380–387. https://doi.org/10.1111/j.1746-1561.2009.00424.x

Magalhães R et al (2021) Habitual coffee drinkers display a distinct pattern of brain functional connectivity. Mol Psychiatry. https://doi.org/10.1038/s41380-021-01075-4

Marmorstein NR (2016) Energy drink and coffee consumption and psychopathology symptoms among early adolescents: cross-sectional and longitudinal associations. J Caffeine Res 6(2):64–72. https://doi.org/10.1089/jcr.2015.0018

Masdrakis VG et al (2008) Caffeine challenge in patients with panic disorder: baseline differences between those who panic and those who do not. Depress Anxiety 25(9):E72–E79. https://doi.org/10.1002/da.20333

Matovu D, Alele PE (2018) Seizure vulnerability and anxiety responses following chronic co-administration and acute withdrawal of caffeine and ethanol in a rat model. J Basic Clin Physiol Pharmacol 29(1):1–10. https://doi.org/10.1515/jbcpp-2017-0018

McLellan TM, Lieberman HR (2012) Do energy drinks contain active components other than caffeine? Nutr Rev 70(12):730–744. https://doi.org/10.1111/j.1753-4887.2012.00525.x

Mioranzza S et al (2014) Prenatal caffeine intake differently affects synaptic proteins during fetal brain development. Int J Dev Neurosci 36(1):45–52. https://doi.org/10.1016/j.ijdevneu.2014.04.006

Naftalovich H, Tauber N, Kalanthroff E (2020) But first, coffee: the roles of arousal and inhibition in the resistance of compulsive cleansing in individuals with high contamination fears. J Anxiety Disord 76:102316. https://doi.org/10.1016/j.janxdis.2020.102316
Nardi AE et al (2007) Caffeine challenge test in panic disorder and depression with panic attacks. Compr Psychiatry 48(3):257–263. https://doi.org/10.1016/j.comppsych.2006.12.001
Nardi AE et al (2009) Panic disorder and social anxiety disorder subtypes in a caffeine challenge test. Psychiatry Res 169(2):149–153. https://doi.org/10.1016/j.psychres.2008.06.023
Nehlig A (2018) Interindividual differences in caffeine metabolism and factors driving caffeine consumption. Pharmacol Rev 70(2):384–411. https://doi.org/10.1124/pr.117.014407
Nicholson SA (1989) Stimulatory effect of caffeine on the hypothalamo-pituitary-adrenocortical axis in the rat. J Endocrinol 122(2):535–543. https://doi.org/10.1677/joe.0.1220535
Nowak D, Jasionowski A (2016) Analysis of consumption of energy drinks by a group of adolescent athletes. Int J Environ Res Public Health 13(8):768. https://doi.org/10.3390/ijerph13080768
O'Neill CE et al (2016) Adolescent caffeine consumption increases adulthood anxiety-related behavior and modifies neuroendocrine signaling. Psychoneuroendocrinology 67:40–50. https://doi.org/10.1016/j.psyneuen.2016.01.030
Okada M et al (1999) Differential effects of adenosine receptor subtypes on release and reuptake of hippocampal serotonin. Eur J Neurosci 11(1):1–9. https://doi.org/10.1046/j.1460-9568.1999.00415.x
Pan H-Z, Chen H-H (2007) Hyperalgesia, low-anxiety, and impairment of avoidance learning in neonatal caffeine-treated rats. Psychopharmacology 191(1):119–125. https://doi.org/10.1007/s00213-006-0613-y
Park C-A et al (2014) The effects of caffeine ingestion on cortical areas: functional imaging study. Magn Reson Imaging 32(4):366–371. https://doi.org/10.1016/j.mri.2013.12.018
Patki G et al (2015) Tempol treatment reduces anxiety-like behaviors induced by multiple Anxiogenic drugs in rats. PLos One 10(3):e0117498. https://doi.org/10.1371/journal.pone.0117498. Edited by A. Kavushansky
Patz MD et al (2006) Modulation of the hypothalamo–pituitary–adrenocortical axis by caffeine. Psychoneuroendocrinology 31(4):493–500. https://doi.org/10.1016/j.psyneuen.2005.11.008
Peng T-I, Jou M-J (2010) Oxidative stress caused by mitochondrial calcium overload. Ann N Y Acad Sci 1201:183–188. https://doi.org/10.1111/j.1749-6632.2010.05634.x
Pennington N et al (2010) Energy drinks: a new health hazard for adolescents. J Sch Nurs 26(5): 352–359. https://doi.org/10.1177/1059840510374188
Richards G, Smith A (2015) Caffeine consumption and self-assessed stress, anxiety, and depression in secondary school children. J Psychopharmacol 29(12):1236–1247. https://doi.org/10.1177/0269881115612404
Rogers PJ et al (2010) Association of the anxiogenic and alerting effects of caffeine with ADORA2A and ADORA1 polymorphisms and habitual level of caffeine consumption. Neuropsychopharmacology 35(9):1973–1983. https://doi.org/10.1038/npp.2010.71
Rorabaugh BR (2021) Does prenatal exposure to CNS stimulants increase the risk of cardiovascular disease in adult offspring? Front Cardiovasc Med 8. https://doi.org/10.3389/fcvm.2021.652634
Savchenko VL, Boughter JD (2011) Regulation of neuronal activation by Alpha2A adrenergic receptor agonist. Neurotox Res 20(3):226–239. https://doi.org/10.1007/s12640-010-9236-5
Seifert SM et al (2011) Health effects of energy drinks on children, adolescents, and young adults. Pediatrics 127(3):511–528. https://doi.org/10.1542/peds.2009-3592
Silva RS et al (2008) Maternal caffeine intake affects acetylcholinesterase in hippocampus of neonate rats. Int J Dev Neurosci 26(3–4):339–343. https://doi.org/10.1016/j.ijdevneu.2007.12.006
Silva CG et al (2013) Adenosine receptor antagonists including caffeine alter fetal brain development in mice. Sci Transl Med 5(197):197ra104. https://doi.org/10.1126/scitranslmed.3006258
Sweeney P et al (2016) Caffeine increases food intake while reducing anxiety-related behaviors. Appetite 101:171–177. https://doi.org/10.1016/j.appet.2016.03.013

Tal O et al (2013) Caffeine-induced global reductions in resting-state BOLD connectivity reflect widespread decreases in MEG connectivity. Front Hum Neurosci 7:63. https://doi.org/10.3389/fnhum.2013.00063

Tchekalarova JD, Kubová H, Mareš P (2014) Early caffeine exposure: transient and long-term consequences on brain excitability. Brain Res Bull 104:27–35. https://doi.org/10.1016/j.brainresbull.2014.04.001

Temple JL, Ziegler AM (2011) Gender differences in subjective and physiological responses to caffeine and the role of steroid hormones. J Caffeine Res 1(1):41–48. https://doi.org/10.1089/jcr.2011.0005

Temple JL et al (2009) Sex differences in reinforcing value of caffeinated beverages in adolescents. Behav Pharmacol 20(8):731–741. https://doi.org/10.1097/FBP.0b013e328333b27c

Trapp GSA et al (2014) Energy drink consumption is associated with anxiety in Australian young adult males. Depress Anxiety 31(5):420–428. https://doi.org/10.1002/da.22175

Tremblay L et al (2015) Selective dysfunction of basal ganglia subterritories: from movement to behavioral disorders. Mov Disord 30(9):1155–1170. https://doi.org/10.1002/mds.26199

Tung R et al (2021) Functional connectivity within an anxiety network and associations with anxiety symptom severity in middle-aged adults with and without autism. Autism Res. https://doi.org/10.1002/aur.2579

Turnbull D, Rodricks JV, Mariano GF (2016) Neurobehavioral hazard identification and characterization for caffeine. Regul Toxicol Pharmacol 74:81–92. https://doi.org/10.1016/j.yrtph.2015.12.002

Turner S et al (2018) Self-medication with alcohol or drugs for mood and anxiety disorders: a narrative review of the epidemiological literature. Depress Anxiety 35(9):851–860. https://doi.org/10.1002/da.22771

van Calker D et al (2019) The role of adenosine receptors in mood and anxiety disorders. J Neurochem 151(1):11–27. https://doi.org/10.1111/jnc.14841

Whalen DJ et al (2007) Caffeine consumption, sleep, and affect in the natural environments of depressed youth and healthy controls. J Pediatr Psychol 33(4):358–367. https://doi.org/10.1093/jpepsy/jsm086

Willson C (2018) The clinical toxicology of caffeine: a review and case study. Toxicol Rep 5:1140–1152. https://doi.org/10.1016/j.toxrep.2018.11.002

Wong CW et al (2012) Anti-correlated networks, global signal regression, and the effects of caffeine in resting-state functional MRI. NeuroImage 63(1):356–364. https://doi.org/10.1016/j.neuroimage.2012.06.035

Xu TJ, Reichelt AC (2018) Sucrose or sucrose and caffeine differentially impact memory and anxiety-like behaviours, and alter hippocampal parvalbumin and doublecortin. Neuropharmacology 137:24–32. https://doi.org/10.1016/j.neuropharm.2018.04.012

Xu Y-L et al (2007) Distribution of neuropeptide S receptor mRNA and neurochemical characteristics of neuropeptide S-expressing neurons in the rat brain. J Comp Neurol 500(1):84–102. https://doi.org/10.1002/cne.21159

Caffeinated Beverages and Diabetes 74

Public Health Concerns and Implications

Muneera Qassim Al-Mssallem and Salah M. Aleid

Contents

Introduction 1592
Applications to Other Areas of Substance Use Disorders 1595
Applications to Public Health 1598
Mini-Dictionary of Terms 1600
Key Facts of Caffeinated Beverage Substances 1601
Key Facts of the Relationship between Caffeinated Beverages and the Risk of Developing T2DM 1601
Summary Points 1601
References 1602

Abstract

Caffeinated beverages are any drink containing caffeine, and the most popular caffeinated beverages worldwide are coffee and tea. Caffeinated beverages have gained their popularity and attractiveness due to their pleasant aromas and psychostimulant impacts, which are mostly attributed to the presence of caffeine. Both beneficial and deleterious impacts of caffeine and its association with developing type 2 diabetes mellitus (T2DM) have been observed. This dual nature of caffeine has been intensively investigated in several prospective cohort and clinical studies. On the other hand, caffeinated beverage constituents other than caffeine have been shown to be the main contributors to increased insulin sensitivity, lowered plasma glucose concentration, and a reduced risk of developing T2DM. These include phytochemicals such as chlorogenic acids and trigonelline. However, other natural and/or artificial additives, such as sucrose, fructose, and cream (saturated and trans fats), can play significant role in reducing insulin sensitivity and affecting glucose metabolism. This chapter discusses the

M. Q. Al-Mssallem (✉) · S. M. Aleid
Department of Food Sciences and Nutrition, College of Agriculture and Food Sciences, King Faisal University, Al-Ahsa, Saudi Arabia
e-mail: mmssallem@kfu.edu.sa; seid@kfu.edu.sa

V. B. Patel, V. R. Preedy (eds.), *Handbook of Substance Misuse and Addictions*,
https://doi.org/10.1007/978-3-030-92392-1_81

beneficial and detrimental effects of caffeinated beverages on human health, particularly in the risk of developing T2DM.

Keywords

Antidiabetics · Antioxidant · Caffeinated beverages · Caffeine · Chlorogenic acids · Diabetes mellitus · Glucose homeostasis · Insulin sensitivity · Oxidative stress · Trigonelline

Abbreviations

cAMP	cyclic adenosine monophosphate
LDL	low-density lipoproteins
T2DM	type 2 diabetes mellitus

Introduction

Various types of caffeinated beverages are available worldwide, including coffee, black tea, green tea, hot chocolate drinks, energy drinks, and caffeinated soft beverages. Coffee and tea are the most popular frequently consumed caffeinated drinks (Frary et al. 2005; Heckman et al. 2010; Oba et al. 2010). The most distinguished features of caffeinated beverages are their pleasant aromas and psychostimulant properties (Ferré 2016). It is well known that the common substance in all of these beverages is caffeine (Fig. 1). Caffeine is a natural chemical constituent present in coffee beans (*Coffea Arabica* and *Coffea robusta*), cacao beans (*Theobroma cacao*), guarana berries (*Paullinia cupana*), tea leaves (*Camellia sinensis*), and kola nuts (*Cola acuminate*). Caffeine is rapidly absorbed from the stomach and metabolized in the liver to form its derivative metabolites, such as 3,7-dimethylxanthine, 1,7-dimethylxanthine, and 1,3-dimethylxanthine (Gan et al. 2018; Heckman et al. 2010). Further demethylation is continued to form paraxanthine, theobromine, and theophylline (Fig. 2). Then these metabolites undergo demethylation and oxidation in the liver (Heckman et al. 2010; Vieira et al. 2020). Certainly, the major source of caffeine in human beverages comes from coffee, and the highest content of caffeine was found in espresso coffee (Fig. 3). In the caffeinated beverages, caffeine exerts various physiological actions, including its impact on developing the risk of type 2 diabetes mellitus (T2DM). In addition to its role in blood glucose homeostasis, caffeine has an effect on cognitive performance, such as increased attention and reaction speed. Moreover, caffeine exhibits stimulant and addictive properties, which are considered the main attractive character for caffeinated beverages (Ferré 2016). In fact, moderate caffeine consumption (<400 mg/day) is not associated with detrimental heath impacts (Mitchell et al. 2014). It is well documented that the biological effect of caffeine must be maintained for an adequate period of time in human tissues and must be at a plentiful concentration (Butt and Sultan 2011; Ludwig et al. 2014).

The other important constituent in caffeinated beverages is chlorogenic acid. Chlorogenic acid is an ester of caffeic acid and quinic acid (Fig. 4). The highest

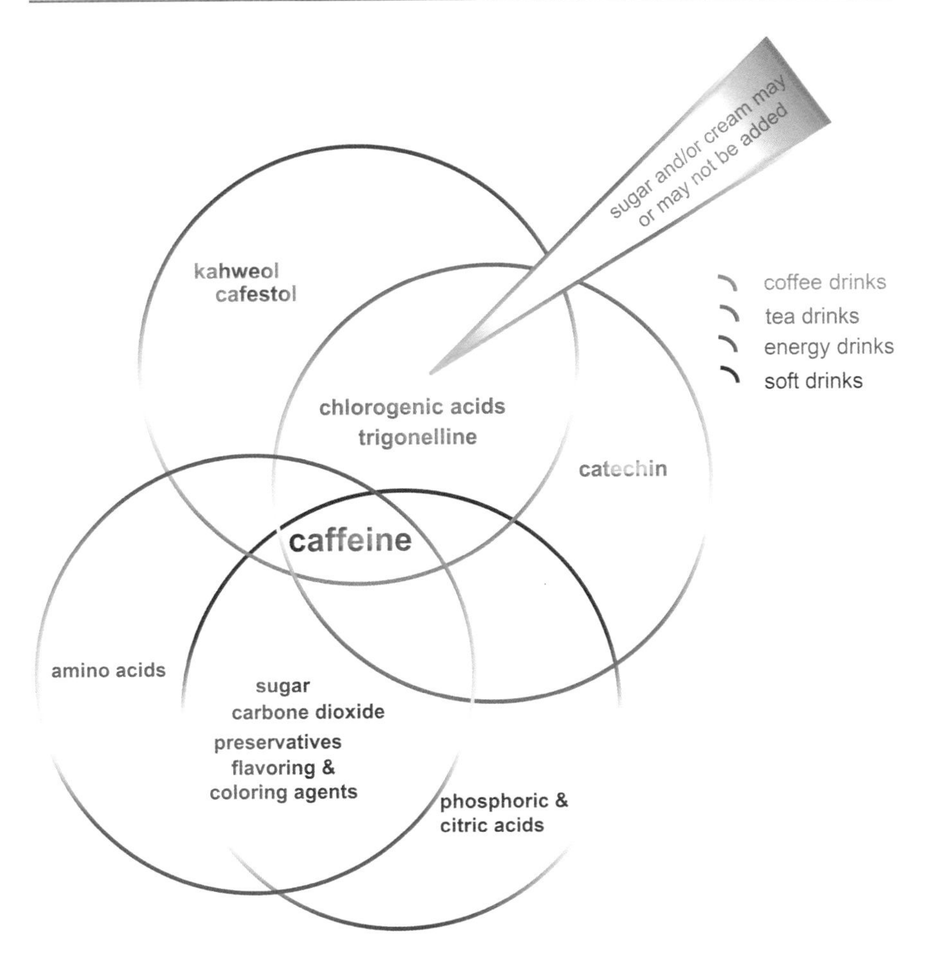

Fig. 1 The most natural and artificial substances of common caffeinated beverages

concentration of chlorogenic acids is found in coffee beans (van Dijk et al. 2009). Chlorogenic acid has an effective role in delaying glucose uptake from small intestines and lowering plasma glucose concentration (Butt and Sultan 2011; van Dijk et al. 2009). Trigonelline is also considered as an important constituent in caffeinated beverages (Fig. 1), which involves lowering the risk of developing T2DM (van Dijk et al. 2009; Zhou et al. 2013).

A combination of genetic and environmental factors is involved in the risk of developing T2DM, including lifestyle and dietary habits. Indeed, dietary habits such as the consumption of caffeinated drinks significantly affect blood glucose and insulin levels among patients with T2DM. Therefore, dietary approach is of paramount importance in preventing the risk of developing T2DM (Forouhi et al. 2018). Investigating habitual consumption of caffeinated beverages is a good approach of studying the interference of their substances with blood glucose absorption and

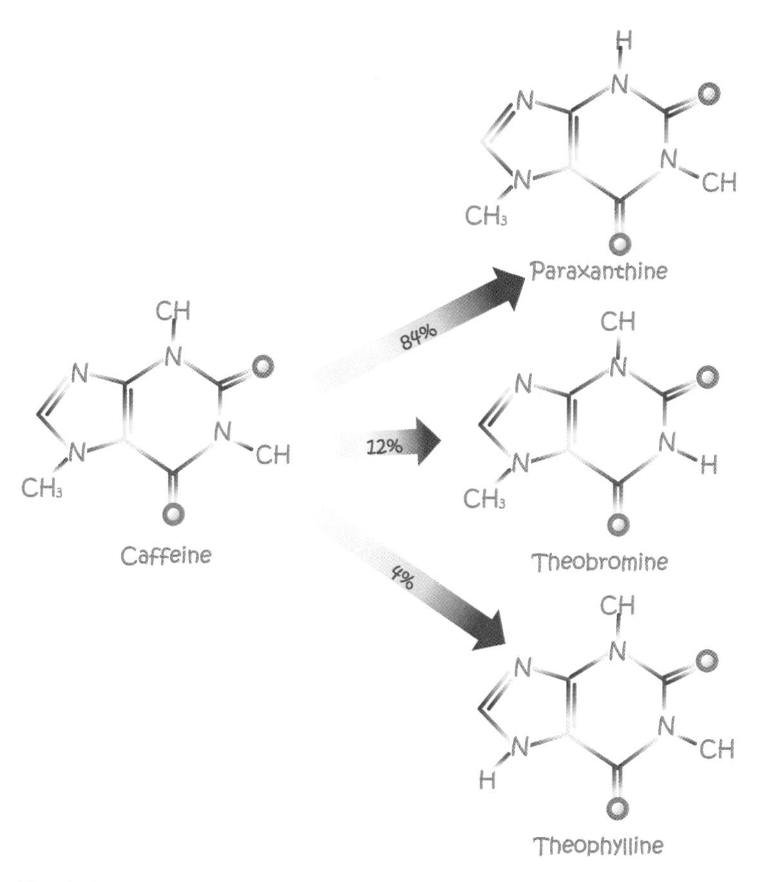

Fig. 2 Chemical structure of caffeine and its metabolites. (From Gan et al. (2018), Heckman et al. (2010))

insulin sensitivity (Ludwig et al. 2014). Therefore, the relationship between the consumption of caffeinated beverages and the risk of developing T2DM has been comprehensively investigated in several cross-sectional and prospective cohort studies. A lower risk of developing T2DM was associated with higher consumption of caffeinated beverages, in particular, coffee drinks. This association has been attributed to the presence of phytochemical compounds, antioxidants, and minerals that may influence insulin sensitivity or insulin secretion (Kim et al. 2020; Oba et al. 2010; Pereira et al. 2006; van Dieren et al. 2009). In contrast, the presence of caffeine in caffeinated beverages has been found to be associated with impaired glucose tolerance and insulin insensitivity (Loopsta-Masters et al. 2011; Ludwig et al. 2014). However, this effect remains controversial, and further investigation of the relationship between a high intake of caffeine and the risk of developing T2DM is required.

Caffeinated soft drinks were first introduced in the late eighteen century. Recently, there has been a massive increase in the consumption of caffeinated soft

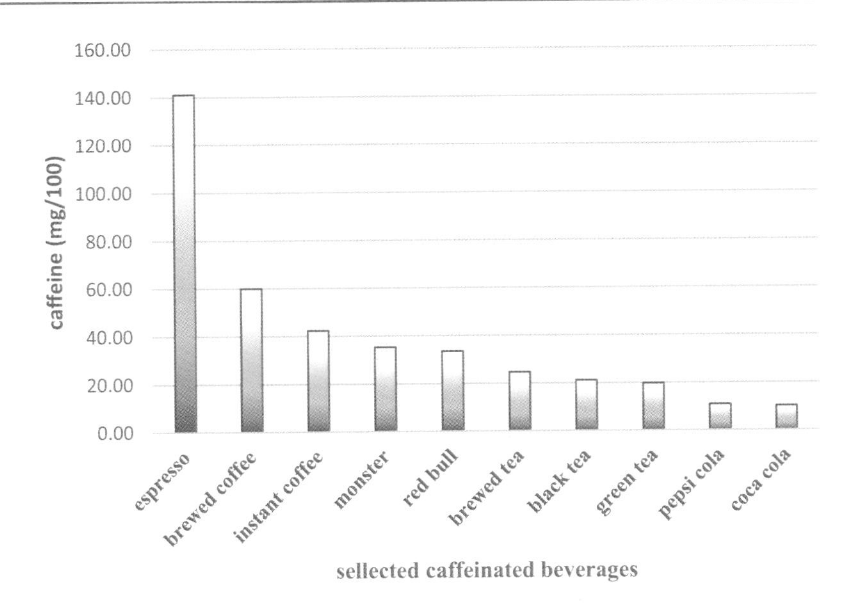

Fig. 3 Caffeine content (mg/100 ml) in a variety of different common caffeinated beverages. (From Heckman et al. (2010))

drinks, such as certain soda drinks and energy drinks (Mitchell et al. 2014). Caffeinated soft drinks contain significant quantity of sugar, which may affect glucose metabolism. High consumption of these types of drinks was linked to an increased risk of developing T2DM and obesity (Imamura et al. 2015). However, other constituents such as catechins, caffeine, and calcium, contribute to preventing weight gain (Rudelle et al. 2007).

Applications to Other Areas of Substance Use Disorders

Most of biological effects of caffeinated beverages can contribute to the presence of phytochemical compounds such as caffeine, chlorogenic acids, trigonelline, cafestol, and kahweol (Table 1). Some of these compounds, more than others, exhibit antioxidant, anti-carcinogenic, anti-cardiovascular, anti-obesity, and antidiabetic activities (Butt and Sultan 2011; Kobayashi et al. 2017; Verzelloni et al. 2011). For instance, chlorogenic acids and trigonelline of caffeinated beverages potentially prevent the risk factors of cardiovascular diseases by reducing blood LDL cholesterol and lipids (Hu et al. 2019; Zhou et al. 2013; Voskoboinik et al. 2019). However, the presence of diterpenes (including cafestol and kahweol) in unfiltered coffee is significantly involved in elevating LDL cholesterol, total cholesterol, and triglycerides, which are considered as risk factors for cardiovascular-related diseases (Cai et al. 2012; Ren et al. 2019).

As mentioned earlier, caffeine plays a role in blood glucose homeostasis, it exerts an addictive effect that is linked to symptoms of restlessness and insomnia (Smit and

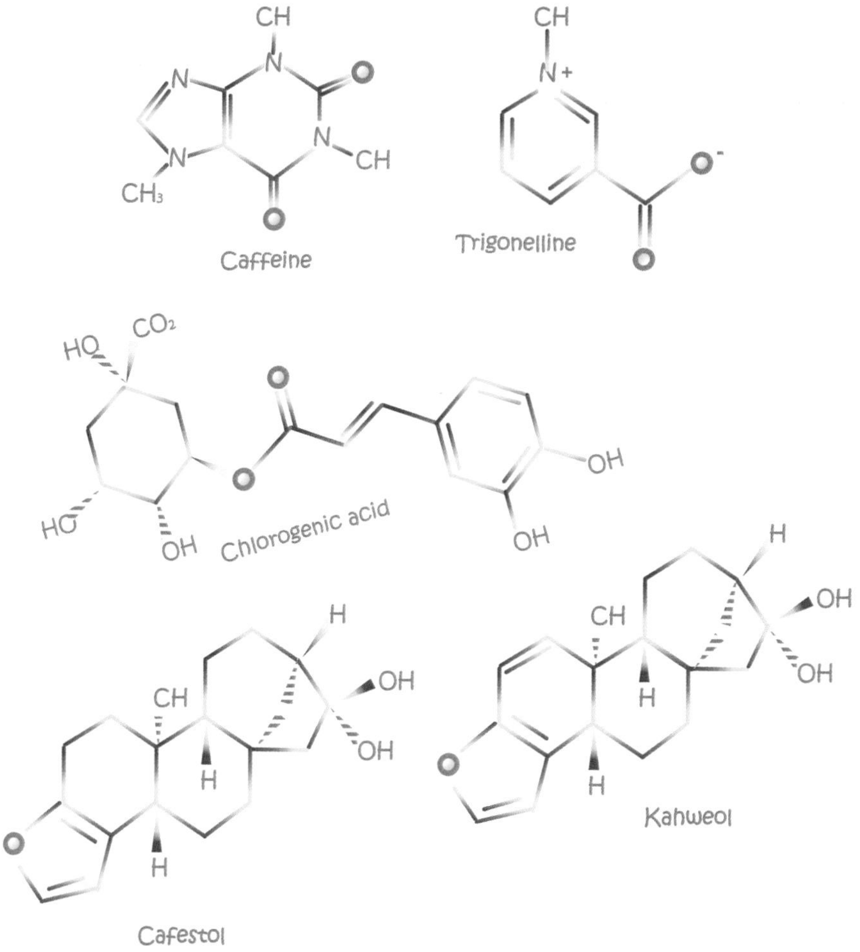

Fig. 4 Chemical structure of the most effective substances in caffeinated beverages (caffeine, chlorogenic acids, trigonelline, cafestol, kahweol). (From Butt and Sultan (2011), Clifford et al. (2003), Gan et al. (2018), Heckman et al. (2010), Ren et al. (2019), Stefanello et al. (2019), Zhou et al. (2013))

Rogers 2000). In addition, high concentrations of caffeine during pregnancy may probably be associated with an increased risk of premature delivery, stillbirth, miscarriage (Chen et al. 2016), and lower birth weight (Rhee et al. 2015).

It is well documented that there is a relationship between obesity and increasing the risk of developing T2DM (Barnes 2011; Hu and Malik 2010). Some beverage additives, such as sugars and cream (saturated and trans fats), often come as part of sweetened caffeinated drinks. There is evidence that the high intake of these sweetened beverages is associated with weight gain, insulin insensitivity, impaired glucose tolerance and consequently increased risk of T2DM (Fagherazzi et al. 2013;

Table 1 Some biological and physiological activities of substances in caffeinated beverages

Biological/ physiological activities	Caffeine	Chlorogenic acids	Trigonelline	Cafestol & Kahweol	Sucrose & Fructose	Saturated & Trans Fats
Risk of diabetes	↑	↓	↓	n/a	↑	↑
Antioxidants	↑	↑	↑	↑	n/a	n/a
Anti-carcinogenic activity	n/a	↑	↑	n/a	↓	↓
Glucose tolerance	↓	↑	↑	n/a	↓	↓
Insulin sensitivity	↓	↑	↑	n/a	↓	↓
LDL cholesterol	n/a	n/a	n/a	↑	n/a	↑
Blood lipids	n/a	n/a	n/a	↑	n/a	↑
Risk of gaining weight	↓	↓	↓	n/a	↑	↑
Risk of premature delivery & miscarriage	↑	n/a	n/a	n/a	n/a	n/a
Risk of stillbirth & lower birth weight	↑	n/a	n/a	n/a	n/a	n/a
Cognitive performance	↑	n/a	n/a	n/a	n/a	n/a
Stimulant and addictive activities	↑	n/a	n/a	n/a	n/a	n/a

↑ = increase; ↓ = decrease; n/a = not applicable.

Hu and Malik 2010; Malik and Hu 2012). However, chlorogenic acids in caffeinated beverages contribute to promoting metabolism of lipid and decreasing low-density lipoproteins (Hu et al. 2019). This effect is also applicable with caffeine which was associated with weight loss through increasing the metabolic rate and stimulating lipid oxidation and thermogenesis (Sarriá et al. 2020). Even though added sugars are associated with reducing insulin sensitivity, this association has not been observed with added cream (saturated and trans fats) or milk as it is applied in small quantities (van Dam and Hu 2005). However, high intake of saturated and trans fats results in impaired glucose tolerance and increased insulin insensitivity (Rivellese and Lilli 2003).

Applications to Public Health

The effective properties of caffeinated beverages are primarily attributed to their natural content of phytochemicals, including caffeine, chlorogenic acids, and trigonelline. The last two substances play a potential role as antidiabetic agents (Butt and Sultan 2011; Kobayashi et al. 2017; Verzelloni et al. 2011), whereas the action exerted by caffeine is controversial. In fact, caffeine is regarded as the main natural component present in caffeinated beverages (Frary et al. 2005). Caffeine has been intensively studied in terms of its association with the risk of developing T2DM and other health conditions. Caffeine has been shown to act as a phosphodiesterase inhibitor, leading to an increase in the level of cyclic adenosine monophosphate (cAMP). Elevated cAMP partially contributes to impaired glucose tolerance (Johnston et al. 2003). Caffeine can also inhibit muscle glucose uptake because it works as an adenosine receptor antagonist (Pettenuzzo et al. 2008). Moreover, caffeine may be involved in reducing insulin sensitivity and increasing plasma free fatty acids (Cherniack et al. 2018). In contrast, as a phytochemical compound, caffeine possesses antioxidant properties and may protect pancreatic beta cells from damage caused by oxidative stress (Pereira et al. 2006). However, the potential role of caffeine in the risk of developing T2DM is still controversial, and further scientific investigations are required.

Even though the common component in all caffeinated beverages is caffeine, there are other components which are specific to certain caffeinated beverages that play a potential role in lowering or elevating the risk of developing T2DM (Table 2). For instance, chlorogenic acids are abundantly found in coffee beans (van Dijk et al. 2009) and play a crucial role in preventing hyperglycemia by inhibiting α-glucosidase activity, which leads to delayed intestinal uptake of glucose and reduced the production of hepatic glucose (Bassoli et al. 2008; van Dijk et al. 2009). Moreover, chlorogenic acids may inhibit glucose-6-phosphatase activity and glucose transporters, which contribute to lowering plasma glucose concentrations (Bassoli et al. 2008; van Dijk et al. 2009). Additionally, chlorogenic acids promote insulin sensitivity because they act as antioxidants to protect pancreatic beta cells from damage

Table 2 The most effective compounds in caffeinated beverages and their association with the risk of developing T2DM

Main caffeinated beverages compound	Possible explanation for elevating the risk of T2DM	Possible explanation for lowering the risk of T2DM	References
Caffeine	impairs glucose tolerance as it plays a role in inhibiting the action of phosphodiesterase, leading to elevating the concentration of cAMP inhibits muscle glucose uptake because it acts as an adenosine receptor antagonist	may promote weight loss through increasing energy expenditures and lipid oxidation	Johnston et al. (2003), Pettenuzzo et al. (2008), Cherniack et al. (2018)
Chlorogenic acids		delays the absorption of intestinal glucose due to inhibiting α-glucosidase activity reduces in plasma glucose output from the liver by inhibiting glucose transporters lowers plasma glucose concentration through impairing the release of glucose from dietary carbohydrates reduces plasma glucose output from the liver by inhibiting glucose-6-phosphatase reduces the production of hepatic glucose via inhibiting the activity of α-glucosidase improves insulin sensitivity through protecting pancreatic beta cells from oxidative stress damages	Bassoli et al. (2008), van Dijk et al. (2009), (Hu et al. (2019), Pereira et al. (2006)
Trigonelline		regulates glucokinase and glucose-6-phosphatase leading to reduced blood glucose and insulin levels	Hu et al. (2019), Zhou et al. (2013)

(continued)

Table 2 (continued)

Main caffeinated beverages compound	Possible explanation for elevating the risk of T2DM	Possible explanation for lowering the risk of T2DM	References
Sucrose & fructose	excessively increases blood glucose and insulin concentrations lowers insulin sensitivity causes fast spike in blood glucose and insulin levels increases in energy intake		Fagherazzi et al. (2013), Hu and Malik (2010), Malik and Hu (2012), Rivellese and Lilli (2003)
Saturated & trans fats	impairs glucose tolerance increases insulin insensitivity raises risk of gaining weight due to increased energy intake		

caused by oxidative stress (Hu et al. 2019; Pereira et al. 2006). There is evidence that increased oxidative stress may be associated with the onset of developing T2DM (Bidel et al. 2008). Chlorogenic acids alleviate oxidative stress due to their ability to induce mRNA and protein expression (Butt and Sultan 2011).

Trigonelline, as one of the main active constituents in caffeinated beverages, contributes to several biological activities (Tables 1 and 2), including reducing the risk of diabetes (Hu et al., 2019). It has been found that ingestion of trigonelline resulted in a significant reduction in glucose and insulin concentrations (van Dijk et al. 2009).

Other caffeinated beverage ingredients, such as added sugar, including sucrose, fructose, and glucose, are involved in elevating the risk of developing T2DM (Malik and Hu 2012). The presence of these mono- and disaccharides in most sweetened caffeinated drinks significantly contributes to the overall carbohydrate intake (Heckman et al. (2010)). This should be taken into account when planning meals, in particularly, for patients with T2DM. In addition to their association with weight gain (Table 1), sugars from sweetened caffeinated beverages are associated with an elevated risk of T2DM due to their capability to influence blood glucose and insulin concentrations and are linked to lower insulin sensitivity (Fagherazzi et al. 2013; Hu and Malik 2010).

Mini-Dictionary of Terms

- **Glycemic homeostasis**. Retaining adequate glucose levels in the blood for survival

- **Hyperglycemia**. High level of blood glucose
- **Impaired glucose tolerance**. Abnormal mild high level of blood glucose
- **Insulin sensitivity**. Response of the body's cells to insulin
- **Oxidative stress**. Imbalance in free radicals and antioxidants
- **Psychostimulant**. A substance with the ability to stimulate the central nervous system
- **Type 2 diabetes mellitus**. A metabolic disorder identified by hyperglycemia and caused primarily by a progressive insulin secretory defect

Key Facts of Caffeinated Beverage Substances

- Caffeinated beverages are basically consumed for their stimulant and hedonistic properties
- Caffeine and chlorogenic acids are the major pharmacologically active constituents in the caffeinated beverages
- Caffeine is rapidly absorbed and metabolized in the liver, where its metabolites undergo demethylation and oxidation
- The primary contributor to caffeine in human diets is coffee
- Some additives in caffeinated beverages, such as sucrose and fructose are associated with reduced insulin sensitivity

Key Facts of the Relationship between Caffeinated Beverages and the Risk of Developing T2DM

- Chlorogenic acids are strongly associated with a lower risk of developing type 2 diabetes mellitus.
- There is a relationship between high consumption of caffeinated sweetened drinks and reduced insulin sensitivity.
- Both chlorogenic acids and trigonelline exhibit antidiabetic and antioxidant activities.
- The role of caffeinated beverages in the risk of developing T2DM remains controversial.

Summary Points

- The most popular caffeinated beverages among adults are coffee and tea, whereas caffeinated soft drinks are more popular among children and adolescents.
- The natural effective compounds in caffeinated beverages are caffeine, chlorogenic acids, and trigonelline.
- Caffeine is associated with impaired glucose tolerance and insulin insensitivity because it acts as a phosphodiesterase inhibitor and an adenosine receptor antagonist.

- Chlorogenic acids inhibit α-glucosidase and glucose-6-phosphatase activities, lowering plasma glucose concentrations and delaying intestinal glucose uptake
- In addition to its role in blood glucose homeostasis, caffeine exhibits a stimulant and addictive properties, which are considered the main attractive characteristics of caffeinated beverages

References

Barnes AS (2011) The epidemic of obesity and diabetes: trends and treatments. Tex Heart Inst J 38 (2):142–144

Bassoli BK, Cassolla P, Borba-Murad GR et al (2008) Chlorogenic acid reduces the plasma glucose peak in the oral glucose tolerance test: effects on hepatic glucose release and glycaemia. Cell Biochem Funct 26:320–328. https://doi.org/10.1002/cbf.1444

Bidel S, Silventoinen K, Hu G et al (2008) Coffee consumption, serum γ -glutamyltransferase and risk of type II diabetes. Eur J Clin Nutr 62:178–185

Butt MS, Sultan MT (2011) Coffee and its consumption: benefits and risks. Crit Rev Food Sci Nutr 51:363–373. https://doi.org/10.1080/10408390903586412

Cai L, Ma D, Zhang Y et al (2012) The effect of coffee consumption on serum lipids: a meta-analysis of randomized controlled trials. Eur J Clin Nutr 66(8):872–877. https://doi.org/10.1038/ejcn.2012.68

Chen LW, Wu Y, Neelakantan N et al (2016) Maternal caffeine intake during pregnancy and risk of pregnancy loss: a categorical and dose-response meta-analysis of prospective studies. Public Health Nutr 19(7):1233–1244. https://doi.org/10.1017/S1368980015002463

Cherniack EP, Buslach N, Lee HF (2018) The potential effects of caffeinated beverages on insulin sensitivity. J Am Coll Nutr 37(2):161–167. https://doi.org/10.1080/07315724.2017.1372822

Clifford MN, Johnston KL, Knight S et al (2003) Hierarchical scheme for LC-MS identification of chlorogenic acids. J Agri Food Chem 51:2900–2911. https://doi.org/10.1021/jf026187q

Fagherazzi G, Vilier A, Saes Sartorelli DS et al (2013) Consumption of artificially and sugar-sweetened beverages and incident type 2 diabetes in the Etude Epidémiologique auprès des femmes de la Mutuelle Générale de l'Education Nationale–European Prospective Investigation into Cancer and Nutrition cohort. Am J Clin Nutr 97(3):517–523. https://doi.org/10.3945/ajcn.112.050997

Ferré S (2016) Mechanisms of the psychostimulant effects of caffeine: implications for substance use disorders. Psychopharmacology 233(10):1963–1979. https://doi.org/10.1007/s00213-016-4212-2

Forouhi NG, Misra A, Mohan V et al (2018) Dietary and nutritional approaches for prevention and management of type 2 diabetes. BMJ 361:k2234. https://doi.org/10.1136/bmj.k2234

Frary CD, Johnson RK, Wang MQ (2005) Food sources and intakes of caffeine in the diets of persons in the United States. J Am Diet Assoc 105(1):110–113. https://doi.org/10.1016/j.jada.2004.10.027

Gan R, Zhang D, Wang M et al (2018) Health benefits of bioactive compounds from the genus Ilex, a source of traditional caffeinated beverages. Nutrients 10(11):1682. https://doi.org/10.3390/nu10111682

Heckman MA, Weil J, De Mejia EG (2010) Caffeine (1, 3, 7-trimethylxanthine) in foods: a comprehensive review on consumption, functionality, safety, and regulatory matters. J Food Sci 75:R77–R87. https://doi.org/10.1111/j.1750-3841.2010.01561.x

Hu FB, Malik VS (2010) Sugar-sweetened beverages and risk of obesity and type 2 diabetes: epidemiologic evidence. Physiol Behav 100(1):47–54. https://doi.org/10.1016/j.physbeh.2010.01.036

Hu G, Wang X, Zhang L et al (2019) The sources and mechanisms of bioactive ingredients in coffee. Food Funct 10(6):3113–3126. https://doi.org/10.1039/C9FO00288J

Imamura F, O'Connor L, Ye Z et al (2015) Consumption of sugar sweetened beverages, artificially sweetened beverages, and fruit juice and incidence of type 2 diabetes: systematic review, meta-analysis, and estimation of population attributable fraction. BMJ 351:h3576. https://doi.org/10.1136/bmj.h3576

Johnston KL, Clifford MN, Morgan LM (2003) Coffee acutely modifies gastrointestinal hormone secretion and glucose tolerance in humans: glycemic effects of chlorogenic acid and caffeine. Am J Clin Nutr 78:728–733. https://doi.org/10.1093/ajcn/78.4.728

Kim AN, Cho HJ, Youn J et al (2020) Coffee consumption, genetic polymorphisms, and the risk of type 2 diabetes mellitus: a pooled analysis of four prospective cohort studies. Int J Environ Res Public Health 17(15):5379. https://doi.org/10.3390/ijerph17155379

Kobayashi M, Kurata T, Hamana Y et al (2017) Coffee ingestion suppresses hyperglycemia in streptozotocin-induced diabetic mice. J Nutr Sci Vitaminol 63(3):200–207. https://doi.org/10.3177/jnsv.63.200

Loopsta-Masters RC, Liese AD, Haffiner SM et al (2011) Associations between the intake of caffeinated and decaffeinated coffee and measures of insulin sensitivity and beta cell function. Diabetologia 54:320–328. https://doi.org/10.1007/s00125-010-1957-8

Ludwig IA, Clifford MN, Lean ME et al (2014) Coffee: biochemistry and potential impact on health. Food Funct 5(8):1695–1717. https://doi.org/10.1039/c4fo00042k

Malik VS, Hu FB (2012) Sweeteners and risk of obesity and type 2 diabetes: the role of sugar-sweetened beverages. Curr Diab Rep. https://doi.org/10.1007/s11892-012-0259-6

Mitchell DC, Knight CA, Hockenberry J et al (2014) Beverage caffeine intakes in the US. *Food* Chem Toxicol 63:136–142. https://doi.org/10.1016/j.fct.2013.10.042

Oba S, Nagata C, Nakamura K et al (2010) Consumption of coffee, green tea, oolong tea, black tea, chocolate snacks and the caffeine content in relation to risk of diabetes in Japanese men and women. Br J Nutr 103(3):453–459. https://doi.org/10.1017/S0007114509991966

Pereira MA, Parker ED, Folsom AR (2006) Coffee consumption and risk of type 2 diabetes mellitus: an 11-year prospective study of 28 812 postmenopausal women. Arch Intern Med 166(12):1311–1316. https://doi.org/10.1001/archinte.166.12.1311

Pettenuzzo LF, Noschang C, von Pozzer TE et al (2008) Effects of chronic administration of caffeine and stress on feeding behavior of rats. Physiol Behav 95(3):295–301. https://doi.org/10.1016/j.physbeh.2008.06.003

Ren Y, Wang C, Xu J et al (2019) Cafestol and Kahweol: a review on their bioactivities and pharmacological properties. Int J Mol Sci 20(17):4238. https://doi.org/10.3390/ijms20174238

Rhee J, Kim R, Kim Y et al (2015) Maternal caffeine consumption during pregnancy and risk of low birth weight: a dose-response meta-analysis of observational studies. PLoS One 10(7): e0132334. https://doi.org/10.1371/journal.pone.0132334

Rivellese AA, Lilli S (2003) Quality of dietary fatty acids, insulin sensitivity and type 2 diabetes. Biomed Pharmacother 57(2):84–87. https://doi.org/10.1016/s0753-3322(03)00003-9

Rudelle S, Ferruzzi MG, Cristiani I et al (2007) Effect of a thermogenic beverage on 24-hour energy metabolism in humans. Obesity 15(2):349–355. https://doi.org/10.1038/oby.2007.529

Sarriá B, Sierra-Cinos JL, García-Diz L et al (2020) Green/roasted coffee may reduce cardiovascular risk in hypercholesterolemic subjects by decreasing body weight, abdominal adiposity and blood pressure. Foods 9(9):1191. https://doi.org/10.3390/foods9091191

Smit HJ, Rogers PJ (2000) Effects of low doses of caffeine on cognitive performance, mood and thirst in low and higher caffeine consumers. Psychopharmacology 152(2):167–173. https://doi.org/10.1007/s002130000506

Stefanello N, Spanevello RM, Passamonti S et al (2019) Coffee, caffeine, chlorogenic acid, and the purinergic system. Food Chem Toxicol 123:298–313. https://doi.org/10.1016/j.fct.2018.10.005

van Dam FB, Hu RM (2005) Coffee consumption and risk of type 2 diabetes. JAMA 294(1):97–104. https://doi.org/10.1001/jama.294.1.97

van Dieren S, Uiterwaal CSPM, van der Schouw YT et al (2009) Coffee and tea consumption and risk of type 2 diabetes. Diabetologia 52:2561–2569. https://doi.org/10.1007/s00125-009-1516-3

van Dijk AE, Olthof MR, Meeuse JC et al (2009) Acute effects of decaffeinated coffee and the major coffee components chlorogenic acid and trigonelline on glucose tolerance. Diabetes Care 32(6):1023–1025. https://doi.org/10.2337/dc09-0207

Verzelloni E, Tagliazucchi D, Del Rio D et al (2011) Antiglycative and antioxidative properties of coffee fractions. Food Chem 124(4):1430–1435. https://doi.org/10.1016/j.foodchem.2010.07.103

Vieira AJ, Gaspar EM, Santos PM (2020) Mechanisms of potential antioxidant activity of caffeine. Radiat Phys Chem 174:108968. https://doi.org/10.1016/j.radphyschem.2020.108968

Voskoboinik A, Koh Y, Kistler PM (2019) Cardiovascular effects of caffeinated beverages. Trends Cardiovasc Med 29(6):345–350

Zhou J, Zhou S, Zeng S (2013) Experimental diabetes treated with trigonelline: effect on β cell and pancreatic oxidative parameters. Fundam Clin Pharmacol 27(3):279–287. https://doi.org/10.1111/j.1472-8206.2011.01022.x

Caffeine as an Active Adulterant: Implication for Drugs of Abuse Consumption

75

Cecilia Scorza, José Pedro Prieto, and Sara Fabius

Contents

Introduction 1606
Caffeine: Mechanism of Action on the Central Nervous System 1606
Interaction Between Adenosinergic and Dopaminergic Receptors: Relevance for Psychostimulant Drugs of Abuse 1610
Adulteration: A Common Phenomenon in the Illicit Drug Market 1610
Caffeine as an Active Adulterant 1611
Applications to Other Areas of Substance Use Disorders 1612
Key Facts 1612
Mini-Dictionary 1613
Summary Points 1613
References 1613

Abstract

Dilution or adulteration processes in the illicit drugs of abuse market are the rule rather than the exception. While diluents are pharmacologically inactive and readily available substances, adulterants are pharmacologically active compounds usually more expensive or less accessible than diluents. Both substances are deliberately added to increase bulk, enhance or mimic a pharmacological effect, or facilitate drug delivery. Active adulterants are substances that could pharmacologically interact with the primary drug, however, their actions are commonly underestimated. This interaction could explain acute or chronic drug intoxication, an increment in drug abuse liability, and even severe health problems in persons who consume drugs. While caffeine is the most widely consumed psychoactive compound worldwide, it is also one of the most frequent active adulterants used in drugs of abuse, particularly psychostimulant drugs. Its psychoactive effect seems apparently to be innocuous; however, depending on the doses and the route

C. Scorza (✉) · J. P. Prieto · S. Fabius
Department of Experimental Neuropharmacology, Instituto de Investigaciones Biológicas Clemente Estable, Montevideo, Uruguay
e-mail: cscorza@iibce.edu.uy; sfabius@iibce.edu.uy

V. B. Patel, V. R. Preedy (eds.), *Handbook of Substance Misuse and Addictions*,
https://doi.org/10.1007/978-3-030-92392-1_82

of administration, it could produce unpleasant effects or even boost the abuse liability of drugs of abuse. This chapter includes data about the neural mechanisms of caffeine on adenosinergic receptors, the interaction between adenosine and dopamine neurotransmissions, and the influence of caffeine as an active adulterant in psychostimulant drugs of abuse.

Keywords

Dopamine · Adenosine · Adulteration · Street drugs · CNS · Addiction · Health

Abbreviations

Cyclic AMP	Cyclic adenosine monophosphate
CPP	Conditioned place preference
DSM-V	Diagnostic and Statistical Manual of Mental Disorders, Fifth Edition
MDA	Methylenedioxyamphetamine
MDMA	3,4-Methylenedioxymethamphetamine
PFC	Prefrontal cortex
VTA	Ventral tegmental area

Introduction

Caffeine, an alkaloid of the xanthine group, is the most popular psychoactive substance in the world. One of the reasons for its popularity lies in its psychostimulant properties and the apparent absence of significant adverse effects after its acute and chronic use (Fisone et al. 2004). However, there are some controversial data. While there are no restrictions on caffeine consumption, some authors have pointed to caffeine as an "atypical drug of abuse" (Daly and Fredholm 1998; Hughes et al. 1998). Accordingly, caffeine intoxication and withdrawal symptoms are included in current diagnostic manuals of psychiatry (Diagnostic and Statistical Manual of Mental Disorders, Fifth Edition, DSM-V). Another controversial issue is that apart from coffee, tea, and other caffeine-containing plant extracts, caffeine is found in many commercially available products, such as energy drinks containing high caffeine content (Reissig et al. 2009). While the acute and long-term effects resulting from chronic consumption of these beverages are not fully known so far, this subject needs particular attention since energy drinks could be consumed combined with other drugs in recreational drug-use settings (Ferré 2016; Vanattou-Saïfoudine et al. 2012).

Caffeine: Mechanism of Action on the Central Nervous System

Caffeine is a competitive nonselective adenosine receptor antagonist and produces a psychostimulant effect by counteracting the tonic effects of endogenous adenosine (Ferré 2016; Fredholm et al. 1999). This action largely depends on the ability of adenosine to modulate the function of multiple neurotransmitter systems, including the dopaminergic (DAergic) system. Adenosine binds to four types of metabotropic receptors (A1, A2A, A2B, and A3), the A1 and A2A receptors being the ones with the highest affinity (Fredholm 2010) and on which caffeine exerts its primary effects (Ferré 2010). These two receptors have opposite pharmacological effects: activation of A1 receptors reduces cyclic AMP levels, while that of A2A receptors increases them (Fisone et al. 2004; Londos et al. 1980). As adenosine decreases neural activity, both arousing and psychomotor activating effects of caffeine depend on its ability to disinhibit the brake that adenosine imposes on the ascending arousal and DA systems. Adenosine is considered one of the principal homeostatic factors for sleep regulation (Basheer et al. 2004; Porkka-Heiskanen et al. 2002); it is a sleep-promoting substance, and by blocking adenosine receptors, caffeine promotes wakefulness. During wakefulness, adenosine increases its concentration in specific brain regions, such as the basal forebrain nucleus, and inhibits its wakefulness-promoting cholinergic neurons (Basheer et al. 2004; Porkka-Heiskanen et al. 2002).

Moreover, Lazarus et al. (2011) proposed that the A2A receptors in the nucleus accumbens (NAc) play a critical role in the arousal effect of caffeine. A1 receptors are widely expressed in the brain; however, A2A expression is limited to brain regions highly innervated by DAergic fibers, such as the striatum (Cauli and Morelli 2005; Fisone et al. 2004; Jarvis et al. 1989). In the striatum, A2A receptors are highly expressed in GABAergic striatopallidal medium-sized spiny neurons co-localized with dopamine D2 receptors. Complexes of A2A-D2 receptor heterotetramers have also been identified, regulating its antagonistic interactions (Ferré et al. 2018; Ferré and Ciruela 2019). This anatomical level shows a close interaction between the adenosine and DA system that can regulate behavior. Caffeine blocked the inhibitory actions of adenosine on DA transmission by A2AR antagonism on GABA neurons, and, consequently, caffeine inhibits the inhibitory actions of GABA neurons on DA neurons (Malave and Broderick 2014). Caffeine stimulates motor activity on these neurons by counteracting the inhibitory control exerted by adenosine A2A receptors on striatal D2 receptors (El Yacoubi et al. 2000; Fisone et al. 2004).

In several reports, the stimulant effect of caffeine on the motor activity of mice and rats was demonstrated in a range of active doses (Antoniou et al. 1998; Antoniou et al. 2005; Nehlig et al. 1992). As an example, Fig. 1 shows the animal response to an intraperitoneal administration of low doses of caffeine. A dose-dependent increment in the distance moved, and the time spent in movement was observed, with a similar pattern of motion to the control group although with more activity. Since it had been described that caffeine could be volatilized (Gostic et al. 2009), we studied the stimulant effect induced by volatilized caffeine (Galvalisi et al. 2017). We passively exposed animals to the fume of caffeine, and the distance moved, the time in movement, and locomotor pattern activity were analyzed. As expected, we observed a dose-dependent stimulant effect induced by volatilized caffeine (Fig. 2). These results are particularly interesting in the drug addiction research since it has been postulated that fast route of administration, like pulmonary inhalation, is one of the main factors which can promote the transition to addiction (i.e., from abuse to compulsive use; Gossop et al. 1992; Samaha and Robinson 2005). Regarding this,

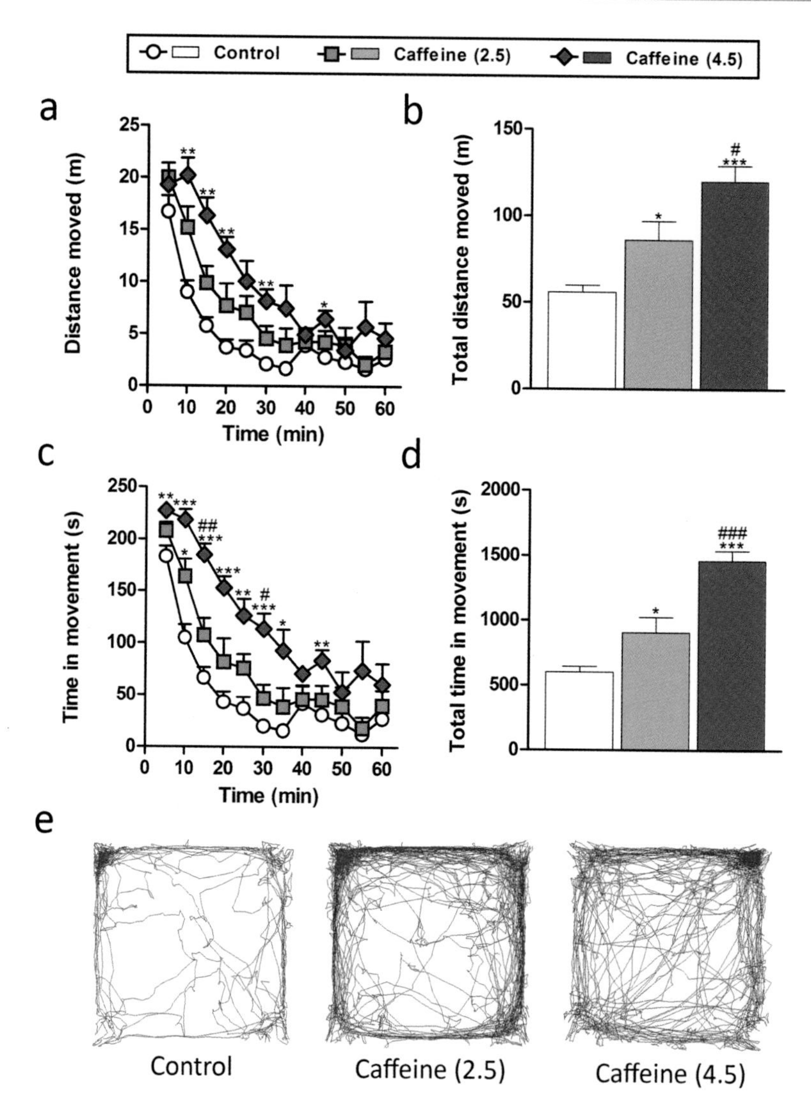

Fig. 1 Behavioral response induced by intraperitoneal administration of caffeine. Representative studies of motor responses induced by the acute intraperitoneal administration of caffeine (2.5 and 4.5 mg/kg). Immediately after the injection of caffeine, animals were placed on an open field, and motor parameters were recorded by the software Ethovision XP 12.0. (**a**) Distance moved (m), (**b**) total distance moved, (**c**) time in movement (sec), (**d**) total time in movement, and (**e**) pattern of movement. Data expressed as mean ±SEM. Two- and one-way ANOVA, followed by Bonferroni and Tukey tests, respectively. * vs. control group; # vs. caffeine group. *,# = $P < 0.05$; **,## = $P < 0.01$; ***, ### = $P < 0.001$. N = 6–8 for each group. (Taken and modified from Lopez Hill et al. (2011))

and taking into account that the psychomotor-activating effect of psychostimulants can predict its reinforcing effects and addiction liability (Wise and Bozarth 1987; Volkow et al. 2015), it can be hypothesized that chronic consumption of a smoked

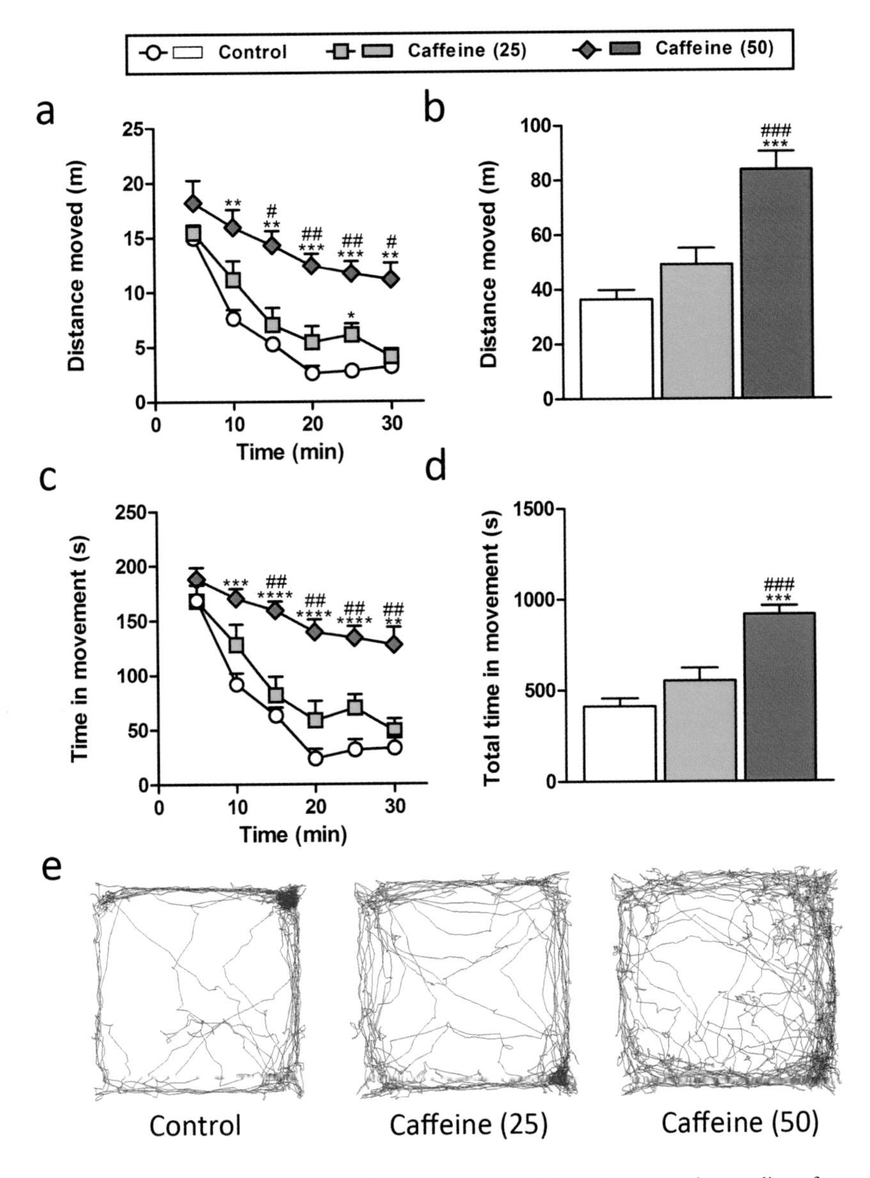

Fig. 2 Behavioral response induced by volatilized caffeine. Representative studies of motor responses induced by the acute and passive exposition of volatilized caffeine (25 and 50 mg). Immediately after the volatilization of caffeine and the animal exposition to the caffeine smoke (10 min, inhalation chamber), animals were placed on an open field, and motor parameters were recorded by the software Ethovision XP 12.0. (**a**) Distance moved (m), (**b**) total distance moved, (**c**) time in movement (sec), (**d**) total time in movement, and (**e**) pattern of movement. Data expressed as mean ± SEM. Two- and one-way ANOVA, followed by Bonferroni and Tukey tests, respectively. * vs. control group; # vs. caffeine group. *,# = $P < 0.05$; **,## = $P < 0.01$; ***, ### = $P < 0.001$. N = 5–7 for each group. (Taken and modified from Galvalisi et al. (2017))

form of caffeine may elicit neuroadaptive processes similar to those initiated by addictive drugs, like cocaine.

Interaction Between Adenosinergic and Dopaminergic Receptors: Relevance for Psychostimulant Drugs of Abuse

Psychostimulants like cocaine and amphetamines constitute one of the most abused classes of illicit drugs in the world. These are drugs whose consumption elicits increased arousal, wakefulness, cardiovascular stimulation, vigilance, and attention, among other effects (Ballesteros-Yáñez et al. 2018). Research on the neurochemical mechanisms underlying psychostimulant addiction has widely focused on the DA system. Using different sites and mechanisms of action (Lüscher and Ungless 2006), the neurochemical mechanism, common to all drugs of abuse in humans, implies a DA increase released from the ventral tegmental area (VTA) to the NAc and the prefrontal cortex (PFC). Both regions define the mesocorticolimbic circuit and are critical brain nuclei in the reward circuitry (Di Chiara and Imperato 1988). This neurochemical alteration has particular relevance since it has been widely recognized that psychostimulants affecting DAergic neurons (as DA reuptake blockers, such as cocaine or DA releasers, like amphetamine) in the limbic reward system underly the rewarding and reinforcing properties of these substances (Drevets et al. 2001; Siciliano et al. 2015; Volkow et al. 1997).

Several comprehensive reviews have been published focused on the close interaction of adenosine and DA neurotransmission in addiction (Ballesteros-Yáñez et al. 2018; Ferré 2016; Filip et al. 2012). Particularly, adenosine neurotransmission has been implicated in the addiction-related behavior of psychostimulants since it has a modulatory function on DA neurotransmission (Fuxe et al. 2010). This modulation is mediated through the direct interaction between adenosine and DA receptors affecting various aspects, including locomotor activity, sensitization, seeking behavior, and reward (Ferre et al. 1997). Anatomical studies have shown that these interactions occur in the striatum, where A2A and D2 receptors and A1 and D1 receptors are co-localized. D1, D2, A1, and A2A receptors are coupled to adenyl cyclase, in addition to other signal transduction pathways (Fredholm 1995). Blocking adenosine receptors (mainly A2A receptors), caffeine can enhance the effects of DAergic stimulation (Ballesteros-Yáñez et al. 2018; Fisone et al. 2004). This effect is a critical factor for the acute rewarding effects of psychostimulant drugs (Koob and Volkow 2010).

Adulteration: A Common Phenomenon in the Illicit Drug Market

Forensic data support that drugs of abuse that are illegally sold are commonly diluted, contaminated, and adulterated (Broséus et al. 2016; Cole et al. 2011; Evrard et al. 2010; Villar Núñez et al. 2018). Depending on the origin of each drug (synthetic, semisynthetic, or natural), a specific process is chosen. Dilution refers to the addition of inert substances (diluents), while contamination refers to the presence of by-products of the drug manufacturing process (contaminants). Adulteration involves the intentional addition of a pharmacologically active substance without the user being aware (adulterants; Broseus et al. 2016; Hoffman et al. 2008). The specific adulterants used are selected depending on the type of drug of abuse and how it is consumed. All these processes occur since illicit drugs are not subjected to sanitary or quality controls. In addition, as drug adulteration involves different stages (i.e., exportation and distribution), the pattern of adulteration could also be used in forensic sciences as a marker of structure and organization of illicit drug markets (Morelato et al. 2019).

Caffeine as an Active Adulterant

Caffeine is one of the substances most frequently found in seized samples of cocaine hydrochloride, methamphetamine, amphetamine derivatives (e.g., MDMA and MDA), and synthetic cathinones (Cole et al. 2011; Kudlacek et al. 2017; Seely et al. 2013; Vanattou-Saïfoudine et al. 2012). Also, it was found in smoked forms of cocaine, like crack and cocaine paste (Abin Carriquiry et al. 2018; Cole et al. 2011; Evrard et al. 2010; Fukushima et al. 2014; Pawlik and Mahler 2001; López Hill et al. 2011; Prieto et al. 2015). Thus, forensic data about the drug purity and the presence of diluents, contaminants, or adulterants is essential to understand overdosage, unexpected side effects (toxicity), putative fatal reactions, or even the abuse liability of a drug. The health risks of illicit drugs of abuse can increase with the frequency and quantity of use, depending on the route of administration, and with the interaction between different substances. However, representative sampling of illegal drug samples is not routinely undertaken to quantify and qualify the extent of adulteration; therefore, the health effects caused by illicit drug adulteration are commonly underestimated (Coomber 1997). A special warning is the smoked psychostimulant drugs, like crack or cocaine paste, since daily cocaine intake may imply several grams in which adulterants may lead to significant toxicologic effects that amplify the effects of cocaine.

It has been reported that habitual caffeine consumption is generally regarded as safe; however, caffeine overdose could be associated with several undesirable effects like gastrointestinal upset, tachyarrhythmias, and seizures (Shannon 1988). Besides, the presence of caffeine as an adulterant has the potential to influence the adverse effects (e.g., cardiovascular, intoxication, seizures) induced by the stimulants like cocaine and amphetamine (Derlet et al. 1992) or even the dangerous effects (e.g., hyperthermia) caused by MDMA consumption (Vanattou-Saïfoudine et al. 2012). Analyzing the chemical content of an extensive series of seized samples of a smoked form of cocaine, we found the caffeine is a very frequent adulterant added to this drug (Abin Carriquiry et al. 2018). Regardless of the mentioned adverse effects of caffeine, we have been focused on studying the influence of caffeine on cocaine behavioral effects related to addiction. We observed that caffeine, at a specific ratio concerning the cocaine content, could boost the stimulant effect of cocaine (López Hill et al. 2011) and potentiate the wakefulness-promoting effect of cocaine (Schwarzkopf et al. 2018). In addition, we found that caffeine facilitated and accelerated the expression of sensitization phenomenon induced by the repeated administration of cocaine in rats. This effect was not observed on cocaine-treated animals under the same protocol schedule (Prieto et al. 2015). In animal studies, the rewarding effect induced by cocaine can be evaluated using the conditioned place preference (CPP) paradigm. Using CPP in rats, we found that caffeine potentiates cocaine reward-associated learning in the conditioning place preference test (Muñiz et al. 2017). It is important to note that many of these effects were induced under a slow route of administration (like intraperitoneal); however, using the intravenous route of administration (i.e., a fast route of administration), we observed that caffeine significantly increased the reinforcing and motivational value of cocaine in the self-administration paradigm (Prieto et al. 2016). Moreover, we reported that caffeine could enhance per se the DA extracellular levels in animals exposed to the smoke of caffeine (Galvalisi et al. 2017), and caffeine can have an additive effect on cocaine-induced stimulant effect and cocaine-induced DA release (Scorza et al. 2021). Either for the oral concomitant consumption of caffeine with drugs (e.g., energy drinks) or as an active adulterant of drugs, the concern on caffeine should be seriously taken into account in the recreational drug-use settings.

Applications to Other Areas of Substance Use Disorders

In this chapter, we have reviewed the relevance of active adulterants in the context of substance use disorders (SUD). Of particular interest was the case of caffeine. Caffeine, the most consumed psychoactive drug globally, becomes particularly important to address psychostimulant use disorder-related problems. Caffeine is commonly found as an adulterant in illicit drugs and energy drinks consumed in combination with psychostimulants or other drugs (e.g., MDMA). All this information has implications from a public health perspective since concomitant consumption of caffeine (as in energy drinks) with recreational psychostimulant drugs of abuse (or other drugs) or as an active adulterant can significantly alter the drug-induced effects and can provoke acute adverse reactions in addition to longer-term consequences. Understanding the pharmacological interactions between caffeine and psychostimulant (or even with other different drugs) will help to define approaches for the clinical management of these side effects and putative toxicity (e.g., hyperthermia, cardiotoxicity, and seizure). Moreover, a comprehensive analysis of the chemical composition of seized psychostimulant drugs by forensic science laboratories, including the regular identification and quantification of diluents and adulterants, should be adopted as a harm reduction policy for SUD.

Key Facts

- Active adulterants are commonly used to mimic or boost the effects of illicit drugs.
- Caffeine is the most popular psychoactive substance in the world consumed under different forms (e.g., coffee, tea, and caffeine-containing plant extracts, energy drinks).

- Caffeine is also one of the most frequent active adulterants used in drugs of abuse, particularly psychostimulant drugs (e.g., cocaine and amphetamines).
- Caffeine is a competitive nonselective adenosine receptor antagonist affecting the adenosinergic neurotransmission.
- Psychostimulant drugs of abuse, like cocaine and amphetamines, increase dopaminergic neurotransmission.
- There is a close pharmacological interaction between brain adenosine and dopamine neurotransmission, which explain caffeine actions as adulterant of psychostimulant drugs of abuse.
- Our focus of interest is to study the influence of caffeine as an active adulterant found in seized samples of a smoked form of cocaine.

Mini-Dictionary

- **Adulteration process**: Adulteration of drugs of abuse involves the intentional addition of pharmacologically active substances in order to use less of the intended product without making the user aware.
- **Adulterant**: Refers to pharmacologically active substances (e.g., caffeine, lidocaine, levamisole, etc.) added to illicit drugs in the process of selling and distribution. An adulterant is added to increase the amount of drug available to be sold but also to mimic or boost the main drug effects.
- **Diluent**: Refers to pharmacologically inactive substances (e.g., mannitol, lactose, etc.). It is added to increase the amount of drug available to be sold.
- **Forensic analysis:** Is the practice to analyze the chemical composition of different drugs, which help us to understand more about adulteration patterns and about impurity/purity levels.
- **Volatilization:** Is the process to heat a volatilized drug from below by a flame until the obtaining of smoke.

Summary Points

- A review of relevant information of illicit drugs of abuse.
- Relevance of adulteration process in illicit drugs of abuse market.
- Caffeine as a main active adulterant in illicit drugs of abuse.
- Summary of brain caffeine mechanisms of action.
- Pharmacological interactions between caffeine and cocaine.
- Identification and quantification of adulterants in drug of abuse should be a regular practice in preclinical and clinical research.

References

Abin Carriquiry JA, Martínez Busi M, Galvalisi M, Minteguiaga M, Prieto JP, Scorza C (2018) Identification and quantification of cocaine and active adulterants in coca-paste seized samples: useful scientific support to health care. Neurotox Res 34:295–304

Antoniou K, Kafetzopoulos E, Papadopoulou-Daifoti Z, Hyphantis T, Marselos M (1998) D-amphetamine, cocaine and caffeine: a comparative study of acute effects on locomotor activity and behavioural patterns in rats. Neurosci Biobehav Rev 23(2):189–196

Antoniou K, Papadopoulou-Daifoti Z, Hyphantis T, Papathanasiou G, Bekris E, Marselos M et al (2005) A detailed behavioral analysis of the acute motor effects of caffeine in the rat: involvement of adenosine A1 and A2A receptors. Psychopharmacology 183:154–162

Ballesteros-Yáñez I, Castillo CA, Merighi S, Gessi S (2018) The role of adenosine receptors in psychostimulant addiction. Front Pharmacol 8:985

Basheer R, Strecker RE, Thakkar MM, McCarley RW (2004) Adenosine and sleep-wake regulation. Prog Neurobiol 73(6):379–396

Broséus J, Gentile N, Esseiva P (2016) The cutting of cocaine and heroin: a critical review. Forensic Sci Int 262:73–83

Cauli O, Morelli M (2005) Caffeine and the dopaminergic system. Behav Pharmacol 16:63–77

Cole C, Jones L, McVeigh J, Kicman A, Syed Q, Bellis M (2011) Adulterants in illicit drugs: a review of empirical evidence. Drug Test Anal 3(2):89–96

Coomber R (1997) Vim in the Veins–Fantasy or fact: the adulteration of illicit drugs. Addict Res 5: 195–212

Daly JW, Fredholm BB (1998) Caffeine – an atypical drug of dependence. Drug Alcohol Depend 51:199–206

Derlet RW, Tseng JC, Albertson TE (1992) Potentiation of cocaine and d-amphetamine toxicity with caffeine. Am J Emerg Med 10:211–216

Di Chiara G, Imperato A (1988) Drugs abused by humans preferentially increase synaptic dopamine concentrations in the mesolimbic system of freely moving rats. Proc Natl Acad Sci U S A 85: 5274–5278

Drevets WC, Gautier C, Price JC, Kupfer DJ, Kinahan PE, Grace AA et al (2001) Amphetamine-induced dopamine release in human ventral striatum correlates with euphoria. Biol Psychiatry 49(2):8196

El Yacoubi M, Ledent C, Menard JF, Parmentier M, Costentin J, Vaugeois JM (2000) The stimulant effects of caffeine on locomotor behaviour in mice are mediated through its blockade of adenosine A2A receptors. Br J Pharmacol 129:1465–1473

Evrard I, Legleye S, Cadet-Taïrou A (2010) Composition, purity and perceived quality of street cocaine in France. Int J Drug Policy 1(5):399–406

Ferré S (2010) Role of the central ascending neurotransmitter systems in the psychostimulant effects of caffeine. J Alzheimers Dis 20(Suppl 1):S35–S49

Ferré S (2016) Mechanisms of the psychostimulant effects of caffeine: implications for substance use disorders. Psychopharmacology 233(10):1963–1979

Ferré S, Ciruela F (2019) Functional and neuroprotective role of striatal adenosine A2A receptor heterotetramers. J Caffeine Res 9:89–97

Ferré S, Fredholm BB, Morelli M, Popoli P, Fuxe K (1997) Adenosine-dopamine receptor-receptor interactions as an integrative mechanism in the basal ganglia. Trends Neurosci 20(10):482–487

Ferré S, Díaz-Ríos M, Salamone J, Prediger R (2018) New developments on the adenosine mechanisms of the central effects of caffeine and their implications for neuropsychiatric disorders. J Caffeine Res 8:121–131

Filip M, Zaniewska M, Frankowska M, Wydra K, Fuxe K (2012) The importance of the adenosine A2A receptor-dopamine D(2) receptor interaction in drug addiction. Curr Med Chem 19: 317–355

Fisone G, Borgkvist A, Usiello A (2004) Caffeine as a psychomotor stimulant: mechanism of action. Cell Mol Life Sci 61:857–872

Fredholm BB (1995) Purinoceptors in the nervous system. Pharmacol Toxicol 76(4):228–239

Fredholm BB (2010) Adenosine receptors as drug targets. Exp Cell Res 316(8):1284–1288

Fredholm BB, Bättig K, Holmén J, Nehlig A, Zvartau EE (1999) Actions of caffeine in the brain with special reference to factors that contribute to its widespread use. Pharmacol Rev 51(1): 83–133

Fukushima AR, Carvalho VM, Carvalho DG, Diaz E, Bustillos JO, Spinosa Hde S et al (2014) Purity and adulterant analysis of crack seizures in Brazil. Forensic Sci Int 243C:95–98

Fuxe K, Marcellino D, Borroto-Escuela DO, Guescini M, Fernández-Dueñas V, Tanganelli S et al (2010) Adenosine-dopamine interactions in the pathophysiology and treatment of CNS disorders. CNS Neurosci Ther 16(3):e18–e42

Galvalisi M, Prieto JP, Martínez M, Abin-Carriquiry JA, Scorza C (2017) Caffeine induces a stimulant effect and increases dopamine release in the nucleus Accumbens Shell through the pulmonary inhalation route of Administration in Rats. Neurotox Res 31(1):90–98

Gossop M, Griffiths P, Powis B, Strang J (1992) Severity of dependence and route of administration of heroin, cocaine and amphetamines. Br J Addict 87(11):1527–1536

Gostic T, Klemenc S, Stefane B (2009) A study of the thermal decomposition of adulterated cocaine samples under optimized aerobic pyrolytic conditions. Forensic Sci Int 187:19–28

Hoffman RS, Kirrane BM, Marcus SM (2008) A descriptive study of an outbreak of clenbuterol-containing heroin. Ann Emerg Med 52(5):548–553

Hughes JR, Oliveto AH, Liguori A, Carpenter J, Howard T (1998) Endorsement of DSM-IV dependence criteria among caffeine users. Drug Alcohol Depend 52(2):99–107

Jarvis MF, Jackson RH, Williams M (1989) Autoradiographic characterization of high-affinity adenosine A2 receptors in the rat brain. Brain Res 484(1–2):111–118

Koob GF, Volkow ND (2010) Neurocircuitry of addiction. Neuropsychopharmacology 35(1): 217–238

Kudlacek O, Hofmaier T, Luf A, Mayer FP, Stockner T, Nagy C, Holy M, Freissmuth M, Schmid R, Sitte HH (2017) Cocaine adulteration. J Chem Neuroanat 83-84:75–81

Lazarus M, Shen HY, Cherasse Y, Qu WM, Huang ZL, Bass CE et al (2011) Arousal effect of caffeine depends on adenosine A2A receptors in the shell of the nucleus accumbens. J Neurosci 31(27):10067–10075

Londos C, Cooper DMF, Wolff J (1980) Subclasses of external adenosine receptors. Proc Natl Acad Sci U S A 77:2551–2554

López Hill X, Prieto JP, Meikle MN, Urbanavicius J, Abin-Carriquiry JA et al (2011) Coca-paste seized samples characterization: chemical analysis, stimulating effect in rats and relevance of caffeine as a major adulterant. Behav Brain Res 221:134–141

Lüscher C, Ungless MA (2006) The mechanistic classification of addictive drugs. PLoS Med 3(11): e437

Malave LB, Broderick PA (2014) Caffeine's attenuation of cocaine-induced dopamine release by inhibition of adenosine. J Caffeine Res 4(2):35–40

Morelato M, Franscella D, Esseiva P, Broséus J (2019) When does the cutting of cocaine and heroin occur? The first large-scale study based on the chemical analysis of cocaine and heroin seizures in Switzerland. Int J Drug Policy 73:7–15

Muñiz JA, Prieto JP, González B, Sosa MH, Cadet JL, Scorza C, Urbano FJ, Bisagno V (2017) Cocaine and caffeine effects on the conditioned place preference test: concomitant changes on early genes within the mouse prefrontal cortex and nucleus Accumbens. Front Behav Neurosci 11:200

Nehlig A, Daval J-L, Debry G (1992) Caffeine and the central nervous system: mechanisms of action, biochemical, metabolic and psychostimulant effects. Brain Res Rev 17(2):139–170

Pawlik E, Mahler H (2001) Smoke analysis of adulterated illicit drug preparations. Toxichem Krimtech 78:200–210

Porkka-Heiskanen T, Alanko L, Kalinchuk A, Stenberg D (2002) Adenosine and sleep. Sleep Med Rev 6(4):321–332

Prieto JP, Galvalisi M, López-Hill X, Meikle MN, Abin-Carriquiry JA, Scorza C (2015) Caffeine enhances and accelerates the expression of sensitization induced by coca paste indicating its relevance as a main adulterant. Am J Addict 24(5):475–481

Prieto JP, Scorza C, Serra GP, Perra V, Galvalisi M, Abin-Carriquiry JA, Piras G, Valentini V (2016) Caffeine, a common active adulterant of cocaine, enhances the reinforcing effect of cocaine and its motivational value. Psychopharmacology 233(15–16):2879–2889

Reissig CJ, Strain EC, Griffiths RR (2009) Caffeinated energy drinks – a growing problem. Drug Alcohol Depend 99(1–3):1–10
Samaha AN, Robinson TE (2005) Why does the rapid delivery of drugs to the brain promote addiction? Trends Pharmacol Sci 26(2):82–87
Schwarzkopf N, Lagos P, Falconi A, Scorza C, Torterolo P (2018) Caffeine as an adulterant of coca paste seized samples: preclinical study on the rat sleep-wake cycle. Behav Pharmacol 29(6): 519–529
Scorza C, Prieto JP, Fabius S, Galvalisi M (2021) Pulmonary inhalation to assess effects of coca-paste on behavior and dopamine neurotransmission. In: Neuromethod. Springer Nature
Seely KA, Patton AL, Moran CL, Womack ML, Prather PL, Fantegrossi WE et al (2013) Forensic investigation of K2, Spice, and "bath salt" commercial preparations: a three-year study of new designer drug products containing synthetic cannabinoid, stimulant, and hallucinogenic compounds. Forensic Sci Int 233(1–3):416–422
Shannon M (1988) Clinical toxicity of cocaine adulterants. Ann Emerg Med 17(11):1243–1247
Siciliano CA, Calipari ES, Ferris MJ, Jones SR (2015) Adaptations of presynaptic dopamine terminals induced by psychostimulant self-administration. ACS Chem Neurosci 6(1):27–36
Vanattou-Saïfoudine N, McNamara R, Harkin A (2012) Caffeine provokes adverse interactions with 3,4-methylenedioxymethamphetamine (MDMA, 'ecstasy') and related psychostimulants: mechanisms and mediators. Br J Pharmacol 167(5):946–959
Villar Núñez MLÁ, Sánchez Morcillo J, Ruíz Martínez MA (2018) Purity and adulteration in cocaine seizures and drug market inspection in Galicia (Spain) across an eight-year period. Drug Test Anal 10(2):381–391
Volkow ND, Wang GJ, Fischman MW, Foltin RW, Fowler JS, Abumrad NN et al (1997) Relationship between subjective effects of cocaine and dopamine transporter occupancy. Nature 386: 827–830
Volkow ND, Wang GJ, Logan J, Alexoff D, Fowler JS, Thanos PK, Wong C, Casado V, Ferre S, Tomasi D (2015) Caffeine increases striatal dopamine D2/D3 receptor availability in the human brain. Transl Psychiatry 5:e549
Wise RA, Bozarth MA (1987) A psychomotor stimulant theory of addiction. Psychol Rev 94: 469–492

Part VIII

Areca and Khat

Areca Nut, Morbidity, and Cardiovascular Disease (Acute Coronary Syndrome): Implications for Policy and Prevention

76

Kashif Shafique and Sumaira Nasim

Contents

Areca Nut ... 1620
Acute Coronary Syndrome (ACS) ... 1621
Primary Features of ACS ... 1622
Signs and Symptoms ... 1622
Medical History ... 1622
Clinical Assessment ... 1622
Biochemical Test ... 1622
Epidemiology of ACS ... 1623
ACS and Areca Nut ... 1623
Consumption of Areca Nut and Risk Factors for ACS ... 1623
Public Health Programs for Prevention and Cessation of Areca Nut Consumption ... 1624
Primary Prevention of ACS ... 1625
Secondary Prevention of ACS ... 1625
Research Implications ... 1626
Research Activities in Asian Countries to Reduce Areca Nut Consumption in Asian Countries ... 1627
Brief Explanation Is as Follows ... 1627
Policies and Legislation ... 1628
Education and Advocacy ... 1628
Surveillance and Research ... 1629
Types of Interventions ... 1629
Product Bans ... 1631
Media Campaign ... 1631
Success Story ... 1632
Mini Dictionary of Terms ... 1633
Summary Points ... 1633
References ... 1633

K. Shafique (✉) · S. Nasim
School of Public Health, Dow University of Health Sciences, Karachi, Pakistan
e-mail: k.shafique@duhs.edu.pk; sumaira.nasim@duhs.edu.pk

V. B. Patel, V. R. Preedy (eds.), *Handbook of Substance Misuse and Addictions*,
https://doi.org/10.1007/978-3-030-92392-1_83

Abstract

The consumption of areca nut is on the rise, particularly among adolescents and population belonging to South Asian countries. The high consumption can mainly be attributed to the lack of knowledge regarding its health hazards, accessibility, and low price. Regular consumption of areca nut can contribute to obesity, hypertension, diabetes, different types of cancers, and heart diseases. This chapter focus on the consumption of areca nut as a public health problem and a contributing factor for the acute coronary syndrome. Moreover, public health initiatives to minimize use of areca nut among different vulnerable groups are discussed.

In order to minimize the consumption of areca nut, initiatives are proposed to be planned and implemented by a multidisciplinary team, which may include public health specialist, cardiologist, psychologist, and social scientists. Moreover, suggested to conduct public health programs in a culturally specific manner, in local language, age and gender specific. The involvement of the influencers such as community and religious leaders, celebrities and use of social media such as Facebook are also recommended.

Keywords

Areca nut · Acute coronary syndrome · High-income countries · Low-middle-income countries · Public health

Abbreviations

ACS	Acute coronary syndrome
HICs	High-income countries
IVR	Interactive voice response
LBW	Low birth weight
LMICs	Low-middle-income countries
SAPHF	South Asian Public Health Forum
UK	United Kingdom
WHO	World Health Organization

Areca Nut

Areca nut is a plant fruit largely grown in South and South-East Asia, and some parts of Africa (Mehrtash et al. 2017; Gupta and Warnakulasuriya 2002; Boucher and Mannan 2002). It is usually 3–5 cm in length and 2–4 cm in diameter and once ripe is yellow-orange in color, slightly bitter, and sharp in taste (Gupta and Warnakulasuriya 2002). It is usually consumed as a whole, or, thinly sliced form, either in raw or processed form such as baked, dried, roasted, or fermented (Karim et al. 2018; Winstock et al. 2000). The type of processing method can affect the color and taste of areca nut.

The areca nut is mainly comprised of polyphenols, steroids, alkaloids, and fatty acids, in different proportions, depending on the geographical locations where it is grown and according to the degree of maturity of the nut (Mehrtash et al. 2017; Peng et al. 2015). According to the cultural practices and preferences, areca nut is used, in addition to its natural form, along with tobacco and other forms of artificial sweeteners and spices like cardamom or cloves in the form of betel quid (Mehrtash et al. 2017).

It is identified as the fourth most commonly used recreational drug after tobacco, ethanol, and caffeine (Gupta and Warnakulasuriya 2002; Gunjal et al. 2020). The global prevalence of areca nut use alone and in its different forms suggest over 600 million users exist globally. Review of literature revealed that 85% of smokeless tobacco consumption with areca nut belong to South Asian countries (Gupta and Warnakulasuriya 2002; Mehrtash et al. 2017; Thakur et al. 2020), which attributes to nearly more than six million Disability Adjusted Life Years (DALYs) and over a quarter of a million deaths occurring each year owing to its consumption (Siddiqi et al. 2015). Moreover, consumption more than once per day is found to be associated with poor oral health-related quality of life (Berhan Nordin et al. 2019). In most of these countries, consumption is socially, culturally, and religiously acceptable, and most importantly, perceived harmless (Peng et al. 2015; Berhan Nordin et al. 2019; Garg et al. 2014). Consumption is mainly in Asian countries such as India, Pakistan, Myanmar, Sri-Lanka, as well as migrants of those countries living in North America, Europe, and African countries (Mehrtash et al. 2017). Areca Nut is also used for its medicinal properties to treat diarrhea, digestive disorders, and parasitic infection (Peng et al. 2015). However, in recent decades, it has been identified as a serious threat to public health particularly in low-middle-income countries (LMICs) since prolonged use of areca nut can adversely affect different vital organs, leading to number of diseases and adverse quality of life (Yen et al. 2006; Mannan et al. 2000; Vedanthan et al. 2014; Lin et al. 2008; Thavarajah et al. 2019). Literature support that regular use of the areca nut is associated with the systemic inflammation, metabolic syndrome, raised blood pressure, certain types of cancers, heart diseases, and weight gain (Karim et al. 2018; Siddiqi et al. 2015; Garg et al. 2014; Thavarajah et al. 2019; Lin et al. 2009; Guh et al. 2006; Yamada et al. 2013; Shafique et al. 2012; Gupta et al. 2016; Javed et al. 2010). For oral cancers, consumption of betel nut can contribute up to 50%, and two-third of this burden of disease belong to low-income countries (LICs) and LMICs (Gupta et al. 2016). Similarly, low birth weight (LBW) and poor pregnancy outcome are also reported (Garg et al. 2014). In 2010, ST use led to 1.7 million disability adjusted life years (DALYs) and 62,283 deaths due to oral, pharyngeal, and esophageal cancers (Berhan Nordin et al. 2019).

All such consequences need to be addressed on an urgent basis by public health professionals and policy makers. This chapter particularly focuses on the link between areca nut and acute coronary syndrome (ACS). It also suggests public health strategies to reduce consumption of areca nut among different vulnerable groups who are at risk of ACS.

Acute Coronary Syndrome (ACS)

Acute Coronary Syndrome (ACS) refers to number of conditions linked to narrowing of coronary arteries, which leads to sudden limited flow of blood to the heart. Prevention and treatment are two main strategies for combating ACS, which includes lifestyle modification of such risk factors such as unhealthy diet, less physical activity, stress, alcohol consumption, and use of tobacco and areca nut, which can contribute to increased risk of certain chronic diseases including ACS (Karim et al. 2018). Since most of the chronic diseases are often preventable through lifestyle modifications, strategies to prevent, minimize, and quitting substance abuse should be one of the leading priority areas for public health system.

Primary Features of ACS

Signs and Symptoms

- Chest pain or discomfort or tightness
- Pain or discomfort in one or both arms, the jaw, neck, back, or stomach
- Shortness of breath
- Feeling dizzy or lightheaded
- Nausea
- Sweating
- Sudden death

Medical History

- History of cardiac diseases or any chronic disease
- Comorbidities such as diabetes, pulmonary diseases

Clinical Assessment

- Pulse
- Blood pressure
- Electrocardiogram
- Echocardiography
- Chest X-ray
- Fluid balance

Biochemical Test

- Complete blood count
- Cardiac enzymes (e.g., CK-MB [creatine kinase MB isoenzyme])
- Cell contents (e.g., troponin I, troponin T, myoglobin)
- Cardiac troponin levels
- Measurement of BNP or NT-proBNP
- Arterial blood gas (ABGs)
- Urea and electrolyte blood test

Epidemiology of ACS

ACS is a major global public health problem, which accounts for 30% of deaths among adults, with more than 80% of this burden in LMICs (Lopez et al. 2006). This burden of disease often leads to societal and economic loses and majority of these diseases are preventable by adapting a healthy lifestyle (Ruff and Braunwald 2011). The incidence of ACS in HICs is on the decline, however immigrants living in high-income countries (HICs) are still at risk due to modifiable and non-modifiable risk factors (Vedanthan et al. 2014). Similarly, due to lifestyle modifications, similar to that seen in the Western countries, the prevalence of ACS in LMICs, particularly at young age, is on the rise (Vedanthan et al. 2014; Ralapanawa and Sivakanesan 2021).

ACS and Areca Nut

Prolong use of areca nut can raise pulse rate and blood pressure. It can act as a vasoconstrictor, effecting the sympathetic nervous system, which results in the secretion of adrenal medullary catecholamine, raised homocysteine levels, and contributes to arterial stiffness (Karim et al. 2018; Lin et al. 2008). Literature reports negative correlation between homocysteine levels and vitamin B-12 levels, whereas regular consumption of areca nut impairs vitamin B-12 absorption. All these factors can contribute to increased risk of ACS, and consumption of areca nut is now identified as a major risk factor for ACS as it can increase risk of developing ACS threefold (Lin et al. 2008). However, unlike alcohol and cigarette smoking, there is limited awareness regarding health hazards of areca nut.

Vitamin D is found to have a protective role in prevention and management of certain heart diseases (Debreceni and Debreceni 2014). The possible mechanism involves the role in reduction of oxidative stress (leads to inflammatory process) produced by the free radicals. However regular consumption of areca nut leads to vitamin D deficiency contributing to reduction of its protective effect (Ogunkolade et al. 2006).

Consumption of Areca Nut and Risk Factors for ACS

An understanding of the consumption of areca nut among different age, sex, and socioeconomic groups is important to understand the facilitation, planning, and implementation of public health programs to minimize risk of ACS related to areca nut use.

Ethnicity: Due to the cultural, religious, and social reasons, high production of areca nut and limited restriction on sale of areca nut contributes to its high consumption among Asians (whether they are living in their own country or as migrant or refugees) as compared to the Western countries (Thavarajah et al. 2019). Moreover, not considering areca nut use as a harmful lifestyle habit results in almost no attempt to quit and most people consider it as a natural product with least or no harm (Thavarajah et al. 2019; Myint et al. 2016; Furber et al. 2013). South Asians, mostly in younger and productive ages are at high risk of ACS as compared to the Caucasian population and with the misconceptions among consumers of areca regarding its health benefits and a relief from various health problems, such as gastrointestinal issues, to cure bad breath and morning sickness during pregnancy, leads to more harm in this population (Mehrtash et al. 2017; Senn et al. 2009).

Gender: Most of the studies reported high consumption of areca nut in men as compared to women (Hussain et al. 2017; Hosein et al. 2015; Oakley et al. 2005; Lee et al. 2011). Relatively excessive use of areca nut among men compared to women is most likely to be attributable to peer pressure and use of areca nut and betel quid by elders especially parents, which silently sends the message that it is not a harmful substance (Berhan Nordin et al. 2019; Hussain et al. 2017). Another possible reason for higher use of areca nut and betel quid among men is the much higher prevalence of smoking among men. These products are used as mouth fresheners and considered as an economical way for this purpose. Lower consumption among women might be attributed to the fact that females are more health literate and mindful about cosmetic issues as consumption of areca nut leads significant staining and damage to lips and teeth (Furber et al. 2013; Hosein et al. 2015). Consumption of areca nut is much diverse with mostly reported among women of reproductive age, anemic or pregnant women (Furber et al. 2013; Placek et al. 2019), and men above 45 years and women above 55 years of age who are obese, suffering from hypertension and diabetes, and are at high risk of ACS (Overbaugh 2009; Dong et al. 2017). The nationally representative Nutrition and Health Survey in Taiwan (1993–1996) reported that consumption of areca nut is independently associated with the heart diseases among women (Guh et al. 2007).

Age: Areca nut consumption may start even as early as in teenage (Hussain et al. 2017; Oakley et al. 2005; Mazahir et al. 2006). This might be due to consumption by either of the parents, friends, or easy availability and marketing in the form of mouth freshener with fancy packaging (Garg et al. 2014). Consumption is reported more among youth belonging to low socioeconomic status as it is considered a cheap form of mouth fresher especially in young male smokers (Hussain et al. 2017; Prabhu et al. 2001). Literature reports that teenagers are more concerned about the effect of areca nut on appearance of the mouth rather than health hazards, thus it can serve as a useful strategy for cessation of areca nut (Prabhu et al. 2001).

Public Health Programs for Prevention and Cessation of Areca Nut Consumption

A multidisciplinary team is required to design and implement public health programs to control areca nut consumption and design programs for primary and secondary prevention of ACS. This may include an epidemiologist, qualitative research experts, cardiologist, psychologist, physiotherapist or exercise physiologist, dietitians, and social workers in such a team.

Designing public health interventions needs to take into account the amount and frequency of consumption, availability and affordability, perceptions toward use, and health literacy. For any public health program aiming to avoid, minimize, or abstain the use of areca nut, the following points should be considered:

1. Identify major stakeholders according to life stage, gender, ethnicity, and religious beliefs.
2. Instead of offering a monetary benefit, encourage the targeted group to voluntarily register for the service.
3. Development of life skills, e.g., confidence building, self-control, communication, and collaboration.

These programs need to be planned and implemented with consultation and involvement of the representatives of the particular vulnerable group. For instance, areca nut consumption is more common among Asians living in HICs. Needs assessments (incorporating quantitative and qualitative approach) can be useful to incorporate health professionals as well as migrant's perspective, and cost-effective health promotion programs can be implemented (Mehrtash et al. 2017).

As mentioned above, literature reports different consumption patterns among gender. Thus, awareness programs need to take into account the trend of areca nut consumption among both genders. For effective prevention and treatment, understanding of a particular culture, sociodemographics; knowledge and perceptions toward areca nut consumption; and attitude toward cessation of intake need to be considered (Winstock 2002). Intake of such a substance is embedded in individual perceptions, family, and social values. Moreover, there are certain triggers that can enhance the intake of areca nut. For instance, in rural areas of India, women consume areca nut to reduce fatigue and enhance work productivity (Placek et al. 2019).

Primary Prevention of ACS

A healthy lifestyle such as healthy diet, exercise, and avoidance of substance abuse such as areca nut can reduce mortality up to 50% (Sanchis-Gomar et al. 2016). For areca nut, primary prevention can include policy to implement a strict ban on sales and marketing, increasing price, or no availability (Berhan Nordin et al. 2019; Thavarajah et al. 2019). In case of both HICs and LMICs, these policies are not as successfully implemented as for other tobacco products (Winstock 2002).

Secondary Prevention of ACS

For ACS, there is a limited concept of secondary prevention. Moreover, patients with ACS have high risk of rehospitalization as compared to nonusers, as a study conducted in Pakistan revealed that consumption of areca nut can significantly increase 30-day rehospitalization rate among ACS patients (Karim et al. 2018).

Similarly, in LMICs, 80.2% of the patients with a history of heart diseases didn't receive medication (Yusuf et al. 2011). These studies show that the concept of secondary prevention, which may include dietary modification; physical activity/ exercise; and quitting of smoking, alcohol, and areca nut should be strengthened in LMICs where prevalence of ACS and areca nut consumption is high. Thus, as a secondary prevention at the time of hospital discharge, education needs to be provided in local language regarding its detrimental effects and to avoid use of areca nut, for instance, development of a booklet or patient education material in local and regional languages. It is suggested that the booklet should have illustrations so that people with limited or no literacy can benefit from it. Health hazards such as ACS can be explained in a simple language.

Healthy dietary practices during pregnancy can improve pregnancy outcome such as birth weight and can prevent adulthood chronic diseases such as ACS (Smith et al. 2016). On the other hand, LBW can be a contributing factor for ACS. In certain ethnic groups, consumption of areca nut during pregnancy (particularly with low hemoglobin levels) is reported to cope with morning sickness, fatigue, and low performance (Senn et al. 2009; Placek et al. 2019). Thus, there is a need to create awareness regarding the hazards of areca nut among pregnant women and their families. Literature reports that regular intake can lead to poor pregnancy outcome such as LBW babies, whereas LBW is associated with ACS. However, nearly 80% of such women have lack of awareness regarding the hazards of areca nut (Senn et al. 2009). Usually, health education programs targeting pregnant women regarding hazards of tobacco, alcohol should also include the hazards of areca nut and be part of the antenatal care.

Areca Nut Quit Helpline: A free-phone service can be helpful to provide valuable information regarding strategies to quit areca nut. This can be useful for migrants living in HICs as they can receive information in native language (with the assistance of an interpreter) without visiting a healthcare center.

Research Implications

In HICs, there has been scientific research and technological advancements regarding hazards of areca nut consumption and its contribution to chronic diseases such as heart diseases, cancers, and impaired dental health. Unfortunately, in LMICs, unlike cigarette smoking and alcohol consumption, there have been limited research activities to explore avenues such as the frequency of areca nut consumption, causes, and consequences. Moreover, there is dearth of literature using mixed-methodology approach, which can be useful as a research tool to assess the areca nut consumption. Development and validation of a questionnaire for a particular ethnic group can be of use. Secondly in research activities, usually healthy adult volunteers participate, who are educated and have better health literacy, and thus have limited intake of areca nut. It is important to identify the slum areas of LMICs, where there is limited literacy (particularly health literacy), availability of areca nut at a low price as compared to the price of healthy food options such as fresh fruits and vegetables (Guo et al. 2013). Moreover, there is a need of collaboration among multidisciplinary team comprised of healthcare professionals from HICs and LMICs using mixed-methodology approach to explore the perception regarding use of areca nut. This will be helpful to design and implement the interventions to reduce consumption. This team may comprise of public health experts, general practitioners, dentist, psychologists, and nutritionists as a part of such healthcare programs and research activities.

Research Activities in Asian Countries to Reduce Areca Nut Consumption in Asian Countries

Keeping in view the extensive use of areca nut in Asian countries, few research activities are initiated. Brief details are as follows:

Asian Betel Quid Consortium (ABC) consortium: This was developed among WHO and six Asian countries (Taiwan, Mainland China, Malaysia, Indonesia, Nepal, and Sri Lanka). The aim of the study was to evaluate the prevalence, practices, consequences, and efforts to reduce consumption among diverse population belonging to selected countries. The data was collected over 8000 adult male and females ($\geq$15 years and above). Prevalence was found from 0.8% to 46.3% and consumption was high among men, belonging to low-income households, less educated, and alcohol drinkers. Adverse effects on oral, mental, and physical health were reported (Lee et al. 2011, 2012, 2018).

ASTRA Study: Similarly, in 2020 Global Health Research Group titled ASTRA (Addressing Smokeless Tobacco Use and Building Research Capacity in South Asia) was developed, which was funded by the UK's National Institute for Health Research (NIHR). Five UK Universities and six partner organizations from Bangladesh, India, and Pakistan are part of this consortium. The aim is to reduce burden of smokeless tobacco such as areca nut in South Asian countries. To achieve this aim, available literature will be reviewed and interventions will be designed and assess feasibility of the interventions particularly for adolescents. It also planned to develop a framework for measure Smokeless Tobacco (ST) control policies (Readshaw et al. 2020).

It is a common observation that people either consume areca nut occasionally or on regular basis, thus dose–response relationship between areca nut consumption and risk of ACS and other chronic diseases can be an area of interest for future research. A number of protocols have been developed for smoking cessation; with a few changes such protocols can be used for areca nut cessation as well (Jayasinghe et al. 2021). A framework for areca nut control, and MPOWER measures, which have been successful in decline of tobacco, can be used to control the use of areca nut (Mehrtash et al. 2017).

Brief Explanation Is as Follows

MPOWER Measures for Areca Nut: MPOWER measures are successful and cost-effective measures for tobacco cessation and can be applied for areca nut as well. For instance, in primary and secondary prevention programs of ACS, use of MPOWER measures can be as follows:

Monitoring areca nut use and prevention policies
Protecting people from areca nut
Offering help to quit areca nut use
Warning about the dangers of areca nut in contributing to ACS
Enforcing bans on areca nut advertising, promotion, and sponsorship
Raising tax on areca nut

Several public health interventions for tobacco cessation are implemented as the 5As (Ask, Advise, Assess, Assist, Arrange) and 5 Rs (Relevance, Risk, Rewards, Roadblocks, Repetition) brief intervention model (Park et al. 2015). A similar model can be developed for prevention and cessation of areca nut among patients at risk of ACS as 6A and 6R as presented in Table 1.

Policies and Legislation

This may include ban of sale (particularly $\leq$18 years), college and university admission criteria, hiring policy of the workplace, no-areca nut consumption policy at public places.

Education and Advocacy

Strategies to promote behavior change: Involve people such as celebrities, social media influencers, religious leaders, and patients and their families who previously consumed areca nut and currently suffering from a chronic disease such as heart disease or mouth cancer.

Table 1 Areca nut cessation: the 6 A's and 6 R's

6'A to help patients to quit areca nut	6A' to increase motivation to quit areca nut and reduce risk of ACS
***A*cute Coronary Syndrome:** Ask about family history of ACS and other modifiable and non-modifiable risk factors for ACS	***R*elevance:** Why quitting areca nut is personally relevant
***A*sk**: Ask amount and frequency of areca nut consumption	***R*isk:** Negative consequences of areca nut and risk of ACS
***A*dvise:** Suggest patient to quit	***R*ewards**: Benefits of areca nut cessations
***A*ssess:** Readiness to quit	***R*oadblocks:** Identify barriers to quitting areca nut, e.g., low price, easy availability, peer-pressure
***A*ssist:** Assist in quit attempt	***R*epetition:** Repeat every time during patient visit
***A*rrange:** Follow-up	***R*educe:** Reduce risk of ACS and other chronic diseases such as oral cancers

Surveillance and Research

There are a number of stakeholders involved in the production, distribution, sale, and consumption of areca nut. Thus, understanding of bio-psycho-socio-economic cultural factors is inevitable to control areca nut consumption (Thavarajah et al. 2019).

Partnerships and Alliances: Partnerships between healthcare professionals, allied health professions, and social scientist can help to jointly plan public health education programs to reduce risk of ACS and promote healthy lifestyle. Moreover, multisite partnerships can be developed between countries where consumption of areca nut and prevalence of ACS is high. Similarly, countries that conducted successful campaigns to curb the use of areca nut can collaborate with countries where intake is still uncontrollable and help to develop effective strategies.

Awareness sessions at educational institutes, particularly schools, are important as peer influence, lack of knowledge regarding use of pocket money to buy healthy snacks, and easy availability of areca nut and related products (such as in school canteen or hawkers outside school) can increase possibility of consumption (Hussain et al. 2017).

In LMICs, ACS is more prevalent among young and productive age (Vedanthan et al. 2014). At the same time, the consumption of areca nut is more common among youth (Hussain et al. 2017; Bhojani et al. 2021). Thus, school-based interventions are required involving school administration, teachers, parents, student canteen owners, and students who are the main stake holders. Moreover, school administration can ensure ban on sale of such products outside the school vicinity. In response to such interventions, success stories of quitting areca nut can be shared on school website or newsletter, which in turn can be motivational for other students as well.

In India, a school-based public health program titled “Lifefirst” was implemented to control the use of tobacco and areca nut among 13–15-year-old school children (Bhojani et al. 2021). This service includes theme-based interactive sessions in groups. Individual sessions were also conducted. The students were equipped with the coping mechanisms and ability to say “no” to peers. All activities were performed in a friendly environment and supplemented with theme-based group activities and role plays. The students were counseled in a child-friendly way with the help of games, activities, role plays, and audiovisual aids. There was a regular follow-up to safeguard the success of the program.

Types of Interventions

mArecaNut Cessation Program to Prevent ACS: Similar to mTobacco cessation, mArecanut cessation program such as text messages and short whatsapp videos in local language can be useful. World Health Organization (WHO) has identified mHealth a useful strategy to prevent or manage a disease, condition, or addiction.

This may include voice messages, Interactive Voice Response (IVR) messages, and videos. mHealth is more focused on self-management as compared to telehealth, which refers to clinician-to-patient approach. Moreover, mHealth can be useful for hard-to-reach population such as individuals living in remote areas, people with language barrier, and low literacy. mHealth is also found to be cost-effective, environment friendly (as less documentation is required), and limited human resource dependent. Thus, the use of social media can be actively utilized with these short videos and entertaining messages.

In order to prevent and control areca nut consumption, there is a need to include different stakeholders such as government officials, nongovernment organizations, community and religious representatives, and multidisciplinary healthcare professionals to engage them all in these preventive strategies.

Community Leaders and Influencers: Involvement of community leaders such as president of a community society, religious leaders, or influencers such as celebrities (actors/actresses, famous players, youtubers, bloggers) can be useful in creating awareness regarding hazards of areca nut.

It is commonly observed that migrants and refuges usually have limited access to healthcare facilities in HICs (Donato-Hunt et al. 2012). Reasons may include: language barriers, lack of awareness, lack of culturally specific healthcare, and limited same gender healthcare professionals. Health promotion programs need to be conducted in a local language or with the facilitation of certified interpreters. Moreover, such programs need to involve all the community and religious leaders of the particular migrant group. Capacity building of health professionals regarding culturally specific strategies is also needed. Community–academic partnership can also be successful as it can enhance good quality research and capacity building of the professionals. Similar to other addictions, areca nut requires continuum of follow-up.

A number of factors can influence the cessation and quitting of the areca nut. Socioecological model can be a useful framework for categorizing these factors into levels of influence, which can be implemented by the Public Health Professionals using print, electronic, and social media campaign. Brief details are as follows:

Intraindividual: Knowledge and perceptions regarding hazards of areca nut, personal choice, and motivation to avoid consumption of areca nut. Keeping track of money spent on areca nut. For instance, a person is consuming areca nut six times a day. So set a goal to consume five times a day for 1 month and follow this pattern for next few months.

Interpersonal: Support and/or influence from peers, family, and teachers to avoid or cease intake of areca nut. Small group education sessions can be conducted involving different stakeholders. For instance, group enrollment, which refers to participation in health promotion program, where two or more than two participants are known to each other and face similar health problems or addiction. Thus, group sessions for pregnancy women at an antenatal clinic in a community can be useful strategy.

Community/organizational: Ban on sale of areca nut at educational institutes and other public places. Creating awareness through media (electronic, print, and social media) and worship places. Most of the organizations are usually providing health insurance to cover the cost of illness. Thus, regular consumption of areca nut and other addiction can increase risk of chronic diseases such as ACS, which is found to be the most expensive for the employers and health insurance companies as compared to other chronic diseases. Thus, promotion of healthy lifestyle such as healthy diet, exercise, and abstinence from alcohol, tobacco, and areca nut can be cost-effective strategies to reduce medical bills, absenteeism, and improve work productivity.

Societal/policy: At the government level, initiatives such as ban on cultivation of areca nut, suggesting and supporting crop substitution, and increasing price of areca nut can be beneficial.

Product Bans

Currently the price of areca nut is extremely low. For instance, in Asian countries, the usual cost is $0.13 for four to six servings. For tobacco control, measures such as taxation, health warning messages on packaging, ban on advertisements and increased price has proven to be quite effective, particularly for LMICs (Mehrtash et al. 2017). Similar measures can be taken for areca nut. Rise in price of areca nut can be a useful strategy to decrease consumption (Thavarajah et al. 2019). However, there are a few limitations that need to be overcome. For instance, in LMICs, areca nut business is mostly owned by the cottage industry, thus usually sale is without packaging making health warning messages and images impossible. Moreover, taxation on cottage industry is difficult to implement (Mehrtash et al. 2017). Therefore, offering alternative business or employment opportunities can be an effective way to reduce areca nut–related business.

Media Campaign

Different types of media can be utilized to create awareness regarding areca nut and ACS. Brief details are as follows:

Print Media: This includes newspapers, newsletters, booklets, patient's education material, and posters for institutions, stickers and leaflets for school vans and for public transport such as buses, airports, and trains (Amarasinghe et al. 2021). All types of print media can be used to create awareness in local languages, illustrations, and religious and cultural demonstrations in simple layman language. Similar to cigarette pack, there should be images and health warning labels of oral cancer and increased risk of ACS on the display of areca nut products.

Electronic Media: This includes the use of television, through teledramas, and the radio. This platform is more suitable for people with limited or no literacy. All such programs should be in local languages and sign language for people with impaired hearing. Moreover, use of cartoon characters can be developed to create awareness particularly for children, to avoid peer-pressure for consumption of areca nut. Short animated videos can capture the attention of targeted audience with limited literacy and youth. These videos can depict in layman's language the mechanism of how areca nut contributes to the pathophysiology of ACS.

Social Media: In the era of social media, the use of facebook, blogs, Linkedin, twitter, youtube, or whatsapp messages and videos can be instrumental in sharing information related to healthcare (Furber et al. 2013). Thus, hazards of areca nut and strategies to avoid and quit can be shared using social media. The choice of social media depends on sociodemographics and psychographics of the target group. For instance, blog and LinkedIn can be useful for people with better literacy, whereas whatsapp and face-book can be useful for youngsters and people with limited or no literacy. Overall, the use of social media can be a cost-effective, available, accessible, affordable, and portable fast method to disseminate information to particularly hard-to-reach population. Social media is also useful as literature reports that use of areca nut is more common among youth and use of social media is more popular among this age group.

The influencers may include community leaders, religious leaders, celebrities, family members of ill or deceased patients who suffered from heart diseases, multidisciplinary Healthcare Professionals such as cardiologist or psychologist. Short videos and messages by such influencers can be an effective way to create awareness about the role of areca nut in the development of chronic diseases such as ACS or cancers. Moreover, such media campaign can be useful on World health Days such as world heart, diabetes, or kidney day.

Success Story

Myanmar is one of the Asian countries where consumption of areca nut is a major public health problem as consumption is above 50% of the population (Myint et al. 2016). Recently, a 6-week media campaign by the title of "War on Cancer" was launched in collaboration with the Ministry of Health and Sports with the collaboration of People's Health Foundation, Myanmar. (A nonprofit, public–private partnership, nongovernmental organization of Myanmar.) Through this campaign, 22.95 million households were targeted to raise awareness regarding areca nut use and related health risk. The targeted age group was 18–55 years of age. The messages were disseminated through television, radio, and different social media platforms to create awareness. The state television and radio channels offered free broadcasting time. For instance, a youtube channel (https://www.youtube.com/watch?v=bT434U8PtIQ&t=10s) was created and interviews of real-world victims were recorded. Similarly, a facebook page titled as #StopArecaMyanmar was created and 5.1 million views were found. The strength of the program was hard-hitting, with culturally appropriate messages engaging different types of media, thus gaining broad coverage. To evaluate the success of the program, focus group discussions were conducted. Similar campaigns can be used to particularly focus on the role of areca nut in increasing risk of the chronic diseases, particularly ACS.

As areca nut consumption and risk of ACS is high in South Asian countries, there is a need for multiregional policy action agenda, advocacy campaign, political commitment, and research activities to create awareness regarding consumption of areca nut and risk of ACS. For instance, South Asian Public Health Forum (SAPHF) is an independent voluntary organization working to prevent and minimize burden of diseases among these countries (Asghar 2006). Thus, a collaborative effort by the SAPHF, particularly public health specialist and cardiologists can take lead to minimize this burden. Similarly, *South Asian Health Foundation* (*SAHF*), UK is a registered charity working for prompting health among migrants from South Asian countries, which can play a vital role in initiating research activities and health promotion programs to reduce areca nut consumption among South Asian migrants residing in the UK. Moreover, it is suggested to include areca nut as a part of global surveillance programs such as Global Tobacco Control Surveillance System and the WHO STEPwise approach to surveillance (Mehrtash et al. 2017).

Mini Dictionary of Terms

Acute Coronary Syndrome: Refers to a range of conditions associated with sudden, limited blood flow to the heart.

Lower Middle-Income economies are those with a GNI per capita between $1,046 and $ 4,095 and high-income economies are those with a GNI per capita of $ 12,696 or more.

Social Media: This is a term used for websites and technology-based applications used for (formal or informal) communication, interaction, and sharing of information.

Influencers: They are individuals who have earned a reputation for their knowledge and competence on a particular subject.

mHealth: Refers to use of any technology-based activity in healthcare. This may include device such as a mobile phone or websites or mobile application.

Summary Points

- All over the world, ACS is a public health problem.
- Consumption of areca nut is an important, however ignored risk factor for ACS.
- Primary and secondary prevention strategies such as culturally specific public health programs should include avoidance of areca nut to reduce ACS and associated factors such as risk of re-hospitalization, morbidity, and mortality.
- Thus, there is a need of advocacy, leadership, research activities, and collaborations with media, educational institutes and community leaders in prevention and cessation of areca nut.

References

Amarasinghe H, Warnakulasuriya S, Johnson NW (2021) Evaluation of a social marketing campaign for the early detection of oral potentially malignant disorders and oral cancer: Sri Lankan experience. J Oral Biol Craniofac Res 11(2):204

Asghar RJ (2006) Promoting regional health cooperation: the South Asian Public Health Forum. PLoS Med 3(5):e108

Berhan Nordin EA, Shoaib LA, Mohd Yusof ZY, Manan NM, Othman SA (2019) Oral health-related quality of life among 11–12 year old indigenous children in Malaysia. BMC Oral Health 19(1):152

Bhojani U, Varma A, Hebbar PB, Mandal G, Gupte H (2021) LifeFirst: impact of a school-based tobacco and supari cessation intervention among adolescent students in Mumbai, India. Popul Med 3(May):1–9

Boucher BJ, Mannan N (2002) Metabolic effects of the consumption of *Areca catechu*. Addict Biol 7(1):103–110

Debreceni B, Debreceni L (2014) Role of vitamins in cardiovascular health and disease. Res Rep Clin Cardiol 5:283–295

Donato-Hunt C, Munot S, Copeland J (2012) Alcohol, tobacco and illicit drug use among six culturally diverse communities in Sydney. Drug Alcohol Rev 31(7):881–889

Dong X, Cai R, Sun J, Huang R, Wang P, Sun H et al (2017) Diabetes as a risk factor for acute coronary syndrome in women compared with men: a meta-analysis, including 10 856 279 individuals and 106 703 acute coronary syndrome events. Diabetes Metab Res Rev 33(5):e2887

Furber S, Jackson J, Johnson K, Sukara R, Franco L (2013) A qualitative study on tobacco smoking and betel quid use among Burmese refugees in Australia. J Immigr Minor Health 15(6):1133–1136

Garg A, Chaturvedi P, Gupta PC (2014) A review of the systemic adverse effects of areca nut or betel nut. Indian J Med Paediatr Oncol 35(1):3

Guh J-Y, Chuang L-Y, Chen H-C (2006) Betel-quid use is associated with the risk of the metabolic syndrome in adults. Am J Clin Nutr 83(6):1313–1320

Guh J-Y, Chen H-C, Tsai J-F, Chuang L-Y (2007) Betel-quid use is associated with heart disease in women. Am J Clin Nutr 85(5):1229–1235

Gunjal S, Pateel DGS, Yang Y-H, Doss JG, Bilal S, Maling TH et al (2020) An overview on betel quid and areca nut practice and control in selected Asian and south east Asian countries. Subst Use Misuse 55(9):1533–1544

Guo S-E, Huang T-J, Huang J-C, Lin M-S, Hong R-M, Chang C-H et al (2013) Alcohol, betel-nut and cigarette consumption are negatively associated with health promoting behaviors in Taiwan: a cross-sectional study. BMC Public Health 13(1):1–8

Gupta P, Warnakulasuriya S (2002) Global epidemiology of areca nut usage. Addict Biol 7(1):77–83

Gupta B, Johnson NW, Kumar N (2016) Global epidemiology of head and neck cancers: a continuing challenge. Oncology 91(1):13–23

Hosein M, Mohiuddin S, Fatima N (2015) Association between grading of oral submucous fibrosis with frequency and consumption of areca nut and its derivatives in a wide age group: a multi-centric cross sectional study from Karachi, Pakistan. J Cancer Prev 20(3):216

Hussain A, Zaheer S, Shafique K (2017) Individual, social and environmental determinants of smokeless tobacco and betel quid use amongst adolescents of Karachi: a school-based cross-sectional survey. BMC Public Health 17(1):913

Javed F, Bello Correra FO, Chotai M, Tappuni AR, Almas K (2010) Systemic conditions associated with areca nut usage: a literature review. Scand J Public Health 38(8):838–844

Jayasinghe RD, Jayasooriya P, Amarasinghe H, Hettiarachchi P, Siriwardena B, Wijerathne U et al (2021) Evaluation of successfulness of capacity building programmes on smokeless tobacco and areca nut cessation. Asian Pac J Cancer Prev 22(4):1287–1293

Karim MT, Inam S, Ashraf T, Shah N, Adil SO, Shafique K (2018) Areca nut chewing and the risk of re-hospitalization and mortality among patients with acute coronary syndrome in Pakistan. J Prev Med Public Health 51(2):71

Lee CH, Ko AMS, Warnakulasuriya S, Yin BL, Zain RB, Ibrahim SO et al (2011) Intercountry prevalences and practices of betel-quid use in south, southeast and eastern Asia regions and associated oral preneoplastic disorders: an international collaborative study by Asian betel-quid consortium of south and east Asia. Int J Cancer 129(7):1741–1751

Lee C-H, Min-Shan Ko A, Warnakulasuriya S, Ling T-Y, Rajapakse PS, Zain RB et al (2012) Population burden of betel quid abuse and its relation to oral premalignant disorders in South, Southeast, and East Asia: an Asian Betel-quid Consortium Study. Am J Public Health 102(3): e17–e24

Lee C-H, Ko AM-S, Yang FM, Hung C-C, Warnakulasuriya S, Ibrahim SO et al (2018) Association of DSM-5 betel-quid use disorder with oral potentially malignant disorder in 6 betel-quid endemic Asian populations. JAMA Psychiatry 75(3):261–269

Lin W-Y, Chiu T-Y, Lee L-T, Lin C-C, Huang C-Y, Huang K-C (2008) Betel nut chewing is associated with increased risk of cardiovascular disease and all-cause mortality in Taiwanese men. Am J Clin Nutr 87(5):1204–1211

Lin WY, Pi-Sunyer FX, Liu CS, Li TC, Li CI, Huang CY et al (2009) Betel nut chewing is strongly associated with general and central obesity in Chinese male middle-aged adults. Obesity 17(6): 1247–1254

Lopez A, Mathers C, Ezzati M, Jamison D, Murray C (2006) Global burden of disease and risk factors. Oxford University Press, New York

Mannan N, Boucher B, Evans S (2000) Increased waist size and weight in relation to consumption of *Areca catechu* (betel-nut); a risk factor for increased glycaemia in Asians in east London. Br J Nutr 83(3):267–275

Mazahir S, Malik R, Maqsood M, Merchant KA, Malik F, Majeed A et al (2006) Socio-demographic correlates of betel, areca and smokeless tobacco use as a high risk behavior for head and neck cancers in a squatter settlement of Karachi, Pakistan. Subst Abuse Treat Prev Policy 1(1):1–6

Mehrtash H, Duncan K, Parascandola M, David A, Gritz ER, Gupta PC et al (2017) Defining a global research and policy agenda for betel quid and areca nut. Lancet Oncol 18(12):e767–e775

Myint SK, Narksawat K, Sillabutra J (2016) Prevalence and factors influencing betel nut chewing among adults in West Insein Township, Yangon, Myanmar. Southeast Asian J Trop Med Public Health 47(5):1089–1097

Oakley E, Demaine L, Warnakulasuriya S (2005) Areca (betel) nut chewing habit among high-school children in the Commonwealth of the Northern Mariana Islands (Micronesia). Bull World Health Organ 83:656–660

Ogunkolade WB, Boucher BJ, Bustin SA, Burrin JM, Noonan K, Mannan N et al (2006) Vitamin D metabolism in peripheral blood mononuclear cells is influenced by chewing "betel nut" (*Areca catechu*) and vitamin D status. J Clin Endocrinol Metabol 91(7):2612–2617

Overbaugh KJ (2009) Acute coronary syndrome. Am J Nurs 109(5):42–52

Park ER, Gareen IF, Japuntich S, Lennes I, Hyland K, DeMello S et al (2015) Primary care provider-delivered smoking cessation interventions and smoking cessation among participants in the National Lung Screening Trial. JAMA Intern Med 175(9):1509–1516

Peng W, Liu Y-J, Wu N, Sun T, He X-Y, Gao Y-X et al (2015) *Areca catechu* L.(Arecaceae): a review of its traditional uses, botany, phytochemistry, pharmacology and toxicology. J Ethnopharmacol 164:340–356

Placek C, Roulette C, Hudanick N, Khan A, Ravi K, Jayakrishna P et al (2019) Exploring biocultural models of chewing tobacco and paan among reproductive-aged women: self-medication, protection, or gender inequality? Am J Hum Biol 31(5):e23281

Prabhu N, Warnakulasuriya K, Gelbier S, Robinson P (2001) Betel quid chewing among Bangladeshi adolescents living in East London. Int J Paediatr Dent 11(1):18–24

Ralapanawa U, Sivakanesan R (2021) Epidemiology and the magnitude of coronary artery disease and acute coronary syndrome: a narrative review. J Epidemiol Glob Health 11(2):169–177

Readshaw A, Mehrotra R, Mishu M, Khan Z, Siddiqui F, Coyle K et al (2020) Addressing smokeless tobacco use and building research capacity in South Asia (ASTRA). J Glob Health 10(1):010327

Ruff CT, Braunwald E (2011) The evolving epidemiology of acute coronary syndromes. Nat Rev Cardiol 8(3):140–147

Sanchis-Gomar F, Perez-Quilis C, Leischik R, Lucia A (2016) Epidemiology of coronary heart disease and acute coronary syndrome. Ann Transl Med 4(13):256

Senn M, Baiwog F, Winmai J, Mueller I, Rogerson S, Senn N (2009) Betel nut chewing during pregnancy, Madang province, Papua New Guinea. Drug Alcohol Depend 105(1–2):126–131

Shafique K, Mirza SS, Vart P, Memon AR, Arain MI, Tareen MF et al (2012) Areca nut chewing and systemic inflammation: evidence of a common pathway for systemic diseases. J Inflamm 9(1): 1–8

Siddiqi K, Shah S, Abbas SM, Vidyasagaran A, Jawad M, Dogar O et al (2015) Global burden of disease due to smokeless tobacco consumption in adults: analysis of data from 113 countries. BMC Med 1(13):1–22

Smith CJ, Ryckman K, Barnabei VM, Howard B, Isasi CR, Sarto GE et al (2016) The impact of birth weight on cardiovascular disease risk in the Women's Health Initiative. Nutr Metab Cardiovasc Dis 26(3):239–245

Thakur N, Sharma AK, Singh H, Mehrotra R (2020) ANDB: development of a database based on a global survey of literature on areca nut and associated health effects. Subst Use Misuse 55(9): 1513–1518

Thavarajah R, Ranganathan K, Joshua E, Rao UK (2019) Areca nut use disorder: a dynamic model map. Indian J Dent Res 30(4):612

Vedanthan R, Seligman B, Fuster V (2014) Global perspective on acute coronary syndrome: a burden on the young and poor. Circ Res 114(12):1959–1975

Winstock A (2002) Areca nut-abuse liability, dependence and public health. Addict Biol 7(1): 133–138

Winstock A, Trivedy C, Warnakulasuriya K, Peters T (2000) A dependency syndrome related to areca nut use: some medical and psychological aspects among areca nut users in the Gujarat community in the UK. Addict Biol 5(2):173–179

Yamada T, Hara K, Kadowaki T (2013) Chewing betel quid and the risk of metabolic disease, cardiovascular disease, and all-cause mortality: a meta-analysis. PLoS One 8(8):e70679

Yen AM-F, Chiu Y-H, Chen L-S, Wu H-M, Huang C-C, Boucher BJ et al (2006) A population-based study of the association between betel-quid chewing and the metabolic syndrome in men. Am J Clin Nutr 83(5):1153–1160

Yusuf S, Islam S, Chow CK, Rangarajan S, Dagenais G, Diaz R et al (2011) Use of secondary prevention drugs for cardiovascular disease in the community in high-income, middle-income, and low-income countries (the PURE Study): a prospective epidemiological survey. Lancet 378 (9798):1231–1243

Carcinogenic Alkaloids Present in Areca Nut 77

How Do They Compare to Tobacco

Nisha Thakur and Ravi Mehrotra

Contents

Introduction 1639
Prevalence of Areca Nut Addiction 1639
Alkaloids of Areca Nut 1640
Tobacco Alkaloids 1641
Health Effects of Areca Nut Alkaloids on Experimental Animals 1642
Carcinogenicity of Areca Nut Alkaloid (Arecoline) on Humans 1643
Areca Nut Dependence 1644
Areca Alkaloids Versus Tobacco Alkaloids 1644
Impact of Age (Young Versus Old) 1645
Impact of Occupation/Socioeconomic Background 1646
Impact on the Societal Fabric 1647
Impact on Divorce and the Family Unit 1647
Impact of Educational Status and Age of Initiation on Addiction 1648
Impact on Medical Care/Effects on Physical Health 1648
Summary Points 1649
Effects on Mental Health 1649
Effects on the Immune System 1650
Prevention: Solving the Problem by Different Means 1650
Current Strategies and Policies 1651
Applications to Other Areas of Substance Use Disorders 1651
Applications to Other Areas of Public Health 1652

N. Thakur
Division of Non-communicable Diseases (NCD), ICMR-National Institute of Research in Tribal Health (NIRTH), Department of Health Research (DHR), Ministry of Health and Family Welfare (Govt. of India), Jabalpur, Madhya Pradesh, India
e-mail: nisha.thakur@gov.in

R. Mehrotra (✉)
Department of Epidemiology, Rollins School of Public Health, Emory University, Atlanta, GA, USA

School of Health Sciences, University of York, York, UK

Centre for Health Innovation and Policy (CHIP) Foundation, Noida, Uttar Pradesh, India
e-mail: ravi.mehrotra@gov.in; ravi.kumar.mehrotra@emory.edu

V. B. Patel, V. R. Preedy (eds.), *Handbook of Substance Misuse and Addictions*,
https://doi.org/10.1007/978-3-030-92392-1_84

Mini-Dictionary of Terms 1652
Key Facts 1652
Summary Points 1653
References 1653

Abstract

Areca nut (AN) and tobacco are widely consumed across the world by ~600 million and 1.3 billion people due to their addictive properties, respectively. Globally, AN is the fourth most common psychoactive substance after caffeine, nicotine, and alcohol. It is not only a psychostimulant and addictive substance, but also a potential carcinogen as per World Health Organization (WHO)-International Agency for Research on Cancer (IARC). There are four major alkaloids present in the areca nut, namely arecoline, arecaidine, guvacine, and guvacoline. Arecoline is the major alkaloid and comparable to the main tobacco alkaloid nicotine due to its analogous addictive effect on the human brain. Chemically, both the alkaloids are tertiary amines and are responsible for the addictive nature of the substance. However, unlike, areca alkaloid arecoline, primary tobacco alkaloid nicotine is not considered a carcinogen.

Prolonged use of AN/tobacco and its products including pan masala, gutkha, and scented supari are responsible for various diseases including oral potentially malignant disorders, oral submucous fibrosis, oral cancer, hypertension, diabetes and cardiovascular disease, etc. Contrary to tobacco control measures, stringent policies are either lacking or not implemented properly against the production, trade and use of AN around the world, especially in the Southeast Asian region, where its use is the most prevalent. Considering the potentially carcinogenic nature of AN alkaloids, well-framed policies to curb the use of AN in favor of public health are urgently warranted.

Keywords

Areca nut · Supari · Betel quid · Chewing · Pan masala · Gutkha · Carcinogenic · Alkaloids · Tobacco · Arecoline · Nicotine

Abbreviations

AN	Areca nut
BQ	Betel quid
IARC	International Agency for Research on Cancer
MAO	Monoamine oxidase
MNPA	N-(methylnitrosamino) propionaldehyde
MNPN	3-(methylnitrosamino) propionitrile
NG	N-nitrosoguvacoline
NGC	N-nitrosoguvacine
NGL	N-nitrosoguvacoline
OPMD	Oral potentially malignant disorder
OSMF	Oral submucous fibrosis
SLT	Smokeless tobacco

Introduction

Areca nut (AN) is the fruit of Areca catechu and has been consumed for centuries mainly in the form of chewing and betel quid (BQ). The use of areca nut in South Asian countries can be traced back to 10,000 BCE (de la Monte et al. 2020). The International Agency for Research on Cancer (IARC) has classified areca nut as a Group I carcinogen. The carcinogenic potential is due to alkaloids present in the areca nut. There is ample scientific evidence available that betel quid causes esophageal and liver cancers (Secretan et al. 2009).

Prevalence of Areca Nut Addiction

According to a report around 600 million people use AN across the world (Gupta and Warnakulasuriya 2002). Prevalence of AN/BQ consumption is remarkably high in the Asia Pacific region including Bangladesh, Sri Lanka, India, Malaysia, Myanmar, Cambodia, Taiwan, Papua New Guinea, and among emigrants of these countries globally (Mehrtash et al. 2017; Gunjal et al. 2020) (Figs. 1 and 2). Epidemiological surveys show that 20–40% of the population in India, Nepal, and Pakistan has used betel quid, while the global average was reported as ~10%. India has the highest number of AN consumers in the world (Sharan et al. 2012). According to a recent report, almost one out of every four adults (~223.79 million) consumes AN in India. The pattern of AN consumption varies widely in different geographical regions of India. BQ with tobacco is primarily consumed in the Northeastern states, whereas betel quid without tobacco in the Southern states of India (Singh et al. 2021). A high prevalence of BQ chewing has been found among Palauans of the West Pacific and inhabitants of the Hunan province of China. In general, men were more likely to use AN in comparison to women. Significantly higher chewing rates were reported among men (10.7–43.6%) than women (1.8–34.9%) from Southeast Asian countries including Nepal, Sri Lanka, Taiwan, and Mainland China; however, higher rates were observed in (29.5–46.8%) Malaysian and Indonesian women than men (9.8–12.0%)

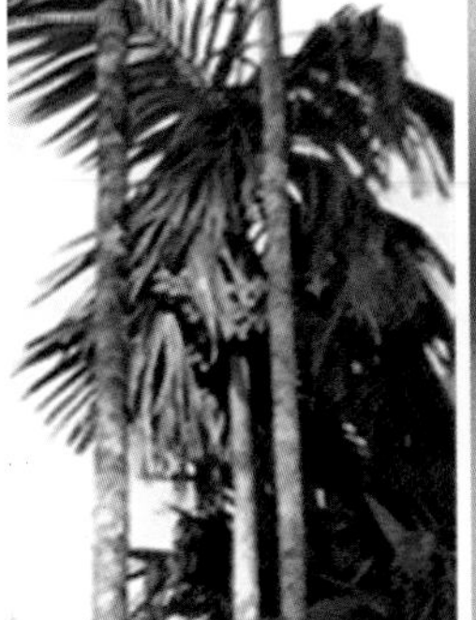

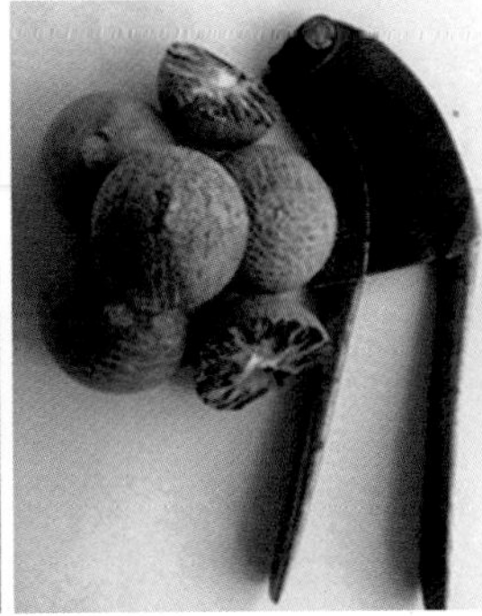

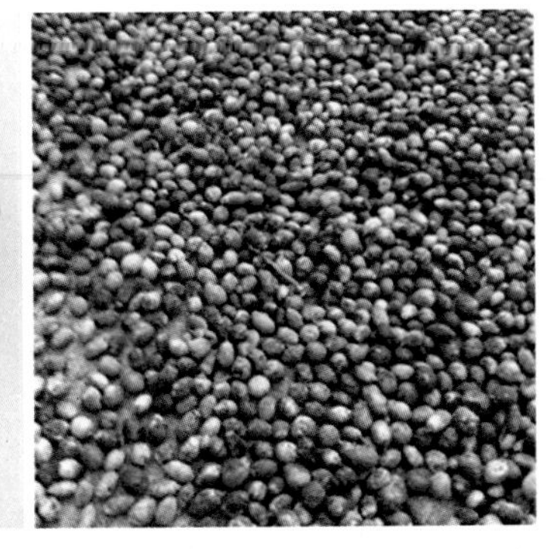

Fig. 1 Areca nut tree and dried areca nut with traditional Indian areca nut cutter (Photo by Ravi Mehrotra, Mihir Singh Rajput & Sudha Thakur)

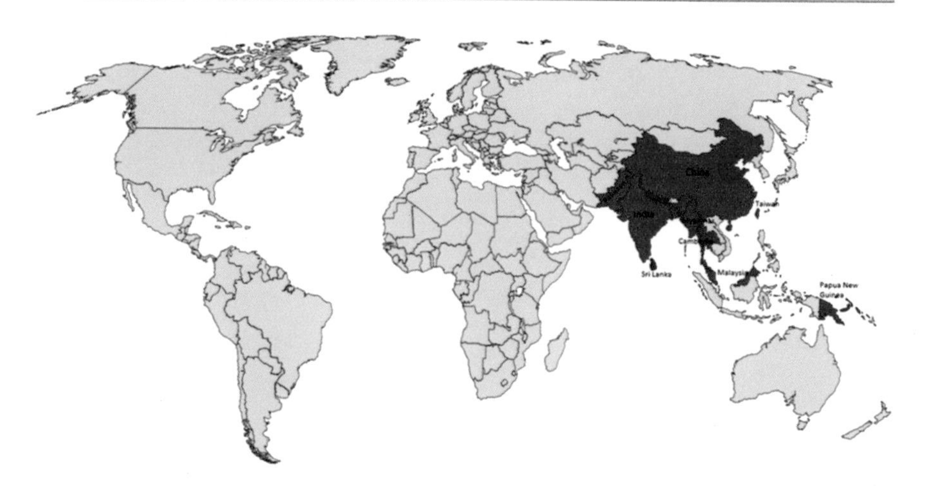

Fig. 2 World map showing the countries with high prevalence of areca nut consumption (highlighted with red color) (Map created by Nisha Thakur)

according to an intercountry Asian Betel-quid Consortium study (ABC study) (Lee et al. 2011). AN addiction has been studied in various populations, including Papua New Guinea, Taiwan, and the UK. Burton-Bradley (1978) and Talonu (1989) have reported addiction to AN in people from Papua New Guinea. A high frequency (17.3 portions/day) of AN consumption was also observed among Taiwanese aborigines (Yang et al. 2001).

Alkaloids of Areca Nut

Alkaloids are biochemically reduced pyridines and their amount varies according to the seasonal and geographical areas. AN alkaloids amount remains unaltered upon cold storage/freeze-drying. However, AN processing reduces the concentration of key areca alkaloid – arecoline – significantly by different methods. (Sharan et al. 2012). High-performance liquid chromatography (HPLC) has shown the presence of various chemical constituents including polysaccharides, protein, fat, crude fiber, polyphenols, alkaloids, and ash in areca nut, among these areca alkaloids are the biologically most important. Biochemical analysis revealed the presence of arecoline, arecaidine, guvacine, and guvacoline in AN (Fig. 3). Arecoline has been detected as the primary areca nut alkaloid. The alkaloid percent contents in fresh AN obtained from Australia were estimated as follows: arecoline (0.30–0.63), arecaidine (0.31–0.66), guvacine (0.03–0.06), and guvacoline (0.19–0.72) by HPLC. The maturity of the fruit and processing methods significantly affects the concentration of arecoline in commercially available nut (0–1.4%). The percentage of arecoline content based on the dry weight was in the slightly higher range in unprocessed ripe areca nut (0.12–0.24) than unripe nut (0.11–0.14) (IARC Monograph Vol. 85).

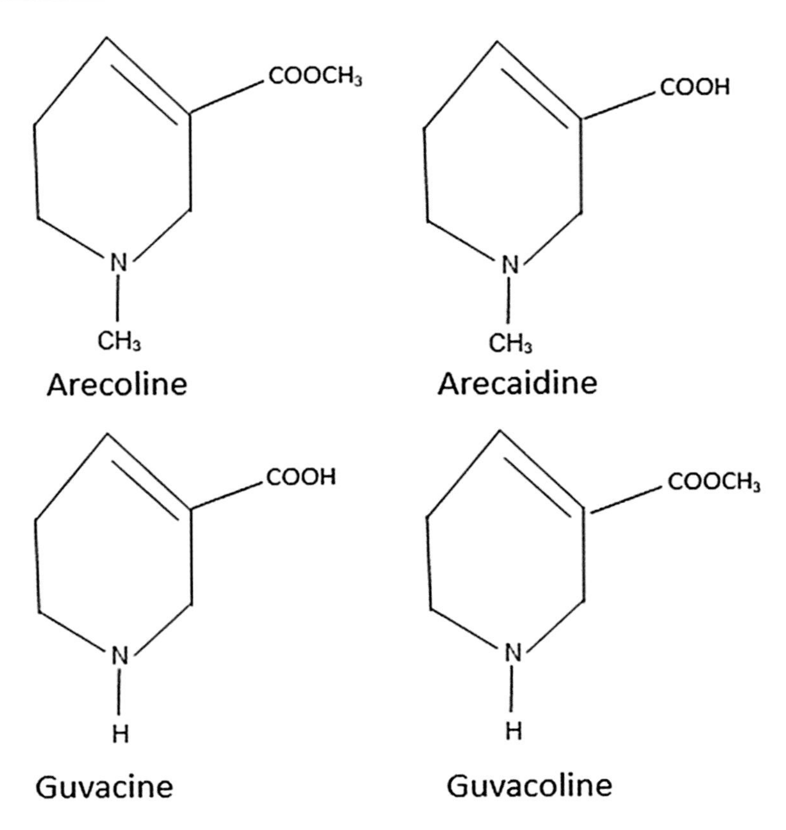

Fig. 3 Chemical structure of areca alkaloids: Arecoline, Arecaidine, Guvacine, and Guvacoline

Of the various constituents of areca nut, alkaloids are mainly responsible for addictive and carcinogenic properties (Volgin et al. 2019). Liquid chromatography-tandem mass spectrometry (LC-MS/MS) analysis demonstrated variation in alkaloids among processed areca nut worldwide (Jain et al. 2017). Variation in addictive and carcinogenic properties is due to the different levels of these alkaloids in areca nut products (Liu et al. 2016). Arecoline, which is a tertiary amine, accounts for the parasympathetic and muscarinic properties of the AN and, consequently, is linked with addictiveness and carcinogenicity of the substance (Lu et al. 2006).

Tobacco Alkaloids

Tobacco is generally mixed with BQ. Tobacco is obtained from the leaves of *Nicotiana rustica* and *Nicotiana tobacum* and is prepared from dried and partially fermented coarsely cut leaves without further processing. Occasionally, it is powdered and mixed with syrup and boiled before use. Tobacco is the most commonly used drug of abuse, currently, there are 1.3 billion tobacco users and 6 million annual

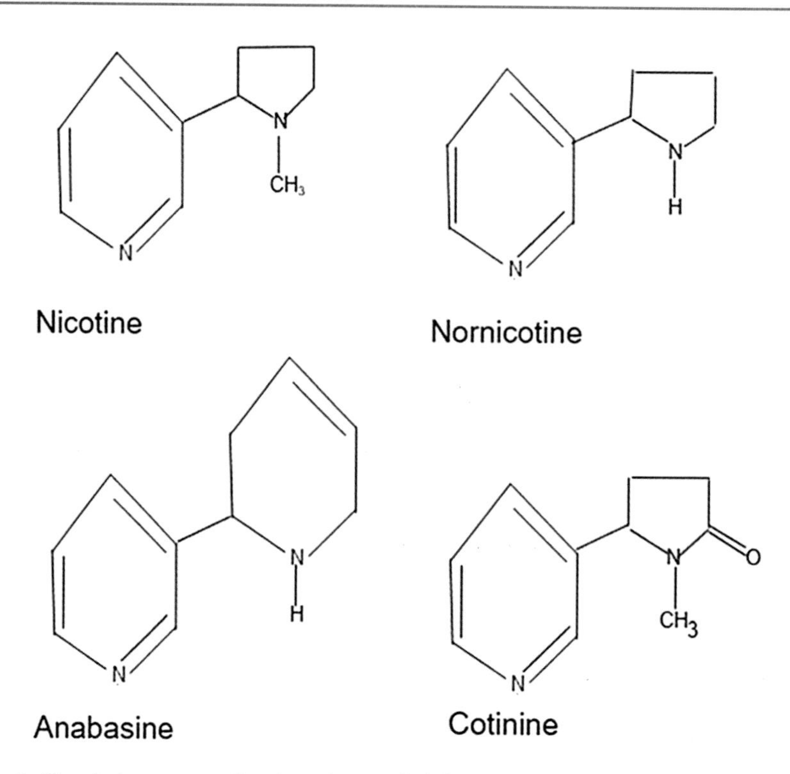

Fig. 4 Chemical structure of major tobacco alkaloids: Nicotine, nornicotine, anabasine, and cotinine

deaths worldwide (The GATS Atlas). According to the Global Adult Tobacco Survey (GATS) conducted in 2016–2017, in India, 42.4% of men, 14.2% of women, and 28.6% (266.8 million) of all adults presently use tobacco (smoked and/or smokeless tobacco) (GATS-2, Facts sheet, India). Nicotine is the principal alkaloid (96–98%) present in the tobacco leaf. While nornicotine, anabasine, anatabine, cotinine, and myosmine constitute the remaining 2–4% of the alkaloid content in tobacco (Fig. 4). These minor tobacco alkaloids exhibit resembling the structure of nicotine and show biologically relevant effects on the brain (Fig. 5). Besides this, nornicotine and cotinine are also involved in nicotine metabolism (Clemens et al. 2009).

Health Effects of Areca Nut Alkaloids on Experimental Animals

Nitrosation of arecoline is the key process in the formation of N-nitrosoguvacoline, 3-(methylnitrosamino) propionitrile (MNPN), 3-(methylnitrosamino) propionaldehyde, and two unidentified N-nitrosamines in model studies. MNPN has been demonstrated as a potent carcinogen, based on observations after subcutaneous injection (1.1 mmoles in 60 doses) in Fischer 344 rats. All 30 (15 M/F each) rats developed tumors within

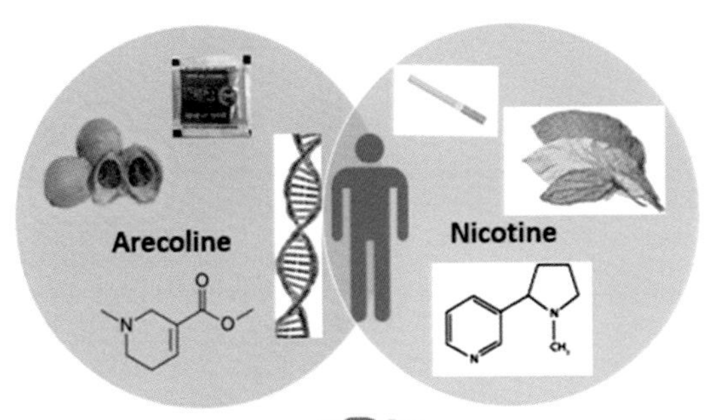

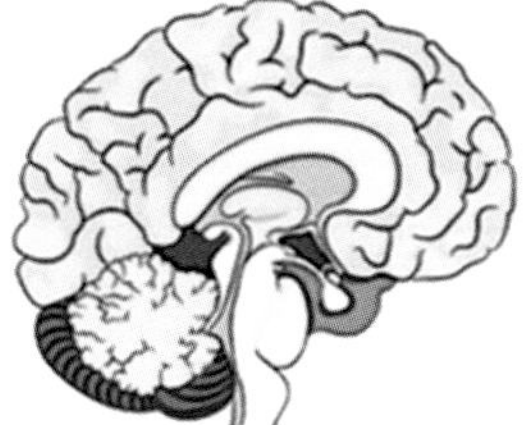

Fig. 5 Addiction mechanism exerted by areca and tobacco alkaloids in the human brain (Pictorial representation by Nisha Thakur)

24 weeks, several tumors (esophagus, nasal cavity, tongue, pharynx, forestomach) were noticed in 26 of them (Wenke et al. 1984). BQ chewing has shown a strong association with oral cancer development. NG is unlikely to be carcinogenic but MNPN is believed to be a strong carcinogen in experimental animals (Wenke and Hoffmann 1983).

Carcinogenicity of Areca Nut Alkaloid (Arecoline) on Humans

In 2004, the AN was classified as a class 1 carcinogen by International Agency for Research on Cancer (IARC). Recently, in 2020, IARC has evaluated the carcinogenicity of "arecoline" a major areca alkaloid and has classified it as "possibly carcinogenic to humans" (Group 2B) based on "strong" mechanistic evidence (IARC Monographs Vol 128 group; 2021). The exact mechanism of carcinogenesis by areca alkaloids is not fully understood so far. Several nitrosamines derivatives are produced in the presence of nitric oxide (Sharan and Choudhury 2010). Four key N-nitroso compounds including N-nitrosoguvacoline (NGL), N-nitrosoguvacine (NGC), N-(methylnitrosamino) propionitrile (MNPN), and N-(methylnitrosamino) propionaldehyde (MNPA) are formed by nitrosation of arecoline (IARC 2004). Various complex compounds, including arecoline N-oxide, arecaidine, arecaidine N-oxide, N-methyl nipecotic acid, N-methyl nipecotylglycine, arecaidinyl glycine, arecaidinyl glycerol, and arecaidine/arecoline/arecoline N-oxide mercapturic acid are formed as products of metabolism in the liver and kidney and were detected in mice urine (Giri et al. 2006). MNPN displayed carcinogenicity *in vitro* and also produces N-(methylnitrosamino) 3-hydroxypropionaldehyde, N-(methanoyl nitrosamino) propionaldehyde, and diazohydroxide derivatives (Garg et al. 2014; Franke et al. 2015). These derivatives were detected in the urine and saliva of areca nut chewers and were associated with carcinogenesis (Nair et al. 1985). According to Giri et al. (2007), arecoline and arecaidine are interconvertible. Arecoline is oxidized to arecoline 1-oxide in rat kidneys, which is further conjugated with glutathione and, ultimately, reduced to mercapturic acids (Boucher and Mannan 2002). AN is frequently consumed with an alkaline agent like slaked lime. Calcium hydroxide present in the slaked lime causes hydrolyzation of areca alkaloids; arecoline and guvacoline to arecaidine and guvacine, respectively. Subsequently, the changed salivary flow and pH make the oral mucosa prone to toxicity in AN chewers (Rooban et al. 2006).

Areca Nut Dependence

Areca nut dependency syndrome was described among the Gujarati community in the UK by Winstock et al. (2000). AN chewing causes relaxation, better concentration, mood upliftment, and satisfaction, while withdrawal symptoms include craving for AN, mood swings, anxiety, irritability disturbed sleep and concentration (Winstock et al. 2000). The mean severity dependence score was reported as 7.3 (range 1–12) which was comparable with the use of amphetamines. Tolerance to the AN effects developed in most of the users (IARC Monograph Vol 85). Areca-derived N-nitrosoguvacoline (NG) has been detected in the saliva (2.2–348 μg/L) of BQ chewers. However, the formation of MNPN has not been established during BQ chewing. Higher levels of NG were found in chewers who mixed tobacco with betel quid. In addition to this, tobacco-specific N-nitrosamines were also present in the saliva of such chewers (Wenke et al. 1984). The salivary presence of most of these derivatives has also been confirmed by other researchers in BQ chewers (Nair et al. 1985). Arecoline level is estimated at ~140 μg/ml at the time of AN chewing and remains at a high level even after 10 min post-chewing in the oral cavity (Venkatesh et al. 2018). Arecoline is one of the best-studied areca alkaloids. AN consumption causes euphoria, alertness, sweating, and salivation in the chewers and these feelings subsequently develop tolerance to areca nut products, which results in dependency syndrome (Mirza et al. 2011). A significant number of (5.6–13.6%) Southeastern men are likely to combine the habit of AN chewing with smoking and drinking (Lee et al. 2011). Betel quid chewing caused milk-alkali syndrome according to Wu et al. (1996) and Lin et al. (2002). This syndrome is reported in patients who chewed 40 betel quid/day and is often characterized by hypercalcemia, metabolic alkalosis, and renal failure. A significant number of patients (44.44%) with prolonged BQ chewing history (up to 35 years) also showed depletion in the level of vitamin B12 in comparison to non-chewers (Winstock et al. 2000).

Areca Alkaloids Versus Tobacco Alkaloids

Major comparisons (similarities and differences) between areca nut (arecoline) and tobacco (nicotine) alkaloids are summarized in Table 1. Some areca nut alkaloids have been reported to have similar effects on the brain as their tobacco counterparts.

Table 1 Comparison between areca nut (arecoline) and tobacco (nicotine) alkaloids

Alkaloids	Arecoline	Nicotine
Characteristics	**Similarities**	
Chemical structure is a tertiary amine	Yes	Yes
Responsible for addictive properties	Yes	Yes
Can cross the blood–brain barrier	Yes	Yes
Rapidly enters into the circulation	Yes	Yes
Effects on central nervous system: Causes feelings of well-being, relaxation, calmness, alertness, euphoria, suppression of pain, appetite, and anxiety	Yes	Yes
Mechanism of action by causing cellular injury, DNA damage, oxidative stress	Yes	Yes
Characteristics	**Differences**	
Elimination Half-life	0.97 h	2–3 h
Stimulation	Via nicotinic acetylcholine receptor (nAChR)	Via muscarinic acetylcholine receptor (mAChR) linked with the release of dopamines
Circulation and distribution	Rapidly enters into the circulation and distributes to various organs including liver and kidney	Absorbs across the epithelium of the lung, the oral mucosa, the nose, and through the skin
Metabolism	Arecoline gets metabolized in the liver mainly by GST enzymes	>80% of the nicotine gets metabolized in the liver by CYP2A6, UDP-glucuronosyltransferase, and monooxygenase

Two AN alkaloids are muscarine acetylcholine, receptor agonists. It has been established that the α4-nicotinic acetylcholine receptor (nAChR) is responsible for tobacco addiction and arecoline is a partial agonist for this receptor (Fig. 5). Hence, this activity of arecoline has the potential to develop new drugs for tobacco cessation, subjected to the identification of promising analogues having nicotinic receptor activity with no muscarinic activity. Iso-arecoline and ethenone are such types of selective partial agonists for α4* nAChR with minimum or undetectable muscarinic activity (Horenstein et al. 2019).

Impact of Age (Young Versus Old)

AN is consumed by all age groups by men, women, and children in South Asian countries. Many studies have been conducted on school children and found that AN, pan masala, and gutkha use generally starts at a younger age under the influence of family or friends (Leghari et al. 2016; Mirza et al. 2011). Various factors like easy accessibility, affordable price, attractive advertisements, and packaging of AN products like gutkha have been responsible for making youth, including children and teenagers addicted in India (Changrani and Gany 2005). In India, AN consumption was higher in men than women, furthermore, people of age group 31–50 years were more frequent users as compared with other age groups (Singh et al. 2021). It is evident from the literature that most of the AN users start the habit during their school years (Huang and Zachar 2020). According to Farrand et al. (2001), adolescents go through various behavior changes before areca nut chewing becomes a habit and the majority of them start the habit out of curiosity (Wang et al. 2003). It is further observed that many young students who initiate the habit become regular chewers by the time they leave the school (Farrand et al. 2001). Likewise, a highest risk of tobacco use is reported among those who initiate the habit at an early age (mean age 8–15 years) half of them become addicted later in their life. According to an Indian study around 70% of boys and 80% of girls ($\leq$15 years) initiate the tobacco use before 11 years of age (Kurupath and Sureka 2018).

Impact of Occupation/Socioeconomic Background

It has also been reported that lower educational and socioeconomic background is particularly associated with a higher risk of consuming AN and other products (gutkha, pan masala, meethi and scented supari, etc.) containing AN. People engaged in labrorious work, long-distance truck drivers, and women laborers are particularly likely to use smokeless tobacco products containing AN either to keep themselves alert or awake during long working shifts or to suppress their hunger (Government of India 2020). Similarly, Javed et al. (2008 and 2010) in Pakistan reported that a significant percentage (8–24%) of adult chewers (between 45 and 64 Years) masticate gutkha to control hunger. According to a report from Sri Lanka, Selvananthan et al. (2018) showed that ~53% rural population – mainly drivers and laborers – use AN to control hunger and tiredness. Low level of school education accompanied by alcohol drinking and tobacco use were identified as factors associated with BQ chewing (Lee et al. 2011). Taiwan is home to >3 million areca nut consumers and this habit is more common in blue-collar workers and less-educated people; however, this trend is shifting toward younger and highly educated people (Huang and Zachar 2020). A cross-sectional survey conducted on secondary school students in Karachi, Pakistan showed that co-education, use of areca nut by parents and peers, lack of awareness on harmful health effects, and easy availability of AN products near schools are the main factors for higher risk of SLT and or areca nut use among adolescents (Hussain et al. 2017). Another study performed on school-aged (4–16 years) children belonging to the fishing community in Baba Island, Karachi showed that 74% of primary school children used areca nut daily in different forms and 95% of them used it in the sweetened form, while 35% of children used betel quid regularly (Table 2) (Shah et al. 2002).

Table 2 Self-reported consumption/prevalence of areca nut use among young/school students

Sl. No.	Category	Percentage	Country	References
1	Adolescent students	10	Taiwan	Wang et al. (2003)
2	Secondary school students	40	Micronesia	Abraham et al. (2018)
3	Secondary school students	40	Pakistan	Hussain et al. (2017)
4	South Asian adolescent	80	Britain	Farrand et al. (2001)
5	School-aged (4–16 years) children	74	Pakistan	Shah et al. (2002)

A cross-sectional study was conducted on 1460 Indian school children >6 years of age to study the prevalence of tobacco use and its relationship with socioeconomic status for a period of 16 months. A significantly higher prevalence of tobacco use was observed in children from the lower socioeconomic background (9.4%) as compared to middle socioeconomic status (5.7%). Additionally, it was also noted that children belonging to the lower socioeconomic status initiated using tobacco at an earlier age than the children with middle socioeconomic background (Kurupath and Sureka 2018). Sreedharan et al. noticed that children of a smoker parent have a higher risk of smoking (Sreedharan et al. 2010).

Impact on the Societal Fabric

The majority of the studies on social factors affecting AN addiction were carried out in Pakistan. Societal pressure plays an important role in the initiation of areca nut use, especially among children. It is evident from the literature that a significant proportion of children (47%) tasted the nut for the first time on the behest of their close relatives (Shah et al. 2002); however, this study may not represent the true population of the country as the sample was taken from a poor fishing community. Similarly, they studied the primary school students in rural Sindh as a part of a World Bank-funded School Nutrition Program (1995) and found that 59% of these children used areca nut on daily basis. Another survey conducted in Karachi in 1981 showed that the prevalence of areca nut consumption among adults was 33% (Shah et al. 2002). The GATS 2016–17 demonstrated the highest percentage (30.2%) of AN consumption among daily laborers in India. Additionally, a high proportion of scheduled tribes (25.6%) and Muslim populations (30.8%) were found to consume AN (Singh et al. 2021).

Impact on Divorce and the Family Unit

Areca nut consumption was observed to increase in children in case of a failed marriage of their parents, lower social background, and parent's AN chewing history (Volgin et al. 2019). In India, nearly 27.1% of widowed, separated, and/or divorced people were reported to consume areca nut in any form (Singh et al. 2021).

The presence of children in the home was found to be associated with lower likelihood of smoking compared to the presence of other family members in China and Japan. Moreover, the presence of younger kids (<2 years) played a highly significant role in reducing the chances of smoking by adults (Lin et al. 2020).

Impact of Educational Status and Age of Initiation on Addiction

Children of less-educated fathers are three-fold more likely to start AN chewing in comparison to the children of more educated fathers (Shah et al. 2002). Similarly, children of literate mothers are less likely to start the chewing habit as compared to children of illiterate mothers. Hence, the educational status of parents plays an important role in AN use in their children (Shah et al. 2002), it is probably due to a higher level of awareness about the harmful effects of the substance. Persons with below the primary level education consumed a higher amount of AN (Singh et al. 2021). The first use of tobacco also starts among adolescents and it is further observed that early age of initiation of the substance abuse is usually associated with higher consumption during later years in life and less likely to quit the addiction. In a study on school children, it was reported that two-thirds of students who start smoking in the 6th grade become regular adult smokers; however, ~46% of the students who start smoking in 11th grade become regular adult smokers. According to the US Department of Health and Human Services report, approximately 90% of the tobacco-dependent adults started smoking at the age of <18 years (Siqueira et al. 2017). Comparable findings were reported with respect to prevalence of areca nut use in a survey carried out among 1500 school students from 1st to 8th grade (mean age 11.8 years) in Gujarat, India, which showed that most of the students started the habit at the age of <14 years and the frequency was higher for boys (33.3%) than girls (22.2%) (Clemens et al. 2009).

Impact on Medical Care/Effects on Physical Health

The four major areca alkaloids arecoline, guvacine, arecaidine, and guvacoline exert harmful effects on human health. Hydrolysed derivatives (guvacine and arecaidine) of guvalcoline and arecoline can stimulate the autonomic and central nervous systems, obstruct the uptake of gamma-aminobutyric acid (GABA) and, subsequently, affect the parasympathetic nervous system. These derivatives affect the release of catecholamines, specifically dopamine, which is a neurotransmitter and responsible for euphoric effects on the brain via the GABA pathway (Lin et al. 2018). Arecoline, a well-established psychoactive areca alkaloid, was found to show an impact on cardiovascular, parasympathetic nervous systems and is also known to induce salivation and sweating. Arecoline is capable of crossing the blood–brain barrier which results in significantly elevated acetylcholine levels in the animal brain (Asthana et al. 1996; Shannon et al. 1994). Due to this property of arecoline, it is similarly addictive to tobacco and alcohol (Chen et al. 2017).

Arecoline can penetrate the brain and, thereby, exert many effects on the central nervous system (Chu 2002). It also acts on nicotinic acetylcholine receptors (nAChR), hence is responsible for addiction (Papke et al. 2015). AN chewing was found to be associated with the impairment of blood sugar levels, blood pressure, and obesity by researchers. Frequent consumption of AN stains the teeth, gums, and mucosa. It is also responsible for abrasion and wearing of the teeth as well as the exposed root surface. Anti-ovulatory and abortion-causing properties of areca nut have also been reported and are associated with lower birth weight and length among newborns. It can also result in cancers of the esophagus, lung, liver, stomach, and cervix (Mehrotra and Yadav 2018). The literature demonstrates that AN nut is a cause of oral submucous fibrosis (OSMF), a potentially malignant lesion, which may progress to oral cancer (Wang et al. 2003). Likewise, prolonged tobacco exposure causes the development of cancer in various organs particularly in the liver, lungs, and pancreas (Clemens et al. 2009). Higher levels of C-reactive protein, which is a marker of inflammation, were estimated in AN chewers with tobacco than areca chewers. The severity of periodontal disease was worse among gutkha consumers than BQ chewer without tobacco.

Summary Points

- Areca nut and tobacco alkaloids including arecoline and tobacco-specific nitrosamines are capable of causing cell injury, DNA damage, oxidative stress, and possibly act synergistically.
- It has been observed that BQ/AN is frequently consumed with tobacco and insufficient research data is available regarding the adverse health effects of the either substance alone.

Effects on Mental Health

Additionally, AN chewing is also responsible for enhanced adrenaline and noradrenaline levels in plasma (Chu 1995). Two of the areca nut alkaloids were reported to inhibit GABA uptake (Johnston et al. 1975; Lodge et al. 1977). Besides stimulant effects, AN is also responsible for relaxation through its anxiolytic effects. These effects are similar to other misused substances and are in line with anecdotal reports claimed by users in support of desirable effects. Areca alkaloids were reported to increase cerebral arousal as well as relaxation by causing higher occipital α and generalized β activity on electroencephalograms (EEG) and reducing θ activity (Joseph and Sitaram 1990; Chu 1994), respectively. Temporary escalation in heart rate due to peripheral stimulation has been noticed by Frewer (1990) after consumption of betel quid. Various researchers observed that people with mental health disorders are more likely to smoke tobacco (Stewart et al. 2020).

Effects on the Immune System

Insufficient data is available on the impact of tobacco on the human immune system. However, nicotine has been found to influence both humoral and cell-mediated immune responses by several researchers (Johnson et al. 1990; Geng et al. 1995, 1996; Kalra et al. 2000). This response is accompanied by reduced inflammation, antibody response, and T-cell-receptor-mediated signaling suggesting that nicotine is a strong immunological agent with respect to T-cell function (Sopori and Kozak 1998).

Similar to tobacco use, areca nut chewing also showed adverse effects on the immune system, as it is found to be associated with elevated high-sensitivity C-reactive protein (hs-CRP), tumor necrosis factor-alpha (TNF-α), leptin, and WBC count thereby (Lin et al. 2018).

Prevention: Solving the Problem by Different Means

Advertisements (paper/television/online modes), promotions (e.g. celebrity endorsement), and sponsorships (e.g. sports events) by the companies manufacturing AN products like Gutkha, pan masala, and scented/meethi supari should be regulated in order to prevent access by minors and those most vulnerable. Additionally, prioritizing research on the topics like the prevalence of spitting in public places and availability of areca products near schools/educational institutions and workplaces to discourage initiation of this addiction and to achieve the goal of the Swacch Bharat Mission launched by the Government of India in its true sense (Mehrotra and Yadav 2018). Increasing the awareness about the harmful effects of AN and products containing it as the main constituent, hiking taxation, involvement of self-help groups/non-governmental organizations/local community, strong pictorial warnings, helpline numbers to quit/cessation programs and not selling in loose/small packets, and ban on sell to minors/children would be helpful to curb this one of the most common addictions. Harmful effects caused by areca nut should be displayed through visual illustration on AN products. All kinds of media promotion including print, movies, music, and other types of media promotion of areca nut products should be strictly banned. The Ministry of Health should play an important role in formulating new policies to control the production, trade, and consumption of areca nut (Goyal and Bhagawati 2016). Recenly, during the COVID-19 pandemic it was noticed that tobacco use/nicotine exposure is a major risk factor for the viral infection, disease severity, and cardiopulmonary vulnerability. Therefore, this pandemic should be considered as an opportunity to encourage the use of well-established cessation methods such as toll-free Quitlines and text messaging through mobiles to quit tobacco/areca nut use in combination with COVID-19 related health programs in order to achieve the much awaited goal of tobacco free world (Gupta et al. 2021).

Current Strategies and Policies

India, despite being the largest producer and consumer of AN, lacks a defined guideline on the use of areca nut. However, it comes under regulations when used as an ingredient in various smokeless tobacco products under the Cigarettes and Other Tobacco Products (COTPA or Prohibition of Advertisement and Regulation of Trade and Commerce, Production, Supply and Distribution) Act, 2003. The government of India also introduced the Food Safety and Standards (Licensing and Registration of Food Businesses) Regulation, 2011, which bans tobacco and nicotine use as an ingredient in food items food including areca nut. In view of the adverse health effects and numerous users, there is an urgent need to formulate guidelines for the production and use of AN and products having AN as an ingredient (Mehrotra and Yadav 2018; Thakur et al. 2020; Gupta et al. 2020; Gunjal et al. 2020).

Conversely, areca nut is widely sold in the market without controlling regulations in Pakistan (Shah et al. 2002). Similarly, no global policy is in place to regulate the use of areca nut like the WHO-Framework Convention on Tobacco Control (FCTC) to restrict tobacco use. Apart from this, interdisciplinary research is warranted to address this fourth most common addiction problem and translate the findings in formulating future policies and guidelines to control AN use globally. A comprehensive understanding of the biology, mechanisms, and epidemiology of areca nut use would help design upcoming cessation programs for AN users and design screening programs for cancers associated with AN use (Mehrtash et al. 2017). Gunjal et al. (2020) noticed a wide variation in the prevalence and interventional policies with respect to BQ and AN use in south, Southeast Asian, and some Western Pacific countries and emphasized the need for improved interventional strategies. Furthermore, it was observed that only 38.5% (5/13) countries specifically Bhutan, Taiwan, Myanmar, Papua New Guinea, and Sri Lanka have BQ policies/interventions in place. The use of tobacco products has been banned at public places in Nepal. Indian railways and many states have enforced the ban on spitting. Similarly, UK, Singapore, and Australia have also been imposed the ban on spitting. Regulations on printing warnings on packages are in place in Taiwan and India (Gunjal et al. 2020).

Applications to Other Areas of Substance Use Disorders

Smokers were found to be eight times more prone to develop dependency syndrome as compared to areca nut users only. Interestingly, this likelihood is two times higher in the case of areca nut users who chew areca nut with tobacco additives (Mirza et al. 2011). The chemical derivatives of arecoline may increase cognitive effects such as drugs having selectivity for muscarinic M1-receptor. In addition to this, research is continuing on arecoline-like compounds for the treatment of other addictions including nicotine, alcohol, and cocaine, owing to their promising secondary cholinergic, GABAergic, and/or neurotransmitter actions (Volgin et al. 2019).

Applications to Other Areas of Public Health

In this review, we have discussed the various aspects of areca nut addiction. Arecoline (areca nut alkaloid) has comparable psycho-addictive effects as nicotine (tobacco alkaloid) on the human nervous system due to the resemblance of their receptors. Evidence-based literature confirms that people from the Asia-Pacific regions and few other diverse backgrounds are the top consumers of areca nut.

Areca nut is consumed in different forms such as raw, ripe, fermented, flavored, with or without tobacco and/or with betel leaves in Southeast Asian countries. Attractive packaging, affordable cost, wide media publicity, advertisement, celebrity endorsement, brand extension, peer pressure, social acceptability, status symbol, beliefs about beneficial health effects, lack of defined regulations/policies, and easy accessibility of areca nut products are the key factors responsible for its increasing rate of consumption among more vulnerable groups like children, adults, people with low socioeconomic and educational level. Due to various positive neural effects of arecoline, its applications can be extrapolated in neurology and psychiatry branches of medicine.

Mini-Dictionary of Terms

- Addiction. The condition of being addicted to a particular substance or activity.
- Abuse. Improper use of something/substance.
- Alkaloids. A class of nitrogenous organic compounds, obtained from plants having physiological effects on humans.
- Areca nut. It is a seed of the areca catechu that mainly grows in Southeast and South Asia, the tropical Pacific including Melanesia and Micronesia and parts of East Africa.
- Arecoline. A major and carcinogenic alkaloid of areca nut.
- Betel quid. Also known as paan in India, it is a mixture of betel leaf, slaked lime, crushed areca nut, spices, and other ingredients. It may be used with or without tobacco.
- Carcinogenesis. The process of transformation of normal, healthy cells into cancerous cells.
- Nicotine. Primary tobacco alkaloid.
- Nornicotine. Minor areca alkaloid affects the brain and induces locomotor activities.
- Misuse. Wrong or improper use of something.
- Tobacco. It is the general term used for any product prepared from leaves of any plant that belongs to Solanaceae.

Key Facts

- Areca nut (AN) is widely consumed across the world by ~10% of the population due to its addictive properties.

- Globally, AN is the fourth most common psychoactive substance after caffeine, nicotine, and alcohol. It is not only a psychostimulant and addictive substance but also a potential carcinogen.
- There are four major alkaloids present in the areca nut, namely arecoline, arecaidine, guvacine, and guvacoline.
- Arecoline is the major alkaloid and comparable to nicotine (tobacco) due to its analogous addictive effect on the human brain.
- Prolonged use of AN and its products including pan masala, gutka, scented supari are responsible for various diseases like hypertension, diabetes, cardiovascular, OPMD, OSMF, and oral cancer.
- Stringent policies are either lacking or not implemented properly against the production, trade and use of AN around the world especially in the Southeast Asia region where its use is the most prevalent.
- Considering the potential carcinogenic nature of AN alkaloids, well-framed policies to curb the use of AN in favor of public health are urgently warranted.

Summary Points

- Areca nut addiction is one of the top four common addictions globally, however a neglected area of research.
- Areca nut has been classified as a potential carcinogen (Group 1) by IARC in 2004. Later, the areca alkaloid – arecoline – has been classified as a possible carcinogen to humans (Group 2B) based on the sufficient experimental data by the working group of IARC Monograph Volume 128 in 2020.
- Arecoline is the key areca nut alkaloid with potential carcinogenic properties; however, the tobacco alkaloid – nicotine is not carcinogenic.
- The addictive nature of areca nut (arecoline) is comparable to tobacco (nicotine) on the basis of its effects on the central nervous system. However, arecoline and nicotine alkaloids stimulate the brain via different acetylcholine receptors: mAChR and nAChR, respectively.
- Areca nut use in most Asian countries has an inverse relationship with education and income.
- Unlike tobacco, for areca nut neither well defined, effective policies are in place nor implemented effectively especially in Southeast Asian countries where substance abuse/misuse is maximum.
- An international policy on areca nut production and consumption is urgently required in order to reduce the growing burden of areca nut associated diseases.

References

Abraham D, Cash HL, Durand AM, Denholm J, Moadsiri A, Gopalani SV, Johnson E (2018) High Prevalence of Non-Communicable Disease Risk Factors among Adolescents in Pohnpei, Micronesia. Hawaii J Med Public Health 77(11):283–288. PMID: 30416871; PMCID: PMC6218683

Asthana S, Greig NH, Holloway HW et al (1996) Clinical pharmacokinetics of arecoline in subjects with Alzheimer's disease. Clin Pharmacol Ther 60:276–282
Boucher BJ, Mannan N (2002) Metabolic effects of the consumption of Areca catechu. Addict Biol 7:103–110
Burton-Bradley BG (1978) Betel chewing in retrospect. Papua New Guinea Med J 21:236–241
Changrani J, Gany F (2005) Paan and Gutka in the United States: an emerging threat. J Imm Health 7. https://doi.org/10.1007/s10903-005-2643-7
Chen PH, Mahmood Q, Mariottini GL et al (2017) Adverse health effects of betel quid and the risk of oral and pharyngeal cancers. Biomed Res Int 2017:3904098. https://doi.org/10.1155/2017/3904098. Epub 2017 Dec 11. PMID: 29376073; PMCID: PMC5742426
Chu NS (1994) Effects of betel chewing on electroencephalographic activity: spectral analysis and topographic mapping. J Formos Med Assoc 93:167–169
Chu NS (1995) Sympathetic response to betel chewing. J Psychoactive Drugs 27:183–186
Chu NS (2002) Neurological aspects of areca and betel chewing. Addict Biol 7:111–114. https://doi.org/10.1080/13556210120091473
Clemens KJ, Caillé S, Stinus L et al (2009) The addition of five minor tobacco alkaloids increases nicotine-induced hyperactivity, sensitization and intravenous self-administration in rats. Int J Neuropsychopharmacol 12:1355–1366. https://doi.org/10.1017/S1461145709000273
de la Monte SM, Moriel N, Lin A et al (2020) Betel quid health risks of insulin resistance diseases in poor young South Asian native and immigrant populations. Int J Environ Res Public Health 17 (18):6690. https://doi.org/10.3390/ijerph17186690. PMID: 32937888; PMCID: PMC7558723)
Farrand P, Rowe RM, Johnston A (2001) Prevalence, age of onset and demographic relationships of different areca nut habits amongst children in Tower Hamlets, London. Br Dent J 190(3):150–154. https://doi.org/10.1038/sj.bdj.4800909
Franke AA, Mendez AJ, Lai JF et al (2015) Composition of betel specific chemicals in saliva during betel chewing for the identification of biomarkers. Food Chem Toxicol 80:241–246. https://doi.org/10.1016/j.fct.2015.03.012
Frewer LJ (1990) The effect of betel nut on human performance. Papua New Guinea Med J 33: 143–145
Garg A, Chaturvedi P, Gupta PC (2014) A review of the systemic adverse effects of areca nut or betel nut. Indian J Med Paediatr Oncol 35(1):3–9. https://doi.org/10.4103/0971-5851.133702. PMID: 25006276; PMCID: PMC4080659
Geng Y, Savage SM, Johnson LJ et al (1995) Effects of nicotine on immune response: I. Chronic exposure to nicotine impairs antigen receptor-mediated signal transduction in lymphocytes. Toxicol Appl Pharmacol 135:268–278
Geng Y, Savage SM, Razani-Boroujerdi S et al (1996) Effects of nicotine on the immune response: II. Chronic nicotine treatment induces T cell anergy. J Immunol 156:2384–2390
Giri S, Idle JR, Chen C et al (2006) A metabolomic approach to the metabolism of the areca nut alkaloids arecoline and arecaidine in the mouse. Chem Res Toxicol 19:818–827. https://doi.org/10.1021/tx0600402
Giri S, Krausz KW, Idle JR et al (2007) The metabolomics of (±)-arecoline 1-oxide in the mouse and its formation by human flavin-containing monooxygenases. Biochem Pharmacol 73:561–573. https://doi.org/10.1016/j.bcp.2006.10.017
Global Adult Tobacco Survey (GATS) (2016–2017) (GATS-2 Facts sheet, India)
Government of India (2020) Smokeless Tobacco (SLT) and Public Health in India, Executive summary. World Health Organization & Ministry of Health and Family Welfare, Government of India. http://origin.searo.who.int/india/tobacco/smokeless_tobacco_and_public_health_in_india.pdf
Goyal G, Bhagawati BT (2016) Knowledge, attitude and practice of chewing gutka, areca nut, snuff and tobacco smoking among the young population in the Northern India population. Asian Pac J Cancer Prev 17(11):4813–4818. https://doi.org/10.22034/APJCP.2016.17.11.4813. PMID: 28030904; PMCID: PMC5454679

Gunjal S, Pateel DGS, Yang YH et al (2020) An overview on betel quid and areca nut practice and control in selected Asian and South East Asian countries. Subst Use Misuse 55(9):1533–1544. https://doi.org/10.1080/10826084.2019.1657149

Gupta AK, Nethan ST, Mehrotra R (2021) Tobacco use as a well-recognized cause of severe COVID-19 manifestations. Respir Med 176:106233. https://doi.org/10.1016/j.rmed.2020.106233

Gupta AK, Tulsyan S, Thakur N et al (2020) Chemistry, metabolism and pharmacology of carcinogenic alkaloids present in areca nut and factors affecting their concentration. Regul Toxicol Pharmacol 110:104548. https://doi.org/10.1016/j.yrtph.2019.104548. Epub 2019 Dec 2

Gupta PC, Warnakulasuriya S (2002) Global epidemiology of areca nut usage. Addict Biol 7(1):77–83. https://doi.org/10.1080/13556210020091437

Horenstein NA, Quadri M, Stokes C et al (2019) Cracking the betel nut: cholinergic activity of areca alkaloids and related compounds. Nicotine Tob Res 21(6):805–812. https://doi.org/10.1093/ntr/ntx187. PMID: 29059390; PMCID: PMC6528145

Huang B, Zachar JJ (2020) Social and behavioural determinants of areca nut consumption in adolescents. Oral Dis 26(8):1820–1826. https://doi.org/10.1111/odi.13467. Epub 2020 Jun 24

Hussain A, Zaheer S, Shafique K (2017) Individual, social and environmental determinants of smokeless tobacco and betel quid use amongst adolescents of Karachi: a school-based cross-sectional survey. BMC Public Health 17:913. https://doi.org/10.1186/s12889-017-4916-1

IARC Monographs Vol 128 group (2021) Carcinogenicity of acrolein, crotonaldehyde, and arecoline. Lancet Oncol 22(1):19–20. https://doi.org/10.1016/S1470-2045(20)30727-0. Epub 2020 Nov 26

IARC Working Group on the Evaluation of Carcinogenic Risks to Humans. Betel-quid and Areca-nut Chewing and Some Areca-nut-derived Nitrosamines. Lyon (FR): International Agency for Research on Cancer (2004) (IARC Monographs on the Evaluation of Carcinogenic Risks to Humans, No. 85). Accessed from https://www.ncbi.nlm.nih.gov/books/NBK316567/

Jain V, Garg A, Parascandola M et al (2017) Analysis of alkaloids in areca nut-containing products by liquid chromatography-tandem mass spectrometry. J Agric Food Chem 65(9):1977–1983. https://doi.org/10.1021/acs.jafc.6b05140

Javed F, Altamash M, Klinge B et al (2008) Periodontal conditions and oral symptoms in gutka-chewers with and without type 2 diabetes. Acta Odontol Scand 66(5):268–273. https://doi.org/10.1080/00016350802286725

Javed F, Chotai M, Mehmood A et al (2010) Oral mucosal disorders associated with habitual gutka usage: a review. Oral Surg Oral Med Oral Pathol Oral Radiol Endod 109(6):857–864., ISSN 1079-2104. https://doi.org/10.1016/j.tripleo.2009.12.038

Johnson JD, Houchens DP, Kluwe WM et al (1990) Effects of mainstream and environmental tobacco smoke on the immune system in animals and humans, a review. Crit Rev Toxicol 20: 369–395

Johnston GAR, Krogsgaard-Larsen P, Stephanson A (1975) Betel nut constituents as inhibitors of γ-aminobutyric acid uptake. Nature 258:627–628

Joseph KC, Sitaram N (1990) Topographical sleep EEG response to arecoline. Psychiatry Res 35: 91–94

Kalra R, Singh SP, Savage SM et al (2000) Effects of cigarette smoke on immune response: chronic exposure to cigarette smoke impairs antigen-mediated signalling in T cells and depletes IP3-sensitive Ca2+ stores. J Pharmacol Exp Ther 293:166–171

Kurupath A, Sureka P (2018) A Study on Tobacco Use Among School Children. Community Ment Health J 54(8):1253–1258. https://doi.org/10.1007/s10597-018-0241-0. Epub 2018 Feb 2. PMID: 29396797.

Lee CH, Ko AM, Warnakulasuriya S et al (2011) Intercountry prevalences and practices of betel-quid use in South, Southeast and Eastern Asia regions and associated oral preneoplastic disorders: an international collaborative study by Asian betel-quid consortium of South and East Asia. Int J Cancer 129(7):1741–1751. https://doi.org/10.1002/ijc.25809. Epub 2011 Mar 8

Leghari MA, Ali S, Maqbool S (2016) The prevalence of use of areca nut on its effect on oral health in school going children in Gadap town, Malir, Karachi, Pakistan. World J Dent 7(1):6–9

Lin TY, Chang HC, Hsu KH (2018) Areca nut chewing is associated with common mental disorders: a population-based study. Soc Psychiatry Psychiatr Epidemiol 53(4):393–401. https://doi.org/10.1007/s00127-017-1460-3

Lin S-H, Lin Y-F, Cheema-Dhadli S et al (2002) Hypercalcaemia and metabolic alkalosis with betel nut chewing: emphasis on its integrative pathophysiology. Nephrol Dial Transplant 17:708–714

Liu Y-JJ, Peng W, Hu M-BB et al (2016) The pharmacology, toxicology and potential applications of arecoline: a review. Pharm Biol 54:2753–2760. https://doi.org/10.3109/13880209.2016.1160251

Lodge D, Johnston GAR, Curtis DR et al (1977) Effects of areca nut constituents arecaidine and guvacine on the action of GABA in the cat central nervous system. Brain Res 136:513–522

Lu SY, Chang KW, Liu CJ et al (2006) Ripe areca nut extract induces G 1 phase arrests and senescence-associated phenotypes in normal human oral keratinocyte. Carcinogenesis 27:1273–1284. https://doi.org/10.1093/carcin/bgi357

Mehrotra R, Yadav A (2018) A Tough nut to crack; The Hindu, 10th March 2018. https://www.thehindu.com/sci-tech/health/a-tough-nut-to-crack/article23036520.ece

Mehrtash H, Duncan K, Parascandola M et al (2017) Defining a global research and policy agenda for betel quid and areca nut. Lancet Oncol 18(12):e767–e775. https://doi.org/10.1016/S1470-2045(17)30460-6

Mirza SS, Shafique K, Vart P et al (2011) Areca nut chewing and dependency syndrome: is the dependence comparable to smoking? A cross sectional study. Subst Abuse Treat Prev Policy 6:23

Nair J, Ohshima H, Friesen M et al (1985) Tobacco specific and betel nut-specific N-nitroso compounds: occurrence in saliva and urine of betel quid chewers and formation in vitro by nitrosation of betel quid. Carcinogenesis 6:295–303

Papke RL, Horenstein NA, Stokes C (2015) Nicotinic activity of arecoline, the psychoactive element of "betel nuts", suggests a basis for habitual use and anti-inflammatory activity. PLoS One 10:e0140907. https://doi.org/10.1371/journal.pone.0140907

Rooban T, Mishra G, Elizabeth J et al (2006) Effect of habitual arecanut chewing on resting whole mouth salivary flow rate and pH. Indian J Med Sci 60(3):95–105. https://doi.org/10.4103/0019-5359.22760

Secretan B, Straif K, Baan R et al (2009) WHO International Agency for Research on Cancer monograph working group. A review of human carcinogens – Part E: tobacco, areca nut, alcohol, coal smoke, and salted fish. Lancet Oncol 10(11):1033–1034. https://doi.org/10.1016/s1470-2045(09)70326-2

Selvananthan S, Sivaganesh S, Vairavanathan S (2018) Betel chewing among bus drivers in Jaffna district. Ceylon Med J 63(2):68–71. https://doi.org/10.4038/cmj.v63i2.8686

Shah SM, Merchant AT, Luby SP et al (2002) Addicted schoolchildren: prevalence and characteristics of areca nut chewers among primary school children in Karachi, Pakistan. J Paediatr Child Health 38(5):507–510. https://doi.org/10.1046/j.1440-1754.2002.00040.x

Shannon HE, Bymaster FP, Calligaro DO et al (1994) Xanomeline: a novel muscarinic receptor agonist with functional selectivity for M1 receptors. J Pharmacol Exp Ther 269:271–281

Sharan RN, Choudhury Y (2010) Betel nut and susceptibility to cancer. In: Environmental 752 factors, genes, and the development of human cancers. Springer, New York, pp 401–428. https://doi.org/10.1007/978-1-4419-6752-7_15

Sharan RN, Mehrotra R, Choudhury Y et al (2012) Association of betel nut with: revisit with a clinical perspective. PLoS One 7(8):e42759. https://doi.org/10.1371/journal.pone.0042759

Singh PK, Yadav A, Singh L et al (2021) Areca nut consumption with and without tobacco among the adult population: a nationally representative study from India. BMJ Open 11:e043987. https://doi.org/10.1136/bmjopen-2020-043987

Siqueira LM, AAP COMMITTEE ON SUBSTANCE USE AND PREVENTION (2017) Nicotine and tobacco as substances of abuse in children and adolescents. Pediatrics 139(1):e20163436

Sopori ML, Kozak W (1998) Immunomodulatory effects of cigarette smoke. J Neuroimmunol 83: 148–156
Sreedharan J, Muttappallymyalil J, Divakaran B (2010) Less demand for tobacco smokers in the marriage market. Tobacco and women. Indian J Cancer 47(Suppl 1):S87–S90. https://doi.org/10.4103/0019-509X.63866
Stewart SB, Bhatia D, Burns EK, Sakai JT, Martin LF, Levinson AH, Vaughn AM, Li Y, James KA (2020) Association of Marijuana, mental health, and tobacco in Colorado. J Addict Med 14(1): 48–55. https://doi.org/10.1097/ADM.0000000000000533
Talonu NT (1989) Observation on betel-nut use, habituation, addiction and carcinogenesis in Papua New Guineans. Papua New Guinea Med J 32:195–197
Thakur N, Sharma AK, Singh H et al (2020) ANDB: development of a database based on a global survey of literature on areca nut and associated health effects. Subst Use Misuse 55(9):1513–1518. https://doi.org/10.1080/10826084.2019.1644523. Epub 2019 Jul 26
The Global Adult Tobacco Survey (GATS) Atlas. Available at http://www.gatsatlas.org. Accessed 24 July 2021
Venkatesh D, Puranik RS, Vanaki SS et al (2018) Study of salivary arecoline in areca nut chewers. J Oral Maxillofac Pathol 22:446–471. https://doi.org/10.4103/jomfp.JOMFP_143_18
Volgin AD, Bashirzade A, Amstislavskaya TG et al (2019) DARK classics in chemical neuroscience: arecoline. ACS Chem Neurosci. https://doi.org/10.1021/acschemneuro.8b00711
Wang SC, Tsai CC, Huang ST et al (2003) Betel nut chewing and related factors in adolescent students in Taiwan. Public Health 117(5):339–345. https://doi.org/10.1016/S0033-3506(03)00082-9
Wenke G, Hoffmann D (1983) A study of betel quid carcinogenesis. 1. On the in vitro N-nitrosation of arecoline. Carcinogenesis 4(2):169–172. https://doi.org/10.1093/carcin/4.2.169
Wenke G, Rivenson A, Brunnemann KD et al (1984) A study of betel quid carcinogenesis. II. Formation of N-nitrosamines during betel quid chewing. IARC Sci Publ 57:859–866
Winstock AR, Trivedy CR, Warnakulasuriya KAAS et al (2000) A dependency syndrome related to areca nut use: some medical and psychological aspects among areca nut users in the Gujarat community in the UK. Addict Biol 5:173–179
Wu KD, Chuang RB, Wu FLL et al (1996) The milk-alkali syndrome caused by betelnuts in oyster shell paste. Clin Toxicol 34:741–745
Yang Y-H, Lee H-Y, Tung S et al (2001) Epidemiological survey of oral submucous fibrosis and leukoplakia in aborigines of Taiwan. J Oral Pathol Med 30:213–219
Lin H, Chang C, Liu Z, Tan H (2020) The effect of the presence of children on adult smoking behaviour: empirical evidence based on China family panel studies. BMC Public Health 20(1): 1448. https://doi.org/10.1186/s12889-020-09543-2. PMID: 32972391; PMCID: PMC7513303

Naturally Occurring Cathinone from Khat, Synthetic Cathinones, and Cytochrome P450

78

Sharoen Yu Ming Lim, Mustafa Ahmed Alshagga, Chin Eng Ong, and Yan Pan

Contents

Introduction 1661
Overview of Khat and Cathinone 1662
The Prevalence of Khat and Cathinone Use 1662
Cathinone Derivatives and Synthetic Cathinone 1663
Consumption and Pharmacokinetics of Khat and Cathinone 1665
Effects of Khat and Cathinone on Mental and Physical Health 1665
Cytochrome P450 (CYP) 1668
Metabolism of Khat and Cathinone Involving CYPs 1668
Inhibition of CYPs by Khat and Cathinones 1672
Impact on Children 1672
Impact on Self and Harm to Others 1674
Anti-cathinone Vaccines 1674
Applications to Other Areas of Addiction 1675
Applications to Public Health 1675
Mini-Dictionary of Terms 1676
Key Facts 1676
Summary Points 1677
References 1677

Abstract

Cathinone is the main euphorigenic compound found in khat plant. It is contro versial to claim that khat use is a form of addiction or abuse as it is social custom and pride for khat-belt countries. Khat and cathinone are often co-administered with medications leading to possible khat-drug and/or cathinone-drug interactions. Despite the belief that khat is effective in relieving tuberculosis and

S. Y. M. Lim · M. A. Alshagga · Y. Pan (✉)
Division of Biomedical Science, School of Pharmacy, University of Nottingham Malaysia, Semenyih, Malaysia

C. E. Ong
School of Pharmacy, International Medical University, Kuala Lumpur, Malaysia

V. B. Patel, V. R. Preedy (eds.), *Handbook of Substance Misuse and Addictions*,
https://doi.org/10.1007/978-3-030-92392-1_85

Parkinson illnesses, khat has negatively impacted the socioeconomic and educational attainment of children, while cathinone abuse is inclined to suicide and fatalities. Continuous modifications are in producing new synthetic cathinones for market demand and to circumvent the legislations, making it a continuous effort to elucidate the mechanism of actions of new cathinones. This chapter rules out prevalence of khat/cathinone abuse, the underlying mechanism of CYPs and synthetic cathinones, current legislation, and the discovery of high affinity anti-cathinone vaccines giving hope for the future to curb cathinone addiction.

Keywords

Addiction · Khat · Cathinone · Cathinone abuse · Cytochrome P450 · CYP · Synthetic cathinones · Bath salts · Legal highs · Metabolism · In vitro · In vivo

List of Abbreviations

α-PBP	Alpha-pyrrolidinobutyrophenone
α-PEP	Alpha-pyrrolidinoenanthophenone
α-PHP	Alpha-pyrrolidinohexanophenone
α-POP	Alpha-pyrrolidinooctanophenone
α-PPP	Alpha-pyrrolidinopropiophenone
α-PVP	Alpha-pyrrolidinopentiophenone
α-PVT	Alpha-pyrrolidinopentiothiophenone
CNS	Central nervous system
CYP	Cytochrome P450
DAT	Dopamine transporter
DDI	Drug-drug interaction
EMCDDA	European Monitoring Centre for Drugs and Drug Addiction
EPH	Ephedrine
IC_{50}	Half maximal inhibitory concentration
KEE	Khat ethanol extract
MAO	Monoamine oxidase
MBDM	3,4-Methylenedioxy-α-ethyl-N-methylphenethylamine
MDEA	3,4-Methylenedioxyethamphetamine
MDMA	3,4-Methylenedioxymethamphetamine
MDPBP	3,4-Methylenedioxy-α-pyrrolidinobutiophenone
MDPPP	3,4-Methylenedioxy-α-pyrrolidinopropiophenone
MDPV	3,4-Methylenedioxypyrovalerone
MEPH	Mephedrone
mg/kg	Milligram/kilogram
MOPPP	4-Methoxy-α-pyrrolidinopropiophenone
MPBP	4-Methyl-α-pyrrolidinobutiophenone
MPHP	4-Methyl-α-pyrrolidinohexiophenone
NADPH	Nicotinamide adenine dinucleotide phosphate
Naphyrone	1-Naphthalen-2-yl-2-pyrrolidin-1-ylpentan-1-one
NET	Norepinephrine transporter

ng/ml	Nanogram/milliliter
NIH	National Institute on Drug Abuse
NPS	Novel psychoactive substances
RH	Substrate hydrocarbon
ROH	Resulting hydroxylated product
SERT	Serotonin transporter
WHO	World Health Organization
3,4-DMMC	3,4-Dimethylmethcathinone
4-CMC	4-Chloromethcathinone
4-MEAP	4-Methyl-α-ethylaminopentiophenone
4-MEC	4-Methylethcathinone

Introduction

The leaves and young shoots of khat (*Catha edulis* Forsk) have been chewed by generations as social gathering snack besides attaining its psychostimulatory effects (Numan 2012). Cathinone and cathine are the major active ingredients of khat plant (Wolfes 1930). They are termed as "natural amphetamines," which are responsible for inducing stimulatory and euphorigenic effect besides warding off fatigue, exerting similar effects as amphetamine (Patel 2000). Khat chewing was mainly practiced in khat-belt countries, for instance, Ethiopia, Kenya, Somalia, and Yemen, due to the difficulty in preserving the cathinone content in fresh khat leaves during transportation. Nevertheless, with the advancement in air transportation, khat usage has been expanded worldwide nowadays (Numan 2012). Khat use considered as drug abuse is opposed by khat users such as the Yemenis because khat confirms identity of the society, social status, and a source of pride (Numan 2012). Over the years, synthetic cathinones are continuously made to evade laws and regulations (Ellefsen et al. 2016). The abuse of synthetic cathinones is extensive; however, continuous efforts are channeled into determining whether the mechanism of action of existing and emerging synthetic cathinones are similar (e.g., inhibitors of dopamine transporter (DAT) and norepinephrine transporter (NET) reuptake) or otherwise (Cheong et al. 2017).

Cytochrome P450 (CYP) is the major phase I drug-metabolizing enzyme responsible for drug-herb interactions. Our previous studies have found that khat ethanol extract (KEE) potentially inhibited major drug-metabolizing CYP isoforms (CYP2C9, CYP2D6, and CYP3A4), leading to delayed drug elimination as well as elevated plasma drug concentrations (Lim et al. 2019). Khat or cathinone users are usually on tuberculosis and Parkinson medications combined with some alcohol usage (Soboka et al. 2020; Caulfield 2015). By inhibition of CYP activities, these khat or cathinone users are at increased risk of developing adverse drug reactions due to higher drug concentrations (Lim et al. 2019). Moreover, synthetic cathinone was found to be metabolized by some major human drug-metabolizing enzymes, namely, CYP1A2, CYP2B6, CYP2C9, CYP2C19, CYP2D6, and CYP3A4 (Manier et al. 2018). Therefore, synthetic cathinone-drug interactions likely resulted from co-administration with clinical drugs.

This chapter offers insights of brief history and background of khat and cathinone including synthetic cathinones, methods of use, possible mechanism of action of cathinones, effects on physical and mental health, dose effects and pharmacokinetics, groups of synthetic cathinones and derivatives, up to the forms of cathinone sold. Furthermore, this chapter also offers an overview of CYP function and role in cathinone metabolism, besides encompassing in silico, in vitro, and in vivo studies of CYPs with khat, naturally occurring and/or synthetic cathinones. Finally, this chapter highlights the possible addiction and abuse of cathinones besides comparing male to female prevalence, existing law and regulations, impact on children's education attainment, impact on self and harm to others, emergence of anti-cathinone vaccines, application to other areas of addiction, and public health.

Overview of Khat and Cathinone

Khat or *Catha edulis* Forsk, classified under plant family called Celastraceae, is a green plant originated from Africa and Arabian Peninsula (Feng et al. 2017). In 1887, an alkaloid termed as "katin" was initially identified, followed by methcathinone in 1928, "cathine" in 1930, and "cathinone" in 1975 (Feng et al. 2017; Banks et al. 2014). The S-enantiomer cathinone is a naturally occurring β-ketone amphetamine analogue and main psychoactive constituent of khat (Wabe 2011; Banks et al. 2014). In khat, cathinone was reported to degrade easily into norpseudoephedrine and norephedrine within days of harvesting (Brenneisen et al. 1986). Cathinone was believed to be unstable and decomposed into dimer called 3,6-dimethyl-2,5-diphenylpyrazine, smaller fragments, and phenylpropanedione, after harvesting, drying, or extracting the plant material (Wabe 2011). As khat plant matured, S-(-)-cathinone was seen to be metabolized into cathine [1S, 2S-(+)-norpseudoephedrine or (+)-norpseudoephedrine] and 1R, 2S-(-)-norephedrine, which share similar structures to amphetamine and noradrenaline (Wabe 2011). Fresh khats are usually wrapped in banana leaves to preserve its psychoactive effects (Wabe 2011). On the other hand, a more recent study consisted of both qualitative and quantitative components demonstrated that dried khat leaves did not lead to the breakdown of cathinone (Nichols et al. 2015). The presence of cathinone was confirmed by presence of cathinone in 3-year-old dried khat leaves (Nichols et al. 2015).

The Prevalence of Khat and Cathinone Use

Naturally occurring or synthetic cathinones are dangerous drugs that may be susceptible to abuse (Schreck et al. 2020). The yearly reports of European Monitoring Centre for Drugs and Drug Addiction (EMCDDA) have recorded an increase of stimulant use, especially cathinones and phenylethylamines (Benedicte et al. 2020). According to the American Addiction Centers, cathinones reinforce binges as the onset and wearing off of effects of cathinones are both quick, thus leading cathinone users to crave, which poses a higher risk of overdose, abuse, and death (https://

americanaddictioncenters.org/synthetic-drugs/cathinone-abuse). It is plausible to take a closer look at khat, as it contains high amount of naturally occurring cathinone. Considering the chemical quantity of cathinones in khat, there is a high probability of induced cathinone use disorder (Schreck et al. 2020). Cathinone abuse was brought about by loss of control due to addiction and the continuation of cathinone use regardless of the negative consequences (Duresso et al. 2016).

The prevalence of khat use was 16.7% among Ethiopian students (Alemu et al. 2020). As of 2019, the pooled prevalence of khat use was 18.85% in Saudi Arabia, 13.04% in Yemen (Ayano et al. 2019), and 36.8% in Kenya (Ongeri et al. 2019). However, the study of khat use prevalence was mostly based on male university students. Another study revealed that the pooled prevalence of khat use in Saudi Arabia, Ethiopia, and Yemen was higher in men at 19.26% as compared in women at 6.41% (Ayano et al. 2019), while Kenya alone had 54.8% more male khat chewers (Ongeri et al. 2019). The lifetime prevalence of khat use was highest in Yemen with 43.27%, 37.32% in Saudi Arabia, and 24.82% in Ethiopia (Ayano et al. 2019). In Norway, prevalence of students' synthetic cathinone consumption varies from 1 to 20% (Bretteville-Jensen et al. 2013). The increase of khat chewing or addiction is highly exacerbated in male (Alemu et al. 2020). The lifetime and current prevalence of khat use among pregnant women were 11.0% and 9.9%, respectively. The odds of being a khat user among women was higher among those who had a khat user partner, consume alcohol, and had mental distress (Mekuriaw et al. 2020). Studies on Yemeni students reported that 42.0%, 50.8%, and 53.8% of students knew that khat effects were similar to amphetamines, khat was addictive, and cathinone was the dependence-producing constituent of khat leaves, respectively (Alshakka et al. 2020).

Synthetic cathinones are addictive (Watterson and Olive 2014); however, the number of users and misuse leading to addiction to these cathinones has not been fully reported. As of February 11, 2020, until date, the trends and statistics of synthetic cathinone use on National Institute on Drug Abuse (NIH) showed no data (https://www.drugabuse.gov/drug-topics/synthetic-cathinones-bath-salts/synthetic-cathinones-bath-salts-trends-statistics).

Cathinone Derivatives and Synthetic Cathinone

Cathinone derivatives vary in two different stereoisomeric forms and their potencies. Cathinone derivatives for instances can be rearranged into dihydropyrazine dimer known as isocathinones, N-alkylated such as hydrochloride salts or 4-methylephedrone, and pyrrolidine derivatives sharing similar structures to pyrovalerone. Most synthetic cathinones are analogues of amphetamine, methamphetamine, or 3,4-methylenedioxymethamphetamine (MDMA) (Banks et al. 2014). Synthetic cathinone is more potent as compared to amphetamine but less potent than methamphetamine. The chemical structure of cathinone is defined by characteristic β-keto group on the side chain of the corresponding phenethylamine and was the model for synthetic cathinone or bath salt

Table 1 Classification of synthetic cathinones

Cathinone class	Selected synthetic cathinones	Reference
Class 1: N-alkylated cathinone derivatives	Anorectics (diethylpropion, dimethylpropion), bupropion, (ephedrine) EPH, methcathinone, ethcathinone, mephedrone (MEPH), flephedrone, 4-methylethcathinone (4-MEC), 4-fluoromethcathinone, buphedrone, pentedrone, 3,4-dimethylmethcathinone (3,4-DMMC), methedrone	(Valente et al. 2014; Gonçalves et al. 2019; Patocka et al. 2020; Schifano et al. 2020)
Class 2: 3,4-methylenedioxy-N-alkylated cathinone derivatives	Methylone, ethylone, butylone, pentylone, 3,4-methylenedioxymethamphetamine (MDMA) or ecstasy, 3,4-methylenedioxyethamphetamine (MDEA), 3,4-methylenedioxy-α-ethyl-N-methylphenethylamine (MBDM)	
Class 3: N-pyrrolidine cathinone derivatives	α-pyrrolidinopentiophenone (α-PVP) or Flakka or zombie drug, pyrovalerone, 4-methyl-α-pyrrolidinobutiophenone (MPBP), 4-methyl-α-pyrrolidinohexiophenone (MPHP), 4-methoxy-α-pyrrolidinopropiophenone (MOPPP)	
Class 4: 3,4-methylenedioxy-N-pyrrolidine cathinone derivatives	3,4-methylenedioxy-α-pyrrolidinobutiophenone (MDPBP), 3,4-methylenedioxypyrovalerone (MDPV), 3,4-methylenedioxy-α-pyrrolidinopropiophenone (MDPPP)	
Second-generation cathinone derivative	Naphyrone (1-naphthalen-2-yl-2-pyrrolidin-1-ylpentan-1-one)	

manufacturing (Costantino et al. 2019). Illicit manufacturers adopt different packaging and distribution of "bath salts" to circumvent the federal act (Banks et al. 2014).

Synthetic cathinone or legal highs or bath salts could be classified into four families (see Table 1). The first class of synthetic cathinones are N-alkylated cathinones at R_1 or R_2 with ring substituents at R_3. The second class of synthetic cathinones have 3,4-methylenedioxy group added to the benzyl ring at R_3 or alkylation at R_1 and R_4. The third class of synthetic cathinones are closely similar to pyrrolidinophenone, with substitution of pyrrolidinyl at the nitrogen atom. The fourth class of synthetic cathinones result from the combination of 3,4-methylenedioxy ring substitution and N-pyrrolidinyl moiety. A second generation of synthetic cathinone called naphyrone contains naphthyl ring, existing in α- and β-isomers (Valente et al. 2014).

Synthetic cathinones are sold in the form of a white or yellowish amorphous or crystalline powder or capsules, weighing approximately 200 mg to 10 g per packet, costing $10 to $20 per gram. Synthetic cathinones can also be purchased in bulk with a discounted price (Valente et al. 2014). For instance, MEPH is commonly found in white or colored hydrochloride salt, sold in racemic mixture of stereoisomeric R and S forms with an unpleasant odor similar to mixture of chlorine, vanilla, and urine, whereas MDPV is commonly found in white light tan powder and emits an odor after exposed to air. Synthetic cathinones are sold in different trade names across the globe either online or smartshops including Explosion, Hagigat, Ivory Wave, Purple Wave, Cloud Nine, Bloom, Bliss, Vanilla Sky, Red Dove, and Blue Silk (Gonçalves et al. 2019).

Consumption and Pharmacokinetics of Khat and Cathinone

Naturally occurring cathinone in khat has been traditionally taken by chewing in khat-belt countries such as Yemen, practiced by both men and women from various social classes for its psychostimulatory effects (Sawair et al. 2007). Khat is usually chewed during khat parties that last for 2–10 h after lunch in special rooms (Sawair et al. 2007). Only leaves and shoots are chewed to release the psychoactive constituents including cathinone and cathine, while the juices are swallowed (Sawair et al. 2007). Synthetic cathinone is commonly taken by swallowing capsules and injection as they are water soluble, but due to lability, cathinones are not suitable for smoking (synthetic cathinone drug profile|www.emcdda.europa.eu). Additionally, "bombing" is a practice wherein powders are consumed through smoking (wrapped in cigarette), nasal insufflation, or snorting (e.g., mephedrone), known as "keying" in which a key is dipped in the powder and then insufflated (Schifano et al. 2011). Other methods of use reported include gingival, sublingual delivery, and rectal administration (faster onset at low dosage). Oral dosage is usually higher than snorting dosage ranging between 150 and 250 mg, while time of onset is 45 min to 2 h, varying based on amount of food contained in the stomach (Schifano et al. 2011). Users prefer to use cathinone on an empty stomach and exploit combination of insufflation and ingestion to achieve faster onset and lasting effects (Schifano et al. 2011).

The contents of naturally occurring cathinone vary in khat from different origins. For instance, the average contents of cathinone is 36–343 mg per 100 g of khat leaves (Wabe 2011). Extraction of khat compounds during khat chewing is primarily absorbed in the oral mucosa followed by the stomach and subsequently the small intestines (Toennes et al. 2003). Nearly 60% of cathinone are efficiently absorbed through the oral mucosa (Toennes et al. 2003). The peak plasma concentration during khat chewing is delayed of 127–138 min versus 72 min when administered as gelatin cathinone capsules (Toennes et al. 2003; Widler et al. 1994a; Brenneisen et al. 1990). Ingested cathinone undergoes first-pass liver metabolism to cathine (S,S (+)norpseudoephedrine) and (R,S(-)norephedrine) (Al-Obaid et al. 1998). The maximum plasma concentration of cathinone attained after ingestion of one dose was 58.9–127 ng/ml reached within 90–210 min per 0.8–1 mg/kg body weight (Toennes et al. 2003; Widler et al. 1994b; Halket et al. 1995).

Effects of Khat and Cathinone on Mental and Physical Health

Several earlier studies were carried out to elucidate the mechanisms of cathinone action on the central nervous system (CNS). It was found that cathinone stimulated release of radioactive label in isolated rabbit caudate nucleus prelabelled with

^{3}H-dopamine, while catecholamine release from rabbit heart tissue prelabelled with ^{3}H-noradrenaline was also observed (Kalix and Khan 1984). As compared to amphetamine, cathinone was, however, threefold less potent in stimulating the release of radioactive label and four times higher affinity to serotonin receptors (Glennon and Liebowitz 1982). Cathinone action is largely activated by serotonin pathways as compared to amphetamine (Babayan et al. 1983). Babayan et al. demonstrated that cathinone effects led to differentiation of visual stimuli in animals (e.g., cat) which are connected to serotonin and dopaminergic systems (Babayan et al. 1983). Cathinone increases dopamine release and reduced dopamine reuptake (Babayan et al. 1983). The activation of serotonin pathways intensifies cathinone effect, while activation of dopamine pathways dampens the cathinone effects (Babayan et al. 1983).

Today, it is believed that (-)-cathinone exerts its psychostimulatory action via central dopaminergic and serotonergic and peripheral noradrenergic storage sites (Pehek et al. 1990; Baumann et al. 2018; Capriola 2013). Cathinones share similar mechanism of action with cocaine and 3,4-methylenedioxymethamphetamine (MDMA) or ecstasy, which involves nonselective inhibition of monoamine reuptake and greater selectivity to dopamine transporter than serotonin transporter (Patel 2000; Kalix and Khan 1984). Furthermore, mechanism of action of amphetamine-like cathinones involves preferential reuptake inhibition of catecholamines and dopamine release, while pyrovalerone cathinones are potent and selective inhibitors of catecholamine reuptake do not release neurotransmitter (Majchrzak et al. 2018). Similarly, synthetic cathinones exert psychostimulatory effects by interacting with monoamine membrane transporters such as dopamine, noradrenaline, and serotonin transporters leading to synaptic concentration increase of these biogenic amines (Gonçalves et al. 2019). The action of cathinone at synaptic level that causes the accumulation of biogenic amines is described in Fig. 1.

Amphetamine-like psychostimulatory effects of cathinone are often observed in humans after khat consumption and are explained by the action of the major constituents, namely, cathinone and cathine, although there is debate on the possibility that cathinone is not the main ingredient exerting those effects. Two studies using human subjects supported the idea that cathinone was the main active constituent of khat and principally accountable for exerting amphetamine-like psychostimulatory effect (Brenneisen et al. 1990; Widler et al. 1994b). The potency of khat-related amphetamine-like effects in dried leaves decreased despite the content of cathine remained unchanged. And most khat users preferred fresh khat, suggesting that khat users were addicted to something contained in fresh khat leaves (Patel 2000). Cathinone is more lipophilic as compared to cathine, which favors its penetration into the CNS, advising that cathinone is the key to CNS stimulation, while peripheral effects are due to stimulation of cathinone and cathine (Patel 2000). The variations in the increase of extracellular dopamine, norepinephrine, and serotonin levels accountable for mood alteration, toxicity, and addiction are manipulated by different types of cathinone (Capriola 2013).

The physical effects of khat use were found mostly sympathomimetic including increased breathing, body temperature, blood pressure, heart rate, and mydriasis

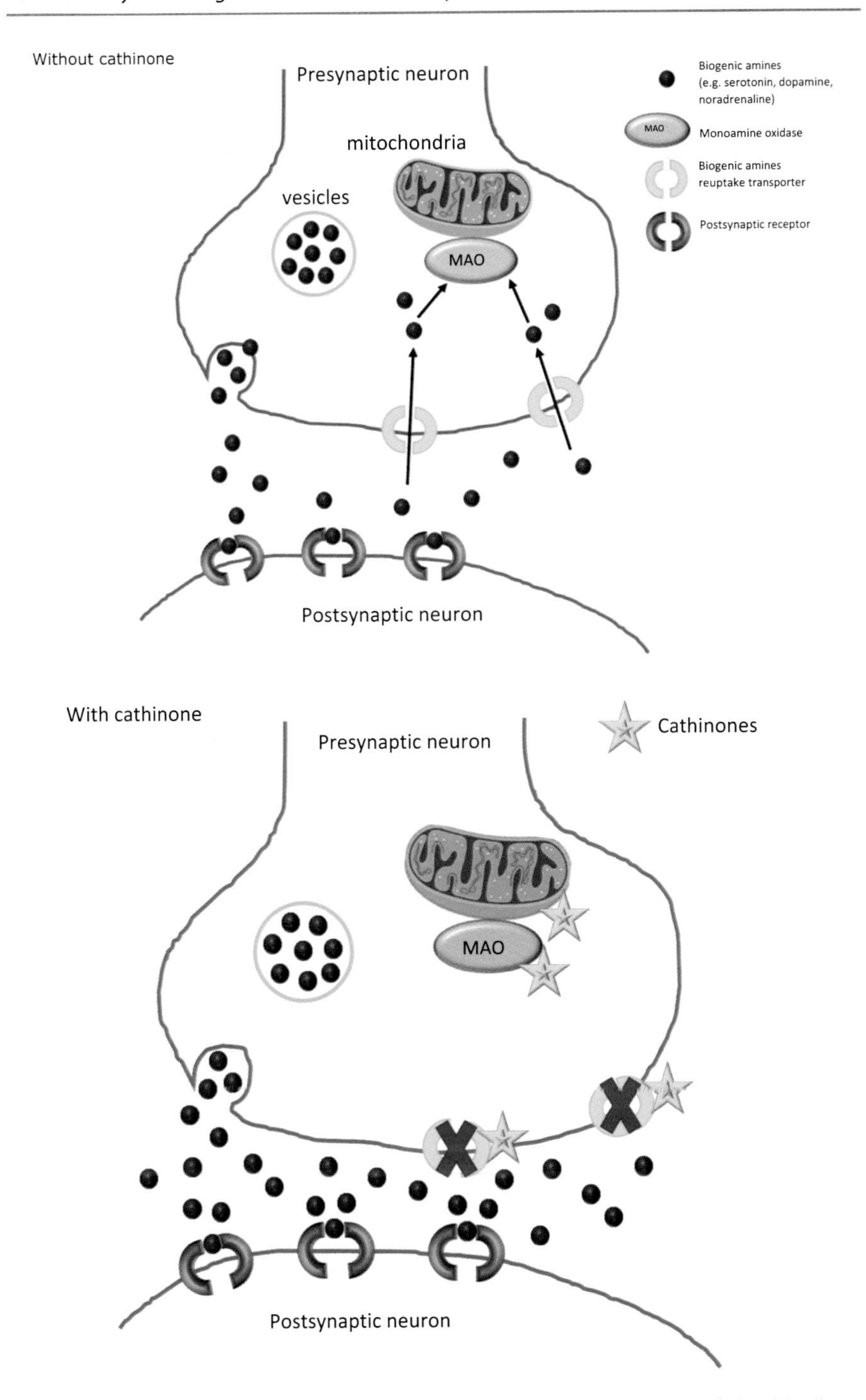

Fig. 1 Mechanism of action in the presence and absence of cathinones at synaptic level leading to an increase of biogenic amine synaptic concentrations

(Patel 2000). Besides, khat usage also has led to insomnia and anorexia, while high dosage of khat has resulted in hyperactivity and excessive talking, hyperthermia, sweating, rhabdomyolysis, tachycardia, hypertension, arrhythmia, cerebral edema, cardiorespiratory depression, myocardial infarction, coma, and even death (Benedicte et al. 2020; Patel 2000; Schifano et al. 2020). Khat intoxication caused several mental complications including anxiety, agitation, confusion, paranoia, hallucinations, psychosis, aggression, violence, manic-like behavior, schizophreniform psychosis or paranoia, psychopathological disturbances, and suicidal behavior (Schifano et al. 2020; Benedicte et al. 2020). Studies have shown that toxicities of cathinones were due to an excessive stimulation of dopaminergic and serotoninergic systems which in turn induced serotonin syndrome or multi-organ failure or both (Benedicte et al. 2020).

Cytochrome P450 (CYP)

CYP is a superfamily of cysteine thiolate-ligated heme monooxygenases which is responsible for oxidative biotransformation of endogenous and exogenous substances including drugs and lipophilic xenobiotics (Zanger and Schwab 2013). The inhibition and induction of CYPs are key mechanisms instigating pharmacokinetic drug-drug interactions (DDIs) (Hakkola et al. 2020). A simplified configuration of inhibition and induction of CYPs is shown in Fig. 2. CYPs can hydroxylize saturated carbon-hydrogen bonds, epoxidize double bonds, and oxidize heteroatoms and aromatics (Meunier et al. 2004). Briefly, upon binding of substrate to CYP enzyme, in the presence of oxygen, CYP inserts one oxygen atom into the substrate and the other one to a water molecule (Lim et al. 2020). Meanwhile, reduced nicotinamide adenine dinucleotide phosphate (NADPH) is used to provide two electrons through a CYP reductase protein and/or cytochrome b5 (Lim et al. 2020). CYPs' conformational adaptations readily offer metabolism of drug and xenobiotic, recognizing structurally diverse substrates (Poulos and Johnson 2005). In addition, substrates of CYPs usually have many oxidation sites, and this in turn reflects that CYPs could bind to more than one orientation, location, or motion of substrates within one active site cavity (Poulos and Johnson 2005).

Metabolism of Khat and Cathinone Involving CYPs

Natural and synthetic cathinones both undergo phase I and II metabolism with only traces of cathinones excreted in urine (Capriola 2013) (see Fig. 3). The phase I metabolism that cathinone undergoes is stereo-selective keto reduction by the liver enzymes to cathine and norephedrine; however, the catalyzing enzyme has yet to be clearly confirmed (Bedada et al. 2018). It was predicted that cathinone, amphetamine, and synthetic cathinones shared similar metabolic pathways involving major drug-metabolizing CYPs (Bedada et al. 2018).

As mentioned previously, cathinones underwent several phases of metabolism including reduction of ketone group to corresponding amino alcohol and is stereo-selective with S-(-)-cathinone metabolized into norephedrine while (+)cathinone into cathine (Gonçalves et al. 2019). Human CYP enzymes including CYP2B6, CYP2C19, CYP2D6, and CYP1A2 were found to be responsible for synthetic cathinone metabolism (Meyer et al. 2010, 2012). Hydroxylation of the propyl side chain of synthetic cathinone, α-PVP, was catalyzed by human CYP2B6, CYP2C19, CYP2D6, and CYP3A4 isoforms (Sauer et al. 2009). Recently, it was reported that synthetic cathinones were mainly metabolized by CYP2D6 (Contrucci et al. 2020). Hence, clinically significant pharmacokinetic interactions could be expected when MDPV or methylone were co-administered with compounds metabolized by CYP2D6 (Contrucci et al. 2020). For instance, high doses of ritonavir interacted with synthetic cathinones as both were metabolized by CYP2D6 (Contrucci et al. 2020). An in vitro study explored the human metabolism of alpha-cathinone-derived drugs, namely, 5 pyrrolidinophenone-derived NPS alpha-pyrrolidinobutyrophenone (α-PBP), alpha-pyrrolidinopentiothiophenone (α-PVT), alpha-pyrrolidinohexanophenone (α-PHP),

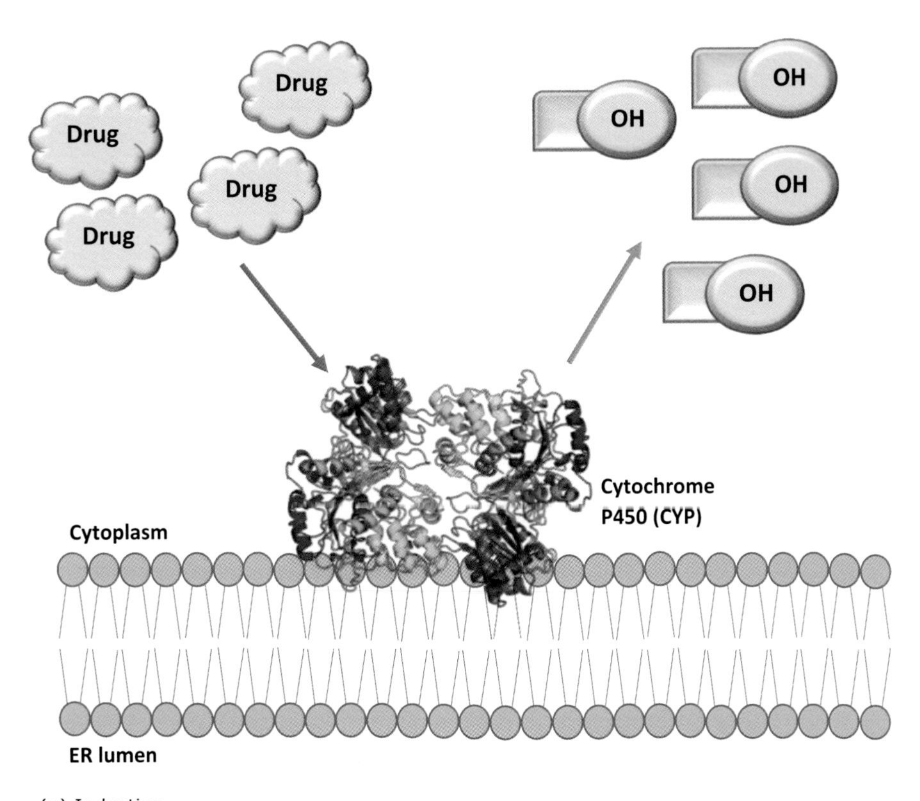

(a) Induction

Fig. 2 (continued)

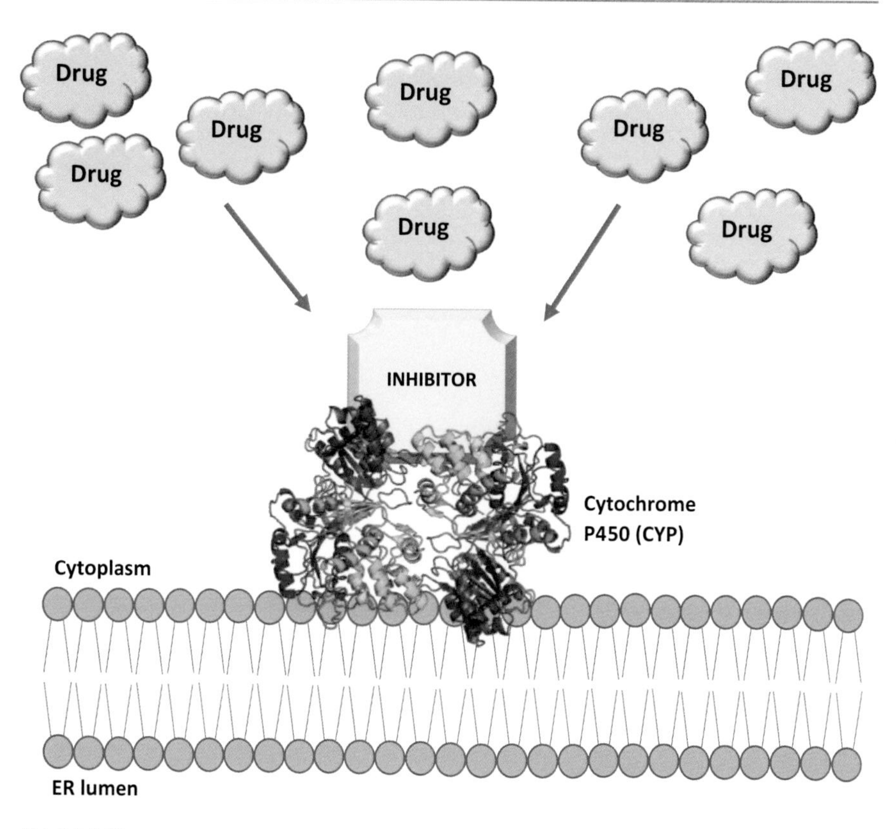

Fig. 2 Overview of inhibition and induction of CYPs. (**a**) During CYP induction, drugs are metabolized by CYPs into oxidized metabolites. (**b**) During CYP inhibition, the inhibitor binding to the CYPs prevented the metabolism process; hence, no metabolites are being produced

alpha-pyrrolidinoenanthophenone (α-PEP, PV8) and alpha-pyrrolidinooctanophenone (α-POP, PV9) (Manier et al. 2018). The initial metabolic steps of these compounds are catalyzed by CYP 1A2, CYP2B6, CYP2C9, CYP2C19, CYP2D6, and CYP3A4 resulting in pyrrolidine, thiophene, or alkyl hydroxy metabolites based on alkyl chain length (Manier et al. 2018). The CYP enzymes increase its affinity with the increase of alkyl chain length. CYP2C19 and CYP2D6 are responsible for metabolizing α-PBP, while CYP1A2, CYP2C9, and CYP2C19 are accountable for metabolizing α-PVT, α-PHP, α-PEP, and α-POP (Manier et al. 2018).

To date, in silico studies of naturally occurring cathinone (from khat) as well as synthetic cathinones with CYPs seemed to be at its infancy stage. Due to the continuous emergence of synthetic cathinones to circumvent laws, there is a need to study metabolic profiles of these drugs to identify their metabolism and adverse effects with regard to abuse. In silico prediction of 4-methoxy-α-PVP using CYP450 liver model found 4-hydroxy-α-PVP as the main metabolite, suggesting that

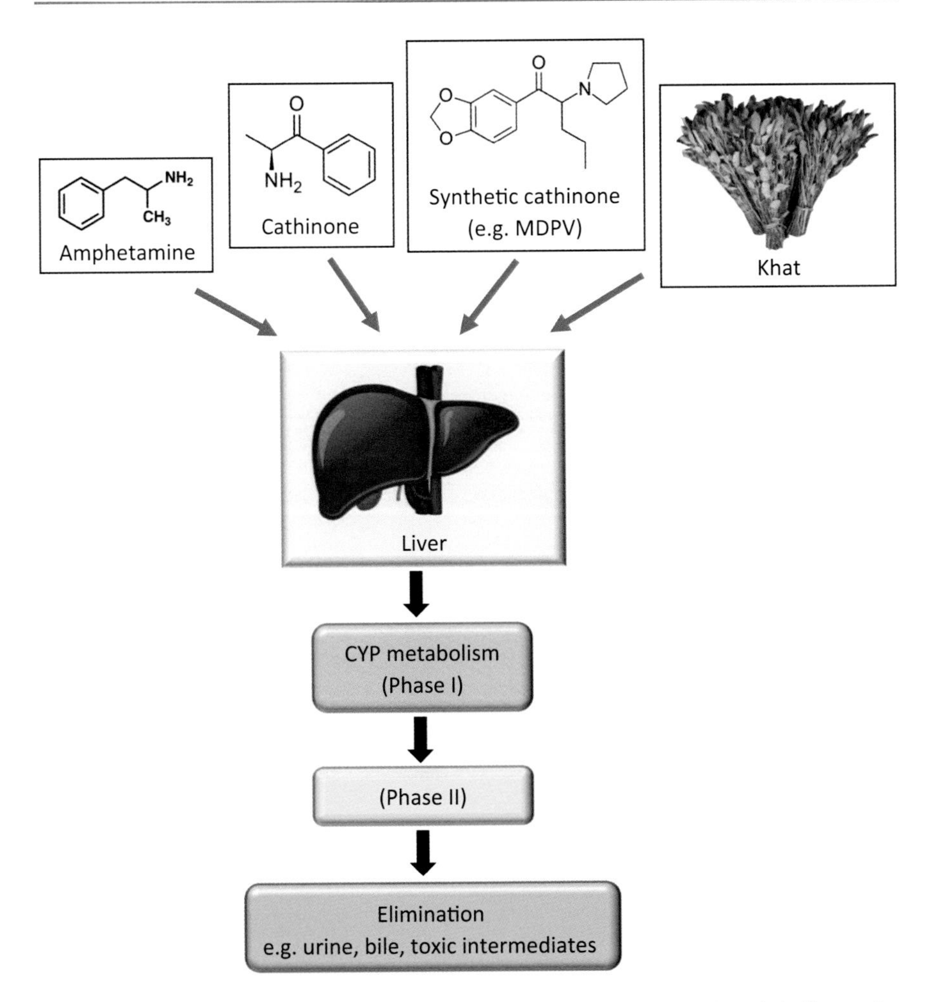

Fig. 3 Amphetamine, khat, cathinone, and synthetic cathinones possibly shared similar mechanism of CYP phase I and phase II metabolism

4-hydroxy-α-PVP is the conducive analytical target in addition to 4-methoxy-α-PVP (parent drug) (Ellefsen et al. 2016). The potential metabolites were analyzed based on 100% probability score, representing the likelihood to be generated (Ellefsen et al. 2016). From the 4-hydroxy-α-PVP generated, second-generation metabolites were subsequently predicted including aromatic hydroxylated metabolite at position C5', metabolite generated from ring opening, and oxidation (Ellefsen et al. 2016). A similar in silico study focuses on docking α-PVP to CYP450 liver model providing sites of metabolism predictions in CYP2C9, CYP2D6, and CYP3A4 (Swortwood et al. 2016). In silico results were compared to in vitro result, but the researchers concluded that MetaSite CYP450 liver model was unsuitable for α-PVP metabolism prediction because only four out of nine predicted metabolites attained probability score more than 20% (Swortwood et al. 2016). Further analytical targets are recommended to focus on α-PVT hydroxythiophenyl, α-PVT dihydroxypyrrolidinyl, α-PVT thiophenol, and α-PVT 2-ketopyrrolidinyl besides the parent drug, α-PVT (Swortwood et al. 2016).

Inhibition of CYPs by Khat and Cathinones

In general, the study of inhibition of CYPs by khat and cathinone is rather limited. An in vitro fluorescence-based study demonstrated that KEE significantly inhibited CYP2C9, CYP2D6, and CYP3A4 (Lim et al. 2019). However, this study showed that cathinone had negligible inhibitory effects on CYP2C9, CYP2D6, and CYP3A4 (Lim et al. 2019). This suggested that other ingredients in khat extract contributed to the inhibition of the three CYPs (Lim et al. 2019). Bedada et al. carried out an in vivo study using 63 male volunteers to determine drug-metabolizing enzyme activities before and after khat abstinence (Bedada et al. 2018). This study found that CYP2D6 was significantly inhibited, CYP3A4 was marginally inhibited, while CYP2C19 and CYP1A2 were genotype-dependently inhibited by khat (Bedada et al. 2018). Based on the CYP2D6 genotype-phenotype correlation with cathinone/phenylpropanolamine ratio, cathinone was implicated as a probable CYP2D6 substrate and inhibitor besides highlighting the potential role of CYP2D6 in cathinone metabolism, and cathinone competitively inhibited CYP2D6 isozyme (Bedada et al. 2018). Additionally, our ongoing study revealed that KEE reversibly inhibited CYP2A6, CYP2B6, CYP2C8, CYP2C19, CYP2E1, CYP2J2, and CYP3A5 but not CYP1A2 (Lim et al. 2021).

Table 2 summarizes naturally occurring and synthetic cathinones metabolized by different CYPs and inhibitory effects on CYPs as reported in in silico, in vitro, and in vivo studies.

Impact on Children

In Yemen, a khat-belt country, children are negatively affected by khat. Khat's grave effects are seen in child khat users including fragile bones and pale skin besides means of schooling that are not provided because family income is spent on khat (Nadia 2012). Families particularly in rural areas tend to ask their children to work in khat farms (Nadia 2012). Children got into the khat chewing habit by watching their elderly and which then progresses to khat addiction (Nadia 2012). Khat consumption paves way to multitude of illiterate generations and risking children's health. From 2010 to 2013, 1328 cumulative cases of pediatric synthetic cathinone exposures in children less than 20 years old were reported and documented by the American Association of Poison Control Centers database (Tekulve et al. 2014). Synthetic cathinone exposures among males are higher as compared to females, with a majority median age between 16.9 and 17.1 years of age (Tekulve et al. 2014). These children experience single or multiple seizures after synthetic cathinone exposure (Tekulve et al. 2014).

Table 2 In silico, in vitro, and in vivo studies of naturally occurring and synthetic cathinones

Type of cathinone	Name	CYP isoform	Type of study	Inhibitory parameters[a]	References
Synthetic cathinone	α-PBP	CYP2B6, CYP2C19 and CYP2D6	In vitro	K_m = 561, 32, 88 μmol/L, and V_{max} = 8E-05, 5.1e-04 PAR/pmol/min respectively	(Manier et al. 2018)
	α-PVT	CYP1A2, CYP2C9, CYP2C19, CYP2D6		K_m = 199, 210, 23, 8 μmol/L, and V_{max} = 2.8e-04, 6.1e-04, 4.2e-04, 9e-05 PAR/pmol/min respectively	
	α-PHP	CYP1A2, CYP2B6, CYP2C9, CYP2C19, CYP3A4		K_m = 50, 65, 1563, 34, 288 μmol/L, and V_{max} = 3.5e-04, 1.2e-04, 3.4e-04, 1e-04, 4e-05 PAR/pmol/min respectively	
	α-PEP	CYP1A2, CYP2B6, CYP2C9, CYP2C19, CYP2D6, CYP3A4		K_m = 49, 36, 88, 43, 63, 122 μmol/L, and V_{max} = 6.8e-04, 2.4e-04, 3.1e-04, 3.3e-04, 5e-05, 2.6e-04 PAR/pmol/min respectively	
	α-POP	CYP1A2, CYP2B6, CYP2C8, CYP2C9, CYP2C19, CYP2D6, CYP3A4		K_m = 28, 17, 681, 8, 8, 3, 66 μmol/L, and V_{max} = 1.21e-03, 1.6e-04, 2.53e-03, 4.3e-04, 6.8e-04, 1.7e-04, 2.8e-04 PAR/pmol/min respectively	
Natural occurring cathinone	Cathinone	CYP2C9, CYP2D6, CYP3A4	In vitro	IC_{50} = negligible	(Lim et al. 2019)
Khat	Khat plant	CYP2D6, CYP3A4 CYP2C19 and CYP1A2	In vivo – human study	Comparing metabolic ratios (MR) before and after khat use using caffeine/paraxanthine (CYP1A2), losartan/losartan carboxylic acid (CYP2C9), omeprazole/5-hydroxyomeprazole (CYP2C19), dextromethorphan/dextrorphan (CYP2D6) and dextromethorphan/3-methoxymorphinan (CYP3A4)	(Bedada et al. 2018)
Synthetic cathinone	4-methoxy-α-PVP	CYP450 liver model	In silico	100% probability score	(Ellefsen et al. 2016)
Synthetic cathinone	α-PVP	CYP450 liver model - predictions in CYP2C9, CYP2D6 and CYP3A4	In silico	CYP450 liver model was unsuitable for α-PVP metabolism prediction – only 4/9 predicted metabolites has probability score > 20%	(Swortwood et al. 2016)

[a]K_m = Michaelis constant, IC_{50} = half maximal inhibitory concentration, MR = metabolic ratios, PAR/pmol/min = product area ratio/picomoles/minute, V_{max} = maximum rate achieved by the system

Impact on Self and Harm to Others

Suicide attempt in Slovenia using a mixture of synthetic cannabinoids and cathinones was reported (Klavž et al. 2016). Upon extraction of the patient's stomach and analysis of urine content, the synthetic cathinones identified were α-PHP, α-PVP, and 4-chloromethcathinone (4-CMC) (Klavž et al. 2016). A subject on MDPV was involved in a domestic dispute with his girlfriend who stabbed him in the stomach with a knife while he was driving (Marinetti and Antonides 2013). Another subject found his wife snorting MDPV and he snorted the bath salt himself to show how she acted while under the influence but was later found to have committed suicide by hanging (Marinetti and Antonides 2013). Other suicide cases including setting themselves on fire and hanging and domestic violence also involve MDPV (Marinetti and Antonides 2013).

Following khat prohibition, it is hoped that occasional, non-dependent users and addictive behaviors be reduced which may resort to criminal use and contact with dangerous illegal drugs. Khat users who developed psychosis are locked up without access to drugs reflecting the lack of professional help for chronic khat addiction (Caulfield 2015). There is evidence that khat usage in countries that banned khat compared to khat-belt countries was still similar implying that the ban did not decrease khat use (Bongard et al. 2015). Nevertheless, social effects of khat ban were not given sufficient consideration as reflected in lack of information to khat market such as adherence, trade regulations, buyers' profile, age restriction, and damage to the economy of many communities relying on khat export (Caulfield 2015).

Anti-cathinone Vaccines

The lack of effective therapeutic interventions for cathinone addiction has promoted the development of novel therapeutic vaccines to target cathinone stimulatory effects on the CNS. Chemical structures of synthetic cathinones are often altered to evade drug laws; thus, researchers aimed to develop a single vaccine that will be effective against more than one synthetic cathinones (European Pharmaceutical Review 2018). Administration of vaccines, namely, α-PVP-KLH and MDPV-KLH, against synthetic cathinones particularly α-PVP and MDPV to rodent models demonstrated efficacy in increasing antibodies against both drugs (Nguyen et al. 2017) (see Table 3). Recently, a bi-specific hapten that produced high affinity antibodies against both MDPV and α-PVP was achieved, which was a racemic vaccine that equally blocked drug disposition into organs especially the brain (McClenahan et al. 2020). The racemic vaccine offered stable immune response more than 16–20 weeks during testing (McClenahan et al. 2020). These studies pave way for further investigations in immune-pharmacotherapies or vaccines for synthetic cathinone drugs.

Table 3 Anti-cathinone vaccines against synthetic cathinones, α-PVP and MDPV

Synthetic cathinones	Vaccine production methods	Immunoconjugates	Vaccination response	References
α-PVP MDPV	Hapten synthesis and protein bioconjugation	α-PVP-KLH MDPV-KLH	Polyclonal antibody response	(Nguyen et al. 2017)
		Bispecific hapten	Blocked drug disposition into organs especially the brain, stable immune response more than 16–20 weeks	(McClenahan et al. 2020)

Applications to Other Areas of Addiction

The practice of slam, sexual intercourse among men, is linked to use of synthetic cathinones with other drugs (Schreck et al. 2020). Approximately all slammers declared a combination of synthetic cathinones with other drugs called polydrug use during slam sessions (Schreck et al. 2020). Polydrug use could affect the users' perception of cathinone's effects leading to overreporting and complicating the cases of cathinone abuse (Schreck et al. 2020). A number of cathinone addicts reported that they reinjected cathinones and binge use over long period of time, due to the short half-life and effects in order to maintain euphoria or psychostimulatory effects (Schifano et al. 2020). A case report by Benedicte et al. described that additional or synergistic effects of two cathinones, namely, MPHP and 4-methyl-α-ethylaminopentiophenone (4-MEAP), led to death after chronic consumption and abuse of these drugs by the patients (Benedicte et al. 2020). Preclinical evidences reported that cathinones such as MDPV and α-PVP were more effective than cocaine or methamphetamine (Gannon et al. 2018). The potency of cathinones depended on its selectivity for DAT, NET, and SERT, with selectivity in descending orders at DAT of α-PVP > α-PPP (α-pyrrolidinopropiophenone) > MDPV > MDPBP > MDPPP > cocaine (Gannon et al. 2018).

Applications to Public Health

Khat use was widely perceived by avid users as food, harmless, beneficial, and medicinal (Douglas et al. 2011). Some Ethiopian khat users also believed that khat use can reduce anti-tuberculosis medication side effects most probably due to their misinterpretation of euphoric mood after taking khat (Soboka et al. 2020). Besides that, khat users usually combine alcohol and khat which leads to development of tuberculosis treatment resistance due to khat's potential impact on patients' immunity and mental health (Soboka et al. 2020). In addition, night shift workers chew khat to stay awake and prevent fatigue, while students use khat to improve mental performance during exam period (Kennedy et al. 1983). Yemeni khat users used khat to treat minor ailments including headaches, colds, body aches, fever, arthritis, and depression (Kennedy et al. 1983). Additionally, khat chewing also serves to cope with traumatic experiences during war by Somali combatants (Odenwald et al. 2009). On the other hand, cathinone significantly reduced catalepsy in animal models with Parkinson disease and could also aid relief in patients with Parkinson disease without neurotoxicity or dyskinesia side effects (Caulfield 2015). In addition, cathinones have demonstrated analgesic properties and self-medication for trauma relief in khat chewers (Caulfield 2015). The effects of khat compounds are poorly understood despite the similar effects observed in cathinone and khat, suggesting that subtle behavioral effects may be overlooked. Khat extracts and cathinone alter weight, fat mass, appetite, lipid biochemistry, and hormonal levels especially dopamine and serotonin over higher dosage and long-term intervention, suggesting their possibilities as anti-obesity treatment (Alshagga et al. 2016). Similar to cathinone, magnitude of khat use could be underestimated because users tend to minimize or deny the quantity and duration of usage (Soboka et al. 2020).

Mini-Dictionary of Terms

- *Cathinone* is the main ingredient found in khat plant and is chemically similar to stimulants such as amphetamine and cocaine.
- *Cytochrome P450* is a group of human liver enzymes important for detoxification and is responsible to metabolize and break down toxic or foreign substances including medicines, herbal products, hormones, and fat molecules.
- *Khat* is a green plant usually grown in shrubs originated from Arabian Peninsula and African countries, in which the natives chew these plants to get its euphoric effect, as a snack during social gatherings besides its use as a traditional medication.
- In silico or molecular docking is a type of study performed on computer using simulation software.
- In vitro is a type of study performed with organisms, cells, or enzymes outside of animal or any living body but instead carried out in laboratory appliances.
- In vivo is a type of study performed using living organisms such as animal, human, and plants.
- *Synthetic cathinones* are a group of man-made drugs with closely similar structures and psychostimulatory effects as naturally occurring cathinone found in khat.

Key Facts

- Naturally occurring cathinone in khat showed negligible in vitro inhibitory effects on CYP2C9, CYP2D6, and CYP3A4.

- Synthetic cathinones are continuously produced under different names and altered chemical structure to circumvent legislative laws.
- Synthetic cathinones are mainly metabolized by CYP1A2, CYP2B6, CYP2C9, CYP2C19, CYP2D6, and CYP3A4.
- There is a debate that cathinone in khat decomposes or otherwise upon harvesting.
- Abuse of synthetic cathinones posed educational, social, economic, criminal, and public health effects to the society particularly in khat-belt countries.
- Khat or cathinone users have misinterpretations that concurrent use of these two substances with drugs or medications is effective to treat some illnesses such as Parkinson disease and tuberculosis with some users also use them together with alcohol.
- Vaccines against synthetic cathinones including MDPV and α-PVP showed promising anti-cathinone effects in rodent (rat) models.
- Little is known regarding the mechanism of the various synthetic cathinones with CYPs, thus paving way to further in silico, in vitro, and in vivo studies.

Summary Points

- Cathinone is the main euphorigenic ingredient present in khat plants.
- It is controversial to claim that khat use is a form of addiction or abuse as compared to synthetic cathinones as khat use is claimed to be a social custom and pride in khat-belt countries.
- Khat and cathinones are often taken together with medications causing possible khat-drug and/or drug-drug interactions.
- Khat is believed as an effective traditional remedy.
- Khat and cathinones have negatively impacted the socioeconomic and educational attainment of children besides increasing the inclination to suicide and fatalities.
- Modifications have been made to produce new synthetic cathinones to be marketed and circumvent the legislations. Hence, continuous effort is needed to elucidate the mechanism of actions of new emerging synthetic cathinones.
- The probable mechanism of synthetic cathinones is increasing biogenic amine (e.g., dopamine, norepinephrine, serotonin) concentration at synapses.
- Anti-cathinone vaccines are capable to produce high affinity antibodies against synthetic cathinones.

References

Alemu WG et al (2020) Prevalence and risk factors for khat use among youth students in Ethiopia: systematic review and meta-analysis, 2018. Ann General Psychiatry 19(16):1–10. https://doi.org/10.1186/s12991-020-00265-8. [Online]

Al-Obaid AM et al (1998) Determination of (S)(-)-cathinone by spectrophotometric detection. J Pharm Biomed Anal 17(2):321–326. [Online]

Alshagga MA et al (2016) Khat (Catha edulis) and obesity: a scoping review of animal and human studies. Ann Nutr Metab 69:200–211. [Online]
Alshakka M et al (2020) Knowledge and attitudes on khat use among yemeni health sciences students. Subst Use Misuse 55(4):557–563. https://doi.org/10.1080/10826084.2019.1688350. [Online]
Ayano G et al (2019) Epidemiology of khat (Catha edulis) consumption among university students: a meta-analysis. BMC Public Health 19(150):1–13. [Online]
Babayan EA et al (1983) Mediator mechanisms of cathinone effects on animal behaviour. Drug Alcohol Depend 12(1):31–35. [Online]
Banks ML et al (2014) Synthetic Cathinones and amphetamine analogues: what's the rave about? J Emerg Med 46(5):632–642. [Online]
Baumann MH et al (2018) Neuropharmacology of synthetic cathinones. Handb Exp Pharmacol 252:113–142. [Online]
Bedada W et al (2018) Effects of Khat (Catha edulis) use on catalytic activities of major drug-metabolizing cytochrome P450 enzymes and implication of pharmacogenetic variations. Sci Rep 8(12726):1–10. [Online]
Benedicte L et al (2020) Case report on two-cathinones abuse: MPHP and N-ethyl-4′methylnorpentedrone, with a fatal outcome. Forensic Toxicol 38(1):243–254. https://doi.org/10.1007/s11419-019-00486-x. [Online]
Bongard S et al (2015) Khat chewing and acculturation in East-African migrants living in Frankfurt am Main/Germany. J Ethnopharmacol 164:223–228. https://doi.org/10.1016/j.jep.2015.01.034. [Online]
Brenneisen R et al (1986) Metabolism of cathinone to(−)-norephedrine and(−)-norpseudoephedrine. J Pharm Pharmacol 38(4):298–300. [Online]
Brenneisen R et al (1990) Amphetamine-like effects in humans of the khat alkaloid cathinone. Br J Clin Pharmacol 30(6):825–828. [Online]
Bretteville-Jensen AL et al (2013) Synthetic Cannabinoids and Cathinones: prevalence and markets. Forensic Sci Rev 25(1–2):7–26. [Online]. Available from: http://www.ncbi.nlm.nih.gov/pubmed/26226848
Capriola M (2013) Synthetic cathinone abuse. Clin Pharmacol Adv Appl 5:109–115. [Online]
Caulfield A (2015) Do the risks of khat-induced dependence and psychosis warrant the 2014 UK ban? Drug Sci Policy Law 2(0):1–8. [Online]
Cheong JH et al (2017) Behavioral evidence for the abuse potential of the novel synthetic cathinone alpha-pyrrolidinopentiothiophenone (PVT) in rodents. Psychopharmacology 234:857–867. [Online]
Contrucci RR et al (2020) Synthetic Cathinones and their potential interactions with prescription drugs. Ther Drug Monit 42(1):75–82. [Online]
Costantino AG et al (2019) Issues of false negative results in toxicology: difficult in detecting certain drugs and issues with detection of synthetic cathinone (bath salts), synthetic cannabinoids (spice), and other new psychoactive substances. Accurate Results in the Clinical Laboratory. 2nd edn. Elsevier. https://doi.org/10.1016/B978-0-12-813776-5.00016-9. [Online]
Douglas H et al (2011) The health impacts of khat: a qualitative study among Somali-Australians. Med J Aust 195(11/12):666–669. [Online]
Duresso SW et al (2016) Is khat use disorder a valid diagnostic entity? Addiction 111(9):1666–1676. [Online]
Ellefsen KN et al (2016) 4-Methoxy-α-PVP: in silico prediction, metabolic stability, and metabolite identification by human hepatocyte incubation and high-resolution mass spectrometry. Forensic Toxicol 34:61–75. [Online]
European Pharmaceutical Review (2018) New vaccine could help people overcome cathinone abuse. Rev Eur Pharm 1–6
Feng LY et al (2017) New psychoactive substances of natural origin: a brief review. J Food Drug Anal 25(3):461–471. https://doi.org/10.1016/j.jfda.2017.04.001. [Online]

Gannon BM et al (2018) The abuse-related effects of pyrrolidine-containing cathinones are related to their potency and selectivity to inhibit the dopamine transporter. Neuropsychopharmacology 43(12):2399–2407. https://doi.org/10.1038/s41386-018-0209-3. [Online]

Glennon RA, Liebowitz SM (1982) Serotonin receptor affinity of cathinone and related analogues. J Med Chem 25:393–397. [Online]

Gonçalves JL et al (2019) Synthetic cathinones: an evolving class of new psychoactive substances. Crit Rev Toxicol 49(7):549–566. https://doi.org/10.1080/10408444.2019.1679087. [Online]

Hakkola, J. et al. (2020) Inhibition and induction of CYP enzymes in humans: an update. Vol. 94. Springer Berlin/Heidelberg. https://doi.org/10.1007/s00204-020-02936-7. [Online].

Halket JM et al (1995) Plasma cathinone levels following chewing khat leaves (Catha edulis Forsk.). J Ethnopharmacol 49(2):111–113. [Online]

Kalix P, Khan I (1984) Khat: an amphetamine-like plant material. Bull World Health Organ 62(5): 681–686

Kennedy JG et al (1983) A medical evaluation of the use of qat in North Yemen. Soc Sci Med 17 (12):783–793. [Online]

Klavž J et al (2016) Suicide attempt with a mix of synthetic cannabinoids and synthetic cathinones: case report of non-fatal intoxication with AB-CHMINACA, AB-FUBINACA, alpha-PHP, alpha-PVP and 4-CMC. Forensic Sci Int 265:121–124. [Online]

Lim SYM et al (2019) Effect of 95% ethanol khat extract and cathinone on in vitro human recombinant cytochrome P450 (CYP) 2C9, CYP2D6, and CYP3A4 activity. Eur J Drug Metab Pharmacokinet 44:423–431. https://doi.org/10.1007/s13318-018-0518-2. [Online]

Lim SYM et al (2020) Cytochrome P450 4B1 (CYP4B1) as a target in cancer treatment. Hum Exp Toxicol 39(6):785–796. [Online]

Lim SYM, Alshagga MA, Alshawsh MA, Ong CE, Pan Y (2021) In vitro effects of 95% khat ethanol extract (KEE) on human recombinant cytochrome P450 (CYP)1A2, CYP2A6, CYP2B6, CYP2C8, CYP2C19, CYP2E1, CYP2J2 and CYP3A5. Drug Metab Pers Ther 37 (1):55–67. https://doi.org/10.1515/dmpt-2021-1000196

Majchrzak M et al (2018) The newest cathinone derivatives as designer drugs: an analytical and toxicological review. Forensic Toxicol 36:33–50. [Online]

Manier SK et al (2018) Different in vitro and in vivo tools for elucidating the human metabolism of alpha-cathinone-derived drugs of abuse. Drug Test Anal 10(7):1119–1130. [Online]

Marinetti LJ, Antonides HM (2013) Analysis of synthetic cathinones commonly found in bath salts in human performance and postmortem toxicology: method development, drug distribution and interpretation of results. J Anal Toxicol 37(3):135–146. [Online]

McClenahan SJ et al (2020) Design, synthesis and biological evaluation of a bi-specific vaccine against α-pyrrolidinovalerophenone (α-PVP) and 3,4- methylenedioxypyrovalerone (MDPV) in rats. Vaccine 38(2):336–344. [Online]

Mekuriaw B et al (2020) Magnitude of Khat use and associated factors among women attending antenatal care in Gedeo zone health centers, southern Ethiopia: a facility based cross sectional study. BMC Public Health 20(110):1–8. [Online]

Meunier B et al (2004) Mechanism of oxidation reactions catalyzed by cytochrome P450 enzymes. Chem Rev 104(9):3947–3980. [Online]

Meyer MR et al (2010) Studies on the metabolism of the α-pyrrolidinophenone designer drug methylenedioxy-pyrovalerone (MDPV) in rat and human urine and human liver microsomes using GC-MS and LC-high-resolution MS and its detectability in urine by GC-MS. J Mass Spectrom 45(12):1426–1442. [Online]

Meyer MR et al (2012) New cathinone-derived designer drugs 3-bromomethcathinone and 3-fluoromethcathinone: studies on their metabolism in rat urine and human liver microsomes using GC-MS and LC-high-resolution MS and their detectability in urine. J Mass Spectrom 47 (2):253–262. [Online]

Nadia M (2012) Yemeni children on qat: an imitation that becomes an addiction. Al Arabiya 1–4

Nguyen JD et al (2017) Active vaccination attenuates the physcostimulant effects of α- PVP and MDPV in rats. Neuropharmacology 116:1–8. [Online]

Nichols T et al (2015) The psychostimulant drug khat (Catha edulis): a mini-review. Phytochem Lett 13:127–133. https://doi.org/10.1016/j.phytol.2015.05.016. [Online]

Numan N (2012) The green leaf: Khat. World J Med Sci 7(4):210–223. [Online]

Odenwald M et al (2009) Use of khat and posttraumatic stress disorder as risk factors for psychotic symptoms: a study of Somali combatants. Soc Sci Med 69(7):1040–1048. https://doi.org/10.1016/j.socscimed.2009.07.020. [Online]

Ongeri L et al (2019) Khat use and psychotic symptoms in a rural Khat growing population in Kenya: a household survey. BMC Psychiatry 19(137):1–10. [Online]

Patel NB (2000) Mechanism of action of cathinone: the active ingredient of khat (Catha edulis). East Afr Med J 77(6):329–332. [Online]

Patocka J et al (2020) Flakka: new dangerous synthetic cathinone on the drug scene. Int J Mol Sci 21(21):1–14. [Online]

Pehek EA et al (1990) Effects of cathinone and amphetamine on the neurochemistry of dopamine in vivo. Neuropharmacology 29(12):1171–1176. [Online]

Poulos TL, Johnson EF (2005) Structures of cytochrome P450 enzymes. In: Ortiz de Montellano, PR (eds) Cytochrome P450. Springer, Boston, MA. https://doi.org/10.1007/0-387-27447-2_3

Sauer C et al (2009) New designer drug α-pyrrolidinovalerophenone (PVP): studies on its metabolism and toxicological detection in rat urine using gas chromatographic/mass spectrometric techniques. J Mass Spectrom 44:952–964. [Online]

Sawair FA et al (2007) High relative frequency of oral squamous cell carcinoma in Yemen: Qat and tobacco chewing as its aetiological background. Int J Environ Health Res 17(3):185–195. [Online]

Schifano F et al (2011) Mephedrone (4-methylmethcathinone; 'meow meow'): chemical, pharmacological and clinical issues. Psychopharmacology 214(3):593–602. [Online]

Schifano F et al (2020) The clinical challenges of synthetic cathinones. Br J Clin Pharmacol 86: 410–419. [Online]

Schreck B et al (2020) Cathinone use disorder in the context of slam practice: new pharmacological and clinical challenges. Front Psych 11(705):1–9. [Online]

Soboka M et al (2020) Magnitude and predictors of khat use among patients with tuberculosis in Southwest Ethiopia: a longitudinal study. PLoS ONE 15(7):1–12. https://doi.org/10.1371/journal.pone.0236154. [Online]

Swortwood MJ et al (2016) In vitro, in vivo and in silico metabolic profiling of α-pyrrolidinopentiothiophenone, a novel thiophene stimulant. Bioanalysis 8(1):65–82

Tekulve K et al (2014) Seizures associated with synthetic cathinone exposures in the pediatric population. Pediatr Neurol 51:67–70. https://doi.org/10.1016/j.pediatrneurol.2014.03.003. [Online]

Toennes SW et al (2003) Pharmacokinetics of cathinone, cathine and norephedrine after the chewing of khat leaves. Br J Clin Pharmacol 56:125–130. [Online]

Valente MJ et al (2014) Khat and synthetic cathinones: a review. Arch Toxicol 88(1):15–45. [Online]

Wabe NT (2011) Chemistry, pharmacology, and toxicology of khat (catha edulis forsk): a review. Addict Health 3(3–4):137–149

Watterson LR, Olive MF (2014) Synthetic cathinones and their rewarding and reinforcing effects in rodents. Adv Neurosci 2014(209875):1–9. [Online]

Widler P et al (1994a) Pharmacodynamics and pharmacokinetics of khat: a controlled study. Clin Pharmacol Ther 55(5):556–562. https://doi.org/10.1038/clpt.1994.69. [Online]

Widler P et al (1994b) Pharmacodynamics and pharmacokinetics of khat: a controlled study. Clin Pharmacol Ther 55(5):556–562

Wolfes O (1930) Über das Vorkommen von d-nor-iso-Ephedrin in Catha edulis. Arch Pharm 268: 81–83

Zanger UM, Schwab M (2013) Cytochrome P450 enzymes in drug metabolism: regulation of gene expression, enzyme activities, and impact of genetic variation. Pharmacol Ther 138:103–141. https://doi.org/10.1016/j.pharmthera.2012.12.007. [Online]

Cognitive Deficits and Synthetic Khat-Related Cathinones

79

Vincent Carfagno, Jonna M. Leyrer-Jackson, and M. Foster Olive

Contents

Introduction 1683
Neuropharmacological Actions of Synthetic Cathinones 1684
Impact on Cognition in Animals 1686
Impact on Cognition in Humans 1688
Cellular Toxicity and Neuroinflammation as Possible Mechanisms of Cathinone-Induced Neurocognitive Dysfunction 1689
Conclusions 1693
Applications to Other Areas of Substance Use Disorders 1694
Applications to Other Areas of Public Health 1694
Mini-dictionary of Terms 1695
Key Facts of Synthetic Khat-Related Cathinones 1696
Key Facts of Cognitive Deficits of Synthetic Khat-Related Cathinones 1696
Summary Points 1697
References 1697

Abstract

The psychoactive shrub *Catha edulis* (khat or qat) has been used by humans for centuries due to the psychoactive properties of its endogenous alkaloid cathinone. In recent years, synthetic derivatives of cathinone, herein referred to as synthetic cathinones and colloquially referred to as "bath salts," have infiltrated drug markets worldwide. As a result, evidence of abuse, dependence, toxicity, and adverse cognitive effects has emerged. In this chapter, we will provide a brief overview of synthetic cathinones and their neuropharmacological mechanisms of action. Next, we will review the adverse cognitive effects of acute and chronic

V. Carfagno
Midwestern University School of Medicine, Glendale, AZ, USA
e-mail: vincent.carfagno@midwestern.edu

J. M. Leyrer-Jackson · M. F. Olive (✉)
Department of Psychology, Arizona State University, Tempe, AZ, USA
e-mail: jmjack22@asu.edu; foster.olive@asu.edu

V. B. Patel, V. R. Preedy (eds.), *Handbook of Substance Misuse and Addictions*,
https://doi.org/10.1007/978-3-030-92392-1_86

exposure to synthetic cathinones in both animals and humans. Finally, we will provide a hypothetic model of potential mechanisms, at the level of both cellular toxicity and neuroinflammation, that may underlie the neurocognitive dysfunction induced by this class of abused substances.

Keywords

Cathinone · Synthetic · Derivative · Psychostimulant · Cognition · Working memory · Object recognition · Fluency · Verbal recall · Oxidative stress · Neuroinflammation

Abbreviations

4-FMC	4-Fluoromethcathinone (flephedrone)
4-MEC	4-Methylethcathinone
4-MMC	4-Methylmethcathinone (mephedrone)
5-HT	5-Hydroxytryptamine (serotonin)
α-PVP	α-Pyrrolidinopentiophenone
α-PVT	α-Pyrrolidinovalerothiophenone
AMPA	α-Amino-3-hydroxy-5-methyl-4-isoxazolepropionic acid
BBB	Blood-brain barrier
DA	Dopamine
DAT	Dopamine transporter
DOPAC	3,4-Dihydroxyphenylacetic acid
GFAP	Glial fibrillary acidic protein
GLT-1	Glutamate transporter 1
Iba1	Ionized binding adapter protein 1
iGluR	Ionotropic glutamate receptor
ILB4	Isolectin B4
LDH	Lactate dehydrogenase
MDMA	3,4-Methylenedioxymethamphetamine
MDMC	3,4-Methylenedioxy-N-methylcathinone
MDPV	3,4-Methylenedioxypyrovalerone
NE	Norepinephrine
NET	Norepinephrine transporter
NMDA	N-methyl-D-aspartate
OCT3	Type 3 organic cation transporter
RNS	Reactive nitrogen species
ROS	Reactive oxygen species
SERT	Serotonin transporter
TAAR1	Trace amine receptor 1
TH	Tyrosine hydroxylase
TNF-α	Tumor necrosis factor α
TPH2	Tryptophan hydroxylase 2
TPSO	18 kDa translocator protein
VMAT2	Vesicular monoamine transporter 2

Introduction

Catha edulis, colloquially referred to as "khat" or "qat," is a perennial shrub indigenous to northeastern areas of Africa as well as the Arabian Peninsula. The plant was first described by Finnish expeditionist Petrus Forskål, and thus the shrub is occasionally referred to *Catha edulis* Forsk (Soares et al. 2021). For centuries, humans residing in regions of indigenous khat growth have utilized the leaves of this shrub, usually in the form of chewing (Alles et al. 1961), for its mild psychostimulant effects. It has been estimated that as many as 80–90% of men in regions such as Yemen are regular users of khat (Patel 2019). The psychostimulant effects of khat desired by its users include increased energy, concentration, libido, and its use as a counterfatigue measure. Such practices are similar to that of chewing of coca leaves by various indigenous peoples of South America.

The psychoactive effects of khat chewing are largely attributable to cathinone (2-amino-1-phenylpropan-1-one), an endogenous amphetamine-like alkaloid in *Catha edulis*. To a lesser degree, the related molecule cathine (2-amino-1-phenyl-propan-1-ol) also contributes to some of the psychoactive effects of khat. The chemical structure of cathinone is highly similar to that of the classical psychostimulant amphetamine, yet contains a β-ketone moiety; thus, cathinones are often referred to as "β-ketone amphetamines." Due to the ease at which they are synthesized, chemical derivatives of cathinone, referred to as "synthetic cathinones," "synthetic cathinone derivatives," or "substituted cathinones," have been pursued for clinical and recreational/illicit use for over a century. In the early to mid-twentieth century, methcathinone was one of the first synthetic cathinones to be synthesized and was developed and marketed as an antidepressant in the former Soviet Union and as an analeptic in the United States (Soares et al. 2021). Subsequent cathinone derivatives were pursued in various countries for use as counterfatigue measures, appetite suppressants, or anti-Parkinsonian treatments. However, for a variety of reasons including a significant abuse potential, most cathinone derivatives are considered illicit controlled substances. Currently, only one synthetic cathinone derivative remains in clinical use – bupropion (2-(tert-butylamino)-1-(3-chlorophenyl)propan-1-one) – which is prescribed as an antidepressant, smoking cessation aid, and appetite suppressant.

In the early to mid-2000s, a large number of illicitly manufactured cathinone derivatives began to infiltrate drug markets worldwide (Winder et al. 2013). These derivatives, usually in crystalline or powder form, were sold in head shops and smoke shops or on the internet in packaging that was intended to disguise them as common household products such as "bath salts," "plant food," "glass cleaner," etc. This attempt to evade attention by drug authorities was paralleled by additional package labelling with verbiage along the lines of "research chemicals" and "not for human consumption," in order for drug manufacturers to minimize their risk of legal prosecution. Although many colloquial terms have been used in the packaging and marketing of cathinone derivatives, "bath salts" has remained the most popular jargon term.

By 2009–2010, an alarming number of cases of toxicity and death emerged in the United Kingdom and other European Union countries which were forensically attributable to the use of the cathinone derivative 4-methylmethcathinone (4-MMC, or mephedrone) (Winstock et al. 2011). While federal authorities were quick to place mephedrone into a controlled substance status, soon thereafter, other cathinone derivatives emerged including 1-(4-methoxyphenyl)-2-(methylamino) propan-1-one (methedrone), 1-naphthalen-2-yl-2-pyrrolidin-1-ylpentan-1-one (naphyrone), 2-(ethylamino)-1-(4-methylphenyl)propan-1-one (4-MEC), and 2-(methylamino)-1-phenylpentan-1-one (pentedrone), and 3,4-methylenedioxy-N-methylcathinone (MDMC, or methylone). In addition, cathinone derivatives with more extended molecular structures, based off of the prescription counterfatigue drug and appetite suppressant 4-methyl-β-keto-prolintane (pyrovalerone), also emerged. Such analogues included 1-phenyl-2-pyrrolidin-1-ylpentan-1-one (α-pyrrolidinopentiophenone, or α-PVP), 2-(pyrrolidin-1-yl)-1-(thiophen-2-yl)pentan-1-one (α-pyrrolidinopentiothiophenone, or α-PVT), and 1-(1,3-benzodioxol-5-yl)-2-pyrrolidin-1-ylpentan-1-one (3,4-methylenedioxypyrovalerone, or MDPV). Most of these synthetic cathinone derivatives have now been placed into controlled substance status in countries across the world. Yet due to the ease at which new analogues can be designed and synthesized, often by as little as a single atom, new cathinone derivatives continue to emerge into drug markets at a rate of approximately 6–8 per year (Majchrzak et al. 2018). To date, over 150 different synthetic cathinones have been identified and detected in drug samples and seizures (Addiction 2021).

A number of factors, including unknown drug potency, adulteration with other drugs of abuse, individual vulnerabilities, prior drug use history, and patterns of polysubstance, synthetic cathinones carry a high risk of inducing clinically significant severe adverse effects. The so-called clinical "toxidrome" of synthetic cathinone use includes symptoms of agitated delirium, psychosis, paranoia, seizures, tachycardia, hypertension, multiple organ failure, and death (Hall et al. 2014; Karila et al. 2018; Zaami et al. 2018). Many of these symptoms are similar in nature to those observed in serotonin syndrome, perhaps due to the affinity of some cathinone derivatives for proteins involved in serotonergic transmission (see below). The incidence of such adverse events appears to be much higher in users of synthetic cathinones as compared to regular users of khat (Karch 2015; Numan 2004; Soares et al. 2021).

Synthetic cathinones are classified under the larger umbrella term novel psychoactive substances (NPS), which also includes synthetic cannabinoids, fentanyl derivatives, novel benzodiazepines, and phenethylamine, piperazine, and ketamine analogues (Baumann and Volkow 2016). Each of these substances is designed to either act substitutes for more traditional abused substances (i.e., marijuana, heroin, methamphetamine, cocaine, ketamine, etc.) or provide a (temporarily) legal alternative to these illicit drugs before local or federal authorities deem it necessary to place them into controlled substance status.

Neuropharmacological Actions of Synthetic Cathinones

Synthetic cathinones have two primary neuropharmacological mechanisms of action, where either they block transporters for dopamine (DA), norepinephrine (NE), or serotonin (5-HT) located on presynaptic terminals (these transporters are referred to as DAT, NET, or SERT, respectively) or they act as a substrates for these transporters as well as the vesicular monoamine transporter 2 (VMAT2), which displaces endogenous monoamines from presynaptic storage and promotes their efflux (Simmler et al. 2013; Simmons et al. 2018). While cathinone itself was originally classified and characterized as an amphetamine-type stimulant (ATS) with monoamine releasing properties (Kalix 1980, 1981, 1982), it was also found to prevent presynaptic DA reuptake (Wagner et al. 1982).

Synthetic cathinone derivatives vary greatly in their affinities for VMAT2, NET, DAT, and SERT. While detailed pharmacological characterization of various cathinone derivatives can be found elsewhere (Baumann et al. 2017; Glennon and Young 2016; Simmler and Liechti 2017; Soares et al. 2021), several examples are worthy of illustration. Pyrovalerone-based cathinone derivatives such as MDPV act in a manner similar to cocaine, with primary affinity for DAT and NET. On the other hand, mephedrone and other cathinone derivatives act a manner to methamphetamine and 3,4-methylenedioxymethamphetamone (MDMA, "ecstasy"), promoting monoamine release as well as blocking presynaptic reuptake. Synthetic cathinones often have affinities for more than one monoamine transporter subtype, and affinities are often reported as a ratio of affinity for DAT:SERT. Higher DAT:SERT ratio values indicate an affinity preference for DAT, which in general is associated with high abuse potential and compulsive intake patterns, whereas lower DAT:SERT ratios indicate a preferential affinity for SERT and tend to be associated with more episodic intake patterns similar to those observed with MDMA (Negus and Banks 2017; Simmler and Liechti 2017; Simmons et al. 2018). It has also been shown that synthetic cathinones with high affinity for DAT induce depolarizing inward sodium currents at this transporter (Kolanos et al. 2013), whereas cathinone derivatives with higher affinity for SERT also produce inward currents, yet have a much slower dissociation rate from the transporter resulting in persistent leak currents (Dolan et al. 2018). One often overlooked phenomenon is the fact that many synthetic cathinones have bioactive metabolites with significant affinity for monoamine transporters (Luethi et al. 2019), which can prolong their effects on these neurotransmitter systems.

In addition to actions at presynaptic monoamine transporters, recent in vitro studies using molecular fingerprinting techniques have shown that synthetic cathinones also exhibit affinity for various monoaminergic receptors (Hondebrink et al. 2018). Specifically, mephedrone shows moderate affinity for 5-HT_1, 5-HT_2, and α-adrenergic receptors, which further increase its effects on noradrenergic and serotonergic tone, whereas it has only limited affinity for all dopamine receptor subtypes. On the other hand, MDPV, α-PVP, and methylone show moderate affinity for D_1, D_2, and D_3 dopamine receptors. Cocaine and ATS have known affinities for the trace amine receptor 1 (TAAR1), and amphetamine (but not cocaine) also acts as a substrate for the type 3 organic cation transporter (OCT3). However, synthetic cathinone derivatives appear to lack any affinity for TAAR1 (Simmler et al. 2016) as well as OCT3 (Mayer et al. 2018). An exception to this was revealed in this latter study by Mayer and colleagues, who showed that while mephedrone and MDPV do not act as OCT3 substrates per se, when NET is fully occupied by MDPV, mephedrone exert substrates releasing effects through OCT3. These studies demonstrate that cathinone derivatives have some non-monoaminergic mechanisms of action when present in combination with substrate releasing analogues.

Glutamate transporter 1 (GLT-1) is the primary transporter responsible for clearing extracellular glutamate, and it has been shown that administration of MDPV to laboratory rats results in a selective downregulation of GLT-1 in the nucleus accumbens (Gregg et al. 2016), an effect also observed following cocaine exposure (Baker et al. 2003). As a result of this downregulation, extracellular levels of glutamate in this region can become elevated by MPDV, potentially inducing excitotoxicity. These effects of MDPV on GLT-1 expression are also implicated in its rewarding effects, since restoration of drug-induced reductions in GLT-1 expression by co-administration of the β-lactam antibiotic ceftriaxone reduces the magnitude of MDPV-induced conditioned reward (Gregg et al. 2016). The conditioned rewarding effects of MDPV also appear to involve chemokine signalling, as they are blocked by antagonism of CXC4R chemokine receptors (Oliver et al. 2018). These latter findings implicate neuroimmune signalling in the central actions of synthetic cathinones such as MDPV. In line with this, a recent study has shown that repeated mephedrone administration to laboratory animals increases expression of matrix metalloproteinase 9, an enzyme that regulates pathological remodelling of the extracellular matrix following neuroinflammation, within the prefrontal cortex and hippocampus (Grochecki et al. 2021). Interestingly, this effect was not observed following amphetamine exposure, highlighting yet another mechanism by which these cathinones diverge from those of other abused stimulants. It is of great interest to determine if any of these non-monoaminergic mechanisms of action of synthetic cathinones contribute to any cognitive dysfunction, neuroinflammation, or neurotoxicity induced by these substances.

Impact on Cognition in Animals

Preclinical studies utilizing rodent animal models and non-human primates allow for in-depth analysis of both acute and long-term effects of synthetic cathinones on cognition in a highly controlled environment. To date, multiple behavioral tasks including the Morris water maze, T- and Y-maze alternations, passive avoidance, sequential operant responding, and novel object recognition tests have been used to assess synthetic cathinone-induced changes in cognition. Many of these studies have yielded conflicting results, especially those that involved acute or repeated low-dose exposure to synthetic cathinones. We have previously reviewed these studies and results in detail (Leyrer-Jackson et al. 2019). Here, we note that there have been several studies that found significant effects of synthetic cathinones on various cognitive measures using moderate to high doses of these drugs, which tend to produce impairments in cognitive functions. Such studies, performed in laboratory rodents, have shown that either repeated administration or extended self-administration of synthetic cathinones such as mephedrone and MDPV impair working recognition memory in an object recognition task (Bernstein et al. 2020;

Motbey et al. 2012; Sewalia et al. 2018) and spatial working memory in a Y-maze task (Daniel and Hughes 2016). These findings are similar to those utilizing psychostimulants such as cocaine, MDMA, and methamphetamine, which also produce impaired cognitive functions following repeated exposure (García-Pardo et al. 2017; Moszczynska and Callan 2017). It is of note that while several studies found impairments in cognitive function induced by synthetic cathinones, some have actually report enhanced cognitive functioning. For example, in male mice, systemic administration of methylone twice a day for 4 days enhanced performance in the probe trial portion of the Morris water maze (den Hollander et al. 2013). In rhesus macaques, repeated administration of mephedrone increased visuospatial memory and learning (Wright et al. 2012). These effects are in line with other studies reporting that amphetamine-type psychostimulants enhance visuospatial components of stimulus associative memory tasks (reviewed in Wood et al. 2014).

Interestingly, synthetic cathinone-induced impairments in cognition have been reported predominantly in male rodents (reviewed in Leyrer-Jackson et al. 2019), perhaps because most behavioral pharmacology studies in rodents still primarily utilize male subjects. However, some exceptions to this have been noted where long-term (30 weeks) administration of mephedrone, as well as a shorter regimen of methylone administration (10 days), increased the number of errors in an operant response sequence task in female rodents and also decreased spatial memory ability in a Y-maze test (Daniel and Hughes 2016; Weed et al. 2014). In the latter study (Weed et al. 2014), it was demonstrated that administration of 17β-estradiol to ovariectomized female rodents produced further decrements in these tasks, suggesting an influence of gonadal hormones on cognitive processes affected by synthetic cathinones. Other than this study, very few have examined sex differences in changes in cognition induced by or the abuse potential of synthetic cathinones.

It should be noted that most studies exploring the effects of synthetic cathinones on cognitive function have examined effects of so-called "first-generation" cathinone derivatives including mephedrone, MDPV, and methylone. As such, effects of other cathinones such as α-PVP have not yet been explored. Given the vast differences in synthetic cathinones with respect to their pharmacological mechanisms of action, additional studies identifying the effects of each synthetic cathinone would likely yield different results in regard to cognition, which may be driven, in part, by their primary molecular affinities. Thus, future studies exploring the effects of other known synthetic cathinones on cognitive function would yield beneficial for exploring such relationships.

In addition to the caveats above, it is also of note that studies exploring the effects of cathinones on cognitive function utilized vastly different dosing procedures, including dosing amounts and the frequency of administration, that would result in different blood and brain levels of the drug. For example, some "binge-like" procedures utilizing bolus doses likely elevate blood and brain levels of the drug far beyond that obtained by voluntarily self-administered drug. Additionally, it is established that experimenter delivered passive drug exposure has substantially different effects on physiological processes and pharmacodynamics than those evoked by voluntary intake (Jacobs et al. 2003; Stuber et al. 2010). Thus, it is likely that passive drug administration, which was most commonly utilized to explore cognitive changes in prior studies, has different effects on cognition than voluntary intake. We argue that although self-administration studies are more difficult and costly to employ, they likely yield more translational effects in terms of blood and brain saturation as well as overall insight into drug-induced cognitive changes. However, studies employing passive administration methods of synthetic cathinones may lend insight into the cognitive and pathophysiological effects that may occur following prolonged voluntary intake. For example, repeated experimenter delivered mephedrone at high doses in rats induces deficits in object recognition memory (Motbey et al. 2012), a result that was also found with long-term binge-like MDPV intravenous self-administration over multiple 96-h access sessions that took place over 5 consecutive weeks (Sewalia et al. 2018). Although these studies utilized different synthetic cathinone derivatives, similarities in cognitive dysfunction were reported. As such, it is important to determine which cognitive deficits are accurately and reliably modelled with both passive and voluntary intake in a number of paradigms to ensure findings are translatable to intake and cognitive impacts in humans.

Impact on Cognition in Humans

Long-term heavy use of traditional psychostimulants such as cocaine or amphetamine-type stimulants has been associated with varying degrees of cognitive dysfunction. These disruptions span multiple cognitive domains including verbal learning, fluency, and recall, visuoperception, psychomotor speed, working memory, attentional and task set-shifting, response inhibition, decision-making, and social functioning (Frazer et al. 2018; London et al. 2015; Potvin et al. 2018). As with all neuropsychiatric studies, however, it is important to keep in mind that oftentimes psychostimulant abuse is accompanied by other psychiatric disorders including attention-deficit hyperactivity disorder, psychosis, depression, and anxiety. Thus, some element of caution should be observed in terms of inferring causality between psychostimulant use and the induction of cognitive deficits, as some level of dysfunction may pre-date initiation of psychostimulant use.

Some studies have shown that habitual khat users, which tend to be predominantly male, exhibit deficits in working memory, psychomotor speed, cognitive set-shifting, and inhibitory control (Ahmed et al. 2021; Colzato et al. 2010, 2011; Hoffman and al'Absi 2013; Khattab and Amer 1995). There is also some evidence of increased risk of psychosis or related disorders in habitual khat users (Ageely 2008; Odenwald et al. 2005, 2009), though not all studies have found such an association (Numan 2004). However, several studies have suggested that cognitive alterations in regular khat use can be exacerbated by concomitant use of tobacco products (Nakajima et al. 2014).

As far as synthetic cathinones are concerned, there is a small but growing literature documenting cognitive deficits in regular users of these substances. One of the first of these examined patients with a history of at least 1 year of prior mephedrone use and found a significant decrease in verbal recall and fluency abilities (Freeman et al. 2012). Similar impairments were observed in users having taken the drug less than 48 h prior to cognitive testing (Herzig et al. 2013). In other studies, regular users of mephedrone (and other NPS) report impairments in executive function, memory, and impulse control (Savulich et al. 2021), although in some studies the specific cognitive domain being assessed is unclear (Homman et al. 2018). Mephedrone intoxication also appears to produce similar impairing effects on some forms of cognition including short-term memory (de Sousa Fernandes Perna et al. 2016), which may be related to the ability of this cathinone derivative to also induce irritability, rapid changes in mood, anxiety, and self-harming behaviors (Mead and Parrott 2020; Ordak et al. 2020; Wood and Dargan 2012). A very recent study examined problem-solving abilities in a cohort of individuals with a history of regular use of methcathinone for either less than or greater than 3 years, and not surprisingly problem-solving deficits were more evident in longer-term users (Zhang et al. 2021).

As with any study assessing potential cognitive impairments in human drug users, the specific contribution of mephedrone use to the observed impairments in verbal recall, fluency, working memory, and inhibitory control is difficult to determine. Many factors could have influenced these observations, such as comorbid neuropsychiatric disorders, polydrug use, reliability of self-report of prior or other drug use, and between-subject comparison (i.e., drug user vs. control subject as opposed to assessment of baseline cognitive function in the user). Further, many synthetic cathinone products contain psychoactive adulterants including caffeine, MDMA, cocaine, or other cathinone derivatives (Palamar et al. 2016). These extraneous factors make it difficult to attribute the use of mephedrone or other cathinone derivatives to any observed cognitive impairment(s).

Cellular Toxicity and Neuroinflammation as Possible Mechanisms of Cathinone-Induced Neurocognitive Dysfunction

Drugs of abuse can activate various cellular processes that contribute to neuronal dysfunction, neurotoxicity, and neuroinflammation, one or more of which may underlie cognitive deficits resulting from long-term drug use. These processes include excitotoxicity, oxidative stress, metabolic compromise, gliosis, neuroinflammation, disruption of integrity of the blood-brain barrier (BBB), and various signalling pathways that lead to cell death. Such phenomenon has been observed following chronic exposure to traditional psychostimulants such as cocaine and amphetamine-type stimulants (Jîtcă et al. 2021; Pimentel et al. 2020; Shaerzadeh et al. 2018), and there is limited evidence for activation of such processes by khat use (Aleryani et al. 2011). Thus, there is a high degree of probability that synthetic cathinone derivatives may also cause neurotoxicity and/or neuroinflammation. Such evidence has recently been reviewed in detail elsewhere (Angoa-Perez et al. 2017; Leyrer-Jackson et al. 2019; Pantano et al. 2017; Riley et al. 2020), and here we summarize some of the existing literature on potential neurotoxic and

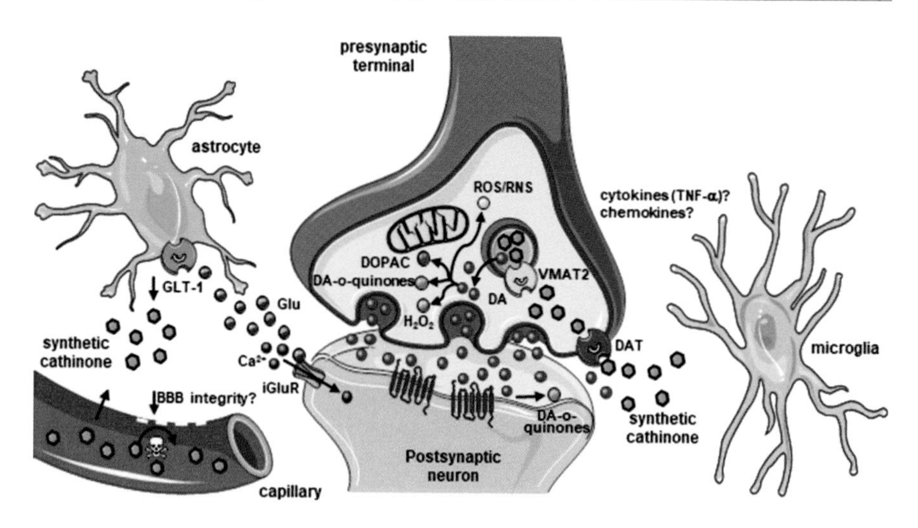

Fig. 1 Hypothetical model of mechanisms underlying synthetic cathinone-induced cytotoxicity and neuroinflammation. Depiction of a hypothetical model by which synthetic cathinones potentially induce cytotoxicity and neuroinflammation, which may contribute to acute or chronic cognitive dysfunction. Synthetic cathinones act as inhibitors and/or substrates of monoamine transporters such as DAT, NET, and SERT, resulting in prolonged accumulation of monoamines in the synaptic cleft as well as in the cytoplasm of the presynaptic terminal. As a result, excess monoamine metabolism, particularly that of DA, promotes the formation of damaging DA-o-quinones, reactive oxygen species (ROS), and reactive nitrogen species (RNS). Nontoxic DA metabolites such as 3,4-dihydroxyphenylacetic acid (DOPAC) and 3-methoxytyramine also accumulate. Aside from affecting monoaminergic transmission, synthetic cathinones can also alter expression of the astrocytic glutamate transporter GLT-1 in astrocytes, resulting in excessive Ca^{2+} influx through ionotropic glutamate receptors (iGluRs), culminating in excitotoxicity. Synthetic cathinones may also exert cytotoxic effects on brain endothelial cells, compromising the function of the blood-brain barrier (BBB). Finally, there is growing evidence that synthetic cathinones produce activation of microglia and increased secretion of chemokines or pro-inflammatory cytokines such as TNF-α. (Reprinted with permission from Leyrer-Jackson et al. (2019)

neuroinflammation induced by synthetic cathinone derivatives. A working hypothetical model of this phenomenon is shown in Fig. 1.

Through their ability to antagonize and/or serve as substrates for presynaptic monoamine transporters (i.e., DAT, NET, and SERT), psychostimulants including synthetic cathinones can induce prolonged accumulation of monoamines in the synaptic cleft (Baumann et al. 2013). Of the three primary monoamines affected (DA, NE, 5-HT), DA has received the most attention as a potential contributor to cytotoxicity, as its overabundance can result in excess DA metabolism which can form cell damaging DA-o-quinones. This process can also generate reactive oxygen species (ROS) such as hydrogen peroxide and reactive nitrogen species (RNS) such as peroxynitrite. These free radicals can also be generated by excitotoxicity induced by excess glutamate release and subsequent excess calcium influx into neurons and other cell types. Other ROS such as superoxides can stem from drug-induced disruption of cellular respiration, which can damage DNA and induces peroxidation of proteins and lipids, culminating in cell death via apoptosis or autophagy (Salim 2017). ROS/RNS production by abused substances is often indirectly measured by changes in levels of endogenous antioxidants such as glutathione. Finally, compromised BBB function can result from chronic drug use via activation of matrix metalloproteinases which disrupt the vascular basement membrane.

The bulk of evidence for potential cytotoxic effects of synthetic cathinones has been derived from in vitro studies assessing effects of various cathinone derivatives on cell viability, ROS/RNS production, glutathione levels, and measures of apoptosis as reviewed elsewhere (Angoa-Perez et al. 2017, Leyrer-Jackson et al. 2019, Pantano et al. 2017, Riley et al. 2020). Cathinone derivatives such as mephedrone, MDPV, methylone, naphyrone, and 3-methylmethcathinone appear to produce evidence of cytotoxicity in a number of neuronal, pulmonary, endothelial, hepatic, smooth muscle, and renal cell lines. Such evidence includes decreases in cell viability, proliferation, mitochondrial function, and oxygen consumption and increases in the reduced form of glutathione. Likewise, cell insult measures such as ROS/RNS production, release of lactate dehydrogenase (LDH, an indicator of cell damage), levels of the oxidized form of glutathione, and lipid peroxidation are increased following exposure to synthetic cathinones. Evidence for various cellular processes leading to cell death have also been observed, such as pro-apoptotic caspase activation, necrosis, pyknotic nuclei formation, chromatin condensation, and autophagy. Potential novel mechanisms of synthetic cathinone-induced cytotoxicity have been reported, including formation of toxic metabolic by-products such as methylbenzamides (den Hollander et al. 2015) and elevated cell death under hypothermic in vitro conditions (Valente et al. 2016). These latter findings are particularly relevant for increased adverse effects and toxicity that result from the body temperature-elevating effects commonly caused by synthetic cathinones.

While this line of research clearly shows cytotoxic effects of various synthetic cathinones, it should be noted that most of these studies found such effects at relatively high cathinone derivative concentrations (i.e., in the range of 10 μm–1 mM) and following extended durations (incubation >24 h). It could be argued that such concentrations are unlikely to be achieved for such a sustained duration following periodic bolus intake in humans. Future studies employing methods that involve fluctuations in applied cathinone derivative concentration that mimic the pharmacokinetics and pharmacodynamics of these substances in vivo are needed.

Evidence for potential cytotoxic effects of synthetic cathinones in vivo are more limited than that generated from in vitro studies. Some investigators have observed reductions in tissue content of presynaptic monoamine transporters (i.e., DAT, SERT, or VMAT2) or rate-limiting monoamine synthesizing enzymes such as tyrosine hydroxylase (TH) or tryptophan hydroxylase 2 (TPH2) in specific brain regions as indirect evidence of neurotoxicity. Rodents exposed to high doses of mephedrone or methylone show reduced DAT and SERT levels in brain regions including the frontal cortex, striatum, and hippocampus (Anneken et al. 2017, 2018; Bernstein et al. 2020; Ciudad-Roberts et al. 2016; Lopez-Arnau et al. 2014a, 2015; Martinez-Clemente et al. 2014). Some of these effects are potentiated by combined exposure to other drugs of abuse such as methamphetamine (Anneken et al. 2018) or ethanol (Ciudad-Roberts et al. 2016). More direct indicators of neurotoxicity, such as increased oxidative DNA damage, lipid peroxidation, and increased glutathione peroxidase levels in the frontal cortex, have been observed in rodents following repeated exposure to mephedrone (Kaminska et al. 2018; Lopez-Arnau et al. 2015). Finally, in rats self-administering MDPV via the intravenous route, it has been demonstrated that this cathinone derivative reduces ventral striatal DAT levels (Bernstein et al. 2020) and produces evidence of neuronal degeneration in the perirhinal and entorhinal cortices as measured by Fluoro-Jade C staining (Sewalia et al. 2018). Both of these studies also found that MDPV self-administering animals exhibited deficits in object recognition memory. Thus, high-dose experimenter administered synthetic cathinones and possibly voluntary self-administration of these substances appear to produce some level of neurotoxicity and alterations in levels of proteins mediating dopaminergic transmission, which may underlie observed dysregulation of cognitive function in users of these drugs.

Neurotoxicity induced by psychostimulants is accompanied by, perhaps even preceded and mediated by, neuroinflammation in monoaminergically innervated brain regions (Lacagnina et al. 2017; Soleimani et al. 2016). For example, it has been shown that cocaine produces an activation of microglia within the ventral striatum that leads to increased production and release of the pro-inflammatory cytokine tumor necrosis factor alpha (TNF-α). A similar phenomenon has been observed following incubation of neuronal (SH-SY5Y) cells with mephedrone in vitro (den Hollander et al. 2015). When rodents are exposed to high doses of cathinone derivatives such as mephedrone, methcathinone, or methylone, increases in astrocyte or microglia number in various brain regions including the frontal cortex, striatum, or hippocampus have been observed as assessed by post-mortem immunohistochemical procedures (Anneken et al. 2018; Lopez-Arnau et al. 2014a, b). However, other studies have shown that repeated administration of these cathinone derivatives fails to produce any evidence of gliosis in these or other regions of the brain (Angoa-Perez et al. 2012, 2014; Lopez-Arnau et al. 2015; Martinez-Clemente et al. 2014; Motbey et al. 2012). Such inconsistent findings likely result from a multitude of factors, such as the use of different dosing paradigms, amount of time elapsed between the end of drug exposure and harvesting of brain tissue, and variations in specific methods or markers used for microgliosis (i.e., immunohistochemistry or immunoblotting for ionized binding adapter protein 1 (Iba1) or isolectin B4 (ILB_4) or radioligand binding to the microglia-specific 18 kDa translocator protein (TSPO)). Finally, a recent study demonstrated that a chemokine CXCR4 receptor antagonist was able to attenuate MDPV-induced conditioned reward and hyperlocomotion (Oliver et al. 2018), providing evidence that synthetic cathinones induce neuroimmune crosstalk that mediates their rewarding effects.

Several key points need to be kept in mind when interpreting either positive or negative results of studies examining neuroinflammatory effects of synthetic cathinones. First, microgliosis and neuroinflammation are highly dynamic processes, often accompanied by transient changes in the synthesis or release of a multitude of cytokines or changes in their gene expression and morphological changes in microglial structure and their localization. Thus, it is possible that neuroinflammatory processes occur as a result of synthetic cathinone exposure that were undetected in these studies. In addition, drug-induced neuroinflammation can occur in the brain to produce alterations in cognition that are not necessarily dependent on any resulting neuronal toxicity (Correia et al. 2020; Pascual et al. 2018). It is now well accepted that neuroinflammatory signalling mediates normal synaptic plasticity, neural circuit development and homeostasis, and learning and memory and that neuron-immune cell crosstalk occurs on second-by-second basis even in the absence of brain insult and inflammation (Bourgognon and Cavanagh 2020; Kopec et al. 2019; Marinelli et al. 2019; Tchessalova et al. 2018; Yirmiya and Goshen 2011). Thus, newer technologies for detecting rapid localized changes in neuroimmune signalling are needed to thoroughly examine neuroinflammation as a potential component of cognitive deficits associated with synthetic cathinone use, either with or without concomitant neurotoxicity.

Conclusions

Like their traditional psychostimulant counterparts, repeated use of or exposure to synthetic cathinone derivatives in animals and humans, as well as the source of their parent molecule (khat), can induce some degree of cognitive impairment. Such impairments include deficits in working and recognition memory, verbal recall and fluency, cognitive flexibility, and inhibitory control. However, clear conclusions as to cause and effect are difficult to make, due to a number of intrinsic and extrinsic factors including the high prevalence of polysubstance abuse, drug adulteration, pre-existing neuropsychiatric conditions, and variability in subject age, educational and socioeconomic background, and baseline cognitive performance. Despite this, evidence from in vitro studies with cell lines, as well as in vivo studies with animals, suggest that synthetic cathinone derivatives exert some cytotoxic effects, which we hypothesize to be a primary result of oxidative stress due to excess dopaminergic transmission. There is also a likelihood that synthetic cathinones have the ability to induce neuroinflammation. Yet here as well, firm conclusions are also difficult to make, since cytotoxicity and lasting alterations in monoaminergic transmission appear to be observed only with prolonged and high doses and/or concentrations of synthetic cathinones and often (but not exclusively) after repeated bolus injections by an experimenter as opposed to after voluntary intake. In addition, the time scale of induction of cytotoxicity and/or neuroinflammation in vivo has not yet been determined.

Another point of concern is the tendency to extrapolate doses and concentrations of synthetic cathinones administered to laboratory animals or in vitro to those used by humans. Many synthetic cathinone products contain psychoactive adulterants and varying levels of purity, and thus self-reported doses may or may not be reliable. Oftentimes, doses of psychoactive substances administered to laboratory animals are scaled up to human equivalents based on body mass, which lead to incorrect assumptions with regard to specific pharmacological aspects such as route of administration, plasma protein binding, drug transport, and the presence of bioactive metabolites (Kenyon 2012; Luethi et al. 2019; Sharma and McNeill 2009).

There is some evidence from in vitro studies that have suggested possible structure-activity relationships (i.e., acyl chain length, presence of methyl groups, and effects of specific stereoisomers) in the abuse potential of cathinone derivatives and their cytotoxicity (Gaspar et al. 2018; Luethi et al. 2018; Negus and Banks 2017; Simmler and Liechti 2017; Valente et al. 2014). Given the varying affinities of synthetic cathinones for monoaminergic transporters and mechanisms of action upon these proteins, it would be specious to suggest that any evidence for cognitive dysfunction, neurotoxicity, or neuroinflammation induced by one particular cathinone derivative would necessarily apply to others. Despite these limited conclusions at present, a thorough scientific understanding of the potential neuroinflammatory and toxic effects induced by use of synthetic cathinone derivatives may provide a basis for novel therapeutics with antioxidant or immunomodulatory mechanisms, which could be aimed at ameliorating cognitive dysfunction in habitual abusers of these novel psychoactive substances.

Applications to Other Areas of Substance Use Disorders

In this chapter, we have provided a brief history of synthetic cathinone derivatives and their neuropharmacological mechanisms of action. We also reviewed existing evidence for the ability of these novel psychoactive substances to induce cognitive dysfunction in both animals and humans, as well as their potential to induce cytotoxicity in the brain and other cell types along with neuroinflammation. There are striking similarities between the mechanisms of action of synthetic cathinones and those of more traditional psychostimulants, such as monoamine reuptake inhibition (cocaine) and/or release facilitation (amphetamine-type stimulants). Therefore, the cognitive domains and processes that are adversely affected by synthetic cathinones are highly relevant to those induced by cocaine and amphetamines. Indeed, the primary cognitive deficits observed in human synthetic cathinone users (i.e., decreases in working and recognition memory function, verbal recall and fluency, cognitive flexibility, and behavioral inhibition) have also been reported in chronic uses of these traditional psychostimulants (Frazer et al. 2018; London et al. 2015; Potvin et al. 2018). Moreover, similar underlying mechanisms for cytotoxic and neuroinflammatory effects of traditional psychostimulants have been proposed and documented (Jîtcă et al. 2021; Pimentel et al. 2020; Shaerzadeh et al. 2018). Thus, the study of synthetic cathinones and the adverse neuropsychological sequelae of their use are highly relevant to psychostimulant use disorders, especially those that involve polysubstance abuse, which is a predominant pattern in users of synthetic cathinones.

Applications to Other Areas of Public Health

Given their euphoric and hallucinogenic effects, synthetic cathinones have recently gained popularity, which has been further facilitated by their ready availability within online markets such as the "dark web" and the use of cryptocurrencies. Further, as their chemical structures are easily manipulated, it is extremely difficult for drug enforcement agencies to implement regulation of these products that are drug specific. As with other NPS, new synthetic cathinone derivatives appear at an increasing rate each year, making them harder to classify and restrict in a timely fashion. Given that these substances have vastly different pharmacological actions that mimic both cocaine and amphetamine-like stimulants, their abuse potential remains high, while their long-lasting effects on the brain and behavior are relatively understudied. Information provided in this chapter highlight the need for additional studies on these compounds to fully understand how use may affect future drug use propensities as well as long-term behavioral deficits that may translate to use other substances and diseases.

Use of synthetic cathinones and other NPS remains a significant threat to public health and imposes a significant strain on healthcare systems. Moreover, since synthetic cathinone overdoses primarily present to first responders, emergency departments, and urgent care facilities, medical professionals at numerous levels need proper training on how to manage patients intoxicated with or overdosed on synthetic cathinones. This is especially important when standard sedation methods are often inadequate to control the agitated delirium and psychosis that patients manifest (Baumann 2014; Gershman and Fass 2012; Karila et al. 2015; Soares et al. 2021). Further, given the high degree of polysubstance abuse in synthetic cathinone users, which includes intravenous drug use, the impact of use of these substances on infectious diseases such as HIV and hepatitis needs to be further evaluated.

Mini-dictionary of Terms

- **Amphetamine-type stimulants (ATS):** Synthetic drugs derived from the central nervous stimulant alpha-methylphenethylamine (amphetamine).
- **Apoptosis:** Programmed cell death; an organized and normal non-inflammatory process occurring in multicellular organisms.
- **Cognitive flexibility:** The ability to transition one's attention, thought patterns, or behavior across different concepts, heuristics, rules, or contexts.
- **Gliosis:** Fibrous glial cell proliferation; a common feature of central nervous system injury or damage.
- **Object memory:** Type of memory assessed in rodents that uses time spent exploring a particular object(s) to measure object recognition, discrimination between similar and dissimilar objects, and spatial placement of the object.
- **Oxidative stress:** A phenomenon resulting from an imbalance between the cellular production of reactive oxygen species and antioxidant levels.
- **Passive avoidance:** A fear-motivated behavioral task used to evaluate cognitive function in which a response, previously "punished" by being paired with an unpleasant stimulus, becomes inhibited so that the aversive stimulus may be avoided.
- **Psychomotor speed:** An evaluation of cognitive processing, defined by the speed at which one can both recognize and respond to a stimulus; similar to reaction time.
- **Response inhibition:** An executive function referring to the ability of an individual to inhibit their own actions or responses.

- **Reuptake inhibitor:** A substance that blocks reabsorption of released neurotransmitters into the presynaptic terminal.
- **Self-administration:** The process of administering a drug substance to oneself.
- **Verbal fluency:** A measure of cognitive and verbal functioning, such as the ease at which an individual can express words.
- **Visuoperceptual memory:** The ability to recognize objects based on visual appearance and characteristics, as well as an individual's perceptual skills.
- **Working memory:** A component of short-term memory that includes the limited capacity to store and manipulate information required to perform a task at hand.

Key Facts of Synthetic Khat-Related Cathinones

- Synthetic cathinones are β-ketone amphetamine-like derivatives of cathinone, a psychoactive alkaloid found in *Catha edulis*.
- Synthetic cathinones typically act in a manner similar to amphetamines as monoamine releasing agents or similar to cocaine as reuptake blockers with varying affinity for presynaptic dopamine, norepinephrine, or serotonin transporters.
- Unlike amphetamines, synthetic cathinones tend to lack affinity for TAAR1, and some may act as substrates for OCT3.
- Users of synthetic cathinones tend to be polysubstance abusers and may have comorbid neuropsychiatric diagnoses.
- Many cathinone derivative products contain adulterants and/or produce bioactive metabolites, which makes cause and effect determinations with regard to cognitive dysfunction, toxicity, and inflammation difficult.
- Multiple distinct cellular processes related to toxicity and inflammation may be induced by synthetic cathinone derivatives, the strongest evidence of which are increases in oxidative stress via excess dopamine metabolism.

Key Facts of Cognitive Deficits of Synthetic Khat-Related Cathinones

- Repeated use of synthetic cathinones, particularly in high doses, may cause deficits in cognition in some users.
- Studies in animals have demonstrated that synthetic cathinones can produce deficits in various cognitive domains including working memory and object recognition; however, there is a high degree of variance in the ability of synthetic cathinones to produce cognitive deficits, likely due to a number of experimental factors.
- 17-β-Estradiol has been shown to potentiate cognitive impairments induced by synthetic cathinones, suggesting a role for gonadal hormones in the deleterious effects of these substances.
- Cognitive deficits in human users of synthetic cathinones include impaired performance in tasks involving verbal fluency and recall, working memory, problem-solving, set-shifting, and behavioral inhibition.

- The possibility of exacerbation of deleterious effects of synthetic cathinones on cognition among tobacco product users.
- Cause and effect relationships between synthetic cathinone use in humans and cognitive impairments are difficult to establish, in light of potential roles of polysubstance abuse and comorbid psychiatric conditions.

Summary Points

- Synthetic cathinones are amphetamine-like novel psychoactive substances derived from the shrub *Catha edulis* (khat or qat), though their mechanisms of action differ slightly from those of classical amphetamines.
- Mechanisms of action for synthetic cathinone derivatives are typically categorized as either presynaptic monoamine reuptake inhibitors or plasma membrane and vesicular monoamine transporter substrates.
- In laboratory animals and humans, exposure to synthetic cathinones, particularly long-term exposure at high doses, produces evidence of deficits in cognitive domains such as working and recognition memory, verbal fluency and recall, cognitive flexibility, and impulse control.
- Changes in tissue monoamines and presynaptic monoaminergic terminal protein content induced by synthetic cathinones in laboratory animals have yielded inconsistent results at low doses, and more consistent changes tend to be found following long-term exposure to higher doses.
- Synthetic cathinones can induce oxidative stress and cell death in a number of neuronal, hepatic, pulmonary, renal, and endothelial cell lines; however, cytotoxicity has been mostly observed after incubation periods >24 h at high (micromolar to millimolar) concentrations, which may be unlikely to take place in vivo.
- Endothelial cell damage has been observed with some synthetic cathinones, potentially contributing to compromised BBB function.
- Neurotoxic effects and cognitive deficits appear more readily when synthetic cathinones are combined with more traditional psychostimulants.
- Evidence of neuroinflammation induced by synthetic cathinones is currently insufficient, but requires further investigation.
- Determination of cytotoxic and neuroinflammatory mechanisms induced by synthetic cathinones may give direction for the development of therapeutic approaches for habitual users for the restoration of cognitive function and recovery from abuse.

References

Ageely HM (2008) Health and socio-economic hazards associated with khat consumption. J Fam Community Med 15:3–11

Ahmed A, Ruiz MJ, Cohen Kadosh K, Patton R, Resurreccion DM (2021) Khat and neurobehavioral functions: a systematic review. PLoS One 16:e0252900. https://doi.org/10.1371/journal.pone.0252900

Aleryani SL, Aleryani RA, Al-Akwa AA (2011) Khat a drug of abuse: roles of free radicals and antioxidants. Drug Test Anal 3:548–551. https://doi.org/10.1002/dta.224

Alles GA, Fairchild MD, Jensen M (1961) Chemical pharmacology of *Catha edulis*. J Med Pharm Chem 3:323–352. https://doi.org/10.1021/jm50015a010

Angoa-Perez M, Kane MJ, Francescutti DM, Sykes KE, Shah MM, Mohammed AM, Thomas DM, Kuhn DM (2012) Mephedrone, an abused psychoactive component of "bath salts" and methamphetamine congener, does not cause neurotoxicity to dopamine nerve endings of the striatum. J Neurochem 120:1097–1107. https://doi.org/10.1111/j.1471-4159.2011.07632.x

Angoa-Perez M, Kane MJ, Herrera-Mundo N, Francescutti DM, Kuhn DM (2014) Effects of combined treatment with mephedrone and methamphetamine or 3,4-methylenedioxymethamphetamine on serotonin nerve endings of the hippocampus. Life Sci 97:31–36. https://doi.org/10.1016/j.lfs.2013.07.015

Angoa-Perez M, Anneken JH, Kuhn DM (2017) Neurotoxicology of synthetic cathinone analogs. Curr Top Behav Neurosci 32:209–230. https://doi.org/10.1007/7854_2016_21

Anneken JH, Angoa-Perez M, Sati GC, Crich D, Kuhn DM (2017) Dissecting the influence of two structural substituents on the differential neurotoxic effects of acute methamphetamine and mephedrone treatment on dopamine nerve endings with the use of 4-methylmethamphetamine and methcathinone. J Pharmacol Exp Ther 360:417–423. https://doi.org/10.1124/jpet.116.237768

Anneken JH, Angoa-Perez M, Sati GC, Crich D, Kuhn DM (2018) Assessing the role of dopamine in the differential neurotoxicity patterns of methamphetamine, mephedrone, methcathinone and 4-methylmethamphetamine. Neuropharmacology 134:46–56. https://doi.org/10.1016/j.neuropharm.2017.08.033

Baker DA, McFarland K, Lake RW, Shen H, Tang XC, Toda S, Kalivas PW (2003) Neuroadaptations in cystine-glutamate exchange underlie cocaine relapse. Nat Neurosci 6:743–749

Baumann MH (2014) Awash in a sea of "bath salts": implications for biomedical research and public health. Addiction 109:1577–1579. https://doi.org/10.1111/add.12601

Baumann MH, Volkow ND (2016) Abuse of new psychoactive substances: threats and solutions. Neuropsychopharmacology 41:663–665. https://doi.org/10.1038/npp.2015.260

Baumann MH, Partilla JS, Lehner KR, Thorndike EB, Hoffman AF, Holy M, Rothman RB, Goldberg SR, Lupica CR, Sitte HH, Brandt SD, Tella SR, Cozzi NV, Schindler CW (2013) Powerful cocaine-like actions of 3,4-methylenedioxypyrovalerone (MDPV), a principal constituent of psychoactive "bath salts" products. Neuropsychopharmacology 38:552–562. https://doi.org/10.1038/npp.2012.204

Baumann MH, Bukhari MO, Lehner KR, Anizan S, Rice KC, Concheiro M, Huestis MA (2017) Neuropharmacology of 3,4-methylenedioxypyrovalerone (MDPV), its metabolites, and related analogs. Curr Top Behav Neurosci 32:93–117. https://doi.org/10.1007/7854_2016_53

Bernstein DL, Nayak SU, Oliver CF, Rawls SM, Rom S (2020) Methylenedioxypyrovalerone (MDPV) impairs working memory and alters patterns of dopamine signaling in mesocorticolimbic substrates. Neurosci Res 155:56–62

Bourgognon JM, Cavanagh J (2020) The role of cytokines in modulating learning and memory and brain plasticity. Brain Neurosci Adv 4:1–13. https://doi.org/10.1177/2398212820979802

Ciudad-Roberts A, Duart-Castells L, Camarasa J, Pubill D, Escubedo E (2016) The combination of ethanol with mephedrone increases the signs of neurotoxicity and impairs neurogenesis and learning in adolescent CD-1 mice. Toxicol Appl Pharmacol 293:10–20. https://doi.org/10.1016/j.taap.2015.12.019

Colzato LS, Ruiz MJ, van den Wildenberg WP, Bajo MT, Hommel B (2010) Long-term effects of chronic khat use: impaired inhibitory control. Front Psychol 1:219. https://doi.org/10.3389/fpsyg.2010.00219

Colzato LS, Ruiz MJ, van den Wildenberg WP, Hommel B (2011) Khat use is associated with impaired working memory and cognitive flexibility. PLoS One 6:e20602. https://doi.org/10.1371/journal.pone.0020602

Correia C, Romieu P, Olmstead MC, Befort K (2020) Can cocaine-induced neuroinflammation explain maladaptive cocaine-associated memories? Neurosci Biobehav Rev 111:69–83

Daniel JJ, Hughes RN (2016) Increased anxiety and impaired spatial memory in young adult rats following adolescent exposure to methylone. Pharmacol Biochem Behav 146–147:44–49. https://doi.org/10.1016/j.pbb.2016.05.003

de Sousa Fernandes Perna EB, Papaseit E, Perez-Mana C, Mateus J, Theunissen EL, Kuypers K, de la Torre R, Farre M, Ramaekers JG (2016) Neurocognitive performance following acute mephedrone administration, with and without alcohol. J Psychopharmacol 30:1305–1312. https://doi.org/10.1177/0269881116662635

den Hollander B, Rozov S, Linden AM, Uusi-Oukari M, Ojanpera I, Korpi ER (2013) Long-term cognitive and neurochemical effects of “bath salt” designer drugs methylone and mephedrone. Pharmacol Biochem Behav 103:501–509. https://doi.org/10.1016/j.pbb.2012.10.006

den Hollander B, Sundstrom M, Pelander A, Siltanen A, Ojanpera I, Mervaala E, Korpi ER, Kankuri E (2015) Mitochondrial respiratory dysfunction due to the conversion of substituted cathinones to methylbenzamides in SH-SY5Y cells. Sci Rep 5:14924. https://doi.org/10.1038/srep14924

Dolan SB, Chen Z, Huang R, Gatch MB (2018) “Ecstasy” to addiction: mechanisms and reinforcing effects of three synthetic cathinone analogs of MDMA. Neuropharmacology 133:171–180. https://doi.org/10.1016/j.neuropharm.2018.01.020

European Monitoring Centre for Drugs and Drug Addiction (2021) European Drug Report 2021: trends and developments. Publications Office of the European Union, Luxembourg. https://doi.org/10.2810/18539

Frazer KM, Richards Q, Keith DR (2018) The long-term effects of cocaine use on cognitive functioning: a systematic critical review. Behav Brain Res 348:241–262. https://doi.org/10.1016/j.bbr.2018.04.005

Freeman TP, Morgan CJ, Vaughn-Jones J, Hussain N, Karimi K, Curran HV (2012) Cognitive and subjective effects of mephedrone and factors influencing use of a “new legal high”. Addiction 107:792–800. https://doi.org/10.1111/j.1360-0443.2011.03719.x

García-Pardo MP, De la Rubia Ortí JE, Aguilar Calpe MA (2017) Differential effects of MDMA and cocaine on inhibitory avoidance and object recognition tests in rodents. Neurobiol Learn Mem 146:1–11. https://doi.org/10.1016/j.nlm.2017.10.013

Gaspar H, Bronze S, Oliveira C, Victor BL, Machuqueiro M, Pacheco R, Caldeira MJ, Santos S (2018) Proactive response to tackle the threat of emerging drugs: synthesis and toxicity evaluation of new cathinones. Forensic Sci Int 290:146–156

Gershman JA, Fass AD (2012) Synthetic cathinones (“bath salts”): legal and health care challenges. P T 37:571–595

Glennon RA, Young R (2016) Neurobiology of 3,4-methylenedioxypyrovalerone (MDPV) and alpha-pyrrolidinovalerophenone (alpha-PVP). Brain Res Bull 126:111–126. https://doi.org/10.1016/j.brainresbull.2016.04.011

Gregg RA, Hicks C, Nayak SU, Tallarida CS, Nucero P, Smith GR, Reitz AB, Rawls SM (2016) Synthetic cathinone MDPV downregulates glutamate transporter subtype I (GLT-1) and produces rewarding and locomotor-activating effects that are reduced by a GLT-1 activator. Neuropharmacology 108:111–119. https://doi.org/10.1016/j.neuropharm.2016.04.014

Grochecki P, Smaga I, Lopatynska-Mazurek M, Gibula-Tarlowska E, Kedzierska E, Listos J, Talarek S, Marszalek-Grabska M, Hubalewska-Mazgaj M, Korga-Plewko A, Dudka J, Marzec Z, Filip M, Kotlinska JH (2021) Effects of mephedrone and amphetamine exposure during adolescence on spatial memory in adulthood: behavioral and neurochemical analysis. Int J Mol Sci 22:589. https://doi.org/10.3390/ijms22020589

Hall C, Heyd C, Butler C, Yarema M (2014) “Bath salts” intoxication: a new recreational drug that presents with a familiar toxidrome. CJEM 16:171–176

Herzig DA, Brooks R, Mohr C (2013) Inferring about individual drug and schizotypy effects on cognitive functioning in polydrug using mephedrone users before and after clubbing. Hum Psychopharmacol 28:168–182. https://doi.org/10.1002/hup.2307

Hoffman R, al'Absi M (2013) Working memory and speed of information processing in chronic khat users: preliminary findings. Eur Addict Res 19:1–6. https://doi.org/10.1159/000338285

Homman L, Seglert J, Morgan MJ (2018) An observational study on the sub-acute effects of mephedrone on mood, cognition, sleep and physical problems in regular mephedrone users. Psychopharmacology 235:2609–2618

Hondebrink L, Zwartsen A, Westerink RHS (2018) Effect fingerprinting of new psychoactive substances (NPS): what can we learn from in vitro data? Pharmacol Ther 182:193–224. https://doi.org/10.1016/j.pharmthera.2017.10.022

Jacobs EH, Smit AB, De Vries TJ, Schoffelmeer ANM (2003) Neuroadaptive effects of active versus passive drug administration in addiction research. Trends Pharmacol Sci 24:566–573

Jîtcă G, Ősz BE, Tero-Vescan A, Vari CE (2021) Psychoactive drugs – from chemical structure to oxidative stress related to dopaminergic neurotransmission. A review. Antioxidants 10:381

Kalix P (1980) A constituent of khat leaves with amphetamine-like releasing properties. Eur J Pharmacol 68:213–215

Kalix P (1981) Cathinone, an alkaloid from khat leaves with an amphetamine-like releasing effect. Psychopharmacology 74:269–270

Kalix P (1982) The amphetamine-like releasing effect of the alkaloid(−)cathinone on rat nucleus accumbens and rabbit caudate nucleus. Prog Neuro-Psychopharmacol Biol Psychiatry 6:43–49

Kaminska K, Noworyta-Sokolowska K, Gorska A, Rzemieniec J, Wnuk A, Wojtas A, Kreiner G, Kajta M, Golembiowska K (2018) The effects of exposure to mephedrone during adolescence on brain neurotransmission and neurotoxicity in adult rats. Neurotox Res 34:525–537

Karch SB (2015) Cathinone neurotoxicity ("the 3Ms"). Curr Neuropharmacol 13:21–25. https://doi.org/10.2174/1570159X13666141210225009

Karila L, Megarbane B, Cottencin O, Lejoyeux M (2015) Synthetic cathinones: a new public health problem. Curr Neuropharmacol 13:12–20. https://doi.org/10.2174/1570159X13666141210224137

Karila L, Lafaye G, Scocard A, Cottencin O, Benyamina A (2018) MDPV and a-PVP use in humans: the twisted sisters. Neuropharmacology 134:65–72. https://doi.org/10.1016/j.neuropharm.2017.10.007

Kenyon EM (2012) Interspecies extrapolation. Methods Mol Biol 929:501–520. https://doi.org/10.1007/978-1-62703-050-2_19

Khattab NY, Amer G (1995) Undetected neuropsychophysiological sequelae of khat chewing in standard aviation medical examination. Aviat Space Environ Med 66:739–744

Kolanos R, Solis EJ, Sakloth F, De Felice LJ, Glennon RA (2013) "Deconstruction" of the abused synthetic cathinone methylenedioxypyrovalerone (MDPV) and an examination of effects at the human dopamine transporter. ACS Chem Neurosci 4:1524–1529. https://doi.org/10.1021/cn4001236

Kopec AM, Smith CJ, Bilbo SD (2019) Neuro-immune mechanisms regulating social behavior: dopamine as mediator? Trends Neurosci 42:337–348

Lacagnina MJ, Rivera PD, Bilbo SD (2017) Glial and neuroimmune mechanisms as critical modulators of drug use and abuse. Neuropsychopharmacology 42:156–177. https://doi.org/10.1038/npp.2016.121

Leyrer-Jackson JM, Nagy EK, Olive MF (2019) Cognitive deficits and neurotoxicity induced by synthetic cathinones: is there a role for neuroinflammation? Psychopharmacology 236:1079–1095. https://doi.org/10.1007/s00213-018-5067-5

London ED, Kohno M, Morales AM, Ballard ME (2015) Chronic methamphetamine abuse and corticostriatal deficits revealed by neuroimaging. Brain Res 1628:174–185. https://doi.org/10.1016/j.brainres.2014.10.044

Lopez-Arnau R, Martinez-Clemente J, Abad S, Pubill D, Camarasa J, Escubedo E (2014a) Repeated doses of methylone, a new drug of abuse, induce changes in serotonin and dopamine systems in the mouse. Psychopharmacology 231:3119–3129. https://doi.org/10.1007/s00213-014-3493-6

Lopez-Arnau R, Martinez-Clemente J, Pubill D, Escubedo E, Camarasa J (2014b) Serotonergic impairment and memory deficits in adolescent rats after binge exposure of methylone. J Psychopharmacol 28:1053–1063. https://doi.org/10.1177/0269881114548439

Lopez-Arnau R, Martinez-Clemente J, Rodrigo T, Pubill D, Camarasa J, Escubedo E (2015) Neuronal changes and oxidative stress in adolescent rats after repeated exposure to mephedrone. Toxicol Appl Pharmacol 286:27–35. https://doi.org/10.1016/j.taap.2015.03.015

Luethi D, Kolaczynska KE, Docci L, Krahenbuhl S, Hoener MC, Liechti ME (2018) Pharmacological profile of mephedrone analogs and related new psychoactive substances. Neuropharmacology 134:4–12. https://doi.org/10.1016/j.neuropharm.2017.07.026

Luethi D, Kolaczynska KE, Walter M, Suzuki M, Rice KC, Blough BE, Hoener MC, Baumann MH, Liechti ME (2019) Metabolites of the ring-substituted stimulants MDMA, methylone and MDPV differentially affect human monoaminergic systems. J Psychopharmacol 33(7):831–841

Majchrzak M, Celinski R, Kus P, Kowalska T, Sajewicz M (2018) The newest cathinone derivatives as designer drugs: an analytical and toxicological review. Forensic Toxicol 36:33–50. https://doi.org/10.1007/s11419-017-0385-6

Marinelli S, Basilico B, Marrone MC, Ragozzino D (2019) Microglia-neuron crosstalk: signaling mechanism and control of synaptic transmission. Semin Cell Dev Biol 94:138–151. https://doi.org/10.1016/j.semcdb.2019.05.017

Martinez-Clemente J, Lopez-Arnau R, Abad S, Pubill D, Escubedo E, Camarasa J (2014) Dose and time-dependent selective neurotoxicity induced by mephedrone in mice. PLoS One 9:e99002. https://doi.org/10.1371/journal.pone.0099002

Mayer FP, Schmid D, Holy M, Daws LC, Sitte HH (2018) "Polytox" synthetic cathinone abuse: a potential role for organic cation transporter 3 in combined cathinone-induced efflux. Neurochem Int. https://doi.org/10.1016/j.neuint.2018.09.008

Mead J, Parrott A (2020) Mephedrone and MDMA: a comparative review. Brain Res 1735:146740. https://doi.org/10.1016/j.brainres.2020.146740

Moszczynska A, Callan SP (2017) Molecular, behavioral, and physiological consequences of methamphetamine neurotoxicity: implications for treatment. J Pharmacol Exp Ther 362:474–488. https://doi.org/10.1124/jpet.116.238501

Motbey CP, Karanges E, Li KM, Wilkinson S, Winstock AR, Ramsay J, Hicks C, Kendig MD, Wyatt N, Callaghan PD, McGregor IS (2012) Mephedrone in adolescent rats: residual memory impairment and acute but not lasting 5-HT depletion. PLoS One 7:e45473. https://doi.org/10.1371/journal.pone.0045473

Nakajima M, Hoffman R, Al'Absi M (2014) Poor working memory and reduced blood pressure levels in concurrent users of khat and tobacco. Nicotine Tob Res 16:279–287. https://doi.org/10.1093/ntr/ntt139

Negus SS, Banks ML (2017) Decoding the structure of abuse potential for new psychoactive substances: structure-activity relationships for abuse-related effects of 4-substituted methcathinone analogs. Curr Top Behav Neurosci 32:119–131. https://doi.org/10.1007/7854_2016_18

Numan N (2004) Exploration of adverse psychological symptoms in Yemeni khat users by the Symptoms Checklist-90 (SCL-90). Addiction 99:61–65. https://doi.org/10.1111/j.1360-0443.2004.00570.x

Odenwald M, Neuner F, Schauer M, Elbert T, Catani C, Lingenfelder B, Hinkel H, Hafner H, Rockstroh B (2005) Khat use as risk factor for psychotic disorders: a cross-sectional and case-control study in Somalia. BMC Med 3:5. https://doi.org/10.1186/1741-7015-3-5

Odenwald M, Hinkel H, Schauer E, Schauer M, Elbert T, Neuner F, Rockstroh B (2009) Use of khat and posttraumatic stress disorder as risk factors for psychotic symptoms: a study of Somali combatants. Soc Sci Med 69:1040–1048. https://doi.org/10.1016/j.socscimed.2009.07.020

Oliver CF, Simmons SJ, Nayak SU, Smith GR, Reitz AB, Rawls SM (2018) Chemokines and "bath salts": CXCR4 receptor antagonist reduces rewarding and locomotor-stimulant effects of the designer cathinone MDPV in rats. Drug Alcohol Depend 186:75–79. https://doi.org/10.1016/j.drugalcdep.2018.01.013

Ordak M, Nasierowski T, Muszynska E, Bujalska-Zadrozny M (2020) The psychiatric characteristics of people on a mephedrone ("bath salts") binge. Subst Use Misuse 55:1610–1617. https://doi.org/10.1080/10826084.2020.1753775

Palamar JJ, Salomone A, Vincenti M, Cleland CM (2016) Detection of "bath salts" and other novel psychoactive substances in hair samples of ecstasy/MDMA/"Molly" users. Drug Alcohol Depend 161:200–205

Pantano F, Tittarelli R, Mannocchi G, Pacifici R, di Luca A, Busardo FP, Marinelli E (2017) Neurotoxicity induced by mephedrone: an up-to-date review. Curr Neuropharmacol 15:738–749. https://doi.org/10.2174/1570159X14666161130130718

Pascual M, Montesinos J, Guerri C (2018) Role of the innate immune system in the neuropathological consequences induced by adolescent binge drinking. J Neurosci Res 96:765–780. https://doi.org/10.1002/jnr.24203

Patel NB (2019) Khat (*Catha edulis* Forsk) – and now there are three. Brain Res Bull 145:92–96. https://doi.org/10.1016/j.brainresbull.2018.07.014

Pimentel E, Sivalingam K, Doke M, Samikkannu T (2020) Effects of drugs of abuse on the blood-brain barrier: a brief overview. Front Neurosci 14:513

Potvin S, Pelletier J, Grot S, Hebert C, Barr AM, Lecomte T (2018) Cognitive deficits in individuals with methamphetamine use disorder: a meta-analysis. Addict Behav 80:154–160. https://doi.org/10.1016/j.addbeh.2018.01.021

Riley AL, Nelson KH, To P, Lopez-Arnau R, Xu P, Wang D, Wang Y, Shen HW, Kuhn DM, Angoa-Perez M, Anneken JH, Muskiewicz D, Hall FS (2020) Abuse potential and toxicity of the synthetic cathinones (i.e., "bath salts"). Neurosci Biobehav Rev 110:150–173

Salim S (2017) Oxidative stress and the central nervous system. J Pharmacol Exp Ther 360:201–205. https://doi.org/10.1124/jpet.116.237503

Savulich G, Bowden-Jones O, Stephenson R, Brühl AB, Ersche KD, Robbins TW, Sahakian BJ (2021) "Hot" and "cold" cognition in users of club drugs/novel psychoactive substances. Front Psychiatry 12:680575. https://doi.org/10.3389/fpsyt.2021.660575

Sewalia K, Watterson LR, Hryciw A, Belloc A, Ortiz JB, Olive MF (2018) Neurocognitive dysfunction following repeated binge-like self-administration of the synthetic cathinone 3,4-methylenedioxypyrovalerone (MDPV). Neuropharmacology 134:36–45. https://doi.org/10.1016/j.neuropharm.2017.11.034

Shaerzadeh F, Streit WJ, Heysieattalab S, Khoshbouei H (2018) Methamphetamine neurotoxicity, microglia, and neuroinflammation. J Neuroinflammation 15:341

Sharma V, McNeill JH (2009) To scale or not to scale: the principles of dose extrapolation. Br J Pharmacol 157:907–921. https://doi.org/10.1111/j.1476-5381.2009.00267.x

Simmler LD, Liechti ME (2017) Interactions of cathinone NPS with human transporters and receptors in transfected cells. Curr Top Behav Neurosci 32:49–72. https://doi.org/10.1007/7854_2016_20

Simmler LD, Buser TA, Donzelli M, Schramm Y, Dieu LH, Huwyler J, Chaboz S, Hoener MC, Liechti ME (2013) Pharmacological characterization of designer cathinones in vitro. Br J Pharmacol 168:458–470. https://doi.org/10.1111/j.1476-5381.2012.02145.x

Simmler LD, Buchy D, Chaboz S, Hoener MC, Liechti ME (2016) In vitro characterization of psychoactive substances at rat, mouse, and human trace amine-associated receptor 1. J Pharmacol Exp Ther 357:134–144. https://doi.org/10.1124/jpet.115.229765

Simmons SJ, Leyrer-Jackson JM, Oliver CF, Hicks C, Muschamp JW, Rawls SM, Olive MF (2018) DARK classics in chemical neuroscience: cathinone-derived psychostimulants. ACS Chem Neurosci 9:2379–2394. https://doi.org/10.1021/acschemneuro.8b00147

Soares J, Costa VM, Bastos ML, Carvalho F, Capela JP (2021) An updated review on synthetic cathinones. Arch Toxicol. https://doi.org/10.1007/s00204-021-03083-3

Soleimani SMA, Ekhtiari H, Cadet JL (2016) Drug-induced neurotoxicity in addiction medicine: from prevention to harm reduction. Prog Brain Res 223:19–41. https://doi.org/10.1016/bs.pbr.2015.07.004

Stuber GD, Hopf FW, Tye KM, Chen BT, Bonci A (2010) Neuroplastic alterations in the limbic system following cocaine or alcohol exposure. Curr Top Behav Neurosci 3:3–27. https://doi.org/10.1007/7854_2009_23

Tchessalova D, Posillico CK, Tronson NC (2018) Neuroimmune activation drives multiple brain states. Front Syst Neurosci 12:39

Valente MJ, Guedes de Pinho P, de Lourdes Bastos M, Carvalho F, Carvalho M (2014) Khat and synthetic cathinones: a review. Arch Toxicol 88:15–45. https://doi.org/10.1007/s00204-013-1163-9

Valente MJ, Araujo AM, Silva R, Bastos Mde L, Carvalho F, Guedes de Pinho P, Carvalho M (2016) 3,4-Methylenedioxypyrovalerone (MDPV): in vitro mechanisms of hepatotoxicity under normothermic and hyperthermic conditions. Arch Toxicol 90:1959–1973. https://doi.org/10.1007/s00204-015-1653-z

Wagner GC, Preston K, Ricaurte GA, Schuster CR, Seiden LS (1982) Neurochemical similarities between d,l-cathinone and d-amphetamine. Drug Alcohol Depend 9:279–284

Weed PF, Leonard ST, Sankaranarayanan A, Winsauer PJ (2014) Estradiol administration to ovariectomized rats potentiates mephedrone-induced disruptions of nonspatial learning. J Exp Anal Behav 101:303–315. https://doi.org/10.1002/jeab.72

Winder GS, Stern N, Hosanagar A (2013) Are “bath salts” the next generation of stimulant abuse? J Subst Abus Treat 44:42–45. https://doi.org/10.1016/j.jsat.2012.02.003

Winstock AR, Mitcheson LR, Deluca P, Davey Z, Corazza O, Schifano F (2011) Mephedrone, new kid for the chop? Addiction 106:154–161. https://doi.org/10.1111/j.1360-0443.2010.03130.x

Wood DM, Dargan PI (2012) Mephedrone (4-methylmethcathinone): what is new in our understanding of its use and toxicity. Prog Neuro-Psychopharmacol Biol Psychiatry 39:227–233. https://doi.org/10.1016/j.pnpbp.2012.04.020

Wood S, Sage JR, Shuman T, Anagnostaras SG (2014) Psychostimulants and cognition: a continuum of behavioral and cognitive activation. Pharmacol Rev 66:193–221. https://doi.org/10.1124/pr.112.007054

Wright MJ Jr, Vandewater SA, Angrish D, Dickerson TJ, Taffe MA (2012) Mephedrone (4-methylmethcathinone) and d-methamphetamine improve visuospatial associative memory, but not spatial working memory, in rhesus macaques. Br J Pharmacol 167:1342–1352. https://doi.org/10.1111/j.1476-5381.2012.02091.x

Yirmiya R, Goshen I (2011) Immune modulation of learning, memory, neural plasticity and neurogenesis. Brain Behav Immun 25:181–213. https://doi.org/10.1016/j.bbi.2010.10.015

Zaami S, Giorgetti R, Pichini S, Pantano F, Marinelli E, Busardo FP (2018) Synthetic cathinones related fatalities: an update. Eur Rev Med Pharmacol Sci 22:268–274. https://doi.org/10.26355/eurrev_201801_14129

Zhang HB, Zhao D, Liu YP, Wang LX, Yang B, Yuan TF (2021) Problem-solving deficits in methcathinone use disorder. Psychopharmacology. https://doi.org/10.1007/s00213-021-05874-z

Khat Use in Defined Population

80

Prisoners

Yimenu Yitayih

Contents

Introduction 1706
Burden of Khat Use 1707
Khat Use and Crime 1708
Addressing Khat Use Inside Prison 1710
Application to Other Areas of Addiction 1711
Application to Other Areas of Public Health 1711
Conclusion on Current Situation and Future Prospects 1712
Mini-Dictionary of Terms 1712
Key Facts of Khat Use Among Prisoners 1713
Summary Points 1713
References 1713

Abstract

Globally, 20 million people chew khat on a daily basis. It is commonly used in East Africa and Arabian Peninsula countries, and nearly ten million people consume khat. Evidence reveals that 59.9% of prisoners have history of khat use. Substance use, particularly amphetamine, is strongly related with violent crimes. Recent qualitative studies have shown that khat use has an association with domestic violence. This chapter provides current literatures khat use with emphasis on providing basic information on the characteristics of khat, magnitude, association with crime, and interventions for khat use inside the prison. First we will deliver crucial information on the burden of khat and how it relates with crime. We also present an overview briefly on addressing khat use inside the prison and conclude by integrative summary and call for further research. In khat belt countries, khat abuse is treated as usually by nonspecific standard psychiatric care treatment. In light of this, prison administrative system provides unique opportunity to intervention for khat users while in prison and after release from

Y. Yitayih (✉)
Department of Psychiatry, Jimma University, Jimma, Ethiopia

V. B. Patel, V. R. Preedy (eds.), *Handbook of Substance Misuse and Addictions*,
https://doi.org/10.1007/978-3-030-92392-1_87

prison in order to disrupt vicious circle of khat use and crime. Only, qualitative studies describe the association of khat use with domestic violence, and yet no studies explore causal link between khat and crime. Whether khat use is thought as facilitator of social communication or as cause for domestic violence, longitudinal research on investigation of the effect of khat use on crime are needed to clarify its causal link.

Keywords

Cathine · Cathinone · Crime · Khat · Prisoners

Abbreviations

ASB	Antisocial behavior
PE	Psychoeducation
USA	United States of America
WHO	World Health Organization

Introduction

Khat (*Catha edulis*, also known as qat, qaad, jaat, or miraa) is stimulant plant tree belonging to the family of Celastraceae, grown in East Africa and Arabian countries. It is mainly cultivated in Ethiopia, Somalia, Kenya, Yemen, and Djibouti as well as in Southern Arabia (Nencini et al. 1989).

Khat leaves are branded, to some extent, as with sweet taste with astringent and aromatic odor (Cox and Rampes 2003). Khat contains different chemical components such as alkaloids, terpenoids, flavonoids, sterols, glycosides, amino acids, minerals, tannins, and vitamins (Cox and Rampes 2003; Nencini et al. 1989; Kalix and Braenden 1985). The main psychoactive alkaloids present in khat leaves are S-(−)-cathinone (s--aminopropriophenone), norpseudoephedrine (cathine), and norephedrine (Engidawork 2017). Fresh khat leaves of 100 mg contains 36 mg of cathinone, 120 mg cathine, and 8 mg norephedrine (Geisshüsler and Brenneisen 1987).

Studies by (Kalix 1988) have shown that cathinone is the main psychoactive alkaloids in khat leaves. In particular, cathinone like amphetamine ingestions has sympathomimetic activity that facilitates the release of endogenous catecholamines from central and peripheral neurons (Patel 2019). Cathinone metabolized into norpseudoephedrine and ephedrine, and these metabolites have weaker central stimulating properties (Toennes et al. 2003). Moreover, cathinone is responsible for CNS effect, whereas norpseudoephedrine is for peripheral effects.

In the 1980s, in the Convention on Psychotropic Substances, cathinone is listed in Schedule I and cathine in Schedule III, while norephedrine is controlled under United Nations Convention against Illicit Traffic in Narcotic Drugs and Psychotropic Substances (Kalix and Toxicology 1992; Widler et al. 1994). However, in 2006, the World Health Organization (WHO) does not recommend khat leaves to be scheduled under international conventions due to paucity of evidences on public health threat to authorize international control over khat leaves (Series 2006).

Khat chewing takes place either in ceremonial form with the company of others or alone and has a religious rituals and cultural and social values, and this was shown previously (Balint et al. 2009).

Chewing fresh leaves of the khat tree is the most common mode of intake, while few users consume it in liquid form by adding dried leaves (Hoffman and Al'Absi 2010). Khat is generally used for its euphoric effects and perceived ability to facilitate interpersonal communication, enhance performance, and fend off fatigue, as well as for its medicinal value in the treatment of headaches and common cold (Wabe and health 2011). Once a person is underway taking substance, they experience psychoactive effect and activates circuits in the brain that will make it more likely that the person will repeat this behavior (Tretter et al. 2009). Substance use, particularly amphetamine, is strongly related with violent crimes (Klee and Policy 2001). Recent qualitative study done by Havell (2004) reveals that khat use has an association with domestic violence (Havell 2004).

Despite, synthetic amphetamine and crime are the two entities that are strongly related, yet little is known about khat and crime. This chapter describes current literatures on khat use among prisoners and its association with crime. First we will deliver crucial information on burden of khat and how it relates with crime. Then, we will overview briefly on addressing khat use in the prison. Finally, we will conclude by integrative summary and call for further research.

Burden of Khat Use

Globally, 20 million people chew khat on a daily basis (Eckersley et al. 2010). It is commonly used in East Africa and Arabian Peninsula countries, and nearly ten million people consume khat (Balint et al. 1991). Evidences revealed that khat is used on a daily basis in East Africa, ranging from 80 to 90% in adult male and 10 to 60% in adult female (Numan 2004; Odenwald et al. 2005). Khat use is highly prevalent in Yemen, with estimated prevalence ranging between 60 and 90% in adult male and 10 and 50% in adult females (Gatter 2012). In Ethiopia, the prevalence of khat use for adult male is 22.6% (Haile and Lakew 2015) and, for reproductive aged women, is 9.1% (Yitayih and van Os 2021). Khat chewing is highest among adults aged 45–49 years compared to youths aged 15–19 years (Haile and Lakew 2015). Those who started to use substance at an earlier age of 14 years or younger were more likely to become addicted than those who started at a later age (Sadock 2011).

Khat use is an important public concern and highly associated with mental health problems such as psychological distress and increased road traffic accidents (Eckersley et al. 2010). People who use khat have higher proportion of mood disturbance, major depression, and suicidal ideation than their counterparts (Bhui et al. 2006; Griffiths et al. 1997; Hassan et al. 2002). They are also more likely to have post-traumatic stress symptoms (Bhui et al. 2003) and to have impairment in working memory (Colzato et al. 2011). Consequently, khat use is associated with exacerbation of psychotic symptoms especially in individuals with preexisting psychotic disorder or family history of psychosis (Odenwald et al. 2012; Teferra et al. 2011).

Though khat use is common among all segments of populations, higher prevalence of khat use is found among prisoners than the general community. Also, community samples are not, however, necessarily reflective of people in custodial settings, where histories of drug and alcohol use are particularly high compared with the general population. The prevalence of substance use among prisoners in England, Kenya, and Ethiopia is 54, 66.1, and 55.9%, respectively (Stewart 2009; Kinyanjui and Atwoli 2013; Yitayih et al. 2018). In 2017 survey done in Ethiopia, 59.9% of prisoners in Jimma correctional center have history of khat use (Yitayih et al. 2020).

In prison, substance use is almost banned but there is possibility of continuing khat use in prison. Prisons are theoretically being an ideal setting for accessing prisoners and preventing and treating addiction, yet there is no addiction care service and it is crucial to consider the mental health implications for those individuals who are addicted. Addicted prisoners' life is troublesome if not given adequate treatment in prison and supervision in the community upon discharge because released inmates have high potential to become re-addicted and commit crime. Treatment program that targets addiction in prison is valuable intervention for prevention of relapse after release and decreasing recidivism in the community.

Khat Use and Crime

Substance use disrupts normal brain function that encourages aggression or violence (Gmel et al. 2003).

According to disinhibition hypothesis, alcohol weakens brain mechanisms that normally restrain impulsive behavior, including inappropriate aggression (Gmel et al. 2003). Alcohol impairs information processing that leads a person misjudging social cues, thereby overacting to a perceived threat (Sharp et al. 2006). Similarly, a narrowing of attention may lead to an erroneous assessment of future risks and acting on an abrupt violent impulse (Cook et al. 1993). Substance use is implicated in substance-related offenses, and now and then, substance users steal money or property to be able to purchase substances (Dorsey et al. 2010). State prisoners (17%) and federal prisoners (18%) in the USA committed crime to get money for their substances (Dorsey et al. 2010). Substance users often commit crime while feeling high by the effect of substances (Pernanen et al. 2000).

The association between substance use and crime can be explained by four causal models (Collins and Lapsley 2008; Pernanen et al. 2000). These are 1) intoxication model, 2) economic-compulsive model, 3) substance defined model, and 4) systematic model. The intoxication model proposes that substance intoxication has direct link to crime committed (Pernanen et al. 2000). The hypothesis is that substance assists the individuals to commit crime; otherwise, crime will not happen if the individual was not under the effect of substances. Many other studies referred this model as disinhibition model or pharmacological model. Especially, on alcohol, perpetrator committed crimes while drinking; it is assumed as caused by alcohol drinking.

The economic-compulsive model or economic means model proposes that crimes are committed to get the looked-for substances, and mainly it is acquisitive crimes (Pernanen et al. 2000). It is linked with intention of getting money or other resources to buy the desired psychoactive substances.

The third model, substance defined model, is not a causal one but explains crimes committed due to the breaking of rule that regulates drug use either in sale, production, or possession in the community (Pernanen et al. 2000).

Crimes are direct result of drug prohibition laws and reveal tautological connection between substance use and crime. In substance defined model, several substance-related crimes are encompassed like drinking and driving, production, smuggling, and trafficking of drugs.

This model suggests drug use is 100% an attributable factor for committed crime.

Finally, systematic models elucidate crimes are correlated to dealing with illegal substances such as crimes allied to trading drugs, collecting drug debts, and conflicting over drug territory. This crime will not take place, if individuals had not been involved with illegal economy transactions linked to illicit substance-derived economy.

Overlap is anticipated between four models, for example, individuals try to collect drug debt in distribution chains using violence to get drugs or an expedient way to buy drugs for personal use. Correspondingly, crime committed under the influence of drug intoxications may be motivated by the intentions of getting more drugs for personal use.

A number of qualitative studies show that khat use is associated with domestic violence (Havell 2004). In Australia study, it was found out that khat withdrawal symptoms, i.e., irritability and depression, lead to violence than direct khat effect (Douglas et al. 2012). Researches revealed that <2% of women experiencing mood swings or temper are khat users' partner, whereas <1% experience violence (Patel et al. 2005). Studies done by Fitzgerald (2010) have shown that not the direct effect of khat use is attributable to domestic violence, whereas the amount of money and time spent on khat chewing are factors for violence (Feigin et al. 2010).

Although researchers have hypothesized that causal relationships exist between khat use and domestic violence, other studies have concluded that there is no evidence that reveals the association between khat use and acquisitive crime (ACMD 2005).

The study done by Patel and policy (2008) shows that there is no association between khat use and acquisitive offending, and this might be due to nonaddictive nature of khat and a cheap cost of bundle of khat (Patel and Policy 2008).

Crime pattern analysis revealed that mafrishi or khat café was safer relatively than other café houses; however, the public fears of khat use leading to crime were not emanated by research (Klein and misuse 2008). The comorbid antisocial behavior (ASB) of khat user may predispose to crime than the direct effect of khat use (Sykes et al. 2010).

Some features of ASB associated with khat users are noise, smoking, urinating, shouting, spitting out of leaves on street, quarrelling among users, and double parking. Similarly in study done in Ethiopia, there is high prevalence of khat abuse (78%) among prisoners with psychopathy (Yitayih et al. 2020).

Khat is cultivated in gardens in Australia, and trespassing to collect khat leaves is considered as crime (Douglas et al. 2012).

In Netherlands, some features of ASB like spitting out khat leaves on the street, shouting, and quarrelling have been reported of khat users. There is no organized crime committed, related to khat trade, where khat is legal (Pennings et al. 2008).

However, in countries where khat is illegal, there is an association between khat trade and organized crime. Moreover, in Sweden, khat is illegal, and transnational crime group was formed and Somali traders have reacted to increase in penalties by diversifying their drug imports into drugs with a substantially higher profit margin like cannabis and cocaine (Jelsma et al. 2012).

Khat use had a multidimensional career, like other substance use. Only, qualitative studies describe the association of khat use with domestic violence, and yet no studies explore causal link between khat and crime. Whether khat use was thought as facilitator of social communication or as cause for domestic violence, longitudinal research on investigation of the effect of khat use on crime are needed to clarify its causal link.

Addressing Khat Use Inside Prison

Substance use disorder in prisoners had negative impacts at individual level and community well-being. Substance use increases criminal behavior and likelihood of arrest by increasing the need to commit crimes. Drug use among prison inmates is worrisome if not treated as released inmates have high potential to become re-addicted and commit another crime. Addressing substance use problems inside the prison yields sole opportunity to threat substance use disorder and decrease associated criminal behavior. There are therapeutic alternatives to incarceration such as treatment merged with judicial oversight in drug courts, prison- and jail-based treatment, and reentry programs intended to help prisoners that are widely used interventional approaches for prisoners who use drugs (Knight and Farabee 2004; Leukefeld et al. 2002). The most commonly used behavioral interventions are cognitive therapies (focus on coping and decision-making skills), contingency management therapy (strengthen abstinence), and motivational therapy (foster the motivation to participate in interventional programs) (Wormith et al. 2007; Prendergast et al. 2002).

In khat belt countries, khat abuse is treated as usually by nonspecific standard psychiatric care treatment. On the other hand, in developed countries, they provide treatment for khat abuse, by integrating into general treatment programs for illicit substances. Similar to treatment for other groups of illegal substance users, in Sweden and the UK, deliver psychosocial support for khat users due to complicated problems that khat users faces. A study done in Somali, adapted version of

ASIST-linked Brief Intervention, shows decrease in khat chewing time and reduction in khat use for individuals without comorbid psychopathology (Widmann et al. 2017). Prisoners with addiction problems can be treated by psychoeducation while in the prison (Taxman et al. 2007). Psychoeducation is a valuable intervention to reduce khat use, yet the intervention should be given in cultural context (Odenwald et al. 2009).

Overall, khat researches are focused on prevalence and to some extent on consequences of khat use, but there is paucity of studies on treatment of khat use disorders. Despite, the prison is ideal setting for treatment of prisoners with khat use problem, and there is no treatment service inside the prison as well as no community supervision after release to the community. Further, only few khat users seek help (Duresso et al. 2016), and in light of this, prison administrative system provides unique opportunity to intervention for khat users while in prison and after release from prison in order to disrupt vicious circle of khat use and crime.

Application to Other Areas of Addiction

In this chapter, we have reviewed studies on khat use among prisoners and its association with crime and interventions in the prison. In a single study done in Ethiopia, more than half of prisoners have lifetime history of khat abuse (Yitayih et al. 2020). Indeed, very few studies reveal as there is association between khat use and domestic violence (Havell 2004), but no studies show association with acquisitive crimes (Patel and policy 2008). Apart from initiatives on the prevalence and qualitative studies on khat use among prisoners, no treatment intervention studies and services for khat abuse are available in the prison. So, this review highlights the need to investigate longitudinally the casual link between khat use and crime. Furthermore, there is a need to establish the addiction health services in prison and implement rehabilitation services after release from the prison. This has implications and application for other addictions. Significantly, psychoeducation (PE) components of intervention for khat users decrease the amount of time spent on using khat and reduce khat use.

Similarly, this PE intervention is widely provided service for addressing alcohol misuse and dependences (Taxman et al. 2007). Further, community-based treatment for khat use helps as well to other addictive substances in addressing difficulties that arise when they return to the community and curbs relapse for addiction. Being involved in community-based treatment fosters the individual capacity to stay in sober that has been made during prison-based treatment.

Application to Other Areas of Public Health

In this review, we reveal the high prevalence of khat use among prisoners before and during imprisonment. This highlights that prisoner with substance use problems needs intervention programs to be integrated between the community and prison. This high prevalence of khat use provides an opportunity to implement interventions that are effective in other situations that can be transferred to prison setting. Undertaking interventions in any stages of imprisonment, i.e., treating withdrawal symptoms immediately during arrival at prison, treatment during stay in prison (Payne-James et al. 2005), and providing integrated treatment after release from prison by linking to the community (Thomas et al. 2016). To tackle consequences of substance use such as premature mortality, recidivism, and subsequent return to prison and prevent the relapse of substance use, there is a need to design comprehensive strategy.

Khat is a traditional drug that has been used for centuries in East Africa and is widely used among large parts of the population. Recently, the (mis)use of khat has become one of the major public health and socioeconomic problems in khat belt countries. As a consequence, a new national strategic action plan (NSAP) for the prevention and control of noncommunicable diseases (NCD) was adopted, after the Brazzaville Declaration on Noncommunicable Diseases in 2011.

One of the main strategies is advocacy, social mobilization, and sensitization for NCD program implementation, with emphasis on major risk factors (substance use, diet, and exercise). These strategies are very important because it potentially enhances quality of life and well-being of individuals.

Conclusion on Current Situation and Future Prospects

The purpose of this chapter was to provide a state of the science review of studies done on khat use among prisoners and its association with crime. Overall, some of work has demonstrated that khat use has association with violence. Taken together, the research on current knowledge base regarding magnitudes of khat use among prisoners and its association with crime is in its infancy, and available studies are limited by a weak methodology, small sample sizes, qualitative studies, lack of follow-up, and a lack of controls. This highlights the critical need for continued research in this area to examine these questions in large samples, with adequate controls and long-term follow-up assessments in order to understand the long-term effects, a major question which still remains.

Future research is needed to evaluate the effectiveness of addiction treatment in prison setting. Indeed, it is a timely need for pertinent stakeholders of khat belt countries to introduce novel khat treatment approaches in the prison to generate financially sustainable programs for the early diagnosis, treatment, and control of khat use through a group of well-trained healthcare providers and awareness creation in the prison.

Mini-Dictionary of Terms

Cathinone. A monoamine alkaloid found in the shrub of khat. This drug acts by facilitating the release of endogenous catecholamines from central and peripheral neurons.

Cathine. Psychoactive drug of the phenethylamine and natural amphetamine, which acts as a stimulant. It is found naturally in khat and it has nearly 7–10% the potency of amphetamine.

Domestic violence. Intimate partner violence, committed by one of the people in an intimate relationship against the other person.

Common names of khat. *Catha edulis* or qat, qaad, and jaat also known as miraa.

Khat. A plant in which the leaf and stem are used as a recreational drug and as medicine.

Key Facts of Khat Use Among Prisoners

- Khat like amphetamine ingestions has sympathomimetic activity that facilitates the release of endogenous catecholamines from central and peripheral neurons.
- Khat is highly prevalent and globally, 20 million people chew khat on a daily basis.
- Cathinone is listed in Schedule I and cathine in Schedule III, while khat is not scheduled under international convention.
- Khat use is associated with domestic violence as shown by qualitative studies.
- Khat contains different chemical components such as alkaloids, terpenoids, flavonoids, sterols, glycosides, amino acids, minerals, tannins, and vitamins.

Summary Points

- Khat use elicits a variety of behaviors such as mood disturbance, major depression, suicidal ideation, post-traumatic stress symptoms, impairment in working memory, and aggression.
- Comorbid antisocial behavior of khat users may predispose to crime than the direct effect of khat use.
- Khat is an important public health problem, and 59.9% of prisoners in Jimma correctional center have history of khat use.
- Crime pattern analysis revealed that mafrishi or khat café was safer relatively than other café houses; however, public fears of khat use leading to crime were not emanated by research.
- In khat belt countries, khat abuse is treated as usually by nonspecific standard psychiatric care treatment.

References

ACMD, KJACOTMOD (2005) Assessment of risk to the individual and communities in the UK

Balint G, Ghebrekidan H, Balint EJEAMJ (1991) Catha edulis, an international socio-medical problem with considerable pharmacological implications. 68:555–561

Balint EE, Falkay G, Balint GAJWKW (2009) Khat–a controversial plant. 121:604–614
Bhui K, Abdi A, Abdi M, Pereira S, Dualeh M, Robertson D, Sathyamoorthy G, Ismail HJSP, Epidemiology P (2003) Traumatic events, migration characteristics and psychiatric symptoms among Somali refugees. 38:35–43
Bhui K, Craig T, Mohamud S, Warfa N, Stansfeld SA, Thornicroft G, Curtis S, McCrone PJSP, Epidemiology P (2006) Mental disorders among Somali refugees. 41:400
Collins D, Lapsley HM (2008) The costs of tobacco, alcohol and illicit drug abuse to Australian society in 2004/05. Department of Health and Ageing, Canberra
Colzato LS, Ruiz MJ, Van Den Wildenberg WP, Hommel BJPO (2011) Khat use is associated with impaired working memory and cognitive flexibility. 6:e20602
Cook PJ, Moore MJJA, Perspectives IVFM (1993) Economic perspectives on reducing alcohol-related violence. 24:193–211
Cox G, Rampes HJAIPT (2003) Adverse effects of khat: a review. 9:456–463
Dorsey TL, Zawitz MW, Middleton PJBOJS (2010) Drugs and crime facts. NCJ, 165148
Douglas H, Pedder M, Lintzeris N (2012) Law enforcement and khat: an analysis of current issues. National Drug Law Enforcement Research Fund (NDLERF)
Duresso SW, Matthews AJ, Ferguson SG, Bruno RJA (2016) Is khat use disorder a valid diagnostic entity? 111:1666–1676
Eckersley W, Salmon R, Gebru MJBOTWHO (2010) Khat, driver impairment and road traffic injuries: a view from Ethiopia. 88:235–236
Engidawork EJPR (2017) Pharmacological and toxicological effects of Catha edulis F.(Khat). 31: 1019–1028
Feigin A, Higgs P, Hellard M, Dietze PJBOTWHO (2010) Further research required to determine link between khat consumption and driver impairment. 88:480–480
Gatter P (2012) Politics of qat: the role of a drug in ruling Yemen. Ludwig Reichert Verlag
Geisshüsler S, Brenneisen RJJOE (1987) The content of psychoactive phenylpropyl and phenylpentenyl khatamines in Catha edulis Forsk. of different origin. 19:269–277
Gmel G, Rehm JJAR, Health (2003) Harmful alcohol use. 27:52
Griffiths P, Gossop M, Wickenden S, Dunworth J, Harris K, Lloyd CJBJOP (1997) A transcultural pattern of drug use: qat (khat) in the UK. 170:281–284
Haile D, Lakew YJPO (2015) Khat chewing practice and associated factors among adults in Ethiopia: further analysis using the 2011 demographic and health survey. 10:e0130460
Hassan NA, Gunaid AA, El-Khally FM, Murray-Lyon IMJSMJ (2002) The effect of chewing Khat leaves on human mood. 23:850–853
Havell CJARBTP (2004) Khat use in Somali, Ethiopian and Yemeni communities in England: issues and solutions
Hoffman R, Al'Absi MJJOE (2010) Khat use and neurobehavioral functions: suggestions for future studies. 132:554–563
Jelsma M, Metaal P, Klein AJTIA (2012) Chewing over Khat prohibition The globalisation of control and regulation of an ancient stimulant
Kalix PJJOSAT (1988) Khat: a plant with amphetamine effects. 5:163–169
Kalix P, Braenden OJPR (1985) Pharmacological aspects of the chewing of khat leaves. 37: 149–164
Kalix PJP, Toxicology (1992) Cathinone, a natural amphetamine. 70:77–86
Kinyanjui DW, Atwoli LJBP (2013) Substance use among inmates at the Eldoret prison in Western Kenya. 13:1–8
Klee SW, Hilary (2001) Violent crime, aggression and amphetamine: what are the implications for drug treatment services? J Drugs: Educ Prevent Policy 8:73–90
Klein AJSU, Misuse (2008) Khat in the neighbourhood – local government responses to khat use in a London community. 43:819–831
Knight K, Farabee D (2004) Treating addicted offenders: A continuum of effective practices. Civic Research Institute, Inc

Leukefeld CG, Tims FE, Farabee DE (2002) Treatment of drug offenders: Policies and issues. Springer Publishing Company
Nencini P, Ahmed AMJD, Dependence A (1989) Khat consumption: a pharmacological review. 23: 19–29
Numan NJA (2004) Exploration of adverse psychological symptoms in Yemeni khat users by the Symptoms Checklist-90 (SCL-90). 99:61–65
Odenwald M, Neuner F, Schauer M, Elbert T, Catani C, Lingenfelder B, Hinkel H, Häfner H, Rockstroh BJBM (2005) Khat use as risk factor for psychotic disorders: a cross-sectional and case-control study in Somalia. 3:1–10
Odenwald M, Hinkel H, Schauer E, Schauer M, Elbert T, Neuner F, Rockstroh BJSS (2009) Use of khat and posttraumatic stress disorder as risk factors for psychotic symptoms: a study of Somali combatants. Soc Sci Med 69:1040–1048
Odenwald M, Lingenfelder B, Peschel W, Haibe FA, Warsame AM, Omer A, Stöckel J, Maedl A, Elbert TJIJOMHS (2012) A pilot study on community-based outpatient treatment for patients with chronic psychotic disorders in Somalia: change in symptoms, functioning and co-morbid khat use. 6:1–18
Patel SLJDE (2008) Attitudes to khat use within the Somali community in England. Prevention & Policy 15, 37–53
Patel NBJBRB (2019) Khat (Catha edulis Forsk) – and now there are three. 145:92–96
Patel SL, Murray R, Britain G (2005) Khat use among Somalis in four English cities. Citeseer
Payne-James J, Wall I, Bailey CJJOCFM (2005) Patterns of illicit drug use of prisoners in police custody in London, UK. 12:196–198
Pennings E, Opperhuizen A, Van Amsterdam JJRT (2008) Risk assessment of khat use in the Netherlands: a review based on adverse health effects, prevalence, criminal involvement and public order. Pharmacology 52, 199–207
Pernanen K, Brochu S, Cousineau M-M, Cournoyer L, Sun FJE, Abuse SCOS (2000) Attributable fractions for alcohol and illicit drugs in relation to crime in Canada: conceptualization, methods and internal consistency of estimates. 53
Prendergast ML, Podus D, Chang E, Urada DJD, Dependence A (2002) The effectiveness of drug abuse treatment: A meta-analysis of comparison group studies. 67:53–72
Sadock B (2011) Kaplan and Sadock's synopsis of psychiatry: behavioral sciences/clinical psychiatry. Lippincott Williams & Wilkins
Series, WECODDJWHOTR (2006) WHO Expert Committee on drug dependence
Sharp D, Atherton SRJIJOOT, Criminology C (2006) Out on the Town: An evaluation of brief motivational interventions to address the risks associated with problematic alcohol use. 50: 540–558
Stewart DJA (2009) Drug use and perceived treatment need among newly sentenced prisoners in England and Wales. 104:243–247
Sykes W, Coleman N, Desai P, Groom C, Gure M, Howarth RJHORLHO (2010) Perceptions of the social harms associated with khat use
Taxman FS, Perdoni ML, Harrison LDJJOSAT (2007) Drug treatment services for adult offenders: the state of the state. 32:239–254
Teferra S, Hanlon C, Alem A, Jacobsson L, Shibre TJTP (2011) Khat chewing in persons with severe mental illness in Ethiopia: a qualitative study exploring perspectives of patients and caregivers. 48:455–472
Thomas E, Spittal M, Heffernan E, Taxman F, Alati R, Kinner SJPM (2016) Trajectories of psychological distress after prison release: implications for mental health service need in ex-prisoners. 46:611–621
Toennes SW, Harder S, Schramm M, Niess C, Kauert GFJBJOCP (2003) Pharmacokinetics of cathinone, cathine and norephedrine after the chewing of khat leaves. 56:125–130
Tretter F, Gebicke-Haerter P, Albus M, An Der Heiden U, Schwegler HJP (2009) Systems biology and addiction. 42:S11–S31

Wabe NTJA, Health (2011) Chemistry, pharmacology, and toxicology of khat (catha edulis forsk): a review. 3:137

Widler P, Mathys K, Brenneisen R, Kalix P, Fisch HUJCP (1994) Pharmacodynamics and pharmacokinetics of khat: a controlled study. Therapeutics 55:556–562

Widmann M, Apondi B, Musau A, Warsame AH, Isse M, Mutiso V, Veltrup C, Ndetei D, Odenwald MJSP, Epidemiology P (2017) Comorbid psychopathology and everyday functioning in a brief intervention study to reduce khat use among Somalis living in Kenya: description of baseline multimorbidity, its effects of intervention and its moderation effects on substance use. 52: 1425–1434

Wormith JS, Althouse R, Simpson M, Reitzel LR, Fagan TJ, Morgan RDJCJ (2007) The rehabilitation and reintegration of offenders: the current landscape and some future directions for correctional psychology. Behavior 34:879–892

Yitayih Y, van Os JJBP (2021) Prevalence and determinants of chewing khat among women in Ethiopia: data from Ethiopian demographic and health survey 2016. 21:1–8

Yitayih Y, Abera M, Tesfaye E, Mamaru A, Soboka M, Adorjan KJBP (2018) Substance use disorder and associated factors among prisoners in a correctional institution in Jimma, Southwest Ethiopia: a cross-sectional study. 18:1–9

Yitayih Y, Soboka M, Tesfaye E, Abera M, Mamaru A, Adorjan KJPO (2020) A cross-sectional study of psychopathy and khat abuse among prisoners in the correctional institution in Jimma, Ethiopia. 15:e0227405

81 Khat Consumption and Household Economies

Zerihun Girma Gudata

Contents

Introduction 1718
Studies on Khat 1721
  Perspective Matter: Producers (Rural) and Traders, Positive Impact Narratives 1721
  Perspective Matter: Urban Consumers, Negative Impact Narratives 1726
  Perspective Matters: Rural Producer plus Urban Consumers, a Balanced View 1729
Conclusion 1731
  Applications to Other Areas of Addiction 1732
  Summary Points 1732
Key Facts of Khat Consumption 1733
Mini-Dictionary 1733
References 1734

Abstract

Khat is one of the most controversial subjects of this day. It is possible to say almost all scholars from different fields studied khat. Works from all disciplines regarding the impact of khat consumption on the economy of a household focus on both positive and negative aspects of khat based on the researcher's perspective. This review indicates how perspective matters in the study of khat. Those studies from the rural or producer and trader perspective highlight the positive impacts of khat on the economy of a household, while those studies from the urban or consumer perspective highlight the negative impacts of khat on the economy of a household. Similarly, on a country level, most studies from Kenya and Ethiopia (producer) focus on the positive side of khat, while studies from Somalia and Djibouti (consumer) stress the negative impacts of khat. In addition, this review concludes by stressing the importance of timing in dealing with chewer respondents.

Z. G. Gudata (✉)
Haramaya University, Hararghe Health Research Project, CHAMPS Ethiopia, Harar, Ethiopia

V. B. Patel, V. R. Preedy (eds.), *Handbook of Substance Misuse and Addictions*,
https://doi.org/10.1007/978-3-030-92392-1_88

Keywords

Chewer/consumer · Economy · Household · Khat · Perspective · Producer · Urban · Rural · Timing

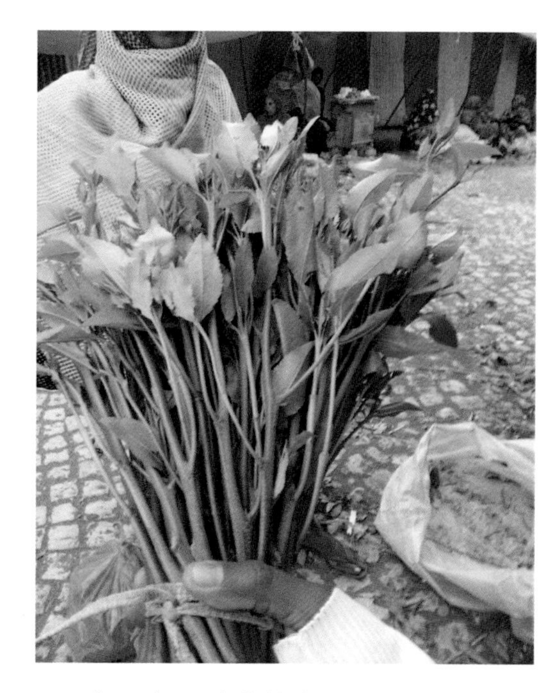

One pack of khat consumed once by one individual. Sold by 300ETB in 2017, although the price fluctuates based on season. This is the time when the price gets low

Introduction

Khat, *chat*, or *qat* (*Catha edulis*) is defined in different ways by different researchers. Gezon (2012, p. 15) put it as "a bushy plant whose leaves when chewed produce a mildly amphetamine-like effect." Others explain it as a plant traditionally chewed to produce a mild stimulant (Cooperative Housing Foundation (CHF) International 2006, p. 13). Ezekiel (2004, p. xi) defined it as a "psychoactive shrub, produced and marketed in the eastern portion of an expansive plateau located in the province of Harerge." There are also other definitions, like, an "evergreen tree cultivated in parts of Ethiopia for of its fresh leaves, which are chewed for their euphoric properties" (Gessesse 2013, p. 7). It is also called "a plant of uncertain and highly controversial status" (Lamina 2010, p. 1). Khat can also be defined as chewable green leaves which have the effect of a euphoric stimulation on the users and consecutive use results in addiction. It has recently emerged as a controversial product due to its economic, social, cultural, and political impacts.

Getahun and Krikorian (1973) indicate that khat originates from Ethiopia. Oral evidence shows that it was first used in the current city of Harar. Accordingly, a group of religious and civic leaders who founded the city of Harar was the first to introduce khat to the region from Yemen to fight the depressing effect of the environment of the area. Nevertheless, Ezekiel (2010a) argues that, similar to opium, coca, tea, coffee, and tobacco which have been used by humans throughout history for medical purposes, khat in the Horn of Africa also first started to be used for treating headaches, diarrhea, depression, muscle aches, and other diseases. Although he did not deny the religious uses of khat, he indicated that making drinks of khat and chewing the leaves possibly first started for medicinal purposes. According to Ezekiel (2012), khat chewing first started in the ancient walled city of Harar and spread to other parts of Ethiopia. After describing the khat trade around Zeyla and Barbara and its popularity in Yemen and parts of Arabia, Burton (1856) in his *First Footsteps in East Africa* indicated that it was Shaikh Ibrahim Abu Zaharbui who introduced khat into Yemen from Abyssinia, refuting the argument that khat was introduced to Harar from Yemen.

Historically, in Ethiopia, Khat was first mentioned during the conflict between Amda Simon (the Christian king who reigned from 1314 to 1344 A.D.) and Sabra Din (a Muslim leader). The latter bragged he would control the capital of the Christian king and "plant there plants of ĉat [or khat]" (Trimingham 1965, p. 228). In the beginning, khat was considered holy and there were a limited number of chewers. A breakthrough in the expansion of khat occurred after the expansion of Menilik to Hararghe, after which the production and consumption widely expanded among the surrounding Oromo (Getahun and Krikorian 1973). Nevertheless, evidence shows that the rise of khat chewing as an important and controversial product on the international level, its widespread consumption among the youth, and the increase in demand for it (not only in Ethiopia but also on the global level) is only a recent development (Ezekiel 2004; Gessesse 2013; Klein 2007).

Khat culture is related to the cultural or ceremonial practices before, during, and after a chewing session. Some writers discuss khat culture (The word "khat culture" was first used by Ezekiel Gebissa in his article entitled "The Culture of Khat." He related the word with *Barcha*, which is becoming a commonplace sight in urban areas of Ethiopia, where "users congregate in a designated room in private houses and lie on their sides on a pile of cushions to meditate, read and engage in the talk of the town." He described how chewers drink water or tea to reduce dryness of the mouth and to assist the extraction of the juice. Some chewers take a pinch of sugar or a sip of Coca Cola to moderate the bitter taste and smoke cigarettes as they chew (Ezekiel 2010). Although more variables are added in the context of this study, these are also some of the features of khat culture. To fully understand khat culture in the context of this study, see the operational definitions) by relating to both the production and consumption of khat. It is mostly related to addiction to khat and consecutive uses. Above all, it involves all the sessions of chewing: starting with *ijabana (eye opener)*, in the morning; followed by *barcha*, in the early afternoon; and *atarora* the last chew session, which takes place before bedtime. In most instances, these sessions especially *barcha* are followed by *chabsi*, a drinking time. As the origin of khat, the people of Harar are most adapt to khat culture (Mekuria 2018; Ezekiel 2010). Khat in Harar society is intertwined with every aspect of life, from entertainment to religion. Generally, khat culture involves all these activities including the equipment used, the time and money spent, and the behavior it produces. The reason for chewing khat varies from relief from stress to use after alcohol consumption (see Fig. 1). This review investigates researcher works done on all these aspects of khat.

The issue of khat is complex and multidimensional; it is not easy to deal with for both politicians and scholars. Governments and policymakers are in a big dilemma on how to deal with khat. According to Cochrane and Negash, policymakers faced a "difficult, and at the same times impossible, task" with khat (2017, p. 144). Research studies also provide a different perspective on khat. There is a great debate among scholars as to whether khat has an impact on the living standards or the economy of a household, becoming a barrier to development and poverty alleviation. The division involves hot arguments supported by research evidence. One group holds that khat chewing leads to loss of work hours, divorce, decreased economic productivity, malnutrition, and diversion of money to buy further khat. They also indicate khat is linked to absenteeism and unemployment, which may, in turn, result in a fall in overall national economic productivity (Cox and Rampes 2003; Girmay et al. 2007; Hassan et al. 2007; Wuletaw 2018; Nakajima et al. 2016). At the same time, others concentrate on its health impacts, which directly affect development and household economy

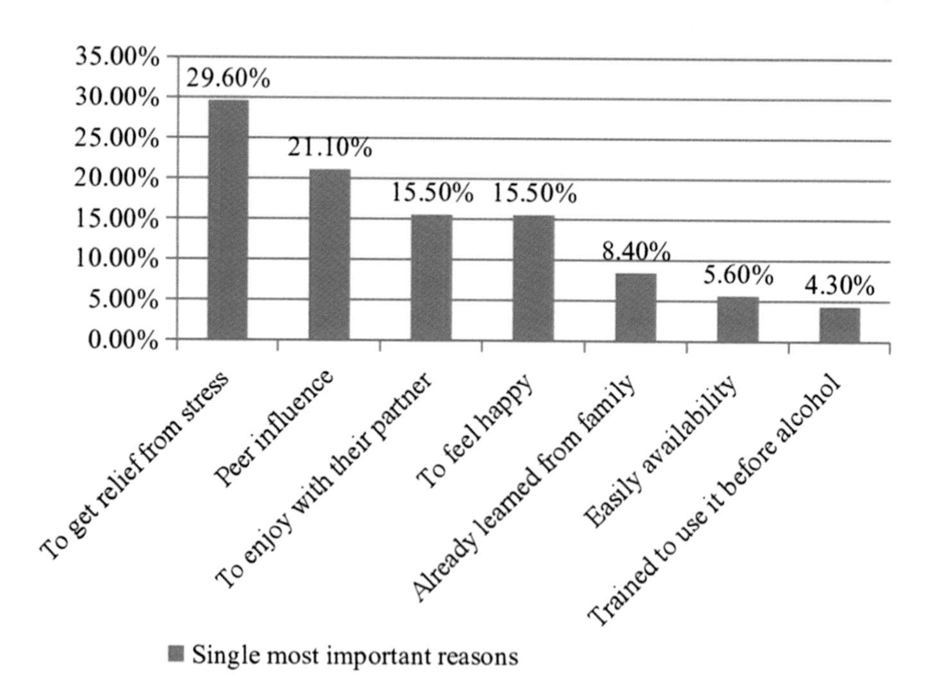

Fig. 1 Reason for consuming khat. (Source: Mekuriaw et al. 2020)

(Fantahun et al. 2012; Manghi et al. 2009), while others hold that khat increases peaceful social coexistence, increases income, promotes productivity, and when chewed "moderately" improves performance and increases work output because it stimulates and postpones fatigue. Consequently, working hours and possibly productivity can decrease when khat is not used because of reduced motivation. They also hold that it doubles the income of khat farmers and boosts their revenue and general living standards (Armstrong 2008; Klein 2014; Ezekiel 2010a, 2012; Beckerleg 2008). As indicated in the following discussion, perspective is the main reason for the debate on khat. Those who focus on urban consumers' economy present the negative impact of khat on chewer, while those who focus their study on rural producers and khat traders stress the positive impact of khat in generating income for a household. Similarly, on a country level, most studies from Kenya and Ethiopia (majority producer) stress the positive side of khat culture, while most studies from Somalia and Djibouti (majority consumer) focus on the negative side of khat. In addition, this review revealed the significance of timing, but most of the researchers on khat did not consider this in dealing with their chewer respondents.

Studies on Khat

Most of the articles and books published on khat first discuss its controversy. Moreover, some of them even reveal the existing controversy in their title, for instance, *The Khat Controversy* (Anderson, et al. 2007); "Should Khat Be Banned?" (Hailu 2007); "Khat: Is It More Like Coffee or Cocaine? Criminalizing a Commodity, targeting a Community" (Ezekiel 2012); *Favouring a Demonised Plant: Khat and Ethiopian smallholder enterprises* (Gessesse Dessie 2013); "Khat in East Africa: Taking Women Into or Out of Sex Work?" (Beckerleg 2008); and "Scourge of Life or an Economic Lifeline? Public Discourses on Khat (Catha edulis) in Ethiopia" (Ezekiel 2008). Others make the issue even more provocative, referring to khat as "Flower of Paradise" (Sikiru 2012) and *the leaf of Allah*, by relating it with religion (Ezekiel 2004). That is why Ference (2009, p. 181) said khat is "the most controversial and ubiquitous stimulant." Other scholars like Wolf (2013) indicated the necessity of studying the impact of khat on the economy of a nation. She raised an important question that served as a topic of discussion for most works on khat: ". . . while khat production is flourishing, it is not yet clear if more users will create less productive Ethiopians." Most of the debates on khat revolve around whether it is good or bad, whether it should be banned or legalized, whether or not it has an impact on the economy of a household, and whether it promotes or demotes development and poverty alleviation.

Perspective Matter: Producers (Rural) and Traders, Positive Impact Narratives

As the place of the origin of khat and also as a major producer and exporter, there are several studies on khat in Ethiopia that focus on its positive aspects for the economy of a household and a nation in general. The work of Ezekiel Gebissa is notable in this aspect. Mostly, he focuses on the cultural significance of khat in the Hararghe region as a recreational material (especially the *barcha* session), a motivator for work as well as its socializing role, and how it maintained cultural cohesion and meditative worship. He says, "khat chewing serves as an essential social lubricant that fosters amity, cooperation, and sociality." He argues that khat chewing is not a waste of time: "the chew sessions are well integrated into the workday." He especially stresses the significance of khat in the religious activities of the Muslim Oromo of Hararghe and why it was regarded as "the leaf of Allah" or "food of the saints." He also discusses the controversy between the Christians and the local Muslims regarding khat that came about after the occupation of the area in the 1880s (Ezekiel 2010).

In his article, "Khat: Is It More Like Coffee or Cocaine? . . .," Ezekiel discussed the expansion of khat chewing from the Horn of Africa to the other parts of the world, particularly to the USA by Oromo migrants from Hararghe. He discussed how khat was regarded first as a "strange immigrant habit" that has no harm, then as a "harmful drug" that should be fought, and finally treated as an "illicit commodity financing terrorism." How this affected the Oromo immigrants in the USA leading to their imprisonment. He stated, for the Oromo immigrant, "chewing khat provides a setting that connects them to the homeland" though chewing is illegal. In this article, Ezekiel also discussed how media and political interest groups shaped the social perception of khat negatively, leading to the implementation of quick policy measures. Above all, besides the rhetoric social cohesive significance of khat, Ezekiel tried to lower the health impact of khat and tried to defend its health importance too. He concluded his article by criticizing the injustice of US laws concerning khat chewers, "[p]owerful cultural and political forces have coalesced to create a political environment in which legislation and policies are formulated based on emotion rather than empirical facts" (Ezekiel 2012).

Ezekiel also published two impressive books frequently cited by scholars who study khat. First, his *Leaf of Allah* was published in 2004. Second, he edited *Taking the Place of Food: Khat in Ethiopia*, which was published in 2010. Both focus on the cultural, economic, and religious significance of khat. His argument in the first book has important implications not only on how someone understands khat but on how one understands the agricultural system in eastern Ethiopia starting from the imperial period until the end of the Darg regime. He discussed how the economic policies of Ethiopia's government encouraged khat trade in the area; the emergence of unofficial trade alongside the official one; the occupation of the area by Menilik and the taking of land from farmers which lead to a shortage of land on the one hand and an expansion of khat on the other hand; and the expansion of transportation system, particularly railroad and air transport which facilitate the expansion of the khat trade, particularly after World War II. He also indicated that the government of Haile Selassie and the Darg encouraged the expansion of the khat trade and tried to control it but were unsuccessful. Besides, he also wrote how the parallel market of khat was essential for the farmer in generating income, providing job opportunities, and serving as a solution for land scarcity and poverty. Nevertheless, he recognizes that the khat trade and farming did not lead to any significant structural change in the area, and he recommends that the government has to listen to what the local farmers say (Ezekiel 2004).

The second study is a kind of compilation of the articles of different scholars like Hussein Ahmed, Daniel Mains, Degol Hailu, Habtemariam Kassa, and others. It is broader in concept than the first one since it discusses developments after the 1990s and khat culture in the other parts of Ethiopia. The focus of the book can broadly be classified into three main themes: the consumption of khat, its production, trade, and policy-related issues. The consumption part shows the widespread use of khat in recent times. It has expanded from traditional ritual culture to wider society including women and men of various economic statuses. Concerning the health and social problems caused by khat, Ezekiel tries to argue that farmers chew khat the same way we might have a cup of coffee in the morning. Regarding youngsters from urban centers who mix khat with alcoholic drinks, he described it as a "bad" consumption habit. Similar to the first book, the positive side of khat is the central part of his theme. The khat trade contributed to the development of infrastructure because of the tax revenues the government earned from farmers; it helped diversify farmers' economic bases; it helped overcome economic hardships due to drought and fluctuations in the global market; it empowered and increased economic significance of women and also enabled farmers to invest in more productive farming. Nevertheless, he also indicates that the productivity and success of khat lead to its expansion into other parts of Ethiopia. Lastly, he raised one important question: will Ethiopia starve itself because farmers are choosing to invest in a more profitable cash crop? He responded "no" because farmers prefer diversity (Ezekiel 2010b). For Ezekiel in general, khat production and consumption had no undesirable consequences for the economy of a household or a nation.

Generally, these two works of Ezekiel and his other articles on khat are foundational works on the subject and very significant. Nevertheless, some points need to be understood cautiously. First, his writing indicates the existence of tension with the then-existing political system. This was observed especially in his first work, the *Leaf of Allah*. As a result, a value judgment is common on some political issues. For instance, he said, "For the Christian 'Amhara' colonists, the consumption of khat was a mark of apostasy" (Ezekiel 2004, pp. xi–xiii). It did not speculate about other forms of socializing and networking agents such as religious organizations and civic-minded groups, which may have the same effect as khat (There is also some contradiction in his works. In his article published in *OGINA*, he strongly asserts that khat chewing first started among the Oromo of Afran Qallo and expanded to other places (Ezekiel 2010). However, contrary to this in another article published by *SciRes*, he said, "khat chewing started among the urban residents of the ancient walled city of Harar in eastern Ethiopia and spread to the surrounding Oromo" (Ezekiel 2012, p. 204)).

Of all research on khat, no one has stressed the importance of khat like Ezekiel. For him, khat has almost no negative impacts on a given community or individual household economy. Although it is not denied that khat plays an important role in bringing different societies together and increasing socialization, increasing the role of women in the economy, and bringing cash for the country as an export product, it also has many negative impacts. Ezekiel does not mention khat's addictive nature that creates dependence on the substance and can disturb health and family. The World Health Organization classifies khat as a "drug whose abuse can produce mild to moderate psychological dependence" (Gessesse 2013, p. 8). Even if someone chews for recreation, it costs a lot of money and time, especially for urban chewers who spent 30% of their income on khat and 10% of their lifetime (Gudata et al. 2019). In general, in his writings, Ezekiel shows his strong support for the expansion of khat not only in Ethiopia but also on a worldwide level. These can be attributed to his methodology. Ezekiel mostly relies on interview data from chewers. He says, "in my interviews in the vicinity of Harar, some Oromo chewers tell me that they use the khat-induced high for work while others do so for pleasure" (Ezekiel 2010, p. 2). Moreover, most of his study is based on and focused on rural farmers and traders.

The Positive Impact: Studies at the National Level

Ezekiel is not the only one who focused on the importance of khat. Several studies from another khat-producing country, Kenya, by Neil Carrier stress the economic, cultural, and social significance of khat (Carrier 2005, 2007). He uses experiential questions and qualitative data to discuss the euphoria of khat. It was an in-depth examination of khat from its harvest to consumption in Meru (equivalent of Awaday in Ethiopia) town, Kenya, where khat production is a major cash crop and export commodity. It also studies the relationships that tie the khat trade network together in Kenya and beyond. Above all, the study is aimed at responding to the negative discourse regarding khat and showed the economic and cultural motivations that drive this far-reaching global trade network. It examined "the social life" of khat and the ritual surrounding its production, inheritance, marketing, and consumption. Besides, it gives a vivid picture of Kenyan social life and networks of economic exchange. Carrier compared khat with an agricultural cash crop like tea and coffee. He gave descriptive details of the lucrative trade in khat, its transportation, and the impressive knowledge of each step of the trade. Kenyan khat consumers and their styles of consumption were also described. He concluded by examining the discourse of the war on drugs and how the Kenyan perception of the "mysterious stimulant" differed to further complicate its regulation and control (Carrier 2007).

In his other study "Miraa is cool: the cultural importance of miraa...," Carrier (2005) discussed how khat, which is controversial, is significant for the Tigania and Igembe youth of Kenya. These communities inherited khat consumption from their ancestors. For the Tigania and Igembe youth, khat are their traditions, heritage, identity, and source of pride. It generates a lot of income and for them, it is a "commercial success." Carrier also compared khat with wine in the "Christians during communion" to show how the perception changed and how the use of wine in secular, everyday contexts does not dilute the importance within a communion. He also compared khat as a source of pride for Meru with a traditional product of Scotland, whisky which is popular throughout the world (Carrier 2005, p. 216, 217). His two other articles, "Is Miraa a Drug?: Categorizing Kenyan Khat" (2009) and "Quasilegality: khat, cannabis and Africa's drug laws" (2018), contributed a lot on the debate on khat whether it is a "drug" and its legal issue. In the first article, he looked at a different view of khat in Kenya: some region strongly disapproves, and the other region strongly approves of khat. In the second paper, he described the vague and flexible laws on khat as "quasilegal."

Throughout his work Carrier proved the argument presented in this review. His early works, in 2005 and 2007, mostly focus on the positive aspects of khat. His study also focuses on the producers only, who feed him with the benefit they are generating from khat. He said "...when I visited the town of Mutuati... I was shown a great pile of high-quality Miraa... The traders were happy to inform me that the pile of Miraa was destined for London" (Carrier 2005, p. 217). Of course, producers and traders are happy to inform any researchers of the benefit they are exaggeratedly gaining from the product. However, if somebody talks to urban chewers, who are spending a large amount of money and time on consuming khat, there is a high possibility of hearing many evils of khat, for instance, family conflict and disintegration, and the overall well-being of a household in urban areas is negatively affected by khat (Gudata 2020). That is what Carrier understood in his later work, 2009 and 2018, in which he discussed the varied perception on khat. In the former work, he looked from both the producer and consumer perspectives and found a polarized view of khat in the same country, Kenya: "strong approval in the Nyambene Hills region where it is cultivated [and] strong disapproval" in the other parts of Kenyan society. In the latter study, he focused on the legal issue of khat and its controversy. Generally, although by focusing on the positive side of khat Carrier becomes the equivalent of Ezekiel in Ethiopia, he is better at demonstrating the importance of perspective in his later study of khat.

A similar study made by David Anderson and his colleagues focuses on the Horn of Africa including Ethiopia and Kenya. By pulling data from these countries, he discusses the global trade of khat. This study examines the pharmacological and social controversy surrounding khat. The writers of the book came together from different fields like sociology, economics, psychology, health, and medicine. The researchers traced the rise of khat production over the last several decades, after which coffee became less profitable in Ethiopia. The returns on khat were much higher than coffee resulting in a shift of agricultural focus to khat as a viable alternative. They indicate how the khat trade has given both young men and women a foothold in the non-agrarian economy and how the complicated and important trade in khat benefits many lives in a wide range of areas like Somalia, Ethiopia, Djibouti, and Kenya. The last part of the book focuses on international trade and trade policies in countries like the UK, Sweden, Australia, and Canada. They argue that the reason khat has not caught on among the wider population in Paris and London is rooted in the ritual and cultural significance of chewing khat as a social function. This cultural practice and perspective complicated the policymakers' claims that khat has largely negative consequences. They also indicated banning khat is removing one more market advantage that small African traders have (Anderson, et al. 2007).

Similar to Ezekiel's work, the above two works argue that khat builds communities and brings people together at home and in the diaspora, the economic and symbolic importance of the substance for people's lives. Especially the latter persuasively argued that khat provides economic security for people that have been victims of neoliberal economic policies, which destroyed coffee and tea markets in Ethiopia and Kenya. Like most of the researchers on khat, they gathered their data from the producers and traders who are benefiting from khat itself. These informants, or those who filled the experiential questions, were influenced by the benefit they were gaining from khat since they are traders and producers who depend on it; they had not experienced any significant side effects of khat.

Perspective Matter: Urban Consumers, Negative Impact Narratives

There are studies on khat that focus on urban chewers; these studies investigate the negative impact of khat on the economy of consumer households. For instance, a study in Jimma by Yeshigeta and Haile-Amlak (2004) on the prevalence and sociodemographic profile of khat chewing and other associated factors relating to the technical staff of Jimma hospital and the academic staff of Jimma University found that the current prevalence of khat chewing was 30.8%. Above all, they found that around 50.4% of khat chewers have one or more times missed their regular work at the university because of chewing and 54.5% of the chewers had come to work late because of chewing khat or left their work early to chew khat. The study concluded that khat has a strong negative impact on service delivery and the teaching-learning process as participants missed their regular work because of chewing (Yeshigeta and Haile-Amlak 2004). This study is one of the works which directly or indirectly assess the negative impacts of khat on society and household economies. The study only focuses on the urban chewers, Jimma University staff.

A similar study was made in Harar city on secondary school students in April 2010 by the staff of Jimma, Haramaya, and Addis Ababa University. The research was entitled "Prevalence and Determinants of Khat (Catha edulis) Chewing among High School Students in Eastern Ethiopia: A Cross-Sectional Study." The high prevalence of khat is discussed as negative, and they recommended measures such as educational campaigns to create awareness among school adolescents and their parents "to reduce the prevalence of the habit and its adverse social and health consequence" (Reda et al. 2012). However, they never specifically mention what is the "adverse social and health consequences" of khat chewing. They do not discuss its impact on the academic achievement of students or their households' economy in general.

Another study by Abiye Girmay and his colleagues deals with the magnitude of khat use by the youth, attitudes, and perceptions toward its utilization and risky sexual behaviors among youth in Asendabo town, South-Western Ethiopia. They indicated that the overall proportion of condom nonusers was very high. Moreover, the study found that khat chewers were twice as likely to have multiple sexual partners. That is, multiple sexual intercourses and substance use such as khat, alcohol, and cigarettes were widely practiced among the studied youth. High proportions of youth were engaged in the consumption of substances and sexual practices with multiple partners. Therefore, they recommended intervention

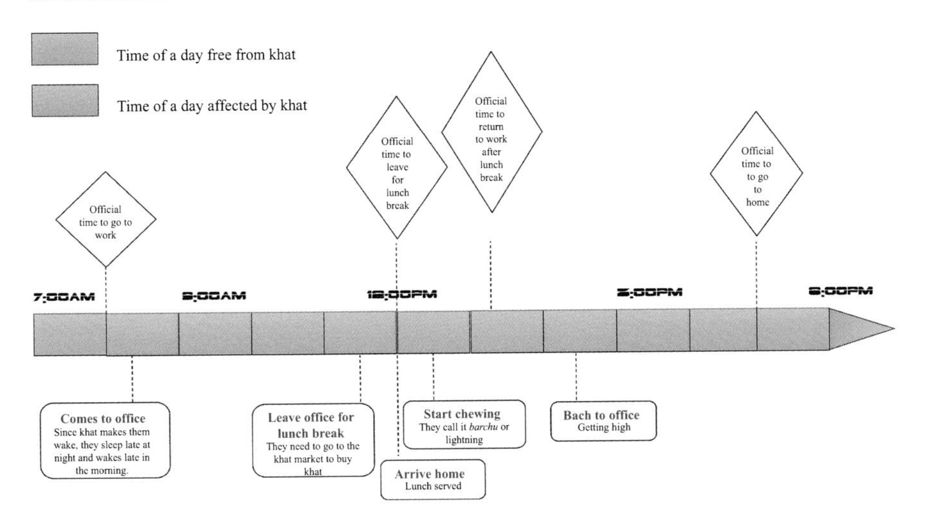

Fig. 2 Time management of khat consumers and how their consumption behavior affects their days. (Source: Girma et al. 2019)

activities to bring about behavioral changes among the youth on the danger of the use of khat, alcohol, and tobacco (Girmay et al. 2007). This study is another work that discusses the negative impacts of khat on household members. Moreover, a work on assessment of khat consumption habit on the economy and family well-being in Harar city clearly presents the impact of khat on urban chewers. The impact includes bad work culture, waste of time, family destabilization, and low living standard. For instance, look at the following diagram to see the time management of chewers in a day (Girma et al. 2019) (Fig. 2).

The Negative Impact: Studies at the National Level

Moreover, a study from Somalia, which always buys and consumes khat from Ethiopia, is one that focuses on the negative imapacts of khat. Michael Odenwald and his colleagues made a cross-sectional study regarding the use of khat and another drug among Somali combatants. Using trained local interviewers, they interviewed 8723 informants. They also engaged local nongovernmental organizations who provided them with interviewers. They assessed the basic socio-demographic information, self-reported khat use, and how respondents perceived the use of khat and other drugs. The study found that drug use among military personnel differed substantially between northern and southern/central Somalia. With a 99% confidence interval total, 36.4% of the respondents reported khat use in the week before the interview. Excessive use of most substances was found in the South of Somalia, a conflict zone suggesting that conflict has been associated with increased substance misuse. They also identified that the self-reported khat use differed substantially from the perceived use in units. According to the perception of respondents, the most frequent form of drug use was khat chewing, on average, 70.1% followed by smoking cannabis. Finally, they recommended, "future disarmament, demobilization, and reintegration (DDR) programs need to be prepared to deal with significant drug-related problems in Somalia" (Odenwald 2007).

Relating to the above study, Kamaldeep Bhui and Nasir Warfa published an article entitled "Drug Consumption in Conflict Zones in Somalia." Their writing revealed the impact of khat on living standards. By quoting different studies on khat, they wrote that when used excessively khat increased the risk of mental illness. Above all, they stated that although there was no clear evidence whether or not khat perpetuates the Somali conflict and is used to finance terrorism, "what is clear is that khat misuse significantly exacerbates poverty levels and has a negative impact on the living standard of the Somali people." They also wrote that 80% of the Somali male population spends around US$4 a day on khat, and they questioned "How could one expect to reduce poverty levels and improve the quality of life" in such conditions. Regarding the target of khat, the paper indicated it was the young people who were most vulnerable (Bhui and Warfa 2007).

Although short and brief, this article tried to indicate how khat could directly affect the living standards and economy of a household. Nevertheless, their study failed in many ways. First, they did not use any primary sources; they have not talked to the local people nor observed the area. They mostly relied on secondary sources, especially that of Michael Odenwald and his colleagues and many studies in Europe. For instance, their sources regarding mental illness and khat came from studies in Europe, which they generalized to the case of Somalia. There was also some conflicting data in their works. For instance, they indicated that 60% of the population of Somalia were living below US$1 a day. At the same time, they wrote that 80% of the Somali male population spends around US$4 a day on khat. Although we took the first statistics as representing the whole community and the latter for only male chewers, it is hard to believe that in a country where the majority of the population live with a daily income of less than 1 dollar, there is around 80 percent of males who can spend 4 dollars a day on khat. Nevertheless, the study reveals how khat consumption can drain the economy of a household.

Other research dealing with Somalis by Axel Klein argued that it was wrong to associate khat with the culture, tradition, and history of the Somali community because it is only a recent development. Thus, it states, the problems associated with khat use are not simply reducible to the pharmacological properties of the drug but need to take into account a new cultural context of its use within the UK. He reviewed different literature and interviewed several informants to reach this conclusion. He also discusses in detail issues like the tradition and history of khat; khat use in the global market; campaigning against khat use by the women who have suffered most from its effects; and khat and the invention of tradition, in which he states that the Somalis who identify khat as part of their culture do so without really understanding the historical origin of this consumption pattern. The study argues that khat was not widely used in Somalia until the 1970s. Thus, the issue of culture and tradition cannot serve as an excuse not to ban khat use (Klein 2007). Nevertheless, at least the historical evidence from Richard Burton's *First Footsteps in East Africa* justifies that the Somalis were using khat in the nineteenth century (Burton et al. 1856). This study indirectly insists khat is bad for a nation and household and needs to be banned.

A recent work on khat from Djibouti, one of a consumer nation like Somalia, by Rachidi S. stresses its negative impacts on the country. The paper raises one basic question, which also served as its title, "'Khat' it Out: Is the Narcotic Plant Holding Back Djibouti's Development?" After highlighting the importance of khat in Djiboutian's life, the paper points out the current difficulties caused by khat. Djibouti is one of the countries which live below the international poverty line; however, people are spending 6 to 11 dollars on khat every day. In addition, khat is negatively affecting the health of the population, since "Many of the country's adult population suffer from cardiovascular disease and diabetes, among other things." However, the government of Djibouti is not taking "serious measures," since it is benefitting from khat both economically and politically. Finally, he asked, "So, does khat hold back the development of Djibouti?" And answers, khat is "Inevitably keeping many members of the small East African country's population trapped in a vicious cycle of addiction, poverty, and political oppression" (Rachidi 2019, pp. 1–6).

Perspective Matters: Rural Producer plus Urban Consumers, a Balanced View

There are also several types of research works that present a balanced view of khat. These studies are inclusive in their methodology. They included both rural (producer) and urban (consumer) chewers in their study. One such study is by Taye Hailu and Jens B. Aune and was conducted in Habro district, western Hararghe, one of the most important khat-producing regions in Ethiopia. They investigated how khat expansion affects the overall farming system in Hararghe and the economic and social impacts of khat production and consumption. The study found that khat production was expanding; the reasons for this include increased market opportunities and favorable prices as khat was 2.7 times more profitable than cereal and a decrease in the productivity of the land. Khat is also less risky to grow than cereals because it is less vulnerable to drought. They showed that although the living standard of khat producers was better than non-khat producers, the food security of khat producers was low. Regarding the negative impacts of khat expansion on the farming system, they stated that khat occupied 55% of the cultivated land in the region and it constituted approximately 70% of a farmer's income. They also directly stated that "khat consumption negatively affects the working capacity of people," because khat consumers showed up late for work, took frequent rests, spent time chewing khat, and were generally more careless. As a result, khat consumers were paid less than non-khat users per day. The consumption of khat has a serious social consequence, and consumers spent a high portion of their income to purchase khat. Concerning health, they wrote that "khat produces mild euphoria and excitement; individuals become very talkative under the influence of the drug and may appear to be unrealistic and emotionally unstable." Finally, they concluded by stating "the expansion of khat production in Ethiopia should be closely observed because further khat expansion harbors considerable social and economic risks" (Taye and Aune 2002, pp. 5–6).

The reason for this balanced view of khat is indicated in their methodology, the "data were collected from informal interviews with khat farmers, traders and users" (Taye and Aune 2002, p. 2). They not only asked the producers or traders about khat but also users or urban chewers, those who always buy and chew khat. This group knows the real effect of khat on their family as it can drain the income of their household. Moreover, although they did not directly indicate the issue of timing in their methodology, they understand the impact of khat on the consumers. As indicated above they showed when chewed khat can make the consumers "unrealistic" (Taye and Aune 2002, p. 5). When they get high, they become optimistic, talkative, unreasonably happy, and excited. If someone talks to a chewer at this time, they will get positive feedback regarding any topic or issue, let alone khat which is making them high.

Another work that presents a balanced view of khat is a study by Gessesse Dessie, *Favouring a Demonised Plant: Khat and Ethiopian smallholder enterprises*. It assesses khat in agricultural landscapes, particularly the spatial flow of the khat trade from its production to its consumption, incorporating discussions on its developments in Europe. The role of khat was analyzed in terms of employment, income generation, and financial flows, and "smallholder-led improvements to khat production" in different agricultural landscapes in Ethiopia. These improvements included technical change, innovations and adaptations, capital investments, and institutions. Harar, Awaday, Gelemso, Adama, Asala, Wondo Genet, Kemise, Bati, Dessie, and others were mentioned as major khat towns, while Jigjiga, Dire Dawa, and Mojo are the major export centers. The paper investigated in detail the agricultural landscapes in all these regions and how farmers produce by mixing with other crops. It also deals with the rising financial income from khat trade at both national and local levels. The involvement of various actors in the khat production process creates job opportunities. The author identified six major activities in both khat production and trade: hauling/feeding, auction/bulk trade, sorting/packing, delivery/transport, retail, and residual. The major challenge faced by farmers in the production and distribution of khat includes moisture, wetlands, slopes, disease, cultivation, management, harvesting, theft, and markets. For each problem, local farmers devised their traditional mechanisms to withstand the problem, which are discussed by the author as technology innovations or adoption, capital, and institution. He also indicates that the income from khat through tax and export can promote the growth of the economy of a nation (Gessesse 2013).

However, unlike Ezekiel, Gessesse did not exclusively focus on the positive role of khat. For instance, he mentioned that children in khat-growing areas do not like to go to school when they can make easy money. Farmers tended to become consumers instead of producing their food and saving. Risks of price volatility existed, which were likely to create food deficits in time, according to him. Continuous income from a perennial crop and frequent harvests of leaves make farmers mainly dependent on khat. Gessesse recommended the "negative health, social and cultural impacts on consumers should not be overemphasized, as it is possible to minimize the impact by controlling the rate of consumption and abuse" (Gessesse 2013, p. 23). But he did not make clear how to control this "rate of consumption." Similar to Taye and Jens,

Gessesse focuses on both urban consumers and rural producers which helped him to come up with a balanced view of khat. He indicates that "It is to be acknowledged that while this [khat] is beneficial to actors involved in khat production, the income of consumers [household] is drained." He also mentioned that although khat has increased peasant's livelihood and the income of the government at a national level, it "spawns corruption and monopolies" (Gessesse 2013, pp. 21–22). He tried to see from both the producers' and the consumers' perspectives.

Conclusion

In general, the issue of khat is one of the most debatable subjects of the twenty-first century. The media, especially from the west, highlights the dangerous health risks (weight loss, lowered immunity, and gum or mouth disease) and addictive qualities of the substance. Socially, some studies also show khat chewing leads to broken families, an idle workforce, and general social deviance. At the same time, other scholars denied all these aspects and stressed the positive side of khat: it brings people together, serves as a source of income, creates job opportunities, forms part of people's culture and tradition, serves in religious rituals and for prayer, increases household economies, etc. Nevertheless, scientific studies on khat show that khat can increase heart rate, decreased appetite, and decreased the need for sleep. These symptoms are apparent and have their negative impacts on health and produce an addicted or dependent household and society. In addition, as shown above, some scholars who focused on the positive aspects of khat did not want to see from other perspectives; they only saw from the producers' and traders' perspectives. However, the question is what about the urban khat chewer? Who did not engage in both production and trade; who are dependent on khat and always buy and consume khat? This addicted urban chewer's family income is drained by khat. Moreover, what about the non-chewer family member who lives with chewers? Who loses a large sum of their income to khat, while their children are hungry or have not gone to school? For that matter, dangerous drugs like cannabis, cocaine, heroin, crystal meth, and others benefit the producers and traders by generating a large amount of income. However, they are banned because of their impact on consumers.

Another reason that contributes to the debate on khat regarding its significance for the economy is the issue of timing in dealing with chewer respondents. Most researchers who focused on the positive side of khat did not consider the issue of timing (from studies reviewed in this paper except for Taye and Aune 2002). They might have interviewed their khat chewer informants when they are high or at a time when they are on *Harara*, a time when they need khat but have not been able to get hold of it. According to studies, chewers reported their subjective experiences of khat use positively when consuming small amounts. They described a feeling of well-being, a sense of euphoria, excitement, increased energy levels, increased alertness, increased ability to concentrate, improvement in self-esteem, a positive outlook of the world, and an increase in libido (Cox and Rampes 2003). Although this only lasts for a maximum of 5 h, it is obvious what to expect if someone asks a question at this high time. Beyond khat, chewers talk enthusiastically about every single minor issue during chewing. Similarly, talking to chewers when they get low, the opposite of what is indicated by Cox and Rampes is true. A paper published by WHO indicates that khat not only creates a state of euphoria, vivid discussions, loquacity, and an excited mood and elation with feelings of increased alertness and arousal, as when not chewed it creates “depressive mood, irritability, anorexia, and difficulty to sleep” (ECDD 2006). Havell also indicates that his study participants acknowledged that “their mood changed – from a positive state of mind during and immediately after chewing, to a negative mood the following day” when not chewing (Havell 2004, p. 40).

Thus, it is important to choose the right time to deal with khat chewers. Most chewers in Harar start chewing in the afternoon. However, the urge and need for khat start at around 11 am. By noon, they reach *Harara*; this is an expression that shows uncomfortableness, boredom, and indifference, needing something but not getting it, being unhappy, being needy, misery, and depression. Chewers do not want to talk at this time. If a researcher knowingly or unknowingly discusses with chewers at that time, there is a high probability of getting a negative outcome. After 2 pm chewers have often already chewed khat; by now their behavior is completely changed. They are another person different from that of 11 am. Now their “feeling of well-being, increased level of energy, mental alertness and self-esteem, sensations of elation and excitement, and enhanced imaginative ability” are increased (Rita Annoni et al. 2009, p. 3). This will continue up to the night. Thus, an appropriate or at least a better time to deal with chewers would be from the morning around 8 am to 10 am. This includes time before they begin chewing and before those who could not find khat felt the negative effects of not consuming it.

Applications to Other Areas of Addiction

This review investigated multiple research works that are conducted on khat and tries to understand the place of study, study participant, and the view and perspective of the writers. Taking into consideration the above issues will be helpful for all studies related to drugs. Thus, the writer believes this understanding can be applied to other similar drugs.

Summary Points

- Khat is an addictive chewable green leaf mostly chewed in Eastern Africa and Saudi Arabia.
- Works from all disciplines regarding the impact of khat consumption on the economy of a household focus on both positive and negative aspects of khat based on the researcher’s perspective.
- Perspective determent in discussing both the positive and negative impacts of khat.

- Those studies from the rural or producer and trader perspective highlight the positive impacts of khat on the economy of a household, while those studies from the urban or consumer perspective highlight the negative impacts of khat on the economy of the household.

Key Facts of Khat Consumption

- Khat consumption is said to be first started in Ethiopia, Harar.
- Currently the consumption of khat is wide spreading from northeast Africa and Saudi Arabia to western countries.
- There are disagreement and debate among scholars regarding the actual impact of khat on the economy of a nation and specifically a household. Some focus on the negative aspect, while others discuss the positive parts.
- Studies that make producer and trader as their target population focus on the positive aspect of khat. How it generates large amount of income for the family and a nation in general.
- Studies that focus on urban consumers deal with the large amount of expense on khat buying and how it physically and psychologically destroys the chewers and destabilizes a family.

Mini-Dictionary

Khat chewer: a person who uses khat more than two times in a week and feels uncomfortable or displays deviant behaviors when not chewing or not finding khat at a time he has to chew.

Atarora: is the last khat-chewing session, mostly at night before bedtime.

Barcha: is a khat-chewing ceremony, mostly in the early afternoon. It is one part of khat culture.

Chabsi: a drinking time after chewing khat to break high stimulation due to khat. It is usually after *barcha*.

Household: is composed of family members that reside in one house or apartment. These family members are economically interdependent and affect one another. This may include husband, wife, their children, and relatives. Accordingly, one building may include more than one household.

Ijabana: a khat-chewing session in the early morning. Literally, it can be translated as *eye opener*.

Kami: the Amharic version of chewer.

Khat culture: involves the ceremony before, during, and after chewing khat; and it includes all the sessions of khat chewing. Frequency of chewing, expenditure, session of chewing, and the integration of khat into the life of the society are some of the indicators of khat culture. In general, it is a situation in which khat becomes a part of one society's culture, economic, political, and spiritual life.

Non-chewer: a person who has never used khat in his life. This can also apply to a person who previously chews khat, but quits for more than a year.

References

Aden A, Dimba EAO, Ndolo UM, Chindia ML (2006) Socio-economic effects of Khat chewing in North Eastern Kenya. East Afr Med J 83(3):69–73

Alfaifi H, Abdelwahab SI, Mohan S, Elhassan Taha MM, Syame SM, Shaala LA et al (2017) Catha edulis Forsk. (Khat): evaluation of its antidepressant-like activity. Phcog Mag 13:S354–S358

Anderson D, Beckerleg S, Hailu D, Klein A (2007) The Khat controversy: stimulating the debate on drugs. Berg, Oxford

Angres KB, Angres DH (2008) The disease of addiction: origins, treatment, and recovery. Dis Mon 54(10):696–721

Armstrong GE (2008) Research note: crime, chemicals, and culture: on the complexity of Khat. J Drug Issues

Baron CE, Hanlon C, Mall S et al (2016) Maternal mental health in primary care in five low- and middle-income countries: a situational analysis. BMC Health Serv Res 16:53. https://doi.org/10.1186/s12913-016-1291-z

Beckerleg S (2008) Khat in East Africa: taking women into or out of sex work? Subst Use Misuse 43(8–9):1170–1185

Bhui K, Warfa N (2007) Drug consumption in conflict zones in Somalia. PLoS Med 4(12)

Bosredon P (2004) Harar, its life history in trade. In: Revault P, Santelli S (eds) A Muslim City of Ethiopia: Harar. Maisonne Uve et Larose, Paris

Burton FR, John SH, William CB (1856) First footsteps in East Africa. Longman, Brown Green, and Longman, London

Carrier N (2005) 'Miraa is Cool': the cultural importance of Miraa (Khat) for Tigania and Igembe youth in Kenya. J Afr Cult Stud 17(2):201–218

Carrier N (2007) Kenyan Khat: the social life of a stimulant. Brill, Leiden

Carrier N (2008) Is Miraa a drug?: Categorizing Kenyan Khat. Subst Use Misuse 43:803–818

Carrier N, Klantschnig G (2018) Quasilegality: Khat, cannabis and Africa's drug laws. Third World Q 39(2):350–365

CHF International (2006) Grassroots conflict assessment of the Somali region, Ethiopia. Addis Ababa, Ethiopia

Cochrane L, Davin O'R (2016) Legal harvest and illegal trade: trends, challenges, and options in Khat production in Ethiopia. Int J Drug Policy 30:27–34

Cochrane L, Negash G (2017) Developing policy in contested space: Khat in Ethiopia. In: Asnake Kefale, Zerihun Mohammed. The multiple faces of Khat. Forum for social studies, pp 143–162

Compendium of OECD Well-Being Indicators (2011) Material living conditions. OECD

Cox G, Rampes H (2003) Adverse effects of Khat: a review. Adv Psychiatr Treat 9

Dhaifalaha I, Santavyb J (2004) Khat habit and its health effect. A natural amphetamine. Biomed Papers 148(1):11–15

ECDD. 2006. Assessment of Khat (Catha edulis Forsk) 34th ECDD 2006/4.4

El-Wajeh YAM, Thornhill MH (2009) Qat and its health effects. Br Dent J 206:17–21

Development Planning and Research Directorate, Ministry of Finance and Economic Development (2012) Ethiopia's Progress towards Eradicating Poverty: An Interim Report on Poverty Analysis Study (2010/11), Addis Ababa

Ezekiel G (2004) Leaf of Allah: Khat and agricultural transformation in Hararge, Ethiopia 1875-1991. James curry Ltd, Oxford

Ezekiel G (2008) Scourge of life or an economic lifeline? Public discourses on Khat (Catha edulis) in Ethiopia. Subst Use Misuse 43(6):784–802

Ezekiel G (2010a) Khat in the horn of Africa: historical perspectives and current trends. J Ethnopharmacol 132(3):607–614
Ezekiel G (ed) (2010b) Taking the place of food: Khat in Ethiopia. Red Sea Press, Asmara
Ezekiel G (2010c) The culture of Khat. OGINA, Oromo arts in Diaspora http://www.ogina.org/issue5/issue5_culture_of_khat_ezekiel.html. April, 2013
Ezekiel G (2012) Khat: is it more like coffee or cocaine? Criminalizing a commodity, targeting a community. Published Online on SciRes Journal
Fantahun A, Tadesse T, Azale T (2012) Alcohol and Khat use as risk factors for HIV infection among visitors to voluntary counselling and testing centres in Northwest Ethiopia. Trop Dr 42:99
Ference M (2009) Book reviews. Soc Hist Alc Drugs *23*(2)
Gebrie A, Alebel A, Zegeye A, Tesfaye B (2018) Prevalence and predictors of Khat chewing among Ethiopian university students: a systematic review and meta-analysis. PLoS One 13(4): e0195718. https://doi.org/10.1371/journal.pone.0195718
Gessesse Dessie (2013) Favouring a demonised plant: Khat and Ethiopian smallholder Enterprise. Nordiska African Institute, Uppsala
Getahun A, Krikorian AD (1973) Chat: Coffee's rival from Harar, Ethiopia. I. Botany, cultivation and use. Econ Bot 27(4):353–377
Gezon L (2012) Drug effects: Khat in biocultural and socioeconomic perspective. Left Cross Print Inc, Walnut Creek
Gibb CTC (1996) In the city of saints: religion, politics and gender in Harar, Ethiopia. Dr. Phil. thesis, University of Oxford
Girmay A, Mariam AG, Yazachew M (2007) Khat use and risky sexual behavior among youth in Asendabo town, South Western Ethiopia. Ethiopia J Health Sci 17(1)
Gudata ZG (2020) Khat culture and economic wellbeing: comparison of a chewer and non-chewer families in Harar city. Cogent Soc Sci 6(1). https://doi.org/10.1080/23311886.2020.1848501
Gudata ZG, Cochrane L, Imana G (2019) An assessment of Khat consumption habit and its linkage to household economies and work culture: the case of Harar city. PLoS One 14(11):e0224606. https://doi.org/10.1371/journal.pone.0224606
Habtamu E (2009) Ethiopia's Khat: opportunity or threat? Ezega Ethiopian News. http://www.Ezega.com, obtained on November 2013
Haile D, Lakew Y (2015) Khat chewing practice and associated factors among adults in Ethiopia: further analysis using the 2011 demographic and health survey. PLoS One 10(6):e0130460. https://doi.org/10.1371/journal.pone.0130460
Hailu D (2007) Should Khat be banned? The development impact. International Poverty Centre (IPC), Number 40
Harrison EL, Samuel HP (eds) (2000) Culture matters: how values shape human Progress. Basic Books, New York
Hassan ANGM, Gunaid AA, Murray-Lyon IM (2007) Khat (Catha edulis): health aspects of Khat chewing. East Mediterr Health J 13(3)
Havell C (2004) Khat use in Somali, Ethiopian and Yemeni communities in England: issues and solutions. A report by Turning Point
Inglehart R, Baker Wayne E (2000) Modernization, cultural change, and the persistence of traditional values. Am Sociol Rev 65
Khawaja M, Al-Nsour M, Saad G (2008) Khat (Catha edulis) chewing during pregnancy in Yemen: findings from a national population survey. Matern Child Health J 12:308–312
Klein A (2007) Khat and the creation of tradition in the Somali diaspora. In: Fountain, Jane and Korf, Dirk J., eds. Drugs in Society: European Perspectives. Radcliffe Publishing Ltd, Oxford. ISBN 978-1-84619-093-3
Klein A (2014) Framing the chew: narratives of development, drugs and danger with regard to Khat (Catha edulis). In: Labate B, Cavnar C (eds) Prohibition, religious freedom, and human rights: regulating traditional drug use. Springer, Berlin/Heidelberg. https://doi.org/10.1007/978-3-642-40957-8_7

Krikorian AD, Getahun A (1973) Chat: Coffee's rival from Harar, Ethiopia. II. Chemical composition. Econ Bot 27(4):378–389
Kuczkowski KM (2005) Herbal ecstasy: cardiovascular complications of Khat chewing in pregnancy. Acta Anaesth Belg 56:19–21
Lamina S (2010) Khat (Catha edulis): the herb with officio-legal, socio-cultural and economic uncertainty. S Afr J Sci 106(3/4)
Lemessa D (2001) Khat (Catha edulis): botany, distribution, cultivation, usage and economics in Ethiopia. UN-Emergencies Unit for Ethiopia, Addis Ababa
Mahamoud HD, Muse SM, Roberts LR et al (2016) Khat chewing and cirrhosis in Somaliland: case series. Afr J Pri Health Care Family Med, ISSN: (Online) 2071–2936, (Print) 2071–2928
Manghi RA, Broers B, Khan R, Benguettat D, Khazaal Y, Zullino D (2009) Khat use: lifestyle or addiction? J Psychoactive Drugs 41(1):1–10
Mekuria W (2018) Public discourse on Khat (Catha edulis) production in Ethiopia: review. J Agric Exten Rural Dev 10(10):192–200
Mekuriaw B, Belayneh Z, Yitayih Y (2020) Magnitude of Khat use and associated factors among women attending antenatal care in Gedeo zone health centers, southern Ethiopia: a facility based cross sectional study. BMC Public Health 20:110
Muluneh Bekele Etana (2018) Economic and social impacts of Khat (Catha edulis Forsk) chewing among youth in Sebeta town, Oromia Ethiopia. Biomed Stat Inform 3(2):29–33
Nakajima M, Dokam A, Saem NK, Alsoofi M, al'Absi M (2016) Correlates of concurrent Khat and tobacco use in Yemen. Subst Use Misuse 51(12). https://doi.org/10.1080/10826084.2016.1188950
Negussie D, Berhane Y, Alem A, Ellsberg M, Emmelin M, Hogberg U, Kullgren G (2009) Intimate partner violence and depression among women in Rural Ethiopia: a cross-sectional study. Clinical Practice and Epidemiology in Mental Health: BioMed Central Ltd
Njoh JA (2006) Tradition, culture and development in Africa: historical lessons for modern development planning. Ashgate Publishing Company, Burlington
Odenwald M (2007) The consumption of Khat and other drugs in Somali combatants: a cross-sectional study. PLoS Med 4(12)
Odenwald M, Hinkel H, Schauer E et al (2009) Use of Khat and posttraumatic stress disorder as risk factors for psychotic symptoms: a study of Somali combatants. Soc Sci Med 69:1040–1048
Orlien S, Ismael Y, Ahmed A et al (2018a) Unexplained chronic liver disease in Ethiopia: a cross-sectional study. BMC Gastroenterol 18:27. https://doi.org/10.1186/s12876-018-0755-5
Orlien S, Sandven I, Berhe N et al (2018b) Khat chewing increases the risk for developing chronic liver disease: a hospital-based case-control study. J Hepatol 68:S168–S169
Rachidi S (2019) "Khat" it out: is the Narcotic plant holding back Djibouti's development? Inside Arabia Online. https://insidearabia.com/khat-it-out-narcotic-plant-holding-back-djiboutis-development/ April 2029
Reda AA, Moges A, Biadgilign S et al (2012) Prevalence and determinants of Khat (Catha edulis) chewing among high school students in eastern Ethiopia: a cross-sectional study. PLoS One 7(3):e33946. https://doi.org/10.1371/journal.pone.0033946
Ruth K (2016) Assessment of the effects of Khat consumption on the wellbeing of families in Meru County, Kenya. A thesis submitted in fulfillment of the requirements for the degree of doctor of philosophy (PhD). Kenyatta University Department of Sociology
Said Sheikh Aden and Ali Yassin Sheikh (2018) Social and economic difficulties caused by Khat usage in Somalia. Int J Humanit Soc Sci 8(8). https://doi.org/10.30845/ijhss.v8n8p21
Sikiru L (2012) Flower of paradise (Khat: Catha edulis): psychosocial, health and sports perspectives. Afr J Health Sci 24:69–83
Solomon T et al (2011) Khat chewing in persons with severe mental illness in Ethiopia: a qualitative study exploring perspectives of patients and caregivers. Transcult Psychiatry 48:455
Sultan Haji Temam (January, 2011) Harari people regional state: programme of plan on adaption to climate change. Environmental Protection Authority of the Federal Democratic Republic of Ethiopia, Harar

Taye H, Aune JB (2002) Khat expansion in the Ethiopian highlands effects on the farming system in Habro District. Noragric. Agricultural University of Norway
The Third Integrated Household Living Conditions Survey (EICV3): Main Indicators Report (2010) National Institute of Statistics of Rwanda
Trimingham JS (1965) Islam in Ethiopia. Frank Cass and Co. Ltd, London
van der Wolf M (April 30, 2013) Chewing Khat increasingly popular among Ethiopians. Reporter for the Voice of America, Addis Ababa
Weber M (1930) The Protestant ethic and the Spirit of capitalism. George Allen & Unwin Ltd, London
Wikipedia the free Encyclopaedia (2014) Living Standard. en.m.wikipedia.org/wiki/Standard_of_living. February 28
Yeshigeta G, Haile-Amlak A (2004) Khat chewing and its socio-demographic correlates among the staff of Jimma University. Ethiop J Health Dev
Yigzaw K (2002) Cigarette smoking and Khat chewing among college students in North West Ethiopia. Ethiop J Health Dev 16(1):9–17

Cytotoxicity and Genotoxicity of Khat (*Catha edulis* Forsk)

82

Maged El-Setouhy and Ashraf A. Hassan

Contents

Summary 1746
Conclusion and Recommendations 1747
References 1747

Abstract

Khat genotoxicity is still a matter of debate especially in human studies. In animal studies, khat administration in different dosages was shown to be associated with different kinds of genotoxicity. This was attributed to its alkaline effect and oxidative stress. These effects were detected in the bone marrow, buccal mucosa, and DNA damage in animals. These results suggested khat relation to cancer but was not proven in humans although some studies showed a statistical relation between khat use and cancer. On the other hand, the number of micronuclei was also found to be higher among khat users which suggested the relation between khat use and oral cancer. However, the combined effect of khat use and smoking should be considered. Still more human studies are needed to prove that the detected genotoxicity of khat in animals is also present in humans with different levels of its use.

M. El-Setouhy (✉)
Department of Family and Community Medicine, Faculty of Medicine, Jazan University, Jazan, Saudi Arabia
e-mail: melsetouhy@jazanu.edu.sa

A. A. Hassan
Department of Medical Laboratory Technology, Faculty of Applied Medical Sciences, Jazan University, Jazan, Saudi Arabia
e-mail: aahassan@jazanu.edu.sa

V. B. Patel, V. R. Preedy (eds.), *Handbook of Substance Misuse and Addictions*,
https://doi.org/10.1007/978-3-030-92392-1_89

Keywords

Khat · Chronic chewing · Genotoxicity · Cytotoxicity · Apoptosis · Cancer · Micronucleus · Reactive oxygen species

Khat is consumed on a daily basis by several million people. Published findings showed that this herb has genotoxic effects in humans which are critical. On the possible link between khat chewing and cancer, epidemiological studies and laboratory experiments are desperately needed. In addition to cancer, the effects of khat on reproduction should be taken into account. Aneuploidy is thought to be responsible for approximately 30% of all spontaneous abortions and 6% of all neonatal deaths. Because khat produces chromosomal abnormalities in mouse sperm cells, it's probable that the same thing happens in khat users' germ cells (Dellarco et al. 1986).

Recent study revealed that the number of micronucleus (MN)-positive buccal mucosa cells was higher in khat consumer groups than controls, and the effects of khat, cigarette, and alcohol were addictive. The largest incidence of khat-induced MN was recorded during the fourth week following use, according to time-kinetics research. Given the growing amount of data linking genetic harm to cancer, their findings suggest that khat usage, particularly when combined with alcohol and tobacco, may increase risk of cancer (Kassie et al. 2001).

The ions or radicals produced by normal cellular metabolic activities are known as reactive oxygen species (ROS). They include radicals such as superoxide anion and hydroxyl radical, as well as non-radicals such as hydrogen peroxide. These molecules play a role in a variety of biological functions, including gene expression, proliferation, and differentiation. Exogenous and endogenous stress can cause an overabundance of reactive oxygen species (ROS), which can harm molecules like nucleic acids, proteins, and lipids. This can lead to cell cycle arrest and premature senescence, as well as the activation of cell death pathways (Fialkow et al. 2007; Dumont et al. 2000; Macip et al. 2002; Huang et al. 2000).

Glutathione (GSH) is an important tripeptide present in mammalian cells, where it regulates thiol redox and detoxifies reactive compounds. GSH deficiency makes cells more susceptible to proapoptotic stimuli and can even trigger apoptosis in the absence of such stimuli. Superoxide dismutase, catalase, and GSH are examples of cellular antioxidant defense systems. They protect cells from oxidative stress by preventing disruptions in ROS homeostasis (Valko et al. 2007).

The oral delivery of khat extract into rats reduced the activities of free radical metabolizing/scavenging enzyme systems, resulting in increased free radical concentration and oxidative stress. This could be related to the alkaloid portion of khat. Sustained oxidative stress caused by khat use has been linked to the development of a number of disorders, including cancer, hepatotoxicity, nephrotoxicity, cardiovascular toxicity, and neurological diseases (Al-Qirim et al. 2002; Carvalho 2003).

In a study conducted by Barkwan et al. (2004), khat extract at 200 ug/ml concentrations caused cytotoxic, genotoxic, and clastogenic effects in a human cell line in vitro. However, two more epidemiological studies on distinct human populations had been conducted, the results of which point to an increased risk of upper gastrointestinal cancer. In the first study, 3064 men and women with a high frequency of tumors of the gastroesophageal junction or cardia were shown to have a high frequency of khat chewing and water pipe smoking (Gunaid et al. 1995). On the other hand, the second study found that long-term khat chewers who were residents of Asir Region, Kingdom of Saudi Arabia, had a higher rate of mouth cancer (Soufi and Kameswaran 1991). These results were supported by animal researches that progressively considered khat as carcinogen agents. The tannins in khat have the propensity to thicken the mucosa of the oropharynx and esophagus in humans, which would lead to cancer in some situations (Drake 1988). Tannins have also been shown to induce nucleosome-size fragmentation in HL-60 cells (Sakagam et al. 1995; Casalini et al. 1999).

There are other components in khat leaves, such as terpenoids, that have been demonstrated to have cytotoxic activity in human tumor cell lines and may have been present in aqueous extract (Zheng 1999).

Our recent research (Hassan et al. 2020) found that chewing khat on a daily basis caused the generation of reactive oxygen species (ROS), which can lead to oxidative damage. Antioxidants, both enzymatic and nonenzymatic, were found to protect against oxidative damage in this study. Chronic khat chewers produced more ROS endogenously, which was associated with a lower level of superoxide dismutase (SOD). In the meantime, increased glutathione reductase (GR) activity indicates the presence of very hazardous substances. Long-term khat chewers are at risk of oxidative toxicity and DNA damage; hence, it is strongly advised that they stop chewing the drug. Our research also discovered a statistically insignificant increase in the levels of 8-hydroxy-deoxy guanosine (8-OHdG) in chronic khat chewers, which could explain why chronic khat chewing plays such a crucial part in the DNA damage process. Chronic khat users were discovered to be at an increased risk of oxidative stress and DNA damage. The carcinogenic process is initiated and accelerated by endogenous oxidative damage to DNA. This finding supports the notion that persistent khat eating poses a health risk. Khat chewers are strongly advised to give up the habit for the sake of their health and quality of life.

Although our earlier investigation found a marginally significant increase in the levels of 8-OHdG in chronic khat chewers (CKCs), the negative influence on the levels of antioxidant enzymes may potentially explain, at least in part, the probable association between CKC and oxidative DNA damage. To our knowledge, no previous research has looked at the association between CKC and the level of 8-OHdG in human blood as a surrogate biomarker of DNA damage (Hassan et al. 2020).

Regarding the effect on the bone marrow, a previous investigation of Khat extract's effect on mouse bone marrow cells found that at doses of 10, 20, and 40 mg/kg, khat extract caused considerably higher frequency of sister chromatid exchanges (SCEs) ($p < 0.001$) in cells treated compared to controls (Abderrahman and Modalla 2008). However, there was no discernible difference between the treated and untreated groups. Das et al. (2004) reported a similar increase in the frequency of SCEs generated by alkaloids in their investigation employing sanguinarine (SG), a benzophenanthridine alkaloid (Das et al. 2004). They discovered that (SG) increased the frequency of sister chromatid exchange. In mouse bone marrow cells, the primary alkaloid in betel nut, arecoline (ARC), was found to cause a high frequency of SCEs after oral administration (OA) and intraperitoneal injection (IP) (Chatterjee and Deb 1999).

It has been suggested that *Catha edulis* (khat) contains mutagenic and potentially carcinogenic substances (Abderrahman and Modalla 2008). Culvenor et al. (1962) offered evidence that alkaloids' effects on cell nuclei are mostly owing to their ability to act as alkylating agents in the cell (Culvenor et al. 1962). The production of several types of chromosomal abnormalities was generated linearly with increasing concentrations of alkaloids and *Catha edulis* (khat) extract. The broken chromosome is the most prevalent anomaly (Abderrahman and Modalla 2008). Chromosomal fractures are caused by interference with DNA synthesis (Evans 1969). The percentages of broken chromosomes rise linearly with the concentrations utilized, and they also increase with time in all situations (Abderrahman and Modalla 2008). This shows that the alkaloidal fraction may contain alkylating substances (S-dependent agents) that cause aberrations through mis-replication (DNA damage caused by DNA replication of a DNA molecule containing lesions) (Palitti 1998). This theory is corroborated by Peter et al. (2002), who discovered a range of genotoxic alkaloids in Asteraceae family of plants (Peter et al. 2002). Various types of chromosome aberrations were induced by *Catha edulis* (khat). The percentage of these abnormalities is increased with the increases of both concentration and exposure time in all treatments (Abderrahman and Modalla 2008).

High concentrations of fresh khat leaf extract (500 and 5000 g/mL) were shown to diminish the mitotic index (MI) significantly ($p < 0.05$) in a recent study by Al-Zubairi AS, 2017, but only the highest concentration (5000 ug/mL) was found to produce chromosomal abnormality. The results of the micronucleus (MN) induction test, on the other hand, revealed no significant micronuclei production after treatment with various doses, although the cytochalasin-B proliferation index (CBPI) was found to be impacted by the highest concentration of fresh khat leaf extract. Only high concentration of fresh khat leaf extract caused chromosomal abnormalities, and the most common types of aberrations were dicentrics, ring chromosomes, breaks, and exchanges (Al-Zubairi 2017).

Formation of dicentric and ring chromosomes in metaphase cells may indicate telomeric loss or telomeric associations, as well as chromatid/chromosome breaks, which initiate the chromosomal breakage-fusion-bridge cycle, which eventually results in the production of mitotically unstable chromosome aberration, such as ring chromosome, dicentric chromosome, or telomeric association (Gisselsson et al. 2000; Lo et al. 2002). Endoreduplication is a mechanism in which DNA is amplification without cell division in eukaryotic cells (Sumner 1998; Sugimoto-Shirasu et al. 2002). Endoreduplication (Sumner 1998; Sugimoto-Shirasu et al. 2002; Pastor et al. 2002; Cortes and Pastor 2003) is formed when DNA topoisomerase II activity is inhibited, and an increase in the number of endoreduplicated cell chromosomes may suggest that the test material is capable of suppressing cell cycle progression.

Oral squamous cell carcinoma (OSCC) develops in participants who use khat, according to a recent study (Alshahrani et al. 2021). Short-term khat users were found to have seven somatic alterations in four of nine cancer-related genes during the study. In addition, nine somatic alterations in five of nine cancer-related genes were discovered in the group of long-term khat users (Fig. 1).

OSCC was diagnosed in both groups of participants. ARID1A, MLH1, PIK3CA, and TP53 were four prevalent cancer-related genes associated with somatic mutations in two sets of respondents. Epidemiological studies have linked mutation processes in specific genes to an increased chance of developing OSCC (Lui et al. 2013; Galot et al. 2020; Husain and Neyaz 2019). In DNA samples from long-term khat users, two landmark mutation processes were discovered in ARID1A and MLH1, whereas only one landmark mutation was found in MLH1 from short-term khat users. By comparing the results to DNA samples from the control group, this was accomplished. Another substitution mutation in ARID2 was discovered and was only found in long-term khat users. Other investigations have suggested that systemic mutations in ARID2 have a role in oral carcinogenesis, which can be induced by NF-B signaling dysregulation (Su et al. 2017; Ma et al. 2017; Er et al. 2015) and vigorous long-term tobacco smoking (Liu and Zhao 2019). TP53 protein expression was positive in all immunohistochemistry oral regions, indicating that both groups had similar rates of OSCC development. Furthermore, all of the affected people had

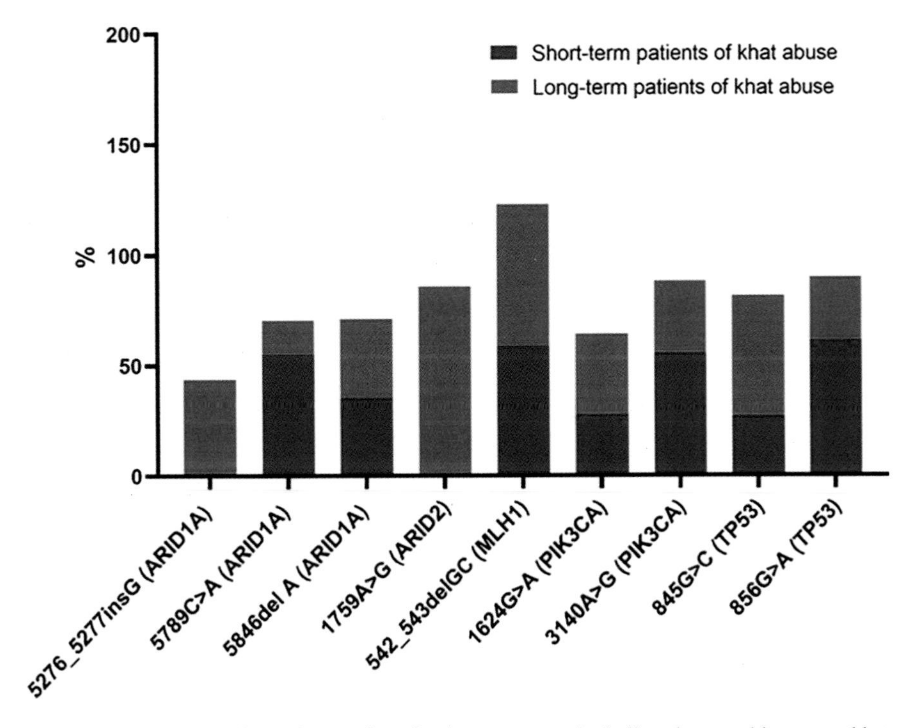

Fig. 1 The incidence of genetic mutations for the two groups including short- and long-term khat users diagnosed with oral squamous cell carcinoma (OSCC) (Alshahrani et al. 2021)

mutations in the TP53 gene, which is one of the most transformative genes in individuals with OSCC (Abrahao et al. 2011; Renzi et al. 2019; Su et al. 2019; Yao et al. 2019). Poorly differentiated cells with an unstable histological structure were also discovered by histopathological examinations. This supports the theory that chewing khat, whether for a short or extended amount of time, causes OSCC.

The viability of several cell types was shown to be decreased by khat therapy, which was found to be significantly increased at higher dosages and after long-term exposure (Al-Qadhi et al. 2021) (Fig. 2).

Microvilli loss, plasma membrane blebbing, pyknosis due to chromatin condensation, cytoplasmic vacuolization, and cell breaking up into apoptotic bodies were all seen in khat-exposed cells under optical and electron microscopes. To corroborate the prior finding and distinguish between the early and late stages of apoptosis, intercalating staining methods were applied. For example, apoptotic fractions were commonly probed using annexin V/propidium iodide (PI) and acridine orange (AO)/ethidium bromide (EB) labeling. Annexin V binding was absent in untreated cells, whereas khat-treated cells had a higher number of annexin V-positive cells (Abid et al. 2013; Murdoch et al. 2011; Lu et al. 2017). Because annexin V binds particularly to the phosphatidylserine (PS) in the inner layer of the plasma membrane, it can detect any breakdown of the phospholipid layer's integrity and so identify apoptotic cells (Logue et al. 2009) (Fig. 3).

In comparison with prior claims (IC50: 33–200 g/mL), the extracts of khat showed significant cytotoxicity on cancer cells, with half-maximal inhibitory

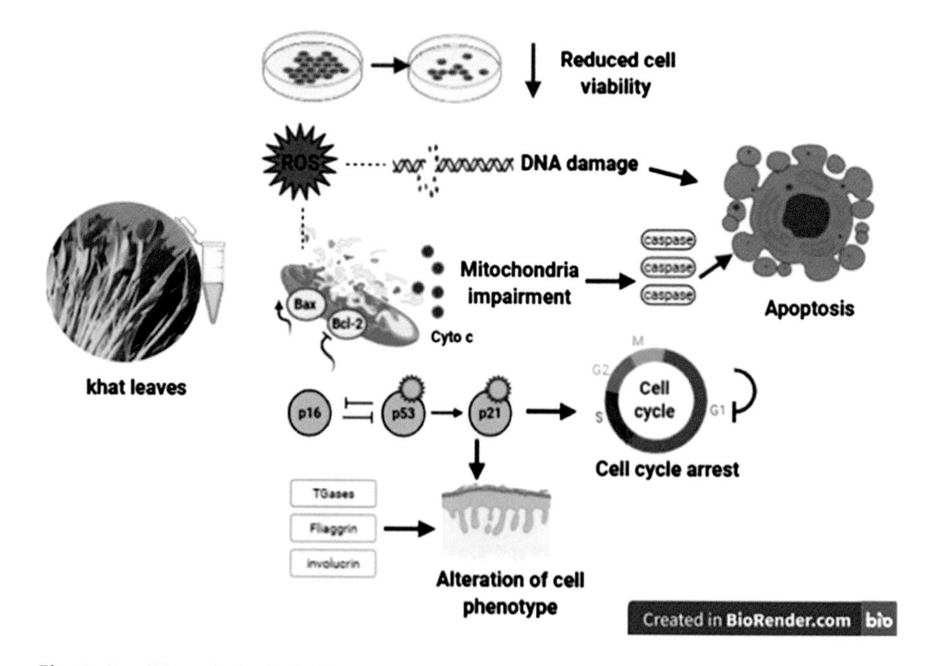

Fig. 2 Possible toxicological effects of khat on cultured cells (Al-Qadhi et al. 2021)

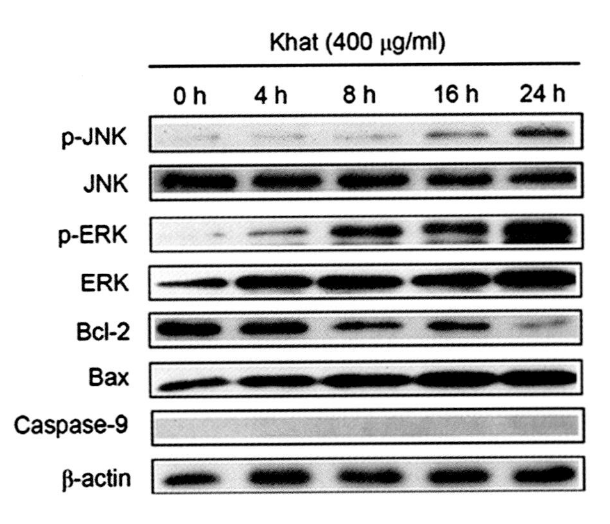

Fig. 3 Expression of apoptosis-associated proteins and MAPKs (p-JNK, JNK, p-ERK, ERK). MDA-MB-231 cells were incubated with 400 μg/ml khat for 4, 8, 16, and 24 h; apoptosis- and MAPK-associated protein expression was detected by Western blotting (Lu et al. 2017)

concentrations (IC50) ranging from 22 to 59 g/mL. Since khat extract showed greater cytotoxicity against normal cells (IC50: 6–41 g/mL) (Alsanosy et al. 2020), cytotoxic effect on normal cells may pose several health problems to khat consumers.

Overall, three pathways are involved in apoptosis, which eventually trigger the caspase cascade, which is responsible for the morphological changes seen after cell death. Receptor-ligand interaction, a mitochondrial-mediated route, and stress in the endoplasmic reticulum are the main processes. These pathways have been linked to the activation of caspases 8, 9, and 12 (Van Cruchten and Van den Broeck 2002; Toshiyuki et al. 2000).

Much research has been conducted to determine caspase activity and Bcl-2/Bax protein expression to better understand the underlying mechanism of khat-induced cell death. The induction of apoptosis by khat impacted most of the cells at the same time and was highly dependent on the dose and duration. The caspase 8 and 9 enzymes were shown to be involved in the cellular mechanisms that led to khat-induced cell death. It's worth noting that Fas expression remained constant throughout the experiment, implying that death signaling molecules, not Fas, were responsible for caspase activation (Abid et al. 2013).

In an in vitro investigation, Al-Qadhi et al. 2021 found that khat decreased the viability and proliferation of a variety of cell types. Khat-exposed cells showed ultrastructural alterations that resembled those seen in apoptosis. This suppression was most likely mediated through the mitochondrial apoptotic pathway, and it was linked to a change in mitochondrial phenotype as well as increased Bax and decreased Bcl-2 protein expression. Similarly, cell death in khat-exposed cells was linked to enhanced ROS generation and subsequent caspase cascade activation. More research is needed to compare the phytochemistry of khat with phytoconstituents from other plants, as well as in vivo and clinical trials (Al-Qadhi et al. 2021).

Khat administration decreased the vitality of MDA MB 231 cells in a time- and dose-dependent manner, according to a recent study of cell viability assay. According to flow cytometric analysis, 400 g/ml of khat caused apoptosis in MDA MB 231 cells in a time-dependent manner, which was compatible with the cell viability experiment (Lu et al. 2017).

In Ethiopia, a recent study looked at the impact of khat consumption during pregnancy on birth outcomes in the year 2020.

A total of 5343 mother-neonate pairings from 15 studies were included in the systematic review and meta-analysis. During pregnancy, alcohol, khat, cigarettes, and narghile were used, and significant poor birth outcomes were observed because of these substances. Khat users were 2.4 times more likely to have congenitally defective neonates (95% CI: AOR 14 2.4; 1.11, 5.19) and 3.1 times more likely to have low birth weight neonates (95% CI: AOR 14 3.19; 1.01, 5.37) than nonusers. Conclusion: In Ethiopia, the detrimental effects of prenatal substance use were prematurity, low birth weight, and congenital deformity. As a result, existing public health activities should be bolstered to assist women in discontinuing their use of these substances. Furthermore, for comprehensive prevention of the problem, raising public awareness about the potential detrimental effects of substance use during pregnancy on birth result is critical (Bayih et al. 2021).

Summary

Our review showed that chronic khat chewing induces ROS production and potentially causes oxidative toxicity. ROS endogenous formation increased in CKCs with a decreased SOD level. Meanwhile, GR activity elevation reflects the presence of highly toxic compounds. Habitually, long-term khat chewers will be susceptible to oxidative toxicity with a possible DNA damage.

On the other hand, fresh khat leaf extract in high concentrations have a genotoxic effect on cultured Chinese hamster cell line that raised the need for further studies to better understand the molecular mechanisms of action of khat leaf extract for a better comprehension.

It was also shown that khat inhibited the viability and proliferation of numerous cell types in in vitro studies. Cells exposed to khat exhibited ultrastructural changes that resemble to apoptosis features. This inhibition was probably mediated via the mitochondrial pathway of apoptosis and associated with an alteration in the mitochondria phenotype as well as increased Bax and decreased Bcl-2 protein expression. In the same way, cell death in khat-exposed cells was associated with increased ROS production and eventual activation of caspase cascades.

One study showed that the adverse neonatal effects of khat, tobacco, alcohol, and narghile use during pregnancy were estimated. Prematurity, low birth weight and congenital malformation were the investigated adverse effects of antenatal substance use. Therefore, the existing public health efforts should be encouraged to help women cease using these substances completely before pregnancy.

Conclusion and Recommendations

- Khat chewers are highly recommended to quit habit of khat chewing for better health and quality of life.
- More studies are required to investigate the role of khat chewing for short and long duration on the genotoxicity and antioxidant defense mechanism.
- Moreover, further studies are required to compare the phytochemistry of khat with phytoconstituents from other plants, and in vivo and clinical reviews are also highly required.
- Increasing public awareness about the potential negative impacts of substance use during pregnancy on birth outcome would be of greatest importance for comprehensive intervention in the prevention of antenatal substance use.

References

Abderrahman SM, Modalla N (2008) Genotoxic effects of Catha edulis (Khat) extract on mice bone marrow cells. Jordan J Biol Sci 1(4):165–172

Abid MDN, Chem J, Xiang M, Zhou J, Chem X, Gong F (2013) Khat (Catha edulis) generate reactive oxygen species and promotes hepatic cell apoptosis via MAPK activation. Int J Mol Med 32:389–395

Abrahao AC, Bonelli BV, Nunes FD et al (2011) Immunohistochemical expression of p53, p16 and hTERT in oral squamous cell carcinoma and potentially malignant disorders. Braz Oral Res 25: 34–41

Al-Qadhi G, Mohammed MMA, Al-Ak'hali M, Al-Moraissi EA (2021) Khat (Catha edulis Forsk) induced apoptosis and cytotoxicity in cultured cells: a scoping review. Heliyon 7:e08466

Al-Qirim TM, Shahwan M, Zaidi KR, Uddin Q, Banu N (2002) Effect of khat, its constituents and restraint stress on free radical metabolism of rats. J Ethnopharmacol 83:245–250

Alsanosy R, Alhazmi HA, Sultana S, Abdalla AN, Ibrahim Y, Al Bratty M, Banji D, Khardali I, Khalid A (2020) Phytochemical screening and cytotoxic properties of ethanolic extract of young and mature Khat leaves. J Chem 2020:1–9

Alshahrani SA, Al-Qahtani WS, Almufareh NA, Domiaty DM, Albasher GI et al (2021) Oral cancer among khat users: finding evidence from DNA analysis of nine cancer-related gene mutations. BMC Oral Health 21:626

Al-Zubairi AS (2017) Genotoxic assessment of fresh khat leaves extract in Chinese hamster ovary cell lines. J Med Sci 17(3):126–132

Barkwan SS, Barnett CR, Barnet YA, Tomkins PT, Fokunang CN (2004) Evaluation of cytotoxic and genotoxic potential of khat (Catha edulis Forsk) extracts on human T lymphoblastoid cell line. J Med Sci 4(2):110–114

Bayih WA, Belay DM, Ayalew MY, Tassew MA, Chanie ES et al (2021) The effect of substance uses during pregnancy on neonatal outcomes in Ethiopia: a systematic review and meta-analysis. Heliyon 7:e06740

Carvalho F (2003) The toxicological potential of khat. J Ethnopharmacol 87:1–2

Casalini C, Lodocivi M, Briani C, Paganelli S et al (1999) Effect of complex polyphenols and tannins fro red wine (WCPT) on chemically induced oxidative DNA damage in rat. Eur J Nutr 38:190–195

Chatterjee A, Deb S (1999) Genotoxic effect of arecoline given either by the peritoneal or oral route in murine bone marrow cells and the influence of N-acetylcysteine. Cancer Lett 139(1):23–31

Cortes F, Pastor N (2003) Induction of endoreduplication by topoisomerase II catalytic inhibitors. Mutagenesis 18:105–112

Culvenor CC, Dann AT, Dick AT (1962) Alkylation as the mechanism by which the hepatotoxic pyrrizidine alkaloids on cell nuclei. Nature 195:570

Das A, Mukherjee A, Chakrabarti J (2004) Sanguinarine: an evaluation of in cytogenetic activity. Mutat Res 563(1):81–87

Dellarco VL, Maurnin KH, Waters MD (1986) Aneuploidy data review committee: summary compilation of chemical data base and evaluation of test methodology. Mutat Res 167:149–169

Drake P (1988) Khat-chewing in the near east. Lancet 331(8584):532–533

Dumont P, Burton M, Chen QM, Gonos ES, Frippiat C et al (2000) Induction of replicative senescence biomarkers by sublethal oxidative stresses in normal human fibroblast. Free Radic Biol Med 28:361–373

Er TK, Wang YY, Chen CC et al (2015) Molecular characterization of oral squamous cell carcinoma using targeted next -generation sequencing. Oral Dis 21(7):872–878

Evans HJ (1969) The induction of chromosome aberration by N-mustard and its dependence on DNA synthesis. Proc R Soc Ser B Biol 173:491–512

Fialkow L, Wang Y, Downey GP (2007) Reactive oxygen and nitrogen species as signaling molecules regulating neutrophil function. Free Radic Biol Med 42:153–164

Galot R, van Marcke C, Helaers R et al (2020) Liquid biopsy for mutational profiling of locoregional recurrent and/or metastatic head and neck squamous cell carcinoma. Oral Oncol 104:104631

Gisselsson D, Pattersson L, Hoglund M, Heidenblad M, Gorunova L et al (2000) Chromosomal breakage-fusion-bridge events cause genetic intratumor heterogeneity. Proc Natl Acad Sci 97: 5357–5362

Gunaid A, Sumairi A et al (1995) Oesophageal and gastric carcinoma in the Republic of Yemen. Br J Cancer 71:409–410

Hassan AA, Hobani YH, Mosbah N, Abdalla S, Zaino M, Mohan S, El-Setouhy M (2020) Chronic khat (Catha edulis) chewing and genotoxicity: the role of antioxidant defense system and oxidative damage of DNA. Pharmacogn Mag 16:S168–S173

Huang C, Zhang Z, Ding M, Li J, Ye J et al (2000) Vanadate induces p53 transactivation through hydrogen peroxide and causes apoptosis. J Biol Chem 275:32516–32522

Husain N, Neyaz A (2019) Molecular diagnostics in head and neck squamous cell carcinoma. In: Molecular diagnostics in cancer patients. Springer, Singapore, pp 165–185

Kassie F, Darroudi F, Kundi M, Schulte-Hermann R, Knasmuller S (2001) Khat (Catha Edulis) consumption causes genotoxic effects in humans int. J Cancer 92:329–332

Liu H, Zhao H (2019) Prognosis related miRNAs, DNA methylation, and epigenetic interactions in lung adenocarcinoma. Neoplasma 66(3):487–493

Lo AWI, Sprung CN, Fouladi B, Pedram M, Sabatier L et al (2002) Chromosome instability as a result of double strand breaks near telomeres in mouse embryonic stem cells. Mol Cell Biol 22: 4836–4850

Logue SE, Elgendy M, Martin SJ (2009) Expression, purification, and use of recombinant annexin V for the detection of apoptotic cells. Nat Protoc 4:1383–1395

Lu Y, Li Y, Xiang M, Zhou J, Chen J (2017) Khat promotes human breast cancer MDAMB-231 cell apoptosis via mitochondria and MAPK-associated pathways. Oncol Lett 14:3947–3952

Lui VW, Hedberg ML, Li H, Vangara BS et al (2013) Frequent mutation of the PI3K pathway in head and neck cancer defines predictive biomarkers. Cancer Disc 3(7):761–769

Ma X, Sheng S, Wu J et al (2017) LncRNAs as an intermediate in HPV16 promoting myeloid -derived suppressor cell recruitment of head and neck squamous cell carcinoma. Oncotarget 8(26):42061

Macip S, Igarashi M, Fang L, Chen A, Pan ZQ et al (2002) Inhibition of p21-mediated ROS accumulation can rescue p21-induced senescence. EMBO J21:2180–2188

Murdoch C, Aziz HA, Fang HY, Jezan H, Musaid R, Muthana M (2011) Khat (Catha edulis) alters the phenotype and anti-microbial activity of peripheral blood mononuclear cells. J Ethnopharmacol 138:780–787

Palitti F (1998) Mechanism if the origin of chromosomal aberration. Mutat Res 20:403–416

Pastor N, Flores MJ, Dominguez I, Mateos S, Cortes F (2002) High yield of endoreduplication induced by ICRF-193: a topoisomerase II catalytic inhibitor. Mutat Res/Genet Toxicol Environ Mutagen 516:113–120

Peter PE, Xia Q, Lin G, Ming WC (2002) Genotoxic pyrrolizidine alkaloids-mechanisms leading to DNA adduct formation and tumorigenicity. Int J Mol Sci 3:945–961

Renzi A, De Bonis P, Morandi L et al (2019) Prevalence of p53 dysregulations in feline oral squamous cell carcinoma and non -neoplastic oral mucosa. PLoS One 14(4):e0215621

Sakagam H, Kuribayashi N, Inda M, Sakagam T et al (1995) Induction of DNA fragmentation by tannin and lignin related substances. Anticancer Res 15(5B):2121–2128

Soufi HE, Kameswaran MT (1991) Khat and oral cancer. J Laryngol Otol 105:643–635

Su SC, Lin CW, Liu YF et al (2017) Exome sequencing of oral squamous cell carcinoma reveals molecular subgroups and novel therapeutic opportunities. Theranostics 7(5):1088

Su W, Sun S, Wang F et al (2019) Circular RNA hsa_circ_0055538 regulates the malignant biological behavior of oral squamous cell carcinoma through the p53/Bcl-2/caspase signaling pathway. J Transl Med 17(1):1–2

Sugimoto-Shirasu K, Stacey NJ, Corsar J, Roberts K, McCann MC (2002) DNA topoisomerase VI is essential for endoreduplication in Arabidopsis. Curr Biol 12:1782–1786

Sumner AT (1998) Induction of diplochromosomes in mammalian cells by inhibitors of topoisomerase II. Chromosoma 107:486–490

Toshiyuki N, Hong Z, Nobuhiro M, En L, Jin X, Bruce AY, Junying Y (2000) Caspase12 mediates endoplasmic reticulum specific apoptosis and cytotoxicity by amyloid-β. Nature 403:98–103

Valko M, Leibfritz D, Moncol J, Cronin MTD, Mazur M et al (2007) Free radicals and antioxidants in normal physiological functions and human disease. Int J Biochem Cell Biol 39:44–84

Van Cruchten S, Van den Broeck W (2002) Morphological and biochemical aspects of apoptosis, oncosis and necrosis. Anat Histol Embryol 31:214–223

Yao Y, Zhou WY, He RX (2019) Down -regulation of JMJD5 suppresses metastasis and induces apoptosis in oral squamous cell carcinoma by regulating p53/NF -κB pathway. Biomed Pharmacother 109:1994–2004

Zheng GQ (1999) Cytotoxic terpenoids and flavonoids from Artemisia annua. J Nat Prod 62: 1518–1521

Khat (*Catha edulis*) and Oral Health

83

Mir Faeq Ali Quadri and Syam Mohan

Contents

Introduction 1752
Khat and Epidemiology of Khat Use 1754
Relationship Between Oral Diseases and Khat Use 1754
Tooth Decay and Khat Use 1754
Periodontal Diseases and Khat Use 1756
Oral Cancer and Khat Use 1758
Influence of Alcohol, Smoking, and Pesticides in Oral Cancers 1760
Applications to Other Areas of Public Health 1761
Conclusion 1761
Key Facts 1762
Summary Points 1762
References 1762

Abstract

Khat chewing is on the rise and has emerged as a public health issue. The longtime consumption of khat has been associated with many health issues such as cardiovascular, gastrointestinal, hepatobiliary, genitourinary, nervous system, respiratory, and oral health (OH)-related problems. Among the OH-related problems, tooth decay, periodontal diseases, and oral cancer are the most prevalent and have been linked with khat use. This chapter introduces OH,

Mir Faeq Ali Quadri and Syam Mohan contributed equally with all other contributors.

M. F. Ali Quadri
Dental Public Health, Department of Preventive Dental Sciences, College of Dentistry, Jazan University, Jazan, Saudi Arabia
e-mail: dr.faeq.quadri@gmail.com; fquadri@jazanu.edu.sa

S. Mohan (✉)
Substance Abuse and Toxicology Research Center, Jazan University, Jazan, Saudi Arabia
e-mail: syammohanm@yahoo.com; smohan@jazanu.edu.sa

V. B. Patel, V. R. Preedy (eds.), *Handbook of Substance Misuse and Addictions*,
https://doi.org/10.1007/978-3-030-92392-1_90

followed by a description of khat and its epidemiology. Then, a review of the evidence relating khat use to oral diseases is presented. It is seen, based on the available reports, that khat use cannot be considered as a causal factor for oral diseases. However, it is possible that cathinone, a prime extract in khat, may cause xerostomia which can aggravate the infection process in an already infected tooth or supporting tissues. Furthermore, with the available literature, the direct relationship between khat alone and oral cancer is also questionable. In few studies, khat seems to be an anticancer agent, but few other studies point to the chances of carcinogenesis associated with a longtime chewing of khat. In conclusion, the effect of khat on oral tissues is not as direct as in case of many other coadministered stuff like sugar or sugared beverages, alcohol, tobacco smoking, smokeless tobacco, and the presence of pesticides.

Keywords

Khat · *Catha edulis* · Oral health · Oral mucosa · Oral cancer · Xerostomia · Periodontal diseases · Tooth decay · Dental caries · Relationship

Abbreviations

FDI	Dental Federation Internationale
GBD	Global Burden of Disease
OH	Oral health
WHO	World Health Organization

Introduction

Oral health (OH) is part of general health. The mouth, which includes the teeth and supporting structures, enables an individual to eat, speak, smile, taste, and carry out fundamental daily activities, thus reflecting one's personality. The World Health Organization (WHO) defined good OH as "a state of being free from mouth and facial pain, oral and throat cancer, oral infection and sores, periodontal (gum) disease, tooth decay, tooth loss, and other diseases and disorders that limit an individual's capacity in biting, chewing, smiling, speaking, and psychosocial wellbeing" (WHO 2016). Recently, the FDI updated the definition and advocated OH as multifaceted, involving the ability to speak, smile, smell, taste, touch, chew, swallow, and convey a range of emotions through facial expressions with confidence and without pain, discomfort, and disease of the craniofacial complex (Glick et al. 2017). Thus, OH represents the very essence of humanity and influences every aspect of our lives.

The prevalence of OH problems continues to pose a significant burden on nations and the individuals residing in them (Nunn 2006). Their impact through pain and suffering hampers the oral functions and daily activities, thus affecting the productivity of the diseased (Petersen et al. 2005a). Data from a developed nation indicates that acute OH problems had accounted for nearly 3.9 million workdays missed by people over 18 years of age and around 1.2 million school days missed by children below 18 years of age (Satcher 2000). Unless prevented or arrested at its initial stage, OH problems may continue to compromise an individual's ability to eat, sleep, socialize, and concentrate, eventually leading to distress and low overall daily performance (Maharani et al. 2017; Nurelhuda et al. 2009, 2010). Tooth decay, gum diseases, and oral cancer are the most prevalent OH problems globally (Peres et al. 2019; Frencken et al. 2017).

The Global Burden of Disease (GBD-2015) study indicates that nearly 3.5 billion people have OH problems and a major proportion of them are reported to be suffering from untreated dental caries, followed by periodontal conditions, edentulism (complete tooth loss), and severe tooth loss (having between 1 and 9 remaining teeth) (G.B.o.D.S. Collaborators 2015). Untreated dental caries of permanent teeth is the most prevalent oral disease, with 35% of the global population, equivalent to 2.4 billion people (data from 2010), being affected (Peres et al. 2021). The global age-standardized prevalence of 35% did not alter much from 1999 to 2010, 28,689 per 1,000,000 person-years in 1990 to 27,257 per 1,000,000 person-years in 2010 (Peres et al. 2021). The GBD-2020 study confirms that it is still the most prevalent oral disease globally (G.D.a.I. Collaborators 2020).

The quality of global epidemiological data for periodontal conditions is not as good as the data for dental caries (Peres et al. 2021). Many reviews are carried out in the past 20 years, but very few of them have addressed the rate of periodontitis (Gjermo et al. 2002; Needleman et al. 2018; Yang et al. 2017; Frencken et al. 2017). However, it is consistently shown that men have a far greater likelihood of suffering from periodontitis than women (Burt 2005; Albandar and Tinoco 2002), which could be attributed to the increased prevalence of established risk factors among the male population. Also, because it is usually a slowly progressing disease, the elderly population demonstrates higher prevalence than the younger ones, and the consequence of such a condition is the early loss of the tooth (Eke et al. 2016).

The next common oral disease is oral cancer. The cancers of the lip and oral cavity are among the 20 most prevalent cancers in the world. In 2018, there were 500,550 newly diagnosed cases, and in the same year, nearly 117,384 people had died due to oral cancer (Bray et al. 2015). These figures, including that of the age-standardized incidence rates, have not changed in 5 years, as demonstrated by the data from Globocan (2021) ("Erratum: Global cancer statistics 2018: GLOBOCAN estimates of incidence and mortality worldwide for 36 cancers in 185 countries" 2020). The data on oral cancer is extensive, and for the ease of obtaining information, the Globocan project summarizes and publishes the data online, which is freely accessible. It is shown that Papua New Guinea has the highest incidence of oral cancer, with 30.3 incident cases per 100,000 people, and more males than females are affected. The Southeast Asian countries of India, Pakistan, Bangladesh, and Kazakhstan have the next highest prevalence rate, ranging from 10.1 to 13.0 per 100,000 inhabitants ("Erratum: Global cancer statistics 2018: GLOBOCAN estimates of incidence and mortality worldwide for 36 cancers in 185 countries" 2020).

Therefore, despite oral diseases being mostly preventable, they continue to pose a substantial burden on the global population. If left untreated, they will negatively impact people, communities, countries, and wider regions of society. One of the widely recognized solutions is identifying common risk factors to diseases and then targeting effective prevention programs. Khat, a plant-based substance, has been studied and is usually regarded as a risk factor for most oral diseases. The following section will describe khat and then provide the current evidence on its relationship with dental caries, periodontal diseases, and oral cancer and intend to address misconceptions.

Khat and Epidemiology of Khat Use

Khat (*Catha edulis*, Celastraceae) is an indigenous plant mostly grown and cultivated in the East of Africa and the Arabian Peninsula. It is a widely accepted viewpoint that Khat originated from Ethiopia and then spread to other nations such as Yemen, Saudi Arabia, Kenya, Somalia, Uganda, Tanzania, Malawi, Congo, Zambia, Zimbabwe, and South Africa (Balint et al. 2009). Because of its citation in New Testament and a belief that it has medicinal benefits, its use is accepted by most of the residents of the abovementioned countries (Balint et al. 2009). The habit of chewing khat is comparable to that of the habit of betel but chewing in the Indian subcontinent.

It is reported that the consumption of khat is strongly associated with many cardiovascular, gastrointestinal, hepatobiliary, genitourinary, nervous system, respiratory, and OH-related problems (Balint et al. 2009). The OH problems associated with khat use include dental caries, periodontal diseases, and oral cancer. The adverse effect of khat on oral tissues was first observed by Laurent in 1962, as reported by Hassan et al. (2007). The findings showed that long-term use of khat resulted in stomatitis and secondary infection. This is mostly attributed to the mechanical strain on the tissues of the oral cavity. The following sections will elaborate on the relationship of khat use with common oral diseases such as dental caries, periodontitis, and oral cancer. These sections would present an argument on the relationship between harmful and harmless state of khat use based on evidence from published literature, because statistical association could be dubious and may not necessarily represent causality.

Relationship Between Oral Diseases and Khat Use

Tooth Decay and Khat Use

Dental caries or tooth decay is a ubiquitous and progressive disease (Zero et al. 2009; Petersen et al. 2005b). It is multifactorial in etiology, with divergent yet interrelated risk factors such as microorganisms, environmental factors, socio-behavioral factors, substrate or host factors, and time (Eriksen and Dimitrov 2003; Kidd et al. 2003; Fejerskov 2004; Xiao et al. 2020). Dental caries shows themselves when a tooth surface becomes demineralized by the acids produced while bacteria ferment food debris, mainly carbohydrates (Selwitz et al. 2007; Kilian et al. 2016). Some studies conducted specifically have shown socio-behavioral and environmental factors to be strong risk indicators for dental caries (Watt and Sheiham 1999; Petersen 2005; Burt 2005).

The overall prevalence of dental caries is a matter of grave concern, even after recent advances made in prevention approaches (Bagramian et al. 2009). Moreover, untreated dental caries has been observed in nations with socioeconomic disparities, low levels of education, and/or poor oral hygiene practices (Edelstein 2006). During the late 1980s and early 1990s, the prevalence of dental caries was especially high in countries that are considered as developed nations (Petersen 2003). A change in this pattern was reported: in the last 10–15 years, caries prevalence came to be higher in developing nations (Glass 1982; Marthaler 2004; Haugejorden 1994; Downer 1994; Petersen and Razanmihaja 1996; Peres et al. 2019), especially upper-middle-income countries, than in developed nations (Frencken et al. 2017).

The relationship between tooth decay and khat chewing is inconsistent among the published literature. Hill and Gibson, in 1987, were the first to investigate the association and suggested a lower likelihood of tooth decay among a sample of Yemeni individuals who chew khat (Hill and Gibson 1987). While discussing the findings, the authors attributed the lower incidence of the disease to the presence of fluoride in the khat leaves (Hill and Gibson 1987). Contrary to this, two studies in different study settings showed that the chances of cervical caries among the khat users were higher in comparison to nonusers (Al-Sharabi A. Oral and para-oral lesions caused by Takhzeen Al-qat(chewing). PhD Thesis. Khartoum: University of Khartoum, 2002) (Nyanchoka I, Dimba E, Chindia M, Wanzala P, Macigo F. The oral and dental effects of khat chewing in the Eastleigh area of Nairobi. J Kenya Dent Assoc. 2008; 1:37–42). It was further reported that the mean caries severity among the users was 8.77 as opposed to the 6.52 in the nonusers. This empirical data is further supported by explanation in other studies (Al Moaleem et al. 2020), whereby it is stated that mechanical and chemical irritation along with xerostomia significantly contributes to tooth decay. Also, the chances of developing extrinsic brown staining, of similar appearance as dental caries, on the teeth surfaces of the chewing side are reported. These grainy-stained surfaces provide favorable inhabitation to streptococci, thus increasing the risk of developing dental caries (Al Moaleem et al. 2020). Another more recent study to the one carried out by Hill and Gibson (1987) in Yemen contradicted their findings and further supported a positive association (El-Wajeh and Thornhill 2009). Yet another study provides evidence that the occlusal caries prevalence at the chewing side and nonchewing side was 39.8% and 32.7%, respectively. Moreover, the findings showed that the relative risk of developing dental caries among the users is nearly two times greater in comparison to nonusers (K.R. Al-Alimi et al. 2018). In this prospective cohort study, 98 khat chewers from Yemen aged 18–35 years were followed for a short time. Bogale et al. (2021) corroborated and asserted that khat chewing was significantly associated with dental caries experience (Bogale et al. 2021). However, in the latest review by Al-Maweri et al. (2018a), khat is described as non-cariogenic, and it is argued that the increased use of soft drinks or sugar among khat users to reduce the bitter taste of the substance is the reason behind high caries incidence (Al-Maweri et al. 2018a).

However, in the same review, the authors present a contradictory argument and suggest that the presence of cathinone in khat results in xerostomia among the users which in turn contributes substantially to the development of dental caries or tooth decay (Al-Maweri et al. 2018a).

Periodontal Diseases and Khat Use

By definition, "periodontal diseases are inherited or acquired disorders of tissues that are investing and supporting the teeth" (Pihlstrom et al. 2005). It initiates due to the infection of gums, characterized by the destruction of tooth-supporting structures, which eventually leads to an untimely loss of a tooth. It is mostly caused by microorganisms inhabiting the oral biofilm that accumulates on the surface of the teeth among individuals with poor oral hygiene practices (Lin and Boynton 2015; Oh et al. 2002). Depending on their nature and progression, periodontal diseases are broadly classified as gingivitis and periodontitis (Albandar 2005). The former is a nondestructive type of disease which is often reversible, while the latter is a more advanced, more destructive form and is irreversible (Albandar 2005; Albandar and Tinoco 2002). At its initial stage, periodontal disease develops as an inflammation affecting mainly the margins of the gingiva; then, it gradually involves the supporting structure of the teeth, leading to loss of connective tissue attachment, bleeding gums, pain, breakdown of alveolar bone, and premature loss of teeth (Clerehugh 2008; Clerehugh and Tugnait 2001). Periodontitis is the second largest OH problem affecting 10–15% of the world's population. While periodontal disease is prevalent among 5–20% of the adult population, calculus and gingival bleeding due to inflammation tend to be more common among adolescents (Petersen and Ogawa 2005).

Khat use can influence the function and proliferation of periodontal cells such as gingival fibroblasts, periodontal membrane cells, periodontal ligament cells, and other cells. Moreover, it can physically harm the tooth-supporting structures or also inhibit the autoimmune defense mechanism and aggravate the inflammation reaction, thus enhancing the destruction of the alveolar bone and other tooth-supporting structures. The relationship between periodontal diseases and khat use is much clearer than that of tooth decay and khat use. The first possible suggestion of an association between khat use and gum diseases was provided as early as 1966 (Rosenzweig and Smith 1966). The study was carried out among the migrants in Israel, and those who migrated from Yemen demonstrated the highest prevalence. The study further suggested that the rate of occurrence of periodontal diseases was greater among the khat users in comparison to nonusers (Rosenzweig and Smith 1966). Similar to this, a study carried out in Yemen indicated that the loss of tooth-supporting structure and also the presence of an abundance of the calculus were significantly greater among those who chew khat (Mengel et al. 1996). These findings are further corroborated by studies that had a comparatively larger sample size (Dhaifullah et al. 2015; Halboub et al. 2009). Some authors attribute the relationship between periodontal diseases and khat use to the change in oral microbiota. Al-hebshi et al. (2010) stated that the likelihood of an increased amount of bacteria is significantly (odds ratio = 20) greater among the khat chewers in comparison to non-chewers; more specifically, *Treponema denticola* was shown to have higher absolute counts in comparison to other bacteria among the users (Al-Hebshi et al. 2010). Contrary to this, another study suggests that khat use has antimicrobial properties, thus indicating that it has protective effects toward periodontal disease (Al-Alimi et al. 2015). This is attributed to the physical mechanism involved in khat chewing which enables effective cleaning of the tooth surface and also its surroundings by means of abrasion. Also, some studies indicate that khat has a chemically active substance (tannins), which is antimicrobial and controls the formation of plaque on the tooth surface (Al-Alimi et al. 2015).

In one study, there was no significant difference in the proportion of khat users and nonusers with regard to the oral hygiene parameters. Nevertheless, the mean oral hygiene index was greater among the users in comparison to nonusers. Therefore, there is a high possibility that the nonsignificant relationship is spurious and that the khat use plays an important role in impaired oral hygiene (Al-Kholani 2010). Earlier, Hill and Gibson stated that khat use is associated with increased gingival bleeding (Hill and Gibson 1987). The friction caused on the oral mucosa and periodontal tissues by the continuous chewing of khat could be the reason for gingival bleeding and progressive periodontitis. Khat is also demonstrated to have alkaloids in addition to certain pesticides that play a causative role in initiating inflammation of gums.

Al-Hebshi et al. (2010) are of the opinion that khat use is protective of gum diseases (Al-Hebshi et al. 2010). In one of their studies, 40 subgingival samples were extracted from ten khat users and an equal number of nonusers, and the findings suggested that the users had a lower median periodontal index, indicating lower damage on tooth-supporting structures. This report is further supported by the findings from one of their another previous reports (Al-hebshi and Al-ak'hali 2010) and also another study carried out much earlier (Jorgensen and Kaimenyi 1990). The authors further state that the users had relatively lower counts of four periodontal pathogens, and they continue to present the argument that these suppressed counts indicate that khat interferes with or slows down the process of periodontitis (Al-Hebshi et al. 2010).

Later, a systematic review analyzed the available evidence to indicate that khat chewing has deleterious effect on the periodontal tissues (Kalakonda et al. 2017). Moreover, increased gingival recession and pocket depths including greater clinical attachment loss were reported by a majority of the studies included in the systematic review (Kalakonda et al. 2017). The authors have attributed this to the intensity and duration of khat chewing which could have possibly resulted in increased damage of tooth-supporting structures. However, in this review, one of the major limitations is that the included studies did not consider the confounding factors and also the use of other risk factors such as smoking, dietary practices, and oral hygiene maintenance. Therefore, the evidence above is inconclusive about khat as a causal factor for periodontal diseases.

Oral Cancer and Khat Use

Khat chewing habit is related to detrimental consequences in many bodily systems. One of the main concerns over the use of khat is the chances of occurrence of oral carcinoma. In this regard, many studies have been carried out. But still, the results of the studies are not in a conclusive stage. Since according to few studies khat is seemed to be an anticancer agent, few other studies point to the chances of carcinogenesis associated with a longtime chewing of khat (Dimba et al. 2003, 2004). There is some evidence of this carcinogenesis behavior, but it is considered as week conclusion due to many associated factors. The drawbacks of these epidemiological studies are coined the weak controls been used in the research. For instance, most of the khat chewers are associated with tobacco chewing, a few are alcoholics, and a few others are associated with another kind of substance of abuse. Hence, without putting suitable control to avoid the chances of getting the effects of such associated factors, khat's carcinogenicity conclusion is always questionable (Kassie et al. 2001). Hence, very limited studies were found to be positively correlating the khat and carcinogenesis.

In a case reported by Fasanmade et al. (2007), a 42-year-old female patient with squamous cell carcinoma of the floor of the mouth, associated with khat chewing, has been presented. The lesion was slowly increasing in size but did not cause any symptoms. She was having the habit of khat chewing for very long under the tongue on the same side as the subsequent lesion. She underwent clinical examination and was referred to pathology studies; the histology report confirmed the diagnosis of well-differentiated squamous cell carcinoma with an invasive front 2 mm deep to the basement membrane. This study (Fasanmade et al. 2007) did not conclude the causative agent for observed cancer to be khat, because it was very unusual to find oral squamous cell carcinoma in younger individuals. And it was of interest to note that she was a chronic alcoholic and tobacco smoker. They have concluded that the observed finding may not be due to the effects of khat alone, but khat may have played a role as precipitating agent and could act as a synergistic agent with other carcinogens present in the tobacco.

It is worth noting a case series published by Soufi et al. (1991); he and colleagues conducted a retrospective study in the Asir region of Saudi Arabia. It is one of the first comprehensive studies reported from southern Saudi Arabia, where khat chewing is spread over the community as it is in Yemen. They used data from 2 years of cases of head and neck cancers presented at the Asir Central hospital, the main and only referral hospital of the region. That study was carried out by using 28 cases of head and neck cancer, both sexes with an average age of 55, where all were using khat for at least 30 years. Eight cases of oral cancers were found among the study population. They all were use to kept the bolus of khat leaves at the same site, where the lesion has been observed for many years. By these findings, their authors expressed strong circumstantial evidence linking the long-term use of khat with increased oral malignancies.

It is difficult to exclude the role of khat in causing oral lesions and probable malignancy. Khat seems to be a responsible agent for changes in the oral mucosa.

Hence it is difficult to exclude the role of khat in causing oral lesions and possible malignancy. (Al-Sharabi 2011) has come to this conclusion from conducting a cross-sectional study, where he and his colleague used 685 khat chewers. Around 95% of the participants had been found to have white patches on the buccal or gingival mucosa of the chewing site; meanwhile, 8% of non-chewers also had shown the same clinical symptoms. Around 4% of the khat chewers were found to have red patches on buccal mucosa. Interestingly, non-chewers had not been found to be associated with red patches. The authors observed that when the study was separated by cigarette usage, the risk persisted among khat chewers demonstrating that white lesions on the oral mucosa would be predominantly induced by khat chewing. There was an important finding observed by the authors that the khat chewers, who were also smokers, had shown white patches on the same site in the buccal cavity, where they used to keep the khat bolus. This suggests that khat has a significant role in such lesion development; otherwise, it should have appeared in any part of the buccal cavity. Similar findings were observed earlier also, whereas Ali et al. (2004) had found that of individuals with keratotic white lesions in the selected study, 26% were khat chews alone, an observation that promoted the potential of associating the chewing of khat with lesion formation. The study also found that the number and severity of these lesions increased as the duration and frequency of khat chewing increased. For instance, 2.6% of the study population were using khat one day a week, and 37% of chewers who were using it every day had oral white lesions, as did 11% of those who used khat for less than 5 years, and 48% of those who used khat for more than 10 years had oral white lesions. In addition, a majority of grade III white lesions developed in people who chewed khat at least ten times a day. It suggests that the severity of these lesions in the buccal cavity of khat chewing is significantly related to the duration of use.

In another cross-sectional investigation, the associations between frequent khat chewing and oral leukoplakia progression among the male population from Yemen were evaluated. Khat chewers, who chewed khat over the last 3 years at least twice a week, and people who did not chew khat were compared. In 39 khat chewers and 9 non-chewers, leukoplakia was detected. Leukoplakia had a substantially greater incidence in the chewing population (95%) in comparison to the nonchewing side (8%). Although more lesions were expected among those who were also smokers, in khat chewers who were smokers (84%) leukoplakia was not significantly different from those who were not smoking (80%); this also supports a possible direct association between leukoplakia development and khat chewing (Yarom et al. 2010). Most of the studies about khat and leukoplakia were subjected to the male population. But there is a cross-sectional study conducted on 162 female participants (Schmidt-Westhausen et al. 2014). In this study, white lesions were detected in the chewing side of the cheek (72%), and the white lesion was found in nonchewing sites only in 5.5% of chewers. The white lesion in the nonchewing site might be due to the large quantity they chew, and this leads to the movement of khat fibers among the sides. Leukoplakia observed in the chewers was statistically significant compared to non-chewers.

According to a study done by Halboub et al. (2009), the sorts of clinical results on the chewing sides differed depending on the duration of khat chewing habit with greater lesions between those with longer chewing periods. He had employed 79 men in the study and found mild or severe corrugation keratosis in all the chewer study population (100%); only 4% of non-chewers had presented with the same symptoms. There was no statistical difference when comparing the clinical results between the left and right sides of the non-chewers, smokers, and nonsmokers, but the difference between the chewing and nonchewing sides of the chews of khat was statistically significant. In addition, they observed that there were statistical differences when comparing khat chewing sides in the buccal cavity with nonchewing, smokers, and nonsmokers on both sides. There was, on the other hand, no statistical difference between the nonchewing sides of khat chewers and the non-chewers on both sides regardless of their smoking custom. The authors found that chewing khat creates oral white lesions on the chewing side and that smoking does not make such lesions worse clinically.

Influence of Alcohol, Smoking, and Pesticides in Oral Cancers

Even though mixed information is available on khat carcinogenesis, some important factors associated with the usage of khat must be taken into account. Because in many instances, the khat users are not taking khat leaves alone; instead, they mix with alcohol or smoking.

Longtime use of alcohol is considered as a modifier risk of cancer, especially with laryngeal and head and neck cancers (Reidy et al. 2011). They have a very close association with oral cancer, and about 75% of all oral cancers arise in association with alcohol and tobacco (Ogden 2005). Alcohol is linked with oral cancer due to its many properties of alcohol. Firstly, increased mucosal penetrability linked with alcohol assist khat related carcinogens in oral mucosa. Then the cellular damage by acetaldehyde present in the alcoholic drink interferes with DNA synthesis. Lastly, alcohol can potentiate genotoxicity and mutagenesis (Reidy et al. 2011). Many of the khat chewers are tobacco users too. Tobacco is a known carcinogen, and it has been used among khat chewers in different forms such as cigarette smoking and pipe smoking (Kassim et al. 2014). There are no dependable controlled studies on the augmented effects when cathinone and nicotine are combined. It has been reported that khat farmers are not following safety measures normally during their cultivation. Extensive use of pesticides is being reported among these farmers. Hence, several incidences of cancers have been reported including oral due to the presence of pesticides (Al-Akwa et al. 2009). Therefore cleaning the khat leaves after collection is very important. It has been reported that all kinds of pesticides used in Yemen are being employed in khat cultivation. Not limited to Yemen, Ethiopia also uses all these pesticides abundantly in khat farming (Daba et al. 2011).

Applications to Other Areas of Public Health

Although the current evidence is inconclusive to indicate the adverse effects of khat use on OH, especially in the case of oral cancer, these findings are not based on high-quality investigations. Moreover, one cannot deny the rise in the prevalence of khat users across the globe (Al-Maweri et al. 2018a). This calls for public health interventions in order to reduce the sale and consumption of khat. Because khat is consumed orally, dental healthcare providers play an essential role in the early diagnosis of the adverse effects of khat. It is of utmost importance that these dental healthcare providers, specifically working in communities where the prevalence of khat use is greater, be skillfully trained to help in the early detection of khat consumption. The diagnosis chart and protocols in the healthcare settings should include the items that record the details on the habits of khat use. Additionally, there is also a need to enlist standardized policies at the government level to regulate the sale of khat and also halt the import of such substances that cause addiction among its users; it is critical because khat consumption impacts the mental health of individuals. Furthermore, as of June 2014, khat has been regarded as a class C drug under the Misuse of Drugs Act.

Awareness among the populations or migrant communities that are prone to khat use is mandatory. This could be achieved by carrying out regular educational campaigns among the targeted communities. Also, harm minimization techniques and motivational interviewing could be adopted to influence the habit of khat use. The impact of these interventions on policymaking could be increased upon having empirical data, and, therefore, high-quality studies and findings from the implementation of prevention strategies should be of utmost priority as they evaluate the effectiveness of each strategy and inform the policymakers. The funds and resources provided by the governmental and nongovernmental agencies also play a crucial role in carrying out high-quality interventions.

Conclusion

Thus, based on the available reports, khat use cannot be considered as a causal factor for oral diseases such as tooth decay and periodontal diseases. However, it is to note that because of the presence of cathinone, which significantly leads to xerostomia, khat use may aggravate the process of tooth decay among the users. Also, because the substance is chewed and not just kept in the buccal mucosa, like tobacco, it may physically damage the tooth-supporting structures among chronic users, thus contributing to gum inflammation.

Furthermore, with the available literature, the direct relationship between khat alone and oral cancer is questionable. But many studies are showing the direct effect of other coadministered stuff like alcohol, tobacco smoking, smokeless tobacco, and the presence of pesticides. In many earlier studies, it has been reported that khat users develop leukoplakia (white patches), especially in the long duration of chewing. It needs further in-depth studies to prove these white patches can be developed into cancer or not. Studies done by Al-Maweri et al. (2018b) observed that these lesions are due to mechanical friction. Thus, contradicting findings are currently available in the relationship of khat and oral cancer. Thus, it warrants large-scale cohort studies, which can prove this relationship with scientific backups.

Key Facts

- The substance of abuse in all forms is considered a severe public health problem, where a multidisciplinary approach always warrants a definitive solution.
- Khat is such a kind of plant legally consumed in some places such as Yemen, but it is fully considered an illegal substance throughout Europe, the USA, and the Middle East.
- Even though users consumed it as a social and pleasant substance, its overall health issues are much more than everybody assumes.
- It affects all bodily parts and can cause mild to moderate diseases in users.
- Involvement from the side of government and other social organizations collectively can cure this social and public issue.

Summary Points

- Khat chewing is on the rise and has emerged as a public health issue.
- Long-term use of khat resulted in stomatitis and attributed to the mechanical strain on the tissues of the oral cavity.
- Rate of occurrence of periodontal diseases was greater among the khat users.
- Chewing khat creates oral white lesions on the chewing side.
- Several incidences of cancers have been reported including oral due to the presence of pesticides in khat.

References

Al Moaleem MM, Porwal A, Al Ahmari NM, Shariff M, Homeida H, Khalid A (2020) Khat chewing induces a floral shift in dental material-associated microbiota: a preliminary study. Med Sci Monit 26:e918219. https://doi.org/10.12659/MSM.918219. https://www.ncbi.nlm.nih.gov/pubmed/31956260

Al-Akwa AA, Shaher M, Al-Akwa S, Aleryani SL (2009) Free radicals are present in human serum of Catha edulis Forsk (khat) abusers. J Ethnopharmacol 125(3):471–473

Al-Alimi A, Taiyeb-Ali T, Jaafar N, Al-hebshi NN (2015) Qat chewing and periodontal pathogens in health and disease: further evidence for a prebiotic-like effect. Biomed Res Int 2015:291305. https://doi.org/10.1155/2015/291305. https://www.ncbi.nlm.nih.gov/pubmed/26351631

Al-Alimi KR, Razak AAA, Saub R (2018) Is khat chewing habit a risk factor for occlusal caries progression? Afr Health Sci 18(4):1036–1045. https://doi.org/10.4314/ahs.v18i4.25. https://www.ncbi.nlm.nih.gov/pubmed/30766570

Albandar JM (2005) Epidemiology and risk factors of periodontal diseases. Dent Clin N Am 49(3): 517–532, v–vi. https://doi.org/10.1016/j.cden.2005.03.003. https://www.ncbi.nlm.nih.gov/pubmed/15978239

Albandar JM, Tinoco EM (2002) Global epidemiology of periodontal diseases in children and young persons. Periodontol 2000(29):153–176. https://www.ncbi.nlm.nih.gov/pubmed/12102707

Al-hebshi NN, Al-ak'hali MS (2010) Experimental gingivitis in male khat (*Catha edulis*) chewers. J Int Acad Periodontol 12(2):56–62. https://www.ncbi.nlm.nih.gov/pubmed/20465033

Al-Hebshi NN, Al-Sharabi AK, Shuga-Aldin HM, Al-Haroni M, Ghandour I (2010) Effect of khat chewing on periodontal pathogens in subgingival biofilm from chronic periodontitis patients. J Ethnopharmacol 132(3):564–569. https://doi.org/10.1016/j.jep.2010.08.051. https://www.ncbi.nlm.nih.gov/pubmed/20816745

Ali AA, Al-Sharabi AK, Aguirre JM, Nahas R (2004) A study of 342 oral keratotic white lesions induced by qat chewing among 2500 Yemeni. J Oral Pathol Med 33(6):368–372

Al-Kholani AI (2010) Influence of khat chewing on periodontal tissues and oral hygiene status among Yemenis. Dent Res J (Isfahan) 7(1):1–6. https://www.ncbi.nlm.nih.gov/pubmed/21448439

Al-Maweri SA, Warnakulasuriya S, Samran A (2018a) Khat (*Catha edulis*) and its oral health effects: an updated review. J Investig Clin Dent 9(1):e12288. https://doi.org/10.1111/jicd.12288. https://www.ncbi.nlm.nih.gov/pubmed/28834423

Al-Maweri SA, Al-Jamaei A, Saini R, Laronde DM, Sharhan A (2018b) White oral mucosal lesions among the Yemeni population and their relation to local oral habits. J Investig Clin Dent 9(2): e12305

Al-Sharabi AK (2011) Conditions of oral mucosa due to takhzeen al-qat. Yemeni J Med Sci 5:6–6

Bagramian RA, Garcia-Godoy F, Volpe AR (2009) The global increase in dental caries. A pending public health crisis. Am J Dent 22(1):3–8. https://www.ncbi.nlm.nih.gov/pubmed/19281105

Balint EE, Falkay G, Balint GA (2009) Khat – a controversial plant. Wien Klin Wochenschr 121(19–20):604–614. https://doi.org/10.1007/s00508-009-1259-7. https://www.ncbi.nlm.nih.gov/pubmed/19921126

Bogale B, Engida F, Hanlon C, Prince MJ, Gallagher JE (2021) Dental caries experience and associated factors in adults: a cross-sectional community survey within Ethiopia. BMC Public Health 21(1):180. https://doi.org/10.1186/s12889-021-10199-9. https://www.ncbi.nlm.nih.gov/pubmed/33478460

Bray F, Ferlay J, Laversanne M, Brewster DH, Gombe Mbalawa C, Kohler B, Piñeros M, Steliarova-Foucher E, Swaminathan R, Antoni S, Soerjomataram I, Forman D (2015) Cancer incidence in five continents: inclusion criteria, highlights from volume X and the global status of cancer registration. Int J Cancer 137(9):2060–2071. https://doi.org/10.1002/ijc.29670. https://www.ncbi.nlm.nih.gov/pubmed/26135522

Burt BA (2005) Concepts of risk in dental public health. Community Dent Oral Epidemiol 33(4): 240–247

Clerehugh V (2008) Periodontal diseases in children and adolescents. Br Dent J 204(8):469–471. https://doi.org/10.1038/sj.bdj.2008.301. https://www.ncbi.nlm.nih.gov/pubmed/18438398

Clerehugh V, Tugnait A (2001) Diagnosis and management of periodontal diseases in children and adolescents. Periodontol 2000(26):146–168. https://www.ncbi.nlm.nih.gov/pubmed/11452903

Collaborators, GBD 2019 Diseases and Injuries (2020) Global burden of 369 diseases and injuries in 204 countries and territories, 1990–2019: a systematic analysis for the Global Burden of Disease Study 2019. Lancet 396(10258):1204–1222. https://doi.org/10.1016/S0140-6736(20)30925-9. https://www.ncbi.nlm.nih.gov/pubmed/33069326

Collaborators, Global Burden of Disease Study 2013 (2015) Global, regional, and national incidence, prevalence, and years lived with disability for 301 acute and chronic diseases and injuries in 188 countries, 1990-2013: a systematic analysis for the Global Burden of Disease Study

2013. Lancet 386(9995):743–800. https://doi.org/10.1016/S0140-6736(15)60692-4. https://www.ncbi.nlm.nih.gov/pubmed/26063472
Daba D, Hymete A, Bekhit AA, Mohamed AMI, Bekhit AE-DA (2011) Multi residue analysis of pesticides in wheat and khat collected from different regions of Ethiopia. Bull Environ Contam Toxicol 86(3):336–341
Dhaifullah E, Al-Maweri SA, Al-Motareb F, Halboub E, Elkhatat E, Baroudi K, Tarakji B (2015) Periodontal health condition and associated factors among university students, Yemen. J Clin Diagn Res 9(12):ZC30-3. https://doi.org/10.7860/JCDR/2015/16435.6964. https://www.ncbi.nlm.nih.gov/pubmed/26813290
Dimba E, Gjertsen BT, Francis GW, Johannessen AC, Vintermyr OK (2003) *Catha edulis* (khat) induces cell death by apoptosis in leukemia cell lines. Ann N Y Acad Sci 1010:384–388
Dimba EAO, Gjertsen BT, Bredholt T, Fossan KO, Costea DE, Francis GW, Johannessen AC, Vintermyr OK (2004) Khat (*Catha edulis*)-induced apoptosis is inhibited by antagonists of caspase-1 and-8 in human leukaemia cells. Br J Cancer 91(9):1726–1734
Downer MC (1994) Caries prevalence in the United Kingdom. Int Dent J 44(4):365–370
Edelstein BL (2006) The dental caries pandemic and disparities problem. BMC Oral Health 6(Suppl 1):S2. https://doi.org/10.1186/1472-6831-6-S1-S2. https://www.ncbi.nlm.nih.gov/pubmed/16934119
Eke PI, Wei L, Thornton-Evans GO, Borrell LN, Borgnakke WS, Dye B, Genco RJ (2016) Risk indicators for periodontitis in US adults: NHANES 2009 to 2012. J Periodontol 87(10):1174–1185. https://doi.org/10.1902/jop.2016.160013. https://www.ncbi.nlm.nih.gov/pubmed/27367420
El-Wajeh YA, Thornhill MH (2009) Qat and its health effects. Br Dent J 206(1):17–21. https://doi.org/10.1038/sj.bdj.2008.1122. https://www.ncbi.nlm.nih.gov/pubmed/19132030
Eriksen HM, Dimitrov V (2003) Ecology of oral health: a complexity perspective. Eur J Oral Sci 111(4):285–290
Erratum: global cancer statistics 2018: GLOBOCAN estimates of incidence and mortality worldwide for 36 cancers in 185 countries (2020) CA Cancer J Clin 70(4):313. https://doi.org/10.3322/caac.21609. https://www.ncbi.nlm.nih.gov/pubmed/32767693
Fasanmade A, Kwok E, Newman L (2007) Oral squamous cell carcinoma associated with khat chewing. Oral Surg Oral Med Oral Pathol Oral Radiol Endodontol 104(1):e53–e55
Fejerskov O (2004) Changing paradigms in concepts on dental caries: consequences for oral health care. Caries Res 38(3):182–191
Frencken JE, Sharma P, Stenhouse L, Green D, Laverty D, Dietrich T (2017) Global epidemiology of dental caries and severe periodontitis – a comprehensive review. J Clin Periodontol 44(Suppl 18):S94–S105. https://doi.org/10.1111/jcpe.12677. https://www.ncbi.nlm.nih.gov/pubmed/28266116
Gjermo P, Rösing CK, Susin C, Oppermann R (2002) Periodontal diseases in Central and South America. Periodontol 2000(29):70–78. https://www.ncbi.nlm.nih.gov/pubmed/12102703
Glass RL (1982) The first international conference on the declining prevalence of dental caries. J Dent Res 61:1304–1383
Glick M, Williams DM, Kleinman DV, Vujicic M, Watt RG, Weyant RJ (2017) A new definition for oral health developed by the FDI World Dental Federation opens the door to a universal definition of oral health. J Public Health Dent 77(1):3–5. https://doi.org/10.1111/jphd.12213. https://www.ncbi.nlm.nih.gov/pubmed/28276588
Halboub E, Dhaifullah E, Abdulhuq M (2009) Khat chewing and smoking effect on oral mucosa: a clinical study. Acta Med (Hradec Kralove) 52(4):155–158
Hassan NA, Gunaid AA, Murray-Lyon IM (2007) Khat (Catha edulis): health aspects of khat chewing. East Mediterr Health J 13(3):706–718. https://www.ncbi.nlm.nih.gov/pubmed/17687845
Haugejorden O (1994) Changing time trend in caries prevalence in Norwegian children and adolescents. Community Dent Oral Epidemiol 22(4):220–225

Hill CM, Gibson A (1987) The oral and dental effects of q'at chewing. Oral Surg Oral Med Oral Pathol 63(4):433–436. https://doi.org/10.1016/0030-4220(87)90255-6. https://www.ncbi.nlm.nih.gov/pubmed/3472143

Jorgensen E, Kaimenyi JT (1990) The status of periodontal health and oral hygiene of Miraa (*Catha edulis*) chewers. East Afr Med J 67(8):585–590. https://www.ncbi.nlm.nih.gov/pubmed/1979771

Kalakonda B, Al-Maweri SA, Al-Shamiri HM, Ijaz A, Gamal S, Dhaifullah E (2017) Is khat (*Catha edulis*) chewing a risk factor for periodontal diseases? A systematic review. J Clin Exp Dent 9(10):e1264–e1270. https://doi.org/10.4317/jced.54163. https://www.ncbi.nlm.nih.gov/pubmed/29167719

Kassie F, Darroudi F, Kundi M, Schulte-Hermann R, Knasmüller S (2001) Khat (*Catha edulis*) consumption causes genotoxic effects in humans. Int J Cancer 92(3):329–332

Kassim S, Rogers N, Leach K (2014) The likelihood of khat chewing serving as a neglected and reverse 'gateway' to tobacco use among UK adult male khat chewers: a cross sectional study. BMC Public Health 14(1):1–11

Kidd EAM, Mejare I, Nyvad B (2003) Clinical and radiographic diagnosis. In: Fejerskov O, Kidd EAM (eds) Dental caries – the disease and its clinical management. Blackwell Munksgaard, Oxford, pp 111–128

Kilian M, Chapple IL, Hannig M, Marsh PD, Meuric V, Pedersen AM, Tonetti MS, Wade WG, Zaura E (2016) The oral microbiome - an update for oral healthcare professionals. Br Dent J 221(10):657–666. https://doi.org/10.1038/sj.bdj.2016.865. https://www.ncbi.nlm.nih.gov/pubmed/27857087

Lin GH, Boynton JR (2015) Periodontal considerations for the child and adolescent. A literature review. J Mich Dent Assoc 97(1):36–40, 42, 74. https://www.ncbi.nlm.nih.gov/pubmed/26285502

Maharani DA, Adiatman M, Rahardjo A, Burnside G, Pine C (2017) An assessment of the impacts of child oral health in Indonesia and associations with self-esteem, school performance and perceived employability. BMC Oral Health 17(1):65. https://doi.org/10.1186/s12903-017-0358-5. https://www.ncbi.nlm.nih.gov/pubmed/28327110

Marthaler TM (2004) Changes in dental caries 1953–2003. Caries Res 38(3):173–181

Mengel R, Eigenbrodt M, Schünemann T, Florès-de-Jacoby L (1996) Periodontal status of a subject sample of Yemen. J Clin Periodontol 23(5):437–443. https://doi.org/10.1111/j.1600-051x.1996.tb00571.x. https://www.ncbi.nlm.nih.gov/pubmed/8783048

Needleman I, Garcia R, Gkranias N, Kirkwood KL, Kocher T, Iorio AD, Moreno F, Petrie A (2018) Mean annual attachment, bone level, and tooth loss: a systematic review. J Periodontol 89(Suppl 1):S120–S139. https://doi.org/10.1002/JPER.17-0062. https://www.ncbi.nlm.nih.gov/pubmed/29926956

Nunn JH (2006) The burden of oral ill health for children. Arch Dis Child 91(3):251–253. https://doi.org/10.1136/adc.2005.077016. https://www.ncbi.nlm.nih.gov/pubmed/16492889

Nurelhuda NM, Trovik TA, Ahmed Ali RW, Ahmed MF (2009) Oral health status of 12-year-old school children in Khartoum state, the Sudan; a school-based survey. BMC-Oral Health 9:15

Nurelhuda NM, Ahmed MF, Trovik TA, Astrom AN (2010) Evaluation of oral health-related quality of life among Sudanese schoolchildren using child-OIDP inventory. Health Qual Life Outcomes 8. https://doi.org/10.1186/1477-7525-8-152

Ogden GR (2005) Alcohol and oral cancer. Alcohol 35(3):169–173

Oh TJ, Eber R, Wang HL (2002) Periodontal diseases in the child and adolescent. J Clin Periodontol 29(5):400–410. https://www.ncbi.nlm.nih.gov/pubmed/12060422

Peres MA, Macpherson LMD, Weyant RJ, Daly B, Venturelli R, Mathur MR, Listl S, Celeste RK, Guarnizo-Herreño CC, Kearns C, Benzian H, Allison P, Watt RG (2019) Oral diseases: a global public health challenge. Lancet 394(10194):249–260. https://doi.org/10.1016/S0140-6736(19)31146-8. https://www.ncbi.nlm.nih.gov/pubmed/31327369

Peres MA, Antunes JLF, Watt R (2021) Oral epidemiology: a textbook on oral health conditions, research topics and methods. Springer Nature

Petersen PE (2003) The World Oral Health Report 2003: continuous improvement of oral health in the 21st century – the approach of the WHO Global Oral Health Programme. Community Dent Oral Epidemiol 31(Suppl 1):3–23. https://www.ncbi.nlm.nih.gov/pubmed/15015736

Petersen PE (2005) Socio-behavioural risk factors in dental caries – international perspectives. Community Dent Oral Epidemiol 33(4):274–279

Petersen PE, Ogawa H (2005) Strengthening the prevention of periodontal disease: the WHO approach. J Periodontol 12:2187–2193

Petersen PE, Razanmihaja N (1996) Oral health status of children and adults in Madagascar. Int Dent J 46:41–47

Petersen PE, Bourgeois D, Ogawa H, Estupinan-Day S, Ndiaye C (2005a) The global burden of oral diseases and risks to oral health. Bull World Health Organ 83(9):661–669. https://doi.org// S0042-96862005000900011. https://www.ncbi.nlm.nih.gov/pubmed/16211157

Petersen PE, Bourgeois D, Ogawa H, Estupinan-Day S, Ndiaye C (2005b) The global burden of oral diseases and risks to oral health. Bull World Health Organ 83(9):661–669

Pihlstrom BL, Michalowicz BS, Johnson NW (2005) Periodontal diseases. Lancet 366(9499): 1809–1820

Reidy J, McHugh E, Stassen LFA (2011) A review of the relationship between alcohol and oral cancer. Surgeon 9(5):278–283

Rosenzweig KA, Smith P (1966) Periodontal health in various ethnic groups in Israel. J Periodontal Res 1(4):250–259. https://doi.org/10.1111/j.1600-0765.1966.tb01869.x. https://www.ncbi.nlm.nih.gov/pubmed/4226588

Satcher DS (2000) Surgeon General's report on oral health. Public Health Rep 115(5):489–490. https://www.ncbi.nlm.nih.gov/pubmed/11236021

Schmidt-Westhausen AM, Al Sanabani J, Al-Sharabi AK (2014) Prevalence of oral white lesions due to qat chewing among women in Yemen. Oral Dis 20(7):675–681

Selwitz RH, Ismail AI, Pitts NB (2007) Dental caries. Lancet 369(9555):51–59. https://doi.org/10.1016/S0140-6736(07)60031-2. https://www.ncbi.nlm.nih.gov/pubmed/17208642

Soufi HE, Kameswaran M, Malatani T (1991) Khat and oral cancer. J Laryngol Otol 105(8): 643–645

Sung, Hyuna, Jacques Ferlay, Rebecca L Siegel, Mathieu Laversanne, Isabelle Soerjomataram, Ahmedin Jemal, Freddie Bray. (2021) Global Cancer Statistics 2020: Globocan Estimates of Incidence and Mortality Worldwide for 36 Cancers in 185 Countries. CA: a cancer journal for clinicians 71(3):209–249

Watt R, Sheiham A (1999) Inequalities in oral health: a review of the evidence and recommendations for action. Br Dent J 187(1):6–12

WHO, World Health Organization (2016) Oral Health Fact sheet: 318. http://www.who.int/mediacentre/factsheets/fs318/en/

Xiao J, Fiscella KA, Gill SR (2020) Oral microbiome: possible harbinger for children's health. Int J Oral Sci 12(1):12. https://doi.org/10.1038/s41368-020-0082-x. https://www.ncbi.nlm.nih.gov/pubmed/32350240

Yang H, Xiao L, Zhang L, Deepal S, Ye G, Zhang X (2017) Epidemic trend of periodontal disease in elderly Chinese population, 1987–2015: a systematic review and meta-analysis. Sci Rep 7: 45000. https://doi.org/10.1038/srep45000. https://www.ncbi.nlm.nih.gov/pubmed/28358004

Yarom N, Epstein J, Levi H, Porat D, Kaufman E, Gorsky M (2010) Oral manifestations of habitual khat chewing: a case-control study. Oral Surg Oral Med Oral Pathol Oral Radiol Endodontol 109(6):e60–e66

Zero DT, Fontana M, Martínez-Mier EA, Ferreira-Zandoná A, Ando M, González-Cabezas C, Bayne S (2009) The biology, prevention, diagnosis and treatment of dental caries: scientific advances in the United States. J Am Dent Assoc 140(Suppl 1):25S–34S. https://doi.org/10.14219/jada.archive.2009.0355. https://www.ncbi.nlm.nih.gov/pubmed/19723928

9783030923914VOL02